STOLEN FROM
JIM NORA

WILLIAMS
OBSTETRICS

This volume represents the Tenth Edition of *Williams* OBSTETRICS, the first six of which were written by the late J. Whitridge Williams, Professor of Obstetrics in Johns Hopkins University, and Obstetrician-in-Chief to the Johns Hopkins Hospital from 1896 to 1931; and the seventh, eighth and ninth of which were prepared by the late Henricus J. Stander, Professor of Obstetrics and Gynecology in Cornell University and Obstetrician and Gynecologist-in-Chief to the New York Hospital from 1931 to 1948.

W I L L I A M S

OBSTETRICS

BY

NICHOLSON J. EASTMAN

Professor of Obstetrics, Johns Hopkins University, and Obstetrician-in-Chief to the Johns Hopkins Hospital

TENTH EDITION

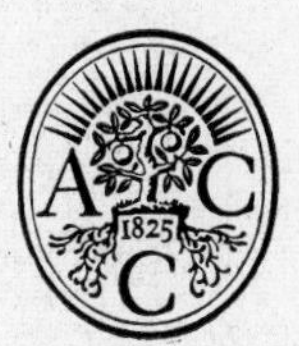

APPLETON-CENTURY-CROFTS, INC.

NEW YORK

PRINTED IN THE UNITED STATES OF AMERICA

TO THE
RESIDENTS, ASSISTANT RESIDENTS AND INTERNES
WHO HAVE SERVED IN THE
DEPARTMENT OF OBSTETRICS
OF THE
JOHNS HOPKINS HOSPITAL
SINCE ITS INCEPTION IN 1896 TO THE PRESENT DAY,
THIS VOLUME IS DEDICATED
WITH AFFECTION AND GRATITUDE.

PREFACE

The purpose of this volume is to set forth in a comprehensive manner the principles and the practice of modern obstetrics for both medical students and practitioners. To achieve this end, extensive changes in the previous edition of Williams Obstetrics have been necessary. In particular, the many important advances in the science and art of obstetrics over the past decade have dictated the inclusion of a large amount of new material and, as a consequence, approximately 55 per cent of the present text and over one third of the illustrations are new.

The first chapter is an especial innovation and represents an attempt to introduce the medical student to obstetrics from the broad viewpoints of vital statistics, public health and medicine in general. Many years of teaching both medical students and nurses have convinced me that such an orientation is at once the most logical and the most stimulating approach to the subject. The long chapter on the toxemias of pregnancy has also been written de novo. It includes a new and simple classification of these disorders which has proved workable in our own clinic and it is hoped that it will prove generally useful. Other major sections which are completely rewritten and brought up-to-date include those dealing with the ovarian and placental hormones, placental transfer, estimation of pelvic size and shape, the forces concerned in labor, analgesia and anesthesia, abortion, clinical aspects of ectopic pregnancy, hydatidiform mole and chorionepithelioma, clinical aspects of placenta previa, treatment of syphilis, diabetes mellitus, the management of uterine inertia, prognosis and management of transverse presentations, prognosis of labor in inlet contraction, midpelvic contraction, rupture of the uterus, postpartum hemorrhage, puerperal infection, apnea neonatorum and hemolytic disease of the newborn. Other sections have been partially rewritten and countless minor alterations made.

In order to make place for new material, substantial deletions in the old text have been obligatory. These consist in part of the omission of those sections which dealt with nineteenth century and early twentieth century issues of a controversial nature. These stemmed mostly from the voluminous German literature of that period and are now only of historical interest. Although the deletion of much material of this kind has seemed desirable, the sections dealing with the major phases of the history of obstetrics have been retained, such as those covering the early annals of cesarean section, forceps, anesthesia and puerperal infection. Likewise, in the bibliographies, the names of some of the great worthies of nineteenth century obstetrics have had to be omitted, but here again references to the great classics such as those of Smellie, Simpson, Semmelweis, Michaelis, Hitschmann and Adler, and Bandl, are still included.

In the belief that the more commonly employed terms in obstetrics need uniformity of definition, a conference was held in September, 1949, in which the following authors participated: Dr. J. P. Greenhill, author of the DeLee-Greenhill Principles and Practice of Obstetrics; Dr. Paul Titus, author of Management of Obstetric Difficulties; Dr. C. O. McCormick, author of Pathology of Labor, the Puerperium and the Newborn; and the author of the present volume. After a thorough discussion it was agreed that the following terms would be defined and classified identically in the four books mentioned: engagement (page 271); primigravida, primipara, multipara, etc. (page 312); toxemias of pregnancy (page 645); placenta previa (page 562); forceps delivery (page 1054); and breech delivery (page 1082). It is hoped that this will reduce the confusion which divergent definitions of these terms have hitherto caused.

The chapter on the toxemias of pregnancy has been read in manuscript form by Dr. William J. Dieckmann, Dr. Leon C. Chesley and Dr. Ernest W. Page, and I wish to acknowledge my great indebtedness to these recognized authorities on the toxemias for their many helpful suggestions. Their kind assistance is much appreciated.

The extensive section on hemolytic disease of the newborn was written by Dr. Milton S. Sacks, Associate Professor of Medicine in the University of Maryland School of Medicine and Director of the Baltimore Rh Typing Laboratory. His vast experience in this field, based on the carefully analyzed observations he has made on more than 75,000 gravidae in respect to Rh type and subsequent course, gives his opinions unusual authority; and I stand heavily in his debt for this lucid survey of an important subject.

The many references to the late Dr. Henricus J. Stander throughout the volume attest my obligations to him for his many contributions to the last three editions. I desire to acknowledge my debt also to several former members of his staff for notable contributions, particularly to Dr. Herbert F. Traut, Dr. R. Gordon Douglas, Dr. Andrew A. Marchetti, Dr. Carl T. Javert, Dr. Katherine Kuder and Miss Elizabeth Brödel.

To members of my own staff I am deeply obligated for assistance of various kinds. To Dr. Eleanor Delfs I am especially grateful, not only for her help in the sections on endocrinology, x-ray pelvimetry, hydatidiform mole and chorionepithelioma, and rupture of the uterus, but also for her kindness in reading the galley sheets for factual errors. Dr. Alan F. Guttmacher has rewritten the chapter on multiple pregnancy and made substantial additions to the section on spontaneous abortion. Dr. Louis M. Hellman has given valuable assistance in the sections devoted to uterine motility, uterine inertia and analgesia and anesthesia, while Dr. Gilbert J. Vosburgh has helped me greatly in bringing up-to-date the discussions of placental transfer and fetal physiology. To Miss Dorothy Vonderwish, who has served as editorial assistant in the preparation of this volume, I am immeasurably indebted, not only for typing the entire manuscript, but also for reading both galley and page proof.

Most of the new illustrations are the work of Miss Ranice Birch, Director of the Department of Art as Applied to Medicine, Johns Hopkins University School of Medicine. Her distinguished drawings are noteworthy contributions to visual education in obstetrics and the book and its author owe her much. I wish also to thank Mr. Leon Schlossberg for a number of drawings, particularly those portraying the Waters and Norton extraperitoneal cesarean section. In addition, I desire to acknowledge the generosity of the J. B. Lippincott Company for permission to use material from their Nurses Handbook of Obstetrics by Louise Zabriskie, R. N., and Nicholson J. Eastman, M. D. The W. B. Prior Company has likewise been very kind in allowing me to include extensive sections from my chapter on puerperal infection in Lewis' Practice of Surgery.

Finally, it is a pleasant duty to acknowledge my indebtedness to Appleton-Century-Crofts, Inc., especially to Mr. George A. McDermott and to Mr. Robert A. Schetty for the meticulous attention which they have given to the preparation of this volume.

NICHOLSON J. EASTMAN

The Johns Hopkins Hospital
Baltimore 5, Maryland

CONTENTS

Section Six: ABNORMALITIES OF PREGNANCY

Section Seven: ABNORMALITIES OF LABOR

Section Eight: ABNORMALITIES OF THE PUERPERIUM

Section Nine: ABNORMALITIES OF THE NEWBORN

Section Ten: OPERATIVE OBSTETRICS

WILLIAMS

OBSTETRICS

Section One: ORIENTATION

1

OBSTETRICS IN BROAD PERSPECTIVE

Definition. *Obstetrics* is that branch of medicine which deals with parturition, its antecedents and its sequels. It is concerned principally, therefore, with the phenomena and management of pregnancy, labor and the puerperium, both under normal and abnormal circumstances. In England, the older term *midwifery* carries the same connotation as obstetrics, and the two words are used synonymously. In the United States, however, owing to inadequate supervision and regulation of midwives, the practice of these attendants has long been conducted rather surreptitiously and, in the main, is held in disrepute. Here, accordingly, "midwifery" carries with it a certain stigma which does not obtain in England and elsewhere. The German word for obstetrics is *Geburtshilfe;* and the French, *obstétrique.*

The word *obstetrics* is derived from the Latin term *obstetrix,* meaning *midwife.* The etymology of obstetrix, however, is obscure. Most dictionaries connect it with the verb *obstare,* which means *to stand by or in front of.* The rationale of this derivation would be that the midwife stood by or in front of the parturient. This etymology has long been attacked by Seligmann, who believed that the word was originally *adstetrix* and that the *ad* had been changed to *ob.* If this etymology is correct, then obstetrix would mean *the woman assisting the parturient.* The fact that on certain inscriptions *obstetrix* is also spelled *opstetrix* has led to the conjecture that it was derived from *ops,* that is, *aid,* and *stare,* and had the meaning of *the woman rendering aid.* According to Temkin, the most likely interpretation is that obstetrix meant *the woman who stood by the parturient.* Whether this alluded merely to the midwife's standing in front of, or near, the parturient, or whether it carried the additional connotation of rendering aid, is not clear.

The term *obstetrics* is of relatively recent usage. Thus, the Oxford English Dictionary gives the earliest example from a book published in 1819; and the same source observes that in 1828 it was necessary to apologize for the use of the word *obstetrician.* Kindred terms are, however, much older. Thus, *obstetricate* occurs in English works published as early as 1623; *obstetricatory,* in 1640; *obstetricious,* in 1645; and *obstetrical,* in 1775. These terms were often used figuratively. As an example of such usage the adjective *obstetric* appears in Pope's *Dunciad* (1742) in the famous couplet:

There all the Learn'd shall at the labour stand,
And Douglas lend his soft, obstetric hand.

The much older term *midwifery* was used instead of *obstetrics* until the latter part of the nineteenth century both in the United States and Great Britain. It is derived from the Middle English *mid,* meaning *with,* plus *wif,* meaning wife in the sense of a *woman;* that is, the "with-woman." The term *midwife* was used as early as 1303; and *midwifery,* in 1483.

The Birth Rate. The magnitude of obstetrics as a branch of medical practice is shown by the number of registered births each year. This figure for the United States was 3,699,940 in 1947 and 3,559,000 (estimated) in 1948. As may be seen in Fig. 1, the birth rate rose sharply during and immediately after World War II from an annual level of about 17 births per 1,000 population before 1940 to a peak of almost 26 per 1,000 in 1947. This was due, in general, to altered economic, social and psycho-

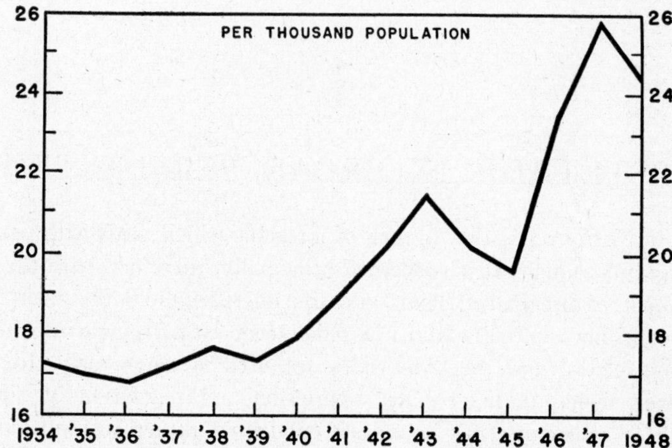

FIG. 1.—BIRTH RATE IN THE UNITED STATES, 1934-1948 INCLUSIVE.
(Based on data from the National Office of Vital Statistics.)

logical circumstances and, more specifically, to a greatly increased marriage rate. The record high marriage rate of 16.3 per 1,000 population set in 1946 was followed by the high birth rate of 25.9 per 1,000 in 1947. This all-time peak in marriage rates,

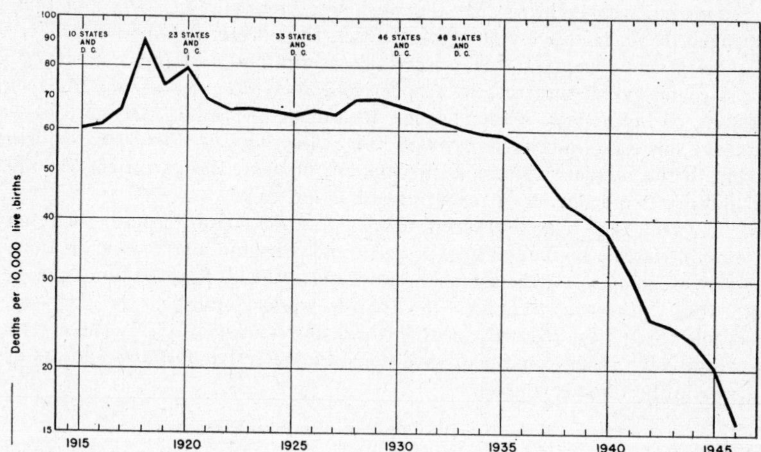

FIG. 2.—MATERNAL MORTALITY RATES IN THE UNITED STATES, 1915-1946.
(Federal Security Agency, U. S. Children's Bureau. Based on data from the National Office of Vital Statistics.)

comparing with only 7.9 per 1,000 in 1932, is attributed to postwar demobilization and favorable economic conditions.

Aims of Obstetrics. The transcendent objective of obstetrics is that every pregnancy culminate in a healthy mother and healthy baby. It strives to reduce to a very minimum the number of women and infants who die as a result of the reproductive process or who are left injured therefrom. It aims further to minimize the discomforts of pregnancy, labor and the puerperium; and, at the same time, so to safeguard and

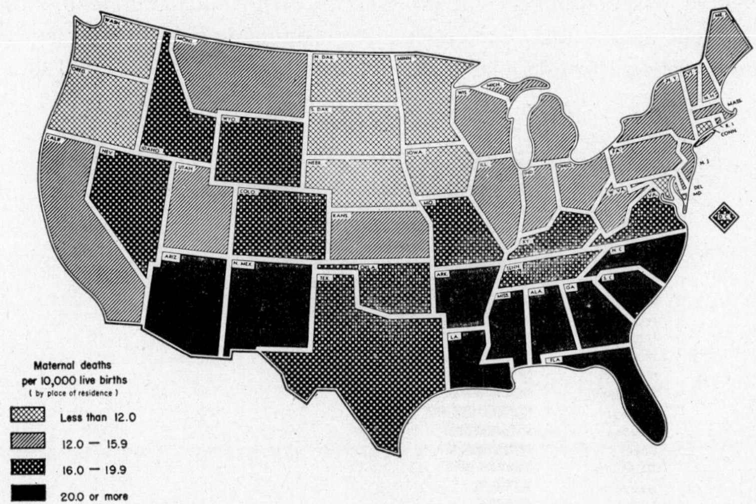

FIG. 3.—MATERNAL MORTALITY ACCORDING TO STATE IN 1946.

(Federal Security Agency, U. S. Children's Bureau. Based on data from the National Office of Vital Statistics.)

ease the whole course that both mother and child will conclude the experience in a healthy state, both physically and mentally. But if it is hoped to reduce the number of mothers and infants who die in the birth process, it first becomes desirable to know

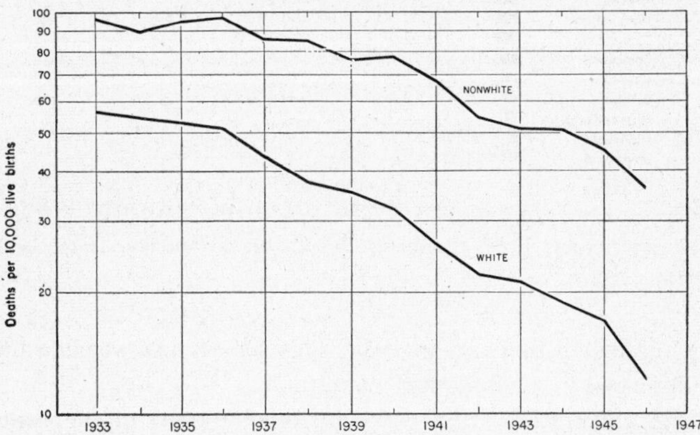

FIG. 4.—MATERNAL MORTALITY AMONG WHITE AND NONWHITE WOMEN, 1933-1946.

(Federal Security Agency, U. S. Children's Bureau. Based on data from the National Office of Vital Statistics.)

how many such deaths take place in this country annually and under what circumstances they occur.

Maternal Mortality. Maternal mortality rates in the United States are expressed officially by the National Office of Vital Statistics in terms of the number of maternal deaths per 10,000 live births. The number of women who died in 1946 as the direct result of childbearing was 5,153 in the course of 3,288,672 live births, giving a mortality rate of 15.7. Perhaps a somewhat better visualization of what was taking place may be had if it be considered that for every 1,000 live births in 1946, 1.57 women died. As may be seen in Fig. 2, there has been a dramatic reduction in maternal mortality during the past two decades from a plateau above 60 before 1930 to a level of

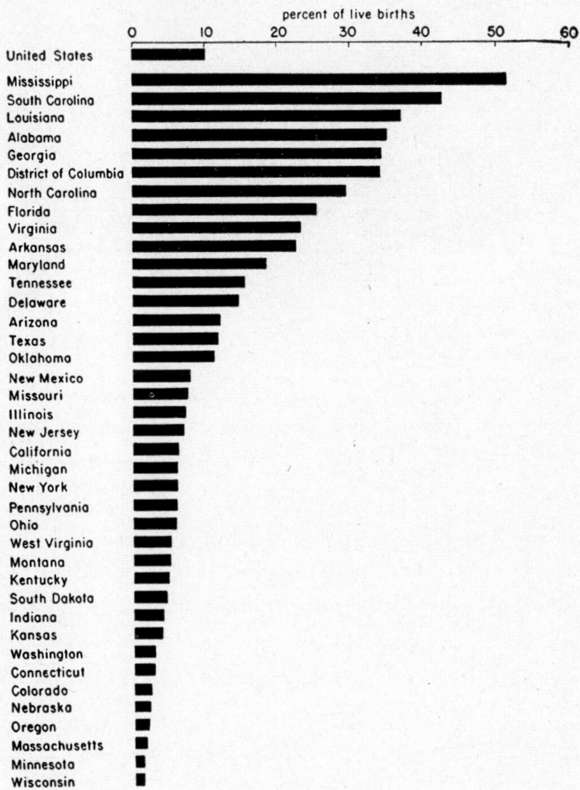

Fig. 5.—Percentage of Live Births that Were Nonwhite in 1946.

(Federal Security Agency, U. S. Children's Bureau. Based on data from the National Office of Vital Statistics.)

approximately one-fourth that rate in 1946. This superb achievement and the reasons for it will be discussed in a subsequent paragraph.

Maternal mortality rates vary greatly in different parts of the United States, as indicated for the year 1946 in Fig. 3. If the specific figures for certain areas are compared, indeed, the differential will be found to be more than threefold. Thus, while Connecticut and Minnesota enjoyed a rate of only 9.2, the corresponding figures for Florida and Mississippi were 30.0 and 31.4. The reason for this difference is made manifest, in part, by Fig. 4, which shows that the mortality rate of nonwhite mothers has long been twice that of white; and in 1946, it was almost three times as great, namely, 35.9 against 13.1. Figure 5 complements the above statement by showing that those states which have the highest maternal mortality figures have also the largest proportion of nonwhite births. For instance, Mississippi heads both lists, while the seven states which follow Mississippi in Fig. 5 (excepting the District of Columbia) all had rates in Fig. 3 over 20.

The principal reason for the high death rates among our nonwhite mothers in southern states is shown in Fig. 6. It now becomes clear that the same states (excepting the District of Columbia) parallel one another in (*a*) a high proportion of nonwhite mothers, (*b*) a high proportion of births with no medical attendant, and

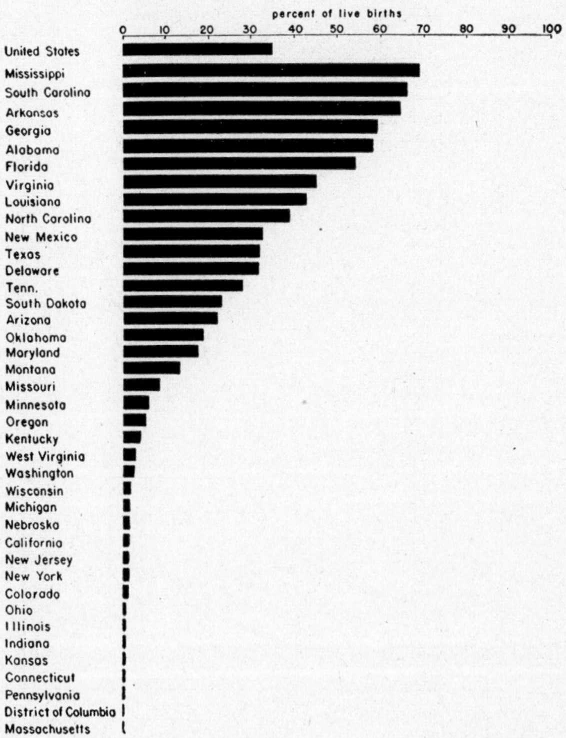

FIG. 6.—PERCENTAGE OF NONWHITE LIVE BIRTHS WITH NO MEDICAL ATTENDANT IN 1946.

(Federal Security Agency, U. S. Children's Bureau. Based on data from the National Office of Vital Statistics.)

(*c*) a high maternal mortality. Let it be noted further that the phrase "birth with no medical attendant" must be construed with its full implications. Almost always, it means also dire poverty, faulty health education, poor hygiene, dietary deficiencies, no prenatal care, and delivery in a shack with no provisions for emergencies and at the hands of an inferior attendant—either the next-door neighbor, or an untrained midwife. In sum, the high maternal mortality rates shown in Fig. 3 for southern states become understandable in view of the large proportion of nonwhites in those areas coupled with the unfavorable environmental conditions and lack of medical attention which they experience. A vigorous attack on this problem is being made by many agencies.

The maternal mortality rate varies also with quite a different type of factor, namely, the age of the mother, as clearly shown in Fig. 7. The extremely high mortality encountered by very young, nonwhite mothers is probably of environmental etiology, since such girls receive notoriously poor care and, in addition, are not infrequently the victims of self-induced abortion. In contradistinction, the tremendous increase in mortality with advancing age, both in whites and nonwhites, can only be explained on the basis of some factor intrinsic in the mother. The increasing frequency of hypertension with advancing years, the higher incidence of uterine neoplasms, and the greater tendency of older uteri to manifest various hemorrhagic

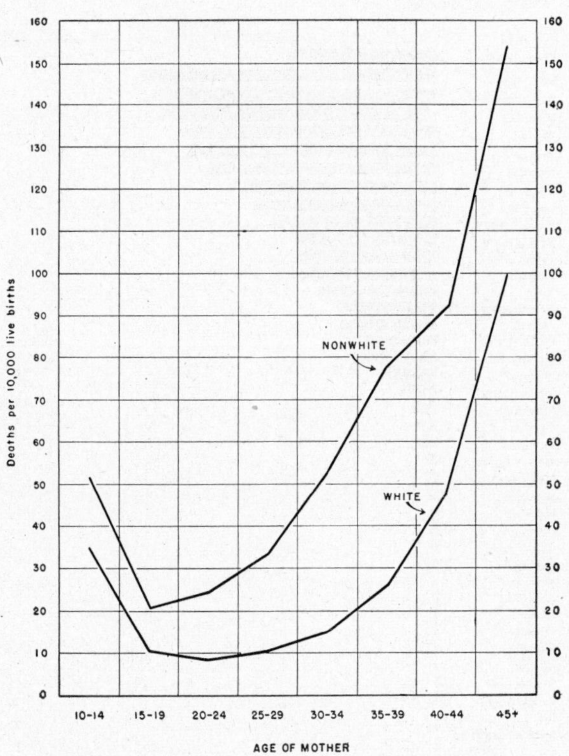

FIG. 7.—MATERNAL MORTALITY RATES ACCORDING TO AGE AND RACE OF MOTHER, IN 1946. (Federal Security Agency, U. S. Children's Bureau. Based on data from the National Office of Vital Statistics.)

complications, all contribute to this effect. As may be seen in Fig. 8, the maternal mortality rises sharply also in women who have eight or more infants. These two factors, advanced age and advanced parity (number of previous births), may occasionally act independently of each other to increase the risk of childbearing, but usually their effects are additive. For example, most women with eight or more children are in the upper-age brackets, while, conversely, the majority of women who bear children during the later reproductive years already have had a number of previous births. In the actual analysis of cases, it is difficult to dissociate these two factors, and hence Fig. 7 as well as Fig. 8 must be interpreted as showing, for the most part, the additive effects of both age and parity.

Finally, in connection with Figs. 7 and 8, let it be emphasized that the lowest maternal mortality rates are encountered in mothers between 20 and 30 years of age. This is also the reproductive period when the outlook for the baby is best. Beyond question, this is the optimum time for childbearing.

Common Causes of Maternal Mortality. The common causes of death in childbearing are hemorrhage, puerperal infection and toxemias of pregnancy. These three complications account for about 90 per cent of all maternal deaths. The causes of obstetric hemorrhage are multiple: uterine bleeding immediately after birth (postpartum hemorrhage); bleeding in association with abortion; bleeding from rupture of the fallopian tube in cases in which the ovum has become implanted there,

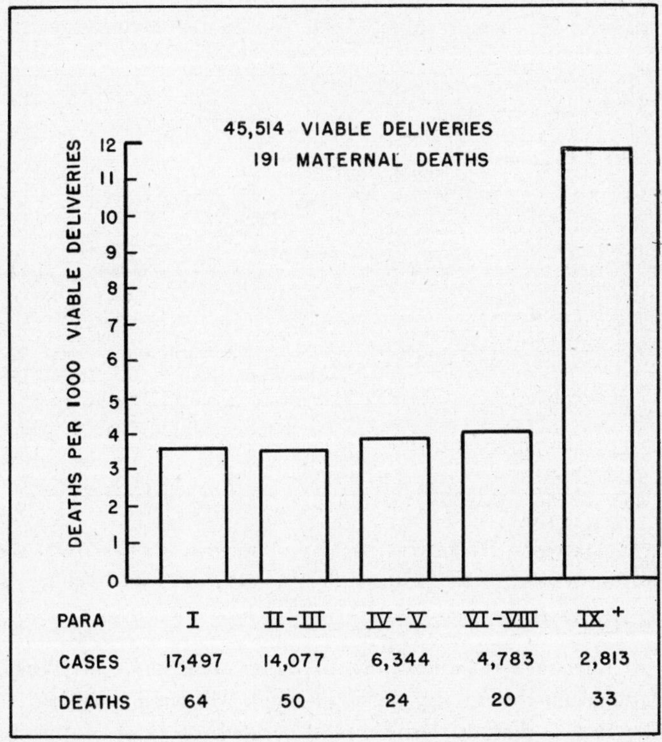

Fig. 8.—Maternal Mortality According to Parity at the Johns Hopkins Hospital, 1896-1939.

rather than in the uterus (extra-uterine, or ectopic, pregnancy); bleeding as the result of abnormal placental location or behavior (placenta previa, abruptio placentae); and bleeding from rupture of the uterus. Puerperal infection is a wound infection of the birth canal, which sometimes undergoes extension to cause peritonitis, thrombophlebitis, bacteremia, and other distant foci of infection. The toxemias of pregnancy are certain disturbances suffered by about five per cent of gravid women which are characterized by hypertension, edema and proteinuria, and in some severe cases by convulsions and coma. The detailed consideration of the nature, prevention and treatment of these conditions constitutes a large portion of the subject matter of obstetrics.

It is apparent from Fig. 9 that there has been a steady decrease in each of these three causes over the 14-year interval shown, and that the decreases have been of about the same degree. Figure 9 indicates also that each of these conditions contributes a similar number of deaths, the exact figures for 1946 being as follows: hemorrhage,

4.8 deaths per 10,000 live births (30.1 per cent of the total maternal deaths); puerperal infection, 5.4 deaths (34.4 per cent); and toxemia, 3.8 deaths (24.2 per cent).

Hemorrhage is listed first among these three causes of maternal mortality for an important reason. In classifying causes of death, it is customary to consider only the *direct* cause, and predisposing causes are necessarily ignored. Thus, if the final and direct cause of death is puerperal infection, it is so classified without further ado. However, a common sequence of events in fatalities from puerperal infection is as follows: the patient suffers a massive but sublethal hemorrhage; her resistance to infection is thereby weakened; then operative procedures are instituted to correct whatever is causing the hemorrhage; these procedures traumatize and devitalize

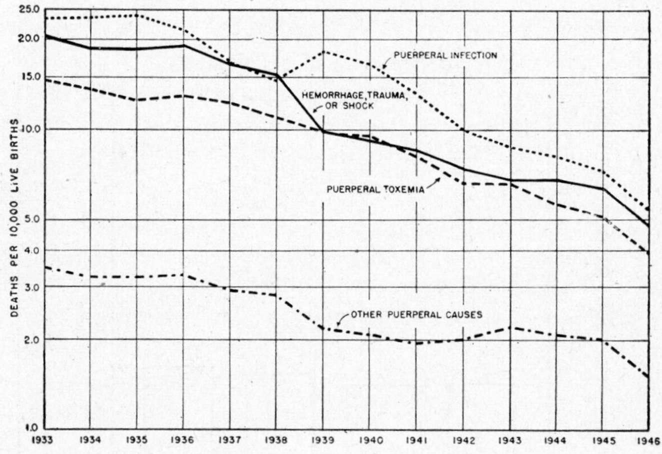

FIG. 9.—MATERNAL MORTALITY FOR MAIN PUERPERAL CAUSES, 1933-1946.

(Federal Security Agency, U. S. Children's Bureau. Based on data from the National Office of Vital Statistics.)

tissues and also introduce infection; death occurs some days or weeks later from puerperal infection, and the fatality is so classified. Although infection is unquestionably the agent which is directly responsible for death in cases of this type, it must be equally clear that the determining cause of such fatalities is hemorrhage abetted by the manipulations made necessary by the bleeding. In varying degrees hemorrhage acts in this manner as a most important predisposing cause of death. But this does not appear in the statistics cited. Only if a woman actually bleeds to death, that is, succumbs to exsanguination and shock, is a death so classified. In view of these circumstances, the total toll which hemorrhage exacts in maternal mortality is much higher than shown in Fig. 9 and, actually, it is the number one killer of childbearing women. This statement is well documented by Gordon's careful study of the Brooklyn statistics for 1944 in which he was able to show that of 62 maternal deaths, 35 were the result of hemorrhage although, officially, most of them were not so assigned.

Reasons for Recent Decline in Maternal Mortality. Many factors and many agencies are responsible for the dramatic fall in the maternal death rate which this country has experienced over the past 15 years (Figs. 2 and 4). Most important perhaps are the widespread training and educational programs in obstetrics which have been developed and which have provided more and better qualified specialists and, at the same time, more competent general practitioners. The American Board of Obstetrics and Gynecology has been especially instrumental in this advance. Although without legal authority, this is the generally endorsed body which certifies specialists in this field. The standards it has set are high. A candidate, after graduation from a Class A medical school and after an interneship, must have had three years of special house-staff training in an acceptable hospital; he must have practiced his specialty for several years thereafter and must submit detailed case reports of the more important cases he has managed personally; and finally, he must pass rigorous written and oral examinations not only in the clinical aspects of the subject but also in obstetrical and gynecological pathology. The 2,500-odd specialists whom the Board has certified have not only established high levels of obstetric care in their own practices, but by example and precept have provided tutelage of high caliber for thousands of medical students, internes and residents.

A unique type of postgraduate instruction for specialists and general practitioners alike was developed by Philip F. Williams in the early 30's—the maternal mortality conference. Begun in Philadelphia, these conferences are now being held in many of our large cities at regular intervals, usually under the sponsorship of the local medical society. They comprise searching analyses of all maternal deaths occurring in a given city, especially from the viewpoint of preventability; that is, was the death due to faulty obstetrics? These meetings are open to the medical profession (including medical students), and the discussions are usually highly informative in respect to the more common and more costly errors in obstetric practice. Such conferences also serve a certain disciplinary function in that practitioners are somewhat more careful in their maternity work and somewhat more likely to call for consultation in difficult cases, if they know that every death will be examined critically at these open meetings.

Postgraduate courses in obstetrics designed especially for general practitioners have been held in such profusion throughout the country that there is scarcely a practitioner who has not had the opportunity of receiving instruction in his own vicinity if he so desired—and the attendance records show that tens of thousands of them have so desired. Even "traveling" postgraduate courses have been instituted in which individual leaders of our specialty have made "one-night stands" in villages to discuss maternity problems with a handful of local physicians. At the other extreme in respect to size, the American Committee on Maternal Welfare has held three huge congresses on obstetrics and gynecology, each of which has been attended by some 5,000 physicians, nurses, public health workers and others interested in the field. The five-day programs of these meetings have been replete with papers, demonstrations and exhibits of the utmost educational and inspirational value. Meanwhile, the Maternity Center Association of New York City and the Frontier Nursing Service have provided a new type of personnel, nurse midwives, who are to be sharply differentiated from the untrained midwife mentioned above. Nurse midwives are graduate nurses who have had extensive postgraduate training in practical obstetrics, and they have contributed greatly to various maternity programs, especially in rural areas.

The *sine qua non* of good work in any field is well-trained personnel. In the ways just mentioned, the personnel available for obstetric work in the United States has been immeasurably improved both in quality and quantity. But this personnel would not have been able to achieve the fine results shown in Figs. 2 and 4 if it had not been for a great expansion in facilities for good obstetric care. Most noteworthy, perhaps, is the extension of facilities for prenatal care. Prenatal care is of American genesis and was first conceived and introduced by the nursing profession. It had its beginning in 1901 when the Instructive Nursing Association in Boston began to pay antenatal visits to some of the expectant mothers who were to be delivered at the Boston Lying-In Hospital. This work gradually spread until in 1906 all these women, prior to confinement, were paid at least one visit by a nurse from the Association. By 1912, this Association was making about three antenatal visits to each patient. In 1907, another pioneer effort in prenatal work was instituted when Mr. George H. F. Schrader gave the Association for Improving the Conditions of the Poor, in New York City, funds to pay the salaries of two nurses to do this work. In 1909, the

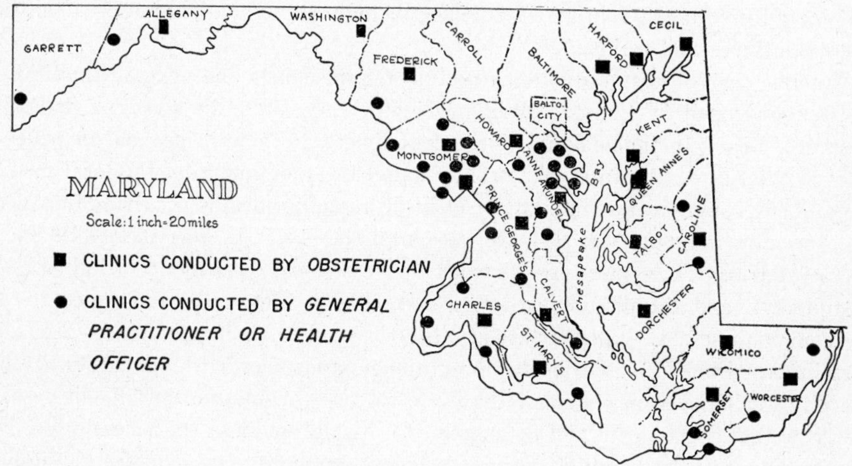

FIG. 10.—PRENATAL CLINICS CONDUCTED BY THE MARYLAND STATE DEPARTMENT OF HEALTH. (Courtesy of Dr. John Whitridge, Jr.)

Committee on Infant Social Service of the Woman's Municipal League of Boston went further: the pregnant women were visited every 10 days, more often if necessary. Thus began the general movement for prenatal care which has probably done more to save mothers' lives in our time than any other single factor.

The past two decades have seen widespread expansion in facilities for prenatal care, particularly in rural areas. As an example may be cited the work of the Maryland State Department of Health as shown in Fig. 10. No less than 55 prenatal clinics are in operation at key points throughout the state; instructions are given to expectant mothers in regard to hygiene, diet, danger signals, and so on; and arrangements are made for competent assistance at deliveries. Patients presenting any abnormalities are carefully screened for referral to well-staffed and completely equipped obstetric clinics for expert care; and, furthermore, a full-time obstetrician is available 24 hours a day for consultation in the event of emergencies. Largely as the result of this program, the maternal mortality rate in the counties of Maryland (excluding Baltimore City) has fallen from 60 maternal deaths per 10,000 live births in 1933 to 10 in 1948.

Similar programs are in operation in other states, with comparable results. They are a great credit to the respective state health departments and to the U. S. Children's Bureau which has sponsored them. The latter organization, through its emphasis on high standards of maternity care, its support of educational programs, its development of obstetric facilities in rural areas and its grants-in-aid for federal and state cooperation in maternal welfare, has played a most important role in providing both better facilities and better personnel.

From the viewpoint of better care during labor, the outstanding advance of the past 15 years has been the great increase in the proportion of hospital deliveries. In 1935, 37 per cent of the live births occurred in hospitals; in 1941, 61 per cent; while in 1946, the percentage had risen to 82.4. In cities of over 100,000, and in 20 states, over 95 per cent of the births take place in hospitals. The multiple safeguards which hospital delivery affords, especially in emergencies, cannot be denied, and this trend alone has accounted for the saving of many maternal lives.

Along with these improvements in personnel and facilities, several major advances in therapy have been introduced. Noteworthy among these is the increased availability and use of blood transfusions, and the employment of sulfonamides and penicillin. Prior to the present decade, many an exsanguinated mother lost her life while the bloods of relatives were being laboriously typed and matched. Now, most maternity services possess blood banks which eliminate these costly delays. They make feasible, moreover, the administration of blood in large quantities which is sometimes essential in massive hemorrhages. The beneficent achievements of the sulfonamides and antibiotics in combating hitherto uncontrollable infections are well known; and in puerperal infection, as in other types, they have saved thousands of lives.

Stillbirths and Neonatal Mortality. The infant mortality which chiefly concerns the obstetrician comprises two groups of cases: those in which the infant dies in utero prior to birth (so-called "stillbirths"); and those in which it dies within the first month after birth (neonatal mortality). This definition of neonatal mortality is that of the National Office of Vital Statistics. The total number of stillbirths in the United States during 1946 was 74,849, while the number of neonatal deaths was 79,079. Of the latter, 69,740 were the direct result of prenatal and natal causes. By adding the stillbirths and those neonatal deaths which were directly the result of antenatal and natal mechanisms, it will be seen that the total infant loss associated with the reproductive process in 1946 was 144,589. During the same year, the total number of deaths in this country from all causes and at all ages was 1,395,617. In other words, the number of infant lives lost in connection with the reproductive mechanism constituted more than 10 per cent of all the deaths in the United States. This same circumstance is observed year after year and indicates the relative magnitude of the infant loss which is associated with pregnancy and parturition.

Almost half of the neonatal deaths occur in the first day of life (Fig. 11). Indeed, the deaths occurring during that 24 hours exceed in number those occurring during the second, third, fourth, fifth and sixth months of life combined. The causes responsible for this huge fetal wastage during the neonatal period are many. However, the most important by far is premature birth (Fig. 12). Thus, of the 79,079 neonatal deaths occurring in 1946, 38,939, or 49.2 per cent, took place in premature infants; that is, in infants who weighed less than 2,500 gm. (5½ pounds) at birth and who, for the most part, were born a month or more early. The factors which are responsible for these premature births, although evident in some cases (toxemia of pregnancy, syphilis, twin pregnancy, and so forth) are completely unknown in 60 per cent of the total. Just why so many gravidae go into labor prematurely and hence give birth to infants who often are unable to cope with extra-uterine conditions is one of the great unsolved problems of obstetrics. The second most common cause of neonatal death is brain injury. Here the word "injury" is used in its broad sense to indicate both

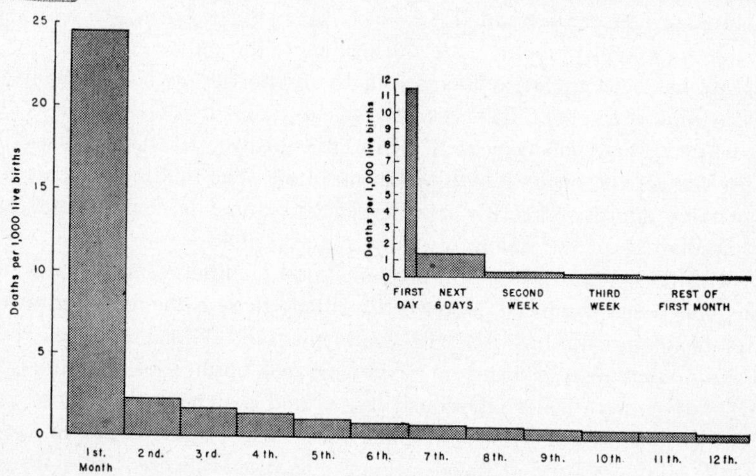

FIG. 11.—INFANT DEATHS ACCORDING TO DAY, WEEK AND MONTH OF LIFE IN 1946.
(Federal Security Agency, U. S. Children's Bureau. Based on data from the National Office of Vital Statistics.)

cerebral injury sustained from anoxia in utero, and traumatic injury to the brain suffered in passing through the birth canal. Many of these deaths could be prevented by more judicious management of labor. Still another but less frequent cause of neonatal death is congenital malformations. Stillbirths may be due to various acci-

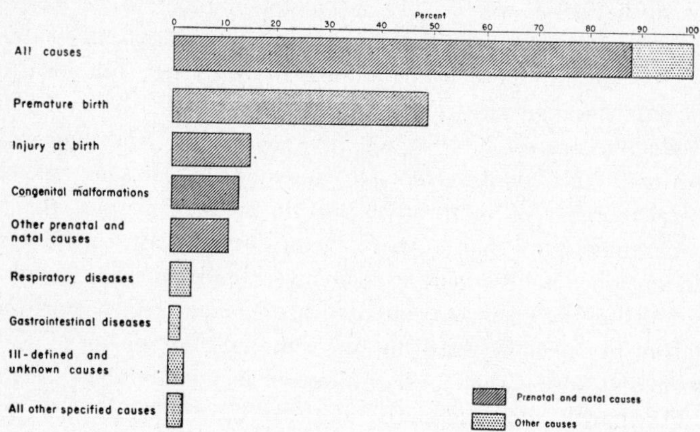

FIG. 12.—DEATHS IN FIRST MONTH OF LIFE, BY CAUSE, IN 1946.
(Federal Security Agency, U. S. Children's Bureau. Based on data from the National Office of Vital Statistics.)

dents which may befall the placental circulation in the course of pregnancy, to certain diseases which may affect the fetus, and also to brain injury sustained during labor. In a large proportion of cases, however, death in utero occurs without demonstrable explanation.

Neonatal mortality rates are expressed by the National Office of Vital Statistics as deaths under one month per 1,000 live births. This figure for 1946 was 24. As may be seen from Fig. 13, there has been a gradual decline in this rate from 32.4 in 1935. The curve for deaths due to prematurity follows a similar course, the rate having fallen from 14.9 in 1935 to 11.8 in 1946. Gratifying as these decreases are, it will be noted that neither is comparable to the fall in maternal mortality, and that both curves have shown a tendency to level off since 1943.

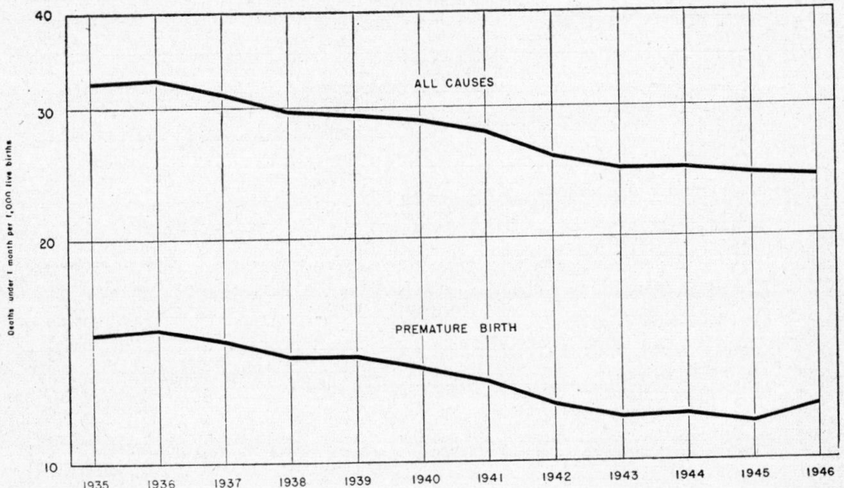

FIG. 13.—NEONATAL MORTALITY RATES FOR ALL CAUSES AND FOR PREMATURE BIRTHS, 1935-1946.

(Federal Security Agency, U. S. Children's Bureau. Based on data from the National Office of Vital Statistics.)

Abortion. Far exceeding stillbirths and neonatal mortality as a cause of fetal wastage is abortion. In medical parlance, abortion connotes both spontaneous and artificial termination of pregnancy prior to the period of viability. Since about 10 per cent of all pregnancies terminate spontaneously in abortion, it may be estimated that the number of these accidents which occur annually in the United States is of the order of 300,000. A large proportion of them are due to faulty germ plasm; many are the result of unsatisfactory environmental conditions, hormonal and otherwise; while still others are of unknown etiology. But if we are to know the total number of potential human lives obliterated each year in this country by abortion, it is necessary to add to these spontaneous abortions a huge but quite unknown number of criminal interruptions of gestation. The sum total is probably not less than one-half million.

The Birth Certificate. Statutes in all 48 states and the District of Columbia demand that a birth certificate (Fig. 14) be filled out on every birth and submitted promptly to the local registrar, municipal or county. After the birth has been duly registered, notification is sent to the parents of the child and a complete report forwarded to the National Office of Vital Statistics in Washington. Most states now require registration of all births, including stillbirths, in which the pregnancy has exceeded 20 weeks in duration; in New York City, however, all births, including abortions, must be reported.

There are many reasons which make the complete and accurate registration of births essential. Individuals need certification of the facts of birth as evidence of age, of citizenship and of family relationships. Thus, in connection with military service and passports, they are indispensable. Moreover, the data they provide are of immeasurable importance to all agencies having to do with human reproduction, be those agencies social, public health, demographic or obstetric. For instance, the data

THIS CERTIFICATE MUST BE FILED WITH THE BUREAU OF VITAL RECORDS WITHIN FOUR (4) DAYS AFTER BIRTH

MARGIN RESERVED FOR BINDING
WRITE PLAINLY WITH UNFADING INK—THIS IS A PERMANENT RECORD.
In case of more than one child at a birth, a SEPARATE RETURN must be made for each, and the number of each in order of birth, stated. Use special certificate for Stillbirth.

BALTIMORE CITY HEALTH DEPARTMENT
CERTIFICATE OF LIVE BIRTH
Registered No.

1. CHILD'S NAME (Type or Print) a. (First) b. (Middle) c. (Last)

2. SEX | 3A. THIS BIRTH SINGLE ☐ TWIN ☐ TRIPLET ☐ | 3B. IF TWIN OR TRIPLET (This child born) 1ST ☐ 2ND ☐ 3RD ☐ | 4A. DATE OF BIRTH | 4B. HOUR M.

5. PLACE OF BIRTH
A. Baltimore City, Maryland
B. FULL NAME OF HOSPITAL OR INSTITUTION (If not in hospital or institution, give street address or location)
C. Length of Mother's stay in Baltimore Yrs. Mos. Days

6. USUAL RESIDENCE OF MOTHER (Where does mother live?)
A. STATE B. COUNTY
C. CITY OR TOWN (If outside corporate limits, write RURAL and give township)
D. STREET ADDRESS (If rural, give location)

FATHER OF CHILD

7. FULL NAME a. (First) b. (Middle) c. (Last) | 8. COLOR OR RACE

9. AGE (At time of this birth) YEARS | 10. BIRTHPLACE (State or foreign country) | 11A. USUAL OCCUPATION | 11B. KIND OF BUSINESS OR INDUSTRY

MOTHER OF CHILD

12. FULL MAIDEN NAME a. (First) b. (Middle) c. (Last) | 13. COLOR OR RACE

14. AGE (At time of this birth) YEARS | 15 BIRTHPLACE (State or foreign country) | 16. CHILDREN PREVIOUSLY BORN TO THIS MOTHER (Do NOT include this child)

17. INFORMANT AND RELATIONSHIP TO CHILD (If different from mother)

a. How many OTHER children are now living? | b. How many OTHER children were born alive but are now dead? | c. How many OTHER children were stillborn (born dead after 20 weeks pregnancy)?

18. I hereby certify to the birth of this child, who was born alive on the date and hour stated above.

Date rec'd by local registrar ________ 19____
Signature ________ Registrar
Given name added ________ by Registrar per ________

Signature ________ M.D.
Physician (or midwife) who attended this birth (Midwife)
or ________ M.D.
Commissioner of Health and Registrar
Address ________ Date

FOR MEDICAL AND HEALTH USE ONLY — CONFIDENTIAL
(*This section MUST be filled out*)

19A LENGTH OF PREGNANCY WEEKS | 19B. WEIGHT OF CHILD AT BIRTH GRAMS OR LBS. OZS. | 20. MOTHER'S NAME AND ADDRESS FOR MAILING REGISTRATION NOTIFICATION:

21. STATE ANY COMPLICATIONS OF PREGNANCY AND LABOR

22 STATE ALL OPERATIONS FOR DELIVERY

23. DESCRIBE ANY BIRTH INJURY

24. DESCRIBE ANY CONGENITAL MALFORMATION

VS 100

FIG. 14.—CERTIFICATE OF LIVE BIRTH USED BY BALTIMORE CITY HEALTH DEPARTMENT. Similar forms are used by other cities and states.

presented in the foregoing paragraphs were culled almost entirely from information which the National Office of Vital Statistics has published on the basis of birth certificates, and these few data represent but a small fraction of the information which might have been obtained from that source. A new birth certificate such as that shown in Fig. 14 provides even more data of direct obstetric importance. Hence, the prompt and meticulous filling out of this certificate after each birth is not only a legal duty but represents also a contribution to the broad field of obstetric knowledge.

Obstetrics and Other Branches of Medicine. Obstetrics is a many-sided subject, and its relations to other branches of medicine are numerous and close. It is most intimately related to the kindred subject of gynecology—so much so that obstetrics and gynecology are generally regarded as constituting one broad specialty. Gynecology has to do with the physiology and the pathology of the female reproductive organs in the nonpregnant state, whereas the distinguishing feature of obstetrics is that it deals with the pregnant state and its sequels. However, since both fields cover the same organs, and since knowledge of the anatomy and physiology of those organs is prerequisite to an understanding of either subject, there is much common ground. Moreover, disorders in either field frequently simulate those in the other, and correct differential diagnosis entails an intimate acquaintance with the clinical syndromes met in both; in addition, the methods of examination and many operative technics are common to both disciplines. For these and other reasons, it is obligatory that every obstetrician should have had extensive experience in gynecology, and vice versa.

The concern of obstetrics in the newborn infant brings the subject in close relationship with pediatrics also. Although in many of our larger medical centers the care of the newborn is turned over immediately to the pediatrician, this is not always feasible the country over; and even in those larger centers, inconvenient hours of birth often impose on the obstetrician the management of the newborn for the first few hours of life—those most critical hours. He must be expert, therefore, in the management of the infant at this time. Since pregnant women are subject to the same diseases, both medical and surgical, as are met in the nonpregnant, the obstetrician is continually encountering the more common diseases in his gravid patients. The clinical picture presented by many of these disorders is altered greatly by pregnancy; and conversely, the disease processes may affect the course of gestation in a decided manner. Thus, in rheumatic heart disease, diabetes, tuberculosis, pyelitis and other common diseases, the whole outlook and management are made different by the fact that the patient is pregnant. The interaction between pregnancy and these intercurrent diseases is very much a part of obstetrics. Psychiatric problems interject themselves more frequently into maternity work than even the obstetrician himself may be aware. As an example, the so-called "morning nausea" of pregnancy has in most cases an important neurotic element which must be treated accordingly.

Among the preclinical sciences, obstetrics is most intimately related perhaps to embryology. Thus, spontaneous abortion may frequently be correlated with anomalies in the development of the early embryo and its trophoblast. Such abortions may also be due to unfavorable environment, such as endocrine imbalance. This and many other hormonal relationships bring obstetrics close to the science of endocrinology. The recently developed concept that the bloods of mother and child are sometimes incompatible (Rh iso-immunization) has shown how immunological factors may interfere with the successful outcome of pregnancy. Obstetrics has its most frequent contacts with general pathology in the field of newborn pathology which is becoming a specialized and most productive field. The important relationships of obstetrics to other preclinical sciences will become more evident as the subsequent chapters of this volume are surveyed; among them are its relationships to bacteriology in connection with puerperal infection, to biochemistry in connection with the toxemias of pregnancy and placental transmission, and to pharmacology in connection with oxytocic and anesthetic agents.

Obstetrics is also related to certain fields which are not strictly medical. Thus, it owes much to the science of nutrition and in time will probably owe more, since many disturbances of pregnancy are suspected of being dietary in origin. In cases of fetal malformation, the science of genetics frequently comes to the fore, because only with its help can any intelligent prognosis for future offspring be established. Since the mother-child relationship constitutes the basis of the family unit, the obstetrician is continually meeting social problems. Not the least of these is the 100,000 illegitimate births which occur in the United States each year. In addition, obstetrics has important legal aspects. This is especially true in cases of criminal abortion, in cases of alleged traumatic abortion (taxicab accidents, for example), and in instances of questionable legitimacy of the child.

The Future. Although the recent decline in maternal mortality has been phenomenal, let no one suppose that the millennium is here or even near at hand. Over 50 per cent of maternal deaths are still preventable, as attested by maternal mortality reports throughout the land. This means that each year some 2,500 women die unnecessarily in the United States as the result of childbearing. Many of these deaths are due to sheer lack of adequate facilities: lack of properly distributed prenatal clinics, lack of suitable hospital arrangements and lack of quickly available blood. Others are due to gross errors of management on the part of the obstetrical attendant. Some of these are errors of omission, such as failure to provide prenatal care, failure to follow the patient carefully throughout labor and for one full hour thereafter, and failure to call consultation. Others are due to errors of commission; among these, unnecessary operative interference looms largest. Today's obstetrics is quite different from that of 20 years ago. Otherwise, we should not have witnessed such a decline in maternal deaths. It stresses conservatism in obstetric surgery and, above all, the avoidance of trauma. Accordingly, the attendant who operates unnecessarily (and, by the same token, often traumatically) practices the obstetrics of a quarter of a century ago and will meet a corresponding mortality.

These several deficiencies in maternity care are obviously the first to be corrected if maternal mortality is to be brought to an irreducible minimum. It can and doubtless will be lowered to approach such a level by the same methods which have proved so efficacious in the past: more and better personnel, more and superior facilities, all more equitably distributed.

But, with our knowledge in its present state, the outlook for reducing the 150,000 infant deaths associated with birth each year and the 300,000 spontaneous abortions—all potential American lives—is less promising. Here new knowledge must be forthcoming if any substantial inroads are to be made. This forecast is based on two considerations. In the first place, over the past 15 years the same caliber of obstetric and pediatric care has been directed toward saving the newborn as toward saving mothers. Nevertheless, the effect of these efforts on stillbirth and neonatal mortality, while appreciable, has been only a small fraction of that which has been exerted on maternal outcome. Hence, while expansion of existing facilities may well be expected to reduce significantly the infant loss associated with birth, this program of itself promises nothing dramatic, if we may judge from past experience.

The second consideration has to do with the obscure causes responsible for these stillbirths, neonatal deaths and abortions. A good example is toxemia of pregnancy, which is responsible for many stillbirths and neonatal losses. But such deaths we are powerless to combat in any effectual way because we do not know the cause and underlying mechanism of this complication. A still larger number of fetal losses is due to the premature onset of labor. What initiates labor prematurely? In most instances, we do not know. In fact, we are even ignorant of what initiates labor at full term. The causes of most abortions are similarly obscure. The same is true of many other diseases which lead to fetal exitus. To unearth the etiologic factors responsible for these many premature labors, these many abortions and the many other complications which threaten the infant as well as the mother, is a Herculean charge, but one which must be met if any great reduction in our fetal losses is to be anticipated. Only with the advent of such knowledge can any true millennium be promised for maternity.

BIBLIOGRAPHY

Adair, F. L. Maternity as the Frontier of Human Welfare. The Mother, 1943, 5:5.

Bryant, R. D., and Assali, N. S. Maternal Mortality. Analysis of Ten Year Period (1937-1946) at the Cincinnati General Hospital. West. J. Surg., 1948, 46:611.

Daily, E. F. Maternal Mortality. J.A.M.A., 1939, 112:2391.

Eastman, N. J. The Hazards of Pregnancy and Labor in the "Grande Multipara." New York State J. Med., 1940, 40:1708.

——— Prematurity from the Viewpoint of the Obstetrician. Am. Pract., 1947, 1:343.

Gordon, C. A. Hemorrhage as the Most Frequent Cause of Maternal Death. An Analysis of the Puerperal Deaths in Brooklyn, 1944. Am. J. Surg., 1945, 70:277.

Maternal Mortality Committee, Minnesota State Medical Association. Minnesota Maternal Mortality Study, Minnesota Med., 1944, 27:475, 577.

Mengert, W. F. Fetal and Neonatal Mortality. Causes and Prevention. Am. J. Obst. & Gynec., 1948, 55:660.

Morton, D. G. Maternal, Fetal and Neonatal Mortality. California Med., 1946, 65:18.

National Office of Vital Statistics. Vital Statistics of the United States, 1946. Part II. Natality and Mortality Data for the United States, Tabulated by Place of Residence. United States Government Printing Office, Washington, D. C., 1948.

Oxford English Dictionary. Oxford at the Clarendon Press, 1933. The statements about the history of the term *obstetrics* were obtained chiefly from this source, as well as the definition of obstetrics as stated in the first sentence of this chapter.

People's League of Health. The Nutrition of Expectant and Nursing Mothers in Relation to Maternal and Infant Mortality and Morbidity. J. Obst. & Gynaec. Brit. Emp., 1946, 53:498.

Seligmann, in Virchow und Hirsch, Jahresbericht über die Leistungen und Fortschritte in der Gesammten Medizin, XIII. Jahrgang, Bericht für das Jahr 1878, Berlin, 1879, erster Band, p. 377.

Stander, H. J. Undergraduate and Graduate Instruction in Obstetrics and Gynecology. Am. J. Obst. & Gynec., 1946, 51:771.

Temkin, O. Personal communication. Dr. Owsei Temkin, Associate Professor of the History of Medicine, Johns Hopkins University School of Medicine, has graciously devoted some time to a study of the etymology of the word *obstetrics,* and the comments on this question are entirely his.

Underwood, F. J. Twenty-Five Years in Maternal and Child Health. Am. J. Pub. Health, 1948, 38:1512.

Williams, P. F. Maternal Welfare and the Negro. J.A.M.A., 1946, 132:611.

Yerushalmy, J., Kramer, M., and Gardiner, E. M. Studies in Childbirth Mortality. I. Puerperal Fatality and Loss of Offspring. J.A.M.A., 1940, 115:568.

Yerushalmy, J., Palmer, C. E., and Kramer, M. Studies in Childbirth Mortality. II. Age and Parity as Factors in Puerperal Mortality. J.A.M.A., 1940, 115:809.

Section Two: ANATOMY AND PHYSIOLOGY OF REPRODUCTION

2

THE ANATOMY OF THE FEMALE REPRODUCTIVE ORGANS

The female organs of reproduction are divided into two groups—the external and the internal. The external organs, together with the vagina, serve more especially for copulation, while the internal organs are directly concerned with the development and birth of the fetus.

THE EXTERNAL GENERATIVE ORGANS

The term *pudenda* is occasionally applied to the external organs of generation, although the more common designation is the *vulva*. This includes everything which is visible externally from the lower margin of the pubis to the perineum—namely, the mons veneris, the labia majora and minora, the clitoris, vestibule, hymen, urethral opening, and various glandular and vascular structures.

Mons Veneris. The mons veneris is the name given to the fatty cushion which rests upon the anterior surface of the symphysis pubis. After puberty the skin over it is covered by a growth of crinkly hair, which is sometimes described as the "*escutcheon*." Generally speaking, the distribution of the pubic hairs differs considerably in the two sexes. In the female they occupy a triangular area whose base corresponds to the upper margin of the symphysis, while a few hairs extend down over the outer surface of the labia majora. In the male, on the other hand, the escutcheon is not so circumscribed, as the hairs composing it extend triangularly upward toward the umbilicus and downward over the inner surface of the thighs. These differences were described in detail by Ploss, and at one time it was believed that they might be of value in determining the sex in doubtful cases. They are, however, not altogether characteristic, the female escutcheon, considered a secondary sex characteristic, not infrequently approaching the male type.

Labia Majora. Extending downwards and backwards from the mons veneris are two rounded folds of adipose tissue covered with skin, the labia majora. They vary in appearance, according to the amount of fat beneath them. They are less prominent after childbearing, and in old age usually assume a shriveled appearance. Ordinarily they measure 7 to 8 cm. in length, 2 to 3 cm. in width, and 1 to 1.5 cm. in thickness. They are somewhat lozenge-shaped, and become narrower at their lower extremities. In children and virginal adults they usually lie in close apposition and completely conceal the underlying parts, whereas in multiparous women they often gape widely. They are directly continuous with the mons veneris above, and fade away into the perineum posteriorly, although in some instances the posterior portions of the labia majora join together to form a transverse fold, the *posterior commissure,* situated directly in front of the fourchet.

Each labium majus presents two surfaces, an outer and an inner. The outer surface corresponds in structure to the adjacent skin, and after the age of puberty is more or less thickly covered with hair. In women who have never borne children the inner surface is moist and resembles a mucous membrane in appearance; whereas in multiparae it becomes more skinlike, but is not covered with hair. It is richly supplied with

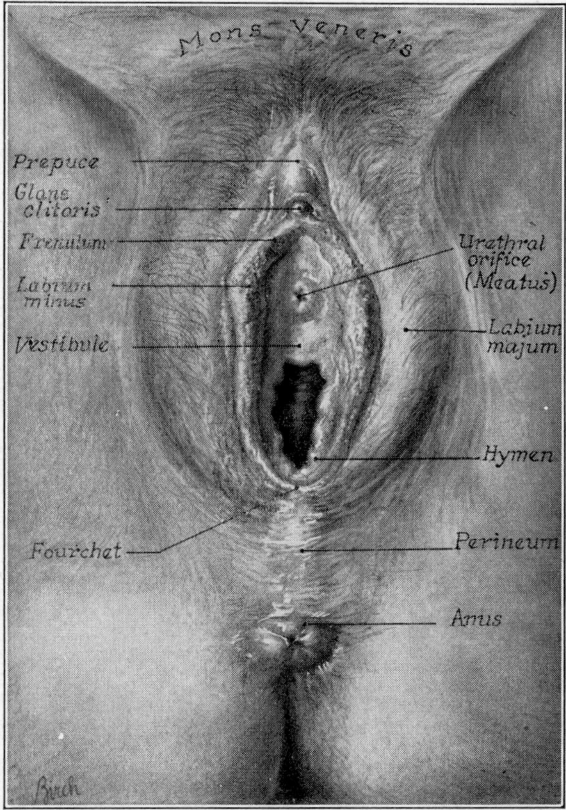

FIG. 15.—THE EXTERNAL ORGANS OF REPRODUCTION.

sebaceous glands. Beneath the skin there is a layer of dense connective tissue, which is rich in elastic fibers and adipose tissue, but does not contain muscular elements. Beneath this layer, which corresponds to the tunica dartos of the scrotum, is a tolerably dense mass of fat, to which the labium owes the greater part of its size. This fatty tissue is supplied with an abundant plexus of veins, which may rupture as the result of external violence or injury sustained during labor, and give rise to an extravasation of blood or hematoma.

The labia majora are analogous to the scrotum in the male, and at their upper ends receive the termination of the round ligaments. Exceptionally, one or both of the inguinal canals, which in the female are designated as the canals of Nuck, may remain patent, so that in rare instances there results a hernial sac which usually contains intestine, but occasionally the tube or ovary, and possibly even the uterus.

Labia Minora. On spreading apart the labia majora, two flat, reddish folds are seen, which meet together at the uppermost portion of the vulva. These are the labia minora or *nymphae,* so called because they were supposed to direct the course of the urine. They vary greatly in size and shape, and in nulliparous women are usually hidden by the labia majora. In multiparae, on the other hand, they project beyond them.

Each labium minus consists of a thin fold of tissue, which when protected presents a moist, reddish appearance, similar to that of a mucous membrane. It is, however, covered by stratified epithelium, into which project numerous papillae. It has no hairs upon it, but contains many sebaceous follicles and occasionally a few sweat glands. The interior of the labial folds is made up of connective tissue, in which are many vessels and a few nonstriated muscular fibers, so that they are classed among the erectile structures. They are extremely sensitive, and are abundantly supplied with the several varieties of terminal nerve endings.

The labia minora converge anteriorly, each dividing toward its upper extremity into two lamellae. Of these the two lower fuse together and form the *frenulum clitoridis,* while the upper ones make the *preputium.* Posteriorly they either pass almost imperceptibly into the labia majora or approach the middle line as low ridges, which fuse together and form the *frenulum labiorum pudendi* or *fourchet.*

Clitoris. The clitoris is a small, cylindrical, erectile body which is situated at the most anterior portion of the vulva, and projects between the branched extremities of the labia minora, which form its prepuce and frenulum. It is the analogue of the penis in the male, from which it differs in not possessing a corpus spongiosum, and in not being perforated by the urethra. It consists of a glans, a corpus, and two crura. According to Temesváry, the glans is made up of spindle-shaped cells, suggesting those of the ovarian stroma; while the corpus contains two corpora cavernosa, in whose walls are nonstriated muscle fibers. The crura are long, narrow structures which arise from the inferior surface of each ischiopubic ramus and fuse together, just below the middle of the pubic arch, to form the body of the clitoris. The clitoris is usually a rudimentary organ and rarely exceeds 2 cm. in length, even when in a state of erection. It is sharply bent on itself, owing to traction exerted upon it by the labia minora. As a result, its free end looks downward and inward toward the vaginal opening. The glans, which rarely exceeds a small pea in size, is covered by squamous epithelium, is richly supplied with nerve endings, and is extremely sensitive. The entire clitoris is very erectile, and its vessels are connected with the vestibular bulbs by means of the pars intermedia. Figure 20 gives a good idea of the relations of the clitoris, its crura, and the vestibular bulbs. The clitoris is regarded as the chief seat of voluptuous sensation.

Vestibule. The vestibule is the almond-shaped area which is inclosed between the labia minora and extends from the clitoris to the fourchet. It is the remnant of the urogenital sinus of the embryo, and is perforated by four openings—the urethra, the vaginal opening, and the ducts of Bartholin's glands. The posterior portion of the vestibule, between the fourchet and the vaginal opening, is called the *fossa navicularis.* This is rarely observed except in nulliparous women, as it usually becomes obliterated after childbirth.

Vestibular Glands. In connection with the vestibule, certain glandular structures—the *glandulae vestibulares majores* and *minores*—are usually described. The former are designated as *Bartholin's glands* (Fig. 16). They are two small compound racemose glands, varying from a pea to a small bean in size, and are situated beneath the vestibule, on either side of the vaginal opening. They lie under the constrictor muscle of the vagina, and in a few instances are found to be partially covered by the vestibular bulbs. Their ducts, from 1.5 to 2 cm. long, open upon the sides of the vestibule just outside the lateral margin of the vaginal orifice. In caliber they are

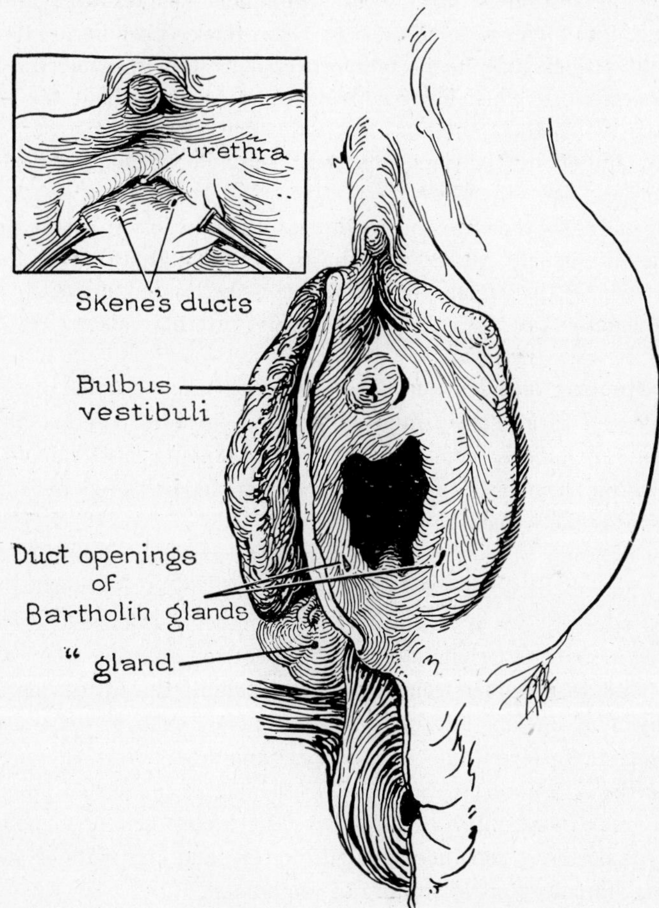

FIG. 16.—THE URETHRA, SKENE'S DUCTS AND BARTHOLIN'S GLANDS.

usually small, and the lumen will admit only a bristle. Under the influence of sexual excitement the glands secrete a small amount of yellowish material. The ducts sometimes harbor gonococci, which may gain access to the gland and cause it to suppurate, so that the entire labium becomes distended by a collection of pus.

The glandulae vestibulares minores are a number of small mucous glands which open upon the upper portion of the vestibule. Their orifices are occasionally several millimeters in diameter, and in such cases they are designated as lacunae.

Urethral Opening. The mouth of the urethra, or urinary meatus, is situated in the middle line of the vestibule, 1 to 1.5 cm. below the pubic arch and a short distance above the vaginal opening. It usually presents a puckered appearance, and its orifice appears as a vertical slit, which on distention is 4 or 5 mm. in diameter. The *para-urethral ducts* open upon the vestibule on either side of the urethra, and occasionally upon its posterior wall, just inside its mouth. They are of small caliber, 0.5 mm. in diameter, of varying length, and in this country are generally known as Skene's ducts (Fig. 16).

Vestibular Bulbs. Lying beneath the mucous membrane of the vestibule, on either side, are the vestibular bulbs. These are almond-shaped aggregations of veins, 3 to 4 cm. long, 1 to 2 cm. wide, and 0.5 to 1 cm. thick. They lie in close apposition to the ischiopubic rami, and are partially covered by the ischiocavernosus and constrictor vaginae muscles. Their lower ends usually terminate about the middle of the vaginal opening, while their anterior extremities extend upward toward the clitoris, where they are united by the pars intermedia through which the blood from them reaches that organ.

Embryologically, they correspond to the corpus spongiosum of the penis. During parturition they are usually pushed up beneath the pubic arch, but, as their posterior ends partially encircle the vagina, they are liable to be injured, and their rupture may give rise to a hematoma of the vulva, or to profuse external hemorrhage if the tissues covering them are torn through.

Vaginal Opening and Hymen. The vaginal opening occupies the lower portion of the vestibule and varies considerably in size and shape in different individuals. In virgins it is entirely hidden from view by the overlapping labia minora, and, when exposed by folding them back, appears almost completely closed by a membranous structure known as the hymen.

The hymen presents marked differences in shape and consistence. In the newborn child it is a redundant structure which projects considerably beyond the surrounding parts, while in adult virgins it is a membrane of varying thickness which closes the vaginal opening more or less completely, and presents an aperture which varies in size from a pin's point to a caliber which will readily admit the tip of one or even two fingers. The hymenal opening is usually crescentic or circular in shape—*hymen semilunaris* or *annularis*. In rare instances it may assume other forms, the most important varieties being the cribriform, septate, and denticulate or fimbriated hymen. The fimbriated variety may be mistaken by an inexperienced observer for a ruptured hymen, so that this type possesses some medicolegal interest, and one must be cautious when making definite statements as to rupture of the hymen.

As a general rule the hymen ruptures at the first coitus, tearing at several points, usually in its posterior portion. The edges of the tears soon cicatrize, and the hymen becomes permanently divided into two or three portions, which are separated by narrow slits extending down to its base. The extent to which rupture occurs varies with the structure of the hymen and the degree to which it is distended, being most marked when it is delicately formed. Although it is generally believed by the laity that its rupture is associated with hemorrhage, this is by no means always the case, though in rare instances such a profuse loss of blood may occur as to require surgical intervention. This idea is probably based upon the Biblical statement that loss of virginity is always associated with loss of blood. In rare instances the membrane may be very resistant and surgical interference be required before coitus can be accomplished. Occasionally instead of giving way in the middle, the hymen may be torn loose from its base in the attempt at coitus, while in other cases the penis may even dilate the urethral canal instead of entering the vagina.

The changes in the hymen following coitus are often of medicolegal interest, as the physician is occasionally called upon to testify as to the virginity of an individual. Unfortunately, however, it is not always possible to arrive at a decisive conclusion as to this point. In occasional instances the hymen may be destroyed in early childhood, either as the result of masturbation or as a consequence of attempting to get rid of seatworms. Among certain Eastern races, again, it is ruptured in early childhood for purposes of cleanliness. On the other hand, the hymen may not be torn, despite repeated coitus; whereas, in other instances, the denticulate or fimbriated type may be mistaken for one which has been ruptured. Haberda stated that he was able to make a positive diagnosis of loss of virginity in only about 50 per cent of the medicolegal cases which he had examined. He believed that in many instances it is impossible to determine whether coitus has taken place or not, unless the individual is seen immediately after the attempt, before the torn surfaces have had an opportunity to unite. Achenbach, in 1890, collected 25, and Kanony, some years later, 43 instances of pregnancy occurring in women with unruptured hymens. We have seen a patient in whom conception had occurred through a hymen which presented only a pinpoint opening, as well as another in whom an elastic hymen had become invaginated sufficiently to admit the penis, but did not rupture until it yielded to the advancing head at labor.

The changes produced by childbirth are much more marked than those following coitus, and, as a rule, are readily recognized. As the result of the distention incident to the birth of the child, the hymen undergoes pressure necrosis in various places, and after the puerperium the remnants are represented by a number of cicatrized nodules of varying size—the *carunculae myrtiformes*. Practically speaking, they are infallible signs of previous childbearing, though occasionally they may follow great distention and long-continued pressure incident to the removal of large tumors through the vagina. In rare instances the hymen may be imperforate, occluding the vaginal orifice completely, and causing retention of the menstrual discharge.

THE VAGINA

The vagina is a musculomembranous tube which extends from the vulva to the uterus, and is interposed between the bladder and the rectum. It serves three important functions: it represents the excretory duct of the uterus, through which its secretion and the menstrual flow escape; it is the female organ of copulation; and, finally, it forms part of the birth canal at labor. Anteriorly, the vagina is in contact with the bladder and urethra, from which it is separated by the vesicovaginal septum. Posteriorly, between its lower portion and the rectum, there is the perineum and rectovaginal septum; in its median portion it lies in close apposition with the rectum, while its upper portion is separated from it by Douglas' cul-de-sac.

Normally, the anterior and posterior walls of the vagina lie in contact, a slight space intervening between their lateral margins. When not distended, the canal presents an H-shaped appearance on transverse section (Fig. 18). The vagina is capable of marked distention, as is manifested at childbirth, or when one attempts to pack it with gauze. The upper end of the vagina ends as a blind vault into which the lower portion of the cervix uteri projects. This vaginal vault, or, as it is usually designated, the *fornix,* for convenience of description, is subdivided into the anterior, posterior, and two lateral fornices. As the vagina is attached higher up upon the posterior than upon the anterior wall of the cervix, the posterior fornix is considerably deeper than the anterior. The fornices are of great clinical importance because, through their thin walls, the internal pelvic organs can usually be palpated without great difficulty. More-

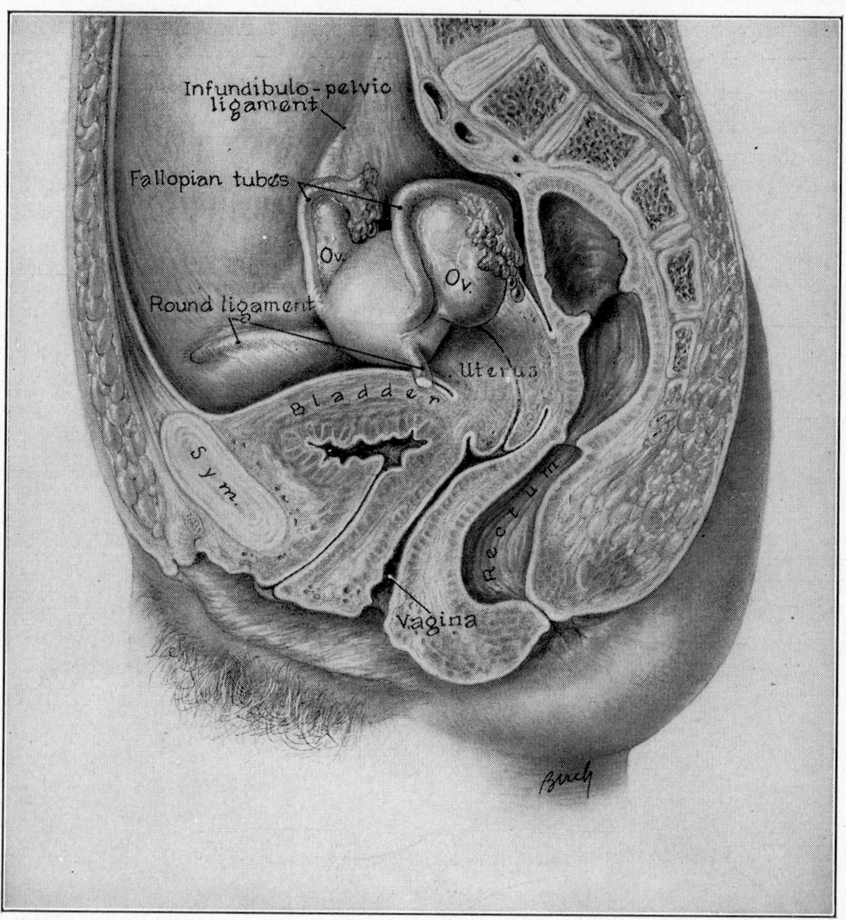

FIG. 17.—CROSS SECTION OF PELVIS SHOWING RELATIONSHIPS OF VAGINA, UTERUS, BLADDER, ETC.

over, the posterior fornix gives ready surgical access to the peritoneal cavity. The vagina presents considerable individual variations in length. Since it is united to the uterus at an acute angle, its anterior is always shorter than its posterior wall—6 to 8, and 7 to 10 cm., respectively.

Projecting from the middle line of both the anterior and posterior walls is a prominent longitudinal ridge—the anterior and posterior vaginal columns, the latter not infrequently being divided into two parts by a longitudinal furrow. In women who have not borne children numerous transverse ridges or *rugae* extend outward from, and almost at right angles to, the vaginal columns, gradually fading away as they approach the lateral walls. They give to the surface a corrugated appearance, which is more marked in the early years of life, and gradually becomes obliterated after repeated childbirth, so that in old multiparae the vaginal walls are often perfectly smooth. The vaginal columns are supposed to represent the remnants of the partition wall separating the ends of the two müllerian ducts, from which the vagina is derived.

The vaginal wall itself is composed of three layers—the mucous, the muscular, and the connective-tissue layers. The mucosa is composed of numerous layers of stratified

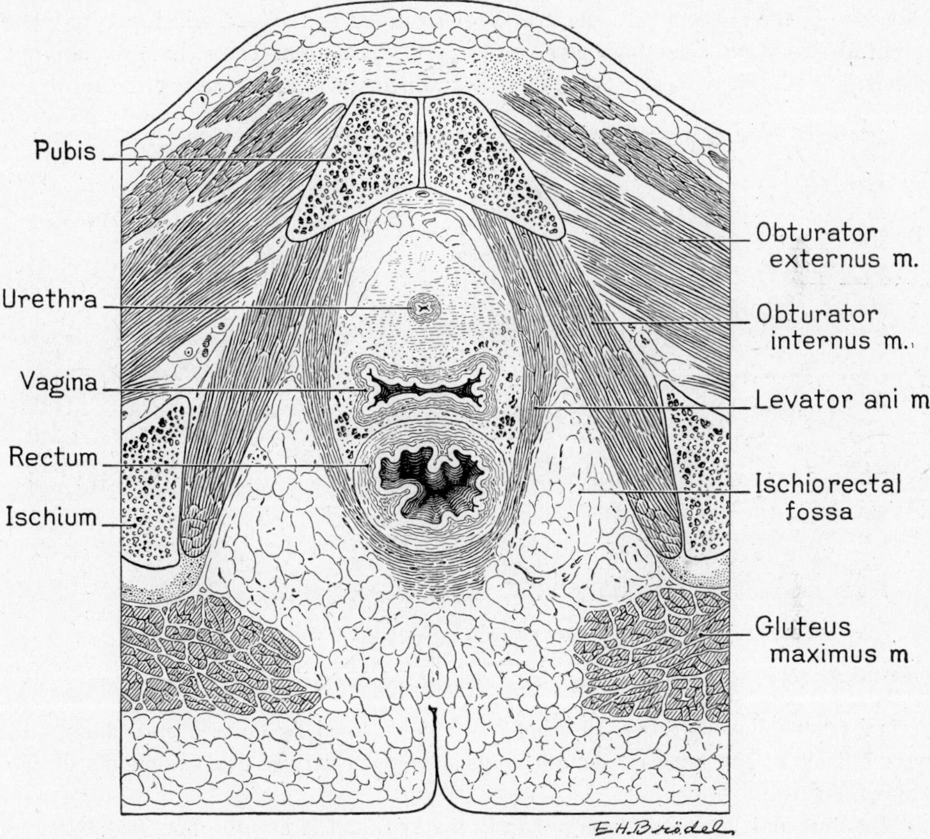

FIG. 18.—CROSS SECTION THROUGH PELVIS SHOWING H-SHAPED LUMEN OF VAGINA. (Adapted from Canton Atlas.)

epithelium, and closely resembles the skin in structure; but, as its surface is not exposed to the air, the horny layer is absent. The lowest layer of epithelium is distinctly columnar in appearance, while the cells immediately above it are polygonal in shape, and gradually become more and more flattened as the free surface is approached. Beneath the epithelium is the submucosa, a thin layer of connective tissue, which is rich in blood vessels. Offshoots from it extend up into the epithelium and form papillae, just as in the skin, and scattered here and there through the submucosa are small lymphoid nodules. The mucosa is very loosely attached to the underlying connective tissue, as is manifested by the ease with which it can be peeled off at operations.

Niderehe, Gragert and all recent investigators have shown that from early infancy until after the menopause, the cells of the superficial layer of the mucosa contain considerable quantities of glycogen. In 1917 Stockard and Papanicolaou demonstrated, by means of their smear method, a definite vaginal histologic cycle in the guinea pig. It is now firmly established that examination of the vaginal contents will permit the recognition of the various stages of the sexual cycle in many lower animals and even in certain primates according to the findings of Heape, Corner and Hartman.

Typical glands lined by cuboidal or cylindrical epithelium are not normal constituents of the vagina. In women who have borne children, one occasionally finds imbedded in the connective tissue masses of stratified epithelium, which may present a central cavity and sometimes give rise to cystic formation. These, however, are not glands, but simply represent tags of mucosa which were buried during the repair of

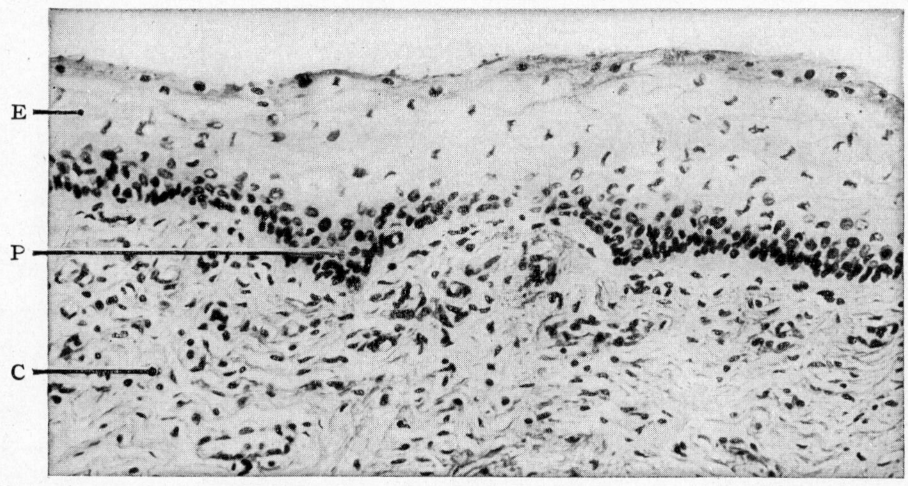

Fig. 19.—Adult Vaginal Mucosa. × 245.
E, epithelium; P, papilla; C, connective tissue.

vaginal tears following labor. In other cases, cysts lined by ciliated epithelium, and lying outside of the mucosa, should be considered as derived from remnants of the wolffian ducts.

The muscular layer is not very sharply marked, and is usually described as being composed of two layers of nonstriated muscle—an outer, longitudinal, and an inner, circular layer. At the lower extremity of the vagina, Luschka described a thin band of voluntary muscle, the constrictor or *sphincter vagina*. This can always be found in perineal dissections, but for practical purposes the levator ani muscle is the real closer of the vagina.

Outside of the muscular layer is a layer of connective tissue which serves to connect the vagina with the surrounding parts. It is rich in elastic fibers, and contains an abundant venous plexus.

In the nonpregnant condition, the vagina is kept moist by a small amount of secretion from the uterus; but in pregnancy a well-marked vaginal secretion is present, which, according to Döderlein and most subsequent observers, normally consists of a dry, white, curdlike material composed of cast-off epithelium and many bacteria, and presents a markedly acid reaction. In regard to the bacterial flora of the vaginal secretion in pregnancy, bacillary forms predominate, though cocci are not infrequently

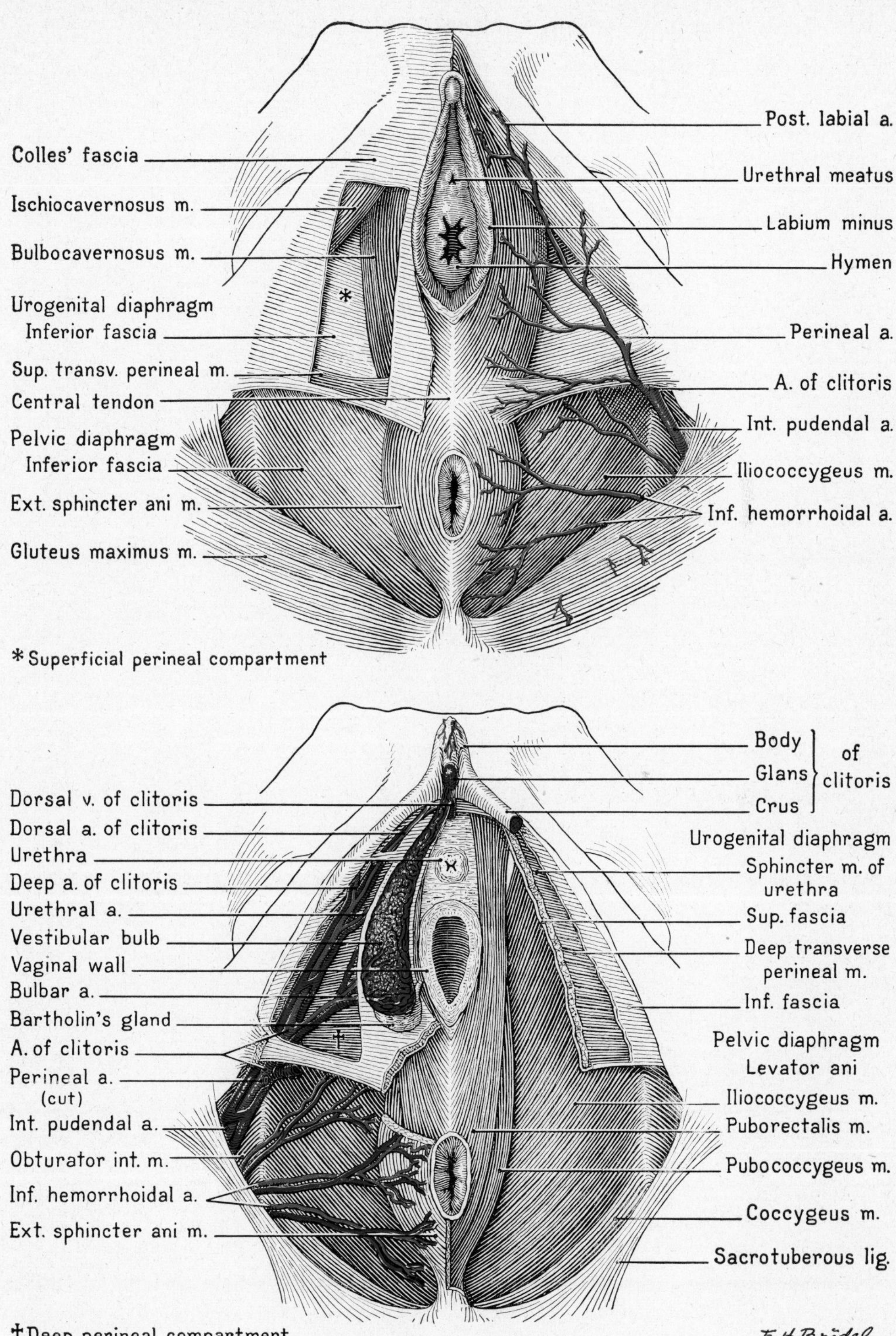
Post. labial a.
Colles' fascia
Urethral meatus
Ischiocavernosus m.
Labium minus
Bulbocavernosus m.
Hymen
Urogenital diaphragm
Inferior fascia
Perineal a.
Sup. transv. perineal m.
A. of clitoris
Central tendon
Int. pudendal a.
Pelvic diaphragm
Inferior fascia
Iliococcygeus m.
Ext. sphincter ani m.
Inf. hemorrhoidal a.
Gluteus maximus m.
* Superficial perineal compartment
Body
Glans
Crus
of clitoris
Dorsal v. of clitoris
Dorsal a. of clitoris
Urogenital diaphragm
Urethra
Sphincter m. of urethra
Deep a. of clitoris
Urethral a.
Sup. fascia
Vestibular bulb
Deep transverse perineal m.
Vaginal wall
Bulbar a.
Inf. fascia
Bartholin's gland
Pelvic diaphragm
A. of clitoris
Levator ani
Perineal a. (cut)
Iliococcygeus m.
Int. pudendal a.
Puborectalis m.
Obturator int. m.
Pubococcygeus m.
Inf. hemorrhoidal a.
Coccygeus m.
Ext. sphincter ani m.
Sacrotuberous lig.
† Deep perineal compartment
E. H. Brödel

FIG. 20.—DIAGRAMS OF THE ANATOMICAL PERINEUM.

seen. The acid reaction has been attributed to the presence of lactic acid, which is supposed to result from the breaking down of the glycogen contained in the mucosal cells by the bacilli of Döderlein.

The H^+ ion concentration of the vagina varies with ovarian activity. Before puberty the pH of the vaginal secretions varies between 6.8 and 7.2, while in the adult it is well below this range, and the Döderlein bacillus is present with greater frequency than before puberty. In a study of 100 normal women, Rakoff, Feo and Goldstein found that the pH of the vagina ranged between 4.0 and 5.0 in all but 3 per cent of their 632 determinations. The pH was lowest at the midcycle and highest at the premenstrual period. They noted correlation between the vaginal pH and flora, the more acid lower range of 3.9 to 5.0 being associated with the presence of Döderlein bacillus only (Grade I); while a higher range, averaging 5.54, was found in the most abnormal flora, consisting of organisms other than Döderlein bacillus (Grade III). The majority of their patients with a Grade II flora (Döderlein bacillus plus other organisms) had a vaginal pH between 4.6 and 5.5. On the other hand, Weinstein and Howard, in a study on the effect of estrogen on the human vagina, found no correlation between the degree of acidity and the frequency of the Döderlein bacillus, and believe that the former may be associated with enzymatic, as well as bacterial action, while the latter is no indication of vaginal acidity.

The vagina possesses an abundant vascular supply, its upper third being supplied by the cervicovaginal branches of the uterine arteries, its middle third by the inferior vesical arteries, and its lower third by the median hemorrhoidal and internal pudic arteries. Immediately surrounding the vagina is an abundant venous plexus, the vessels from which follow the course of the arteries and eventually empty into the hypogastric veins. The lymphatics from the lower third of the vagina empty into the inguinal lymph glands, those from its middle third into the hypogastric, and those from its upper third into the iliac glands.

THE PERINEUM

The perineum consists of the muscles and fascias of the urogenital and pelvic diaphragms. The urogenital diaphragm lies across the pubic arch above Colles' fascia and consists of the deep transverse perineal muscles, and the constrictor muscle of the urethra. The pelvic diaphragm consists of the coccygeus and levator ani muscles, the latter consisting of three portions: the iliococcygeus, the pubococcygeus, and the puborectalis muscles. These muscles form a sling-like support for the pelvic structures and between them pass the urethra, vagina and rectum. The puborectalis and pubococcygeus muscles serve to constrict the vagina and rectum, and form an efficient functional sphincter for the latter (Fig. 20). The median raphe of the levator ani muscles between the anus and the vagina is reinforced by the central tendon of the perineum to which three pairs of muscles converge: the bulbocavernosus, the superficial transverse muscles of the perineum, and the external sphincter ani. These structures constitute the *perineal body* and form the main support of the perineal floor, and are often lacerated during delivery (Figs. 294 and 295). The ischiocavernosus muscles enclose the crura of the clitoris and facilitate erection of that organ (see Figs. 241-247, inclusive).

THE UTERUS

The uterus is a muscular structure, partially covered by peritoneum, and presents a cavity lined by mucous membrane. It is the organ of menstruation, and during pregnancy serves for the reception, retention, and nutrition of the ovum, which it expels at the time of labor by its contractions.

The nonpregnant uterus is situated in the pelvic cavity between the bladder and rectum, its inferior extremity projecting into the vagina. Almost its entire posterior wall is covered by peritoneum, the lower portion of which forms the anterior boundary of Douglas' cul-de-sac; only the upper portion of the anterior wall is so covered, its lower portion being united to the posterior wall of the bladder by a tolerably thick layer of connective tissue.

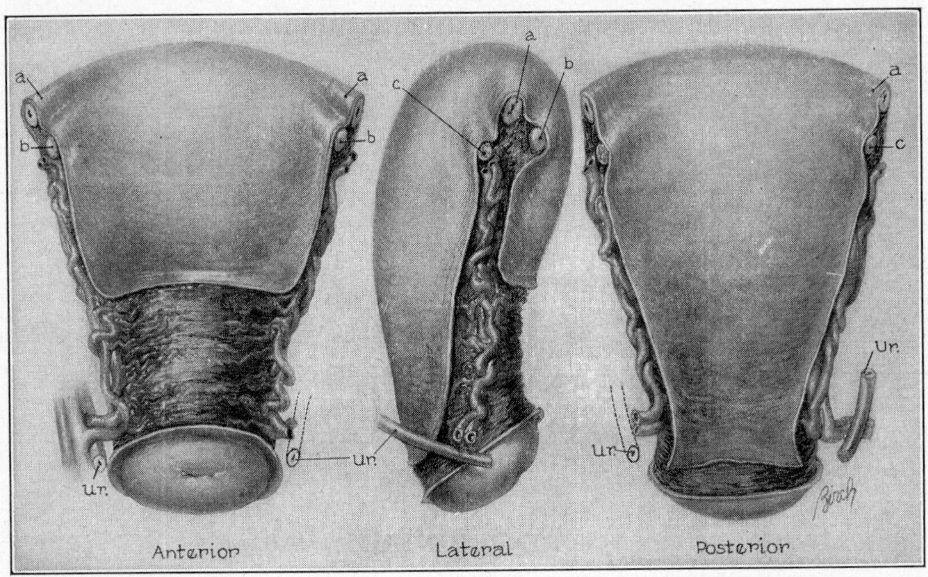

Fig. 21.—Anterior, Lateral and Posterior Aspects of Uterus.
a, fallopian tube; *b,* round ligament; *c,* ovarian ligament; *ur.,* ureter.

Roughly speaking, the uterus resembles a flattened pear in appearance, and consists of two unequal parts: an upper triangular portion—the *corpus*—and a lower, cylindrical, or fusiform portion—the *cervix.* The anterior surface of the corpus is almost flat, while its posterior surface is distinctly convex. In view of the fact that the former, which looks downward and forward, rests upon the bladder, while the latter is in contact with the intestines, His has suggested that the surfaces be described as vesical and intestinal, instead of anterior and posterior, respectively. The fallopian tubes come off from the *cornua* of the uterus on either side, *i.e.,* at the junction of the superior and lateral margins; the convex upper margin between their points of insertion is called the *fundus uteri.* The lateral margins extend from the insertion of the fallopian tubes on either side to the pelvic floor. They are not covered by peritoneum, but receive the attachments of the broad ligaments.

The uterus presents marked variations in size and shape, according to the age of the individual, and whether or not she has borne children. The infantile organ varies from 2.5 to 3 cm. in length; that of adult virgins measures from 5.5 to 8, 3.5 to 4, and 2 to 2.5 cm. in its greatest vertical, transverse, and anteroposterior diameters, respectively, as compared with 9 to 9.5, 5.5 to 6, and 3 to 3.5 cm. in multiparous women. Virginal and parous uteri also differ considerably in weight, the former ranging from 40 to 50, and the latter from 60 to 70 gm. The relation between the length of the corpus and that of the cervix likewise varies widely. In the young child the former is only half as long as the cervix; in young virgins the two are of equal length, or the corpus may be slightly longer. In multiparous women, on the other hand, the relation is reversed, and the cervix represents only a little more than one third of the total length of the organ.

On sagittal section, it is seen that the great bulk of the uterus is made up of muscular tissue, and that the anterior and posterior walls of its body lie almost in contact, the cavity between them appearing as a mere slit. By comparison, the body of the cervix is fusiform in shape with a small opening above and below—the *internal os* and the *external os*. On frontal section, the cavity of the body of the uterus presents a triangular appearance, while that of the cervix retains its fusiform shape. After the childbearing period, the triangular appearance becomes less pronounced as its margins become concave instead of convex, as in the virginal condition. At the menopause, the organ atrophies, becoming smaller in size with a decrease in the amount of muscle tissue, and the endometrium becomes senile.

In 1905, Aschoff pointed out that the lowermost portion of the uterine cavity forms a narrow canal—the *isthmus uteri*—and that the histological internal os is situated at the junction of its lower extremity with the cervical canal. The isthmus is of great obstetrical significance because in pregnancy it expands to become the lower part of the uterine cavity in which the fetus lies—the lower uterine segment.

Cervix Uteri. The cervix is the portion of the uterus which lies below the isthmus and the internal os. On the anterior surface of the uterus its upper boundary is roughly indicated by the point at which the peritoneum is reflected on to the bladder.

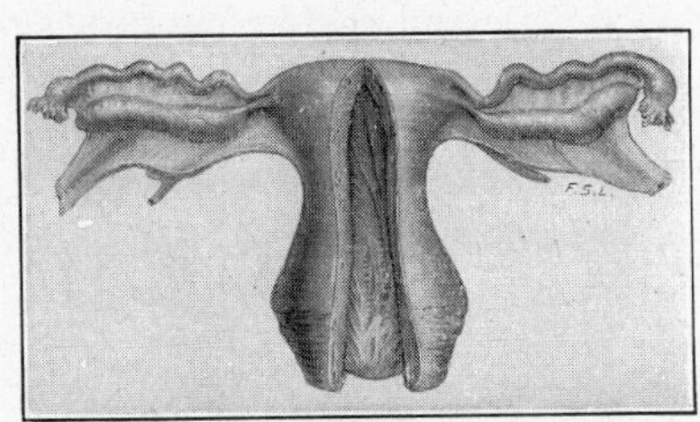

FIG. 22.—UTERUS AND APPENDAGES OF YOUNG CHILD. × ⅔.

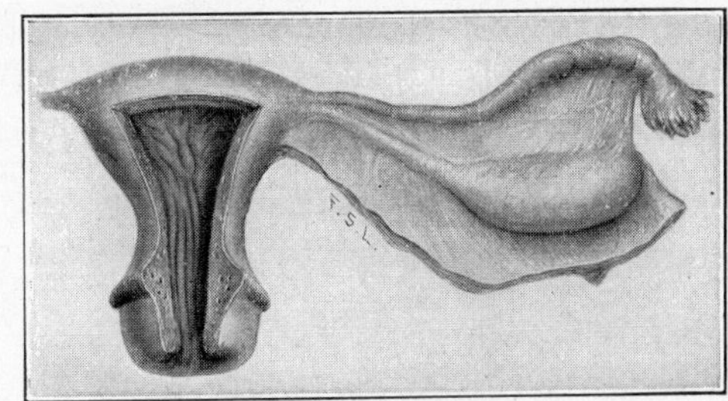

FIG. 23.—UTERUS AND APPENDAGES OF FOURTEEN-YEAR-OLD GIRL. × ⅔.

It is divided, by the attachment of the vagina, into two parts: the supravaginal and infravaginal portions of the cervix. The former is covered on its posterior surface by peritoneum, while its lateral and anterior surfaces are in contact with the connective tissue of the broad ligaments and bladder.

The infravaginal portion of the cervix, which is usually designated as the *portio vaginalis,* projects into the vaginal fornix, and at its tip presents the external os, a small, transverse opening bounded in front and behind by the so-called anterior and posterior lips of the cervix. Owing to the fact that the posterior fornix of the vagina is deeper than the anterior, the posterior lip appears longer than the anterior.

The external os may vary greatly in appearance. In the virgin it is a small, oval opening resembling a tench's mouth, whence the name, *os tincae*. On vaginal examina-

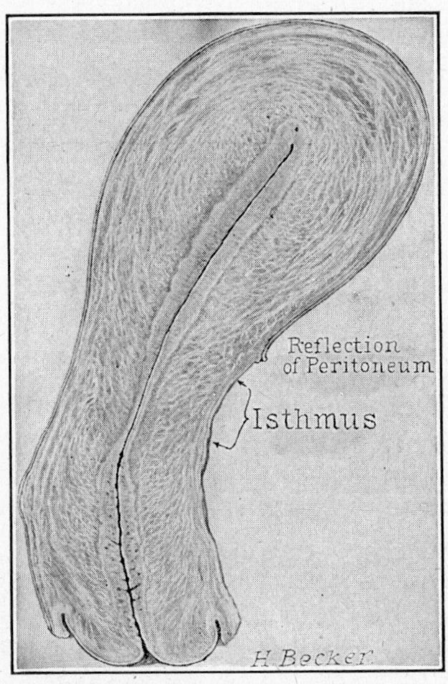

Fig. 24.—Sagittal Section of Normal Adult Uterus. × 1.

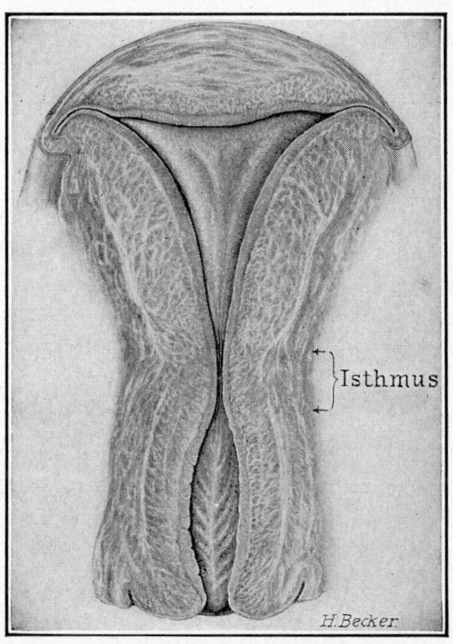

Fig. 25.—Frontal Section of Normal Adult Uterus, showing Shape of Cavity and Isthmus. × 1.

tion it gives a sensation similar to that obtained on feeling the cartilage at the end of one's nose. After childbirth the orifice becomes converted into a transverse slit, and when the cervix has been deeply torn during labor it may present an irregular nodular or stellate appearance. These changes are very characteristic and enable one to assert with tolerable accuracy whether a woman has borne children or not (Figs. 26 and 27).

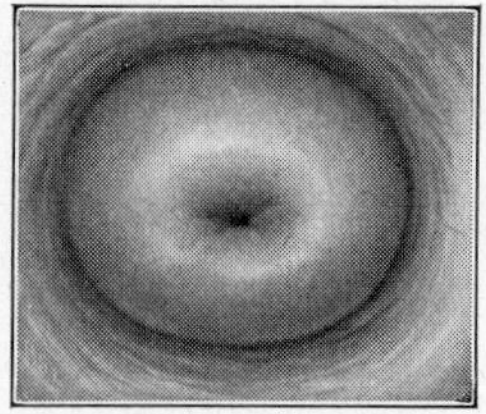

Fig. 26.—Virginal External Os.

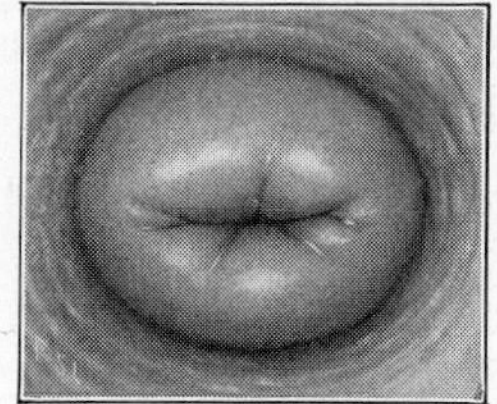

Fig. 27.—Parous External Os.

The cervix is composed mostly of connective tissue in which are many nonstriated muscle fibers, many vessels and a certain amount of elastic tissue, a large part of its distensibility being due to the presence of the latter. Recent studies by David Danforth have shown that about 85 per cent of the cervix is made up of fibrous connective tissue. The transition from the fibrous to the muscular tissue of the lower uterine segment is generally abrupt but may be gradual, extending over the space of 10 mm.

The mucosa of the cervical canal, embryologically speaking, is a direct continuation of the lining of the uterine cavity, but has become differentiated from it and possesses a characteristic appearance, so that sections through the canal present a honeycomb-like structure (Fig. 28). The mucosa is composed of a single layer of very high and narrow columnar epithelium, which rests upon a thin basement membrane. The oval nuclei are situated near the base of the columnar cells, the upper portions of which present a clear, more or less transparent appearance due to the presence of mucus. These cells are abundantly supplied with cilia.

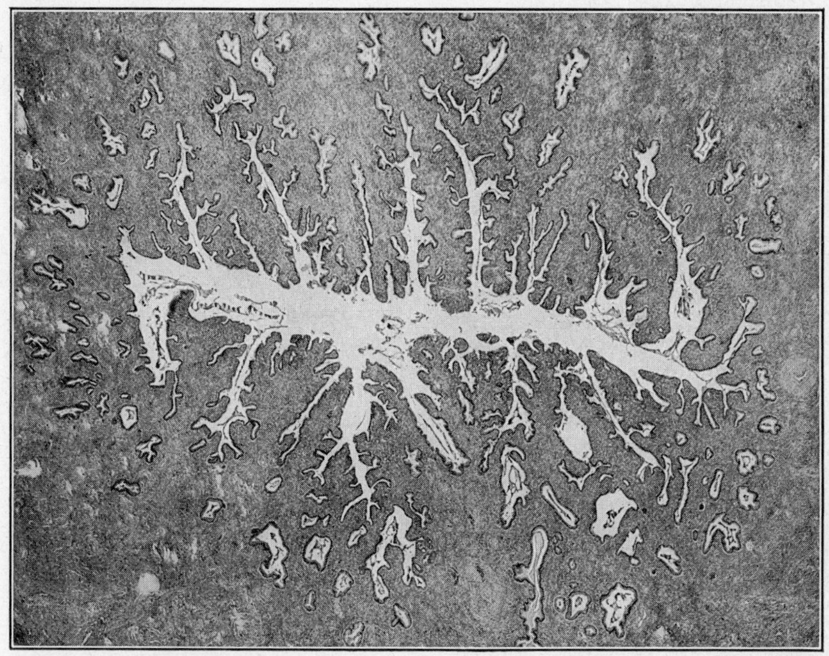

Fig. 28.—Cross Section through Cervical Canal. × 14.

The cervical glands extend down from the surface of the mucosa into the stroma. They are of the branching, racemose variety, and are merely reduplications of the surface epithelium, being lined by epithelium of the same character. The mucous cells of this epithelium furnish the thick, tenacious secretion of the cervical canal. There is no submucosa in the cervix, the mucosa resting directly upon the underlying stroma of connective tissue.

The mucosa covering the vaginal portion of the cervix is directly continuous with that of the vagina, and, like it, consists of many layers of stratified epithelium. Normally, there are no glands beneath it, but occasionally those from the cervical canal may extend down almost to its surface, and, if their ducts are occluded, may become converted into retention cysts, which shimmer through it and appear as rounded protuberances the size of small peas. These are the so-called *nabothian follicles* or *ovula Nabothi.*

Normally, the stratified epithelium of the vaginal portion and the cylindrical epithelium of the cervical canal meet abruptly at the external os. This, however, is the case only in early life, as in older persons the stratified epithelium gradually extends up the cervical canal until its lower third, and occasionally its lower half, is covered by it. This change is more especially marked in multiparous women, in whom the lips of the cervix are not infrequently markedly everted; and occasionally, in cases of this character, almost the entire cervical canal may be lined by stratified epithelium. In rare instances the junction of the two varieties of epithelium may be upon the vaginal portion, outside the external os. This condition is designated as *congenital ectropion.*

According to Wollner there are distinct cyclical changes in the cervical mucosa dependent upon hormonal influences accompanying the menstrual cycle. This is discussed in connection with the endometrial cycle on page 97.

Corpus Uteri. The wall of the uterine body is made up of three layers: serous, muscular and mucous. The serous layer is formed by the peritoneum covering the uterus, to which it is firmly adherent except just above the bladder and at the margins, where it is deflected to the broad ligaments.

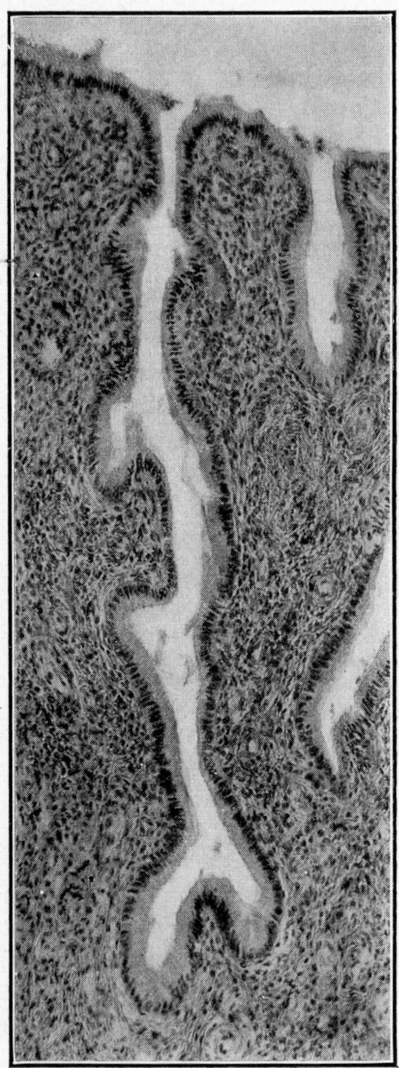

Fig. 29.—Cervical Glands. × 150.

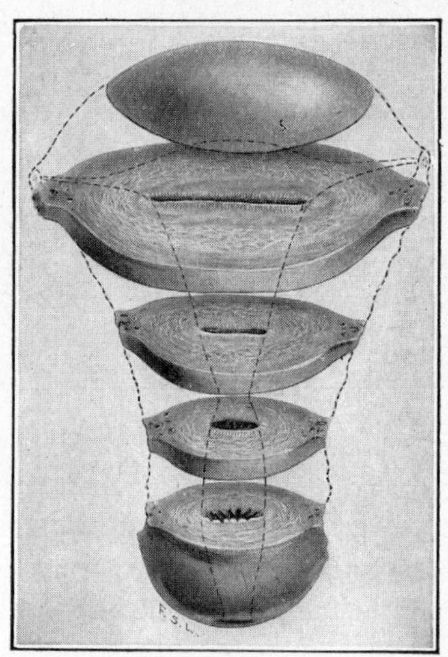

Fig. 30.—Reconstruction of Uterus, showing Shape of its Cavity and Cervical Canal. × ¾.

Endometrium. The innermost or mucous layer, which serves as a lining for the uterine cavity, is commonly known as the endometrium. It is a thin, pinkish, velvety membrane, which on close examination is seen to be perforated by large numbers of minute openings—the mouths of the uterine glands. On account of the constant cyclical changes to which it is subject during the sexual life of woman, the endometrium varies greatly in thickness, and may measure anywhere from 0.5 to 3 or 5 mm. without being necessarily abnormal. It consists of a surface epithelium, glands, and interglandular tissue, in which are found numerous blood vessels and lymphatic spaces. The normal endometrium of the presecretory phase is shown in Fig. 31.

As the endometrium does not possess a submucosa, it is attached directly to the underlying muscular layer in such a manner that its outer boundary presents irregularities in outline corresponding with the interstices between the muscle bundles. This arrangement is of considerable importance in connection with the operation of curettage;

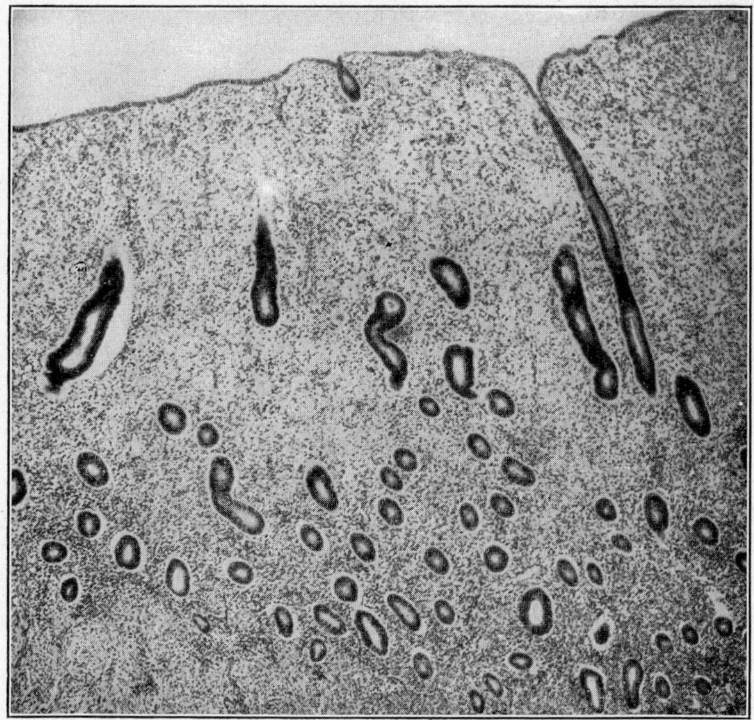

Fig. 31.—Normal Endometrium Shortly after Menstruation. × 50.

for it is from the portions between the muscle bundles that the endometrium is regenerated after that procedure.

The surface epithelium of the uterine mucosa is composed of a single layer of high columnar ciliated cells, which are closely packed together. The oval nuclei are situated in the lower portions of the cells, but not so near their bases as in the cervix. Beneath the epithelium is a thin basement membrane with narrow, spindle-shaped nuclei.

The existence of *cilia* has been demonstrated in all mammals (Fig. 33). The researches of Meyer show that the time of their first appearance is variable, as they may be present at birth, but sometimes do not appear until much later. They are not present upon all cells, but the ciliated cells occur in discrete patches, while the secretory activity appears to be limited to nonciliated cells. The cilia persist throughout the entire period of sexual activity and disappear 8 or 10 years after the menopause. The ciliary current in both the tubes and the uterus is in the same direction, and extends downward from the fimbriated end of the tubes to the external os.

Projecting down from the surface of the endometrium are large numbers of small tubular glands—the *uterine glands*. These must be regarded as invaginations of the surface epithelium and, in the resting state, resemble the fingers of a glove, though

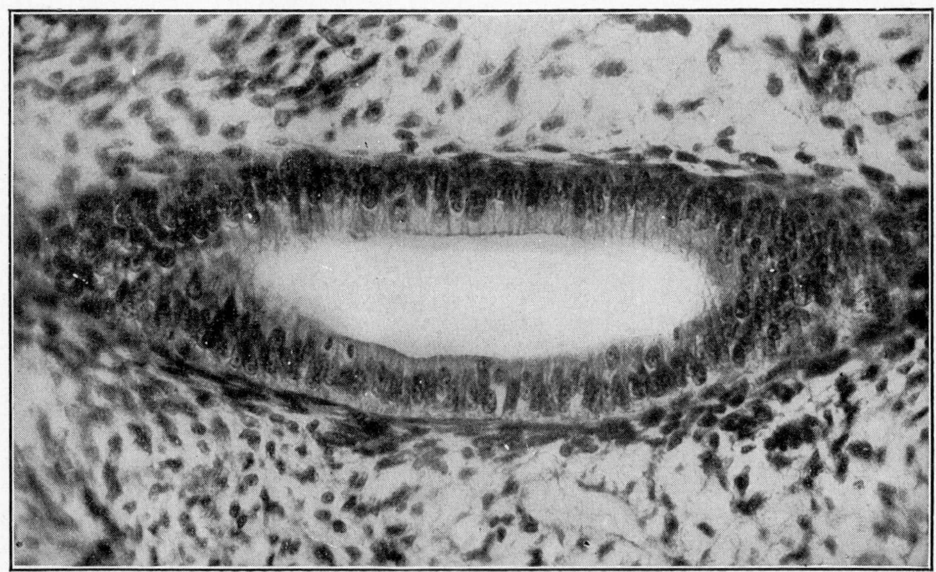

FIG. 32.—GLAND AND STROMA, PROLIFERATIVE ENDOMETRIUM. × 250.

occasionally they branch slightly at their deeper extremities. They extend through the entire thickness of the endometrium to the muscular layer, which they occasionally penetrate for a short distance. They present the same histological structure as the surface epithelium, and are lined by a single layer of high columnar ciliated epithelium,

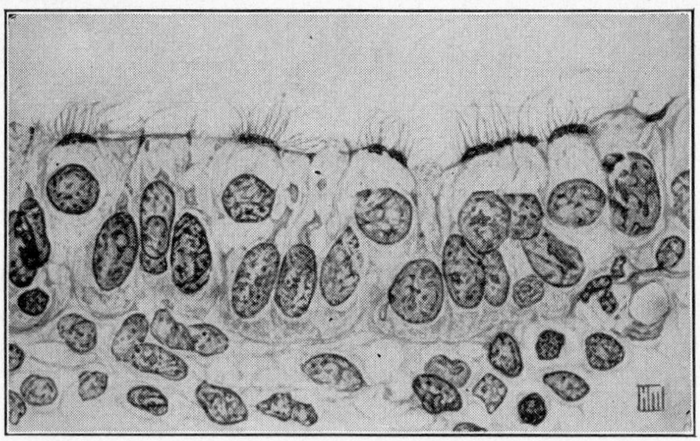

FIG. 33.—CROSS SECTION OF UTERINE GLAND SHOWING CILIATED CELLS. × 535.
(Courtesy of Dr. George N. Papanicolaou.)

which rests upon a thin basement membrane. They secrete small quantities of a thin, alkaline fluid which serves to keep the uterine cavity moist (see Figs. 31 and 33).

Following the appearance of the epoch-making monograph of Hitschmann and Adler in 1908, much work has been done upon the anatomy of the endometrium. The consensus is that it is undergoing constant change during each menstrual cycle, and that three fundamental phases may be observed every 28 days: menstruation, proliferation, and a period of secretory activity. These changes will be considered in detail in the section upon menstruation, and here it will suffice to say that immediately

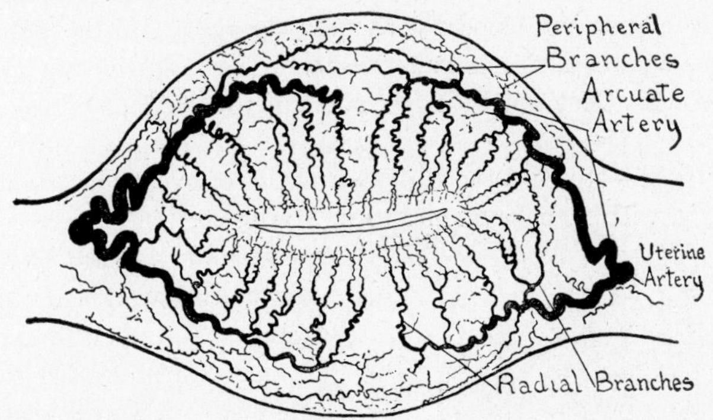

FIG. 34.—COMPOSITE TRACING OF RADIOGRAPHS OF THIN CROSS SECTIONS OF UTERUS, SHOWING ARTERIAL SYSTEM. (Sampson.)

after menstruation the normal membrane is quite thin and contains relatively few tubular glands; while it increases rapidly in thickness during the period of premenstrual swelling, and then contains many convoluted or corkscrew-like glands. At the menopause the entire endometrium undergoes atrophic change; its epithelium becomes

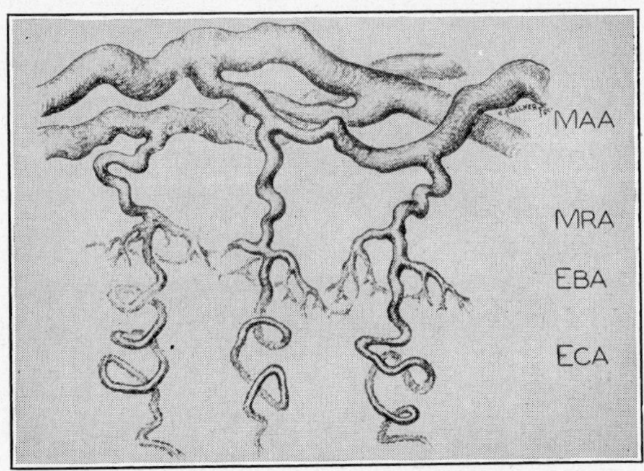

FIG. 35.—STEREOGRAPHIC REPRESENTATION OF MYOMETRIAL AND ENDOMETRIAL GROUPS IN THE MACAQUE MONKEY.

Above are shown parts of myometrial arcuate arteries (*MAA*) from which proceed myometrial radial arteries (*MRA*) toward the endometrium, in which two types of arteries are found: the larger endometrial coiled arteries (*ECA*) and the smaller endometrial basal arteries (*EBA*). (From Okkels and Engle, *Acta path. et microbiol. Scandinav.*, 1938, 15:150.)

flatter, its glands gradually disappear, and its interglandular tissue takes on a more fibrous appearance.

The portion of the endometrium lying between the surface epithelium and the underlying muscle, which is not occupied by glands, is filled by an *interglandular* tissue or stroma of an embryonic type. In the postmenstrual stage, under the microscope (Figs. 31 and 32), it is seen to be made up of closely packed oval and spindle-shaped nuclei, around which there is very little protoplasm. When the tissues are spread apart by edema it is readily seen that the cells present a stellate appearance, with branching protoplasmic processes which anastomose one with another. The cells are more closely packed around the glands and blood vessels than elsewhere. On the other hand, during the premenstrual stage they become larger and more vesicular in character, and closely resemble decidual cells. Occasionally larger or smaller collections of round cells may be seen among them.

The vascular architecture of the endometrium is of great importance since it has a close relationship with menstruation and also with certain phenomena observed in pregnancy. Arterial blood is carried to the uterus by the uterine and ovarian arteries and their branches. As these branches, penetrating the uterine wall obliquely inward, reach its middle third, they ramify on a plane parallel to the surface and are known as the *arcuate arteries.* From these arcuate arteries, radial branches extend at right angles toward the endometrium, as shown in Fig. 34. The endometrial arteries are of two sorts: *spiral arteries,* which represent essentially a continuation of these radial arteries; and *basal arteries,* which branch from the radial arteries at a sharp angle, as shown in Fig. 35. The spiral arteries, which are characterized by their coiled state, supply most of the middle and all the superficial third of the endometrium. Their walls have been shown by Okkels and Engle to be quite sensitive to hormonal influences, especially to vasoconstricting effects, and for this reason they probably play some part in the mechanism of menstrual bleeding, as explained on page 93. The basal, or straight, endometrial arteries are smaller both in caliber and length than the spiral. They extend only into the basal layer of the endometrium or at most a short distance into the middle layer. The basal arteries, in contradistinction to the spiral, are not affected by hormonal influences.

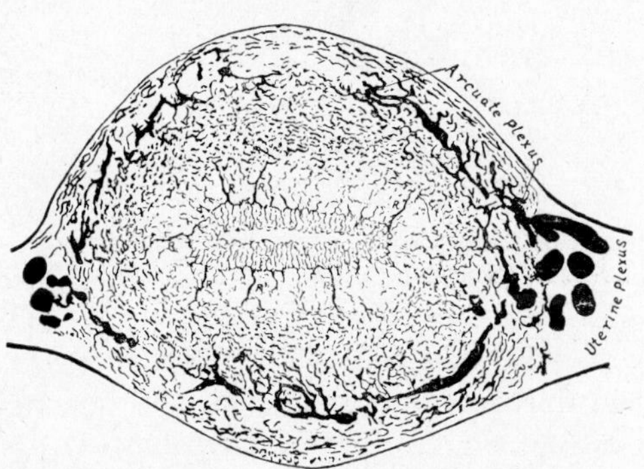

Fig. 36.—Composite Tracing of Radiographs of Thin Cross Sections of Uterus showing Venous System. (Sampson.)

Musculature of the Uterus. The major part of the uterus is made up of bundles of nonstriated muscle, which are united by a greater or lesser amount of connective tissue, in which are found many elastic fibers. On section, the nonpregnant uterine wall presents a thick, felt-like structure, in which definite layers cannot be distinguished.

Ligaments of the Uterus. Extending from either half of the uterus are three ligamentous structures—the broad, round, and uterosacral ligaments (ligamenta lata, teretia, and uterosacralia).

The *broad ligaments,* or *ligamenta lata,* are two winglike structures which extend from the lateral margins of the uterus to the pelvic walls, and serve to divide the pelvic cavity into an anterior and a posterior compartment. Each broad ligament consists of a fold of peritoneum inclosing various structures within it, and presents four margins for examination—a superior, lateral, inferior, and median. The superior margin, for its inner two thirds, is occupied by the fallopian tube, while its outer third, extending from the fimbriated end of the tube to the pelvic wall, is known as the *infundibulo-pelvic ligament*—the suspensory ligament of the ovary (Henle)—and serves to transmit the ovarian vessels. The portion of the broad ligament beneath the fallopian tube is called the *mesosalpinx,* and consists of two layers of peritoneum which are united by a small amount of loose connective tissue, in which is embedded the *parovarium* or organ of Rosenmüller.

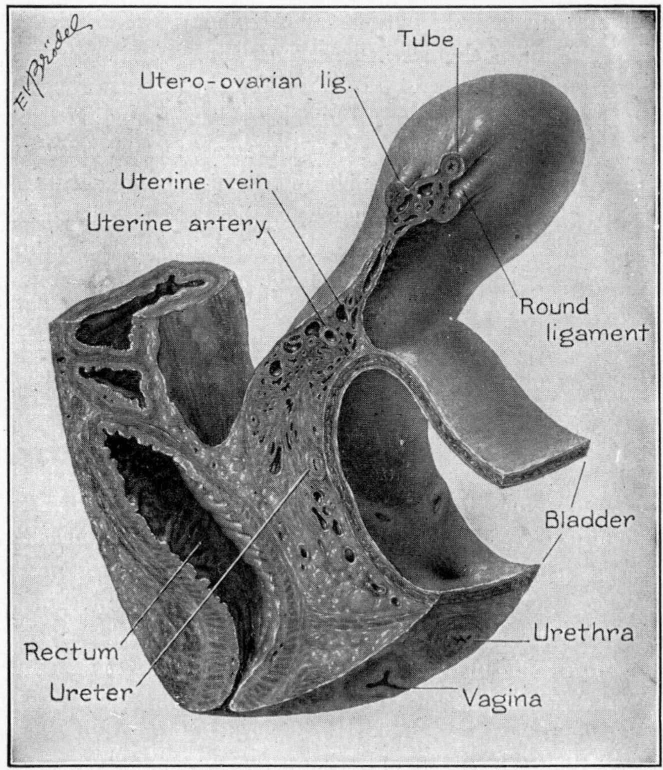

Fig. 37.—Section through Uterine End of Broad Ligament. × ⅔.

The parovarium consists of a number of narrow vertical tubules, lined with ciliated epithelium, which connect by their upper ends with a longitudinal duct, which extends just below the tube to the lateral margin of the uterus, in whose muscular wall it ends blindly at about the region of the internal os. This canal is the remnant of the wolffian duct, and in the female is designated as Gartner's duct. The parovarium corresponds to the epididymis and is usually considered as the remains of the wolffian body. Waldeyer, in 1870, however, showed that it represents only the cranial portion of the latter, and designated it as the epoophoron, and suggested the term paroophoron for its caudal portion.

The latter is the analogue of the organ of Giraldès, and according to Rieländer is situated near the free end of the broad ligament between the terminal branches of the ovarian artery just before they enter the ovary. The paroophoron consists of a small number of slightly convoluted tubules, lined by nonciliated epithelium. The organ tends to disappear with advancing years; and is of interest only from the fact that it occasionally gives rise to tumor formations.

Hofbauer in 1926 showed that in the connective tissue at the sides of the uterus, as well as at the base of the broad ligament, there are always a certain number of clasmatocytes. He believes that in the presence of infection or of other irritation they increase greatly in number and serve to engulf bacteria, so that he has designated the phenomenon as a defensive mechanism.

At the lateral margin of the broad ligament, the peritoneal covering is reflected upon the side of the pelvis. The inferior margin, which is quite thick, is continuous with the connective tissue of the pelvic floor. Through it pass the uterine vessels. Its lower portion—the cardinal ligament of Kocks, the *ligamentum transversale colli* of Mackenrodt, or the *retinaculum uteri* of Martin—is composed of dense connective tissue which is firmly united to the supravaginal portion of the cervix. The median margin is connected with the lateral margin of the uterus, and incloses the uterine vessels; through it certain muscular and connective tissue bands extend from the uterus into the broad ligament.

A vertical section through the uterine end of the broad ligament is triangular in shape, with the apex directed upward, while its base is broad and contains the uterine vessels; it is widely connected with the connective tissue of the pelvic floor, which is designated as the *parametrium*. A vertical section through the middle portion of the broad ligament shows that its upper part is made up mainly of three branches in which the tube, ovary, and round ligament are situated, while its lower portion is not so thick as in the previous section.

The *round ligaments,* or *ligamenta teretia,* extend on either side from the anterior and lateral portion of the uterus, just below the insertion of the tubes. Each lies in a fold of the broad ligament and runs in an upward and outward direction to the inguinal canal, through which it passes, to terminate finally in the upper portion of the labium majus. The round ligament varies from 3 to 5 mm. in diameter; it is composed of nonstriated muscle, which is directly continuous with that of the uterine wall, and a certain amount of connective tissue. In the nonpregnant condition it appears as a lax cord, but in pregnancy it undergoes considerable hypertrophy and seems to act as a stay for the uterus. It can be palpated during pregnancy, and by its varying position aids in diagnosing the location of the placenta.

The *uterosacral ligaments* are two structures which extend from the posterior and upper portion of the cervix, encircle the rectum, and are inserted into the fascia covering the second and third sacral vertebrae. They are likewise composed of connective tissue and muscle, and are covered by peritoneum. They form the lateral boundaries of Douglas' cul-de-sac and play a small part in retaining the uterus in its normal position by exerting traction upon the cervix.

Position of the Uterus. The normal position of the uterus is one of slight anteflexion. With the woman standing upright, it occupies an almost horizontal position and is somewhat bent upon its vesical surface, the fundus resting upon the bladder, while the cervix is directed backward toward the tip of the sacrum, with the external os about on the level of the ischial spines. The position of the organ varies markedly according to the degree of distention of the bladder and rectum, but when these are empty the uterus tends to resume the position described.

The completely normal uterus is a movable organ within certain limits. The cervix

NOTE

The following two illustrations are presented face to face in order to provide better visualization of the anatomy of the uterine blood supply. The first of these (Fig. 38) shows the blood vessels of the pelvis in their general relation to the major organs of the female pelvis. Figure 39 depicts the more minute relationships of the blood vessels which supply the uterus, ovaries and fallopian tubes. In the latter illustration the close proximity of the uterine artery to the ureter is particularly worthy of note.

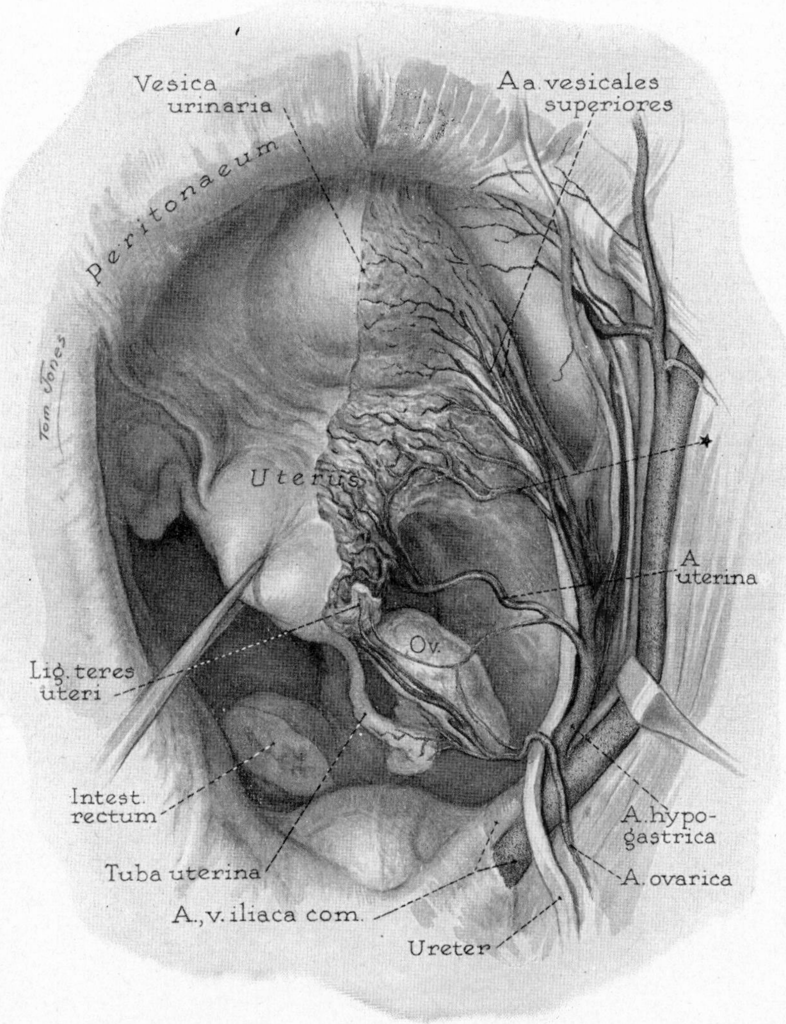

FIG. 38.—BLOOD VESSELS OF THE UTERUS AND PELVIS.

(From Curtis, Anson, Ashley and Jones, *Surg. Gyn. Obst.*, 1942, 75:421-423. By permission of Surgery, Gynecology and Obstetrics. Copyright, 1942, by The Surgical Publishing Co. of Chicago.)

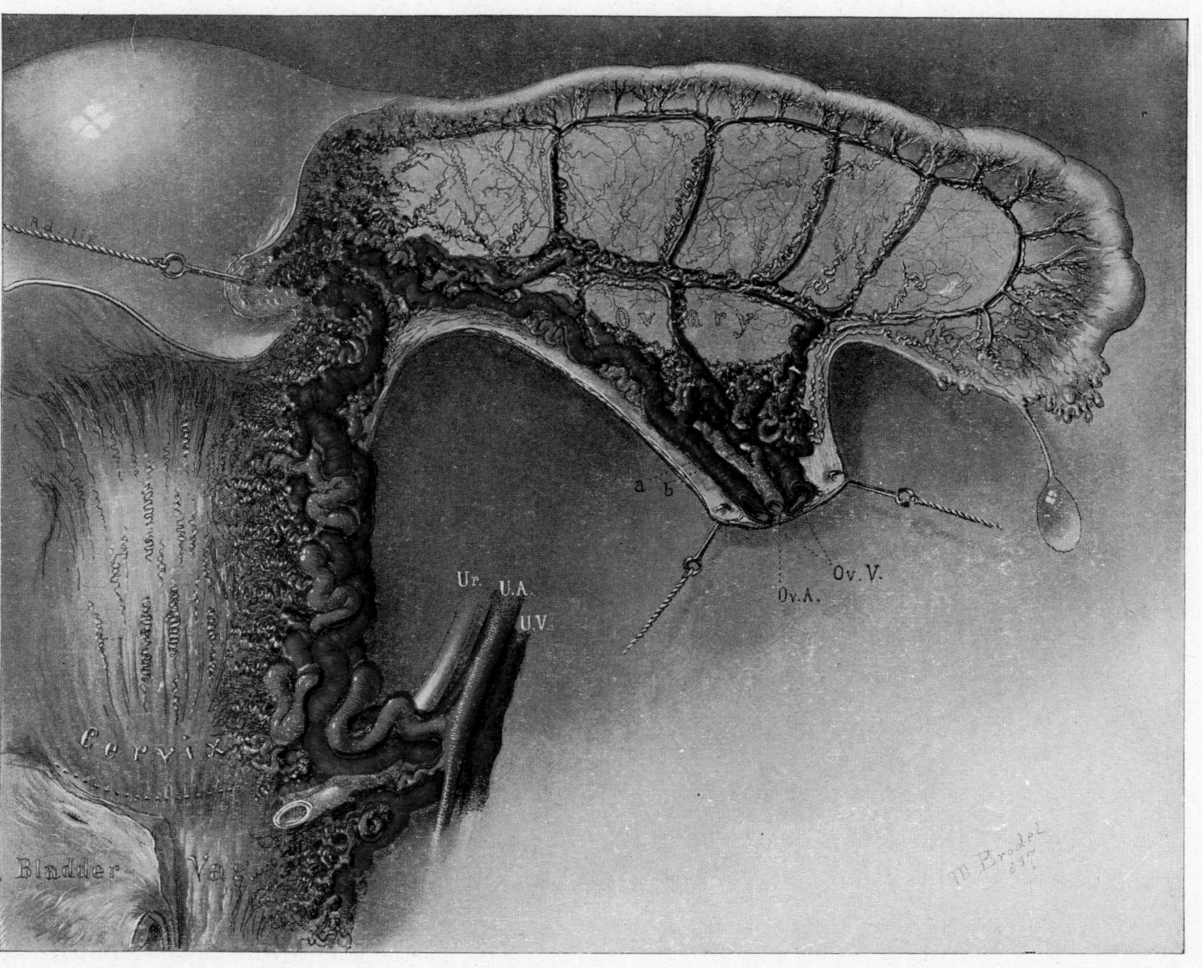

FIG. 39.—BLOOD SUPPLY OF UTERUS, TUBES AND OVARIES. (From Kelly, *Gynecology*, D. Appleton Co.)

is anchored, but the body of the uterus is free to move in the anteroposterior plane. As might be expected under these circumstances, posture and gravity play an important role in the position of the uterus, as has been demonstrated very convincingly by Mengert. He showed that 13 (65 per cent) of 20 women with normal pelvic viscera, confined to bed with pulmonary tuberculosis, had retroverted uteri. However, if these 13 patients lay most of the time on their abdomens, a change of position to the anterior was effected in 90 per cent of cases over a period of 1 to 5 days. The action of gravity on the uterus would seem, therefore, definite, though slow. In Mengert's opinion, the fact that the uterus is anterior in the majority of women is due to the forward tilt of the pelvis in the erect position, in which women spend a majority of their waking hours. As a consequence, the uterine body has a tendency to gravitate anteriorly rather than posteriorly.

As noted previously, the base of the broad ligament contains dense connective tissue which is reflected laterally upon the side of the pelvis and medially is firmly united to the supravaginal portion of the cervix. This parametrial connective tissue, usually called the *cardinal ligament,* is of the utmost importance, because it serves to support the uterus. The upper portion of the broad ligament appears to have no influence upon the position of the uterus, since Mackenrodt, as well as Mengert, has demonstrated that the upper ligament can be cut through without occasioning any descent of the uterus even in the presence of downward traction. Such occurs only when its deeper portion, the cardinal ligament or parametrial tissue, is divided. Recently, Mengert has shown that the paravaginal connective tissue shares with the parametrial tissue this important function.

Blood Vessels of the Uterus. The vascular supply of the uterus is derived from two sources: principally from the uterine, and to a lesser extent from the ovarian, arteries. The uterine artery is the main branch of the hypogastric, which, after descending for a short distance, enters the base of the broad ligament, crosses the ureter, and makes its way to the side of the uterus. Just before reaching the supravaginal portion of the cervix, it divides into two branches, the smaller—the cervicovaginal artery—supplying the lower portion of the cervix and the upper portion of the vagina. The main branch turns abruptly upward and extends as a very convoluted vessel along the margin of the uterus, giving off a branch of considerable size to the upper portion of the cervix, and numerous smaller ones, which penetrate the body of the uterus. Just before reaching the tube it divides into three terminal branches—the fundal, tubal and ovarian—the last of which anastomoses with the terminal branch of the ovarian artery; the second, making its way through the mesosalpinx, supplies the tube, while the fundal branch is distributed to the upper portion of the uterus.

After traversing the broad ligament, the uterine artery reaches the uterus approximately at the level of the internal os. About 2 cm. to the side of the uterus, it crosses over the ureter, as shown in Figs. 21 and 39. This close proximity of the uterine artery to the ureter at this point is of the utmost importance in the operation of hysterectomy because, unless proper precautions are observed, the ureter may be injured or ligatured in the process of clamping and tying the uterine vessels.

The ovarian or internal spermatic artery is a branch of the aorta and enters the broad ligament through the infundibulopelvic ligament. On reaching the hilum of the ovary it breaks up into a number of smaller branches which enter that organ, while its main stem traverses the entire length of the broad ligament and makes its way to the upper portion of the margin of the uterus, where it anastomoses with the ovarian branch of the uterine artery.

It is generally stated that there is very little communication between the vessels on the two sides of the uterus, but the experiments of Clark have demonstrated that such is not the case. This observer found that when the uterine artery on one side was injected the fluid escaped from the opposite uterine artery before it began to flow from the veins, thus indicating the presence of numerous arterial anastomoses in the substance of the uterus. Figure 34 affords additional evidence of this fact, and shows how the radial branches of the arcuate arteries extend from the outer portion of the uterine wall to supply the endometrium.

The veins of the uterus are very abundant and pursue a course the reverse of that of the arteries. When the uterus is contracted their lumens are collapsed, but in injected specimens the greater part of the uterine wall appears to be composed of venous sinuses, as was pointed out by Sampson. The arcuate veins unite to form the uterine vein on either side, which then empties into the hypogastric vein, which makes its way into the internal iliac. The blood from the ovary and upper part of the broad ligament is collected by a number of veins, which form a large plexus within the broad ligament—the *pampiniform plexus*—the vessels from which terminate in the ovarian vein. The right ovarian vein empties into the vena cava, while the left empties into the renal vein.

Lymphatics. The endometrium is abundantly supplied with lymph spaces, but possesses no true lymphatic vessels. Immediately beneath it in the muscularis a few lymphatics may be found, which become better defined as the peritoneum is approached, and form an abundant lymphatic plexus just beneath it, especially on the posterior wall of the uterus, and to a lesser extent on the anterior surface.

The lymphatics from the various portions of the uterus are connected with several sets of glands—those of the cervix terminating in the hypogastric glands, which are situated in the spaces between the external iliac and hypogastric arteries. The lymphatics from the body of the uterus are distributed to two groups of glands, one set of vessels making their way to the hypogastric glands, while another set, after joining certain lymphatics from the ovarian region, terminate in the lumbar glands, which, in turn, are situated in front of the aorta at about the level of the lower portion of the kidneys.

Innervation. The uterus possesses an abundant nerve supply, whose function, however, appears to be regulatory rather than primary. This is shown by the fact that in experimental animals labor can progress satisfactorily after all nerves going to the uterus have been severed, and especially by the fact that the human uterus, from the latter part of intra-uterine life until after the menopause, will contract rhythmically for hours after excision if immersed in warm Locke's solution and plentifully supplied with oxygen.

The nerve supply is derived principally from the sympathetic nervous system, but partly from the cerebrospinal and parasympathetic system. The parasympathetic or autonomic system is represented on either side by the pelvic nerve, which consists of a few fibers derived from the second, third and fourth sacral nerves, and loses itself in the ganglion of Frankenhäuser. The sympathetic system gains access to the pelvis by means of the hypogastric plexus, which arises from the forking of the aortic plexus just below the promontory of the sacrum, and after descending on either side also enters the Frankenhäuser plexus. This plexus consists of ganglia of varying size,

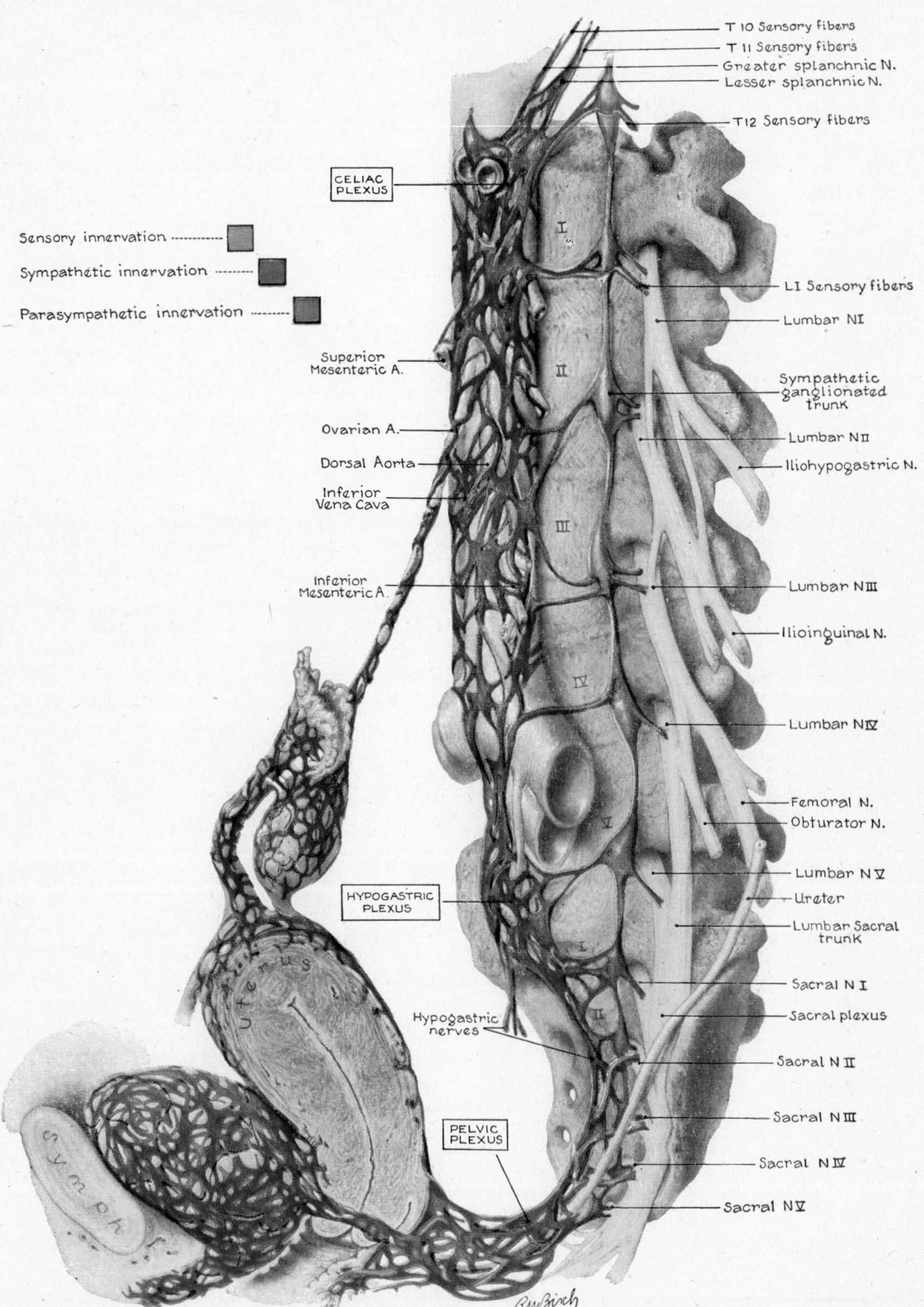
T 10 Sensory fibers
T 11 Sensory fibers
Greater splanchnic N.
Lesser splanchnic N.
T12 Sensory fibers
CELIAC PLEXUS
Sensory innervation
Sympathetic innervation
Parasympathetic innervation
LI Sensory fibers
Lumbar NI
Superior Mesenteric A.
Sympathetic ganglionated trunk
Ovarian A.
Lumbar NII
Dorsal Aorta
Iliohypogastric N.
Inferior Vena Cava
Inferior Mesenteric A.
Lumbar NIII
Ilioinguinal N.
Lumbar NIV
Femoral N.
Obturator N.
Lumbar NV
HYPOGASTRIC PLEXUS
Ureter
Lumbar Sacral trunk
Uterus
Sacral N I
Hypogastric nerves
Sacral plexus
Sacral N II
Sacral NIII
PELVIC PLEXUS
Sacral NIV
Symph.
Sacral NV
RuBirch

Fig. 40.—Nerve Supply of the Uterus.

but particularly of a large ganglionic plate situated on either side of the cervix just above the posterior fornix and in front of the rectum. In their excellent gross anatomical study, Latarjet and Rochet state that in reality Frankenhäuser's ganglion lies posterior to the cervix and occupies the base of the uterosacral ligament.

Branches from these plexuses supply the uterus, bladder and upper part of the vagina, and are made up of both medullated and nonmedullated fibers. Some of them terminate by free endings between the muscle fibers, while others make their way toward the free surface of the endometrium. It has not yet been determined whether or not ganglionic cells are present in the walls of the uterus or tubes.

Both the sympathetic and parasympathetic nerve supplies contain motor and a few sensory fibers. The functions of the nerve supply of the two systems are in great part antagonistic; the sympathetic causes muscular contraction and vasoconstriction, the parasympathetic inhibits contraction and leads to vasodilatation. As the Frankenhäuser plexus is derived from both sources it is apparent that it must partake of the properties of both types of nerves. From the actions of various drugs on the uterine contractions in parturient women, Mahon concludes that the sympathetic nerves maintain the tonus and the parasympathetic control the intermittent contractions of the uterus.

Since 1926, the nerve supply of the genitalia has assumed a definitely practical interest, as Segonod, Cotte and others have shown that various painful pelvic affections may be permanently relieved by severing the hypogastric plexus, which they designate as the *nerf presacré*. The eleventh and twelfth thoracic nerve roots carry sensory fibers from the uterus, transmitting pain of uterine contractions to the central nervous system; the sensory nerves from the cervix and upper birth canal pass through the pelvic nerves to the second, third and fourth sacral, while those from the lower birth canal pass through the ilioinguinal and pudendal nerves.

Development of the Uterus. It is universally admitted by embryologists that both the tubes and the uterus are derived from the müllerian ducts. According to His, the first signs of their development can be noted in embryos having a body length of from 7 to 7.5 mm., when a thickening may be noticed in the celomic epithelium on the outer margin of each wolffian body. These gradually become converted into two epithelial ducts, which converge and eventually meet together in the middle line, terminating in the urogenital sinus.

The müllerian ducts reach the urogenital sinus in embryos having a body length of 2.5 to 3.5 cm. Their upper ends form the fallopian tubes, while their lower portions fuse together to form the uterus and vagina. The fusion of the müllerian ducts is usually completed at about the third month, though the point at which the process is to occur is indicated at a much earlier period by the position of the round ligaments.

THE FALLOPIAN TUBES

The fallopian or uterine tubes are more or less convoluted muscular canals which extend from the uterine cornua to the ovaries, and represent the excretory ducts of the latter, as it is through them that ova gain access to the uterine cavity. They are more or less cylindrical in shape, vary from 8 to 14 cm. in length, are covered by peritoneum, and possess a lumen lined by mucous membrane.

For ease of description, each tube may be divided into the interstitial portion, isthmus, ampulla, and infundibulum. The *interstitial* portion is included within the muscular wall of the uterus, and extends from the cornu to the upper angle of the uterine cavity. Its lumen is so small that it will admit only the finest probe. The *isthmus* is the narrow portion of the tube immediately adjoining the uterus, and gradually passes into the wider lateral portion or *ampulla.* The *infundibulum,* or fimbriated extremity, is the funnel-shaped opening of the lateral end of the tube, the margins of which present a dentate appearance (see Figs. 41 and 42).

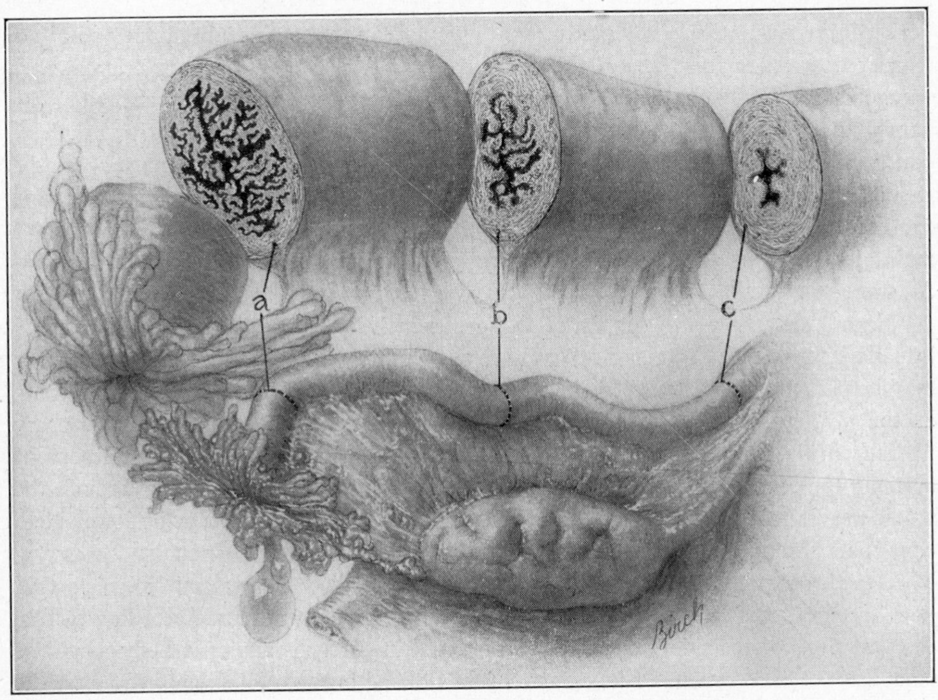

Fig. 41.—The Fallopian Tube in Cross Section Showing the Gross Structure of the Epithelium in Several Portions: (a) Infundibular, (b) Ampullar and (c) Isthmic.

The tube varies considerably in thickness, the narrowest portion of the isthmus measuring from 2 to 3 mm., and the widest portion of the ampulla from 5 to 8 mm. in diameter.

With the exception of its uterine portion, the tube, throughout its entire length, is included within the upper margin of the broad ligament; it is completely surrounded by peritoneum except at its lower portion, corresponding to the mesosalpinx. The fimbriated extremity opens freely into the abdominal cavity, and one of its fimbriae—the *fimbria ovarica*—which is considerably longer than the others, forms a shallow gutter which extends almost to or quite to the ovary.

Generally speaking, the musculature of the tube is arranged in two layers—an inner, circular, and an outer, longitudinal layer. In its uterine portion a third layer, lying between the circular layer and the mucosa, and composed of longitudinal fibers, may be distinguished. In the lateral portion of the tube the two primary layers become less marked, and in the neighborhood of the fimbriated extremity are replaced by an interlacing network of muscle fibers. Williams was the first to call attention to the presence of the inner longitudinal layer, and his observations have been generally confirmed. Seckinger and Snyder, in 1926, showed that the tubal musculature is constantly undergoing rhythmic contractions, whose rate varies with the several phases of the sexual cycle. The contractions occur with greatest frequency and intensity at the time when ova are descending the tube, and are slowest and weakest during pregnancy. Cella and Georgescu, in 1937, corroborated these findings and observed the peristaltic rhythm to be from four to six times per minute, starting at the ampulla. They believe

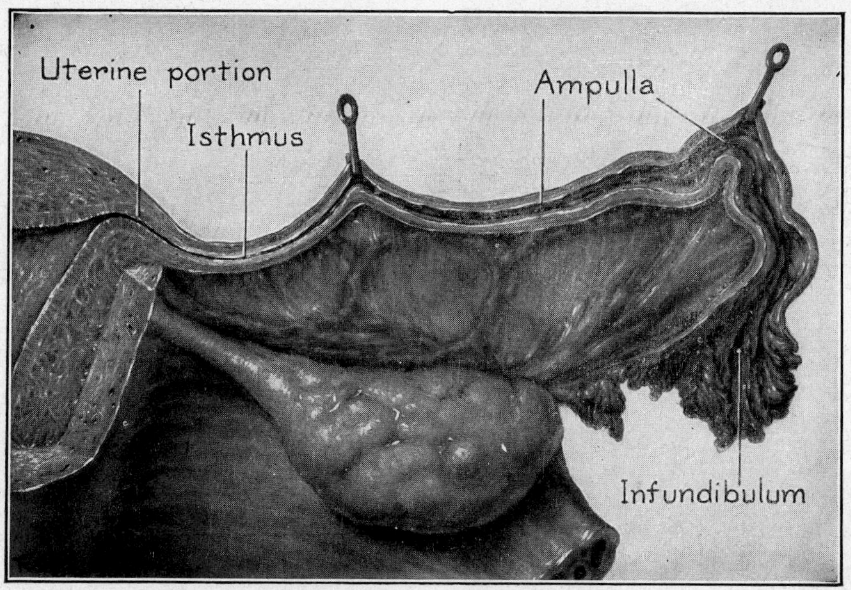

FIG. 42.—THE FALLOPIAN TUBE IN LONGITUDINAL SECTION.

This shows the variation in the size of the tubal lumen, the longitudinal folds and the relationships of the tube to the mesosalpinx, the uterine cornu and ovary.

this peristalsis to be dependent upon both the muscular coat and the intramural ganglion cells of the tubes. The lumen of the tube is lined with a mucous membrane whose epithelium is composed of a single layer of high columnar cells, which rest upon a thin basement membrane (Fig. 43). According to Snyder, Novak and Everett, and others, only a portion of the cells are ciliated. These are arranged in discrete patches, while the nonciliated cells are supposed to be secretory. Grosser, on the other hand, contends that the great majority are ciliated. There is no submucosa, the epithelium being separated from the underlying muscle by a layer of connective tissue of varying thickness.

The mucosa is arranged in longitudinal folds which become more complicated as the fimbriated end is approached. Consequently, the appearance of the lumen varies according to the portion of the tube examined. In cross sections through the uterine portion four simple folds are seen, which together make a figure resembling a Maltese cross. In the isthmic portion a more complicated appearance can be noted; while in the ampulla the lumen is almost completely occupied by the arborescent mucosa, which upon careful examination is seen to be made up of four very complicated treelike folds.

In Figs. 41 and 42 are shown the longitudinal folds of the various portions of the tubal mucosa.

The current produced by the cilia of the tube is directed from the fimbriated extremity toward the uterus. Indeed, minute foreign bodies introduced into the abdominal cavity of animals eventually appear in the vagina, after making their way down the lumen of the tubes and the cavity of the uterus. Contrary to the teaching of many

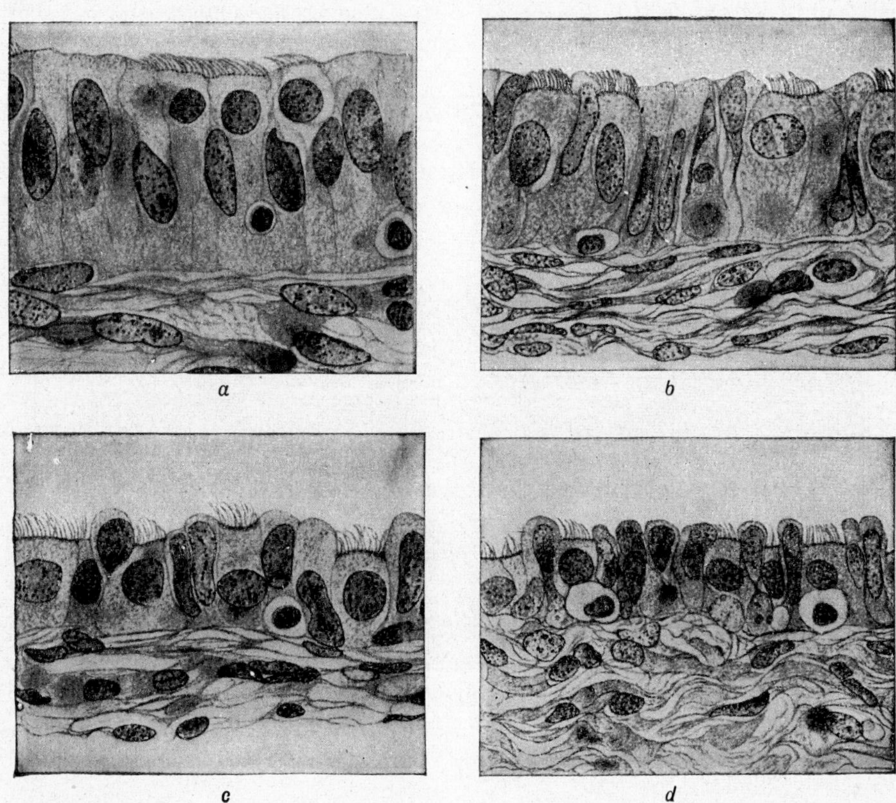

Fig. 43.—Epithelium of Human Fallopian Tube showing Cyclic Changes.

a, early proliferative; b, advanced proliferative; c, premenstrual; d, pregnancy. × 700.

Note: Two chief types of cells, ciliated or nonsecretory and nonciliated or secretory. (From Snyder in *Johns Hopkins Hospital Bulletin.* Drawings by J. F. Didusch.)

that peristaltic muscular contraction is the main factor concerned in the downward passage of the ovum, Grosser contends that the ciliary current plays the principal part.

The tubes are richly supplied with elastic tissue, blood vessels and lymphatics, and the latter sometimes become so dilated as to fill up almost entirely certain folds of the mucosa.

Diverticula may occasionally extend from the lumen of the tube for a variable distance into its muscular wall, and reach almost to its peritoneal covering. The suggestion that they might play a part in the production of tubal pregnancy would seem plausible, inasmuch as a fertilized ovum, which might chance to make its way into such a diverticulum, would be arrested at its end and there develop, if suitable conditions existed.

Many investigators, including Tröscher, Snyder, as well as Novak and Everett, have demonstrated that the tubal mucosa undergoes cyclic histological changes similar to those seen in the endometrium. Although these cyclical changes are not as marked as those in the endometrium, these investigators were able to observe characteristic histological changes in the tubal epithelium in each of the four menstrual phases, as shown in Fig. 43. The postmenstrual phase is associated with a low epithelium which rapidly increases in height. During the proliferative phase the cells are tall, the ciliated ones being broad with nuclei near the margin, and the nonciliated narrow, with more deeply placed nuclei. In the premenstrual phase the secretory cells project beyond the ciliated cells, due to a shortening of the latter. There is also extrusion of the nuclei of the secretory cells. In the menstrual phase these changes become even more marked. The secretory cells become shorter, being emptied of their cytoplasm, some assuming a "peg" appearance. Binder suggests that these cyclical changes in the tubal mucosa are coordinated with alterations in the contractibility of the tubal musculature.

THE OVARIES

General Anatomy. The ovaries are two flattened, more or less almond-shaped organs, whose chief functions are the development and extrusion of ova, and the elaboration of internal secretions. They may vary considerably in size, and during the childbearing period measure from 2.5 to 5 cm. in length, 1.5 to 3 cm. in breadth, and 0.6 to 1.5 cm. in thickness. After the menopause they diminish markedly in size, and in old women are often scarcely larger than peas.

Normally, the ovaries are situated in the upper part of the pelvic cavity, one surface of each ovary resting in a slight depression in the upper portion of the inner surface of the obturator muscle—the *fossa ovarica* of Waldeyer. With the woman standing, the long axes of the ovaries occupy an almost vertical position, which become horizontal when she is on her back. Their situation, however, is subject to marked variations, and it is rare to find both ovaries at exactly the same level.

Each ovary presents for examination two surfaces, two margins, and two poles. The surface which is in contact with the ovarian fossa is called the lateral, and the one directed toward the uterus is known as the median surface. The margin which is attached to the mesovarium is more or less straight, and is designated as the hilum, while the free margin is convex and is directed backward and inward toward the rectum. The extremities of the ovary are termed the upper and lower or tubal and uterine poles, respectively, the latter being directed toward the uterus.

The ovary is attached to the broad ligament by the *mesovarium,* which forms the posterior leaf of that structure. The *ovarian ligament* extends from the lateral and posterior portion of the uterus, just beneath the tubal insertion, to the uterine or lower pole of the ovary. It is usually several centimeters long and 3 to 4 mm. in diameter. It is covered by peritoneum, and is made up of muscle and connective-tissue fibers, which are continuous with those of the uterus. The *infundibulo-pelvic* or *suspensory ligament* of the ovary extends from its upper or tubal pole to the pelvic wall. It represents the portion of the upper margin of the broad ligament which is not occupied by the tube, and through it the ovarian vessels and nerves gain access to the broad ligament.

For the most part the ovary projects freely into the abdominal cavity, and is not covered by peritoneum except near its hilum, where a narrow band may be observed which is continuous with the peritoneum covering the mesosalpinx. It follows, therefore, that over its lower portion only can be noted the glistening appearance characteristic of peritoneum, while the greater part of its surface is of a dull white color and it looks moist.

The exterior of the ovary varies in appearance according to the age of the individual. In young women the organ presents a smooth, dull white surface, through which glisten a number of small, clear vesicles—the graafian follicles. As the woman grows older it takes on a more corrugated appearance, which in the aged may become so marked as to be suggestive of the convolutions of the brain.

The general structure of the ovary can best be studied in cross sections, when the organ is seen to be made up of two portions: the *cortex* and *medulla,* or *zona parenchymatosa* and *zona vasculosa.* The cortex, or outer layer, varies in thickness according to the age of the individual, becoming thinner with advancing years. In this layer the ova and graafian follicles are situated. It is composed of spindle-shaped connective-tissue cells, through which are scattered primordial and graafian follicles in various stages of development, which become less numerous as the woman grows older. The most external portion of the cortex presents a dull whitish appearance, and is designated as the *albuginea,* though it is not analogous with the similarly named structure in the testicle; on its surface is a single layer of cuboidal epithelium—the ovarium epithelium of Waldeyer.

The medulla or central portion of the ovary is composed of loose connective tissue, which is continuous with that of the mesovarium. It contains large numbers of blood vessels, both arteries and veins, and also a small number of nonstriated muscle fibers.

Kraul has shown that both sympathetic and parasympathetic nerves supply the ovaries, and that their coordination is essential to perfect functioning. The sympathetic nerves are derived in great part from the plexus which accompanies the ovarian vessels—the so-called ovarian plexus—while a few are derived from the plexus surrounding the ovarian branch of the uterine artery. The ovary is very richly supplied with nonmedullated nerve fibers, which for the most part accompany the blood vessels, and are merely vascular nerves; whereas others form wreaths around normal and atretic follicles and give off many minute branches, which have been traced up to, but not through, the membrana granulosa.

Accessory Ovaries. Waldeyer, in 1870, directed attention to the occasional presence of accessory bodies which are sometimes found on the broad ligament in the neighborhood of the main ovary. These structures are usually small, although in rare instances they may attain a considerable size. Occasionally they result from faulty development, but more frequently are to be attributed to inflammatory changes occurring during fetal life, as a consequence of which small portions of the ovary have been cut off from the body of the organ.

Development of the Ovary. In 1870 Waldeyer published his monograph on the ovary and ovum (Eierstock und Ei) and, although subsequent investigation has invalidated many of his conclusions, it must be regarded as the foundation of our knowledge of the subject. His work, which was based in great part upon the embryology of the chicken, showed that by the fourth day of development the celomic epithelium covering the inner surface of the wolffian body becomes differentiated from the surrounding tissue, its cells becoming larger and more cuboidal in shape, and some of them assuming a considerable size. Within a short time the epithelium proliferates to such an extent as to form a distinct elevation, which indicates the situation of the future ovary. This epithelium Waldeyer designated as *germinal epithelium* and the large, clear cells found within it as *primordial ova*. As proliferation continues, a mass of cells is formed consisting of large primordial ova and smaller epithelial cells. By the upward growth of the connective tissue and blood vessels from the wolffian body, the epithelial masses become divided into smaller portions, the so-called egg-nests or Pflüger tubes,

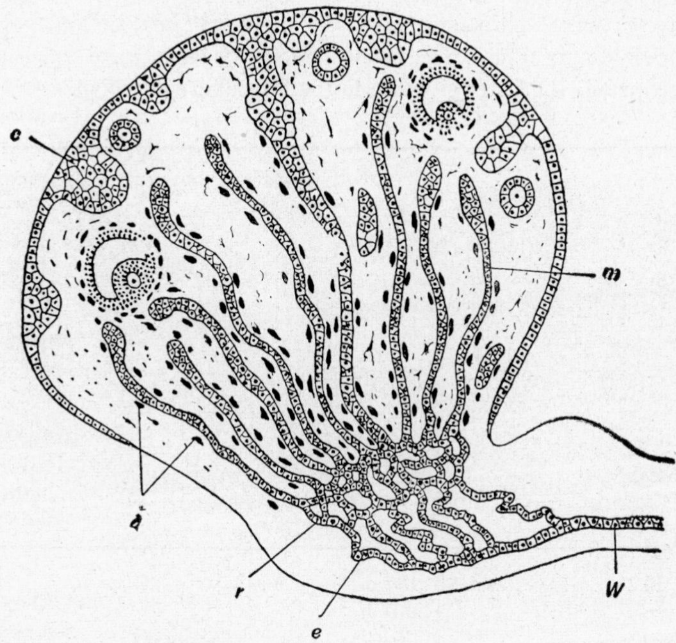

FIG. 44.—DEVELOPMENT OF OVARY.

C, cortical substance with formation of follicles; M, medullary cords, derivatives of the sex cords, homologues of the seminiferous tubules in the testis; I, interstitial cells; R, rete ovarii; E, epoophoron; W, Wolffian duct. Redrawn after Kohn. (From Maximow and Bloom, *Textbook of Histology,* W. B. Saunders Co., Philadelphia.)

which in turn become broken up into smaller and smaller masses, until, eventually, isolated primordial ova are found, which are surrounded by a single layer of more or less flattened epithelium. These represent the primordial follicles, containing the primordial ova.

In either sex, the first trace of the sexual glands is found in a thickening of the epithelium on the inner surface of the wolffian body. These primitive sex cells rapidly proliferate and give rise to a distinct elevation, made up of closely packed undifferentiated epithelial cells, which are covered by a single layer of cuboidal cells arranged perpendicularly to the surface of the mass. The latter correspond to the future ovarian epithelium but take no part in the formation of ova and follicles.

The cells of the primitive sex gland proliferate rapidly and invade the underlying stroma of the wolffian body, so that a cortical and medullary portion can be distinguished at an early period. The epithelial cells soon become broken up into irregular masses by the upgrowth of connective tissue and have little or no connection with the surface epithelium. The most deeply lying cells do not become differentiated, but extend downward as solid cords—the medullary cords. These terminate in a series of epithelial tubes—the so-called *rete ovarii,* which in turn communicate with the wolffian body tubules. In the female this is a transient condition, which disappears early in fetal life, but in the male it is permanent and affords a ready explanation for the utilization of the wolffian ducts as the efferent channels of the testicles (Fig. 44). The more superficial cells become arranged in irregularly shaped masses, continue to proliferate, and soon show signs of differentiation. Many become large cells with prominent, clear nuclei, whose chromatin takes on a different arrangement, while others retain their original appearance. The former are the oogonia, from which the ova are to be developed, while the latter give rise to the follicular epithelium.

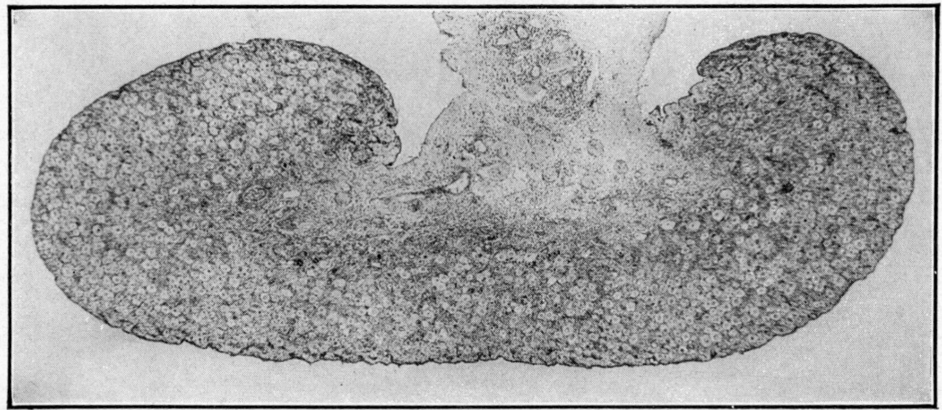

Fig. 45.—Transverse Section of Ovary of Newborn Girl. × 40.

After a certain period the oogonia cease proliferating, when the resulting cells become larger, and their chromatin undergoes a series of complicated changes, which eventually lead to the formation of the reticulated nucleus of the primordial ovum or oocyte of the first order. By the continued growth of connective tissue the masses of oocytes and undifferentiated epithelial cells become still further broken up, so that eventually each oocyte is surrounded by a single layer of flattened cells, thus giving rise to a primordial follicle.

At birth the greater part of the ovary consists of the cortex, which is made up of closely packed primordial follicles, which are separated from one another by very thin bands of connective tissue, although occasionally small groups of follicles may be in direct contact (Figs. 45 and 46). At this period the surface of the ovary is covered by a single layer of cuboidal epithelium which shows no signs of proliferation.

All authorities agree that the primordial ova are derived from the primary sex cells, but there is still considerable discussion as to the origin of the latter. Certain authorities hold with Boveri that they represent a specialized type of cell, which is a direct descendant from one of the early blastomeres of the segmenting ovum. Later these cells find their way to the vicinity of the developing ovary—the so-called "Keimbahn." Most investigators, however, believe that the primary sex cells develop in situ.

Microscopic Structure of Ovary. From the first stages of its development until after the menopause, the ovary is undergoing constant change. According to Waldeyer, each ovary at birth contains at least 100,000 oocytes, the majority of which disappear before the age of puberty; so that at that time only 30,000 to 40,000 remain, and these disappear during the following thirty years. That this is a moderate estimate is shown by the fact that Häggström was able to count 400,000 follicles in the ovaries of a woman 22 years old. As only one ovum is ordinarily cast off each month, it is apparent that a few hundred ova would suffice for the purposes of reproduction. The mode by which the others disappear will be considered when we take up the study of the corpus luteum and follicular atresia.

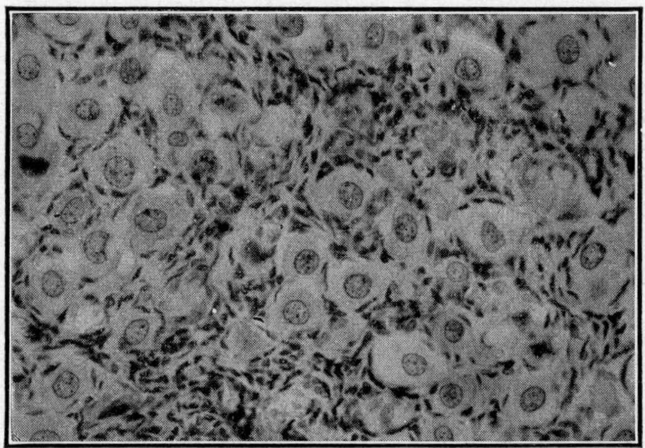

FIG. 46.—CORTEX OF OVARY OF NEWBORN GIRL SHOWING PRIMORDIAL FOLLICLES. × 250.

Since this huge store of primordial follicles present at birth more than suffices the woman for her reproductive life, it has long been maintained that no more are formed. In other words, the concept has been held that this large initial store is gradually exhausted during the period of sexual maturity. During the past two decades various evidence has been advanced to show that not only before birth but also during the time of sexual maturity, new ova and follicles are being formed. Proponents of this theory believe that oogenesis is a rhythmic process and, moreover, that all the ova reaching maturity are of recent origin, being, at the most, in the human only a few weeks old and not from 15 to 40 years old as suggested by the storage theory. The new hypothesis would bring the ova more in line with the male germ cells, the spermatozoa, which are being produced continually. Although the monograph of Evans and Swezy presents convincing evidence in support of this new concept, it has not been generally accepted, particularly as it applies to the higher mammals, including man.

In the young child the greater portion of the ovary is composed of the cortex, which is filled with large numbers of closely packed primordial follicles, those nearest the central portion of the ovary showing the most advanced stages of development. In young women the cortex is relatively thinner, but still contains large numbers of primordial follicles separated by bands of connective tissue cells with spindle-shaped or oval nuclei. Each primordial follicle consists of an oocyte and its surrounding single layer of epithelium. The cells composing the latter are small and flattened, spindle-shaped, and are somewhat sharply differentiated from the still smaller spindle-shaped cells of the surrounding stroma.

The oocyte is a single large cell, more or less round in shape, with a clear protoplasm and a tolerably large nucleus occupying its central portion. The nucleus presents a marked reticulated network and at one point a well-defined nucleolus, as well as numerous accessory nucleoli, which are formed at the intersections of the nuclear threadwork. These primordial ova, or oocytes of the first order, measure from 48 to 69 microns; and their nuclei, from 29 to 32 microns in diameter.

BIBLIOGRAPHY

ABEL, W., and MCILROY, A. L. The Arrangement and Distribution of the Nerves in Certain Mammalian Ovaries. Proc. Roy. Soc. Med. (Gynec. & Obst. Sect.), 1913, 6:240.

ACHENBACH. 25 Fälle von Schwangerschaft und Geburt bei undurchbohrtem Hymen. D. I., Marburg, 1890.

ANSON, B. J. Anatomy of the Female Genitalia and Pelvic Soft Parts. In Obstetrics and Gynecology, edited by Curtis. W. B. Saunders Co., Philadelphia, 1933, 1:195.

ASCHOFF, L. Zur Cervixfrage. Monatschr. f. Geburtsh. u. Gynäk., 1905, *22*:611.

AYKROYD, O. E., and GATENBY, J. B. Cytology of Human Uterine Glands in Gravid and Non-Gravid Phases. Quart. J. Micr. Sci., 1941, 82:541.

VON BAER, K. E. De Ovi Mammalium et Hominis Genesi. Leipzig, 1827.

BARTELMEZ, G. W., and BENSLEY, C. M. Human Uterine Gland Cells. Cowdry's Special Cytology, 1932, 3:1525.

BINDER, A. Experimentelle Untersuchungen über den Einfluss der Keimdrüsenhormone auf die Motilität der Eileiter; die Wirkung des Follikelhormons. Arch f. Gynäk., 1939, 168:545.

CELLA, C., and GEORGESCU, I. D. Experimentelle Untersuchungen über die Physiologie und Pharmakodynamik des Eileiters. Arch. f. Gynäk., 1937, 165:36.

CLELAND, J. G. P. Paravertebral Anesthesia in Obstetrics. Surg., Gynec. & Obst., 1933, 57:51.

——— and TAIT, J. Nervous Connections of the Mammalian Spleen Including an Account of Certain Viscero-Motor and Other Abdominal Reflexes. Quart. J. Exper. Physiol., 1927, 17:179.

CORNER, G. W. Cytology of the Ovum, Ovary and Fallopian Tube. Cowdry's Special Cytology, 1928, Vol. 2, p. 1111.

DANFORTH, D. N. The Fibrous Nature of the Human Cervix and its Relation to the Isthmic Segment in Gravid and Non-Gravid Uteri. Am. J. Obst. & Gynec., 1947, 53:541.

DAVIS, A. A. The Innervation of the Uterus. J. Obst. & Gynaec. Brit. Emp., 1933, 40:481.

——— The Surgical Anatomy of the Presacral Nerve. *Ibid.*, 1934, 41:942.

DIERKS, K. Der normale mensuelle Zyklus der menschlichen Vaginalschleimhaut. Arch. f. Gynäk., 1927, 130:46.

——— and MÜNSTER, C. Polarisationsoptische Studien am menschlichen Vaginalepithel. Arch. f. Gynäk., 1933, 152:1.

DÖDERLEIN, A. Das Scheidensekret. Leipzig, 1892.

EVANS, H. M., and SWEZY, O. Ovogenesis and Normal Follicular Cycle in Adult Mammalia. Mem. Univ. Calif., 1931, 9:119.

GELLHORN, G. Anatomy, Pathology and Development of the Hymen. Tr. Am. Gynec. Soc., 1904, 29:405.

GEMMELL, A. A. A Method of Demonstrating the Ganglia of the Cervix Uteri. J. Obst. & Gynaec. Brit. Emp., 1926, 33:259.

GRAGERT, O. Ueber das Glykogen in der fetalen Vagina. Arch. F. Gynäk., 1926, 128:43.

GROSSER, O. Ovulation und Implantation und die Funktion der Tube beim Menschen. Arch. f. Gynäk., 1919, 110:297.

HABERDA, A. Ueber den anatomischen Nachweis der erfolgten Defloration. Monatschr. f. Geburtsh. u. Gynäk., 1900, 11:69.

HARRIS, L. J., MENGERT, W. F., and PLASS, E. D. Mechanics of Uterine Support and Position. II. Factors Influencing Uterine Position (an Experimental Study). Am. J. Obst. & Gynec., 1936, 31:1009.

HARTMAN, C. G. The Homology of Menstruation. New Observations of Intermenstrual Bleeding in the Monkey. J.A.M.A., 1929, 92:1992.

——— How Large Is the Mammalian Egg? Quart. Rev. Biol., 1929, 4:373.

HEAPE, W. The Menstruation and Ovulation of Monkeys and the Human Female. Med. Press. & Circ. Lond., 1898, 65:378.

HIS, W. Die anatomische Nomenclatur. Leipzig, 1895.

HITSCHMANN, F., and ADLER, L. Der Bau der Uterusschleimhaut des geschlechtsreifen Weibes, etc. Monatschr. f. Geburtsh. u. Gynäk., 1908, 27:1.

HOFBAUER, J. The Defensive Mechanism of the Parametrium during Pregnancy and Labor. Bull. Johns Hopkins Hosp., 1926, 38:255.

HUFFMAN, J. W. The Detailed Anatomy of the Paraurethral Ducts in the Adult Human Female. Am. J. Obst. & Gynec., 1948, 55:86.

KRAUL, L. Der Einfluss der Innervation auf den Eierstock. Arch. f. Gynäk., 1928, 131:600.

KUNTZ, A. The Autonomic Nervous System, 2nd Ed. Lea and Febiger, Philadelphia, 1934, p. 340.

LATARJET, A., and ROCHET, P. Le Plexus Hypogastrique chez la Femme. Gynéc. et obst., 1922, 6:225.

LUSCHKA, H. Die Anatomie des menschlichen Beckens. Tubinden, 1861.

MACKENRODT, A. Ueber die Ursachen der normalen und path. Lagen des Uterus. Arch. f. Gynäk., 1895, 48:393.

MCILROY, A. L. The Development of the Germ Cells in the Mammalian Ovary. Proc. Roy. Soc. Edinb., 1910, 31:151.

MAHON, R. Les Ruptures Extra-peritoneales du Dome Vesical d'Origine Obstétricale. Gynéc. et obst., 1939, 39:19.

MENGERT, W. F. Mechanics of Uterine Support and Position. I. Factors Influencing Uterine Support (an Experimental Study). Am. J. Obst. & Gynec., 1936, 31:775.

MEYER, R. Zur Frage der Entwicklung der menschlichen Vagina. Teil I, Arch. f. Gynäk., 1934, 158:639; Teil II, *ibid.*, 1937, 163:205; Teil III, *ibid.*, 1937, 164:207; Teil IV, *ibid.*, 1938, 165:504; Teil V, *ibid.*, 1938, 167:306.

——— Zusammenfassende Bemerkungen über die Entwicklung des distalen Endes der Vagina und des Hymens beim Menschen; ein Beitrag zur konstitutionellen Embryologie. Zentralbl. f. Gynäk., 1937, 61:2846.

NOVAK, E., and EVERETT, H. Cyclical and Other Variations in the Tubal Epithelium. Am. J. Obst. & Gynec., 1928, 16:499.

NOVAK, J. Anatomie u. Physiologie des weiblichen Genital-nervensystems, in Halban-Seitz, Die Biologie und Pathologie des Weibes, 1928, Bd. V, Teil 4, ff. 1373.

OKKELS, H., and ENGLE, E. T. Studies on Finer Structure of Uterine Blood Vessels of Macacus Monkey. Acta path. et microbiol. Scandinav., 1938, 15:150.

PAPANICOLAOU, G. N. The Sexual Cycle in the Human Female as Revealed by Vaginal Smears. Am. J. Anat., 1933, 52:519.

PUCCIONI, L. Modificazioni Istologiche della Vagina della Donna in Rapporto con le Varie Fasi del Ciclo Funzionale dell' Ovaio. Riv. ital. di ginec., 1927, 6:544.

RAKOFF, A. E., FEO, L. G., and GOLDSTEIN, L. The Biologic Characteristics of the Normal Vagina. Am. J. Obst. & Gynec., 1944, 47:467.

SAMPSON, J. A. The Escape of Foreign Material from the Uterine Cavity into the Uterine Veins. Am. J. Obst., 1918, 78:161.

SCHROEDER. The Condition of the Hymen and its Remains after Cohabitation, Childbearing, etc. Tr. Edinburgh Obst. Soc., 1878.

SECKINGER, D. L., and SNYDER, F. F. Cyclic Changes in the Spontaneous Contractions of the Human Fallopian Tube. Bull. Johns Hopkins Hosp., 1926, 39:371.

SIMKINS, C. S. Development of the Human Ovary from Birth to Sexual Maturity. Am. J. Anat., 1932, 51:465.

SKENE, A. J. C. The Anatomy and Pathology of Two Important Glands of the Female Urethra. Am. J. Obst., 1880, 13:265.

SMOUT, C. F. V. Gynaecological and Obstetrical Anatomy. Williams and Wilkins Co., Baltimore, 1948.

SNYDER, F. F. Changes in the Human Oviduct during the Menstrual Cycle and Pregnancy. Bull. Johns Hopkins Hosp., 1924, 35:141.

STIEVE, H. Die Enge der menschlichen Gebärmutter und ihre Bedeutung. Ztschr. f. mikr.-anat. Forsch., 1928, 14:549.

TEMESVÁRY, N. Die Regio Clitoridis. Arch. f. Gynäk., 1924, 122:102.

TRAUT, H. F., BLOCH, P. W., and KUDER, A. Cyclical Changes in the Human Vaginal Mucosa. Surg., Gynec. & Obst., 1936, 63:7.

TRÖSCHER, H. Über den Bau und die Funktion des Tubenepithels beim Menschen. Monatschr. f. Geburtsch. u. Gynäk., 1917, 45:205.

WALDEYER, H. W. G. Eierstock und Ei. Leipzig, 1870.

WILSON, K. M. Origin and Development of the Rete Ovarii and the Rete Testis in the Human Embryo. Carnegie Inst. of Wash., 1926, Publ. 362.

3

THE OVARIAN CYCLE AND ITS HORMONES

Orientation. This and the subsequent chapter are devoted to the closely integrated and beautifully synchronized series of phenomena which normally take place in the ovary and endometrium of the nonpregnant woman each month during her reproductive years. The main objective of the ovarian cycle is to provide an ovum for fertilization, while the purpose of the endometrial cycle is to furnish a suitable bed in which the fertilized ovum may implant and develop. Since, however, the endometrial changes are governed entirely by certain processes inherent in the ovarian cycle—namely, the production of the ovarian hormones—the two cycles are so closely related as to be essentially one: the female sexual cycle. Nevertheless, for the sake of clarity, the ovarian cycle and its endocrinology will be discussed separately in the present chapter, while in the next, attention will be given to the endometrial cycle, followed by a consideration of the intimate relationships between the two, especially in respect to causation and timing.

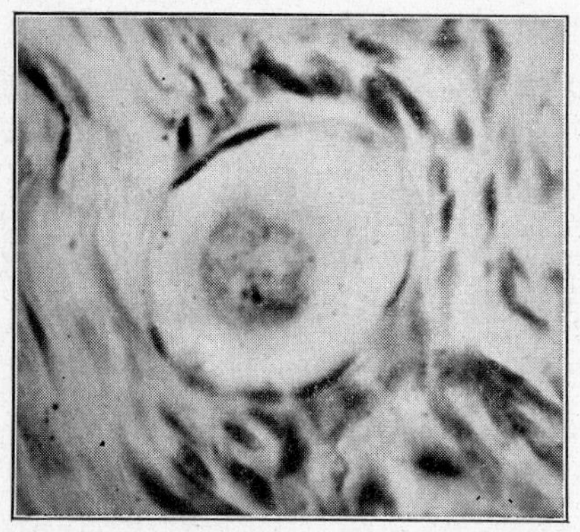

Fig. 47.—Primordial Follicle Just Beginning to Develop. × 700.

Both the ovarian and menstrual cycles are dated from the first day of one menstrual flow to the first day of the next. Thus, if we speak of a phenomenon as occurring on the seventeenth day of either cycle, we mean day 17 in reference to the first day of menstrual bleeding as day 1. As will be discussed in detail subsequently, the average duration of the sexual cycle in woman is 28 days, but variations are common.

Development of the Primordial Follicle. Throughout the reproductive years of a woman, and also in childhood to a lesser degree, certain primordial follicles show evidence of growth and development. First, the epithelium becomes converted into a single layer of cuboidal cells (Fig. 48). Nuclear figures soon make their appearance, and the cells begin to proliferate rapidly, so that in a very short time the ovum becomes surrounded by a number of layers of epithelial cells. Certain of these undergo degeneration, and vacuolated areas are not infrequently observed between them. This process continues until a considerable portion of the follicle becomes filled with fluid, which is formed partly by the degeneration of the follicular cells and partly by transudation from the surrounding vessels. With the development of fluid among the follicular cells, and the consequent formation of an antrum, this vesicular follicle becomes known as a *graafian follicle,* being named for the Dutch physician, Regner de Graaf, who first described it in 1672.

Coincident with the development of the fluid, the so-called *liquor folliculi,* the ovum becomes pushed to one side of the follicle, where it is surrounded by a mass of cells—the *discus proligerus* or *cumulus oophorus*—while the rest of the epithelium is arranged in a number of layers around the interior of the follicle, and is known as the *membrana granulosa* (Fig. 51).

While these changes are taking place, the ovum itself becomes larger, and important changes take place in its nucleus preparatory to the formation of the first polar

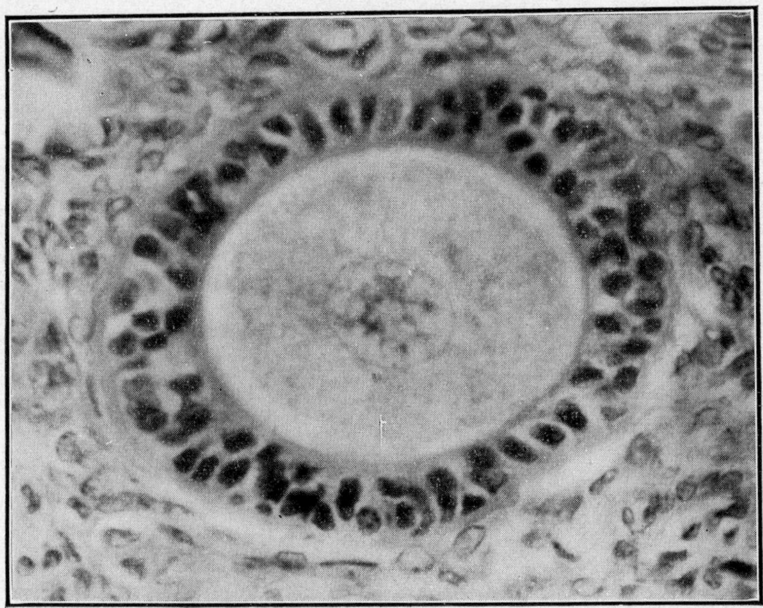

FIG. 48.—DEVELOPING FOLLICLE. × 700.

body: yolk granules, or deutoplasm, are deposited in its protoplasm, and a thin, transparent structure—the *zona pellucida*—appears about its periphery. At the same time, the stroma immediately surrounding the growing follicle becomes vascular, and its cells show marked evidences of proliferation. The membrana granulosa is separated from the stroma by a thin basement membrane consisting of a single layer of flattened, spindle-shaped, connective-tissue cells. Just between the basement membrane and the outermost layer of the membrana granulosa there not infrequently appears a thin, transparent layer. This, like the zona pellucida, is a species of exudate from the granulosa cells.

Mature Graafian Follicle. From birth until the cessation of sexual life, graafian follicles are constantly being developed. Before the age of puberty, they are found only in the deeper portions of the cortex, and do not reach the surface of the ovary. Later, however, they develop in the superficial portions of the cortex, and each 28 days or so, one makes its way to the surface, where it appears as a transparent vesicle, varying from a few to 10 or 12 mm. in diameter. As the follicle approaches the surface of the ovary, its walls become thinner and more abundantly supplied with vessels, except in its most prominent projecting portion, which appears almost bloodless and is designated as the *stigma,* the spot where rupture is to occur.

From without inward, the mature graafian follicle consists of a connective-tissue covering—the theca folliculi; an epithelial lining—the membrana granulosa; the ovum;

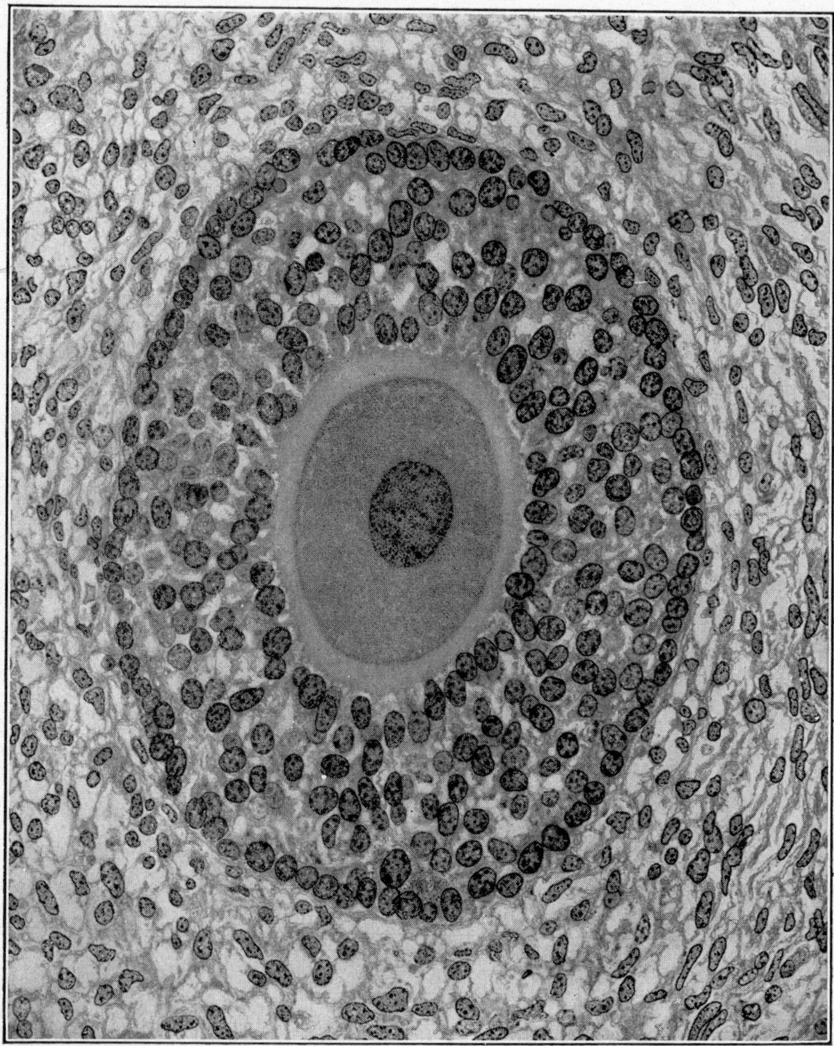

FIG. 49.—DEVELOPING FOLLICLE. × 700.

and the liquor folliculi. The theca folliculi is readily divided into two layers: an outer, the tunica externa, and an inner, the tunica interna. The tunica externa consists of the ordinary ovarian stroma, which is arranged concentrically about the follicle, while the connective-tissue cells of the tunica interna have undergone marked change.

Almost as soon as the primordial follicle shows signs of development, nuclear figures appear in the stroma immediately surrounding it, and a considerable multiplication of cells occurs. These become considerably larger than the surrounding connective-tissue cells, and as the follicle increases in size assume a granular appearance, which is due to the presence of fat and of a yellowish pigment. These cells are designated as *theca lutein cells* and, as will be seen later, play an important part in the formation of the corpus luteum, as well as in the process of follicular atresia. In most hardened specimens the fatty matter has been dissolved out, and the cells appear not unlike those of the suprarenal capsules (see *T.I.*, Fig. 51). At the same time there is a marked

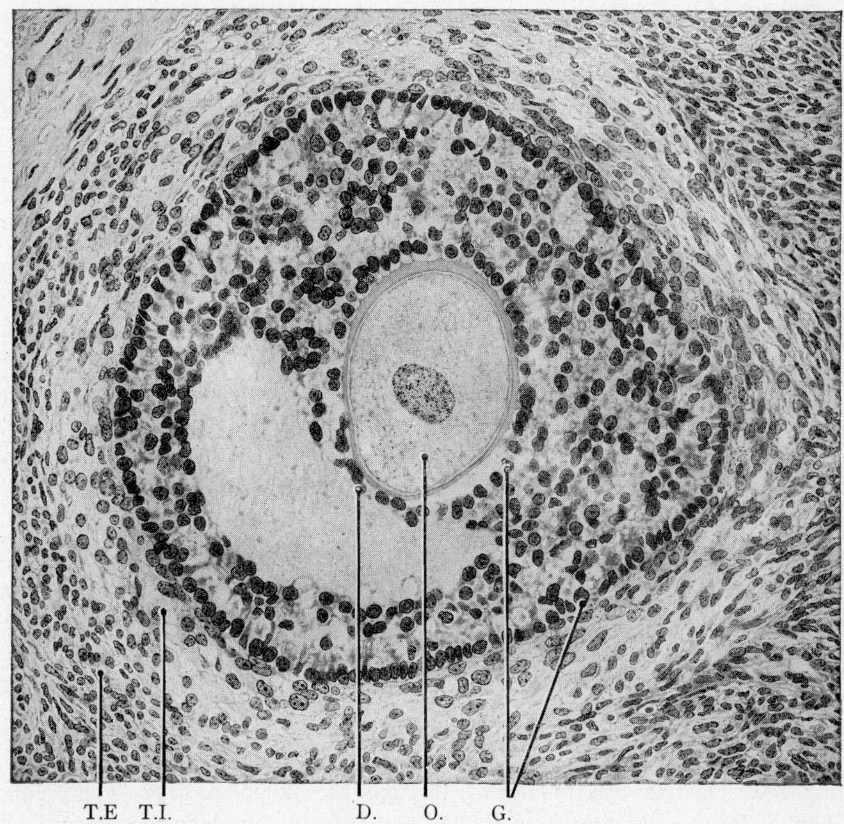

FIG. 50.—GRAAFIAN FOLLICLE APPROACHING MATURITY. × 250.

G., granulosa cell layer; O., ovum; D., discus proligerus; T.I., tunica interna; T.E., tunica externa.

increase in the vascularity of the theca, and numerous lymphatic spaces make their appearance.

The epithelial lining of the follicle, or membrana granulosa, consists of a number of layers of small polygonal or cuboidal cells, with round, darkly staining nuclei, which are arranged in fewer layers the larger the follicle. At one point the membrana granulosa is much thicker than elsewhere, and forms a more or less pyramidal mound in which the ovum is included. This is the discus proligerus, or oophorus, and while the follicle is developing it is situated at the portion farthest removed from the surface of the ovary. However, according to Strassmann, as the follicle approaches maturity the discus proligerus tends to move toward the surface, eventually assuming a position corresponding to the numerals 10 or 2 on the face of a clock. The follicle is filled with a clear, albuminous fluid, the liquor folliculi, which is partly the product of the degenerated follicular epithelium and partly a transudate from surrounding vessels. The liquor contains the specific internal secretion of the ovary—estrogen. As the follicle approaches its highest development, its epithelium undergoes fatty degeneration, as can be demonstrated by appropriate technic.

As the ovum approaches maturity, it becomes the largest cell in the body and measures from 150 to 250 microns (0.2 mm.) in diameter, as compared with 48 to 69 microns in its primordial condition. In 1928, Allen and his associates succeeded in

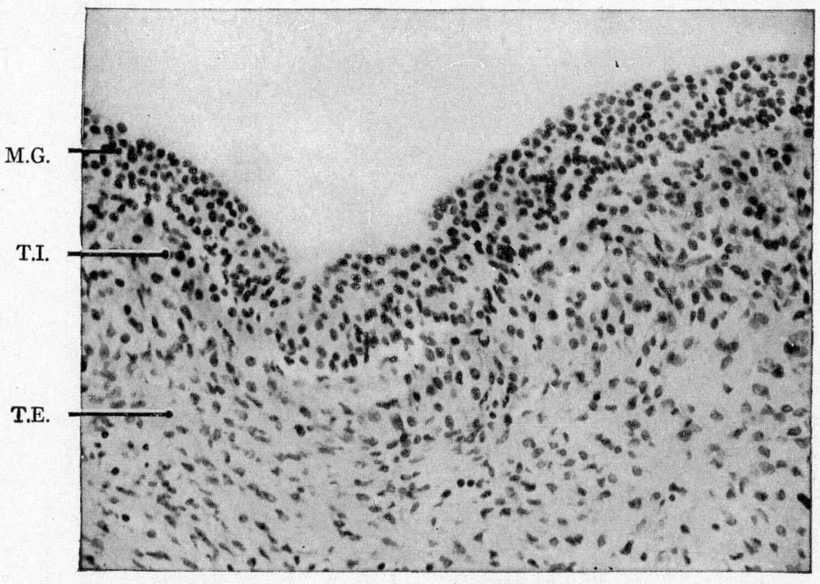

Fig. 51.—Section through Wall of Mature Follicle. × 245.
M.G., membrana granulosa; T.I., tunica interna; T.E., tunica externa.

isolating seven human ova in transit through the fallopian tube. They differed considerably in size, varying from 0.084 to 0.184 mm. in diameter. According to Hartman, the average size of the human ovum varies from 0.130 mm. to 0.140 mm. in diameter.

If the nearly mature ovum is examined in the liquor folliculi or in normal salt solution, the following structures may be distinguished in and about it: (*a*) a corona radiata; (*b*) a zona pellucida; (*c*) a perivitelline space; (*d*) a small clear zone of protoplasm; (*e*) a broad, finely granulated zone of protoplasm; (*f*) a central, deutoplasmic zone; (*g*) the germinal vesicle with its germinal spot; and, if appropriately stained, (*h*) a centriole, and (*i*) many mitochondria.

The *corona radiata* consists of a number of layers of follicular epithelium which adhere to the ovum. Inside of the corona radiata is a narrow, transparent zone—the zona pellucida—which is a product of the granulosa cells, and does not belong to the ovum itself. Separating the ovum from the zona pellucida is a clear, narrow space, the *perivitelline space,* within which the ovum is freely movable, so that no matter what position it may assume, its germinal vesicle will always point upward. Inside of the perivitelline space is the ovum proper, which differs from the primordial oocyte, not only by its increased size, but more especially by the presence of a yolk or deutoplasm, which fills the greater part of its interior.

The *deutoplasm* occupies the central portion of the ovum, and is made up of large numbers of irregularly shaped, highly refractive granules. As it develops it pushes the germinal vesicle to one side, so that the latter always assumes an eccentric position in the ovum. Outside of the deutoplasm is a narrow zone of finely granular protoplasm, which owes its peculiar appearance to the presence of very small yolk granules;

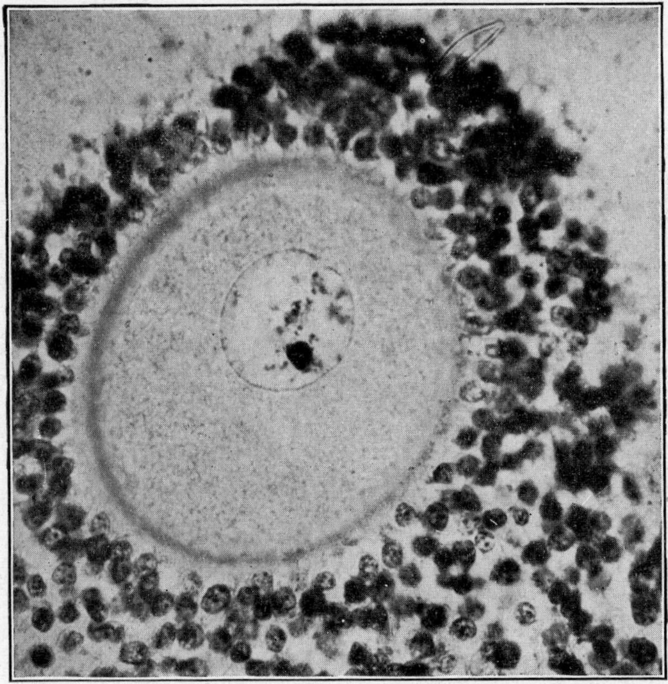

FIG. 52.—MATURE HUMAN OVUM. × 480. (Carnegie Laboratory.)

external to this, again, is a still narrower zone of clear protoplasm. Corner, however, believes that this statement is incorrect, and that the human ovum is almost devoid of yolk granules. The microscopic structure of the human ovum is shown in Figs. 52 and 53.

The *nucleus,* or *germinal vesicle,* presents a distinct reticular, nuclear network, the intersections of which appear as very darkly staining points. The *nucleolus,* or *germinal spot,* is much larger than in the primordial ovum and is believed to present ameboid movements. Mitochondria are present in large numbers in the ova, and after fertilization pass into the blastomeres and thus to all cells of the embryo. An ovum presenting the above characteristics is generally described as mature, but is not capable of fertilization and further development until it has undergone certain changes, which are designated as maturation, and manifested by the formation and casting off of the polar bodies.

Graafian follicles, as we have already pointed out, develop throughout childhood, and occasionally attain a considerable size; but they rarely rupture at this time on account of their position in the depths of the ovary, and undergo atresia in situ. In adults, on the other hand, the developing follicle usually makes its way to the surface, and when it has attained its highest development ruptures and extrudes its ovum into the peritoneal cavity or the tube, where it may be fertilized.

Ovulation. As the graafian follicle grows to a size of 10 to 15 mm. in diameter, it gradually reaches the surface of the ovary and finally protrudes above it. Due to continued production of liquor folliculi, the internal pressure is considerable since, if the follicle is punctured with the point of a knife, the fluid will spurt a short distance. The internal pressure of the follicle, however, is not the principal factor governing its rupture, since certain necrobiotic changes in the overlying tissues play an equally important role. These consist of a thinning out of the cells at the exposed tip of the follicle to the extent that this area becomes thin and transparent. The thinnest clear area then bursts, and the liquor folliculi, carrying with it the detached ovum, wells out —the process of ovulation. The actual rupture of the follicle is not an explosive phenomenon but a gradual opening. The discharge of the ovum with its zona pellucida and attached follicular cells is expedited by the fact that, just prior to rupture, the ovum with the surrounding structures becomes separated from the follicle wall as the result of the generative changes in the discus, and hence floats freely in the liquor.

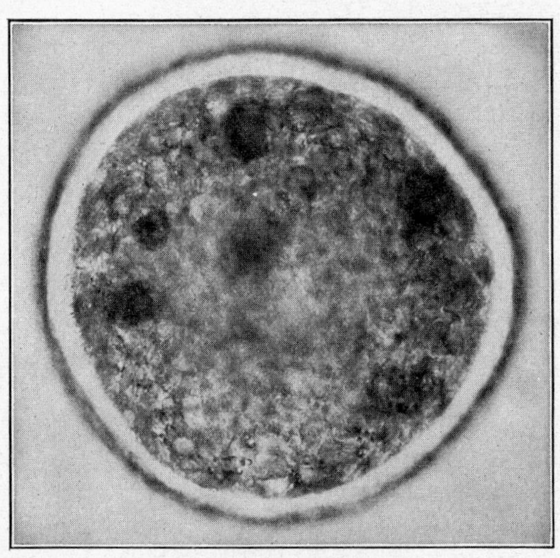

FIG. 53.—HUMAN OVUM WASHED FROM TUBE. FRESH SPECIMEN. × 405.

Protoplasm is enclosed by semitransparent zona pellucida and consists largely of lipoid masses. (Carnegie Col. 6289. Dr. W. H. Lewis.)

The exact time of ovulation each month is of the utmost importance for several reasons. In the first place, since the life span of both the spermatozoon and the unfertilized ovum is limited to a day or so, fertilization must take place within some 24 hours after ovulation if conception is to occur that month. In cases of female sterility, the determination of the time of ovulation and adjustment of coitus to that time, is one of the most important steps in therapy. In the second place, if it is desired to avoid conception, coitus can be limited to that part of the cycle which is some days distant from the time of ovulation; this is the basis of the concept of the "Safe Period." Finally, ovulation marks the important midpoint of both the ovarian and menstrual cycles. Thus, in respect to the ovarian cycle, the period from the first day of menstrual bleeding to ovulation is sometimes referred to as the pre-ovulatory phase of the cycle, but is more commonly designated, for understandable reasons, as the *follicular phase*. In an approximate way, this follicular phase represents the first half of the ovarian cycle, while the second half is known as the *luteal phase* for reasons which will become clear presently. The point to be emphasized here is that the phenomenon of ovulation divides the ovarian cycle into two main phases.

Various methods have been employed to ascertain the time of ovulation in women, the most dependable of which is the direct recovery of ova from the fallopian tube at operation. Allen, Newell, Pratt, and Bland were the first (1928) to recover mature unfertilized ova from the fallopian tube. They recovered eggs from the fallopian tube on the twelfth, fifteenth, and sixteenth days of the cycle, and concluded that ovulation occurs approximately on day 14 of a 28-day cycle. Other dependable methods for the determination of ovulation time are examination of fertilized ova and also evaluation of the changes which have taken place at the site of the ruptured follicle. In other words, how old is the corpus luteum? Investigations by these technics have demonstrated two important facts: (1) While it is true that ovulation occurs on the thirteenth or fourteenth day of the cycle in the majority of cases, there is considerable variation

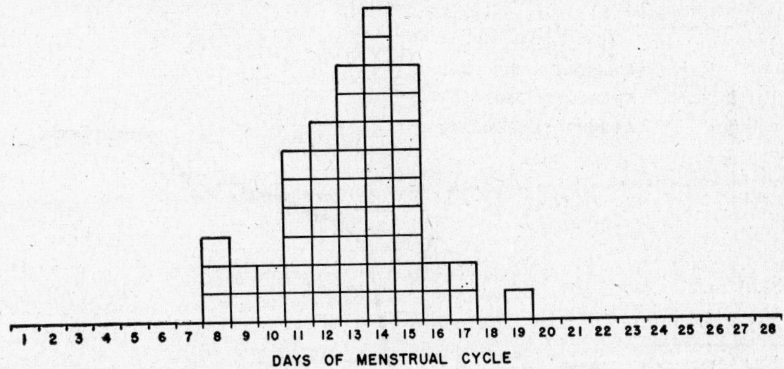

Fig. 54.—Day of Ovulation in 54 Women.

Each block represents an observation on one woman. (Modified, with permission, from Brewer and Jones.)

and it is not uncommon for ovulation to take place at any time between the eighth and twentieth days. This is shown in Fig. 54, which is based on a study by Brewer and Jones of the age of the corpus luteum in 54 women undergoing gynecologic surgery. (2) Ovulation bears a more exact time relationship to the next menstrual period than to the previous one and occurs approximately 14 days before the first day of the succeeding menstrual flow. Thus, data collected by Rock and Hertig on three unfertilized and 11 fertilized ova showed that the postovulatory phase of the cycle was 14 $\pm$ 2 days, whereas the pre-ovulatory phase varied by one to three days.

Still another method for ascertaining the time of ovulation, and one widely employed in cases of sterility, is the demonstration of a certain shift which the body temperature undergoes at that time. During the follicular phase of the cycle, the temperature is relatively low, while in the luteal phase it is relatively high. A fall in temperature occurs in association with the onset of menstruation followed at the midmenstruum, or at the time of ovulation, by a rather abrupt rise. A basal body temperature curve characteristic of follicle rupture is shown in Fig. 55.

A test for ovulation has been devised by Farris, based upon the observation that the urine of sexually mature women contains, during a period of about four days before ovulation, a gonadotrophic substance, presumably of pituitary origin, which produces hyperemia of the ovaries of immature rats when it is administered by hypodermic injection. In 39 women studied by Corner, Farris, and Corner, the Farris urinary rat test for ovulation was done, and the date of ovulation was estimated subsequently by histological examination of the ovaries and endometria obtained at operation. In 26 of the cases, the dating by the test and by histological examination agreed within one day, or with a difference of only one day. In four cases, there were differences of two, three, or four days. The frequency distribution of ovulation in the cycle resembled closely that found by various other methods of estimating the time of ovulation. Ovulation occurred between days 8 and 20 of the cycle, but most frequently from days 11 to 14, with the peak on day 13.

Ovulation does not necessarily occur alternately in the two ovaries. Thus, Van Wagenen and Morse have found in the monkey that one ovary sometimes ovulates repeatedly for as many as five cycles.

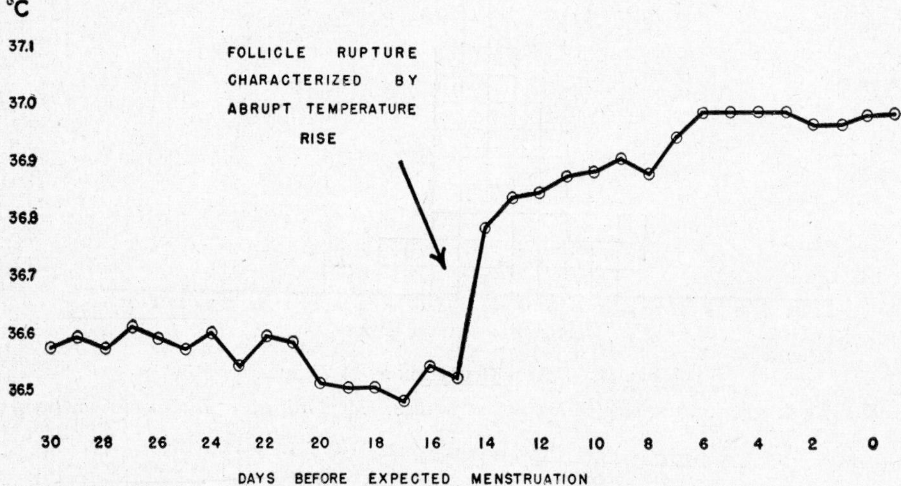

Fig. 55.—Basal Temperature Shift Characteristic of Follicle Rupture. (Palmer.)

Corpus Luteum. The corpus luteum is a structure which is formed at the site of a ruptured follicle. When the mature follicle ruptures, the ovum, liquor folliculi, and a considerable portion of the degenerated membrana granulosa make their escape, and the walls of the empty follicle collapse. In a short time, however, its cavity becomes filled with blood, which is derived partly from the vessels at the point of rupture, but principally from those of the tunica interna of the theca.

The corpus luteum, therefore, in its earliest stages is simply a ruptured follicle filled with blood, outside of which is a narrow yellow ring formed by the theca lutein cells. It is now generally believed that the granulosa cells, which are not cast off at the time of rupture, proliferate rapidly and invade the blood-filled follicle, forming a festooned layer about its central blood clot (Fig. 56). This layer is yellowish in color, whence the term "corpus luteum." As the structure becomes older, the yellow ring becomes thicker and thicker, until at last it almost entirely fills the interior of the follicle, the central blood clot remaining being now quite small.

At its period of greatest development, the corpus luteum may measure 10 to 20 mm. in diameter and sometimes occupies as much as one third of the entire ovary.

Microscopic sections through a well-developed example show that its center is occupied by a compressed blood clot, immediately outside of which is a thin layer of newly formed connective tissue. The greater part of the structure, however, is occupied by the festooned yellow ring, which is made up of large, polygonal, epithelioid cells, with small, round, somewhat faintly staining nuclei. These are the *lutein cells,* whose protoplasm presents a granular or vacuolated appearance, resulting from the disappearance of neutral fat and various lipids which have been dissolved out by the substances used in the fixation of the tissue or in the preparation of the microscopic slides. The yellow color, characteristic of the fresh state of the corpus luteum, is believed to be due to the presence of the pigment *carotene.* The layer of lutein cells is transversed by numerous radiate, moderately thick, connective-tissue partitions,

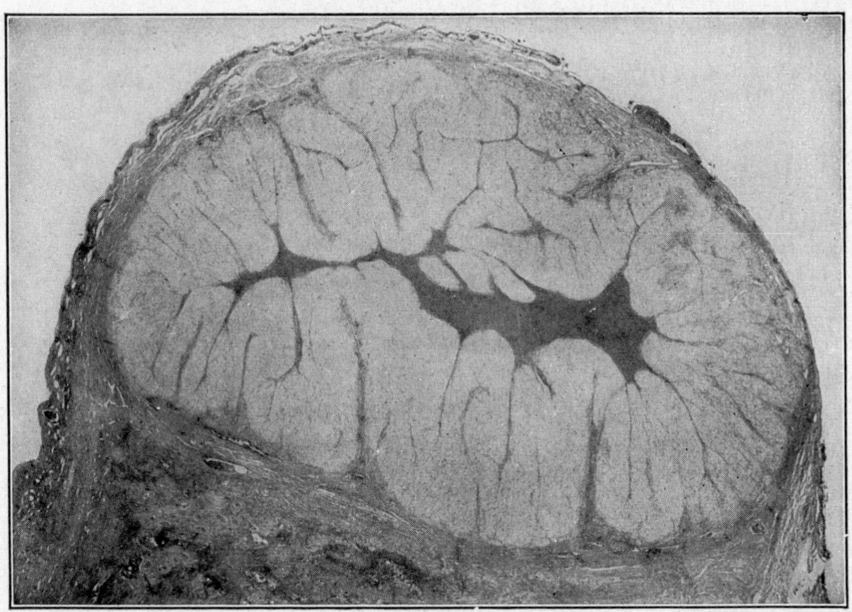

FIG. 56.—CORPUS LUTEUM OF PREGNANCY. LOW POWER. (See Fig. 57.)

growing up from the theca, to which it owes its festooned appearance. They are richly supplied with blood vessels and lymphatics (Fig. 57).

As the cavity of the follicle is encroached upon by the growing lutein cells, the blood clot becomes more and more compressed, and vascular loops extend into it and soon cause its organization. At the same time, the blood pigment is removed by leukocytes, which can be found in the surrounding tissue with their bodies filled with particles of it. Occasionally, hemorrhage does not take place into the ruptured follicle, and a corpus luteum is formed without a central blood clot. This is the exception in human beings, but the rule in many of the lower animals.

After the cavity of the follicle has become obliterated by the ingrowth of the lutein cells and connective tissue, degenerative changes soon make their appearance in the former, some of which undergo hyaline, and others fatty degeneration. In young women, in whom the circulation is active, the degenerated lutein cells are rapidly absorbed, so that in a short time the corpus luteum becomes replaced by newly formed connective tissue which corresponds closely in appearance to the surrounding ovarian stroma. But in more advanced life, when the ovarian circulation has become impaired, absorption goes on less rapidly; and not infrequently the degeneration extends to the intervening connective tissue and blood vessels until the entire structure is converted into an almost homogeneous mass of hyalin in which only a few connective-tissue cells and degenerated blood vessels can be seen (Fig. 58). These structures—the so-called *corpora fibrosa* or *albicantia*—present on fresh section a dull white appearance, somewhat suggestive of old scar tissue. They are, however, gradually invaded by the surrounding stroma, and become broken up into smaller and smaller hyaline masses, which

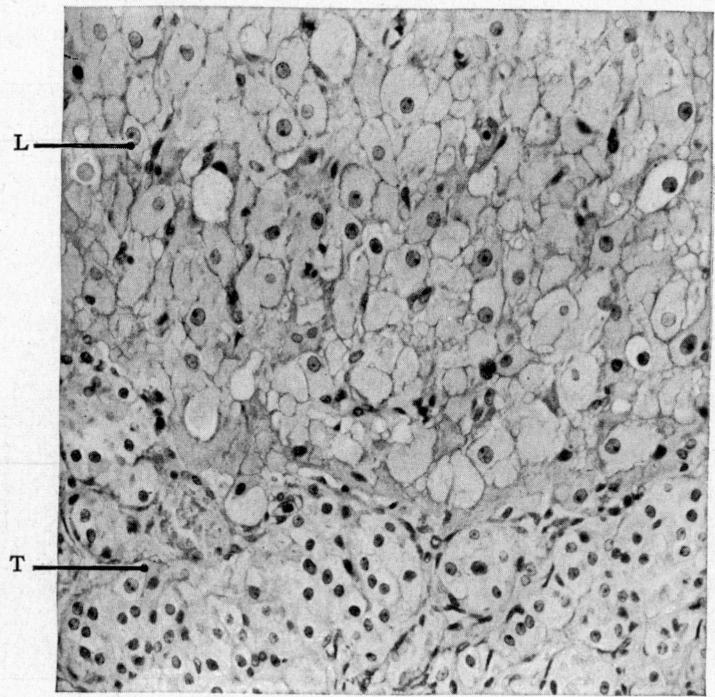

FIG. 57.—CORPUS LUTEUM OF PREGNANCY. HIGH POWER.
L., lutein cells; T., theca-lutein cells.

are eventually absorbed, the site of the original follicle being indicated only by an area of slightly thickened connective tissue. When the circulation is very defective, absorption takes place much more slowly, so that it is not uncommon to find the ovaries of women near the menopause almost filled by corpora fibrosa of varying size. Frequently the small hyaline bodies resulting from the breaking up of these structures assume peculiar and bizarre forms, and very often present a curved and twisted appearance suggestive of a degenerated artery. Similar structures are sometimes left after the obliteration of nonruptured follicles.

If, as in the majority of cases, fertilization does not take place, the corpus luteum is spoken of as the *corpus luteum of menstruation*. If, on the other hand, fertilization does occur, the degenerative changes just described are postponed for about six months and, under such circumstances, the structure is called the *corpus luteum of pregnancy*. The active life span of the corpus luteum of menstruation, as demonstrated by the careful studies of Brewer and other evidence, is about eight days. It is at the end of this period that degenerative changes first make their appearance; and simultaneously the secretory activity of the corpus luteum—namely, the manufacture of the hormone *progesterone*—also begins to wane. It will be noted that this critical point in the life of the structure occurs about eight days after ovulation and approximately six days prior to the onset of the next menstruation. As will be explained subsequently, these time relationships are of the utmost importance. (See pages 95 and 97.)

Practically all authorities are agreed as to the life history of the corpus luteum, and the only point which still remains unsettled deals with the *origin of the lutein cells.* As indicated in the collective review of Asdell (1928), three main views have been

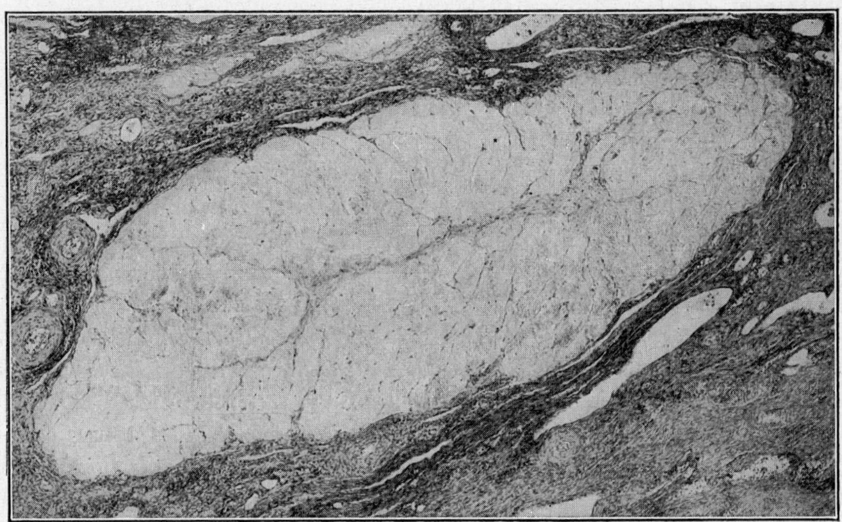

FIG. 58.—CORPUS FIBROSUM. × 150.

advanced: (*a*) that the lutein cells are of connective-tissue origin and are derived from the cells of the theca interna; (*b*) that they are derived from the proliferation of the cells composing the membrana granulosa; and (*c*) that they are derived from both sources, when one has to deal with a mixture of connective tissue and of epithelial cells. The first view is thought to be incorrect. The second view is supported by a constantly increasing number of investigators who have shown that, following the rupture of the follicle, the cells of the membrana granulosa, instead of being exfoliated as was previously taught, rapidly proliferate, soon fill the cavity and become the true lutein cells. The third view was particularly advocated by Corner, Evans and others, but has found only limited acceptance.

The consensus favors the granulosa origin of the characteristic cells of the human corpus luteum. Attention has already been directed to the changes which occur in the cells of the tunica interna of the theca during the growth of the follicle, and in every well-developed corpus luteum groups of such cells can be demonstrated about the periphery of the corpus luteum and often in the strands of connective tissue invading it, so that theca cells in many instances may become admixed with granulosa lutein cells. Generally speaking, however, the two types of cells are sharply differentiated, the granulosa lutein cells being larger, more vacuolated and provided with a smaller nucleus, while the theca lutein cells are somewhat smaller, stain more deeply and have a relatively larger nucleus.

On the other hand, the theca lutein cells play a prominent part in the life history of follicles which degenerate in situ without rupture. This process, which is designated as *follicular atresia,* is particularly pronounced during pregnancy, as will be noted later. In such circumstances, after the follicle has attained a certain size, the ovum undergoes cytolysis, the membrana granulosa degenerates, is cast off into the liquor folliculi, and eventually is absorbed. While these changes are in progress, the theca lutein cells proliferate and form a tunic many layers thick about the follicle, which frequently assumes a yellowish coloration. Eventually, as the liquor folliculi disappears, the walls of the follicle collapse and the theca cells composing it undergo fatty and hyaline change, so that finally an irregularly hyaline body results, which cannot be distinguished from a similar structure derived from a corpus luteum, or even from a degenerated vessel.

It should be remembered that atresia is the fate of the vast majority of follicles which develop beyond the primordial stage, and that the process begins during intrauterine life and continues until after the menopause, while corpora lutea develop only from the comparatively small number of follicles which rupture after reaching maturity. The earlier observers considered that the changes in the corpus luteum were analogous to the organization of a blood clot, but at present such a view is only of historical interest. Possibly, one of the less important functions of the corpus luteum is to bring about the obliteration of the spaces left by the ruptured follicles without the formation of cicatricial tissue; for if they healed by the latter process it is evident that in a very short time the entire ovary would be converted into a mass consisting of nothing but scar tissue, the very nature of which would effectually prevent further ovulation.

THE OVARIAN HORMONES

Estrogen

For many years it has been suspected that the ovary is responsible for internal secretions which have numerous functions, such as: (1) the onset of puberty; (2) secondary sex characteristics; (3) cyclical changes associated with the menstrual function; (4) the maintenance of pregnancy; and (5) lactation. An important tool for the study of this question was provided by Stockard and Papanicolaou when, in 1917, they demonstrated the cyclical changes in the vaginal smear of the guinea pig. In 1922 Allen and Doisy made practical use of this discovery in their experiments with the follicular fluid of the sow's ovary. They found that 48 hours after this fluid was injected into ovariectomized mice and rats, the vaginal smear changed from the castrate to the estrous type (cornification of vaginal epithelium) in every way similar to that of animals with intact ovaries. In other words, they had discovered in the ovary of one animal, a hormonal substance which was capable of producing estrous response or "heat" in another.

Allen and Doisy continued their work and found that the histological changes in the uterus and vagina of spayed rats, injected with follicular hormone, corresponded to the estrous phases of normal animals. To Frank belongs the credit of demonstrating the estrus-producing hormone in the circulating blood. Many tissues and body fluids were then assayed, and the hormone was found in the venous and menstrual blood of women, the titer varying with the phases of the menstrual cycle. It was also discovered in the blood and urine of pregnant women, as well as in the amniotic fluid and in the placenta. Subsequent investigation has revealed a very wide distribution of this substance in the feces, bile and liver, and in the testes, blood and tissues of males, as well as in many plants.

The results of Allen and Doisy were promptly confirmed by many workers, and each applied a name to the follicular substance. Thus, the literature for a time became confused by a varied nomenclature all referring to the same substance. A few of these are estrin, folliculin, theelin, amniotin, oophorin, feminin, the female sex hormone, menformon and progynon. In 1936 the Council on Pharmacy and Chemistry of the

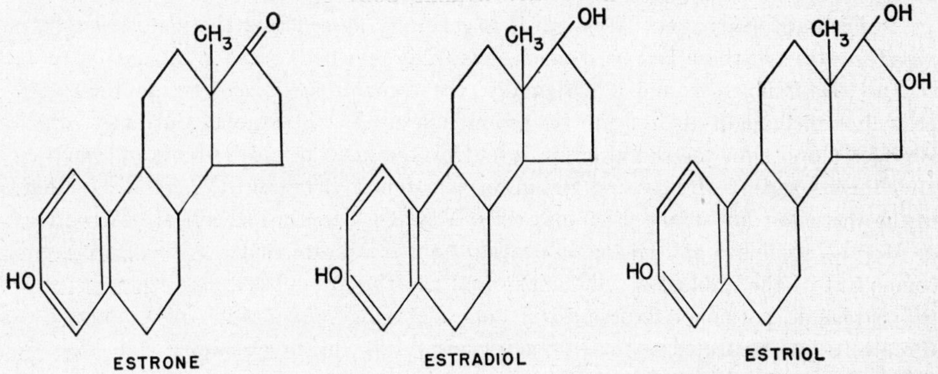

ESTRONE ESTRADIOL ESTRIOL

FIG. 59.—STRUCTURAL FORMULAS OF ESTRONE, ESTRADIOL AND ESTRIOL.

American Medical Association adapted the term *estrogen* as the collective term for all substances, regardless of chemical composition or source, which are capable of producing the typical changes of estrus or "heat" (enlargement of uterus, cornification of vagina, and mating) in immature or spayed adult animals. Synonymous terms are "the estrogenic hormone" and "the estrogens."

Chemistry of the Estrogens. The most important naturally occurring estrogens are estrone, estriol and estradiol, the chemical formulas of which are shown in Fig. 59. They are steroid compounds, with a phenanthrene nucleus, related to such sterols as cholesterol, the bile acids, ergosterol, calciferol and the androgens. They are essentially lipoid soluble, their solubility in water being comparatively low.

Of the three naturally occurring estrogens, estradiol is the one actually formed in the ovary and is much more potent than the other two. Estrone is found chiefly in the urine and is presumably an end product of estradiol. Estriol, the least active of the three, is found in greatest concentration in the placenta.

The estrogens were first standardized in terms of rat and mouse units. These were defined as the least amount of substance which, when given in three doses at four-hour intervals to a spayed adult female rat or mouse, will produce a full change from the negative to the estrous vaginal smear in 48 to 56 hours after the first injection. It soon became evident that numerous factors influence the minimal effective dose, so that even minor variations in technic may result in wide discrepancies. To insure uniformity, an international unit was established in 1932 and defined as the specific estrus-producing activity contained in 0.1 gamma (0.0001 mg.) of the international standard ketohydroxyestratriene (estrone), preserved at the National Institute for Medical Research in London. It has been estimated that one international unit is equivalent to from one third to one tenth of a rat unit, depending on the method of bio-assay used.

Synthetic Estrogens. A number of synthetic estrogens have been prepared, of which the best known and most widely employed is diethylstilbestrol. The Council on Pharmacy and Chemistry of the American Medical Association has adopted the term *stilbestrol* for the mother substance, 4,4′-dihydroxystilbene, and for its more potent derivative, 4,4′-dihydroxy-α:β-diethylstilbene, the term *diethylstilbestrol.* This latter substance is employed extensively in obstetrics and gynecology and simulates almost completely the action of the normally occurring estrogens.

Sources of Estrogen. Although it is generally agreed that the maturing follicle secretes estrogen, there has been much debate as to whether the granulosa or theca cells of the follicles secrete it. Originally, the recognition of estrogen in the liquor folliculi was thought to indicate its production by the granulosa. Currently, much stronger support for the thecal origin is lent by the histochemical studies of Dempsey and Bassett and of McKay and Robinson who found characteristic steroid reactions in the theca but not in the granulosa cells. Moreover, the histochemical observations of McKay, Robinson and Hertig on ovarian tumors indicate that it is the "theca-cell" component of the granulosa cell tumor—and not the granulosa cells—which secretes the estrogenic hormone. Experimental data involving implantation of granulosa or theca cells into castrated animals (Zondek and Aschheim, Bell) showed endocrine activity associated with the theca only. Likewise, ovarian irradiation with destruction of the granulosa and proliferation of the theca resulted in persistence of estrogenic activity (Hüssey and Wallart). As will be stressed later, in pregnancy the placenta is an all-important source of estrogen.

Actions of Estrogen. Estrogen is essentially a growth hormone with selective affinity for tissues derived from the müllerian ducts, this group including the endometrium, the musculature of the uterine body, the cervix, and the upper part of the vagina. These specific growth effects as well as other more widespread actions may be enumerated as follows:

1. *Effects on Uterus.* In the intact immature and in the spayed adult monkey (as in lower species), estrogen causes hypertrophy of the uterine musculature and marked proliferation of the endometrium. Associated with these changes is an increased blood supply. The spiral arteries respond to the growth stimulus of estrogen even more actively than the rest of the endometrium, and as a result their tips approach more and more to the epithelial surface. In addition, estrogen affects the activity of the cervical epithelium in such a way that the cervical mucus increases in quantity and pH, attains a clear fluid state and is more readily penetrated by spermatozoa.

Estrogen possesses no oxytocic powers per se, but its presence is an important prerequisite to normal myometrial activity. The uterus of animals, including monkeys, manifests active contractility only at the time of estrus or ovulation; that is, when estrogen production is at its height. During other phases of the cycle it is quiescent. The uterus of ovariectomized animals, moreover, is regularly quiescent, but the myometrial activity may be restored by transplantation of ovarian tissue, or by the injection of estrogen. Although these observations may suggest a direct oxytocic action of estrogen, the fallacy of any such deduction is demonstrated by the following facts: (1) estrogen is inactive on the uterus in vitro; (2) when estrogen is administered to the ovariectomized animal, there is a very long latent period of 8 to 10 hours before myometrial activity ensues; (3) even the most massive doses of estrogen do not initiate labor in pregnant women or monkeys. As Reynolds has pointed out, these seemingly contradictory findings are adequately explained if it is borne in mind that the primary action of estrogen is on the metabolic processes and vascular alterations in the uterus associated with growth, and that the attainment of rhythmic, coordinated activity of the myometrium represents simply a stage in the train of these anabolic processes.

2. *Effects on Vagina*. Estrogen produces proliferation and cornification of the vaginal epithelium, causing it to change in castrate monkeys as well as in castrate women from a thin structure which is only two or three cells deep to one which is multicellular in depth. Thus, in castrate women, Shorr has shown that the administration of estrogen results in a vaginal epithelium which is densely packed with thick layers of compressed cells.

3. *Effects on Fallopian Tubes*. Estrogen stimulates growth of the fallopian tubes and appears to influence also the activity of the tubal musculature. In experimental animals tubal contractions reach their height at estrus. Their dependence on estrogen is indicated by the fact that they disappear following ovariectomy and can be restored by administration of estrogen. Likewise, in women, tubal contractions increase at the time of ovulation.

4. *Effects on Breasts*. The administration of estrogen to the immature or castrate animal, in which the mammary glands are rudimentary or atrophic, causes an extension of the ducts comparable to that seen in the sexually mature, nulliparous animal. The type of growth varies in different species. In some, as in the human and monkey, partial lobule-alveolar growth is induced, as well as duct development. In others, the action is solely on the ducts, and the simultaneous action of the corpus-luteum hormone is necessary for the proliferation of the lobule-alveolar system.

5. *Effects on Other Secondary Sex Characteristics*. Estrogen is responsible for all the secondary sex characteristics which make their appearance at puberty including mammary growth and the characteristic rounding of the body contour.

6. *Sex Effects of Estrogen on Mating Behavior*. In the lower animals estrogen plays an important role in libido, or sexual desire, as evidenced by the fact that the female will generally accept the male only at the time of estrus. On the other hand, the human female appears to be little influenced in this regard by the cyclic variations in estrogen production. Thus, Davis interviewed 2,200 women by means of questionnaires and found that less than 20 per cent were conscious of regular periods of sex desire.

Cyclic Estrogen Levels in Blood and Urine. Blood estrogen increases from a very low level after the menses to a peak at about the time of ovulation; this is followed by a slight decline and subsequently by a secondary premenstrual rise. Frank and Goldberger were able to recover a mouse unit of the hormone from an extract of 40 cc. of the blood as early as the seventh day after the beginning of the menstrual flow; 2 mouse units were obtained on the fourteenth day; and 3 mouse units from 40 cc. of blood during the last week of the menstrual cycle. Thus they demonstrated a gradual increase of estrogen in the menstrual cycle from the seventh to the twenty-fifth day. Fluhmann, on the other hand, found the highest level of estrogen in the blood at or near the time of ovulation. Cyclic fluctuations in the elimination of estrogen in the urine corresponded generally to these changes in the hormone content of the blood. As may be seen in Fig. 60, the total excretion of estrogen on the seventh day of the cycle is of the order of 50 mouse units, rises to about 150 mouse units at the time of ovulation, declines slightly, and then rises again to a level of about 175 mouse units around the twenty-first day of the cycle. During the four or five days prior to the next menstrual period, it declines rapidly. Most of the estrogen excreted

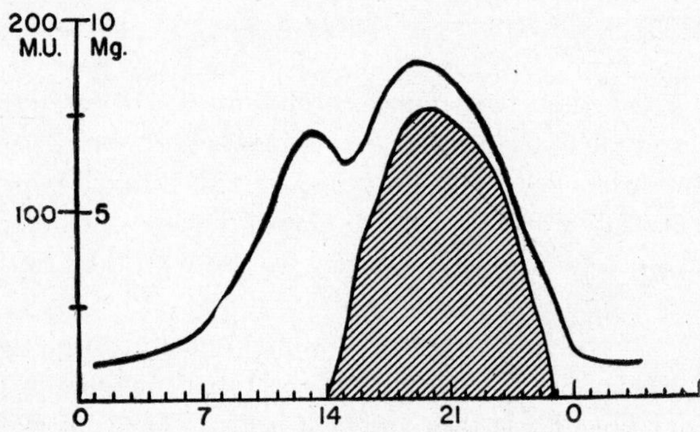

FIG. 60.—EXCRETION OF ESTROGEN AND PREGNANEDIOL SHOWING TIME RELATIONSHIPS TO CYCLE. Shaded area shows pregnanediol; black line, estrogen (Venning).

in the urine is in chemical combination which renders it inactive, but about one third is excreted simply as estrone and estriol. Since, when estrogen is administered perorally or parenterally to castrate or totally amenorrheic women, no more than 20 per cent is excreted, it has been estimated that the total amount of this hormone produced by the ovaries in the course of a menstrual cycle must be of the order of 5,000 rat units or 20,000 mouse units. The fate of the 80 per cent of administered estrogen which does not appear in the urine is not definitely known, but most of it is presumably inactivated by the liver. Recent studies by Twombly and his associates indicate that large amounts of estrogen may be excreted in the feces.

PROGESTERONE

During the post-ovulatory phase of the ovarian cycle, an extremely important hormone, progesterone, is manufactured by the corpus luteum. The name of this hormone stems from the fact that its main function is to produce certain endometrial changes essential for the nidation of the fertilized ovum; that is, it favors gestation. As Courrier has well said: "In general, estrogen is the *hormone of the woman*: it assures the development of the genital and mammary apparatus; progesterone is the *hormone of the mother*: it is indispensable for reproduction."

Chemistry of Progesterone. The chemical formula for progesterone is shown in Fig. 61 where it may be seen that, like the estrogens, progesterone is a sterol with a phenanthrene nucleus and that there is a striking chemical kinship to those hormones. Like the estrogens, it is fat soluble. The chemical configuration of progesterone is also very similar to that of the male sex hormone testosterone (the testicular hormone), and to androsterone (the male urinary hormone substance).

When the body metabolizes progesterone it is converted into another substance called pregnanediol, the chemical formula of which is shown beside that of progesterone in Fig. 61. As may be seen, the conversion takes place by the addition of six atoms of hydrogen. Pregnanediol is an inert substance as far as hormone action is concerned. Its great importance lies in the fact that it can be assayed in the urine as pregnanediol glycuronidate, and since one molecule of this waste product in the urine means that at least one molecule of progesterone has been produced, it is a most valuable index of corpus luteum function.

Progesterone was first standardized on the basis of its ability to induce progestational modifications in the estrogen-primed endometrium of the rabbit. A unit, as defined by Corner and Allen, is the minimum dose which, given in five equal doses on

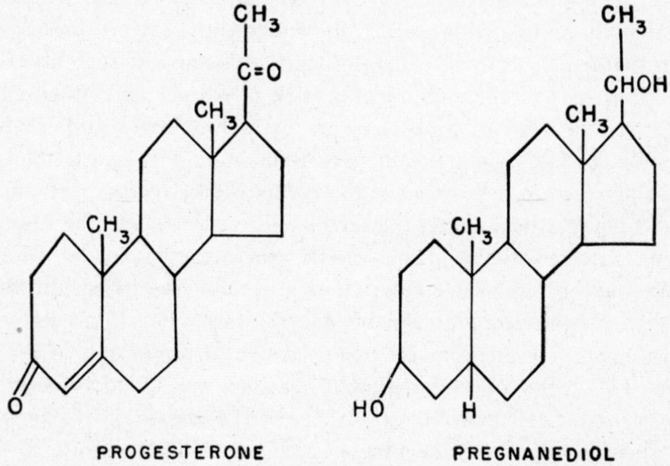

Fig. 61.—Structural Formulas of Progesterone and Pregnanediol.

five successive days to adult female rabbits castrated when in heat, will produce by the sixth day progestational modifications of the uterine mucosa equivalent to those seen on the eighth day of gestation. A Clauberg unit, estimated to equal from one half to one fifth of a Corner-Allen unit, is the amount of active substance required to induce progestational mucosal changes in the immature intact rabbit, weighing 600 gm. and previously primed with estrogen. In 1935 the Standardization Committee of the League of Nations adopted an international unit which is defined as the progestational activity present in one milligram of beta-progesterone. This equals approximately one Corner-Allen unit.

Effects of Progesterone. The main action of progesterone is to produce secretory activity of the endometrial glands, together with certain effects upon the stromal and vascular elements. These effects, together with other actions, may be enumerated as follows:

1. *Effects on Endometrium.* Before it can respond to progesterone, the endometrium must first be primed by the administration of estrogen, the so-called "one-two sequence." Upon such an endometrium, progesterone produces manifold evidences of secretory activity, especially the conversion of the straight glandular pattern characteristic of the pre-ovulatory phase to a tortuous, corkscrew glandular picture. The stroma becomes edematous and loose-textured, especially in its superficial layer, and its constituent cells undergo hypertrophy with an increased amount of cytoplasm. This suc-

culent progestational epithelium, characteristic of progesterone effect, will be discussed in more detail in connection with the menstrual cycle.

2. *Effects on Maintenance of Pregnancy.* By producing, with the aid of estrogen, the type of endometrium just described, progesterone creates in the uterine mucosa nutritive conditions favorable for the nidation and retention of the ovum. If, owing to progesterone deficiency, such a fetal bed collapses, any product of conception implanted therein becomes loosened from its attachments and is aborted. In many lower animals, such as the rat, mouse, goat, ground squirrel and opossum, the presence of the corpus luteum seems to be necessary throughout pregnancy, since its removal at any stage invariably leads to abortion. In the pregnant rabbit castration or destruction of all the corpora lutea before the eighteenth day of the 31-day gestational period, regularly causes abortion; after the eighteenth day, it usually does. The demonstration that a deficiency of progesterone is the cause of such abortions constituted an important part of the monumental work of Corner and Allen on the corpus luteum in the late 20's. By administering an extract of sow's corpora lutea, these workers were able to maintain pregnancy to term in rabbits ovariectomized shortly after mating. They further found that if the corpora lutea of the pregnant rabbit are excised 14 to 18 hours after mating, the fertilized ova develop to the blastocyst stage and are then transported to the uterine cavity where they soon die. More recently, Pincus and Werthessen have shown that if ovariectomy is carried out shortly after copulation, ovum growth stops at the blastocyst stage; but if progesterone is administered postoperatively, it promotes ovum growth in proportion to the amount of hormone given. The degree of ovular growth observed was found to be in proportion to the degree of endometrial proliferation achieved. Since these workers could also promote growth of such ova by keeping them in a suitable culture medium, they concluded that the arrest of ovular growth which regularly follows oophorectomy in the rabbit was due to the absence of special uterine conditions. In other words, progesterone maintains pregnancy through its protective action on the fetal bed.

On the other hand, in the human as well as the monkey, pregnancy may continue to a normal conclusion despite corpus luteum ablation performed after the first few weeks of gestation. Asdell, in a review of the literature to 1928, found only four abortions among a group of 34 cases subjected to bilateral oophorectomy some time between the first and seventh months of gestation. DeWit and Oppers collected 131 cases in which only 23.7 per cent aborted following removal of the corpus luteum during the first four months of gestation. Hartman and Corner state that in the monkey, with a gestational period of 165 days, the twenty-fifth day marks the approximate time after which the corpus luteum is no longer necessary. The corresponding figure for the human would be about six weeks, or around the time of the second missed period. There is evidence that in the human the corpus luteum may be removed even earlier than this without interfering with the successful continuation of pregnancy. Perhaps the record in this regard is the case of Pratt who removed a corpus luteum on the twenty-first day after the onset of the last menstruation. The patient had come for treatment for sterility and was operated upon for retroversion and other complicating circumstances. It seemed safe on account of the recent menstruation to remove the corpus luteum for study. The patient did not menstruate following the removal of the corpus luteum but continued through a normal pregnancy and lactation. Both ovaries had been carefully inspected to insure that no other corpus luteum was present. Jones and Weil record removal of the corpus luteum as early as the fifty-eighth day after the last menstrual period without abortion taking place.

But this ability of the human female to carry pregnancy to completion without the presence of the corpus luteum is in no way indicative that progesterone is unnecessary. It means simply that the human placenta (which normally produces progesterone and estrogen in large quantities throughout the last six months of pregnancy) is able to manufacture these hormones very early in gestation and in sufficient

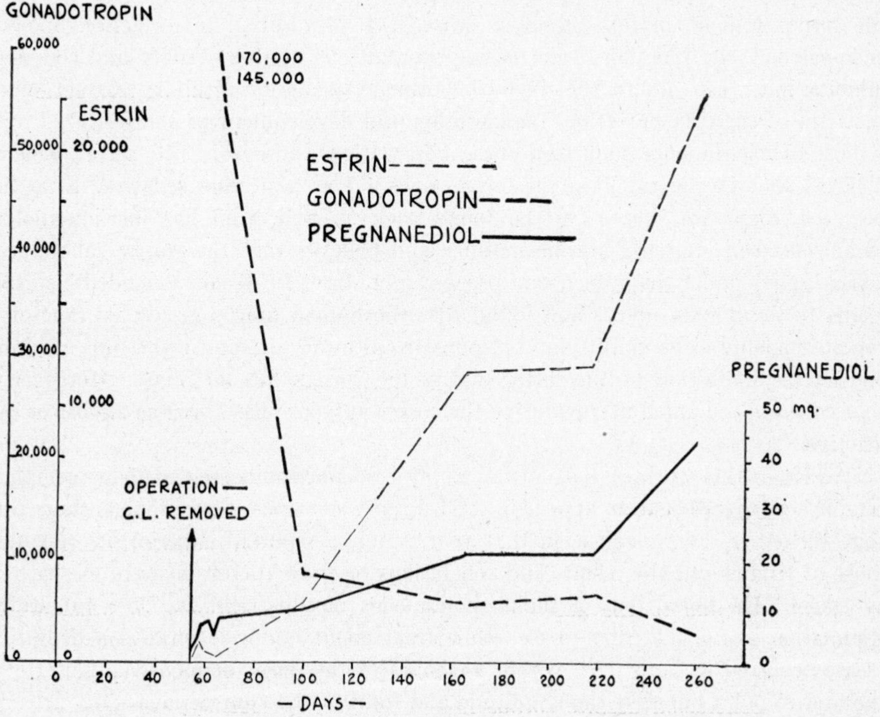

FIG. 62.—EXCRETION OF PREGNANEDIOL COMPLEX AND ESTROGEN DESPITE REMOVAL OF THE CORPUS LUTEUM IN VERY EARLY HUMAN PREGNANCY (Venning).

quantities to substitute for the corpus luteum in such cases. This fact has been demonstrated in many instances by pregnanediol studies following ablation of the corpus luteum in pregnancy. As an example may be cited Venning's case in which the ovary containing the corpus luteum had to be removed for therapeutic reasons at the fifty-fourth day after the last menstrual bleeding. As shown in Fig. 62, there was a slight fall in pregnanediol excretion immediately after the operation, but 10 days postoperatively it had risen to 10 mg. a day and continued to increase thereafter. Likewise, the excretion of estrogen continued to augment in normal fashion. This manufacture of estrogen and progesterone is one of the most important of placental functions and is discussed in more detail on page 162. The transfer of the site of formation of estrogens and progesterone from ovary to placenta is probably a gradual one, being completed between the second and third month. The time at which the early rise in excretion of pregnanediol takes place is an indication of the increasing activity of the placenta. It varies in different cases, but is frequently seen by the sixty-fifth or seventieth day, although in some apparently normal pregnancies this may not occur until the eightieth or ninetieth day.

3. *Effect on Uterine Motility.* Although it has long been held that progesterone inhibits uterine contractility, recent observations have raised serious questions about this tenet. The original understanding about progesterone was that it acts as a uterine sedative, and it has long been so employed in the treatment of threatened abortion, dysmenorrhea and after-pains. This attitude toward the hormone dates back to a series of experiments by Knaus in 1926 on rabbits, which led him to the belief that the corpus luteum, in this species at least, had, in addition to its action upon the endometrium, the function of decreasing spontaneous uterine activity and completely inhibiting its response to the oxytocic hormone, posterior pituitary extract, during the term of the transportation, implantation and development of the fertilized ovum. A host of experiments confirmed these observations, and it is still rather generally believed that in the rabbit progesterone does act as a uterine sedative. Even here, however, there are skeptics to be found such as Bell, who has incriminated the technic used in studying uterine motility and believes that the empty rabbit uterus is very active under the influence of progesterone. In 1929, Knaus extended his experiments to the human uterus and found that the human uterus resembled that of the rabbit in spontaneous motility and response to pituitary extract in the follicular phase and in the inhibition of the latter during the corpus luteum phase. Moreover, he showed that the human uterus during the corpus luteum phase became almost or quite inactive.

Although this work of Knaus was amply confirmed and seemed to be completely established, there began to appear in 1931 a series of papers by various authors which contradicted it. For instance, in that year Schultze reported experiments resembling those of Knaus, but the results and conclusions he drew therefrom were in sharp disagreement. He found only a slight spontaneous motility and response to pituitary stimulation in the follicular phase, while from about midcycle onward a definite increase occurred in both until within 24 hours of the onset of menstruation. He was the first to point out that the amplitude and form of the contractions were characteristic of the phase of the cycle in which they were recorded, and that the response to pituitary extract increased progressively toward the end of the cycle and reached a maximum between the twentieth day and 24 hours before the onset of the next period. Likewise, in 1934, Moir using an intra-uterine bag found that the contractions were much stronger in the second half of the cycle and even more forceful during menstruation, when they came at two-minute intervals. In both the premenstrual phase and the menstrual phase of the cycle pituitary extract caused "spasmodic contractions."

After reviewing this whole problem extensively several years ago, Henry and Browne reached the conclusion on the basis of their own as well as others' work that the spontaneous activity of the human uterus and its sensitivity to pituitary extract are greatest in the luteal phase of the cycle and, by the same token, that progesterone is not a uterine sedative. The question is hence a moot one, but the consensus among most clinicians, contrary to the findings of Henry and Browne, is that progesterone does exert an appreciable degree of relaxing action on the myometrium.

4. *Effect on Fallopian Tubes.* As already indicated, histological studies show that the tubal mucosa undergoes cyclic changes in the course of the menstrual cycle. During the luteal phase of the cycle it shows changes which indicate secretory activity. This

interpretation is substantiated by Joel's observation that the glycogen and ascorbic acid content of the human tubal mucosa reaches its height during the luteal phase and that its lipoid content is highest at the beginning of this phase. That the progestational hormone is responsible for the tubal modification seen during the luteal phase has been demonstrated in the rabbit by Westman and Caffier. Cyclic variations in the activity of the tubal musculature have also been ascribed to progesterone. Rhythmic contractions occur, the amplitude of which is greatest at the height of the follicular phase and least during the luteal phase of the cycle, and the relative quiescence in the latter phase is attributed to progesterone action. Recent studies suggest that the relative quiescence of the tubal musculature induced by progesterone is purposeful and plays an important part in transport of the fertilized ovum to the uterine cavity.

5. *Effect on the Cervix.* As already stated, the cervix is known to undergo cyclic changes in respect to the type of cervical mucus produced. During the premenstruum, the secretions are scanty, viscid, full of leukocytes and impermeable to spermatozoa—a quite different state of affairs from that which exists under the influence of estrogen alone. These changes are presumably the result of progesterone action.

6. *Effect on Ovulation.* Progesterone inhibits ovulation and follicular maturation, so that, generally speaking, these are in abeyance in the presence of an actively functioning corpus luteum. Thus, during pregnancy ovulation does not take place.

7. *Effect on Breasts.* Progesterone is believed to be largely responsible for the acinose and lobular growth seen in the latter part of the cycle, thus complementing the action of estrogen. These two hormones then, by dual action, are capable of bringing about complete mammary development, estrogen acting chiefly on the duct system and progesterone on the lobule-alveolar apparatus. Whether these hormones act directly on the mammary tissue, or whether they exert their effects through the mediation of the pituitary body is a moot question. After reviewing the evidence, Astwood reaches the conclusion that both estrogen and pituitary extract are capable of exerting a growth effect upon the mammary gland, and that the normal situation probably entails an action of both hormones. The estrogen stimulus is a direct one in his opinion, which is more fully and completely expressed in the presence of a normally functioning hypophysis. In Astwood's opinion, the pituitary is not essential to complete lobular development induced either by active corpora lutea or by the placenta.

8. *Effect on Pelvic Ligaments (Relaxin).* Either progesterone or a separate hormone secreted by the corpus luteum possesses the power of causing extraordinary softening and separation of the symphysis pubis in certain mammals, especially the guinea pig. After reviewing the available evidence, Hoffman reaches the conclusion that this action is produced by a specific luteal hormone distinct from the progestational principle. Hisaw has given this hormone the name "relaxin." This hormone has been demonstrated in the blood of pregnant women, but its significance is not entirely clear. As pointed out by Abramson, Hurwitt and Lesnick, pregnancy is associated with a thickening, softening and increased vascularization of tissues in and about the pelvic joints, but whether these alterations are produced by relaxin has not been established.

Pregnanediol Excretion. As shown in Fig. 60, no pregnanediol is excreted during the pre-ovulatory phase of the cycle. According to Corner, pregnanediol appears in the urine a day or two after ovulation. The excretion becomes greatest about a week before menstruation and usually disappears entirely a few days before the onset of bleeding. The curve of excretion of pregnanediol thus parallels the life history of the corpus luteum. At the peak of the luteal phase, pregnanediol excretion is of the order of 5 to 10 mg. per 24 hours, a total excretion of 30 to 60 mg. being considered normal for one cycle. Menstruation occurs within one to three days following the disappearance of pregnanediol from the urine.

THE PITUITARY GONADOTROPHIC HORMONE

With occasional exceptions, the ovarian cycle becomes established at about the thirteenth year and then, with amazing periodicity, makes its measured rounds for some three decades, to subside between the forty-fifth and fiftieth years of life. What initiates and what controls this rhythmic process? The directing forces come presumably from the anterior lobe of the hypophysis, which has been called the "master clock of the gonads."

Removal of the hypophysis inhibits the development of the genital organs in the immature and produces regression of these organs in the mature animal. From ablation procedures on the posterior lobe, as well as from injections of posterior-pituitary extracts, it is apparent that only the anterior hypophysis is concerned in these effects upon the reproductive organs. In 1933, Fevold, Hisaw, Hellbaum and Hertz succeeded in fractionating gonadotrophic extract of the hypophysis into the follicle-stimulating hormone (FSH) and the luteinizing hormone (LH). The evidence to date indicates that these two hormones are separate chemical substances.

At the present time, the generally accepted theory with regard to these gonadotrophic hormones from the anterior pituitary may be epitomized as follows: The follicle-stimulating hormone, also called thylakentrin, is responsible for the growth of the follicle with its production of estrogen, which brings about the proliferative phase of the menstrual cycle. The luteinizing hormone is responsible for the changing of the follicle into the corpus luteum, which secretes progesterone, which in turn produces the progestational or luteal phase of the cycle. In regard to the manner in which these two hormones cause ovulation, the evidence has been summarized by Hoffman as follows: Ovulation is not due to a distinct ovulation hormone, but depends upon the interaction of the follicle-stimulating and luteinizing hormones. To insure the occurrence of ovulation, the following requirements must be fulfilled: (1) The ovary must contain antra-bearing follicles capable of responding normally to the follicle-stimulating principle. (2) Follicle-stimulating extracts, practically free from luteinizer, must be supplied in adequate amounts and for long enough to develop the follicle to the fully mature stage. (3) Luteinizing hormone must be permitted to supplement the follicle stimulator at the time when the follicle reaches this stage, and must be supplied in an exact amount which bears a certain relationship to the quantity of follicle stimulator available.

A third pituitary gonadotrophic hormone, luteotrophin, has been demonstrated by Astwood to control the secretory function of the corpus luteum in experimental animals. This substance is apparently identical with prolactin. Hisaw has shown it to be a secretory stimulator for the corpus luteum of the monkey, but such function has not yet been demonstrated in the human.

Although the anterior pituitary appears to be the controlling force in gonadal function, a certain reciprocal action is observed. Thus, when estrogen acts upon the hypophysis, the follicle-stimulating hormone production decreases, while that of the luteinizing hormone increases. Again, when estrogen is absent, the hypophysis produces an increasing amount of the follicle-stimulating hormone, with a lowered output of the luteinizing hormone. Furthermore, progesterone probably inhibits the production of the luteinizing hormone, but does not influence the secretion by the anterior lobe of the follicle-stimulating hormone. The vast literature on this general problem has been succinctly reviewed by Hoffman.

BIBLIOGRAPHY

Abramson, D., Hurwitt, E., and Lesnick, G. Relaxin in Human Serum as a Test of Pregnancy. Surg., Gynec. & Obst., 1937, 65:335.

Abramson, D., Roberts, S. M., and Wilson, P. D. Relaxation of the Pelvic Joints in Pregnancy. Surg., Gynec. & Obst., 1934, 58:595.

Allen, E., and Doisy, E. A. An Ovarian Hormone. J.A.M.A., 1923, 81:819.

——— Ovarian and Placental Hormones. Physiol. Rev., 1927, 7:600.

Allen, E., Hisaw, F. L., and Gardner, W. U. The Endocrine Functions of the Ovaries. In Allen, Danforth and Doisy, Sex and Internal Secretions, 2nd Ed. Williams and Wilkins Co., Baltimore, 1939, p. 452.

Allen, E., Pratt, J. P., and Doisy, E. A. The Ovarian Follicular Hormone. J.A.M.A., 1925, 85:399.

Allen, E., Pratt, J. P., Newell, Q. U., and Bland, L. J. Recovery of Human Ova from the Fallopian Tubes. J.A.M.A., 1928, 91:1018.

Allen, W. M. Biochemistry of the Corpus Luteum Hormone, Progesterone. In Allen, Danforth and Doisy, Sex and Internal Secretions, 2nd Ed. Williams and Wilkins Co., Baltimore, 1939, p. 901.

——— The Preparation of Purified Progestin. J. Biol. Chem., 1932, 98:591.

——— and Corner, G. W. Physiology of the Corpus Luteum. VII. Maintenance of Pregnancy in the Rabbit after Very Early Castration by Corpus Luteum Extracts. Proc. Soc. Exper. Biol. & Med., 1930, 27:403.

Asdell, S. A. The Growth and Function of the Corpus Luteum. Physiol. Rev., 1928, 8:313.

Astwood, E. B. The Regulation of Corpus Luteum Function by Hypophyseal Luteotropin. Endocrinol., 1941, 28:309.

Bell, G. H. The Movements of the Unloaded Rabbit Uterus. J. Physiol., 1939, 95:8.

Bell, W. B. The Sex Complex, 2nd Ed. William Wood and Co., London, 1920.

Brewer, J. I. Studies of the Human Corpus Luteum. Evidence for the Early Onset of Regression of the Corpus Luteum of Menstruation. Am. J. Obst. & Gynec., 1942, 44:1048.

——— and Jones, H. O. The Time of Ovulation. Am. J. Obst. & Gynec., 1947, 53:637.

Caffier, P. Über die hormonale Beeinflussung der menschlichen Tubenschleimhaut und ihre therapeutische Ausnutzung. Zentralbl. f. Gynäk., 1938, 62:1024.

Corner, G. W. On the Origin of the Corpus Luteum of the Sow from both Granulosa and Theca Interna. Am. J. Anat., 1919, 26:117.

——— Cyclic Changes in the Ovaries and Uterus of the Sow. Carnegie Inst. of Wash., 1921, Publ. 276:117.

——— Physiology of the Corpus Luteum. 1. The Effect of Very Early Ablation of the Corpus Luteum upon Embryos and Uterus. Am. J. Physiol., 1928, 86:74.

——— The Hormones in Human Reproduction. Princeton University Press, 1942.

——— Development, Organization and Breakdown of the Corpus Luteum in the Rhesus Monkey. Carnegie Inst. of Wash., 1945, Publ. 204, Contrib. to Embryology, 557:117.

——— and Allen, W. M. Physiology of the Corpus Luteum. Production of a Special Uterine Reaction (Progestational Proliferation) by Extracts of the Corpus Luteum. Am. J. Physiol., 1929, 88:326.

Corner, G. W., Sr., Farris, E. J., and Corner, G. W., Jr. The Dating of Ovulation and Other Ovarian Crises by Histological Examination in Comparison with the Farris Test. Am. J. Obst. & Gynec., March, 1950.

Council on Pharmacy and Chemistry. Nomenclature of Endocrine Principles (Estrogen). J.A.M.A., 1936, 107:1221.

——— Diethylstilbestrol. J.A.M.A., 1942, 119:632.

Courrier. Quoted by Corner, G. W., in the Hormones in Human Reproduction. Princeton University Press, 1942.

Davis, K. B. Factors in the Sexual Life of 2,200 Women. Harper & Brothers, New York, 1929.

Dempsey, E. W., and Bassett, D. L. Observations on the Fluorescence, Birefringence and Histochemistry of the Rat Ovary during the Reproductive Cycle. Endocrinol., 1943, 33:384.

DeWit and Oppers. Quoted by Hoffman, J., in Female Endocrinology. W. B. Saunders Co., Philadelphia, 1944.

Doisy, E. A. Estrogenic Substances. Harvey Lectures for 1933-34. 1935, p. 158.

Evans, H. M., and Swezy, O. Ovogenesis and the Normal Follicular Cycle in Adult Mammalia. Mem. Univ. Calif., 1931, 9:119.

Farris, E. J. The Prediction of the Day of Human Ovulation by the Rat Test As Confirmed by Fifty Conceptions. Am. J. Obst. & Gynec., 1948, 56:347.

Fevold, H. L., Hisaw, F. L., Hellbaum, A., and Hertz, R. Sex Hormones of Anterior Lobe of Hypophysis: Further Purification of Follicular Stimulating Factor and Physiological Effects on Immature Rats and Rabbits. Am. J. Physiol., 1933, 104:710.

Fluhmann, C. F. A New Procedure for the Demonstration of Estrin in the Blood of Women. Endocrinol., 1934, 18:705.

Frank, R. T., and Goldberger, M. A. The Female Sex Hormone. J.A.M.A., 1926, 86:1686.

——— Improvement in Female Sex Hormone Blood Test in Cyclical Menstruating Women and in Pregnancy Blood. Proc. Soc. Exper. Biol. & Med., 1935, 32:1663.

Hamblen, E. C. Endocrine Gynecology. Charles C Thomas, Springfield, Ill., 1939.

Hartman, C. G. How Large Is the Mammalian Egg? Quart. Rev. Biol., 1929, 4:373.

——— Time of Ovulation in Women. A study on the Fertile Period in the Menstrual Cycle. Williams and Wilkins Co., Baltimore, 1936.

——— and Corner, G. W. Removal of the Corpus Luteum and of the Ovaries of the Rhesus Monkey during Pregnancy: Observations and Cautions. Anat. Rec., 1947, 98:539.

Henry, J. S., and Browne, J. S. L. The Contractions of the Human Uterus during the Menstrual Cycle. Am. J. Obst. & Gynec., 1943, 45:927.

Hisaw, F. L. Corpus Luteum Hormone: Experimental Relaxation of Pelvic Ligaments of Guinea Pig. Physiol. Zoöl., 1929, 2:59.

Hisaw, F. L., and Astwood, E. B. The Physiology of Reproduction. Ann. Rev. Physiol., 1942, 4:503.

Hisaw, F. L., Meyer, R. K., and Fevold, H. L. Production of a Premenstrual Endometrium in Castrated Monkeys by Ovarian Hormones. Proc. Soc. Exper. Biol. & Med., 1929, 27:400.

Hisaw, F. L., Zarrow, M. X., Money, W. L., Talmage, R. V. N., and Abramowitz, A. A. Importance of the Female Reproductive Tract in the Formation of Relaxin. Endocrinol., 1944, 34:122.

Hoffman, J. Female Endocrinology. W. B. Saunders Co., Philadelphia, 1944.

Hüssy, P., and Wallart, J. Interstitielle Drüse und Röntgenkastration. Ztschr. f. Geburtsh. u. Gynäk., 1915, 77:177.

Joël, K. The Glycogen Content of the Fallopian Tubes during the Menstrual Cycle and during Pregnancy. J. Obst. & Gynaec. Brit. Emp., 1939, 46:721.

——— The Lipoid Content of the Fallopian Tubes during the Menstrual Cycle and during Pregnancy. J. Obst. & Gynaec. Brit. Emp., 1939, 46:731.

Jones, H. W., and Weil, P. G. The Corpus Luteum Hormone in Early Pregnancy. Report of a Case in Which There Was Early Removal of the Corpus Luteum. J.A.M.A., 1938, 111:519.

Knaus, H. Eine neue Methode zur Bestimmung des Ovulationstermines. Zentralbl. f. Gynäk., 1929, 53:2193.

——— The Action of Pituitary Extract Upon the Pregnant Uterus of the Rabbit. J. Physiol., 1926, 61:383.

McKay, D. G., and Robinson, D. Observations on Fluorescence, Birefringence and Histochemistry of Human Ovary during Menstrual Cycle. Endocrinol., 1947, 41:378.

——— and Hertig, A. T. Histochemical Observations on Granulosa-cell Tumors, Thecomas and Fibromas of the Ovary. Am. J. Obst. & Gynec., 1949, 58:625.

Moir, C. Recording Contractions of Human Pregnant and Nonpregnant Uterus. Tr. Edinburgh Obst. Soc., 1934, 54:93.

Palmer, A. The Diagnostic Use of the Basal Body Temperature in Gynecology and Obstetrics. Obst. & Gynec. Surv., 1949, 4:1.

Pincus, G., and Werthessen, N. T. Quantitative Method for Bioassay of Progestin. Am. J. Physiol., 1937, 120:100.

Pratt, J. P. Human Corpus Luteum. Arch. Path., 1935, 19:380.

——— Discussion of Paper by K. M. Wilson. Am. J. Obst. & Gynec., 1937, 34:986.

Reynolds, S. R. M. Physiology of the Uterus with Clinical Correlations, 2nd Ed. Paul Hoeber, New York, 1949.

Rock, J., and Hertig, A. T. Information Regarding the Time of Human Ovulation Derived from a Study of 3 Unfertilized and 11 Fertilized Ova. Am. J. Obst. & Gynec., 1944, 47:343.

Schultze, G. K. F. Die Reaktion der nicht schwangeren menschlichen Gebärmutter auf Hypophysenhinterlappenextrakte. Zentralbl. f. Gynäk., 1931, 55:3042.

Shorr, E. Discussion of Paper by A. E. Rakoff. Problems of Human Fertility. George Banata Publishing Co., Menasha, Wisconsin, 1943, p. 119.

SMITH, GEO. VAN S., SMITH, O. W., and PINCUS, G. Total Urinary Estrogen, Estrone and Estriol during a Menstrual Cycle and a Pregnancy. Am. J. Physiol., 1938, 121:98.

SMITH, P. E., and ENGLE, E. T. Experimental Evidence Regarding the Role of the Anterior Pituitary in the Development and Regulation of the Genital System. Am. J. Anat., 1927, 40:159.

STOCKARD, C. R., and PAPANICOLAOU, G. N. The Existence of a Typical Oestrous Cycle in the Guinea Pig, with a Study of Its Histological and Physiological Changes. Am. J. Anat., 1917, 22:225.

STRASSMANN, E. O. Theca Interna Cone and Its Role in Ovulation. Surg., Gynec. & Obst., 1938, 67:299.

——— The Theca Cone and Its Tropism toward the Ovarian Surface, a Typical Feature of Growing Human and Mammalian Follicles. Am. J. Obst. & Gynec., 1941, 41:363.

TOMPKINS, P. The Use of Basal Temperature Graphs in Determining the Date of Ovulation. J.A.M.A., 1944, 124:698.

TRAUT, H. F., and MARCHETTI, A. A. A Consideration of So-Called "Granulosa" and "Theca" Cell Tumors of the Ovary. Surg., Gynec. & Obst., 1940, 70:632.

TWOMBLY, G. H., MCCLINTOCK, L., and ENGELMAN, M. Tissue Localization and Excretion Routes of Radioactive Dibromestrone. Am. J. Obst. & Gynec., 1948, 56:260.

VAN WAGENEN, G., and MORSE, A. H. The Frequency and Position of Ovulation in the Monkey Ovary. Am. J. Physiol., 1937, 119:416.

VENNING, E. H. Excretion of Various Hormone Metabolites in Normal Pregnancy. Obst. & Gynec. Surv., 1948, 3:661.

——— and BROWNE, J. S. L. Studies on Corpus Luteum Function. I. The Urinary Excretion of Sodium Pregnanediol Glucuronidate in the Human Menstrual Cycle. Endocrinol., 1937, 21:711.

WESTMAN, A., JORPES, E., and WIDSTRÖM, G. Untersuchungen über den Schleimhautzyklus in der Tuba uterina, seine hormonale Regulierung und die Bedeutung des Tubensekrets für die Vitalität der befruchteten Eier. Acta obst. et gynec. Scandinav., 1931, 11:279.

ZONDEK, B., and ASCHHEIM, S. Hypophysenvorderlappen und Ovarium. Beziehungen der endokrinen Drüsen zur Ovarialfunktion. Arch. f. Gynäk., 1927, 130:1.

4

THE ENDOMETRIAL CYCLE AND MENSTRUATION

Orientation. As described in the previous chapter, a sequence of endocrine phenomena is inherent in the ovarian cycle which may be summarized as follows: (1) During the pre-ovulatory or follicular phase of the cycle, estrogen is produced in increasing quantity. (2) During most of the postovulatory or luteal phase of the cycle, progesterone is produced in addition to estrogen. (3) During the last days of the luteal phase, the corpus luteum regresses and both these hormones are withdrawn. Consequent upon these three hormonal states and roughly concurrent with them, are the three main phases of the endometrial cycle, as follows: (1) phase of proliferation due to estrogen stimulation; (2) phase of secretion due to combined progesterone and estrogen action; and (3) phase of menstruation due to withdrawal of these hormones and collapse of the endometrial bed which they have built up. Since the phase of proliferation is a progressive one, it is helpful to divide it into an early proliferative and an advanced proliferative phase. Since the secretory phase is likewise a progressive one throughout most of its course until, a few days before menstruation, it undergoes regression, it becomes desirable to divide it into an early secretory, an advanced secretory, and a premenstrual phase. From what has been said, it must be clear that menstrual bleeding, which is simply an objective manifestation of the breakdown of the endometrial bed, is actually the terminal rather than the beginning phase of the cycle.

Early Proliferative Phase. The early proliferative stage of the endometrial cycle is shown in Fig. 63. The endometrium is thin, scarcely 2 mm. in depth. The glands are straight, narrow, tubular structures pursuing almost a straight line from the surface toward the basal layer. The glandular epithelium is low columnar and the gland lumens are so narrow that the epithelial cells of the opposite sides appear to be touching each other. The nuclei, which tend to be round, are situated basally. In the deeper part of the endometrium, the stroma is rather dense while the nuclei are deep-staining and small. In the superficial regenerating layer, the stroma is looser while the nuclei are rounder, more vesicular and larger than in the deeper layers; and here, mitotic figures may be seen. Although the blood vessels are numerous and may be as large as the glands, there is no extravasated blood or lymphocytic infiltration at this stage.

Advanced Proliferative Phase. As shown in Fig. 64, the proliferative changes become more marked. The thickness of the endometrium increases so that it may measure 3 mm. in depth. The glands are less straight, showing slight infolding of the walls in places, and the gland lumens are becoming capacious. The nuclei tend to become oval or long and to assume a more central position in the cell. Meanwhile, the glandular epithelium has become gradually taller and reaches its maximum height near the time of ovulation.

Early Secretory Phase. The total thickness of the endometrium becomes increased over the proliferative type and approximates 4 to 5 mm. in depth (Fig. 65).

At this stage, it becomes possible to differentiate three layers, the *basalis*, the *spongiosa* and the *compacta*. The basalis (adjoining the myometrium) remains characteristically inactive throughout the cycle. The spongiosa constitutes the middle layer and is so called because of its lacy, labyrinthine appearance caused by the large, dilated and tortuous uterine glands with little stroma between them. It is in these sacculated, corkscrew glands that the secretory phase of the endometrial cycle exhibits its most characteristic pattern. In the compacta, or superficial layer, the glands are straighter and narrower, but their lumens are often filled with secretion. The stroma becomes edematous and loose-textured, and its constituent cells undergo hypertrophy, with an increased amount of cytoplasm. In pregnancy these stromal cells, under the further influence of progesterone, hypertrophy still more to become the decidual cells, as described on page 137.

Advanced Secretory Phase. This stage represents an exaggeration of the previous phase and must be regarded as the final objective of the endometrial cycle, since the endometrium is now extremely vascular, succulent, rich in glycogen and ideal for nidation of the ovum. It is now 5 to 6 mm. thick, and the honeycomb pattern of the corkscrew glands has reached its height. However, there is no extravasation of blood and as yet no evidence of infiltration of white cells.

From the above description it is evident that the cyclic changes in the endometrium are manifestations of the compacta and spongiosa, and together these two layers have been called the *functionalis*. The basalis, on the other hand, is the layer responsible for regeneration of the endometrium following menstruation.

A further characteristic feature of the advanced secretory phase is the striking development of the spiral arterioles which pass through the mucous membranes in a corkscrew manner and break up into capillaries below the surface. During the first week of the menstrual cycle the arteries extend only about half way through the endometrium, although the arterioles which arise from them are longer. Since they lengthen more rapidly than the endometrium thickens, their distal ends approach nearer and nearer to the surface of the endometrium. This unequal growth causes a disproportion between the length of the arterioles and the thickness of the endometrium, in consequence of which they become more and more coiled.

Premenstrual Phase. The premenstrual phase of the cycle occupies the last two or three days prior to menstruation and may be regarded as that stage when the endometrium is beginning to show signs of corpus luteum regression. As shown by Novak and TeLinde, Bartelmez and others, the chief histologic characteristic of this phase of the endometrial cycle is infiltration of the stroma by white blood cells. These may be either polymorphonuclear or mononuclear leukocytes, and they produce a pseudo-inflammatory appearance. Concurrently with this infiltration, the reticular framework of the stroma disintegrates, and as a result the thickness of the endometrium is often decreased by half during the two days before menstruation (Fig. 66).

In one of the classics of modern research, Markee has studied extensively the vascular changes which take place prior to menstruation, by means of intra-ocular

Fig. 63.—Endometrium in Early to Mid-proliferative Phase. The Glands Are Tubular and Relatively Straight.

Fig. 64.—Endometrium in Advanced Proliferative Phase. The Glands Are Still Tubular; the Mucosa Is Higher Than in Fig. 63.

(From Papanicolaou, Traut and Marchetti, *The Epithelia of Woman's Reproductive Organs*, The Commonwealth Fund, New York.)

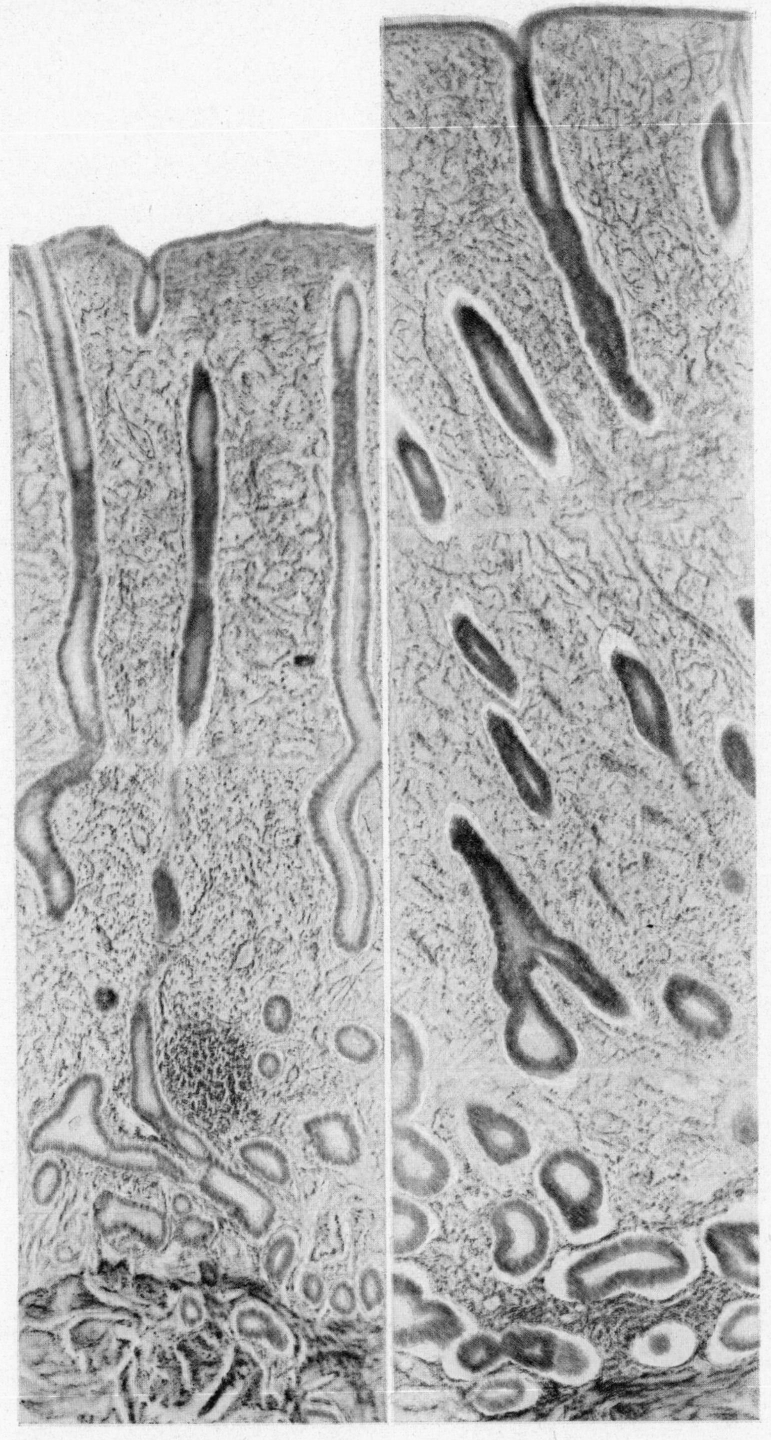

Fig. 63. Fig. 64.

FIG. 65.—ENDOMETRIUM IN MID-SECRETORY PHASE. THE GLANDS ARE MORE TORTUOUS AND APPEAR TO BE MORE NUMEROUS THAN IN FIG. 64.

FIG. 66.—ENDOMETRIUM IN ADVANCED SECRETORY PHASE (COMMONLY DESIGNATED AS THE PRE-MENSTRUAL STAGE).

Note the beginning of hemorrhagic extravasations and disintegration in the superior layer. Diffuse leukocytic infiltration is apparent.

(From Papanicolaou, Traut and Marchetti, *The Epithelia of Woman's Reproductive Organs*, The Commonwealth Fund, New York.)

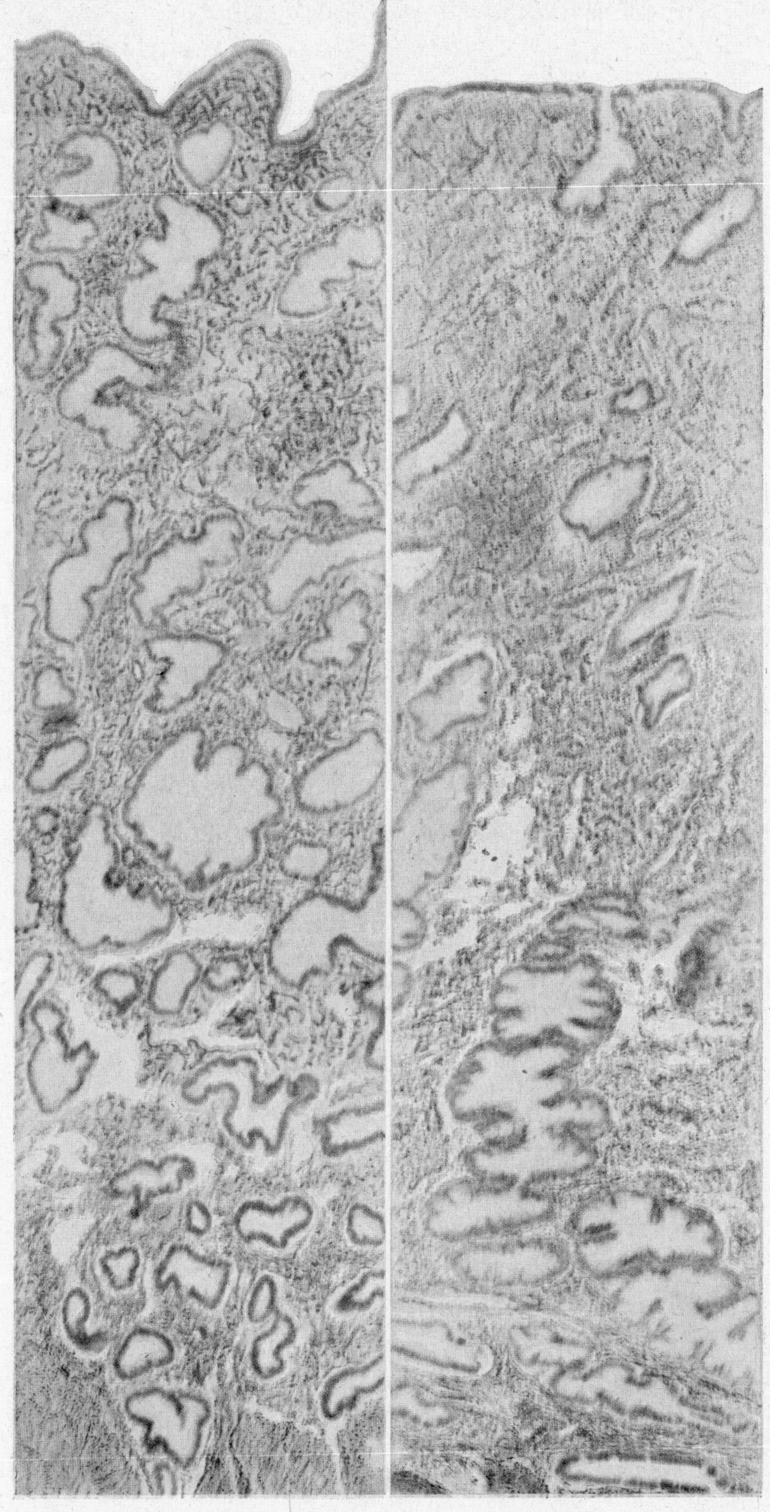

Fig. 65. Fig. 66.

transplants of endometrium in the Rhesus monkey. He finds that, as the result of the compression of the endometrium just mentioned, the coiled arterioles manifest additional coils at this time (as many as eight appeared during the 24 hours before the onset of menstruation), and he explained this on the grounds that the coiled arteries are being compressed endwise. Although the coils may be fairly regular before this phase of the cycle, they now become quite irregular and appear even to be knotted.

In addition to the changes in the spiral arteries, Markee's work has shown that two entirely different vascular phenomena are seen in endometrial transplants a few days preceding menstrual bleeding. Beginning one to five days before the onset of menstruation, there is a period of slowed circulation, or relative stasis, during which vasodilatation may occur. This is followed by a period of vasoconstriction beginning 4 to 24 hours before the escape of any blood. The period of stasis is extremely variable, ranging from less than 24 hours to 4 days. In Markee's opinion, the slowing of the circulation leading to stasis is caused by the increased resistance to blood flow offered by the coiled arteries. As more coils are added, the blood flow becomes slower and slower.

A period of vasoconstriction of the coiled arteries precedes every menstrual period and begins 4 to 24 hours before the onset of bleeding. After the constriction has begun, the superficial half to two thirds of the endometrium receives no adequate blood supply during the remainder of that menstrual cycle, the anemic appearance of the functional zone being in striking contrast to that of other tissues. When, after a period of constriction, an individual coiled artery relaxes, hemorrhage occurs from that artery or its arteriole or capillary. Then, in succession, one after another of these constricted arteries exhibits relaxation and hemorrhage; and this succession of small hemorrhages from individual arterioles or capillaries continues throughout the period of menstrual bleeding. Although this sequence of vasoconstriction, relaxation and hemorrhage appears to be well established, the mechanism which actually brings about the escape of blood from the vessels remains an enigma.

Menstrual Phase. Menstrual bleeding may be either arterial or venous, with the former predominating. It usually occurs as the result of rhexis of a coiled artery with consequent hematoma formation, but occasionally it takes place by diapedesis. When a hematoma is formed, the superficial endometrium is bulged outward and ruptures. Fissures subsequently develop in the surrounding functionalis, and tissue fragments of various sizes become detached and admixed with the blood. Markee describes the disintegration of the mucosa as a crumbling process which occurs after bleeding in any given area ceases. In this way the greater part of the functionalis undergoes destruction and escapes through the cervix and vagina as part of the menstrual discharge. In most instances only the deepest layer of the mucosa (the basalis) remains, from which the functionalis of the next cycle will be regenerated. Hemorrhage stops when the coiled artery returns to a state of contraction. A greater part of the coiled arteries is shed with the functionalis, and new coiled arteries develop from the straight arteries in the basalis. Regeneration of the mucosa, as described by Markee, occurs from growth of the flanges or collars which form from the everted free ends of what remains of the uterine glands. These flanges increase in diameter very rapidly, and the continuity of the epithelium is effected by the fusion of the edges of these proliferating masses.

Phase	Menstrual	Early Follicular or Early Proliferative	Advanced Follicular or Advanced Proliferative	Ovulation	Early Luteal or Early Secretory	Advanced Luteal or Advanced Secretory	Premenstrual
Days	1-3 to 5	4 to 6-8	9-13	14	15-18	19-25	26-28
Ovary	Involution of corpus luteum	Growth and maturation of graafian follicle		Ovulation	Active corpus luteum		Involution of corpus luteum
Estrogen	Diminution	Progressive increase in blood and urine		High concentration	Secondary rise		Decreasing
Progesterone	Absent				Present		Decreasing
Endometrium	Menstrual Desquamation	Early Proliferation	Advanced Proliferation		Early Secretory	Advanced Secretory	Premenstrual (Regressive)
	Regeneration						

TABLE 1. CORRELATION OF THE OVARIAN AND ENDOMETRIAL CYCLES.

The Endometrial Cycle in Retrospect. The relationship between the ovarian cycle, its hormones, and the endometrial cycle, together with the action of the pituitary gonadotrophic hormones, is summarized in Table 1 and in Fig. 67. For the sake of clarity the endometrial cycle has been considered as exhibiting three main phases, the proliferative, the secretory and the menstrual. In regard to the first and last of these, this attitude would seem to be entirely justifiable, as, even if the proliferative phase be subdivided into early and advanced, it is clear that we are dealing here simply with a progressive difference in degree. However, the situation in regard to the last

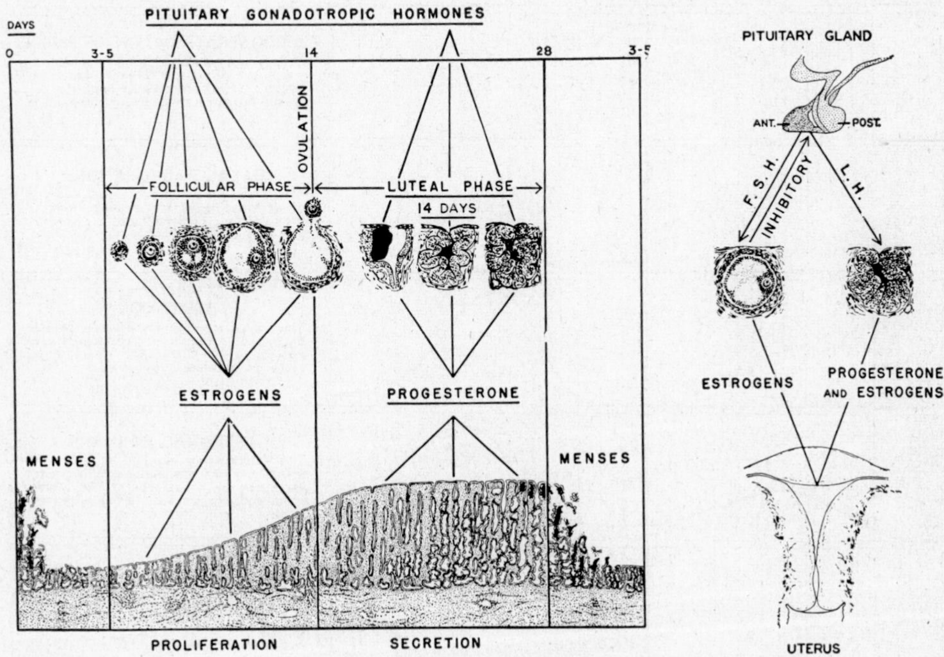

Fig. 67.—Diagram Illustrating the Hormonal Relationships of the Pituitary Gland, Ovaries and Endometrium in the Menstrual Cycle. (After W. F. Gemmill.)

three days or so of the secretory phase is quite another one, because here the picture is rather special, being one of abrupt regression corresponding to and following shortly after the regression of the corpus luteum. It is well to think, therefore, of the secretory phase of the cycle as lasting from the time of ovulation to some three days before menstruation, as being subdivided into early and advanced phases, and as being followed by a true premenstrual phase which is regressive in character. This is shown in Fig. 68. Further details of the histological changes which the endometrium undergoes in its cycle are set forth in Table 2. So characteristic are these alterations that an experienced pathologist can "date" an endometrium very accurately from its microscopic appearance.

Although many details of the mechanism which causes menstrual bleeding are obscure, there is general agreement that menstruation is due essentially to the withdrawal of the hormones progesterone and estrogen. Thus, the menstrual cycle may be mimicked both in castrate women and in castrate monkeys by administering these

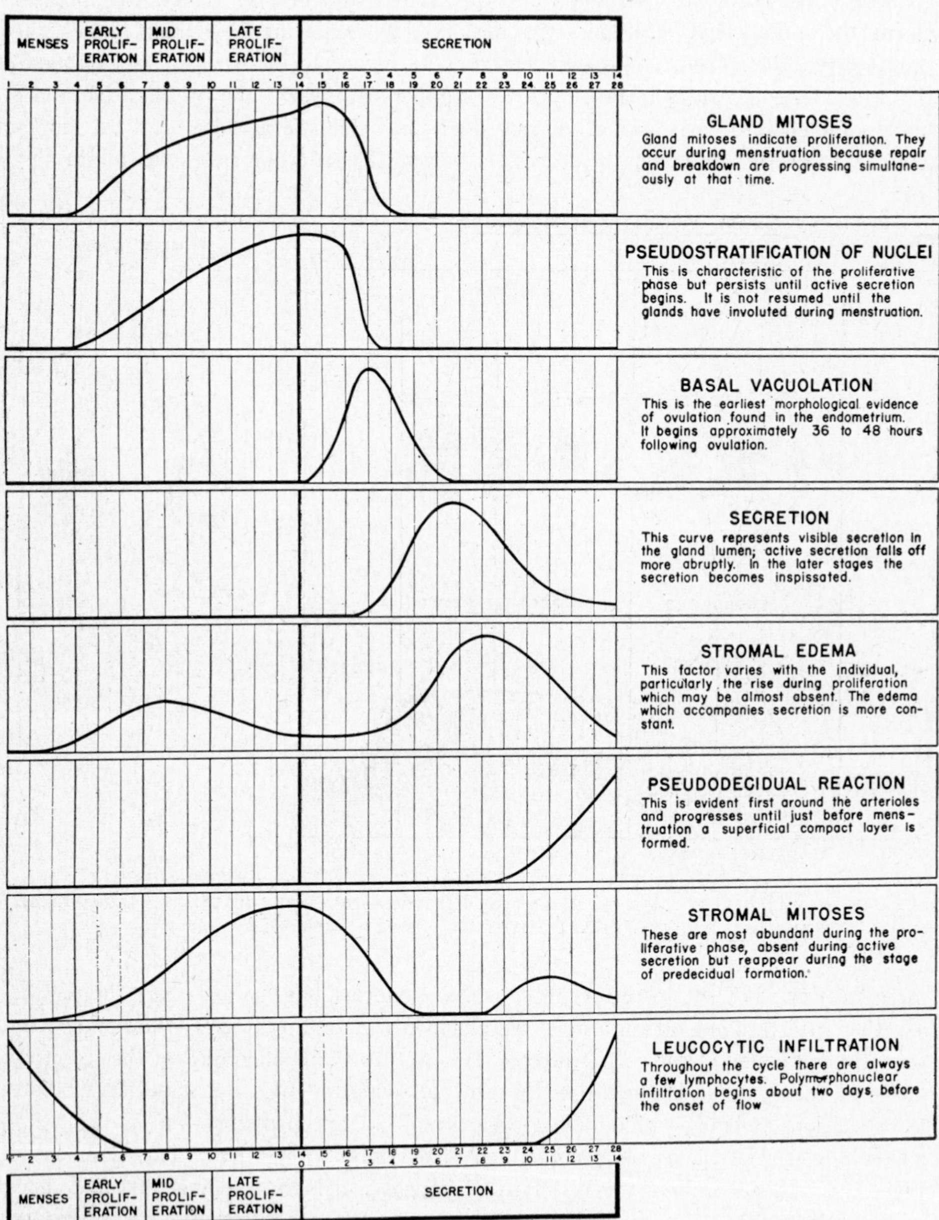

TABLE 2.—DATING THE ENDOMETRIUM. CORRELATION OF IMPORTANT MORPHOLOGICAL FINDINGS. (Courtesy of Dr. Arthur T. Hertig.)

hormones for certain periods and then withdrawing them abruptly. Bleeding follows the withdrawal. Although there has been much debate as to whether progesterone or estrogen is the more important in this deprivation process, Hoffman, after reviewing the extensive literature, reaches the conclusion that bleeding from a progestational endometrium is due to a withdrawal of progesterone and, to a lesser degree, to withdrawal of estrogen. Here, as in other connections, these two hormones appear to behave synergistically.

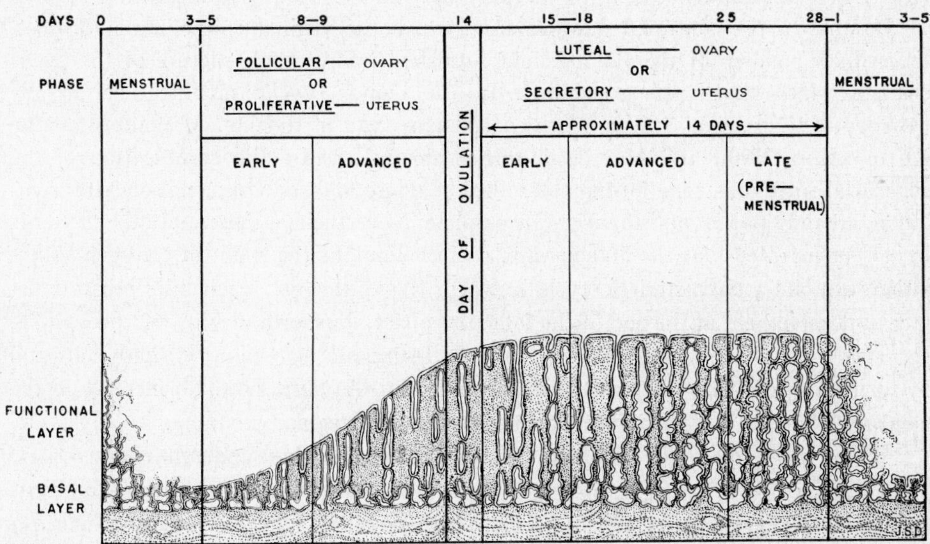

FIG. 68.—DIAGRAM ILLUSTRATING PHASES OF MENSTRUAL CYCLE.

From what has been said, it is self-evident that the purpose of the endometrial cycle is to provide a bed for any ovum that happens to have been fertilized during that cycle. Its whole objective centers on that four- or five-day period in the secretory phase (between days 19 and 25 of the cycle) when the lush, succulent endometrium offers optimum conditions for ovular implantation and nutrition. If no fertilized egg appears to take advantage of this bed, the bed disintegrates and is cleared out in preparation for the provision of another such bed in the succeeding cycle. In other words, as Hoffman has well said, menstruation represents frustration of a physiologic effort to achieve fertility.

The Cervical, Vaginal and Tubal Cycles. As described and beautifully illustrated in the monograph of Papanicolaou, Traut and Marchetti, cyclic changes occur in the endocervical glands, especially during the follicular phase of the cycle. During the early follicular phase, the glands are only slightly tortuous and the secretory cells are not very tall. Mucous secretion is meager. The late follicular phase is characterized by pronounced tortuosity of the glands, deep invaginations, tumescence of the epithelium, high columnar cells and abundant secretion. The connective tissue acquires a looser texture and shows better vascularization.

Ovulation is followed by regression. The increasing secretory activity of the endocervical glands, reaching its height about the time of ovulation, is the result of estrogen stimulation, as shown by the studies of Sjövall, and is designed to facilitate penetration of the spermatozoa into the uterine cavity. Only at that time, in most women, is the cervical mucus of such consistency as to permit passage of the spermatozoa. As pointed out by Papanicolaou, Traut and Marchetti, the synchronization of the height of secretory activity in the cervical and endometrial cycles is beautifully precise and purposeful. In the cervical cycle, where it facilitates passage of the spermatozoa, it occurs when the ovum is just ready to be fertilized. In the endometrial cycle, where the purpose is to provide a luxuriant bed for the fertilized ovum, it occurs some six days later when the ovum is in the uterine cavity and just ready to implant.

Because of the continual desquamation which the vaginal epithelium undergoes, the cellular makeup of the vaginal fluid furnishes a dependable picture of the cyclic changes which that surface exhibits. In the human, cyclic modifications in the cytology of the vaginal fluid are less conspicuous than in rodents. As pointed out by Papanicolaou, Traut and Marchetti, this is chiefly because the cornification of the superficial squamous zone during the follicular phase and its desquamation after ovulation, are only partial and therefore incomplete. Nevertheless, these and other authors have demonstrated that the human vaginal epithelium, as the result of estrogen stimulation, exhibits a characteristic cycle in which the epithelium reaches its greatest degree of development at the end of the follicular phase. As shown in Figs. 69 through 72, this stage is characterized by enlargement, flattening and spreading of these cells and by relative leukopenia, whereas the smear in the luteal phase shows an increase in the number of basophilic cells and leukocytes, as well as irregular grouping.

As has been discussed on page 53, the fallopian tubes undergo characteristic cyclic changes both in respect to their epithelium and muscular activity. The most characteristic morphologic variation that the epithelial cells of the tubal mucosa undergo is a change in height. Snyder carefully measured this difference and showed that in the follicular phase the height of the epithelium is over 30 microns, while in the luteal phase it averages not more than 20 microns.

CLINICAL ASPECTS OF MENSTRUATION

Menstruation may be defined as a periodic, physiologic discharge of blood, mucus, and cellular debris from the uterine mucosa which normally occurs at fairly regular intervals, except during pregnancy and lactation, from the time of puberty to the menopause.

The Menarche and Puberty. The average age at which menstruation begins is between the thirteenth and fourteenth year, but in a small minority of cases its onset may be observed as early as the tenth or as late as the seventeenth year and still be within normal limits. In Engle and Shelesnyak's study of 250 Jewish girls in whom the date of birth and onset of menstruation were accurately known, the average age at which menstruation began was 13.53 years. The term *menarche* (from the Greek, *men,* month, and *arche,* beginning) is used to indicate the onset of the first menstruation. On the other hand, the term *puberty* (from the Latin, *pubertas,* adulthood) has a much broader connotation and refers to the whole transitional stage between childhood and maturity. The menarche, hence, is just one sign of puberty during which the appearance of the secondary sex characteristics and the development of sex consciousness are other equally important manifestations.

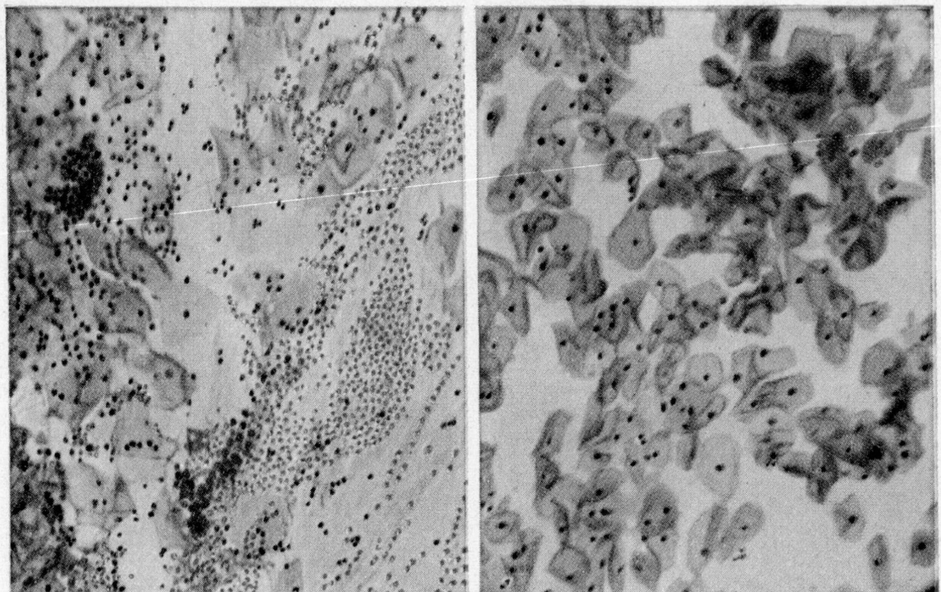

Fig. 69.—Menstrual Phase.

Fig. 70.—Early Proliferative Phase.

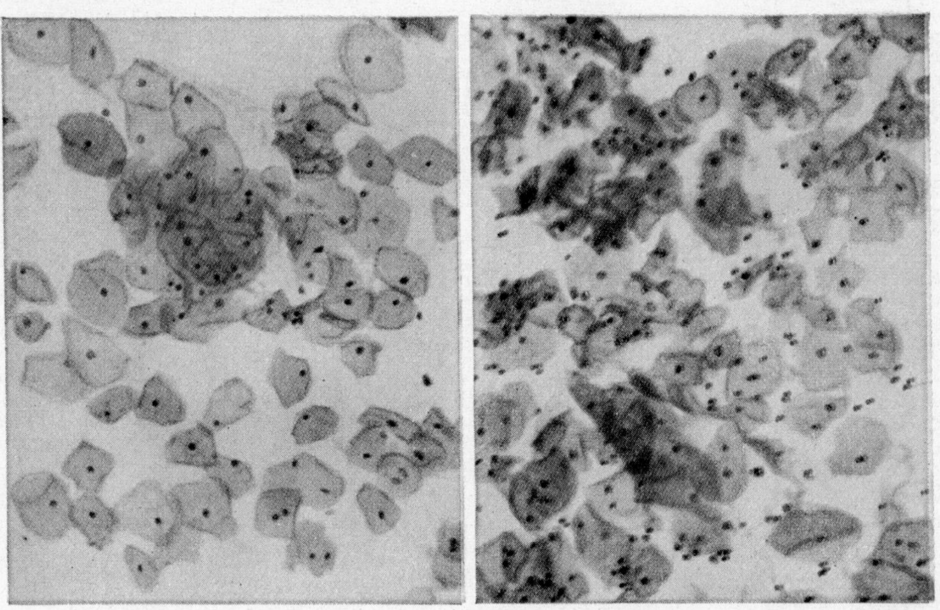

Fig. 71.—Advanced Proliferative Phase.

Fig. 72.—Secretory Phase.

Vaginal Smears in Normal Menstrual Cycle.

Smears stained with OG6-EA36, acidophilic cells red, basophilic cells blue green. Photomicrographs colored by H. Murayama. × 150. (Courtesy of Dr. George N. Papanicolaou.)

The Menopause or Climacteric. The term *menopause* (from the Greek, *men,* month, and *pausis,* cessation) may be defined as the final cessation of menstrual function. This occurs, on the average, at 47 years, but there are wide variations as shown by the following generalization: About one half of all women cease menstruating between 45 and 50; about one quarter stop before 45, and another one quarter continue to menstruate until past 50. The term *climacteric* is a synonym for menopause. Coming from the Greek, *klimacter,* rung of a ladder, it refers to the fact that the woman has reached a critical period in her life. The laity uses the phrase *change of life* in referring to the menopause.

Interval. Although the average interval at which menstruation occurs is 28 days, there is great variation among women in general as well as in the cycles of any individual woman. Arey has analyzed 12 different studies comprising some 20,000 calendar records from 1,500 women and girls and reached the conclusion that there is no evidence pointing to perfect regularity for even a single individual studied, thus supporting Fraenkel's statement that the only regularity of menstruation is its irregularity. In a study of 479 normal British women studied by Gunn, Jenkin and Gunn, the typical difference between the shortest and longest cycle was eight or nine days; in 30 per cent, it was over 13 days; in no case was it less than two or three days. Arey found that an average adult woman must expect one third of all her cycles to depart more than two days from her mean cycle length. Arey's analysis of 5,322 cycles in 485 normal white women gave an average interval of 28.4 days; his figure for the average cycle in pubertal girls was longer, namely, 33.9 days. Haman surveyed 2,460 cycles in 150 housewives attending a maternal consultation clinic where especial attention was directed to recording accurately the length of the menstrual cycles. Haman's data and Arey's figures on white women are superimposed in the distribution curves shown in Fig. 73. It will be noted that the findings in the two series are almost identical.

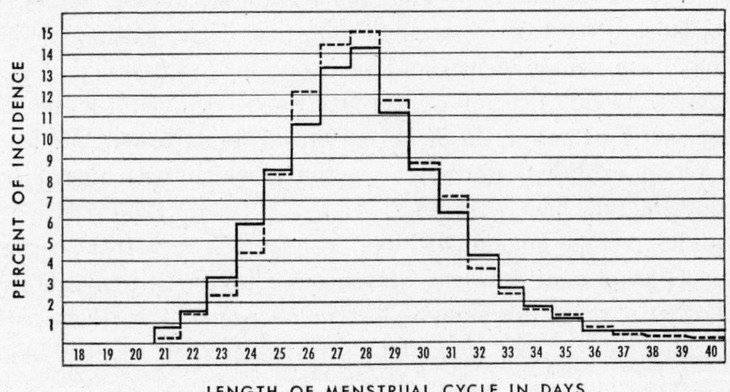

Fig. 73.—Duration of Menstrual Cycle Based on Distribution Data of Arey (Continuous Line) and of Haman (Broken Line).
(Courtesy of Eli Lilly and Co.)

Duration. The duration of menstrual flow is also variable, the usual duration being four to six days, but lengths between two and eight days are considered physiologic. In any one woman, however, the duration of the flow is usually fairly uniform.

Character of Menstrual Discharge. The menstrual flow consists of blood mixed with mucus, and castoff fragments of endometrium. It contains fewer red cells and more lymphocytes than does the circulating blood. It also possesses a toxic substance, the nature of which is as yet unknown. Attention was directed to this fact in 1920 by Schick who demonstrated that if flowers had contact with a menstruating woman they withered promptly, whereas no effect was noted if the woman was not menstruating. Macht and Lubin demonstrated that the legume *lupinus albus* would sprout luxuriantly when placed in a vessel of water, but that the addition of a few drops of menstrual blood would result in a striking inhibition of growth. This they attributed to the action of a toxic substance, which they have designated as *menotoxin.* Smith and Smith have likewise found the normal menstrual discharges to be highly toxic to rats.

One of the most interesting aspects of menstrual blood is its apparent incoagulability. Recent studies indicate that it actually does clot but then undergoes intra-uterine liquefaction because of certain fibrinolytic enzymes. Thus, Huggins, Vail and Davis have shown that fresh human menstrual blood contains proteases capable of dissolving clots of peripheral blood. Proteolytic activity as determined by the dissolution of fibrin was observed by them in 36 of 38 menstrual fluids tested. All fresh specimens of menstrual blood exhibited fibrinolytic activity which was absent only in those cases where putrefaction had occurred.

Amount. The average amount of blood lost in each menstrual period is approximately 50 cc. (Barker and Fowler; Stevenson, Culver, Stinson and Kuehne). In Barker and Fowler's series the amount lost in 50 per cent of their patients ranged between 23.2 and 68.4 cc. The amount of iron represented by this blood loss is of interest for reasons which will appear shortly. Taking 50 cc. as the usual blood loss, assuming a high normal hemoglobin content of 14 gm. per 100 cc. of blood and employing Butterfield's figure of 3.35 mg. of iron for each gm. of hemoglobin, the amount of iron lost at each period may be calculated as being on the average 23.5 mg. In Barker and Fowler's series, 75 per cent of the cases lost less than 20 mg. of iron per period. Since a pregnant woman does not menstruate, it can be stated on the basis of the above figures that she saves approximately 200 mg. of iron in the course of nine missed menstrual periods. As will be noted in connection with the causation of anemia in pregnancy, the amount of iron required by the fetus and growing uterus is several times this figure.

BIBLIOGRAPHY

Arey, L. B. The Degree of Normal Menstrual Irregularity. An Analysis of 20,000 Calendar Records from 1,500 Individuals. Am. J. Obst. & Gynec., 1939, 37:12.

Barker, A., and Fowler, W. The Blood Loss during Normal Menstruation. Am. J. Obst. & Gynec., 1936, 31:979.

Bartelmez, G. W. Human Uterine Mucous Membrane during Menstruation. Am. J. Obst. & Gynec., 1931, 21:623.

——— Histological Studies on the Menstruating Mucous Membrane of the Human Uterus. Carnegie Inst. of Wash., 1933, Publ. 443, Contrib. to Embryology.

——— Menstruation. Physiol. Rev., 1937, 17:28.

——— Menstruation. J.A.M.A., 1941, 116:702.

——— Corner, G. W., and Hartman, C. G. Phases of Menstrual Cycle in the Macaque Monkey. Anat. Rec., 1946, 94:512.

Brewer, J. I., and Jones, H. O. Studies on the Human Corpus Luteum. Histologic Variations in Corpora Lutea and in Corpus Luteum; Endometrial Relationships at the Onset of Normal Menstruation. Am. J. Obst. & Gynec., 1947, 54:561.

Butterfield, E. E. Ueber die Lichtextinktion, das Gasbindungsvermögen und den Eisengehalt des menschlichen Blutfarbstoffs in normalen und krankhaften Zuständen. Ztschr. f. physiol. Chem., 1909, 62:173.

CORNER, G. W. The Nature of the Menstrual Cycle. Medicine, 1933, 12:61.

——— The Ovarian Hormones and Experimental Menstruation. Am. J. Obst. & Gynec., 1939, 38:862.

DARON, G. H. Arterial Pattern of the Tunica Mucosa of the Uterus in Macacus Rhesus. Am. J. Anat., 1936, 58:349.

ENGLE, E. T. Current Views on the Causation of Menstruation. Am. J. Obst. & Gynec., 1939, 38:600.

ENGLE, E. T., and SHELESNYAK, M. C. First Menstruation and Subsequent Menstrual Cycles of Pubertal Girls. Human Biol., 1934, 6:431.

ENGLE, E. T., SMITH, P. E., and SHELESNYAK, M. C. The Role of Estrin and Progestin in Experimental Menstruation, with Especial Reference to the Complete Ovulatory Cycle in Monkeys and Human Beings. Am. J. Obst. & Gynec., 1935, 29:787.

FLUHMANN, C. F. Menstrual Disorders. W. B. Saunders Co., Philadelphia, 1939.

——— The Period of Puberty and the Inception of Menstruation. Am. J. Obst. & Gynec., 1936, 31:573.

GUNN, D. L., JENKIN, P. M., and GUNN, A. L. Menstrual Periodicity; Statistical Observations on a Large Sample of Normal Cases. J. Obst. & Gynaec. Brit. Emp., 1937, 44:839.

HAMAN, J. O. The Length of the Menstrual Cycle. A Study of 150 Normal Women. Am. J. Obst. & Gynec., 1942, 43:870.

HARTMAN, C. G. Studies in the Reproduction of the Monkey Macacus (Pithecus) Rhesus with Special Reference to Menstruation and Pregnancy. Carnegie Inst. of Wash., 1932, Publ. 23, Contrib. to Embryology.

HITSCHMANN, F., and ADLER, L. Der Bau der Uterusschleimhaut des geschlechtsreifen Weibes mit besonderer Berücksichtigung der Menstruation. Monatschr. f. Geburtsh. u. Gynäk., 1908, 27:1.

HOFFMAN, J. Female Endocrinology. W. B. Saunders, Philadelphia, 1944.

HUGGINS, C., VAIL, V. C., and DAVIS, M. E. Fluidity of Menstrual Blood, a Proteolytic Effect. Am. J. Obst. & Gynec., 1943, 46:78.

KENNEDY, W. P. Menarche and Menstrual Type, Notes on 10,000 Case Records. J. Obst. & Gynaec. Brit. Emp., 1933, 49:792.

LAMAR, J. K., SHETTLES, L. B., and DELFS, E. Cyclic Penetrability of Human Cervical Mucus to Spermatozoa in Vitro. Am. J. Physiol., 1940, 129:234.

MACHT, D. I., and LUBIN, D. S. A Phytopharmacological Study of Menstrual Toxin. J. Pharmacol. & Exper. Therap., 1924, 22:413.

MARKEE, J. E. Menstruation in Intra-Ocular Transplants in the Rhesus Monkey. Carnegie Inst. of Wash., 1940, Publ. 177, Contrib. to Embryology, 518:219.

NOVAK, E., and TELINDE, R. W. The Endometrium of the Menstruating Uterus. J.A.M.A., 1924, 83:900.

O'LEARY, J. L. Form Changes in the Human Uterine Gland during the Menstrual Cycle and in Early Pregnancy. Am. J. Anat., 1929, 43:289.

PAPANICOLAOU, G. N. The Sexual Cycle in the Human Female as Revealed by Vaginal Smears. Am. J. Anat. (Supp.), 1933, 52:519.

———TRAUT, H. F., and MARCHETTI, A. A. The Epithelia of Woman's Reproductive Organs. Commonwealth Fund, New York, 1948.

RANDALL, L. M., and POWER, M. H. Amounts of Glycogen in the Endometrium. Proc. Staff Meet. Mayo Clin., 1942, 17:158.

SCHICK, B. Das Menstruationsgift. Wien. med. Wchnschr., No. 19, 1920, Vol. 33.

SCHROEDER, R. Anat. Studien zur normalen und path. Physiologie des Menstruationzyklus. Arch. f. Gynäk., 1915, 104:27.

SECKINGER, D. L., and SNYDER, F. F. Cyclic Changes in the Spontaneous Contractions of the Human Fallopian Tube. Bull. Johns Hopkins Hosp., 1926, 39:371.

SJÖVALL, A. Untersuchungen über die Schleimhaut der Cervix uteri. Acta obst. et gynec. Scandinav. (Supp.), 1938, 18:3.

SMITH, O. W., and SMITH, G. V. Menstrual Discharge of Women. I. Its Toxicity in Rats. Proc. Soc. Exper. Biol. & Med., 1940, 44:100.

SPYKER, M. A., and FIDLER, R. S. Glycogen Studies on Human Endometrium. J. Clin. Endocrinol., 1942, 2:365.

STEVENSON, R. A., CULVER, G. A., STINSON, J. C., Jr., and KUEHNE, B. A. The Quantity of Menstrual Flow. Texas Rep. Biol. & Med., 1945, 3:371.

STURGIS, S. H., and MEIGS, J. V. Endometrial Cycle and Mechanism of Normal Menstruation. Am. J. Surg., 1936, 33:369.

TRAUT, H. F., BLOCH, P. W., and KUDER, A. Cyclical Changes in the Human Vaginal Mucosa. Surg., Gynec. & Obst., 1936, 63:7.

WESTMAN, A. Studien über den Sexualzyklus bei Makakus, Rhesus, Affen, nebst einigen Bemerkungen über den menstruellen Blutungsmechanismus. Acta. obst. & gynec. Scandinav., 1932, 12:282.

5

THE PHYSIOLOGY AND DEVELOPMENT OF THE OVUM

Migration of the Ovum. The mechanism by which the ovum gains access to the tube after escaping from the ruptured follicle is a question of extreme interest, and one which has given rise to a great deal of discussion, and has been exhaustively studied in the rabbit by Westman. The process is readily understood in those animals in which the ovaries are completely inclosed in a peritoneal sac into which the tube opens; but in women, and in animals in which the ovary projects freely into the peritoneal cavity, the question presents greater difficulties and has not as yet received a thoroughly satisfactory solution.

The fimbriated extremity of the tube lies in the neighborhood of the ovary, but is not necessarily in direct contact with it, the only organic connection between the two structures being furnished by the *fimbria ovarica,* which is attached to the upper or tubal pole of the ovary.

Numerous theories have been advanced to explain the manner in which the ovum enters the tube. All experimental evidence to date points to two factors, which are probably involved in this transfer of the ovum, tubal ciliary current and ovarian and tubal movement due to muscular action. It is generally believed that the cilia upon the fimbriated end of the tube give rise to a current in the capillary layer of fluid lying between the various pelvic organs. Thus, it is known that the tubal cilia are capable of transferring foreign particles, such as cinnabar, as well as *Ascaris* ova, from the body cavity to the uterus.

The movements of the tube and ovary have been particularly studied by Westman, who has shown not only that the infundibulum of the tube moves in the direction of the ovary but also that the latter may actually rotate on an axis parallel to its longitudinal plane. He injected drops of lipiodol beneath the tunica albuginea of the ovary at laparotomy thus enabling him to study subsequently the relative positions of the ovary, the tube and the uterus by means of utero-salpingography. These experiments in the woman, corroborating his earlier findings in the rabbit and the monkey, indicate that the smooth muscle fiber contained in the ligaments of the adnexa and in the adventitia of the veins may play an important role in bringing about a movement of the tube toward the ovary, as well as a rotary and linear movement of the ovary, so that transfer of ova from ovary to tube is greatly enhanced.

After the ovum has gained access to the tube its transit to the uterus may be effected in part by the ciliary current and in part by contraction of the tubal musculature. Hartman, in an excellent survey of the extensive literature on the subject of the transport of ova through the uterine tubes, sums up the experimental evidence as follows: contractions are always present in the tubes, being of greatest intensity at the time of follicle ripening. Although these contractions do not constitute definite peristalsis, the progress of successive contractions is in the direction of the uterus, as shown by Mikulicz-Radecki by means of both direct observation through abdominal windows and by photographic recording of the waves as measured by delicate levers placed upon different portions of the tube. The follicular hormone is probably the activating agent in this peristalsis, while the corpus luteum hormone may have an opposite effect. In general, most observers are of the opinion that the tubal contractions may be an important factor in the transport of the ovum through the tube.

The period of greatest activity of the tube appears to be at the time of passage of the ova. Wislocki and Snyder found that the time required for the transit of ova through the tube may be shortened in rabbits in which a second ovulation has been induced early in pregnancy. Their observations, as well as those of Corner, suggest that corpora lutea may play an important role in determining the physiological state of the tubes. Burdick and Whitney have since shown that the follicular hormone estrogen hastened the passage of ova through the tubes. There can be little doubt that the cyclic changes in motility of the tubes are closely related to the ovarian hormones.

In all animals so far studied the passage of the ovum through the tube requires from three to three and a half days. It is generally assumed that in man the ovum does not reach the uterine cavity until about three to four days after fertilization.

In animals possessing bicornuate uteri one frequently finds that the corpora lutea are in one ovary, while the embryos are developed in the uterine horn on the opposite side. In such cases the fertilized ova come from the ovary in which the corpora lutea are found, and make their way into the cornu of the opposite side, instead of into the one corresponding to the ovary from which they came. This process is called *migration of the ovum.*

Such an occurrence in women might be brought about in two ways: either by the ovum's making a circuit through the pelvic cavity and thus gaining access to the opposite tube, or by the ovum's passing down one tube, traversing the uterine cavity, and then making its way up the opposite tube. The former is designated as external, the latter as internal, migration of the ovum.

External migration of the ovum is frequently observed, while internal migration is probably a very rare occurrence in women. We are unable to ascertain how frequently external migration takes place in normal uterine pregnancies, though it is probably much more common than is generally believed. Its occurrence has been repeatedly demonstrated in cases of bicornuate uteri, and in those presenting a rudimentary horn; and frequently in normal uteri, when the fimbriated extremity of one tube is occluded, as in cases of hydrosalpinx or inflammatory lesions, while that of the other tube is patent.

External migration of the ovum has been produced experimentally in animals by excising one ovary and the opposite tube, and in a number of such cases the animals became pregnant after the operation. A very convincing case has been reported by Kelly, who removed the diseased left ovary and the right tube from a patient, leaving the normal right ovary and left tube behind. Fifteen months later she was delivered at term, and seventeen months subsequently the remaining tube was removed for a ruptured extra-uterine pregnancy.

In many specimens of extra-uterine pregnancy, we find incontrovertible evidence of external migration of the ovum, the corpus luteum being in the ovary of one side and the pregnancy in the opposite tube. Allen and his associates adduced conclusive evidence of the occurrence of external migration in normal genitalia by finding an ovum in the right tube 12 days after the onset of the last period, while the corpus luteum was situated in the left ovary.

Corner has demonstrated the occurrence of *internal migration* in sows by showing that the number of embryos in the two horns of the uterus is not the same as the number of corpora lutea in the corresponding ovary. For example, if four embryos are found in either horn, while the right ovary contains two and the left six corpora lutea, he assumes that the right horn originally contained two and the left horn six embryos, but that as they grew larger two embryos were forced mechanically from the left to the right horn. Kinney in 1924 reported that internal migration of the ovum does not occur in the guinea pig. Kelly on the other hand concludes that internal migration probably occurs in all forms in which there is free access from one uterine cornu to the other through the uterine body, and where there are sufficient fertilized ova to require such spacing. Cases of internal migration in the human have been reported by Andrews, Schlink and others. From these authors' descriptions of the findings at laparotomy we may conclude that satisfactory evidence in favor of the occurrence of internal migration has been adduced for women.

Sperm Transport. During coitus the semen is deposited in the vagina, and the question arises: How do the spermatozoa contained in it make their way into the uterus, and when and where do they come in contact with the ovum?

In a study of 22 normal fertile men, Hotchkiss found the average volume of ejaculate to be 2.6 cc. with a spermatozoa count of 135,960,000 per cc., or a total average count of 312,180,000, of which 87.6 per cent are oval or normal forms. These figures agree substantially with his earlier findings.

Although various theories have been advanced to explain how the spermatozoa gain access to the fallopian tubes, it is probable that in the majority of cases they make their way thither by their own activity. Plausibility is lent to such a view by the instances of pregnancy following imperfect coitus, and particularly those which have been observed in women with unruptured hymens. Furthermore, all recent observations show that mammalian spermatozoa move at quite a rapid rate, probably about 3 mm. per minute. In experiments on excised human uteri and tubes, Brown found that spermatozoa traversed an average distance of 2.7 mm. per minute and calculated the average time required to reach the ovum in women to be from 65 to 75 minutes.

After the spermatozoa gain access to the tubes, fertilization usually occurs in the lateral half. Consequently, practically every pregnancy is primarily tubal, so that the question to be solved is how the fertilized egg gains access to the uterus. It is generally assumed that it is carried down by the ciliary current, but when it is realized how relatively large the egg is in comparison to the free space between the folds of the tubal mucosa, it may well be that muscular peristalsis plays a more important part.

MATURATION, FERTILIZATION, AND DEVELOPMENT OF THE OVUM

We shall not attempt to trace the development of the ovum through all its stages, but shall consider only those changes which are directly concerned in the formation of the fetal membranes and the placenta. For detailed information concerning the general development of the embryo the student is referred to the standard works upon embryology.

As stated in an earlier section, ova are produced by a proliferation of the primitive germ cells from the ovarian germinal epithelium. It has been generally assumed

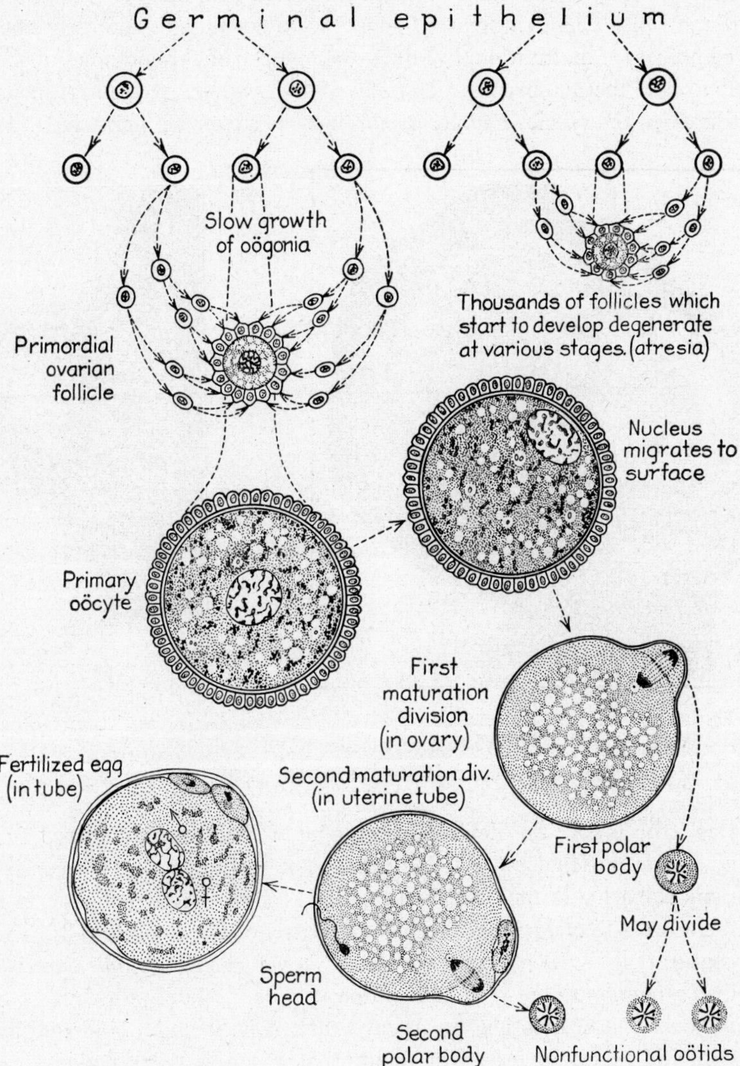

FIG. 74.—FORMATION OF POLAR BODIES AND FERTILIZATION OF MATURE MAMMALIAN EGG. (From Hartman and Patten in Curtis, *Obstetrics and Gynecology,* W. B. Saunders Co., Philadelphia.)

that some of the primordial follicles present at birth begin to grow after puberty is reached and that certain of these periodically progress to maturity. A more recent theory is to the effect that none of the primordial follicles seen at birth ripen in later life, but that all functioning ova arise from the germinal epithelium. The processes involved in the development of the mature ovum are known as *oogenesis,* while the corresponding growth in sperm-formation is *spermatogenesis*. In each three definite stages take place, (1) cell proliferation or repeated primitive germ cell division, (2) growth as shown by enlargement of these cells, and finally (3) maturation.

Maturation of Ovum. In the ovary and testis there are many primitive germ cells undergoing mitotic division. The chromatin in these cells appears in condensed bundles or bodies of different form and size, quite unlike the chromatin granules in other gland cells. These chromatin bodies in the gonad cells represent the chromosomes. The process of maturation, by which the number of chromosomes of the gametes is reduced to half the number characteristic of the species, is essential in order that, after fertilization, the species number of chromosomes may be maintained. The ovum,

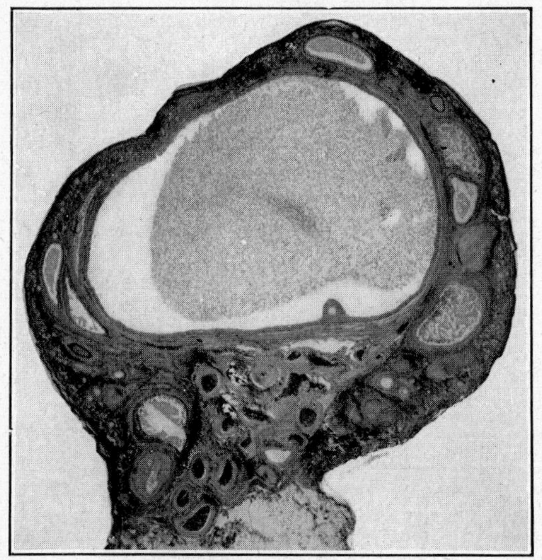

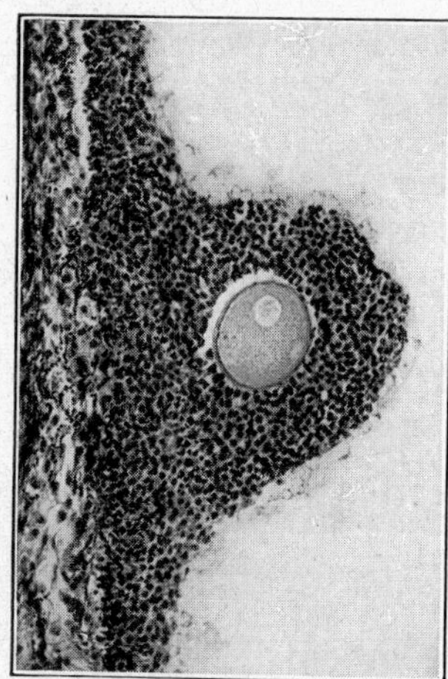

Fig. 76.—Same Ovum. × 100.

Fig. 75.—Transverse Section of Macaque Ovary Showing Ovum in Almost Fully-grown 5 mm. Follicle. × 10.
(Macaque No. 100, Collection of Dr. G. W. Corner.)

therefore, as it occurs in the developing graafian follicle, must undergo further development, or maturation, before it is adapted for fertilization. This consists in the formation and extrusion of the polar bodies; this process effects reduction in the number of chromosomes to one half of that characteristic of the somatic cells. The various stages in maturation of the human ovum have, as yet, not been fully observed. Stieve has described a human oocyte with maturation spindle, probably the first, in a 14-mm. graafian follicle. The description by Allen, Pratt, Newell and Bland of human ova, discovered in the tubes, leaves slight doubt that the first polar body is cast off in the ovary, as is the case in all other mammals studied, with the exception of the dog. The changes involved in maturation probably begin just before rupture of the follicle and are completed while the ovum is in the upper portion of the tube.

As the follicle grows under the influence of the anterior pituitary stimulating hormone, the oogonium, surrounded by small follicle cells, increases in size to an extent of about sevenfold, the full-grown oogonium measuring 0.135 mm. in diameter, according to Hartman, as compared to the original oogonium of 0.019 mm. diameter. When the process of maturation of this large cell, the primary oocyte, is about to begin, the germinal vesicle approaches the surface of the ovum, and appears to become

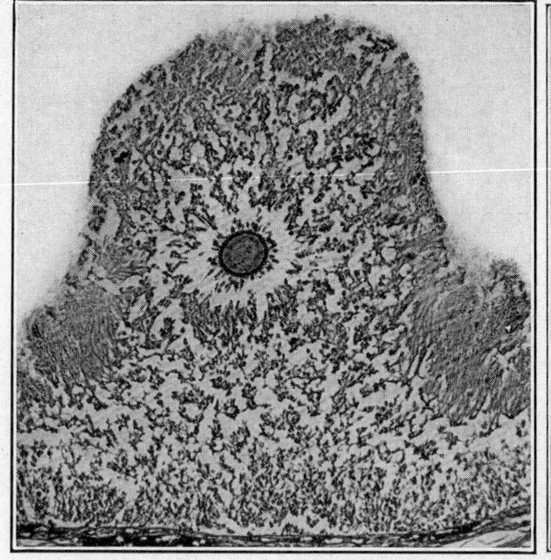

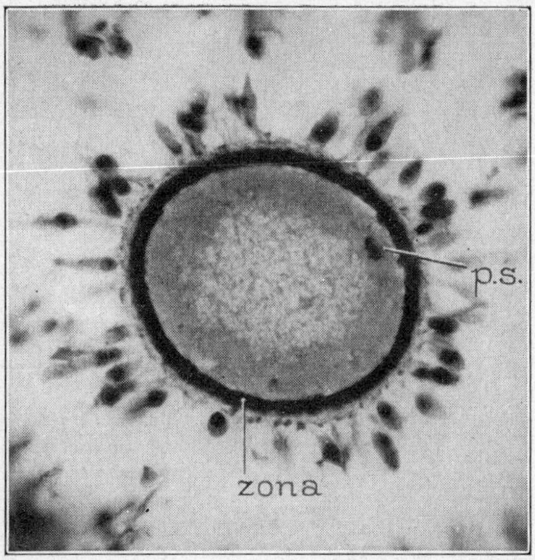

Fig. 77.—Ovum in Mature 7 mm. Follicle. × 50.

Note loosening up of cells of cumulus oophorus. (Macaque No. 109. Collection of Dr. G. W. Corner.)

Fig. 78.—Same Ovum Containing 1st Polar Spindle, p.s., and Surrounded by Corona Radiata. × 385.

(Macaque No. 109. Collection of Dr. G. W. Corner.)

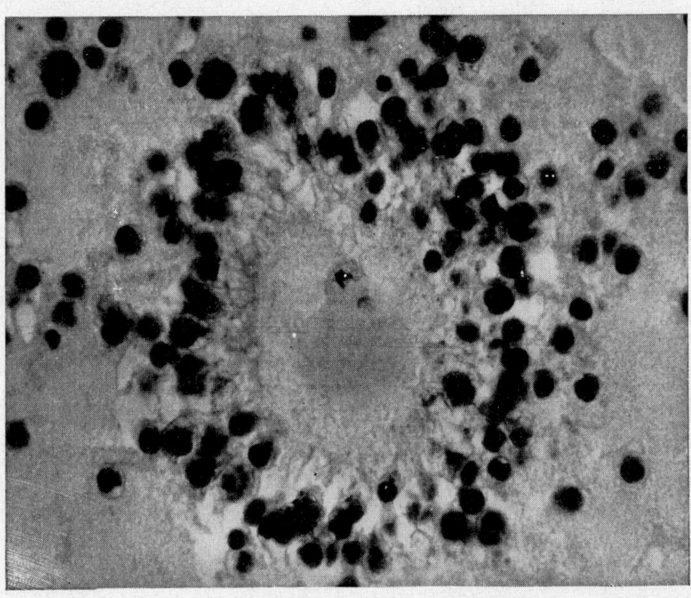

Fig. 79.—A Human Follicular Egg in the Late Anaphase of the First Maturation Division.

Note the mitotic figure close to the center of the field. (From Hertig and Rock, *American Journal of Obstetrics and Gynecology.*)

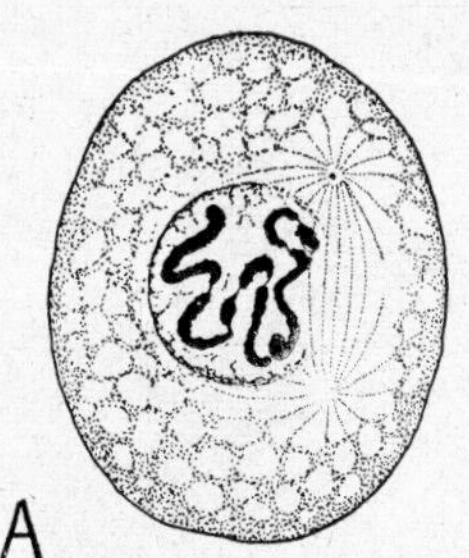
A.
Prophase
Chromosomes being formed from the spireme thread.

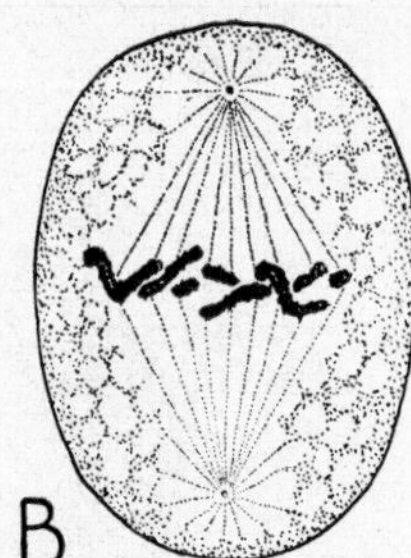
B.
Equatorial Plate
Members of the chromosomal pairs not together

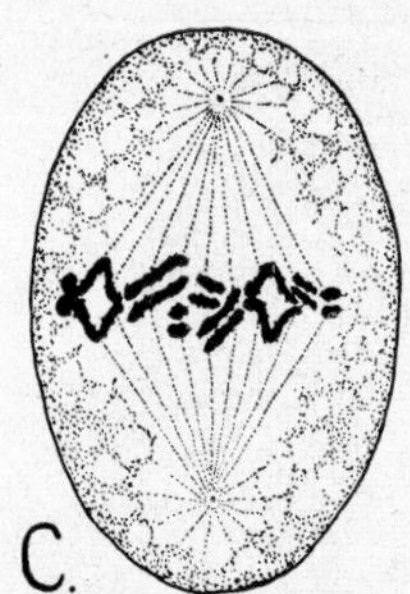
C.
Early Anaphase
Daughter chromosomes begin moving toward poles of spindle

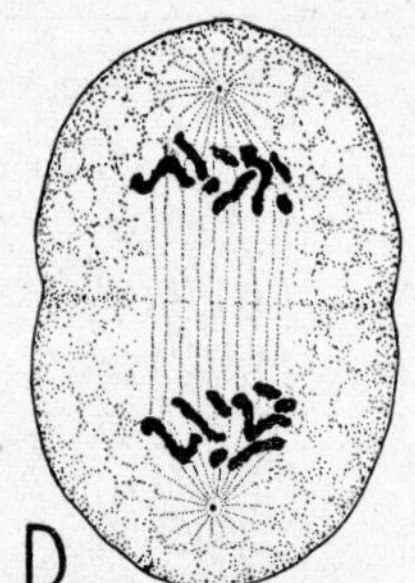
D.
Late Anaphase
Full species number of chromosomes to each daughter cell.
Ordinary Mitotic Division

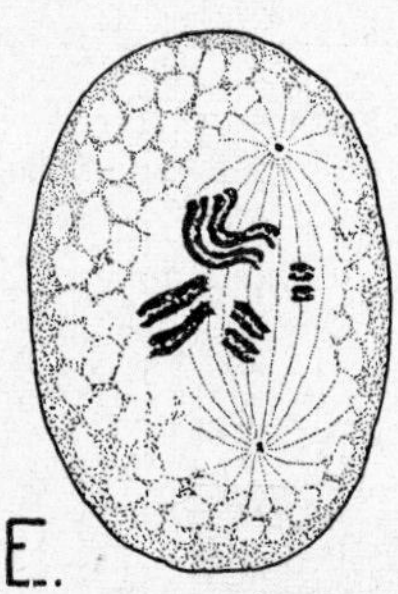
E.
Prophase
Members of chromosomal pairs approach each other.

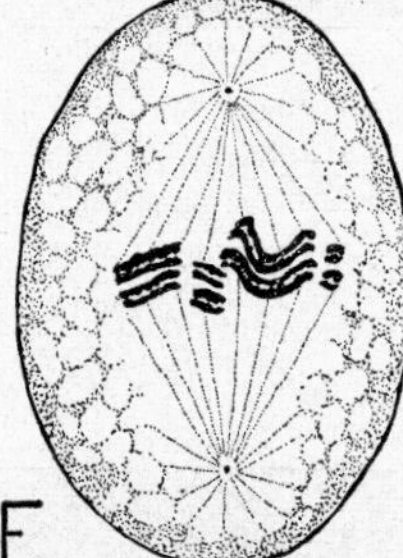
F.
Equatorial Plate
Chromosomes on spindle in synaptic pairs.

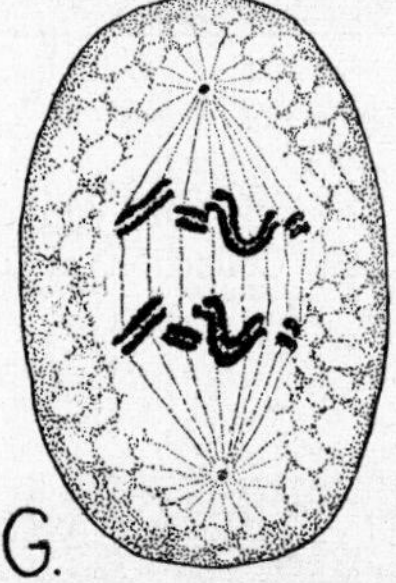
G.
Early Anaphase
Members of synaptic chromosomal pairs move apart.

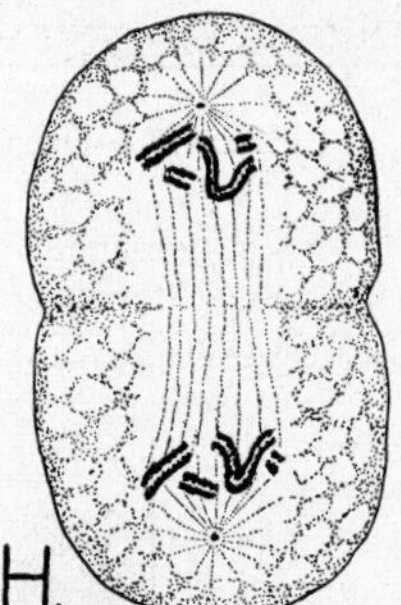
H.
Late Anaphase
One member of each pair goes to each daughter cell.
First Maturation Division

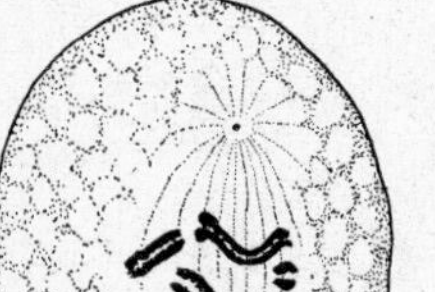
I
Prophase
Second maturation division follows without resting stage.

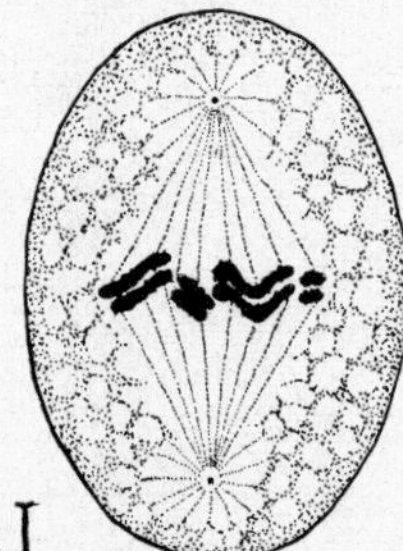
J.
Equatorial Plate
Already split chromosomes at equator of spindle.

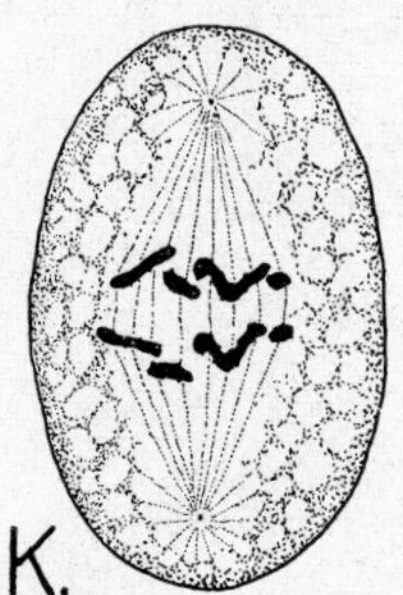
K.
Early Anaphase
Daughter chromosomes begin moving to poles of spindle.

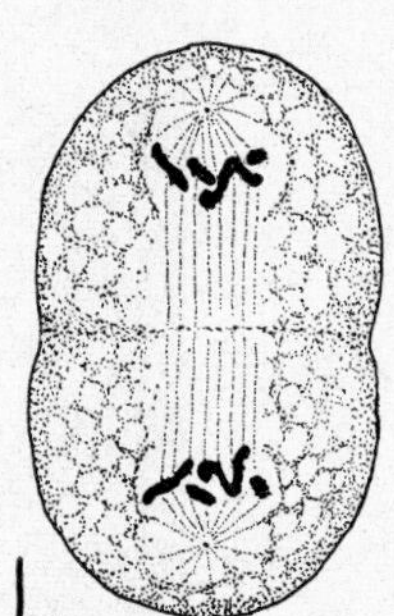
L.
Late Anaphase
Half species number of chromosomes to each matured gamete.
Second Maturation Division

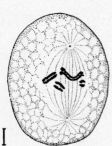

FIG. 80.—THE MATURATION DIVISIONS.

(Prepared by Bradley M. Patten for his "Human Embryology." Courtesy of The Blakiston Company.)

smaller, while at the same time its membrane disappears. It gradually becomes less and less distinct, until finally its situation is indicated by a clear area surrounded by deutoplasm, which is traversed by many radiating lines. In a short time this becomes transformed into a typical karyokinetic or mitotic figure, which undergoes the usual changes and soon become spindle-shaped. The spindle, when it first appears, is situated tangentially to the surface of the ovum, but later turns and becomes perpendicular to it. The chromatin of the spindle then becomes rearranged and a typical dyaster is formed (Fig. 74). Division rapidly ensues, and the new nucleus nearest the surface, with the portion of protoplasm surrounding it, is cut off from the bulk of the ovum and comes to lie between it and the vitelline membrane. In this way is formed the first *polar body* and the oocyte of the second order. As the process is a typical cell division, with a preliminary cleavage of the chromosomes, the nucleus of both the polar body and of the oocyte will contain the typical number of chromosomes.

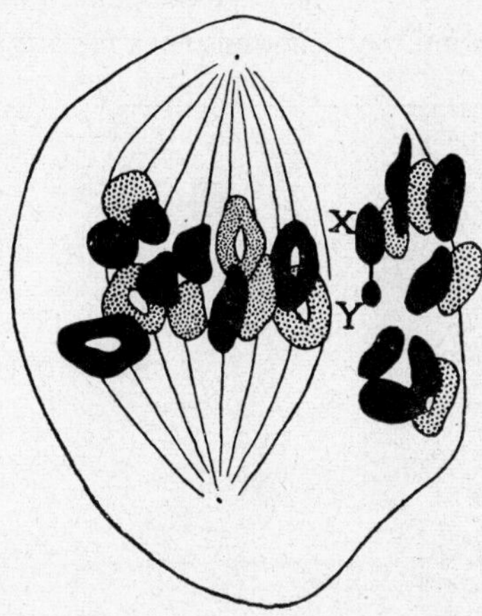

Fig. 81.—Primary Spermatocyte Spindle with 24 Chromosomes.

Note X Y chromosome consisting of two unequal parts. (From Evans and Swezy, *The Chromosomes in Man*. Courtesy of University of California Press, 1929, Vol. 9, No. 1.)

Almost immediately a new spindle appears in the oocyte, and division occurs without preliminary cleavage of the chromosomes, so that two cells are formed, each of which has only one half of the number of chromosomes characteristic of the species. The smaller of these is cast off as the second polar body, while the remaining large cell is the mature ovum, whose nucleus is then designated as the female pronucleus.

As the first polar body is formed by typical division, it must be regarded as homologous with the oocyte, from which it differs only by its smaller size. On the other hand, the second polar body is homologous with the mature ovum, and contains only

A

B

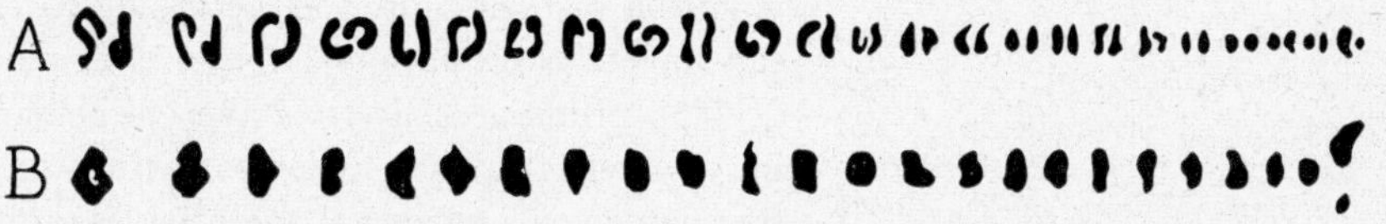

Fig. 82.—A, Twenty-four Chromosome Pairs of a Human Spermatogonium; the X and the Y Chromosomes are at the End of the Series.

B, Twenty-three Tetrads and the X-Y Combination from the Primary (reductional) Spermatocytic Division.

(From Evans and Swezy, *The Chromosomes in Man*. Courtesy of University of California Press, 1929, Vol. 9, No. 1.)

one half the number of chromosomes characteristic of the body cells. It would therefore appear that in the process of maturation six cells may develop from the original oocyte of the first order: by the nonreducing division, the oocyte of the second order and the first polar body; while by the reducing division the oocyte gives rise to the mature ovum and the second polar body, and the first polar body to two cells homologous with the second polar body, as is shown in Fig. 80. The stimulus to the final step in maturation, the reduction division, taking place after ovulation, is probably the entrance of the spermatozoon. At the conclusion of maturation, the ripe ovum or ootid, with its nucleus reduced in size and known as the female pronucleus with half the number of the original chromosomes and with the centrosome disappeared, is ready to unite with the male pronucleus of the spermatozoon.

Maturation is essentially a means of reducing the number of chromosomes. As the number of chromosomes for any given species is constant, it is apparent that maturation makes possible the introduction of paternal chromosomes into the ovum without increasing the number of the species, as must inevitably occur were some such mechanism not provided. In such manner, it is possible to maintain the continuity of the germ plasm of both parents. It is now generally accepted that the number of chromosomes in the human, in both male and female cells, is 48. During maturation this number is reduced to 24.

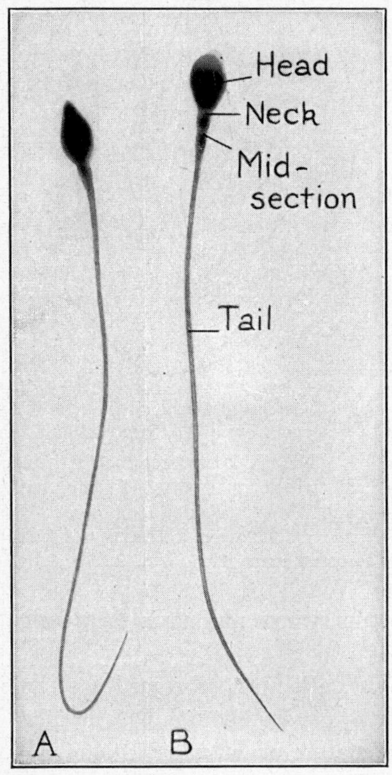

Fig. 83.—Human Spermatozoa. Retouched Photomicrographs. × 2100.

Head viewed in profile in A and from flat surface in B. The head contains the deeply staining nucleus above which is the light cap. (Courtesy of Dr. R. S. Hotchkiss, New York Hospital.)

Fertilization. By fertilization is understood the union of a spermatozoon and a mature ovum. Penetration of the ovum by the spermatozoon and the fusion of the male and female pronuclei are essential to successful fertilization. Each *spermatozoon* must be regarded as a distinct cell, and consists of three portions—the head, which contains the nuclear material; the tail; and an intermediate portion. The head is somewhat triangular in shape and flattened from side to side. Between it and the long tail is a small cylindrical body, the intermediate portion (Fig. 83). The spermatozoa are endowed with marked motility, derived undoubtedly from the rapid vibration of their tails, and, according to Henle, can traverse a distance of 1 cm. in three minutes.

The primitive cells from the epithelium lining the testis tubules undergo division to form spermatogonia. As sexual maturity is attained, each spermatogonium divides into two cells, the primary spermatocyte and a mother spermatogonium from which come later generations of germ cells. In spermatogenesis, changes are observed analogous to those occurring in the maturation of the ovum, and it has been clearly shown that each spermatocyte of the first order, or primary spermatocyte, divides into two cells, each of which in turn gives rise to two others containing only one half of the number of chromosomes characteristic of the species (Fig. 84). These latter are the spermatids, which later become the spermatozoa. Each spermatozoon, therefore, must be regarded as analogous with the mature ovum and the second polar body. Figure 81, from the monograph of Evans and Swezy, shows that the human spermatocyte contains 48 chromosomes; consequently, each spermatozoon must contain 24.

As has already been pointed out, the spermatozoon and ovum usually come together in the lateral portion of the tube, although in rare instances the meeting may take place on the surface of the ovary or even in a graafian follicle, as is demonstrated by the occurrence of ovarian pregnancy.

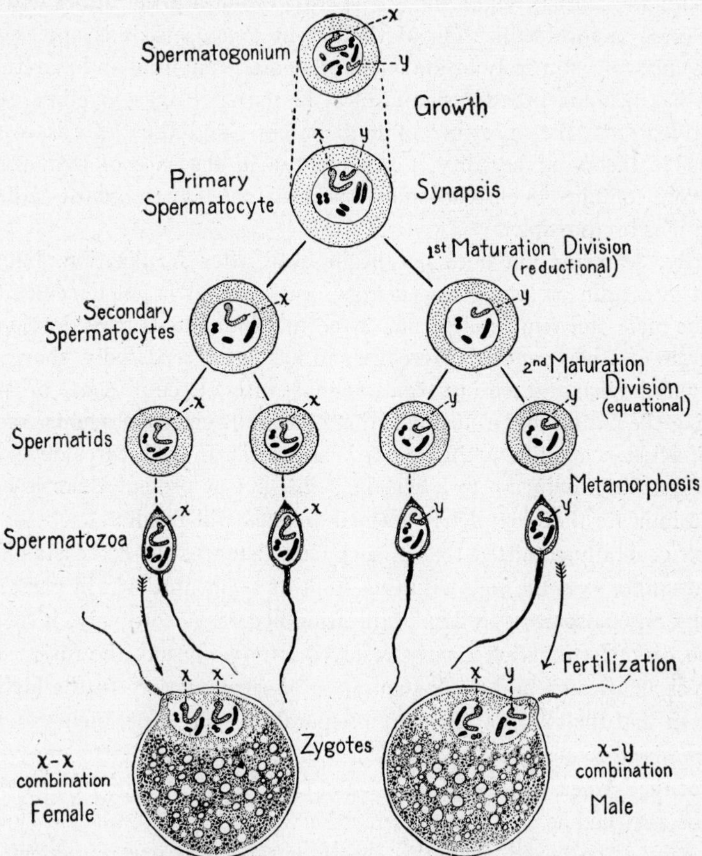

FIG. 84.—SCHEMATIC DIAGRAM SHOWING THE SEPARATION OF THE MEMBERS OF THE SEX CHROMOSOME PAIR IN MATURATION, AND THEIR RECOMBINATIONS IN FERTILIZATION.

It is assumed that the species number of chromosomes is eight and that it is the male which produces gametes of different potentialities with regard to sex determination. The sex chromosomes are stippled; other chromosomes are drawn in solid black. (From Patten, *Embryology of the Chick,* P. Blakiston's Son & Co., Inc.)

In the lower animals in which the process of fertilization has been studied, the ovum is found in the lateral end of the tube, surrounded by a considerable number of spermatozoa, as many as 60 having been counted about a single ovum. These rapidly penetrate the vitelline membrane, but it appears that normally only one of them makes its way into the ovum, and that after its entry the superficial portion of the latter becomes impervious to other spermatozoa.

After the head has entered the ovum the tail rapidly disappears, and in a short time nothing is left of the original spermatozoon but a small spindle-shaped mass, the *male pronucleus.* This rapidly makes its way to the center of the ovum, where it meets and fuses with the female pronucleus to form the segmentation nucleus.

As the male and female pronuclei each contains one half the number of chromosomes characteristic of the species, their union restores the normal number. Thus, in *Ascaris,* two of the chromosomes of the segmentation nucleus are of paternal and two of maternal origin, while in man 24 come from each cell. Moreover, as the chromosomes of both the mature ovum and the spermatozoon are the direct descendants of those concerned in the fertilization of the parent organisms, it is apparent that the process does not consist merely in the union of so many paternal and maternal chromosomes, but has a much broader significance, in that it brings together nuclear substances derived from the ancestors of both parents, and thus affords a basis for a comprehensible theory of heredity. Consequently, in the case of man in which the fertilized ovum contains 48 chromosomes, it is apparent that an almost endless number of combinations are possible.

Ordinarily, segmentation does not begin until after fertilization, but it is well known that in certain invertebrates (insects, crustacea) it is not dependent upon the fusion of the male and female elements, as normal individuals may develop from unfertilized ova—parthenogenesis. Moreover, it has been repeatedly shown that segmentation may be inaugurated in various animals without the presence of spermatozoa by subjecting the mature ovum to the action of various chemical agents, such as weak solutions of acids or alkalis—artificial parthenogenesis. In such cases development appears to progress normally up to a certain point, but at present there is no evidence available to indicate that completely formed animals will result.

It is now generally admitted that in such circumstances the egg casts off two polar bodies, as usual, so that the cells resulting from its segmentation will possess only one half as many chromosomes as when fertilization occurs. Accordingly, it would appear that the process of fertilization may be resolved into two parts—the fusion of the male and female chromosomes, and the inauguration of segmentation. In the higher animals it would seem that the two functions are inseparable, while experiments upon artificial parthenogenesis in some of the lower species indicate that the latter may occur independently of the former. In view of such facts, Loeb, in 1909, stated that the spermatozoon may be regarded as an activator which serves to stimulate nuclein synthesis.

It is generally believed that the centrosome—the structure which apparently presides over the act of cell division—disappears from the ovum during the last phases of maturation, and accordingly the mature ovum cannot begin to segment until the lacking structure has been restored by means of the male pronucleus. This can only be accepted as a universal rule if in parthenogenesis there is formation of only one polar body with no subsequent chromosome reduction division in the secondary oocyte. This appears to be quite probable.

General Development of Ovum. Soon after the appearance of the segmentation nucleus, karyokinetic changes take place within it and give rise to a typical nuclear spindle, which is soon converted into a dyaster, to be speedily followed by the division of the ovum into two cells (Fig. 85). Each of these in turn divides, giving rise to four cells, though one of the original cells may divide earlier than the other, so that we next may have three cells. This process of cell division or segmentation goes on until the original ovum becomes converted into a mass of cells, which is designated as the morula, or mulberry mass.

During this division, according to Streeter, the cells become segregated into two

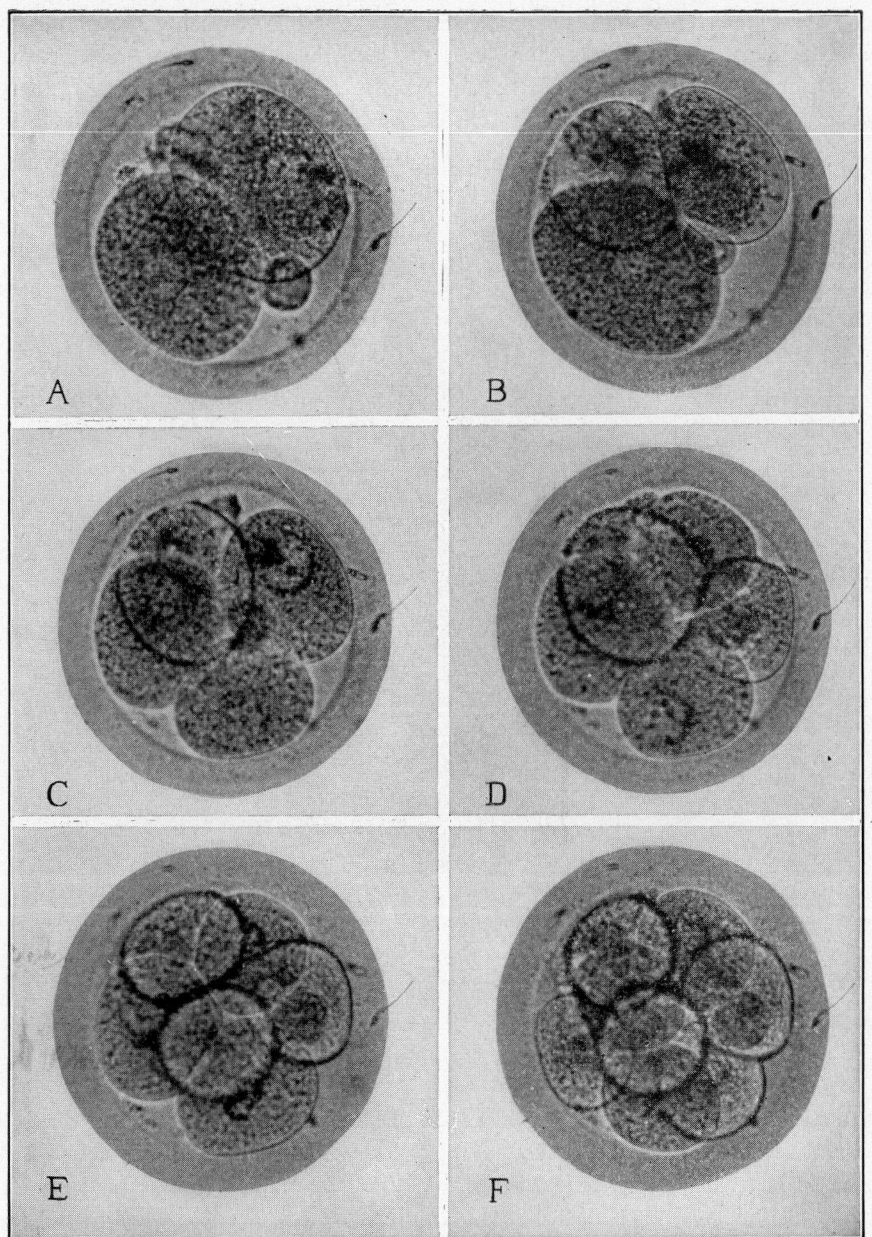

FIG. 85.—PHOTOMICROGRAPHS (× 300) OF LIVING MONKEY OVUM SHOWING ITS CLEAVAGE DIVISIONS.

The fertilized ovum was washed out of the tube, cultivated in plasma, and its growth changes recorded as micromoving pictures. The illustrations are enlargements from single frames of the film. A, Two-cell stage, twenty-nine hours and thirty minutes after ovulation. B, Three-cell stage, thirty-six hours and four minutes after ovulation. C, Four-cell stage, thirty-seven hours and thirty-five minutes after ovulation. D, Five-cell stage, forty-eight hours and thirty-nine minutes after ovulation. E, Six-cell stage, forty-nine hours and no minutes after ovulation. F, Eight-cell stage, forty-nine hours and forty-eight minutes after ovulation. (After Lewis and Hartman, *Contributions to Embryology,* Carnegie Institution.)

groups or types, the formative and the auxiliary. The latter being more precocious divide at first at a greater rate than the former and thus form a single-celled covering for the formative cells, from which the embryo itself is to develop. Fluid soon appears, probably secreted from the auxiliary cells on the periphery, and collects in the interior of the mulberry mass, thus giving rise to a vesicular structure consisting of a single layer of cells which surround a cavity filled with fluid—the segmentation cavity. The

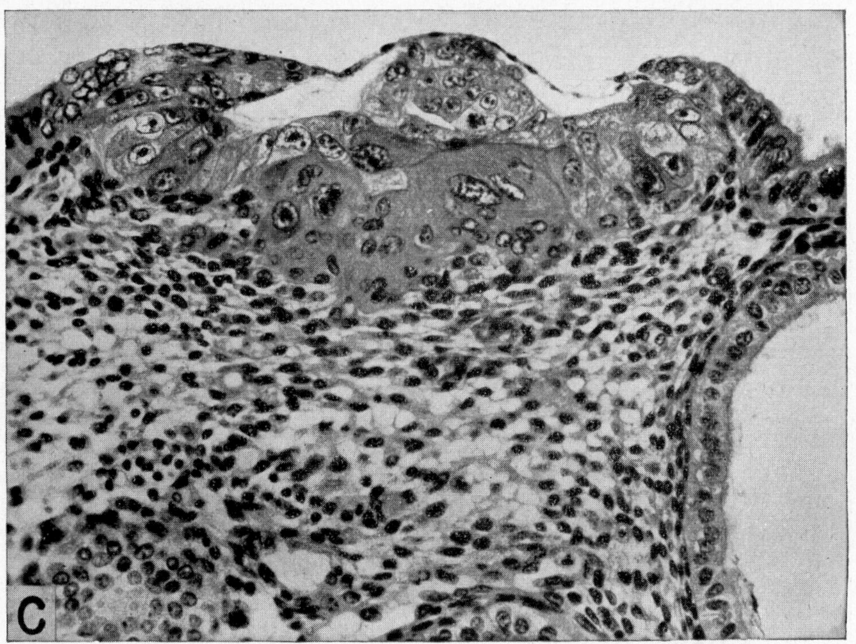

Fig. 86.—Youngest Human Ovum (about 7½ days). × 300.

Carnegie col. Mu—8020. Implantation is still shallow so that the characteristics of the collapsed blastocyst wall continue to be in evidence. However, ovum is well anchored to the endometrium by its trophoblast. The embryo is the small globular mass situated between the blastocyst wall above and the proliferating trophoblast underneath it. (From Hertig and Rock, *American Journal of Obstetrics and Gynecology.*)

entire structure at this time is known as the blastodermic vesicle, which in the rabbit and many other animals is still surrounded by the vitelline membrane, whereas in the mouse the latter disappears before the formation of the mulberry mass. In the monkey the blastodermic vesicle or blastula has been observed as early as the eighth and ninth days after ovulation (Fig. 87).

As the fluid collects in the vesicle the formative cells become crowded to one side and with the other cells of that region form the embryonic pole of the ovum. This embryonic pole is generally known as the inner cell mass, while the single layer of cells forming the remaining part of the wall of the vesicle is pure trophoblast though it is sometimes spoken of as the primitive chorion. As the result of improved methods of washing out ova from the tubes, this process has been demonstrated in large numbers of animals, and it is interesting to note that Warren H. Lewis in 1928 succeeded in demonstrating it by tissue-culture methods in the case of the rabbit, and consequently was able to demonstrate vividly the process, in all its detail, by means of moving pictures.

Lewis and Hartman have succeeded in taking photomicrographs of the living monkey ovum showing the cleavage division. They washed the fertilized ovum out of the fallopian tube, were able to cultivate it in plasma and noted by means of micro-moving pictures, the changes from the one-cell to the eight-cell stage. These are shown in Fig. 85.

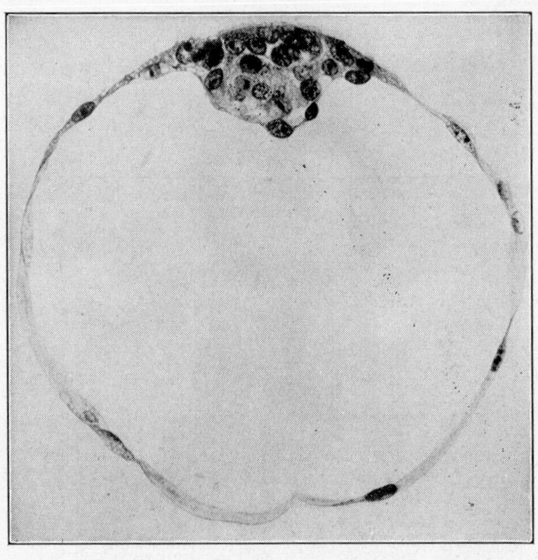

Fig. 87.—Section through Blastula of Monkey. × 300.

C 522, Carnegie Collection, Ovulation Age 9 Days. The delicate trophoblast forms the outer wall of the segmentation cavity; the embryo develops from the inner cell mass at the pole uppermost in this figure. (Retouched photomicrograph.) (From Streeter, *Contributions to Embryology,* Carnegie Institution.)

When viewed by transmitted light the embryonic pole appears darker than the rest of the surface of the blastodermic vesicle, and hence is called the macula embryonalis. Sections made through it at this point show that it is composed of several layers of cells, those nearest the exterior being the trophoblast cells by which this egg will attach itself, those nearest the segmentation cavity being the primitive entoderm.

In all mammals studied a segmentation cavity is formed by cleavage, so that the solid cell mass is converted into a vesicle, known as a "blastocyst." As Streeter and his associates have shown that in the monkey likewise a pre-implantation blastocyst stage exists, it is probable that the same is true for the human. In other words, the egg does not become implanted as a solid spherule of cells, as formerly taught, but as a fluid-filled vesicle or blastocyst.

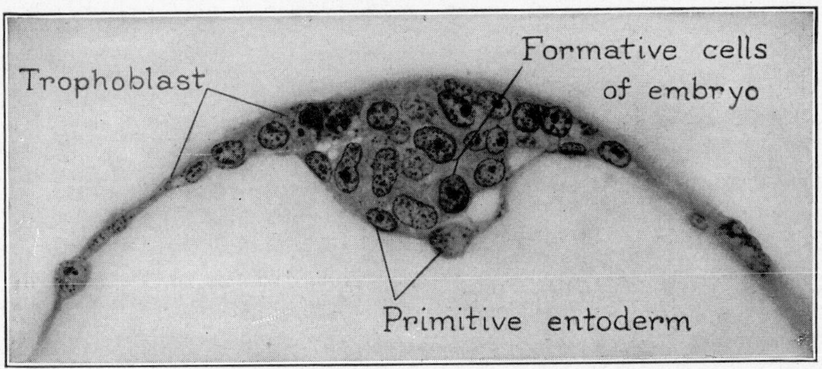

Fig. 88.—Section through Embryonic Area of Monkey.

Blastula shown in Fig. 75. × 500. (Retouched photomicrograph.) (From Streeter, *Contributions to Embryology,* Carnegie Institution.)

These changes, from fertilization to blastocyst formation, take place while the ovum is making its way through the tube and while lying free in the uterine cavity before implantation ensues. It was assumed, from observations on the monkey, that, for completion of the above changes, the human ovum requires eight to nine days, three to four of which are spent in the tube and the remainder in the upper uterine cavity. However, Rock and Hertig, as a result of having recovered from one of their series of excised uteri the youngest human ovum yet reported (estimated age between seven and eight days old), state that the human blastocyst probably implants itself during the late sixth or early seventh day of its development.

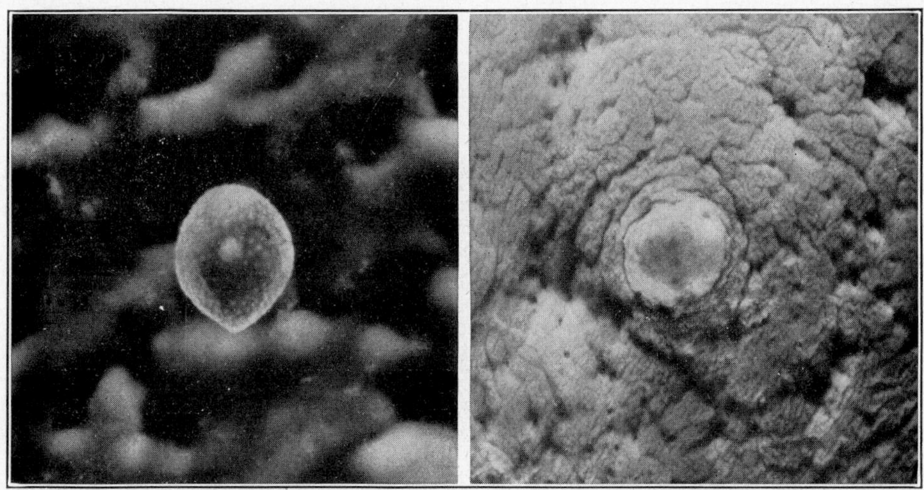

Fig. 89 Fig. 90

Fig. 89.—Monkey Blastocyst Beginning to Implant on Surface of Endometrium. × 45.
Age 9 days. Carnegie Col. C 610. White opaque mass inside is embryo. Note orifices of glands. (From Heuser and Streeter, *Contributions to Embryology*. Courtesy of Carnegie Institution, Baltimore.)

Fig. 90.—Human Ovum Partially Submerged in Endometrium (about 11 days). × 12.
Carnegie Col. 7700. Same ovum shown in Fig. 80. (From Hertig and Rock, *Contributions to Embryology*. Courtesy of Carnegie Institution, Baltimore.)

In 1938 Streeter described the characteristics of four primate eggs immediately preceding implantation. The blastocyst, of ovulation age eight days, is still surrounded by a thin envelope, the zona pellucida, which must disappear before implantation can occur. At this stage an embryonic pole of many cells can be seen, while the trophoblast cells are the most differentiated, those composing the greater part of the blastocyst wall being arranged in a single layer. These cells produce the accumulation of fluid, changing the blastula into a blastocyst. At the embryonic pole three types of cells can be seen: the larger "formative" cells; small irregular cells, arranged among and over the former, trophoblastic cells which will provide the means of attachment to the uterine wall; and cells (primitive endoderm) forming a single-layered membrane, separating the other two types of cells from the cavity. It should be noted that while the small irregular cells at the embryonic pole and the flattened layers of cells constituting the major portion of the wall of the blastocyst are regarded as trophoblast, their functions are different, as indicated above. During the next day the blastocyst, ovulation age nine days, reaches its maximum size, completing its primary differentiation. At the embryonic pole one observes a nodal center of active proliferation. The superficial cells, trophoblasts, are ready for invasion of the endometrium or implantation (Fig. 89) while the deeper cells will form the embryo.

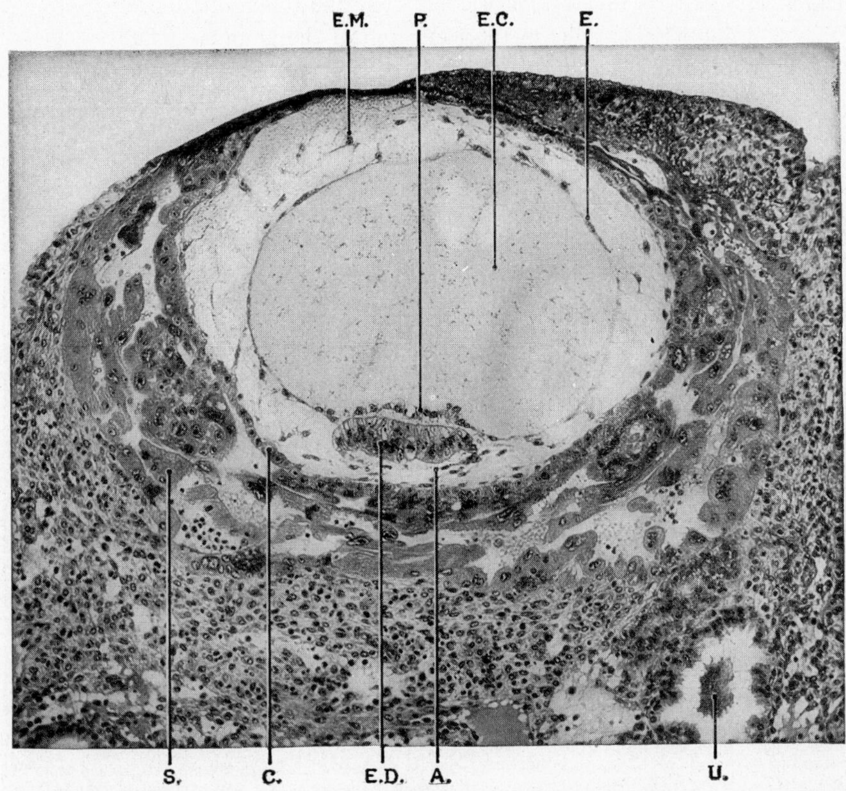

FIG. 91.—HUMAN OVUM OF PREVILLOUS STAGE (about 11 days). × 120.

Carnegie Col. 7700. Reticular cells are delaminating from inner surface of trophoblast around its entire circumference, forming amnion adjacent to germ disc. E.D., embryonic disc; P., primitive entoderm; A., amnion; E., exocelomic membrane; E.C., exocelomic cavity; C., cytotrophoblast; S., syncytium; E.M., extra-embryonic mesoblast; U., uterine gland. (From Hertig and Rock, *Contributions to Embryology*. Courtesy of Carnegie Institution, Baltimore.)

At about this stage in the development we can turn from the monkey to man, as the earliest human embryo is a blastocyst imbedded in the uterine wall. These early embryos reveal great proliferation of the trophoblast, by virtue of which the uterine wall is invaded and implantation occurs. Brewer and Fitzgerald, in describing six presomite human eggs, state that the vascular changes in the endometrium preceding implantation are similar to those accompanying the normal menstrual cycle, namely vasodilatation, vasoconstriction, extravasation of blood, congestion and actual necrosis in the superficial layer. In addition to these changes, which are evidently for the preparation of a site for implantation, the trophoblastic cells invade the maternal tissue, destroying maternal capillaries, venous sinuses, stroma, glands and reticulum. They, furthermore, demonstrated phagocytic activity on the part of the trophoblast. By these two means, then, the vascular changes occurring in the endometrium and the activity of the trophoblast, the blastocyst becomes imbedded and implanted in the endometrium. The maternal epithelium soon heals over the point of entrance of the egg, so that the embryo becomes surrounded by maternal tissues. The trophoblastic wall surrounds the embryo (Fig. 90), providing for its nourishment.

The inner cell mass now begins segmentation and differentiation, as well as a readjustment in its position. Due to the formation of the amnion and the yolk sac the cells at the embryonic pole take on the form of two vesicles, the amniotic vesicle and

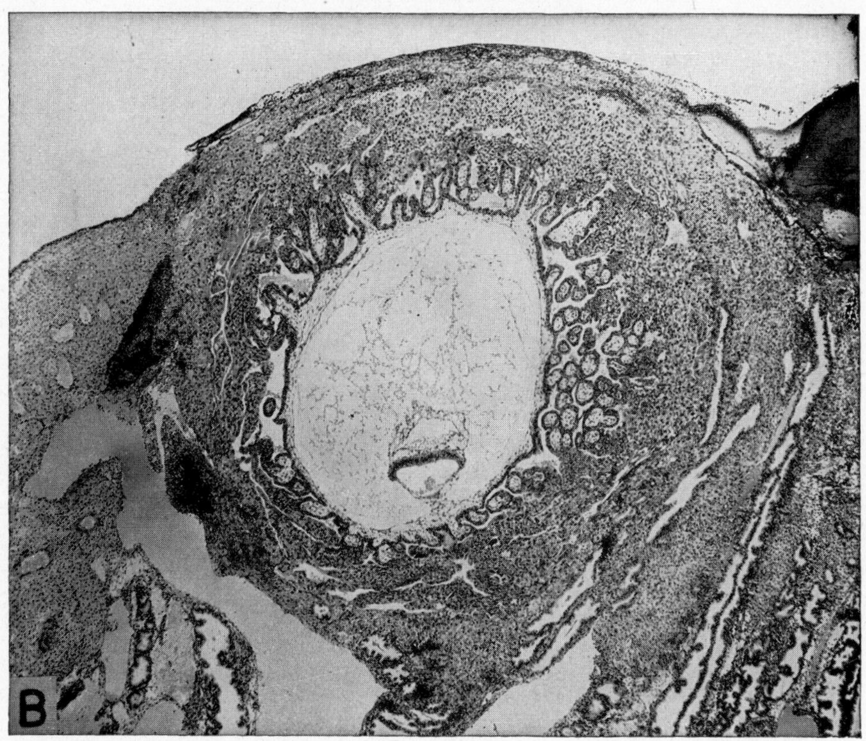

FIG. 92.—HUMAN OVUM OF VILLOUS STAGE (16½ days).

Carnegie Col. Bu—7802. Showing development of yolk sac and early branching villi. (From Hertig and Rock, *American Journal of Obstetrics and Gynecology.*)

the yolk-sac vesicle. These two vesicles become flattened against each other, forming the two-layered bilaminar plate or primordium of the embryo. Not only do the cells of the disk differentiate but they also interact upon one another, forming new types of cells. Soon a third layer (mesoblastic cells) is seen between the other two layers. Later the mesoderm becomes thickened at one end, the site of formation of the body-stalk, which is the main component of the future umbilical cord.

The embryonic area soon becomes slightly elevated, and forms what is known as the embryonic shield (Fig. 91). Later a darker zone appears at one end of the shield and soon exceeds it in size. This is the mesodermic tissue which spreads as an embryonic connective tissue between the embryonic ectoderm and entoderm (Fig. 97).

A little later there appears in the middle of the embryonic area a slight longitudinal depression—the primitive groove—which is bounded on either side by a slight elevation—the primitive folds. Shortly afterward a second depression—the medullary groove—appears in front of the primitive groove. It is bounded on either side by an elevated fold—the medullary ridges—which converge anteriorly to form the cranial end of the embryo. The medullary groove is in the same line with the primitive streak, but never unites with it; while the medullary folds diverge posteriorly and inclose the

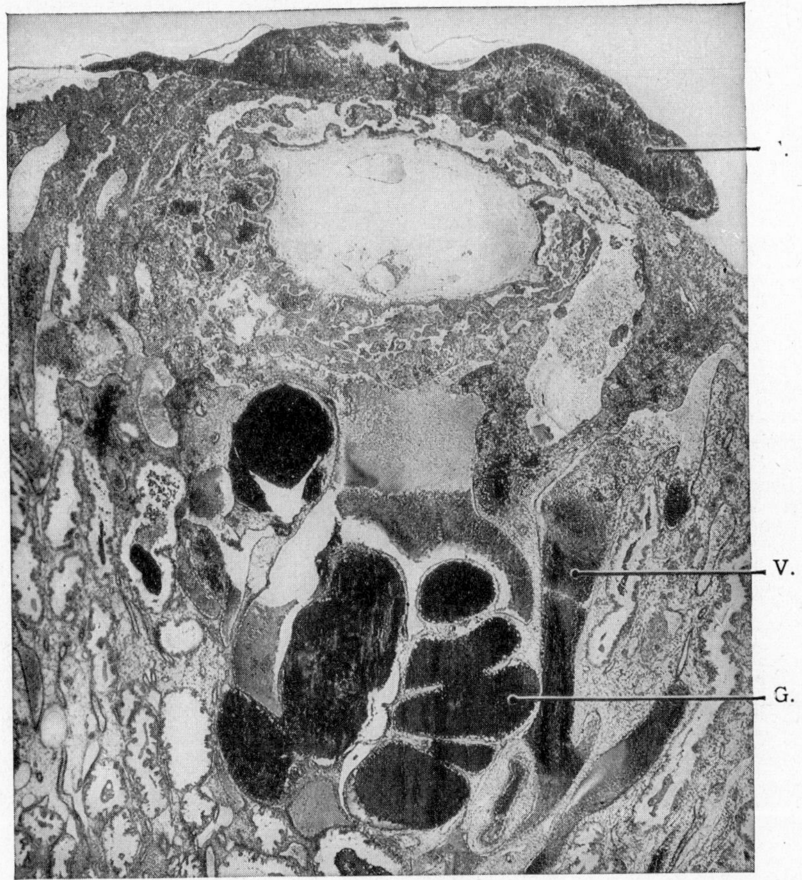

Fig. 93.—Edwards-Jones-Brewer Ovum. × 20.

Stage of primitive unbranched villi. Embryo is attached to chorion at its basal pole and has a definite yolk sac, which is smaller than the amniotic cavity. Note blood in sinuses underlying ovum and distending uterine glands. G., gland; V., vein; C., coagulum on surface. (From Brewer and Fitzgerald, *American Journal of Obstetrics and Gynecology.*)

anterior end of the primitive streak. As the ovum becomes older, the medullary groove and folds, which result from proliferation of the neural ectoderm and later give rise to the central nervous system, rapidly increase in size; while the primitive streak remains stationary, so that in a short time it occupies only an insignificant portion of the embryonic area (Figs. 100-102).

While these changes are taking place on the surface of the embryonic area, others of no less importance are going on in its depth; these result in the formation of the mesodermic structures. On either side of the medullary canal can be observed a slight thickening—the segmental layer—outside of which is a thinner layer—the parietal zone. The segmental layer soon becomes divided into a number of more or less cuboidal masses of tissue on either side of the medullary groove, which are variously designated as protovertebrae, primary segments, or mesoblastic somites; from these the musculature of the dorsal portion of the body is developed. The parietal zone, which is also made up of mesoderm, soon becomes divided into two layers which inclose a cavity, the celom. The outer layer is covered by ectoderm, and is designated as the somatopleure, while the inner is lined by entoderm and is called the splanchnopleure. From a

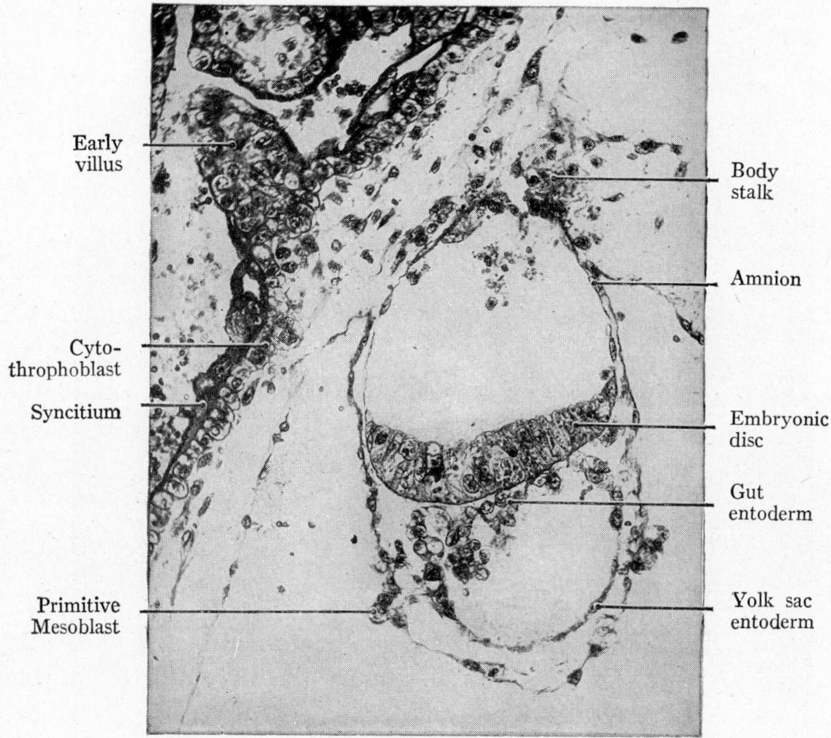

Fig. 94.—Embryo Shown in Fig. 82. Higher Power. × 180. (Photograph loaned by Dr. J. I. Brewer.)

part of the former the anterior and lateral abdominal walls are developed, while in many animals its greater portion gives rise to the chorion and amnion.

From the ectoderm are developed the central nervous system and the cutaneous structures; from the mesoderm are derived the muscular and circulatory portions of the body, the reproductive organs and the connective tissue framework of the various other organs; the entoderm gives rise to the digestive tract and the organs which are more or less intimately connected with it.

Implantation of the Human Ovum. As has already been indicated, the human ovum has not as yet been observed during the process of segmentation nor in the earliest stages of implantation. The studies of Streeter and his group, as well as those of Brewer and Fitzgerald, referred to previously, indicate that implantation depends upon the vascular changes occurring in the endometrium, similar to those seen in the menstrual cycle, as well as the invasive and phagocytic activity of the trophoblastic cells. As a result the ovum gradually sinks into the endometrium and comes to lie beneath its surface. Following this the margins of the opening coalesce, so that the ovum is eventually buried in the uterine stroma and has no communication with the uterine cavity. Such a procedure does not imply so radical a destruction of tissue as one might suppose, since it involves an area only the width of a few epithelial cells (Figs. 93, 94).

Following the appearance of Peters' monograph, a number of still earlier fertilized ova in situ have been described, and some of these must be mentioned. These new ova range in size from less than 1 mm. to 5 mm. in diameter and vary from seven and one-half days to the end of three weeks after ovulation. In each instance the ovum is imbedded in the

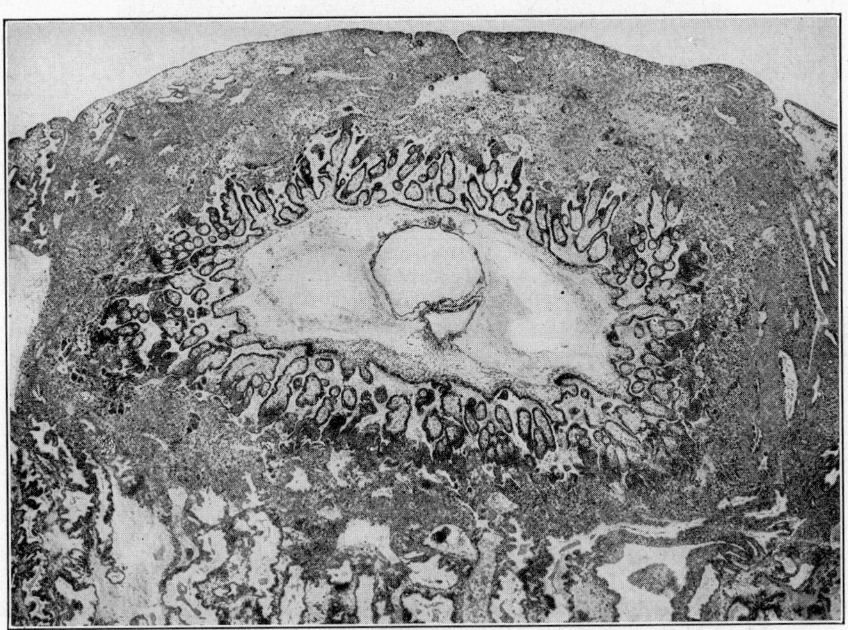

FIG. 95.—JONES-BREWER I EMBRYO. × 16.

Stage of early branching of villi. Note decidual reaction in surrounding tissues. Yolk sac is larger than amniotic cavity. (From Brewer and Fitzgerald, *American Journal of Obstetrics and Gynecology*.)

superficial portion of the endometrium and is separated from the uterine cavity by a definite, but thin, layer of epithelium and, when the entire uterus is available for study, appears as a minute vesicular structure whose upper pole projects somewhat beyond the general surface of the mucosa. In many instances, a funnel-shaped defect apparently marks the point of ingress of the ovum which, in a certain number of specimens, is covered by a mushroom-shaped mass of fibers infiltrated with leukocytes, while in still other specimens the tissue in this locality presents so complicated a structure that Teacher has designated it as the operculum.

Thus far, the youngest human ovum observed is estimated to be between seven and eight days old and was reported by Hertig and Rock in 1942. Among other previllous ova that have been described and reported, and which have not been noted to be older in general than 13 days, should be mentioned several of Hertig and Rock, in addition to those of Miller (Streeter), West and Dible, Werner (Stieve), Müller, and Marchetti. Young villous ova ranging between the thirteenth and seventeenth days of their development have been described by Heuser, Hertig and Rock, Brewer, Wilson, Ramsey, and Peters.

Formation of the Chorion and Amnion. In the early ova, it is seen that the center of the ovum consists of very loosely reticular mesodermic tissue—primitive mesoderm—containing at its embryonic pole a small mass of cells, to which reference will soon be made. Outside of this there is a thick capsule of epithelioid tissue—the trophoblast—in which two types of cells can be distinguished. The first, immediately adjoining the mesodermic tissue, consists of a single layer of cells with sharply marked

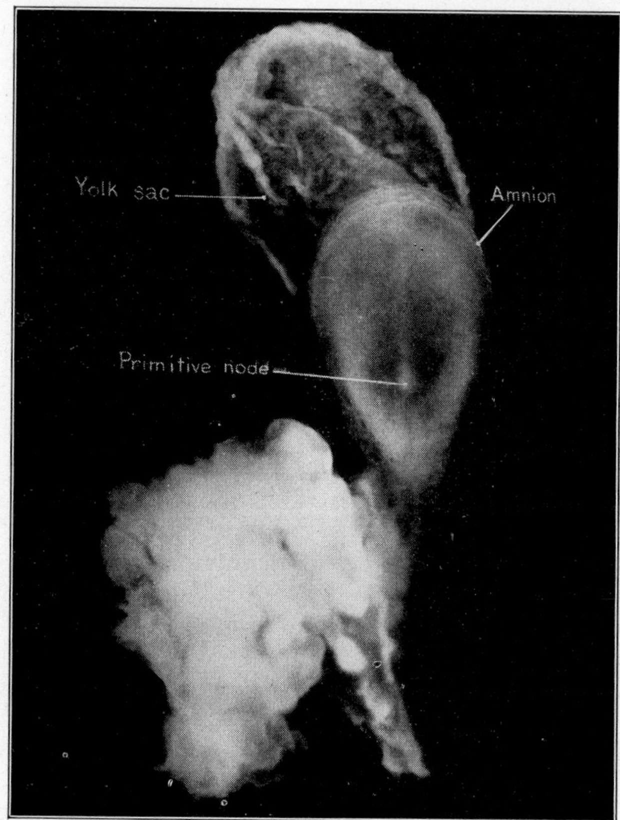

FIG. 96.—PHOTOGRAPH OF DORSAL VIEW OF PRESOMITE HUMAN EMBRYO. × 25.

No. 5960, Carnegie Collection; Ovulation Age 19 days, estimated by Dr. G. L. Streeter. At lower left is a mass of primitive villi. (From Heuser, *Contributions to Embryology,* Carnegie Institution.)

outlines; while the second is a syncytium and is characterized by the presence of masses and bands of protoplasm containing nuclei, but not divided into individual cells. The trophoblastic capsule, which is the most characteristic feature of the ovum at this time, varies greatly in thickness and, in its several portions, is actively invading the surrounding maternal tissue and opening up its blood vessels and gland spaces.

In the Edwards-Jones-Brewer ovum (Fig. 93), the mesodermic tissue appears immediately inside of the trophoblast, while from its periphery outgrowths extend into the latter and represent the earliest stage in the formation of chorionic villi. At this period the trophoblast with its mesodermic lining constitutes the chorion, while the cavity included within it is designated as the extra-embryonic celom.

In Hertig's ovum the small collection of cells at the basal portion of the mesodermic core represents the embryonic mass, while in the slightly older ova, such as the Jones-Brewer one, two cavities surrounded by mesoderm are present, and represent the amnion and the yolk sac. In the lining of the former, two types of ectodermal cells may be distinguished—first, a single layer of flattened cells, which constitute the amniotic epithelium, and second, several layers of larger cells, which constitute the embryonic plate or shield, which, however, at this time shows no sign of further differentiation. In the Hertig specimen there is some question as to whether a yolk sac is present or not. In the Jones-Brewer, however, the yolk sac is definitely laid down.

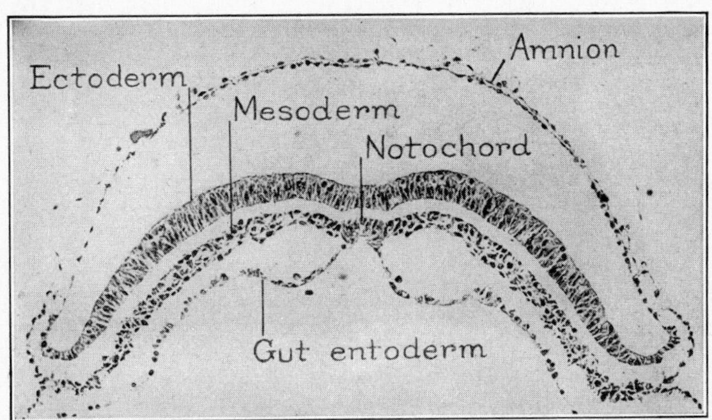

FIG. 97.—PHOTOMICROGRAPH OF TRANSVERSE SECTION THROUGH PRESOMITE HUMAN EMBRYO. × 125. No. 5960 Carnegie Collection. (From Heuser, *Contributions to Embryology*, Carnegie Institution.)

In other words, these early ova already present the first evidences of the differentiation of the three primary germ layers, ectoderm, mesoderm and entoderm, and consist of a relatively highly developed chorion with its mesodermic and trophoblastic layers inclosing a relatively large celomic cavity and of a small flattened amniotic cavity, one side of which is occupied by the embryonic shield, which as yet presents no sign of the future embryo. It is, therefore, apparent that in man the chorion and amnion do not develop in the same manner as in the chick, rabbit or dog, as in them there is no sign of amnion until the embryo has taken on a distinct form, when it appears as folds of somatopleure which arch over the embryo and eventually meet and fuse. Furthermore, in the early human ovum, the mesodermic tissue has attained a degree of development far out of proportion to that observed in those animals.

In the early ova the amnion and embryonic area are broadly attached to the basal portion of the inner surface of the chorionic membrane, or, in other words, toward the side which is richest in blood supply and where the placenta will subsequently form. At first the embryonic disk grows as a tissue culture. The trophoblast wall collects the food and transmits it to the exocelomic cavity which "conditions" it for the purposes of the embryo. Later the body stalk and umbilical cord take over the transportation of nutritive material.

Moreover, while none of the early ova are entirely spherical, they tend to become lenticular in outline with increasing age, so that by the end of the fourth week the longitudinal diameter greatly exceeds the vertical. Likewise, there is a marked change in the relative size of the yolk sac. In very early ova it is smaller than the amnion and embryonic area, but within a short time the relations become reversed, so that it becomes so large that the amnion and embryonic shield sit upon it as a mere protuberance. This, however, is a transient phenomenon, as the increase in size soon ceases, while the embryo continues to grow, so that at the end of pregnancy the yolk sac constitutes only a minute fraction of the entire product of conception. It is, however, important to remember that, aside from the chorion, the yolk sac is the most imposing constituent of the early ovum during the third and fourth weeks of development, which must indicate that at that time it fulfils some important function.

In the early ova thus far considered, the embryonic shield is merely a smooth plate of ectodermal cells, whose margins are continuous with the flattened cells which line the interior of the amnion. The first change indicative of the formation of the embryo is the appearance of the primitive groove toward the latter part of the third week. This is well exemplified in Figs. 98 and 99. This measured 9 by 8 by 3.5 mm. and was ob-

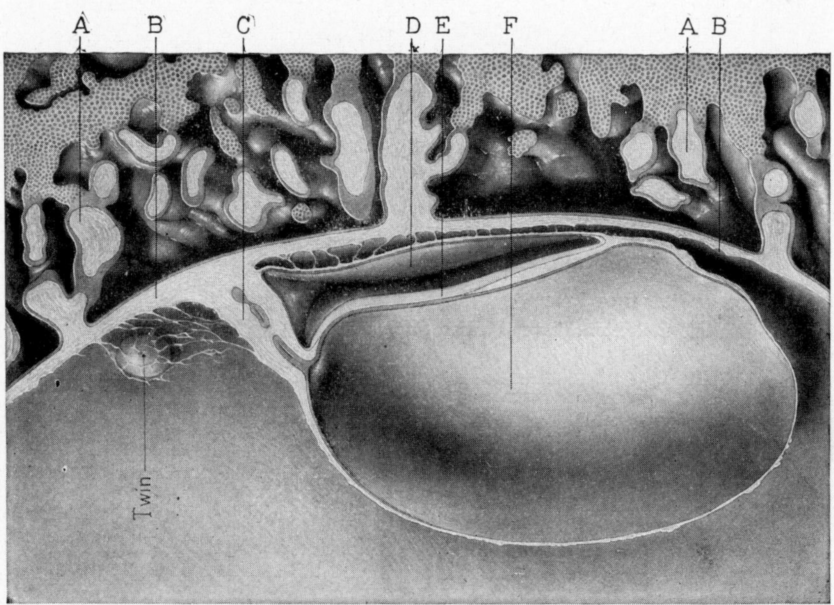

FIG. 98.—MEDIAN VIEW OF WAX RECONSTRUCTION OF MATEER OVUM, SHOWING THE AMNIOTIC CAVITY AND ITS RELATIONS TO CHORIONIC MEMBRANE AND YOLK SAC (Streeter). × 50.

A., chorionic villi; *B.*, chorionic membrane; *C.*, body stalk with allantois; *D.*, flattened amniotic cavity; *E.*, embryonic area; *F.*, yolk sac.

tained at operation 11 days after the failure of menstruation to appear. Figure 98 represents a portion of the chorionic membrane, to which the embryo, consisting of the flattened amniotic cavity, the embryonic shield, and the relatively large yolk sac, is attached by the abdominal pedicle, which contains in its interior a tubule lined by entoderm, which represents all of the allantois that is formed in man. Figure 99 represents a surface view of the same ovum, showing the large yolk sac, with the embryonic plate resting upon it and outlined by the cut edges of the amnion. The primitive groove extends forward from the cut end of the abdominal pedicle or body stalk. These specimens once more emphasize the fact that in man the amnion cannot originate from the folds of the somatopleure as in the chick.

The Streeter ovum (Fig. 98) shows clearly the relations of its various parts. The embryo is attached to the inner surface of the chorionic membrane by the abdominal pedicle, and its greater portion is occupied by the yolk sac, from one end of which a small process, lined by entoderm, which must be considered as a rudimentary allantois, extends into the pedicle. Occupying one side of the pedicle is a small cavity lined by a single layer of epithelium, which represents the amnion. On one side of this, again, is a mass of cells arranged in several layers—the embryonic area—in which a primitive streak can be distinguished. The three germ layers are well developed. Each of them, with the exception of the entoderm, consists of several layers of cells.

In the slightly older egg, the embryo is attached to the inner surface of the chorion by the abdominal pedicle, and is still made up in great part of the yolk sac. The embryonic area is oval in shape and presents a definite medullary groove and prim-

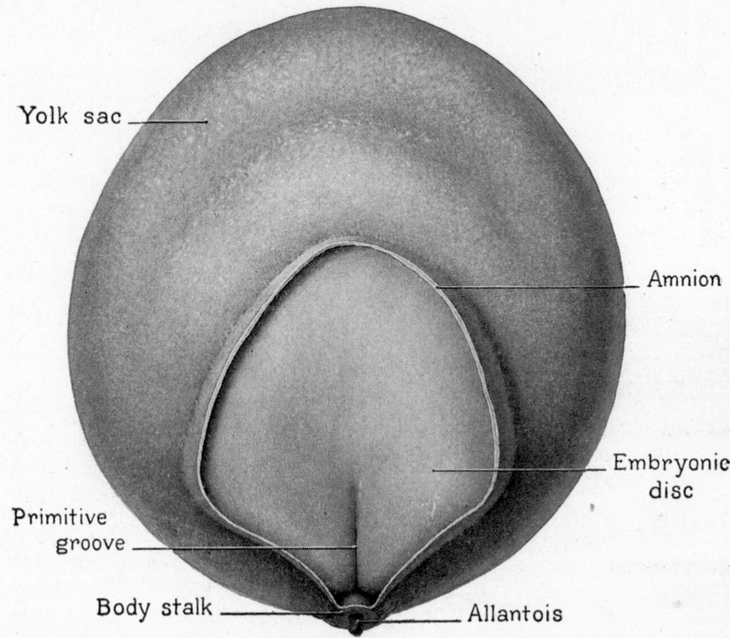

Fig. 99.—Dorsal View of Ovum Shown in Fig. 98, Shield-shaped Embryonic Area, with Primitive Groove, Resting upon the Relatively Large Yolk Sac. × 60.

The band-like structure bounding the embryonic area represents the basis of the amnion, whose major portion has been cut away. The structure at the more pointed extremity of the amnion represents the severed body stalk, with the allantois in its center. (After Streeter, Carnegie Col., 1399.)

itive streak. The two are not in the same plane, but the latter is bent almost at right angles to the former and occupies the inferior end of the embryonic area. Between the two is a small opening, the neurenteric canal, which serves to connect the ectoderm with the entoderm. The chorion now is well developed with typical villi, while the amnion is a small sac closely applied over the beginning embryo. Three germ layers and a well-developed somatopleure and splanchnopleure are now readily observed. By the folding in of the former it can be understood how the body walls are formed, and by that of the latter how the primitive gut becomes differentiated from the yolk sac.

In studying early human ova, two fundamental facts should be borne in mind. In the first place, several phases should be distinguished in the growth of the trophoblast, which appears to present two stages of proliferation: a first and temporary one, which is primarily concerned in the fixation or implantation of the ovum; and a second or more permanent one, which has to do with the ectodermal covering of the chorionic villi. Accordingly, Teacher, Streeter, and Grosser distinguish between implantation

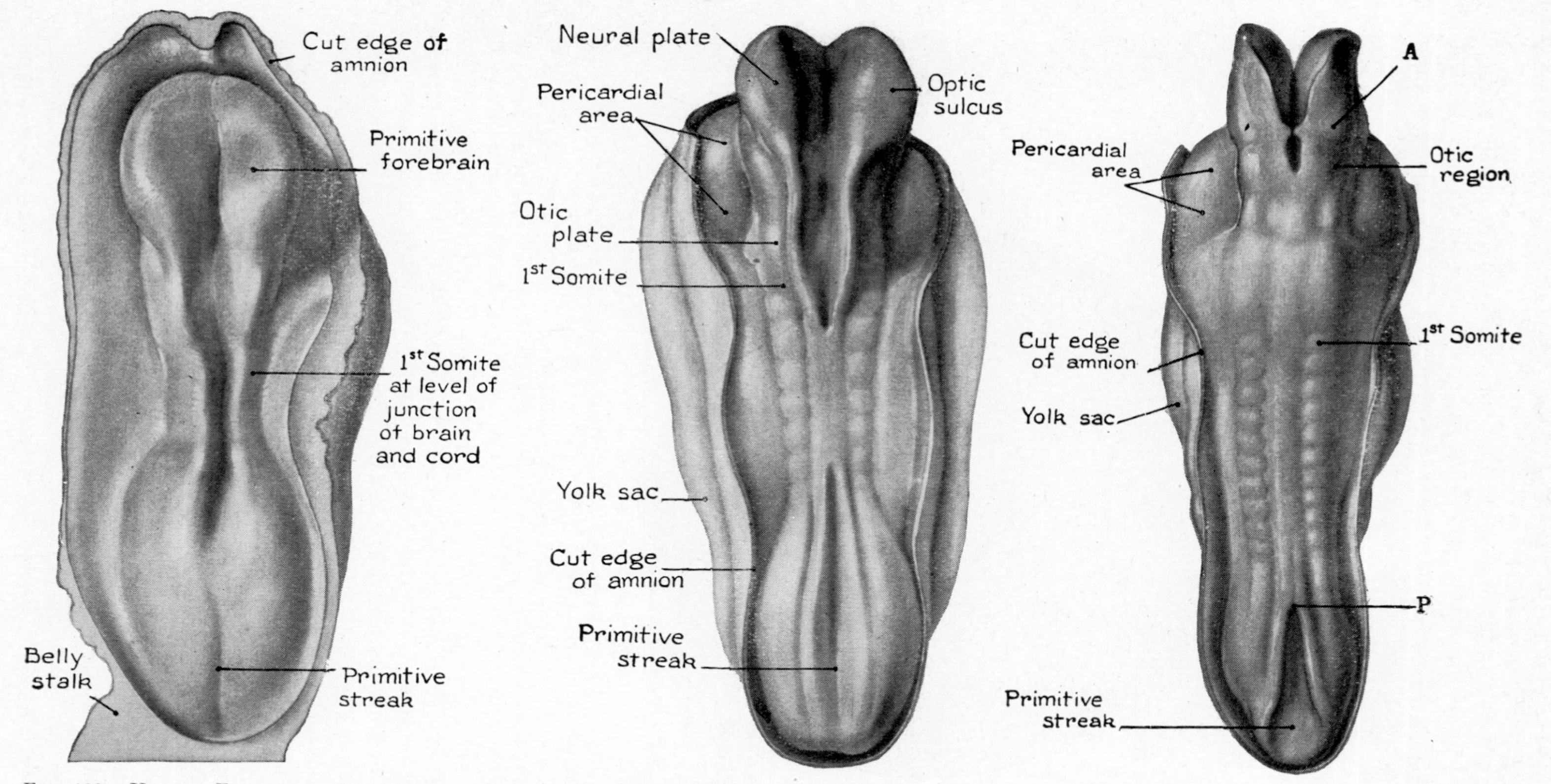

FIG. 100.—HUMAN EMBRYO AT BEGINNING OF SEGMENTATION. × 67.

Embryo No. 1878, Carnegie Collection. Dorsal View of Model Showing Open Neural Groove. (After Ingalls, *Contributions to Embryology*, Carnegie Institution.)

FIG. 101.—7–SOMITE HUMAN EMBRYO. × 45.

No. 4216, Carnegie Collection. Estimation of Ovulation. Age, 21 days (Streeter). Note closure of Neural Tube in Middle Region. (After Payne, *Contributions to Embryology*, Carnegie Institution.)

FIG. 102.—10–SOMITE HUMAN EMBRYO. × 25.

No. 5074, Carnegie Collection. A and P mark superior and inferior limits of neural tube closure. (After Corner, *Contributions to Embryology*.)

(From Streeter, *The Scientific Monthly*. Drawings by Didusch.)

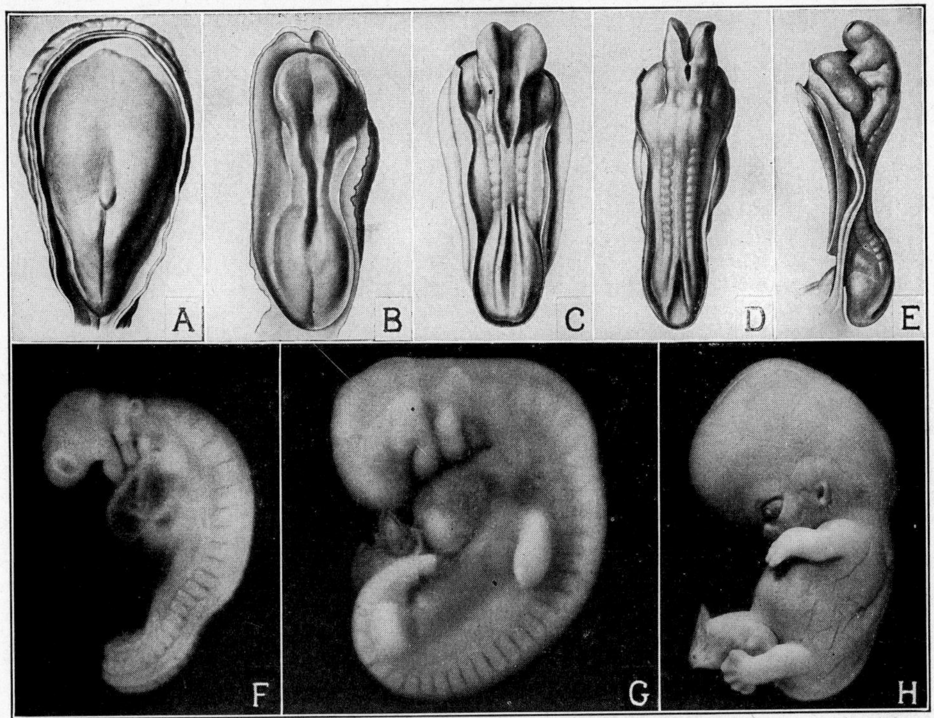

FIG. 103.—HUMAN EMBRYOGENESIS. (Carnegie Col.)

A., Heuser, × 30, 19 days; B., Ingalls, × 28; C., Payne, × 23; D., Corner, × 23; E., Atwell, × 15.5, 21 to 22 days; F., × 12, fourth week; G., × 8.5, fifth week; H., × 2.5, eighth week. (From Streeter, *Scientific Monthly*. Courtesy of Science Press, New York.)

and placental cytotrophoblast. Indeed, the latter goes so far as to enumerate five stages in its differentiation. In the second place, the so-called primitive mesoblast, which at first fills, and later lines, the celomic cavity, differs essentially from the extra-embryonic mesoblast occurring in other animals, as well as from that taking part in the formation of the human embryo itself. As has already been indicated, the latter arises from the under surface of the embryonic shield as a derivative of the primitive streak, while the former is well developed before the embryonic shield becomes distinguishable. For these reasons, Streeter sharply distinguished between the body and primitive mesoderm and was inclined to believe that the latter is derived from the trophoblast.

BIBLIOGRAPHY

ALLEN, E., PRATT, J. P., NEWELL, Q. U., and BLAND, L. J. Recovery of Human Ova from the Uterine Tubes. J.A.M.A., 1928, 91:1018.

——— Human Tubal Ova; Related Early Corpora Lutea and Uterine Tubes. Carnegie Inst. of Wash., 1930, Publ. 414, Contrib. to Embryology, 22:45.

ANDREWS, H. R. A Case of Simultaneous Intra-uterine and Extra-uterine Pregnancy with Probable "Internal Wandering" of the Ovum. Proc. Roy. Soc. Med., 1912-13, 6:52.

BREWER, J. I. A Human Embryo in the Bilaminar Blastodisc Stage (the Edwards-Jones-Brewer Ovum). Carnegie Inst. of Wash., 1938, Publ. 496, Contrib. to Embryology, 27:85.

——— and FITZGERALD, J. E. Six Normal and Complete Pre-Somite Human Ova. Am. J. Obst. & Gynec., 1937, 34:210.

BROWN, R. L. The Rate of Transport of Spermia in Human Uterus and Tubes. Am. J. Obst. & Gynec., 1944, 47:407.

BRYCE, T. H., and TEACHER, J. H. Early Development and Imbedding of the Human Ovum. Glasgow, 1908.

CARY, W. H. The Duration of Sperm Cell Migration in Uterine Secretions. J.A.M.A., 1936, 106:2221.

CORNER, G. W. Internal Migration of the Ovum. Bull. Johns Hopkins Hosp., 1921, 32:78.

GROSSER, O. Frühentwickelung, Eihautbildung, und Plazentation des Menschen und der Säugetiere. Munich, 1927.

HAMILTON, W. J., BOYD, J. D., and MOSSMAN, H. W. Human Embryology. The Williams and Wilkins Co., Baltimore, 1945.

HARTMAN, C. G. Migration of Ovum. In Allen, Danforth and Doisy, Sex and Internal Secretions, 2nd Ed. Williams and Wilkins Co., Baltimore, 1939.

——— and BALL, J. On the Almost Instantaneous Transport of Spermatozoa through the Cervix and the Uterus in the Rat. Proc. Soc. Exper. Biol. & Med., 1930, 28:312.

HERTIG, A. T., and ROCK, J. On the Development of the Early Human Ovum with Special Reference to the Trophoblast of the Previllous Stage: a Description of 7 Normal and 5 Pathologic Human Ova. Am. J. Obst. & Gynec., 1944, 47:149.

——— Two Human Ova of the Previllous Stage, Having a Developmental Age of about 7 and 9 Days Respectively. Carnegie Inst. of Wash., 1945, Publ. 557, Contrib. to Embryology, 31:65.

HEUSER, C., HERTIG, A. T., and ROCK, J. Two Human Embryos Showing Early Stages of the Definitive Yolk Sac. Carnegie Inst. of Wash., 1945, Publ. 557, Contrib. to Embryology, 31:85.

HOTCHKISS, R. S., BRUNNER, E. K., and GRENLEY, P. Semen Analyses of 200 Fertile Men. Am. J. Med. Sc., 1938, 196:362.

KELLY, G. L. Additional Observations on Internal Migration of the Ovum in the Sow and in the Guinea Pig. Anat. Rec., 1928, 40:365.

KINNEY, P. B. Internal Migration of the Ovum in the Guinea Pig. Am. J. Obst. & Gynec., 1924, 8:198.

LEWIS, W., and HARTMAN, C. G. Early Cleavage Stages of the Egg of the Monkey, Macacus (Pithecus) Rhesus. Carnegie Inst. of Wash., 1933, Publ. 443, Contrib. to Embryology, 24:187.

MARCHETTI, A. A. A Previllous Human Ovum Accidentally Recovered from a Curettage Specimen. Carnegie Inst. of Wash., 1945, Publ. 557, Contrib. to Embryology, 31:107.

MILLER, J. W. Corpus luteum und Schwangerschaft. Das jungste operativ erhaltene menschliche Ei. Berl. klin. Wchnschr., 1913, B.D. 50:865.

MOELLENDORF, W. Ueber einen jungen, operativ gewonnenen menschlichen Keim. Ztschr. f. d. ges. Anat., 1921, 62:406.

MULLER, S. Ein jungtes menschliches Ei. Ztschr. f. mikr.-anat. Forsch., 1930, 20:175.

NITABUCH. Beitrag zur Kenntnis der menschlichen Placenta. D. I. Bern, 1887.

PAINTER, T. S. Studies in Mammalian Spermatogenesis. II. The Spermatogenesis of Man. J. Exper. Zool., 1923, 37:291.

PETERS, H. Ueber die Einbettung des menschlichen Eier. Wien, 1899.

RAMSEY, E. M. The Yale Embryo. Carnegie Inst. of Wash., 1938, Publ. 496, Contrib. to Embryology, 27:67.

SCHLINK, H. H. A Clinical Contribution on Internal and External Migration of the Ovum, etc. M. J. Australia, 1924, 1:555.

STIEVE, H. Ein 13½ Tage altes, in der Gebärmutter erhaltenes und durch Eingriff gewonnenes menschliches Ei. Arch. f. mikr.-anat. Forsch., 1926, 7:295.

——— Ein ganz junges, in der Gebärmutter erhaltenes menschliches Ei. Ztschr. f. mikr.-anat. Forsch., 1936, 40:281.

STREETER, G. L. Developmental Horizons in Human Embryos. Carnegie Inst. of Wash., 1945, Publ. 541, p. 211; Publ. 557, p. 27.

——— A Human Embryo of the Presomite Period. Carnegie Inst. of Wash., 1920, Publ. 272, Contrib. to Embryology, 9:389.

——— The "Miller" Ovum—The Youngest Normal Human Embryo Thus Far Known. Carnegie Inst. of Wash., 1926, Publ. 363, Contrib. to Embryology, 18:31.

TEACHER, J. H. On the Implantation of the Human Ovum and the Early Development of the Trophoblast. J. Obst. & Gynaec. Brit. Emp., 1924, 31:166.

THOMSON, A. The Maturation of the Human Ovum. J. Anat., 1919, 53:172.

WEST, C. M., and DIBLE, J. H. A Very Early Human Ovum. J. Anat., 1939, 74:139.

WESTMAN, A. A Contribution to the Question of the Transit of the Ovum from Ovary to Uterus in Rabbits. Acta obst. & gynec. Scandinav., 1926, 5:Suppl. 1.

——— Investigations into the Transit of Ova in Man. J. Obst. & Gynaec. Brit. Emp., 1937, 44:821.

WILSON, K. M. A Normal Human Ovum of About 16 Days Development (The Rochester Ovum). Carnegie Inst. of Wash., 1945, Publ. 557, Contrib. to Embryology, 31:101.

WISLOCKI, G. B., and SNYDER, F. F. The Experimental Acceleration of the Rate of Transport of Ova through the Fallopian Tube. Bull. Johns Hopkins Hosp., 1933, 52:379.

YOUNG, J. A Study of an Early Human Ovum. Tr. Edinburgh Obst. Soc., 1926, 46:113.

6

THE PLACENTA AND ITS HORMONES

DEVELOPMENT AND ANATOMY OF THE PLACENTA

The placenta may be defined as the organ by which intimate union is effected between the mucosa of the maternal generative tract and the embryonic adnexa, particularly the chorion, for the purpose of facilitating the transfer of the nutritive material from the mother to the fetus, and of excrementitious material in the reverse direction.

In the various species of animals the placenta exhibits such pronounced differences in the mode of union between fetal and maternal tissues, in intimate structure, as well as in gross appearance, that it is safe to say that no other organ in the animal economy, which serves a single function, presents such marked variations. For example, the liver or kidney is practically identical in all mammalia, yet the placenta of swine differs so radically from that of the guinea pig that the casual observer would hesitate to conclude that he had to deal with the same organ, were it not obvious that it serves a similar function in each animal. For this reason, it is unsafe to apply to a given animal conclusions which have been drawn from the study of the placenta of any other species, even though closely related. Consequently, in considering the human placenta, it is essential that our conclusions be based entirely upon the study of placentation in human beings. Before taking up a detailed study of the placenta, it would seem advisable to consider separately certain points concerning the anatomy of the three parts which enter into its composition—namely, the chorion, amnion and decidua.

Structure of the Chorion. In its very earliest stages the chorion probably consists of the single layer of ectodermal cells forming the wall of the blastodermic vesicle. Soon after the implantation of the ovum, however, the chorionic epithelium rapidly proliferates and invades the surrounding decidual tissue, forming the many-layered trophoblast, which is lined internally by the primitive mesoderm. In a short time buds from the latter make their way into the trophoblast and give rise to rudimentary villi. Within a short time the entire periphery of the chorion becomes covered by villi, which rapidly increase in size and complexity and give it a shaggy appearance—chorion frondosum or "leafy chorion" (Fig. 104). In an ovum from the latter part of the third week Stieve was able to count 942 individual villi.

Figure 105 represents a section through a portion of the periphery of a three weeks' pregnancy and shows the relations between the chorion and the underlying decidua. Above is the chorionic membrane with rudimentary villi projecting from it. The membrane consists of two layers—the inner of connective tissue, the outer of epithelium. The former is composed of spindle-shaped and star-shaped cells embedded in a mucoid intercellular substance and at this period does not contain blood vessels. The latter is arranged in two layers: an inner, adjoining the connective tissue, which is composed of cuboidal or roundish cells with clear protoplasm and lightly staining vesicular nuclei —*Langhans' layer*—and an outer layer made up of coarsely granular protoplasm, which shows no signs of division into cells, and through which are scattered irregularly shaped, darkly staining nuclei—the *syncytium*.

Each villus arises from the chorionic membrane as a single stem which later gives origin to numerous branches which assume an arborescent form, the complexity of which increases with advancing age. The villi consist of a connective tissue stroma and an epithelial covering, each of which is continuous with the corresponding tissue of the chorionic membrane. At this time they do not contain blood vessels. It will be noted that most of the villi extend directly from the chorionic membrane to the decidua, to which they are attached by proliferating trophoblast. At the tips of the villi the cells are generally of the Langhans' type, while in other places buds and masses of syncytium are seen invading the decidua and opening up its vessels. A few villi do not reach the decidua, but project into spaces lying between the chorionic membrane and decidua—the so-called placental or intervillous space. Projecting here and there from the surface of the villi are epithelial buds, consisting of syncytium, which, when seen in cross or tangential section, resemble giant cells. These buds indicate proliferation of the outer layer of the chorionic epithelium, and may represent the first stage in the development of new villous branches.

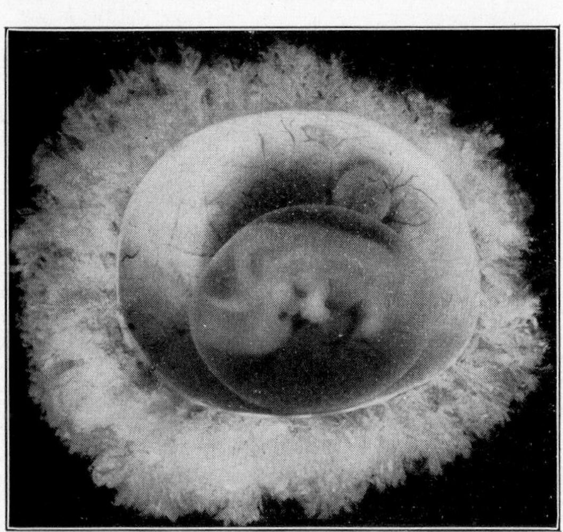

Fig. 104.—Human Chorionic Vesicle. × 2.
Carnegie No. 8537. Ovulation age, 40 days. Carnegie Institution of Washington, Dept. of Embryology.

In early ova, the embryo is connected with the connective-tissue layer of the chorion by a mesodermic structure, the *abdominal pedicle*, or body stalk, and is the forerunner of the umbilical cord. Through this, umbilical vessels of the embryo eventually make their way to the chorionic membrane and there fuse with blood vessels which have originated in situ. In this way, the fetal circulation gains access to the villi and makes possible the exchange of substances between the maternal and fetal blood.

In early pregnancy the villi are fairly equally distributed over the periphery of the chorionic membrane (chorion frondosum), but soon the greater part of them, which are in contact with the decidua capsularis, cease to grow and eventually undergo almost complete degeneration, while those in contact with the decidua basalis proliferate and form the fetal portion of the placenta. After the greater part of the surface of the chorion has become denuded of villi, it is designated as the chorion laeve or bald chorion.

A certain proportion of the villi forming the placenta extend from the chorionic membrane to the underlying decidua, attaching the ovum to it, and hence are designated as *fastening villi*. The majority, on the other hand, are arborescent structures whose free endings do not reach the decidua. In early pregnancy the villi are short and plump and represent simply the main stems, but later they give off numerous branches and assume an arborescent appearance. Thus, sections through a young

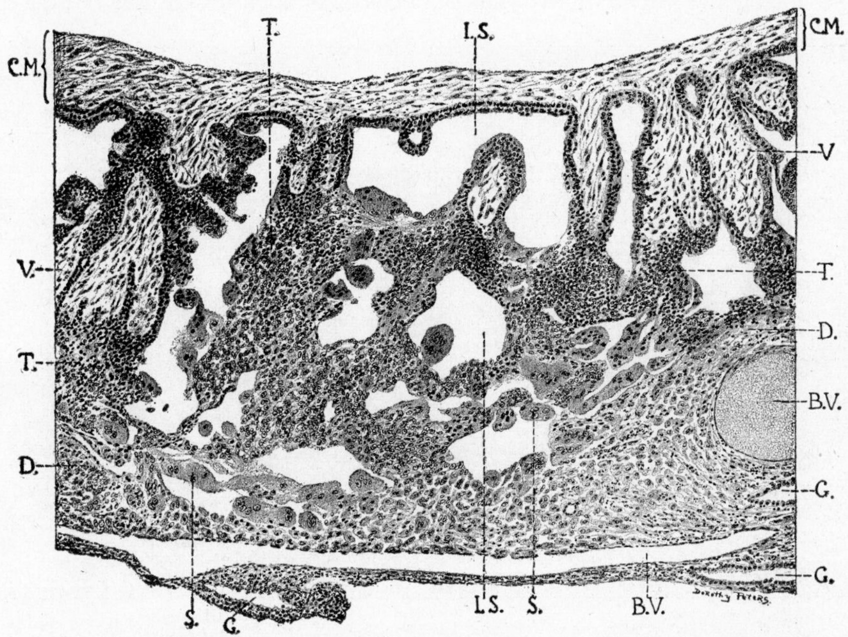

Fig. 105.—Section through Three Weeks' Human Ovum, Showing Chorion, Decidua, and Intervillous Spaces.

B.V., maternal blood vessel; *C.M.*, chorionic membrane; *D.*, decidua; *G.*, uterine gland; *I.S.*, intervillous space; *S.*, syncytium; *T.*, trophoblast; *V.*, villus.

chorion show only a few large villi, while those through an older one are filled with a multitude of smaller branches. This change in appearance may be compared to what takes place in a clump of trees, which at an early period consist of a number of almost isolated trunks, each of which later gives off innumerable branches and twigs. These differences have been particularly emphasized by de Loos, who has shown that with a little practice one can roughly estimate the age of the chorion by its appearance on section. (See Fig. 106.)

The stroma of the villi also varies in appearance according to the age of the chorion. In the earlier stages the cells are branching in shape, and are separated from one another by a large amount of mucoid intercellular substance; later on they become more spindle-shaped and more closely packed together, so that the stroma assumes a denser appearance. Another type of cell also occurs in the stroma—the so-called plasma or Hofbauer cells. These are roundish cells with vesicular nuclei and very granular or vacuolated protoplasm. In fresh specimens Warren H. Lewis has shown that their granules stain so characteristically with vital stains that he is inclined to classify them as clasmatocytes or histiocytes. They are present in all stages of pregnancy, but are most abundant during the early months. Hofbauer showed that they are particularly abundant when the fetus is defective or in the presence of infectious processes.

After the third week, but before there is any sign of the fetal heart, blood islands appear in the mesodermic tissue of the chorion, and vascular walls soon appear around them. These coalesce to form larger vessels, and soon lead to complete vascularization of the chorion and its villi. Indeed, this is a favorite location for the study of the spon-

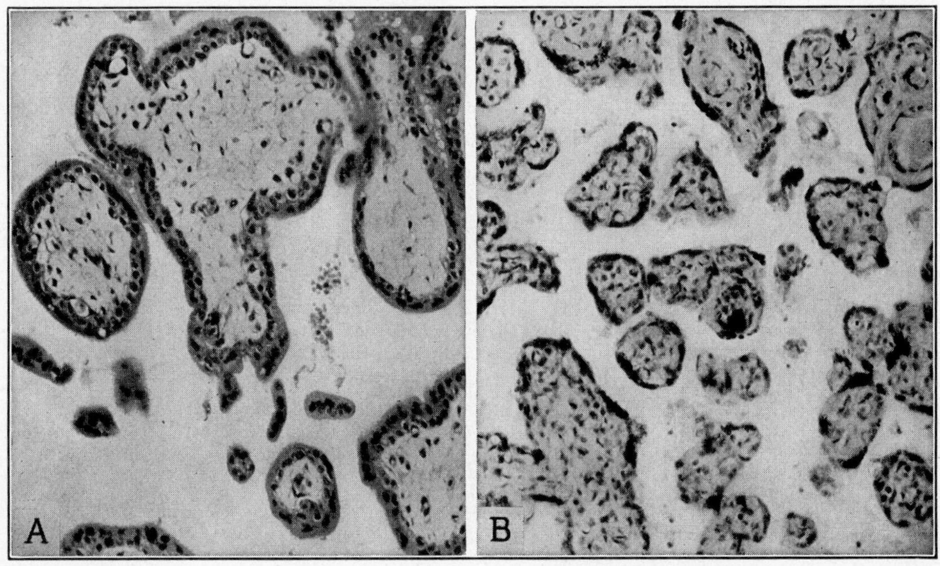

Fig. 106.—Comparison of Chorionic Villi in Early and Late Pregnancy. × 245.

A. Two months gestation. Note inner Langhans' cells and outer syncytial layer. B. Term Placenta. Syncytial layer persists. Langhans' cells are absent.

taneous development of blood cells and blood vessels, and the isolated blood islands with their nucleated red cells and delicate endothelial walls present a striking picture. It is important to remember that in man the chorionic vessels originate in situ and are not derived from the allantois, as is often taught. The villous vessels soon become very abundant, and in the later months of pregnancy almost displace the stroma. The arteries and veins extend to the tips of the villi, where they break up into capillaries, but there is no anastomosis between the vascular supply of the various villi, any more than there is connection between the branches of different trees in a forest.

During the first half of pregnancy the Langhans' and syncytial layers of the villus are readily distinguished, but later the former becomes more and more indistinct, so that during the second half the villi are covered only by a single layer of syncytium. Careful examination of properly prepared specimens shows that the syncytial layer presents a vacuolated structure, and that its outer marking does not present a smooth surface, but is made up of a vertically arranged pseudopodia-like protoplasmic process. These structures are too coarse to be considered as cilia, and are designated as bristle-like processes.

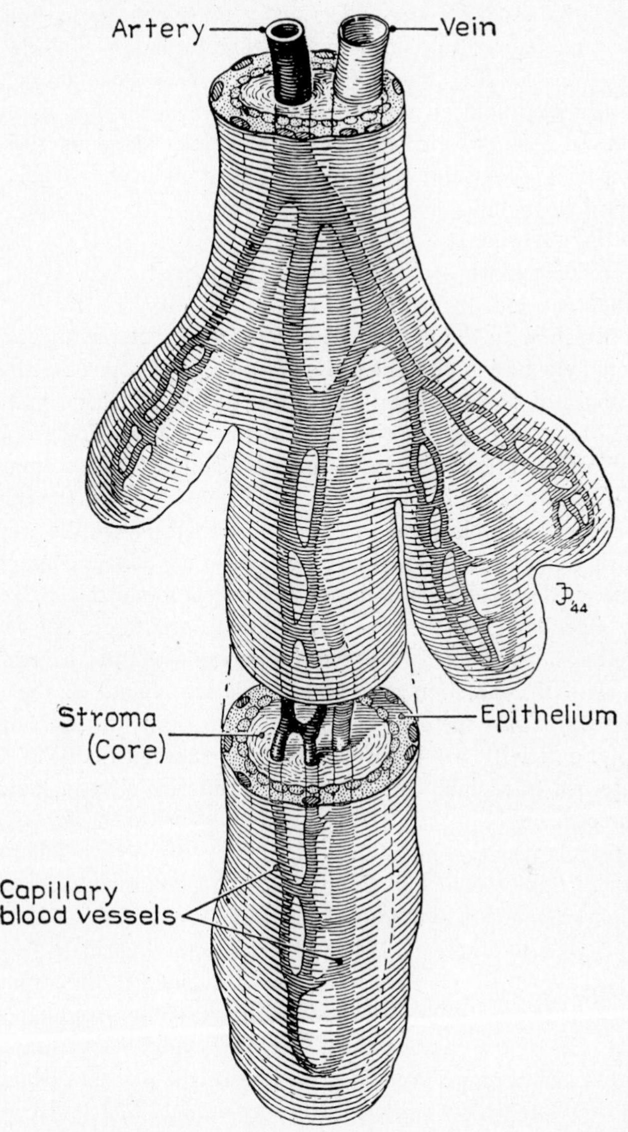

FIG. 107.—PART OF A FULLY FORMED VILLUS OF THE HUMAN PLACENTA, SHOWING COURSE OF BLOOD VESSELS AND ARRANGEMENT OF EPITHELIAL COVERING. MAGNIFIED ABOUT 160 DIAMETERS. (From *Ourselves Unborn* by Dr. George W. Corner, Yale University Press.)

The trophoblast, which is the parenchyma of the placenta, provides for the nutrition of the embryo by the destruction and absorption of parts of the uterine decidua and by the absorption of metabolites from the maternal blood circulating in the intervillous space. The trophoblast also serves as an avenue of excretion for a variety of waste products. The transfer of various metabolites as well as the destruction of parts of the decidua is mediated by a variety of enzymes and chemical processes, some of which it is possible to study by histochemical means. In addition to these various functions, it has become evident in recent years from endocrinological and chemical investigations that the placenta is an important endocrine organ which forms and secretes both steroid and chorionic gonadotrophic hormones. The formation of these lipid and protein bodies involves complex metabolic synthesis. Experimental and histochemical methods have also shed light on the probable sites of localization of these substances in the placenta. In a noteworthy series of monographs based on these newer histochemical technics, Wislocki and his associates have adduced a whole new canon of knowledge regarding the finer histology and functions of the placenta, as summarized very briefly in the following two paragraphs.

The cytotrophoblast, which corresponds to Langhans' "cell layer," and the syncytium play different and distinctive roles in respect to these various functional activities of the placenta. In the first months of pregnancy the cytotrophoblast appears to produce proteolytic and cytolytic substances capable of attacking the endometrium. In the early stages of normal gestation in primates, hemorrhage in the decidua coincides with the erosion of the uterine mucosa by the advancing trophoblast. It has been generally assumed that the extravasated blood originates from the maternal vessels whose walls are actually invaded by the trophoblast. On the other hand, there is reason to believe that a chemical substance is elaborated by the trophoblast which can initiate such changes in decidual tissue which is not yet in contact with the egg. In the macaque, evidence of such a chemical factor is found in the fact that the epithelium at the secondary implantation site begins to proliferate before erosion of the uterine surface has taken place. In a previllous human ovum of 11 days' ovulation age, moreover, an area of congestion and hemorrhage was found in the opposite endometrial surface which had merely been in close proximity to the implantation site. Similar proteolytic activity has been demonstrated experimentally in the presence of fertilized mouse ova transplanted to various extra-uterine sites including the anterior chamber of the eye.

The syncytium is very rich in cytoplasmic ribonucleoproteins. The presence of such a great amount of this substance in the early part of gestation suggests that the syncytium is an important site of synthesis of the proteins required by the growing embryo at that time. Glycogen occurs widely in the placenta but little is present in the syncytium or in Langhans' cells themselves. Some is found in the stroma of the chorionic villi, and it is demonstrable in large quantities in the glandular epithelium and in the decidual cells of the endometrium. Dempsey and Wislocki have expressed the opinion that glycogen occurs especially in regions of the placenta which are relatively avascular and therefore poorly supplied with oxygen, and that under anaerobic conditions it may provide a readily available source of oxygen. In the cytotrophoblast of hydatidiform moles unusually large amounts of glycogen are encountered, in keeping with the relative avascularity apparent in these pathological villi (page 528). Finally, Wislocki and his associates have adduced histochemical evidence which indicates that the syncytium is the site of formation of the placental steroid hormones (estrogen and progesterone), whereas the cytotrophoblast, or Langhans' layer, produces chorionic gonadotrophin (page 156).

Structure of the Amnion. In the very earliest stages of pregnancy, as we have already shown, the amnion is a minute vesicle; later it forms a small sac which covers only the dorsal surface of the embryo, and eventually becomes larger and completely surrounds it. At first the amnion occupies only a minute portion of the entire ovum, but as pregnancy advances it increases in size, until eventually it comes in contact with the interior of the chorion and obliterates the extra-embryonic portion of the celom. When the outer surface of the amnion has applied itself to the inner surface of the chorion, the two membranes become slightly adherent, but are never very intimately connected, for even at the end of pregnancy, they can be readily separated from one another.

From its earliest stages the amnion consists of two layers: an outer layer of mesoderm and an inner layer, made up of cuboidal or flattened, ectodermal cells. The mesodermic layer eventually becomes converted into mucoid-like tissue which does not contain blood vessels, while the ectodermal portion is represented by a single layer of epithelial cells which vary considerably in shape but tend to be cuboidal. As the amniotic epithelium is homologous in origin with the cells making up the embryonic shield, they may be regarded as simply an extension of the skin of the embryo. This relationship is accentuated by the fact that in somewhat more than one half of all placentas, at term, small, rounded plaques may be observed upon the amnion, particularly in the neighborhood of the attachment of the umbilical cord. Upon microscopic examination they are found to be made up of stratified epithelium, which bears a close resemblance to that of the skin. They are designated as *amniotic caruncles*, and will be considered more fully in the section on the pathology of the ovum.

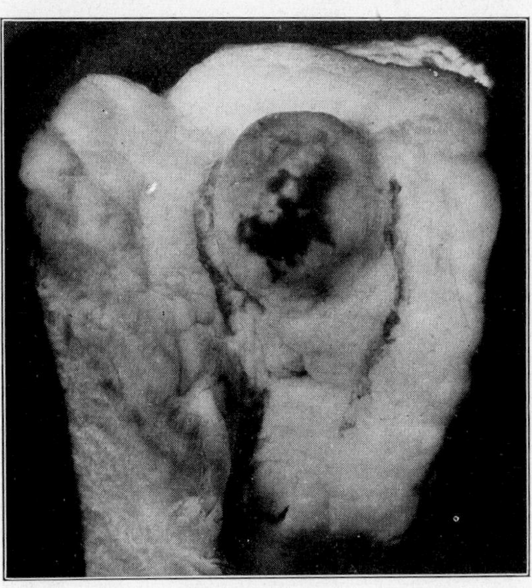

Fig. 108.—Early Ovum in Situ. × 1.5.

Carnegie Col. 5960. Note blood beneath decidua capsularis. See Figs. 96, 103 A. (From Heuser, *Contributions to Embryology*. Courtesy of Carnegie Institution, Baltimore.)

Soon after its formation, a certain amount of clear fluid—the amniotic fluid—collects within the amniotic cavity and increases in quantity as pregnancy advances. The amount varies within wide limits but averages about 600 cc. at the end of pregnancy, although under abnormal conditions it may vary from a few cubic centimeters to many liters. Its specific gravity ranges from 1.007 to 1.025, and it contains a certain amount of albumin, urea, creatinine, and various salts. Its origin and function will be considered when we take up the physiology of the fetus.

Decidua. The decidua is the mucous membrane of the pregnant uterus which has already undergone certain changes, under the influence of the ovulation cycle, to fit it for the implantation and nutrition of the ovum. It is so named from the fact that it is cast off after labor.

The conversion of the uterine mucosa into decidua occurs shortly after the fertilization of the ovum, though we are unable to state exactly when the process commences, inasmuch as the premenstrual swelling is accompanied by changes in structure, which must be regarded as pregravid or predecidual in character.

After conception the hypertrophic premenstrual or progestational endometrium grows still thicker and eventually attains a thickness of from 5 to 10 mm., while its surface becomes indented by furrows of considerable depth, which give the entire membrane a mamelonated appearance. Under the magnifying glass numerous small

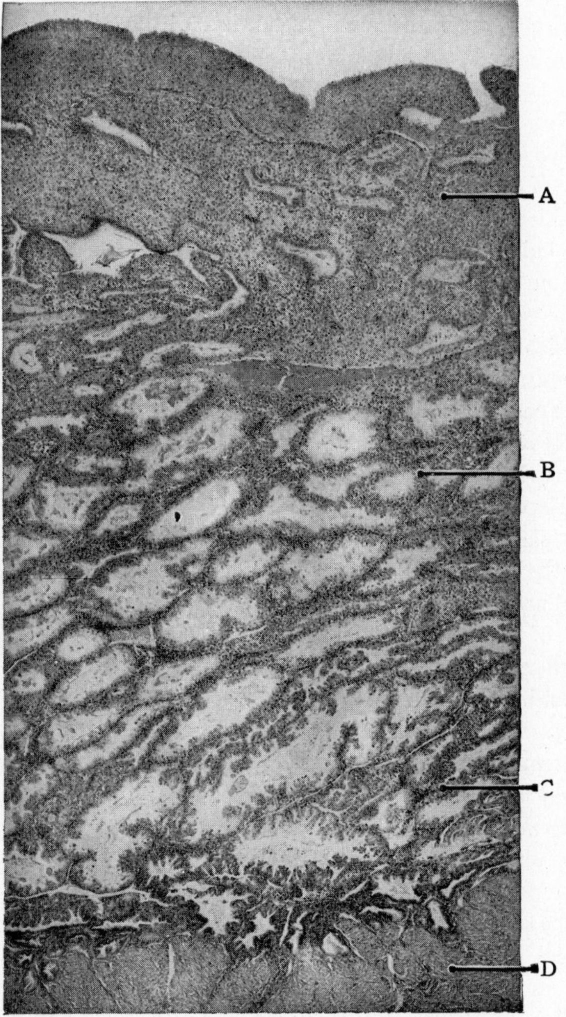

FIG. 109.—EARLY DECIDUA VERA. × 50.

A., compact layer (see Fig. 110); B., spongy layer; C., functional layer; D., muscularis. (Compare with Figs. 65 and 66.)

openings can be distinguished which are the mouths of the uterine glands. The decidual formation is limited to the body of the uterus, and does not extend below the internal os.

For purposes of description the decidua is divided into three portions: that lining the main cavity of the uterus being designated as the *decidua vera;* that beneath the ovum as the *decidua basalis;* while that portion which surrounds the ovum and shuts it off from the rest of the uterine cavity is known as the *decidua capsularis.*

Decidua Vera. The decidua vera is composed of two portions: a *compact* layer superimposed upon a *spongy* or *glandular* layer, the latter adjoining the muscular wall of the uterus, and forming the main thickness of the membrane. The compact layer is made up of the *decidual cells,* large, round, oval or polygonal cells with large, lightly staining, vesicular nuclei, while the spongy layer is composed of dilated and hyperplastic uterine glands.

The decidua vera increases markedly in thickness during the first three or four months of pregnancy, so that at the end of that time it may attain a thickness of about

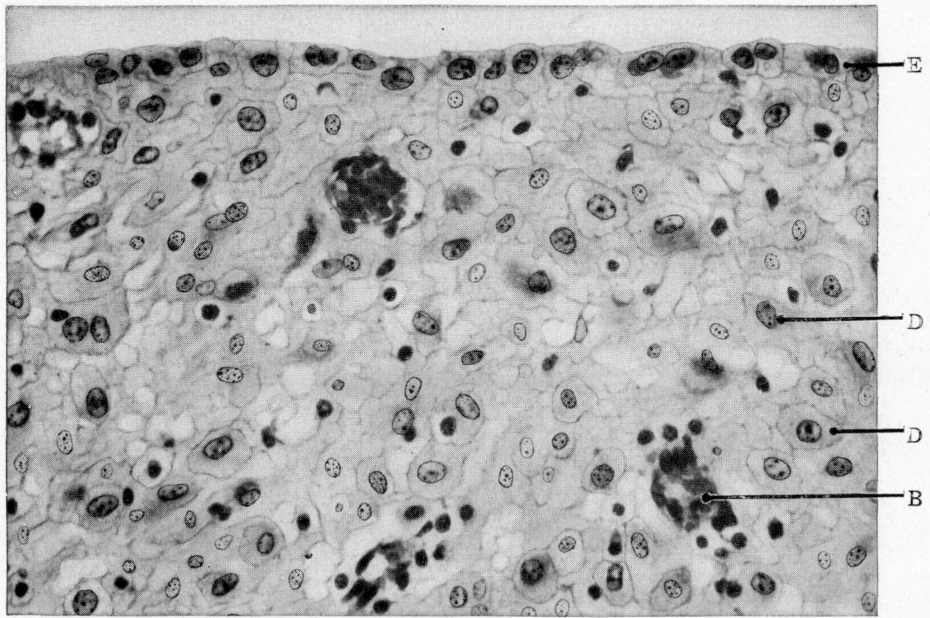

FIG. 110.—DECIDUA VERA, COMPACT LAYER. × 360.
D, decidual cells; E, epithelium; B, blood vessel.

1 cm. After the fourth month, owing to the distention of the uterus, the vera gradually becomes thinner, so that at term it is rarely more than 1 or 2 mm. thick.

Under the microscope the compact layer is seen to be made up of closely packed, large, oval, or polygonal cells, which are distinctly epithelioid in appearance and possess round, vesicular nuclei which stain but slightly with the ordinary reagents. When the tissue has been distended by hemorrhage or edema, it is seen that many of the decidual cells present a stellate appearance, and are provided with long protoplasmic outgrowths which anastomose with similar processes from neighboring cells. Particularly in the early months of pregnancy, one sees scattered among the typical decidual cells a considerable number of small round cells, whose bodies are almost entirely filled by the nucleus. Such cells were formerly considered as lymphoid in character, but Marchand contended that they are forerunners of new decidual cells, basing his contention upon the fact that they frequently contain mitotic figures and that all gradations may be observed between them. In the early months of pregnancy the ducts of the uterine glands may be seen traversing the compact layer, but they soon disappear, so that in the later months all trace of them is lost.

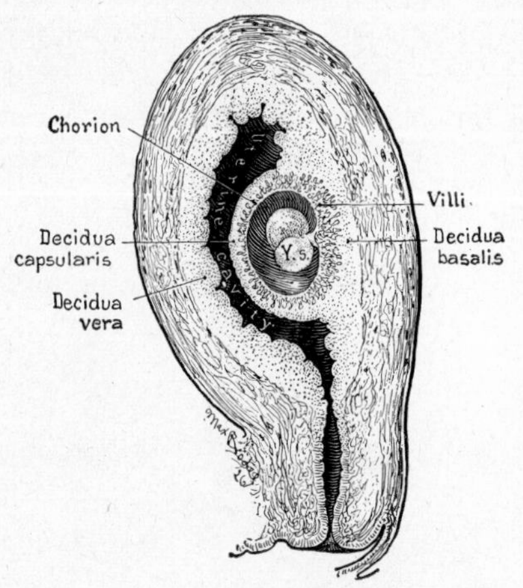

Fig. 111A.—Diagram Showing Chorion Frondosum of Early Pregnancy and Beginning Chorion Laeve (decidua capsularis). (From Williams, *American Journal of Obstetrics and Gynecology.*)

The spongy layer is made up of the distended and hyperplastic glands of the endometrium, which are separated from one another by a minimal amount of stroma. In many instances the glandular hyperplasia is so marked that the spongy layer suggests an adenoma in appearance. At first the glands are lined by typical cylindrical uterine epithelium, which presents evidence of abundant secretory activity. The material secreted probably serves as a pabulum for the ovum pending the establishment of the placental circulation. Later the epithelium gradually becomes cuboidal, or even flattened, in shape and, undergoing fatty degeneration, is cast off in great part into the lumens of the glands. Particularly toward the muscularis, the stroma between the dilated glands undergoes but little change, and closely resembles that of the nonpregnant uterus. For this reason, certain authorities divide the decidua into three layers—compact, functional, and basal—and it is from the basal that the endometrium is regenerated during the first month following labor.

Under the influence of pregnancy, the surface epithelium covering the decidua soon loses its cylindrical shape and becomes cuboidal or flattened, sometimes even resembling endothelium.

Figure 110 represents a section through the compact layer of the decidua vera at the fourth month, while Fig. 32 shows a gland with its surrounding stroma from a nonpregnant endometrium. On comparing them, it is readily seen that the decidua differs from the latter by a marked increase in size of the stroma cells, and by a decrease in size of the epithelial cells. It is now universally held that the decidual cells are derived from the stroma cells of the endometrium, which have undergone marked increase in size but only slight increase in number.

Decidua Capsularis. Except for the first few hours after its entry into the uterus, the ovum is shut off from the rest of the uterine cavity by the decidua capsularis, which forms a capsule of decidual tissue around it. Figure 111A shows an early pregnancy in which the capsularis is quite apparent, and Fig. 111B, a later pregnancy in which it is well developed.

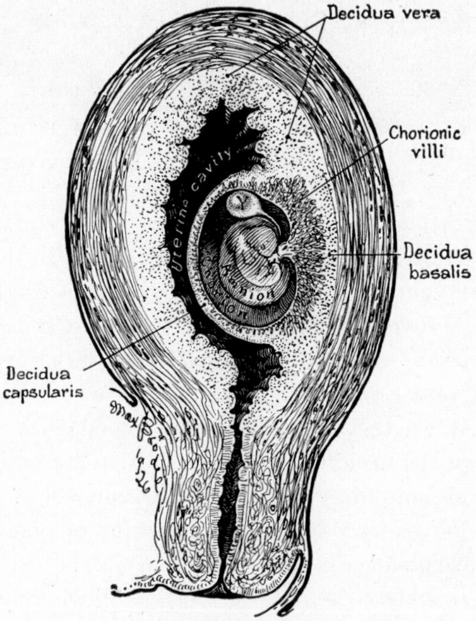

Fig. 111B.—Diagram Showing More Advanced Pregnancy, Atrophic Chorion Laeve, and Chorion Frondosum (chorionic villi) Proliferating into Decidua Basalis. (From Williams, *American Journal of Obstetrics and Gynecology.*)

During the early months of pregnancy the decidua capsularis does not entirely fill the uterine cavity, so that a space of varying size exists between it and the vera. This is shown well in Fig. 113 which represents an eight weeks' pregnant uterus. At the fourth month of pregnancy, however, the growing ovum entirely fills the uterine cavity, so that the capsularis and vera are brought into intimate contact, and the part of the uterine cavity which had remained unoccupied up to that time becomes obliterated. In a short time the two structures fuse together, and then the capsularis gradually degenerates and disappears.

The decidua capsularis usually attains its greatest thickness at about the second month. Sections through it at this time show that it is made up of decidual cells and is covered on its exterior by a single layer of flattened epithelial cells, while internally it is in contact with the fetal villi, and at no time shows any trace of uterine epithelium. In its lowest portion, where it is connected with the vera, a few glands may be found, whose ducts, when present, are seen to open only upon the outer surface of the membrane.

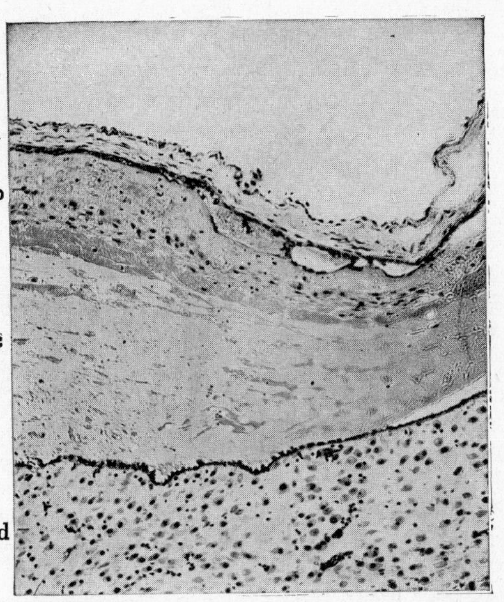

Fig. 112.—Unfused Decidua Vera and Capsularis.

Section through 10-week pregnant uterus, showing that the decidua vera and capsularis have not yet fused. × 1. *a,* amnion and chorionic membrane; *b,* degenerated decidua capsularis; *c,* uterine cavity; *d,* decidua vera.

Decidua Basalis. The decidua basalis is the portion of the decidua which lies immediately beneath the ovum; from it the maternal portion of the placenta is developed. Broadly speaking, it presents the same general structure as the decidua vera, except that it has been invaded by fetal tissue, so that its superficial portions are composed of fetal ectoderm, as well as decidual cells, and frequently of fibrinous degenerative areas to which reference will be made later. Compare Figs. 110 and 117. Giant cells appear in the basalis about the middle of pregnancy. These so-called giant cells are not of decidual origin but represent portions of trophoblast which have invaded the decidua. Fig. 117, representing a section through the decidua basalis in the last month of pregnancy, shows clearly that its superficial portions are composed of a mixture of both fetal and maternal cells.

In the decidua basalis large numbers of blood vessels are observed. The arteries pursue a spiral course and usually penetrate the entire thickness of the membrane while many of the veins become markedly dilated and form large sinuses. These small vessels, after pursuing their course through the superficial layer of the serotina, open into the intervillous spaces of the placenta. The consideration of the vascular connections between the fetus and the uterus, however, will be deferred until we take up the study of the placenta.

Structure of the Placenta in the Early Months. The mode of implantation of the ovum has already been described, and it is generally believed that it usually occurs upon the upper portion of either the anterior or posterior wall of the uterus and only exceptionally upon its lower portion. The ovum is very rarely implanted at the fundus or in the angles, since in these locations the decidual reaction is much less pronounced than elsewhere. After the ovum has burrowed into the depths of the

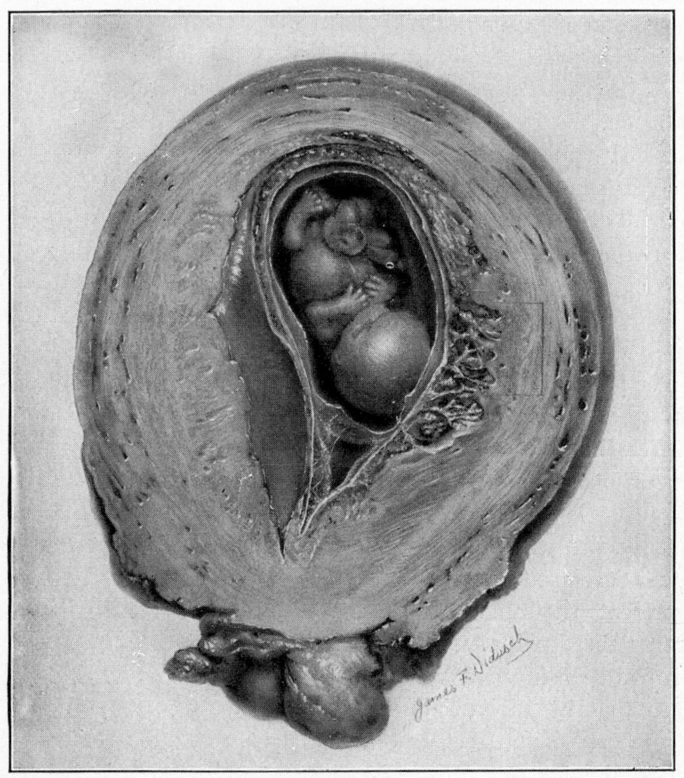

FIG. 113.—SAGITTAL SECTION OF AN EIGHT WEEKS' PREGNANT UTERUS, SLIGHTLY TO ONE SIDE OF THE MIDDLE. × 1.

Note the early placenta on right and thick decidua vera on left side. The embryo lies in the amniotic cavity, outside of which is the chorion and the decidua capsularis. The remnant of the uterine cavity lies between the decidua vera and capsularis. (Carnegie Col. 782.)

decidua, the portion separating it from the uterine cavity is known as the capsularis, and that beneath it as the basalis. It undoubtedly becomes implanted as a blastocyst, in a manner similar to that observed in the monkey. The outer covering of this blastocyst, now designated as the trophoblast, at once begins to proliferate and invade the surrounding decidual tissue. As it does so, it breaks through the walls of maternal capillaries, from which the blood escapes and forms cavities which are bounded partly by trophoblast and partly by decidua (Fig. 118). As the process goes on more vessels are opened up, so that in a short time the trophoblast presents a sievelike appearance, due to the presence of large numbers of blood spaces filled with maternal blood. As a result, the trophoblastic cells become compressed into irregularly shaped masses of varying size, some of which extend from the surface of the ovum to the surrounding decidua and afford the epithelial basis from which the fastening villi are developed.

The maternal blood spaces established in this manner represent the earliest stages in the formation of the *intervillous blood spaces* of the future placenta and are abundantly present in the early ova recently studied. Coincidentally with their formation, the trophoblastic masses are invaded by connective-tissue offshoots from the

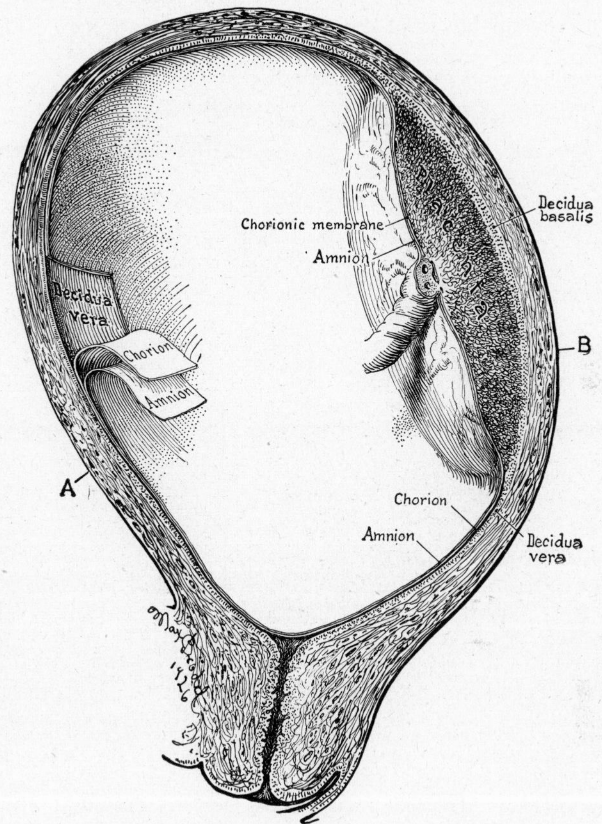

FIG. 114.—DIAGRAM OF UTERUS IN PREGNANCY, SHOWING NORMAL PLACENTA IN SITU.
A, location of section shown in Fig. 115; B, location of section shown in Fig. 116. (From Williams, *American Journal of Obstetrics and Gynecology.*)

chorionic membrane and are thus converted into villi whose epithelial covering becomes arranged in the characteristic two layers.

During the early weeks of pregnancy branching villi project from the entire periphery of the ovum, as is shown well in Fig. 104. They come in contact not only with the decidua basalis, but also with the capsularis, so that for a time intervillous blood spaces surround the entire ovum. As the chorionic villi are devoid of blood vessels for the first few weeks, the ovum must be nourished during that period by osmosis from the maternal fluids.

As pregnancy advances, the blood supply of the decidua basalis becomes more and more abundant, while that of the capsularis diminishes; as a consequence the villi in contact with the former are better nourished and grow more luxuriantly, and it is these which take part in the formation of the placenta. Over the rest of the surface of the ovum the villi develop less rapidly, and eventually atrophy, giving rise to the *chorion laeve* (bald chorion). As the ovum increases in size, the intervillous spaces in the chorion laeve become smaller and smaller, and by the fourth month, when the decidua reflexa has come in contact with the vera, they become obliterated, and the corresponding villi undergo degeneration, but do not completely disappear. For, even at term, sections through the uterine wall (Fig. 115) show that the chorion laeve consists of several layers of chorionic epithelium, through which are scattered

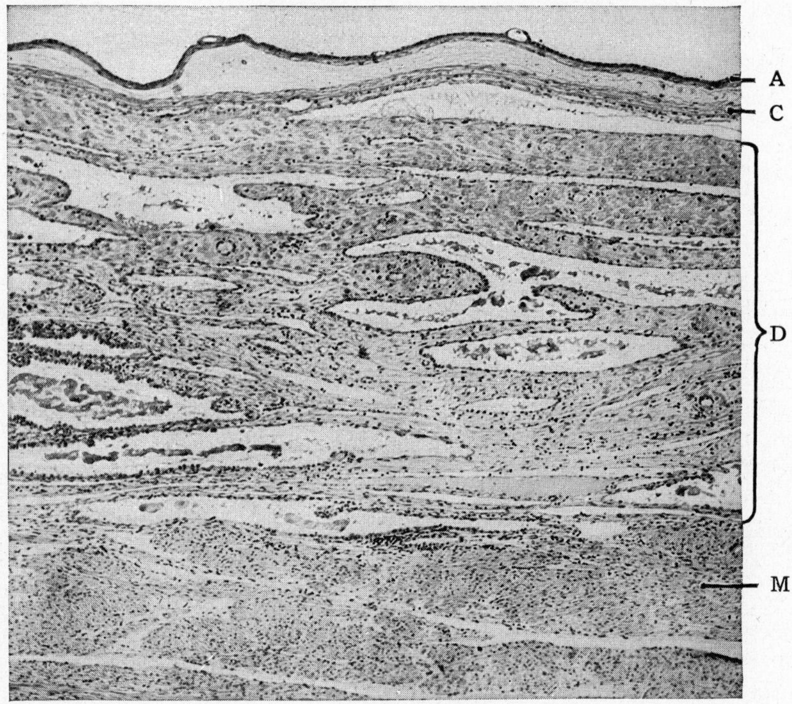

FIG. 115.—SECTION OF FETAL MEMBRANES AND UTERUS OPPOSITE PLACENTAL SITE AT A IN FIG. 114. A, amnion; C, chorion; D, decidua vera; M, muscularis.

round or oblong hyaline bodies, in which a few spindle-shaped nuclei can be distinguished. These are the remains of the earlier villi. At the same time degenerative changes take place—even where the chorionic epithelium comes in contact with the decidual tissue—which result in the formation of fibrin-like material which will be considered in detail later. On the other hand, the villi of the chorion frondosum increase in size and number, and the blood vessels which originate within them connect with branches of the umbilical vessels of the embryo, so that after the first few weeks the fetal circulation extends to the tips of the smallest villi.

The placenta is formed by the union of the chorion frondosum and the decidua basalis, and therefore is composed of both fetal and maternal tissues. It soon constitutes a distinct structure, although its site is indicated at a still earlier period by the point of attachment of the abdominal pedicle to the inner surface of the chorionic membrane.

One can probably best understand the structure of the placenta by studying sections through it at various periods of pregnancy. One from the fourth month shows that the organ is made up in great part of chorionic villi whose stroma presents a somewhat mucoid appearance and contains spindle-shaped and star-shaped connective-tissue cells, between which well-developed arteries, veins and capillaries may be observed. At this stage the villous epithelium is arranged in two layers —Langhans' layer and the syncytium—and from the latter many buds protrude, which, when examined in cross or tangential section, appear as giant cells lying free in the intervillous spaces.

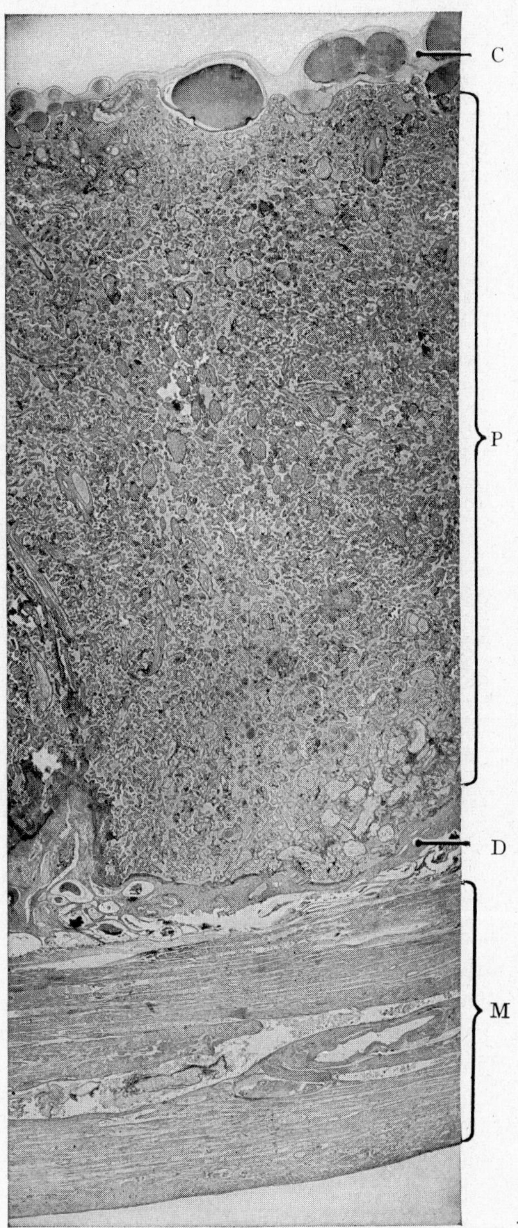

FIG. 116.—SECTION OF PLACENTA AND UTERUS AT B IN FIG. 114. × 7.

C, chorionic plate; P, placental villi; D, decidua basalis; M, muscularis.

The decidua basalis, with which are connected some of the fastening *villi,* extends from the chorionic membrane through the entire thickness of the placenta. At their ends can be noted a marked proliferation of ectodermal cells which invade the underlying decidua, giving rise to the *cell nodes* or *cell columns* and corresponding to the trophoblastic proliferation of the early days of pregnancy. The cell nodes are composed almost exclusively of Langhans' cells, as the syncytium does not follow them down into the depths of the decidua. The great majority of the villi, however, do not reach the decidua but end freely in the intervillous space. The space between the chorionic membrane on the fetal side and the decidua basalis on the maternal side, which is not occupied by villi, is designated as the placental or intervillous space. These spaces are filled with maternal blood and their walls are lined by syncytium. Scattered through them are isolated giant cells—the so-called placental giant cells—whose origin has already been considered. Here and there are seen a few large areas composed of cuboidal or polygonal cells with vesicular nuclei, which frequently present signs of degeneration. These are the so-called trophoblastic islands, which represent masses of trophoblast which have not received a core of connective tissue and therefore have not developed into typical villi. As they contain no vessels and are nourished solely by osmosis from the maternal blood contained in the intervillous spaces, they are very prone to degenerative changes and play a considerable part in the production of placental lesions, which will be considered in their appropriate place. They were formerly called decidual

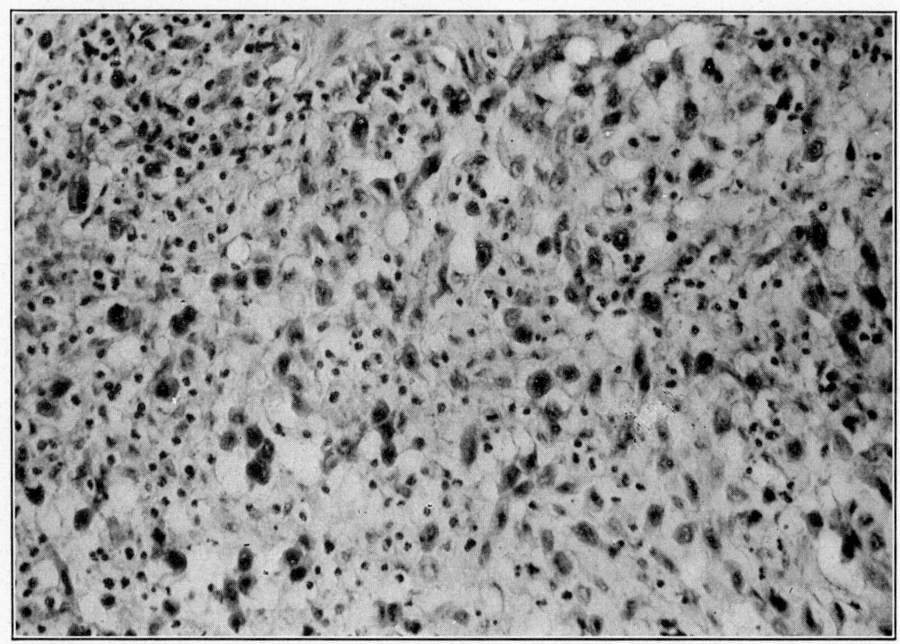

Fig. 117.—Decidua Basalis Showing Mixture of Fetal Giant Cells and Maternal Decidual Cells. × 245.

islands, and were supposed to represent sections through decidual septa, which projected from the decidual basalis toward the chorionic membrane. With our present knowledge of the development of the placenta such a view is no longer tenable.

At the junction between the fetal and decidual tissue, areas are noted which stain deeply with eosin, and which, on closer examination, are seen to be made up of fibrinoid material, honeycombed in various directions by small spaces—*canalized fibrin*. This results from the degeneration of both fetal and decidual cells, and is known as Nitabuch's layer, from the author who first called attention to its presence in the decidua. It would seem that degenerative changes of this type occur wherever fetal and maternal tissues come in contact, and the phenomenon suggests that a very important function of the decidua is to protect the maternal organism against invasion by fetal cells. That this is not a fanciful conception is shown by the fact that whenever the decidual reaction is defective or lacking the growing villi may invade the maternal tissues almost like a malignant growth. This is observed in tubal pregnancy, in placenta accreta, as well as in certain rare cases of spontaneous rupture of the uterus.

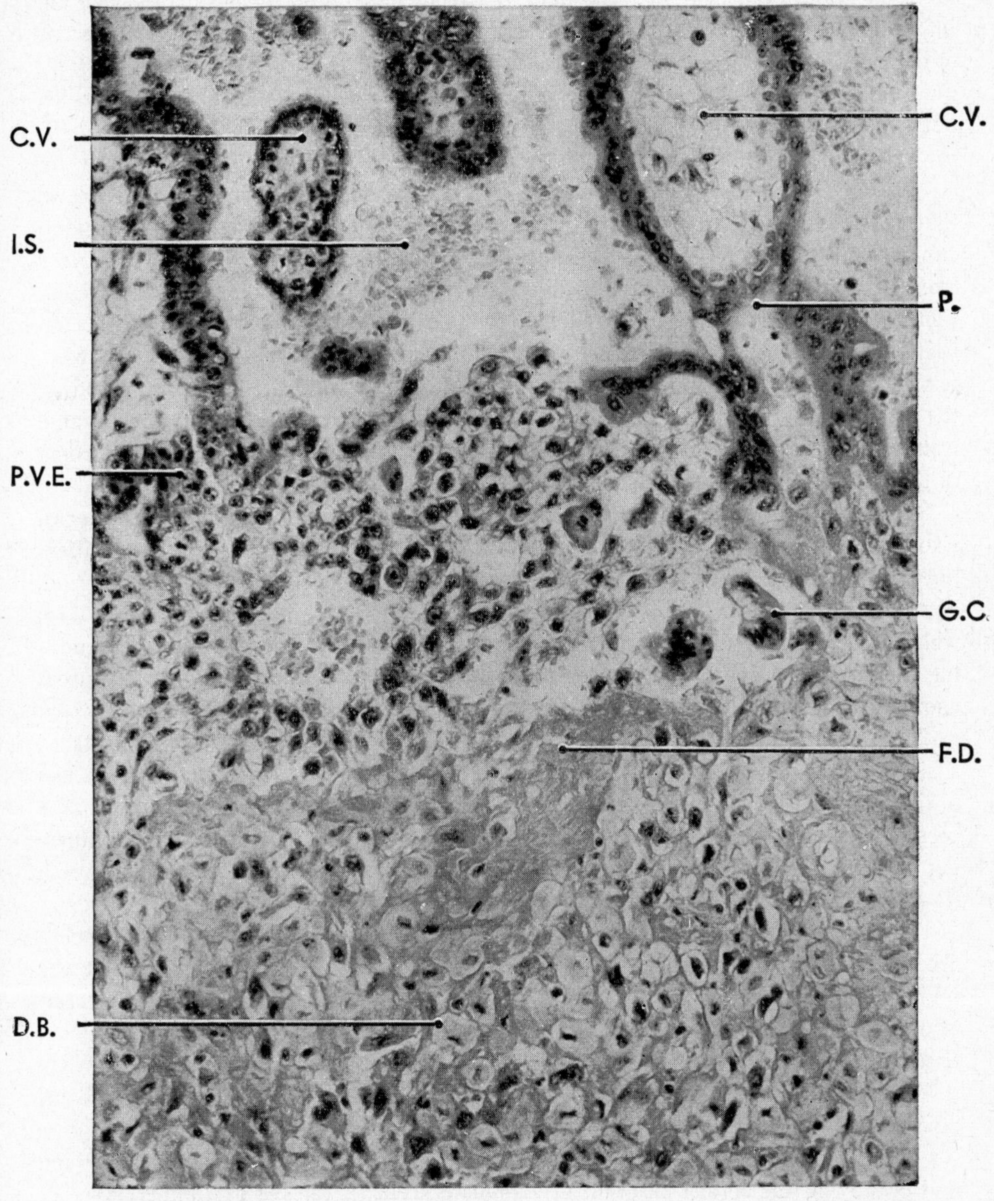

FIG. 118.—SECTION THROUGH JUNCTION OF CHORION AND DECIDUA BASALIS. FOURTH MONTH OF GESTATION. × 245.

CV, chorionic villi; D.B., decidua basalis; I.S., intervillous space containing maternal blood; F.D., fibrinoid degeneration; G.C., giant cell; P.V.E., proliferating villous epithelium; P., tip of villus projecting into a maternal blood vessel.

It has long been held that the maternal blood flows very sluggishly through the intervillous spaces, but the extremely rapid rate at which heavy water, radioactive sodium and other isotopes pass back and forth across the placenta would raise some question about this old tenet. At one point in Fig. 118 a maternal vessel is seen opening directly into the intervillous space, with the tip of the villus marked "P." projecting into its lumen. This is not uncommon, as the ends of villi may grow for a considerable distance into vessels. In such circumstances it has long been known that portions of villi may become broken off, and thus gain access to the general circulation. In the course of such breaking off and deportation of villi, it is very likely that minute amounts of fetal blood may gain access to the maternal circulation along with the villi. This possibility will be important to bear in mind in connection with the modern theory of Rh iso-immunization (page 1011). Otherwise, fetal blood in the chorionic vessels at no time mixes with the maternal blood in the intervillous spaces, and during the first half of pregnancy the two are separated from each other by the double layer of chorionic epithelium, a portion of the stroma of the villus, and the vessel walls.

Structure of Placenta in Latter Half of Pregnancy and at Full Term. Except in its increased size, the placenta in the second half of pregnancy differs but slightly from that of the fourth month. Microscopic sections at this period, however, show certain points of difference. These are well illustrated in Fig. 116, which represents a section through a term placenta and the adjacent decidua. Studying it from above downward, we see that it is composed of the following structures: chorionic plate, placental villi, and decidua basalis.

The amnion covers the inner or fetal surface of the placenta, and consists of a single layer of cuboidal epithelium, below which comes a layer of more or less fibrillar connective tissue containing no blood vessels. The chorionic membrane presents essentially the same structure as in the earlier months of pregnancy, differing only in the presence of a large amount of canalized fibrin immediately beneath its epithelium, as well as in the presence of larger vessels.

The great bulk of the placenta is made up of chorionic villi, whose branches are much more abundant, but at the same time considerably smaller, than at the fourth month. Their stroma, which is made up of spindle-shaped cells, is denser, is occupied in great part by blood vessels, and differs materially from the mucoid tissue of the earlier months. These changes have already been referred to.

The epithelium covering the villi has also undergone marked change; Langhans' layer has disappeared and there remains only a thin layer of syncytium, which gives rise to fewer buds than previously. In many villi immediately under the epithelium, and occupying the former position of Langhans' cells, a thicker or thinner layer of canalized fibrin may be observed. This was first described by Langhans, is of constant occurrence in the latter half of pregnancy, and is probably indicative of senility of the organ. At the same time, many of the arteries present all stages of an obliterating endarteritis, to which, in part, the formation of the tissue in question should be attributed.

The superficial portion of the decidua at this period is covered by a layer of canalized fibrin of varying thickness, which probably results from the necrosis following the contact of fetal trophoblast with maternal decidua. In the deeper layers numerous giant cells are observed, which occasionally extend deeply into the connective-tissue septa between the muscle fibers. They are of various shapes and represent portions of trophoblast which have wandered down into the decidua.

From the free surface of the decidua numerous elevations of varying shape and size extend for a greater or lesser distance toward the chorionic membrane. These are the trophoblastic or, as formerly designated, the decidual septa. They are composed of cuboidal or polygonal cells with round, vesicular, deeply staining nuclei and represent masses of trophoblast which have not been converted into villi. Owing to the absence of blood vessels they are very prone to degenerative change and tend to become converted into canalized fibrin, or to lead to the formation of small cystic structures.

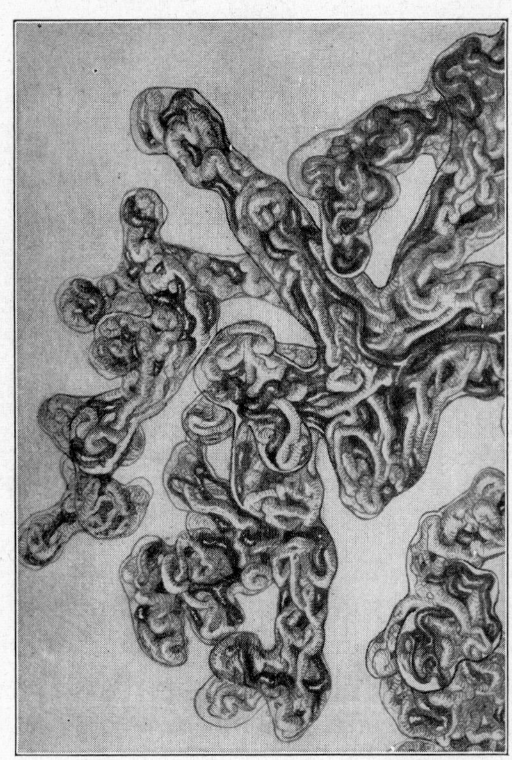

FIG. 119.—BLOOD VESSELS OF CHORIONIC VILLUS.

The space between the chorionic membrane and the free surface of the decidua basalis is designated as the *placental space;* into this the chorionic villi dip, thereby subdividing it into myriads of irregularly shaped cavities which communicate freely with one another — the intervillous spaces. These are lined throughout by syncytium, except where it has given place to canalized fibrin. The syncytium is thinner than in the earlier months, and under suitable magnification its protoplasm presents a vacuolated appearance, which, according to Marchand, is due to the glycogen normally contained in it having been dissolved out by the fluids used in hardening the tissue.

The intervillous spaces are at no time lined by endothelial cells, and it is probable that what had formerly been described as such, in reality, represents thinned-out syncytium. Hence, it would appear that the intervillous spaces are lined entirely by fetal tissue, and that the maternal blood, which is circulating through them, lies outside of the maternal tissues. The maternal blood gains access to the placental space by branches of the uterine arteries, which pursue a convoluted course through the decidua basalis and, after their walls have gradually become reduced to a single layer of endothelium, open upon the sides of the decidual septa. The blood escapes from the intervillous spaces through more or less funnel-shaped openings upon the surface of the decidua, which can be traced directly into large venous sinuses in its depths. Consequently, there must be a distinct circulation through the intercommunicating intervillous spaces, though it is said to be very sluggish. Grosser believes that it is maintained entirely by the intermittent contractions of the uterine muscle, as he holds that the terminal ends of the uterine arteries are so thinned out that a *vis a tergo* cannot be concerned.

In view of these facts, then, the placenta must be regarded as a collection of maternal blood, included between the chorionic membrane and the decidua basalis, into which the villi dip and by which they are surrounded. The injection studies of Kearns reveal that the placenta is capable of reconstruction of portions of its vascular system affected by senile or sclerotic changes, should functional demands require increased circulation. Jonen states that the capacity of the intervillous space

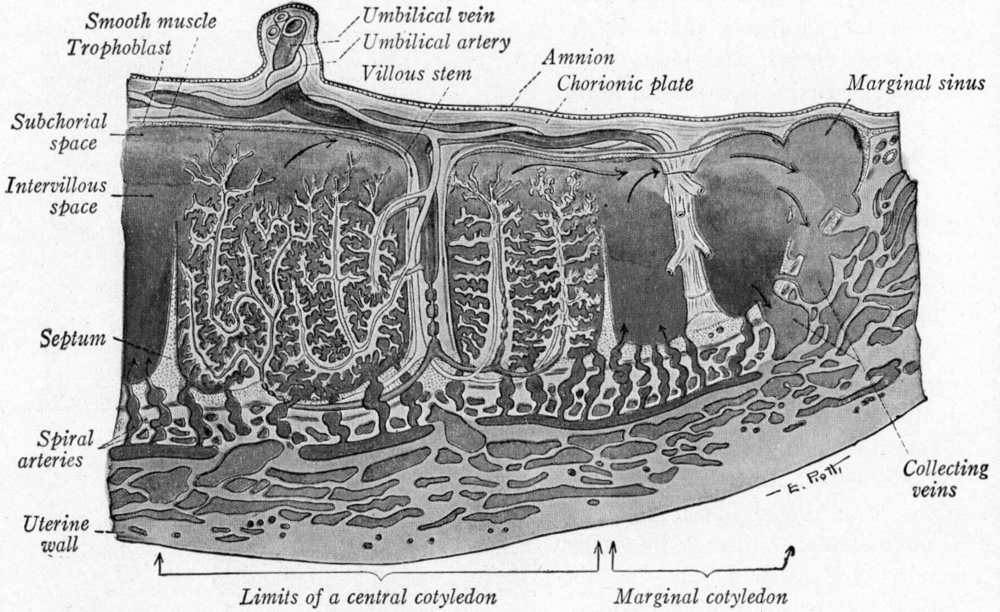

Fig. 120.—Scheme of Circulation in the Human Placenta, as Shown in Vertical Section.

For diagrammatic purposes the half of the placenta shown here is represented as bearing just one chorionic villus and the stump of another extending into the intervillous spaces of the cotyledons. (From Arey, *Developmental Anatomy,* 5th edition, W. B. Saunders Company, Philadelphia.)

varies greatly, and places the lower and upper limits at 90 and 330 cc., respectively. It would appear that the complicated arrangement of the villi is a device by which the greatest possible area of chorionic tissue can be exposed to the maternal blood within a small space. Dodds and Rech have calculated that the exposed surface of the villi equals an area of approximately 7.0 and 6.3 square meters, respectively, findings in agreement with this theory.

The After-birth. The placenta, as it is cast off from the uterus after the birth of the child, is a flattened, roundish, or oval organ—15 to 20 cm. in diameter, and 2 to 3 cm. in height at its thickest part—from the margins of which the membranes extend. Ordinarily its weight is about one sixth of that of the fetus, so that when the latter is normally developed the placenta weighs from 500 to 600 gm.

It presents for examination two surfaces and a margin—the surface which was in contact with the decidua basalis being designated as the maternal or outer, and that directed toward the cavity of the ovum as the fetal or inner surface. The

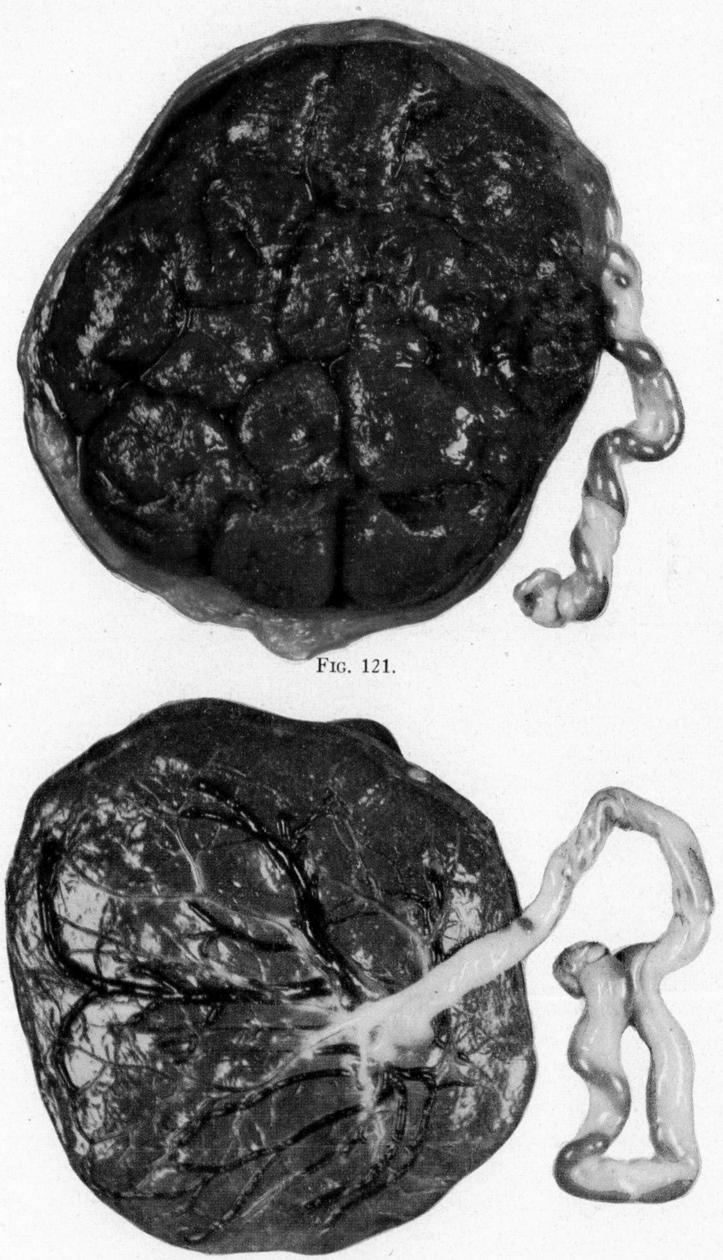

Fig. 121.

Fig. 122.

Fig. 121.—Maternal Surface of Normal Mature Placenta. Fig. 122.—Fetal Surface of Same Placenta.

outer is covered by a thin layer of decidua and presents a ragged, torn appearance, being divided by depressions of varying depth into a number of irregularly shaped areas, the so-called *cotyledons,* which vary considerably in number, as many as 20 being sometimes observed. On careful examination of the decidual surface, numerous vessels may be seen which have been torn through when the placenta was separated.

The fetal or inner surface presents a glistening appearance, owing to the fact that it is covered by amnion, which, however, is only slightly adherent. When the latter is removed it leaves a coarsely granular surface, upon which the umbilical cord is usually inserted somewhat eccentrically, though it may be just at the center of the organ or near its margin. The various modes of insertion will be considered when we take up the abnormalities of the placenta.

The vessels composing the umbilical cord spread out beneath the amnion and rapidly divide, but the main branches remain upon the fetal surface of the placenta until its margin is reached. In many instances a large vein, which is known as the circular sinus, extends around a portion of the periphery of the placenta, but only rarely completely encircles it.

The *fetal membranes* extend from the margins of the placenta, and consist of the amnion, chorion, and a thin layer of decidua. The amnion, the innermost of the membranes, is a thin, transparent, glistening structure, which is rarely thicker than a sheet of writing paper. Its outer surface is closely applied to the chorion, from which, however, it can usually be separated without difficulty. The chorion is more opaque and thicker than the amnion, though it rarely exceeds 1 mm. in thickness. It represents the chorion laeve of the early months, and under the microscope is seen to possess a number of degenerated villi. Clinging to its outer surface are a few shreds of decidual tissue, which is all that is cast off immediately after the birth of the child. Figure 115 represents a section through the fetal membranes and the uterine wall outside of the placental site and gives a good idea of their composition.

Umbilical Cord. The umbilical cord, or funis, extends from the navel of the child to the fetal surface of the placenta. Its exterior presents a dull white, moist appearance, and through it shimmer the umbilical vessels—two arteries and a vein. It varies from 1 to 2.5 cm. in diameter and averages about 55 cm. in length, though in extreme cases it may vary from 0.5 to 198 cm. The average length of 1,000 cords, which Williams measured, was 55 cm., the shortest being less than 1 and the longest 100 cm.

A cord frequently presents a twisted appearance, the coiling usually being from left to right. As the vessels are usually longer than the cord, they are frequently folded upon themselves, thus giving rise to nodulations upon the surface which are designated as *false knots.*

The cord is covered by a sheath of amnion which is closely adherent to it. Under the microscope, the covering epithelium usually consists of a single layer of flattened cells, although occasionally it is arranged in several layers resembling those of the skin. Except for the large vessels, the interior of the cord is made up of a watery connective tissue called *Wharton's jelly.* In the opinion of Reynolds, this jelly-like substance, which surrounds the umbilical vessels, may play an important role in the propulsion of blood through them. The usual concept of the blood vessels in the umbilical cord is shown in Fig. 123. This is a section of a human umbilical cord showing the two umbilical arteries and the single vein surrounded by a large amount of Wharton's jelly. However, the relative magnitude of the arteries and vein cannot be judged from such a picture inasmuch as the tissues were fixed after the blood vessels were empty. In Fig. 124, a section of the same cord is shown from a segment which had not been emptied of blood, and here an entirely different impression is obtained. This shows that the arteries are smaller in diameter than the vein and that all three are of considerable size. Moreover, the Wharton's jelly has now been stretched excessively around the blood vessels with the result

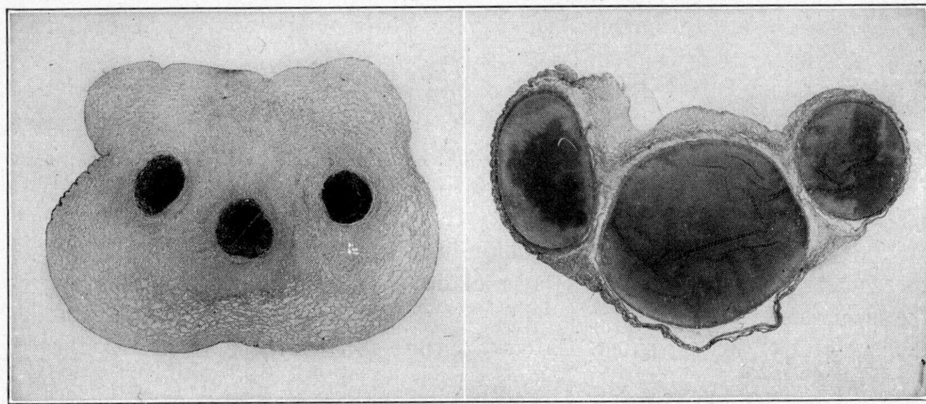

FIG. 123.—CROSS SECTION OF UMBILICAL CORD FIXED AFTER BLOOD VESSELS HAD BEEN EMPTIED.

The umbilical vein, carrying arterial blood to the fetus, is in the center, and, on either side, are the two umbilical arteries which carry venous blood from the fetus to the placenta (Reynolds).

FIG. 124.—CROSS SECTION OF SAME UMBILICAL CORD AS SHOWN IN FIG. 123, BUT FROM A SEGMENT IN WHICH THE BLOOD VESSELS HAD NOT BEEN EMPTIED.

This probably represents the conditions which actually exist in utero (Reynolds).

that this jelly, which occupies a small space when the blood vessels are distended, must exert in the living condition a force tending to make the blood vessels collapse. It is important, therefore, that an adequate pressure be maintained in both the arteries and vein if flow of blood is to be maintained within them. As a consequence, in Reynolds' opinion, the living umbilical cord is a semirigid structure. Wharton's jelly has another important function, namely, through its high water content, to facilitate easy dessication of the cord after birth. This dessication of the cord is the chief factor in the dropping off of the cord stump early in neonatal life.

The umbilical cord proper contains no demonstrable nerves, but Spivack has recently demonstrated nonmedullated nerve fibers in the abdominal portion of the umbilical arteries. Hence, there is no neurological connection whatsoever between mother and fetus. This fact is important to note in connection with the old and erroneous notion that psychological disturbances in the mother may "mark" the fetus—the doctrine of "maternal impressions." All experience, moreover, contradicts this old idea.

On microscopic examination of sections through any portion of the cord, one generally finds near its center a small, darkly stained area, which under higher magnification appears as a small duct lined by a single layer of cuboidal or flattened epithelial cells and surrounded by a zone of relatively dense connective tissue. This is the duct or stalk of the umbilical vesicle. On the other hand, in sections taken just beyond the umbilicus of the fetus, one occasionally finds a second duct, which represents the remnant of the allantois, but this is never found at the maternal end of the cord.

Formerly it was taught that the cord was derived from the allantois, but since the researches of His it has been generally recognized that such is not the case in man. In the youngest human ova, in which the embryo consists merely of a minute amnion and yolk sac, it is connected with the inner surface of the chorionic membrane by a thick mass of mesodermic or connective tissue, which His designated as the abdominal pedicle or body stalk, and which, after increasing in length and receiving a covering of amnion, becomes converted into the umbilical cord. Furthermore, the allantois in man at no time develops into the imposing organ which it becomes in many animals, but always remains a rudimentary structure, being represented by an entodermal tubule at the fetal end of the abdominal pedicle.

A section through the abdominal pedicle of one of the early embryos studied by His clearly shows its analogy with the embryonic area. The great bulk of the structure is made up of mesodermic tissue in which the umbilical vessels and the allantois are embedded; its dorsal surface is covered by a single layer of ectoderm, showing at its middle a slight depression which represents a continuation of the medullary groove, while arching over it is the amnion. In its further development, the amnion, corresponding to the somatopleure, extends downward and inward, eventually inclosing a small portion of the celom in a way similar to that in which the abdominal walls are formed in the embryo itself. In this cavity the stalk of the umbilical vesicle or yolk sac is included.

Umbilical Vesicle. The yolk sac, or, as it becomes later, the umbilical vesicle, is a very prominent organ at the beginning of pregnancy, and is present in all ova. In its earliest stages it represents the largest and most striking structure connected with the embryo, but as the latter develops, it becomes relatively smaller, and, as we have already shown, is taken up in great part to form the intestinal canal, so that after the formation of the abdominal walls it protrudes from the umbilicus into the celomic cavity as a rounded sac with a distinct stalk. As pregnancy advances the sac becomes smaller and its stalk longer.

The structure persists through pregnancy, and can frequently be found at full term, when it is represented by a flattened oval sac, 3 to 5 mm. in diameter, which usually lies on the fetal surface of the placenta, between the chorion and amnion, but occasionally in the membranes just beyond the placental margin. It is connected with the umbilical cord by a fine pedicle, the *stalk,* which, as has been already indicated, may be seen in sections through the cord at term. Schultze in 1861 was able to demonstrate the umbilical vesicle in 146 out of 150 mature placentas examined. Meyer has found that the vesicle may sometimes exceed the usual proportions, and measure as much as 10 to 15 mm. in diameter.

The intra-abdominal portion of the duct of the umbilical vesicle, which extends from the umbilicus to the intestine, usually atrophies and disappears, but occasionally it remains patent, forming what is known as *Meckel's diverticulum,* which sometimes plays a very important pathological part in later life.

In animals whose ova possess a large amount of yolk, the umbilical vesicle is the main source of nutrition for the embryo; but in humans its significance is not so clear, since the proportion of yolk is exceedingly small. In some of the lower animals it affords a means of vascularizing the chorion, while in still others it takes part in the formation of an accessory placenta, in addition to the main one which is vascularized by vessels originating primarily in the chorionic membrane. It must, however, play an important part in the economy of the human embryo, as it develops a considerable circulation, and, as Selenka has shown, forms numerous crypts from its entodermal lining.

THE PLACENTAL HORMONES

Chorionic Gonadotrophin

At least as early as the sixtieth day of pregnancy, as stated in Chapter 3, the placenta begins to produce estrogen and progesterone, and it continues to provide these hormones in increasing amounts until the very end of pregnancy. At an even earlier date, within 10 days after ovulation, the trophoblast elaborates still a third hormone, a special hormone of its own, chorionic gonadotrophin. This substance was discovered in the urine of pregnant women by Aschheim and Zondek in 1928 and was at first thought to be of pituitary origin. However, it was promptly found to differ decidedly from the pituitary gonadotrophic hormones, and to derive from the epithelium of the chorionic villus, probably Langhans' layer.

Chemistry. Despite extensive investigation the specific chemical nature of chorionic gonadotrophin is unknown. It appears, however, to be a glycoprotein with a large molecular weight of at least 80,000. The original method of standardization made use of its effect, via the ovary, on the vaginal epithelium of the immature rat. A rat unit is defined as the amount required to induce cornification of the vaginal epithelium in the immature rat. Obviously, the use of this procedure necessitates the exclusion of any estrogenic substance from the material tested. Since the chorionic hormone exerts its effect through its action on the ovary (follicle development, luteinization, estrogen production, and so on), it will not induce estrus in the spayed animal. It may also be assayed by means of its action through the ovary on the uterine weight of immature rats as in the test employed by Delfs. The specific gonadotrophic action of 0.1 mg. of an arbitrarily adopted standard prepared in dried form and deposited at the National Institute of Health, London, has been accepted as the international unit. The international unit is equal approximately to one rat unit.

Actions. The action of chorionic gonadotrophin on the rodent ovary and on the ovary of the human must be sharply differentiated. In the immature female rodent it induces maturation of follicles, followed by ovulation and corpus luteum formation. Since in hypophysectomized mature animals it does not induce maturation of the follicles or their conversion into true corpora lutea, but causes simply theca luteinization with estrogen secretion, chorionic gonadotrophin must be regarded predominantly as a luteinizing hormone with no intrinsic follicle-stimulating powers. The latter effects, when produced in the intact animal, are presumably due to the activation of the animal's own hypophysis by this hormone. From a practical viewpoint, the effects which chorionic gonadotrophin exerts on the rodent ovary are of great importance, for they constitute the basis of the more commonly employed tests for pregnancy (page 243).

In the human as well as the monkey, chorionic gonadotrophin causes neither follicular maturation nor luteinization, but rather degenerative changes. Thus, if administered during the follicular phase of the cycle in the adult female monkey, atretic involution with suppression of estrogen secretion ensues. Likewise, in the immature female monkey, Engle has shown that the chorionic hormone causes atresia of the large follicles and hyalinization of the small ones. Various attempts have been made to study the action of chorionic gonadotrophin on the human ovary by injecting extracts of this hormone into women for several days to several weeks prior to pelvic surgery. The studies of Geist, of Hamblen and of Pratt all agree in showing that chorionic gonadotrophin, when injected into women, does not stimulate ovulation or corpus luteum formation, but tends rather to promote follicular atresia. On the other hand, Hamblen believes that this hormone is capable of augmenting and extending the function of an already existing corpus luteum. This he bases on his observation that the administration of chorionic gonadotrophin in women in the luteal phase of the cycle is followed by a rise in pregnanediol excretion and prolongation of the luteal phase. Confirmation of the latter action is found in the work of Browne and Venning, who showed that if chorionic gonadotrophin is given to women after the luteal phase of the cycle has begun, this phase could be extended as long as 17 days. In sum, it would appear that the main effects of chorionic gonadotrophin in women are the promotion of follicular atresia and, in all probability, the augmentation and prolongation of function of an already existing corpus luteum.

Function of Chorionic Gonadotrophin in Human Pregnancy. It will be recalled that the corpus luteum of menstruation has a life span of about 8 to 10 days and then, if conception has not taken place, it degenerates. If, however, a fertilized ovum has embedded itself (and let it be remembered that implantation occurs about the sixth day of the luteal phase), the corpus luteum does not degenerate but continues to flourish as the corpus luteum of pregnancy. In other words, during the two days after implantation, the fertilized ovum does something which forestalls degeneration of the corpus luteum and promotes its continuation. Although it is difficult to prove, the circumstantial evidence as stated above indicates that the embedded ovum is able to effect continuation of the corpus luteum through its manufacture of chorionic gonadotrophin and through the action of the latter on an already existing corpus luteum. The extension of the life of the corpus luteum and the continued production of progesterone and estrogen which result, prevent, in turn, the collapse of the endometrial bed. As a consequence, menstruation does not ensue, and the thick, secretory endometrium continues to thrive as a suitable nidation place for the growing ovum (Fig. 125).

Contrast between Chorionic and Hypophyseal Gonadotrophins. The chorionic and hypophyseal gonadotrophins are two entirely different substances, as demonstrated by several facts. For instance, in hypophysectomized animals, the former can in no wise substitute for the latter. Thus, in the hypophysectomized rodent, the administration of pituitary gonadotrophin completely repairs the gonadal atrophy which has been produced, causing a resumption of follicular growth and a resumption of estrus; contrariwise, the administration of chorionic gonadotrophin produces only a slight effect on the interstitial tissue and nothing else. As already

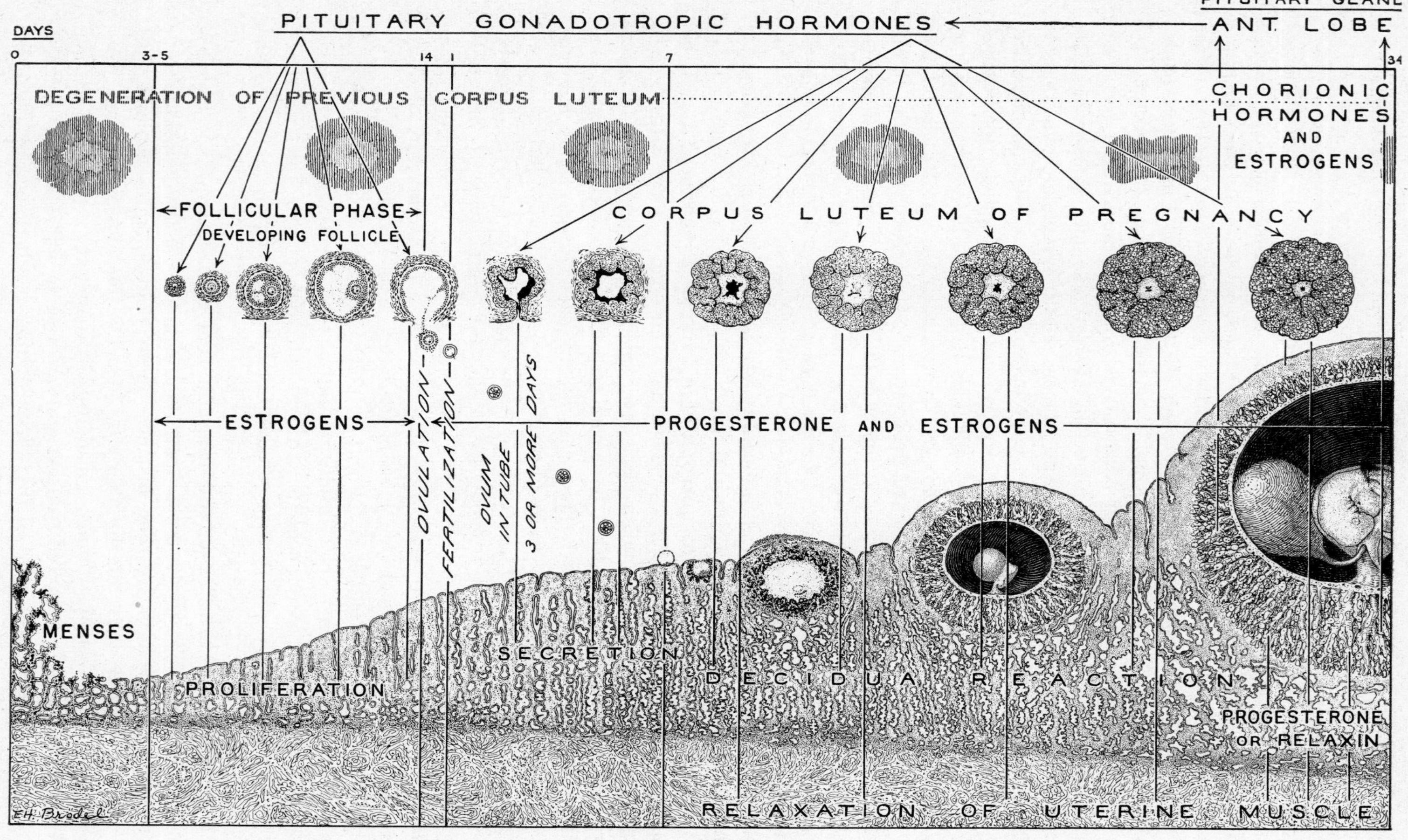

FIG. 125.—THE OVARIAN CYCLE, THE ENDOMETRIAL CYCLE, DECIDUAL DEVELOPMENT AND RELATED HORMONE ACTION IN A CYCLE IN WHICH CONCEPTION OCCURRED.

noted, chorionic gonadotrophin causes retrogressive changes in the ovaries of immature monkeys; on the other hand, hypophyseal gonadotrophin produces follicle development and estrogen production as evidenced by reddening of the sexual skin (Engle). Among other differences between the two substances are their respective effects on ovarian weight in rodents. When increasing doses of hypophyseal gonadotrophin are administered to immature rats and mice, the ovaries show a corresponding augmentation in weight to a point where a 300 per cent increase may be observed. On the other hand, if the same experiment is repeated with chorionic gonadotrophin, some increase in ovarian weight is observed, but it soon reaches a plateau.

Source of Chorionic Gonadotrophin. The source of chorionic gonadotrophin is the epithelial covering of the chorionic villus; that is, the trophoblast which must be regarded as the parenchyma of the placenta. Gey, Jones and Hellman, and Jones, Gey and Gey have demonstrated that tissue cultures containing actively growing trophoblast produce appreciable amounts of chorionic gonadotrophin even after repeated transplantation over a period of several months. Furthermore, these observations, as well as the previous ones of Sengupta, indicate that it is the Langhans' layer, or the cytotrophoblast, that survives and proliferates in these tissue cultures. In this connection many observers have emphasized that the curve of excretion of gonadotrophic hormone in the pregnant woman parallels approximately the rise and decline of the Langhans' layer, or cytotrophoblast, rather than the slow, steady increase in the amount of syncytial trophoblast.

Blood and Urine Values. The range of blood levels of chorionic gonadotrophin which are encountered in pregnancy are shown in Figs. 126 and 127, taken from the studies of Jones, Delfs and Stran. When it is noted that the concentration of the hormone in the latter chart is plotted on a logarithmic scale, it becomes evident that the most conspicuous feature of the curve is a stupendous increase in blood levels between the fiftieth and sixty-fifth days of pregnancy, counting from the first day of the last menstrual period. The peak averages over 120,000 and may rise as high as a half million international units per liter, a fact to be borne in mind in connection with the high levels also encountered in certain pathological conditions; notably, hydatidiform mole and chorionepithelioma (page 532). The urinary excretion of chorionic gonadotrophin follows a similar curve. According to the investigations of Venning, chorionic gonadotrophin appears in the urine within a few days after implantation of the ovum, that is, between the twenty-second and twenty-fifth days of the cycle. The excretion values augment gradually until the thirty-second day after the last menstrual period, when they vary between 200 and 500 rat units per liter. It may be noted parenthetically that these concentrations, which are reached shortly after the first missed period, are just beginning to be of sufficient degree to give a positive reaction to the commonly employed hormonal tests for pregnancy. Prior to the first missed period, the amount of chorionic gonadotrophin in the urine, although detectable by refined methods, is not usually enough to give a positive reaction to the ordinary tests. Subsequently, the excretion increases with extreme rapidity to reach a peak between the fifty-second and sixty-fifth days of 133,000 to 400,000 rat units per liter per 24 hours. The peak lasts only a few days. After the sixty-seventh day a sharp decline occurs down to values of about 40,000 rat units per liter; after the one-hundred-twentieth day, the values range between 1,000 and 10,000 rat units per liter.

The mechanism and significance of this extraordinary blood and excretion curve are not understood but, as indicated, it probably parallels the growth and activity of the Langhans' layer. Following delivery, chorionic gonadotrophin normally disappears from the blood and urine within 3 to 10 days.

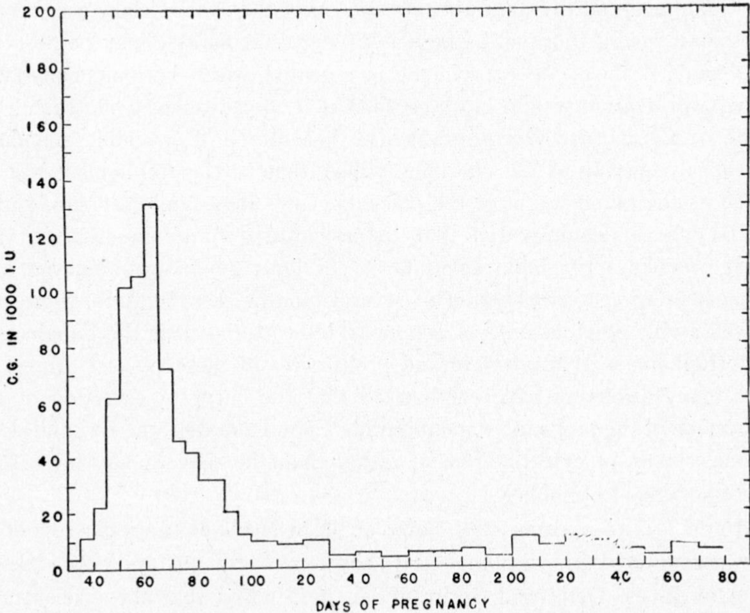

FIG. 126.—AVERAGE CONCENTRATION OF SERUM GONADOTROPHIN AT VARIOUS TIMES IN NORMAL PREGNANCY, BASED ON 24 CASES (Delfs).

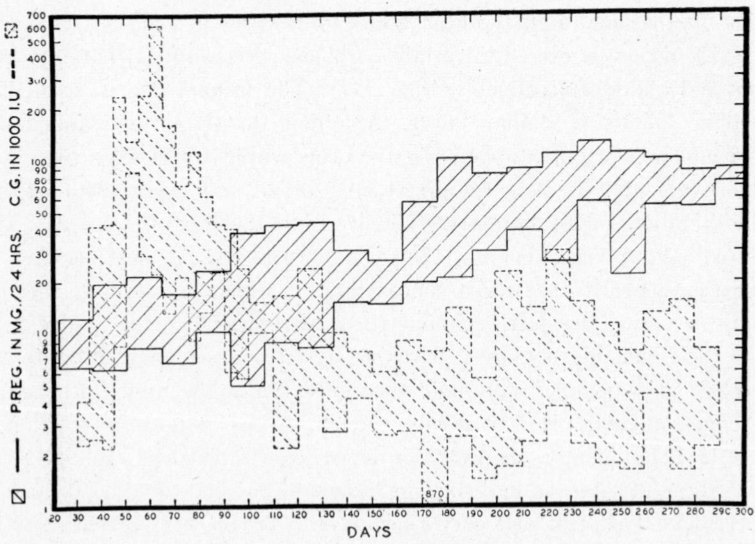

FIG. 127.—RANGE OF CONCENTRATION OF SERUM GONADOTROPHIN AND RANGE OF DAILY EXCRETION OF PREGNANEDIOL AT VARIOUS TIMES IN NORMAL PREGNANCY, BASED ON 19 CASES (Delfs).

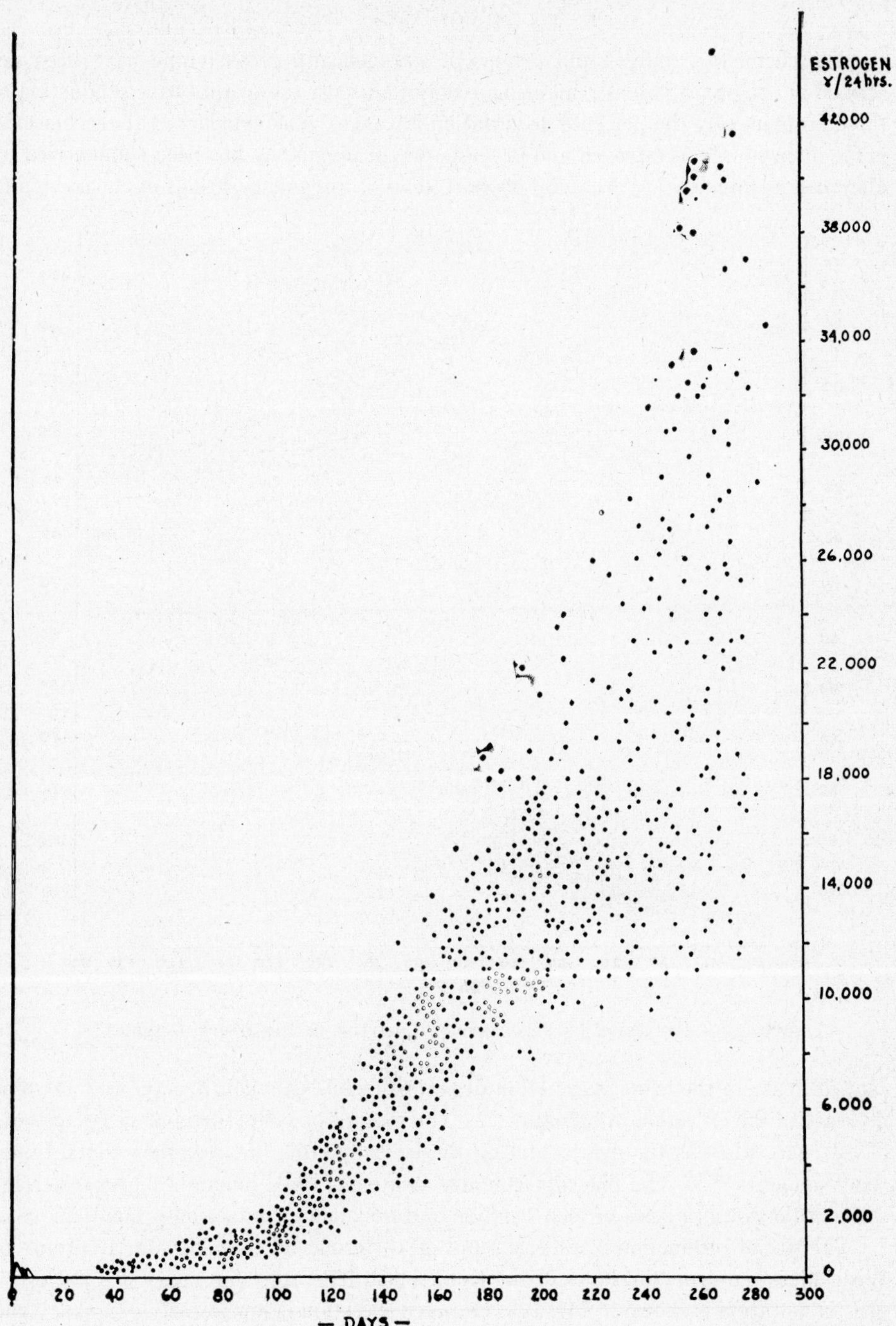

Fig. 128.—Excretion of Total Estrogens in Pregnancy (Venning).

Estrogen and Progesterone

The chemistry, sources and actions of estrogen and progesterone have been described in Chapter 3, and it remains here only to discuss the quantitative production of these hormones by the placenta as gestation advances. The evidence that the placenta is the main source of estrogen and progesterone in pregnancy has been summarized by Hamblen as follows: (1) Bilateral oophorectomy in pregnancy brings about no significant decrease in the urinary excretion of pregnanediol, although it may produce some decrease in the excretion of estrogen. (2) The mature placenta contains large amounts of estrogen, whereas the ovaries during the latter months of pregnancy contain only small amounts. (3) The placenta contains relatively large amounts of progesterone, whereas the corpora lutea of menstruation and pregnancy contain only small amounts.

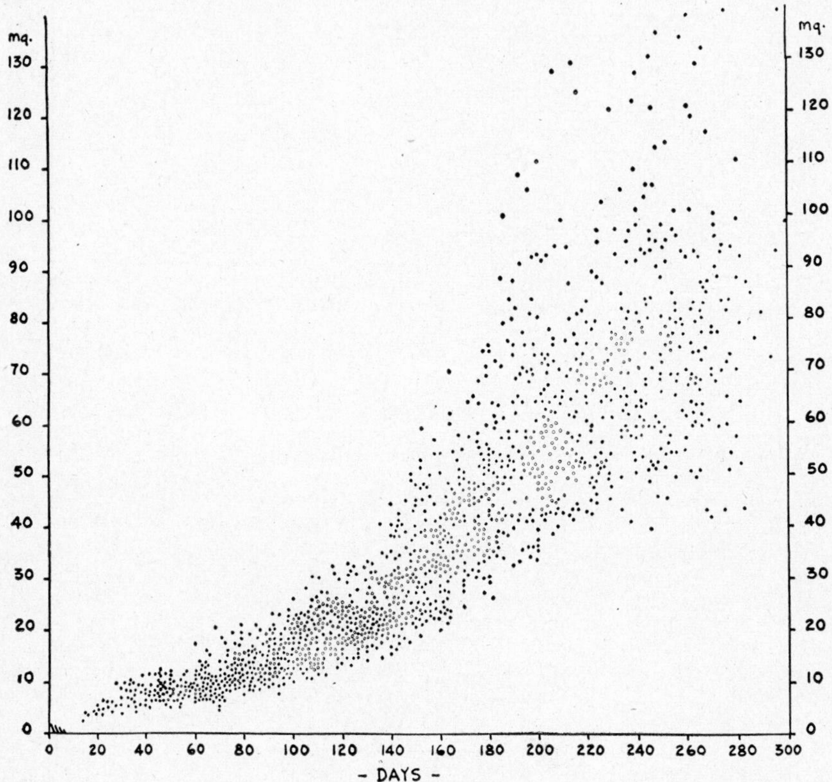

Fig. 129.—Excretion of Pregnanediol Complex in Pregnancy (Venning).

The site of production of estrogen and progesterone by the placenta, according to Wislocki, is the syncytial layer of the trophoblast. The excretion curve of total estrogens in gestation is shown in Fig. 128. Estrogen excretion is low in early pregnancy and does not appear to increase significantly until the one-hundredth day, after which it rises rapidly. The excretion curve of pregnanediol is shown in Fig. 129. Unlike the excretion curve of estrogen which continues to rise up until the time of delivery, progesterone excretion appears to level off in a plateau around the two-hundredth day. Although some observers have claimed that progesterone production decreases a few days before the onset of labor and that this withdrawal is a factor in the onset of labor, the factual evidence for any such relationship is contradictory. Thus, Venning finds that labor may start in on a rising pregnanediol excretion. On the other hand, Lyon has reported that the onset of labor is preceded for several days by a marked decline in the excretion of pregnanediol. The composite of 68 urinary assays performed on patients near term showed a steady decline from an output of 30 mg. of sodium pregnanediol glucuronidate four days before delivery to an average output of 19.5 mg. 48 hours preceding labor and 14.8 mg. one day prior to the onset of labor. On the basis of these findings, it is Lyon's opinion that very little progesterone is available at the onset of labor, and it is implied that the concentration of progesterone at the onset of labor is insufficient to maintain and continue pregnancy. Following delivery, both estrogen and pregnanediol disappear rapidly from the urine.

BIBLIOGRAPHY

Aschheim, S., and Zondek, B. Die Schwangerschaftsdiagnose aus dem Harn durch nachweis des Hypophysenvorderlappenhormons. Klin. Wchnschr., 1928, 7:1404.

Browne, J. S. L., and Venning, E. H. The Effect of Intramuscular Injection of Gonadotrophic Substances on the Corpus Luteum Phase of the Human Menstrual Cycle. Am. J. Physiol., 1938, 123:26.

Corner, G. W. Ovulation and Menstruation in Macacus Rhesus. Carnegie Inst. of Wash., 1923, Publ. 323, p. 73.

Delfs, E. An Assay Method for Human Chorionic Gonadotropin. Endocrinol., 1941, 28:196.

Dempsey, E. W., and Wislocki, G. B. Observations on Some Histochemical Reactions in the Human Placenta, with Special Reference to the Significance of the Lipoids, Glycogen and Iron. Endocrinol., 1944, 35:409.

Dodds, G. S. The Area of the Chorionic Villi in the Full Term Placenta. Anat. Rec., 1923, 24:287.

Engle, E. T. Gonadotropic Substances of Blood, Urine and Other Body Fluids. In Allen, Danforth and Doisy, Sex and Internal Secretions, 2nd Ed. Williams and Wilkins Co., Baltimore, 1939, p. 1003.

——— Ovarian Responses. Differences Elicited by Treatment with Urine from Pregnant Women and by Freshly Implanted Anterior Lobe. J.A.M.A., 1929, 93:276.

——— Experimentally Induced Descent of the Testis in the Macacus Monkey by Hormones from the Anterior Pituitary and Pregnancy Urine. Endocrinol., 1932, 16:513.

Evans, H. M., Kohls, C. L., and Wonder, D. H. Gonadotrophic Hormone in the Blood and Urine of Early Pregnancy; Normal Occurrence of Transient Extremely High Levels. J.A.M.A., 1937, 108:287.

Geist, S. H. Reaction of the Mature Human Ovary to Antuitrin-S. Am. J. Obst. & Gynec., 1933, 26:588.

Gey, G. O., Jones, G. E. S., and Hellman, L. M. The Production of a Gonadotrophic Substance (Prolan) by Placental Cells in Tissue Culture. Science, 1938, 88:306.

Grosser. Frühentwickelung, Eihautbildung, und Plazentation des Menschen und der Säugetiere. München, 1927.

Hamblen, E. C. Endocrine Gynecology. Charles C Thomas Co., Springfield, Ill., 1939.

Hertig, A. T., and Rock, J. On the Development of the Early Human Ovum, with Special Reference to the Trophoblast of the Previllous Stages: a Description of 7 Normal and 5 Pathologic Human Ova. Am. J. Obst. & Gynec., 1944, 47:149.

His, W. Bauchstiel und Nabelstrang, Anatomie menschlicher Embryonen. 1885, 3:222.

——— Die Umschleissung der menschl. Frucht während der frühesten Zeiten der Schwangerschaft. Arch. f. Anat. u. Physiol., Anat. Abth., 1897, p. 399.

Hisaw, F. L., and Astwood, E. B. The Physiology of Reproduction. Ann. Rev. Physiol., 1942, 4:503.

Hofbauer, J. Biologie d. menschlichen Plazenta. Wien, 1905.

——— The Function of the Hofbauer Cells of the Chorionic Villus Particularly in Relation to Acute Infection and Syphilis. Am. J. Obst. & Gynec., 1925, 10:1.

Hunter, W. Anatomy of the Human Gravid Uterus. London, 1774.

Jonen, P. Untersuchungen über die Kapazität des intervillösen Raumes der menschlichen Plazenta. Arch. f. Gynäk., 1927, 129:610.

Jones, G. E. S., Delfs, E., and Stran, H. Chorionic Gonadotropin and Pregnanediol Values in Normal Pregnancy. Bull. Johns Hopkins Hosp., 1944, 75:359.

JONES, G. E. S., GEY, E., and GEY, M. K. Hormone Production by Placental Cells Maintained in Continuous Culture. Bull. Johns Hopkins Hosp., 1943, 72:26.

KEARNS, P. J. Changes in the Uterine and Placental Circulations during Different Stages of Pregnancy. Am. J. Obst. & Gynec., 1939, 38:400.

LANGHANS, T. Untersuchungen über die menschliche Placenta. Arch. f. Anat. u. Entwckngsgesch., Leipzig, 1877, pp. 188-276.

——— Ueber die Zellschicht des menschlichen Chorions. Beitr. z. Anat. u. Embryol., als Fest. Jacob Henle, Bonn, 1882.

LYON, R. Pregnanediol Excretion at the Onset of Labor. Am. J. Obst. & Gynec., 1946, 51:403.

MAYER, A. Biologie der Placenta. I. Physiol. Teil., Arch. f. Gynäk., 1929, 137:1.

MEYER, A. On the Structure of the Human Umbilical Vesicle. Am. J. Anat., 1904, 3:155.

NITABUCH. Beitrag zur Kenntnis der menschlichen Plazenta. D. I., Bern, 1887.

RECH, W. Untersuchungen über die Grösse der Zottenoberfläche der menschlichen Plazenta. Ztschr. Biol., 1924, 80:349.

REYNOLDS, S. R. M. Unpublished data on the hemodynamics of the umbilical cord.

RUNGE, H. Ueber die Funktion der Nabelschnur und des Amnions. Zentralbl. f. Gynäk., 1927, 51:46.

SENGUPTA, B. Plazenta in Gewebekultur. Arch. f. exper. Zellforsch., 1935, 17:281.

SPIVACK, M. On the Presence or Absence of Nerves in the Umbilical Blood Vessels of Man and Guinea Pig. Anat. Rec., 1943, 85:85.

STOECKEL, W. Zwei Fragen über den Intervillösen-Raum. Zentralbl. f. Gynäk., 1928, 52:2578.

TEACHER, J. H. On the Implantation of the Human Ovum and the Early Development of the Trophoblast. J. Obst. & Gynaec. Brit. Emp., 1924, 31:165.

VENNING, E. H. Excretion of Various Hormone Metabolites in Normal Pregnancy. Obst. & Gynec. Surv., 1948, 3:661.

WAGNER, G. A. Der intervillöse Raum. Arch. f. Gynäk., 1929, 137:699.

WISLOCKI, G. B., and BENNETT, H. S. The Histology and Cytology of the Human and Monkey Placenta with Special Reference to the Trophoblast. Am. J. Anat., 1943, 73:335.

WISLOCKI, G. B., and DEMPSEY, E. W. The Chemical Histology of the Human Placenta and Decidua with Reference to Mucoproteins, Glycogen, Lipids and Acid Phosphotase. Am. J. Anat., 1948, 83:1.

WISLOCKI, G. B., DEMPSEY, E. W., and FAWCETT, D. W. Some Functional Activities of the Placental Trophoblast. Obst. & Gynec. Surv., 1948, 3:604.

WISLOCKI, G. B., and STREETER, G. L. On the Placentation of the Macaque (Macaca mulatta), from the Time of Implantation until the Formation of the Definitive Placenta. Carnegie Inst. of Wash., 1938, Contrib. to Embryology, 27:1.

7

THE DEVELOPMENT AND PHYSIOLOGY OF THE FETUS

The Fetus in the Various Months of Pregnancy. It is important that the physician be able to tell approximately the age of embryos and prematurely born children; hence the following short description of the fetus at its various periods of development.

During the first two weeks of pregnancy the product of conception is designated as the ovum; from the third to the fifth week—the period during which the various organs are developed and a definite form is assumed—it is known as the embryo; after the fifth week it is called the fetus.

First Two Weeks. The earliest human ova with which we are acquainted (third week after fertilization) were enumerated in the preceding chapter. They are vesicular structures whose main feature is the chorionic vesicle, to one side of whose interior is attached the future embryo, so small a body that its component parts can be distinguished only with the aid of the microscope. In each instance the embryonic area is covered by a well-developed amnion, and the most imposing constituent of the embryo consists of the yolk sac.

Third Week. The embryonal period begins with the third week, in the latter part of which can be detected the beginning formation of the medullary groove and canal, soon to be followed by the appearance of the head folds. At this stage of development the abdominal pedicle is seen coming off from the tail end of the embryo, and lying almost in the same axis with it. The embryo is concave on its dorsal surface, and is made up, in great part, of the yolk sac.

A little later the formation of the double heart may be noted; the cerebral and optic vesicle soon appear, as well as the visceral arches and cleft. The yolk sac becomes more and more constricted, and is connected with the ventral surface of the embryo by a broad pedicle. At the very end of the third week (about the twenty-first day) the limbs make their appearance as small buds upon the surface of the embryo (Figs. 130 and 131).

Fourth Week. This week is characterized by a great increase in the size of the embryo, which becomes markedly flexed upon its ventral surface, so that its head and tail ends come almost in contact. The rudiments of the eyes, ears, and nose now make their appearance, and the umbilical vesicle becomes still more pedunculated. At the end of the first lunar month, the anlagen for all the organs have become differentiated and the embryo measures from 7.5 to 10 mm. in length.

Second Month. In the first half of the second month the human embryo does not differ essentially in appearance from that of other mammals. It is still markedly bent on itself, and the visceral clefts and arches are the most prominent characteristics of its cephalic region, while the extremities are in a rudimentary condition. In the latter part of the month, owing to the development of the brain, the head becomes disproportionately large, and assumes a certain resemblance to that of a human being. At the same time the nose, mouth, and ears become relatively less prominent and the extremities more developed, so that it can be seen that each is made up of three portions.

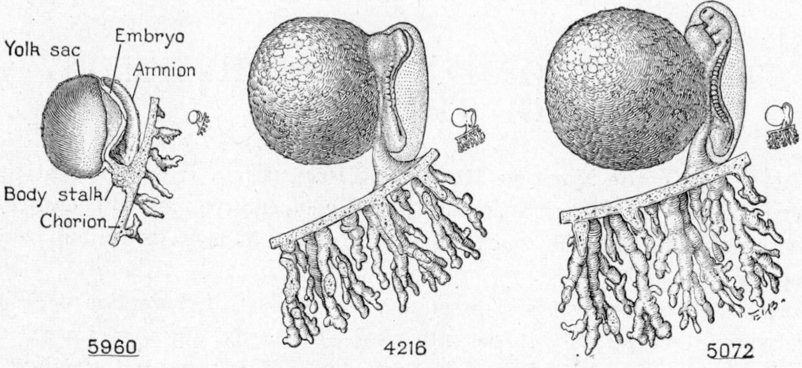

Fig. 130.—Early Human Embryos. × 7.5.

Small outline to right of each embryo gives its actual size. Ovulation Ages: No. 5960, Carnegie Collection (Presomite), 19 Days; No. 4216 (7 Somites), 21 Days; No. 5072 (17 Somites), 22 Days. (After drawings and models of the Carnegie Institution.)

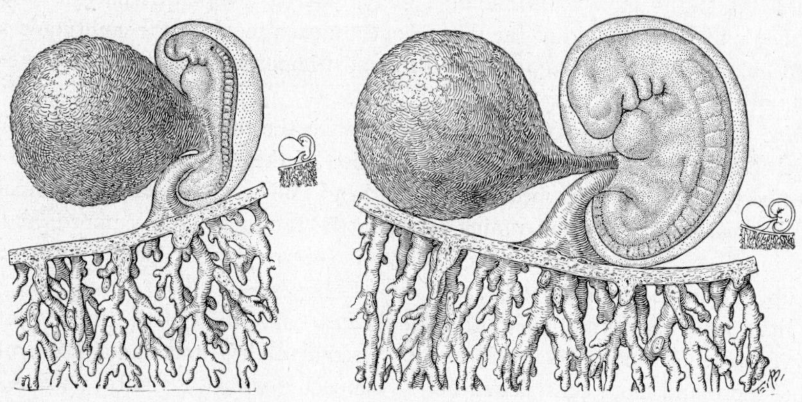

Fig. 131.—Early Human Embryos. × 7.5.

Small outline to right of each embryo gives its actual size. Ovulation Ages: No. 2053, Carnegie Collection, 22 Days; No. 836, 23 Days. (After drawings and models of Carnegie Institution.)

The external genitalia also make their appearance in the latter part of this month, and at its end the fetus has attained a length of 2.5 cm.

Third Month. At the end of this month the embryo is 7 to 9 cm. in length. Centers of ossification have appeared in most of the bones; the fingers and toes have become differentiated and are supplied with nails; the external genitalia are beginning to show definite signs of sex. A fetus born at this time may make spontaneous movements if still within the amniotic sac or if immersed in warm saline solution.

Fourth Month. By the end of the fourth month the fetus is from 10 to 17 cm. long, and weighs about 120 gm. Casual examination of the external genital organs will now definitely reveal the sex.

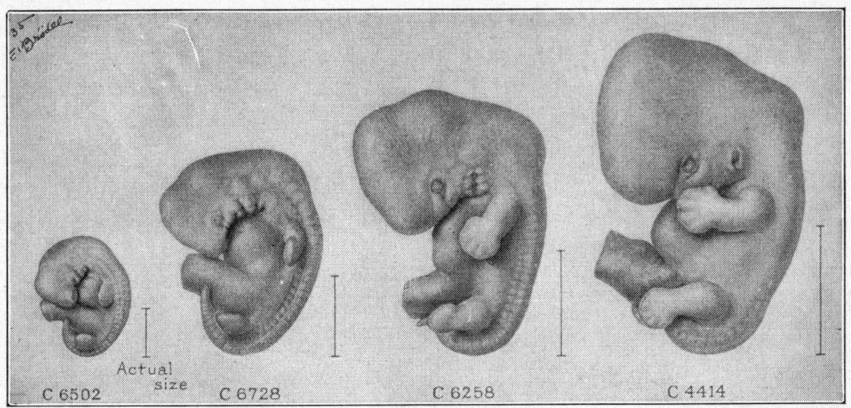

Fig. 132.—Human Embryos, 4 to 5.5 Weeks, Ovulation Age. × 2.5.

Ovulation Ages: No. 6502, Carnegie Collection, 28 Days; No. 6728, 31 Days; No. 6258, 38 Days; No. 4414, 39 Days.

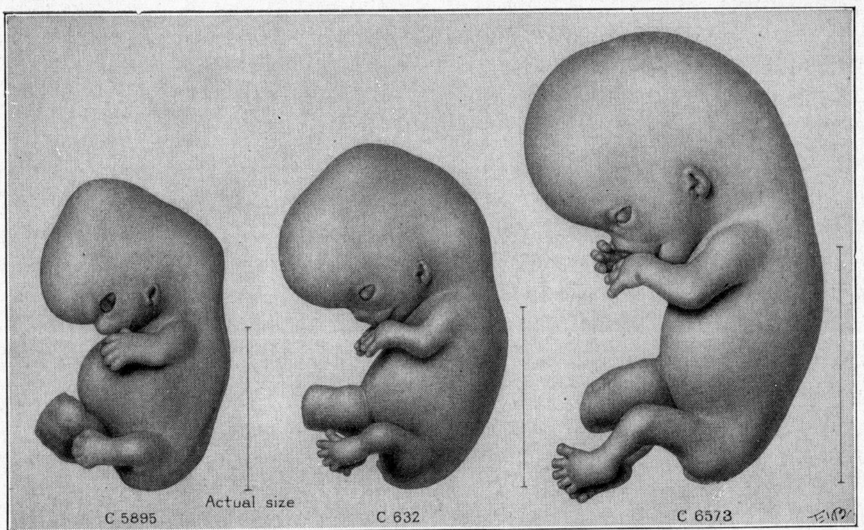

Fig. 133.—Human Embryos, 8 to 8.5 Weeks, Menstrual Age. × 1.9.
(Numbers refer to embryos in the Carnegie Collection.)

Fifth Month. The fetus varies from 18 to 27 cm. in length and weighs about 280 gm. Its skin has become less transparent, a down covering—lanugo—is seen over its entire body, while a certain amount of typical hair has made its appearance on the head.

Sixth Month. At the end of the sixth month the fetus varies from 28 to 34 cm. in length, and weighs about 634 gm. The skin presents a characteristically wrinkled appearance, and fat begins to be deposited beneath it; the head is still comparatively quite large. A fetus born at this period will attempt to breathe, but almost always perishes within a short time.

Seventh Month. The length during this month varies from 35 to 38 cm., and the fetus attains a weight of over 1,200 gm. The entire body is very thin; the skin is reddish and covered with vernix caseosa. The pupillary membrane has just disappeared from the eyes. A fetus born at this period moves its limbs quite energetically and cries with a weak voice. As a rule, it cannot be raised, but occasionally expert care is rewarded by a successful outcome.

It is generally believed among the laity that a child born at the end of the seventh month has a better chance of living than when it comes into the world four weeks later. This idea is a remnant of the old Hippocratic doctrine and is altogether erroneous, as the more developed the child the greater are its chances for life.

Eighth Month. At the end of the eighth month the fetus has attained a length of 42.5 cm. and a weight of about 1,900 gm. The surface of the skin is still red and wrinkled and the child resembles an old man in appearance. Children born at this period may live if properly cared for, although their chances are not very promising.

Ninth Month. At the end of the ninth month the fetus is 46 cm. long and weighs about 2,500 gm. Owing to the deposition of subcutaneous fat, the body has become more rotund and the face has lost its previous wrinkled appearance. Children born during this month have a very good chance of life if properly cared for.

Tenth Month. Full term is reached at the end of this month. The fetus is now fully developed, and presents the appearances which we shall consider in detail when the newborn child is described.

The fetus grows relatively much faster in the early than in the later months of pregnancy. Hartman, in a review of available statistics, states that the human ovum probably has an average measurement of between 130 and 140 microns, being the largest mammalian egg. According to Jackson, the weight of the mature ovum is 0.000004 gm., which increases to 0.04 gm. by the end of the first month after fertilization—an increase of 9,999 times, or practically one million per cent. In the second and third months the rate of increase has fallen to 74 and 11 times respectively, and gradually falls to 0.3 times in the last month. Even this comparatively slow rate is not maintained after birth, for if it were, the child would weigh about 160 pounds by the end of the first year.

Lunar Month	Sitting Height, Centimeters	Weight, Grams
Second	0.23	1.1
Third	6.1	14.2
Fourth	11.6	108.0
Fifth	16.4	316.0
Sixth	20.8	630.0
Seventh	24.7	1,045.0
Eighth	28.3	1,680.0
Ninth	32.1	2,478.0
Tenth	36.2	3,405.0

TABLE 3. AVERAGE SITTING HEIGHT AND WEIGHT OF THE FETUS AT THE END OF VARIOUS LUNAR MONTHS OF PREGNANCY. (Streeter.)

Owing to inequalities in the length of the legs and the difficulty of maintaining them in extension during mensuration, the determination of the sitting height (crown-rump) is more accurate than that of the standing height. The average sitting height and weight of the fetus at the end of the various lunar months, as determined by Streeter from 704 specimens, is shown in Table 3.

Such figures possess only an approximate value, and generally speaking the length affords a more accurate criterion of the age of a fetus than its weight. Haase has suggested that for clinical purposes the length of the embryo in centimeters may be approximated during the first five months by squaring the number of the month to which the pregnancy has advanced; in the second half of pregnancy, by multiplying the month by five, as is shown in Table 4.

At the end of the first month	1 × 1,	1 cm.
At the end of the second month	2 × 2,	4 cm.
At the end of the third month	3 × 3,	9 cm.
At the end of the fourth month	4 × 4,	16 cm.
At the end of the fifth month	5 × 5,	25 cm.
At the end of the sixth month	6 × 5,	30 cm.
At the end of the seventh month	7 × 5,	35 cm.
At the end of the eighth month	8 × 5,	40 cm.
At the end of the ninth month	9 × 5,	45 cm.
At the end of the tenth month	10 × 5,	50 cm.

TABLE 4. HAASE'S RULE FOR ASCERTAINING APPROXIMATELY THE DURATION OF PREGNANCY FROM THE LENGTH OF THE FETUS, AND VICE VERSA.

The Child at Full Term. The child at full term is about 50 cm., or 20 inches long (36 cm., or 14 inches sitting height), and weighs approximately 3,250 gm., or 7 pounds. The skin is smooth and polished in appearance, and shows no lanugo, except occasionally about the shoulders. Over the entire surface is spread a whitish, greasy material, the *vernix caseosa,* which is a mixture of epithelial cells, lanugo hairs, and the secretion of the sebaceous glands. The head is usually covered by darkish hairs 2 to 3 cm. in length, and the cartilages of the nose and ears are well developed. The fingers and toes possess well-developed nails, which project beyond their tips. In male children the testicles are usually found within the scrotum; in girls the labia majora are well developed and are in contact with one another, and usually conceal the rest of the genitalia. The bones of the head are well ossified, and are in close contact at the various sutures. The eyes possess a uniformly slate color, so that it is impossible to predict their final tone.

The time of appearance of certain of the ossification centers is sometimes of auxiliary aid in establishing the maturity, or degree of prematurity, of infants after birth. Of the several centers, the inferior femoral epiphysis is the most useful for this purpose. Basing their conclusions on 1,717 observations, Adair and Scammon found this center of ossification to be present in one case in 20 in the eighth fetal month, in one case in three in the ninth month, in six cases in seven in the tenth month and in about 19 cases in 20 at term. The time of appearance of the ossification centers is affected greatly by race and sex, as demonstrated by Christie's study of 1,112 newborn which included 298 white boys, 267 white girls, 271 Negro boys and 276 Negro girls. In Christie's infants with weight of less than 2,000 gm., the distal epiphysis of the femur was present in 9.1 per cent of white boys, 50 per cent of white girls, 18.2 per cent of the Negro boys and 50 per cent of the Negro girls. In the 2,000 to 2,499 gm. weight group, the distal epiphysis of the femur was present in 75 per cent of the white boys, 91.7 per cent of the white girls, 88.5 per cent of the Negro boys, and 93.8 per cent of the Negro girls. In the 3,000 to 3,499 gm. weight group, the distal epiphysis of the femur was present in 85.3 per cent of the white boys, 98 per cent of the white girls, 90.7 per cent of the Negro boys and 99 per cent of the Negro girls. In the weight groups of less than 2,000 gm., the proximal epiphysis of the tibia was not present in any white boy, white girl, or Negro boy, but was demonstrable in 14.3 per cent of the Negro girls. Its presence in white boys is an almost certain sign of maturity, but its absence in any of the race-sex groups means little, since even in term infants, it is present in only 52.9 per cent of white boys, 75.5 per cent of white girls, 62.7 per cent of Negro boys and 76.7 per cent of Negro girls, according to Christie's statistics. He finds that the order of appearance of the ossification centers is as follows: calcaneous, talus, distal epiphysis of the femur, proximal epiphysis of the tibia, cuboid bone, head of the humerus, capitatum, hamate bone, third cuneiform bone, and head of the femur.

Negro babies at birth differ somewhat in appearance from white children, but not so much as one might expect. Their skin presents a dusky, bluish-red hue, but does not at all suggest the darker color which it will assume in the course of a few weeks. Where there is a considerable admixture of white blood, the dusky hue may be entirely absent, and the only certain evidence of Negro ancestry will be found in an increased pigmentation about the external genitalia and at the matrix of the nails.

Weight of the Newborn. The average infant at birth weighs about 3,200 gm. (7 pounds), boys being usually 100 gm. (3 ounces) heavier than girls. Marked variations are frequently observed; these are dependent upon the race and size of the parents, the number of children which the mother has borne, her mode of life, and her nutrition and general condition during the later months of pregnancy. In 18,160 full-term white children born at the Woman's Clinic of the New York Hospital it was found that the average length was 50.8 cm., and the average weight 3,224.6 gm., the smallest child being 1,660 gm. in weight and 49 cm. in length, and the largest 6,280 gm. in weight and 62 cm. in length.

Colored children weigh considerably less on the average. In 915 full-term colored children in the New York Hospital, the average length was 49.9 cm., and the weight 3,078.1 gm., a difference of 146.5 gm. in favor of the white race.

Perfectly healthy full-term children may vary from 2,500 to 5,000 gm. (5.5 to 11 pounds) in weight. It is, however, customary to designate them as excessive in size whenever 4,500 gm. (10 pounds) is exceeded; yet actual dystocia is rarely encountered unless the weight exceeds 5,000 gm., provided, of course, that the pelvis and fetal presentation are normal.

It is not uncommon to hear of children much heavier than 5,000 gm. and sometimes almost fabulous weights are reported. Most of these must be regarded as apocryphal, and careful inquiry will usually show that the weight has been only roughly estimated by lifting the child in one hand, and was not based upon accurate determination. In 31,932 deliveries in the New York Hospital there were 63 infants that weighed 5,000 gm. or over. The largest infant weighed 6,280 gm. and measured 62 cm. in length. The statistics of the Johns Hopkins Hospital are similar, but since approximately one-half our patients are colored, the incidence of very large babies is somewhat less. Thus, in 23,662 deliveries between 1936 and 1948, no baby weighed more than 6,000 gm. (13.2 pounds), and only 36, or 1 in 657, weighed more than 5,000 gm. (11.0 pounds). Presumably the largest baby recorded in the literature is that described by Belcher of a stillborn female weighing 11,340 gm. (25 pounds). In spite of these exceptional cases, one should be extremely skeptical in accepting reports concerning phenomenally heavy children, unless convinced that the reporter is a truthful person and that he has weighed the newborn child upon an accurate balance.

On the other hand, healthy full-term children frequently weigh less than 3,250 gm. and sometimes as little as 2,300 gm. (5 pounds), although, when the weight falls below 2,500 gm., the child should be considered as premature.

The Head of the Child. From an obstetrical point of view the head of the child is its most important part, as the essential feature of labor is a process of adaptation between it and the various portions of the birth canal through which it passes. An accurate knowledge of its characteristics and size is therefore of capital importance.

Only a comparatively small part of the head of the child at term is represented by the face, the rest being composed of the firm, hard skull, which is made up of two frontal, two parietal, two temporal bones, the upper portion of the occipital, and the wings of the sphenoid. These bony portions are not firmly united together, but are separated from one another by spaces filled with membrane—the *sutures*. Of these the most important are the *frontal,* between the two frontal bones; the *sagittal,* between the two parietal bones; the *coronal,* between the frontal and parietal bones; and the *lambdoid* suture, between the posterior margins of the parietal bones and the upper margin of the occipital bone. All these sutures can be felt during labor; whereas the *temporal* suture, which is situated on either side between the inferior margin of the parietal and the upper margin of the temporal bones, is covered by soft parts and cannot be felt on the living child.

Where several sutures meet together an irregular space is formed, which is closed by a membrane and designated as a *fontanel.* Four such structures are usually distinguished: the greater and lesser, and the two temporal fontanels. The *greater* or *anterior fontanel* is a lozenge-shaped space situated at the junction of the sagittal and the coronal sutures. The *lesser* or *posterior fontanel* is represented by a small triangular area at the intersection of the sagittal and lambdoid sutures. The *temporal* or *gasserian fontanels* are situated at the junction of the lambdoid and temporal sutures. The first two are readily felt during labor, and their recognition gives important information concerning the presentation and position of the child; the temporal or gasserian fontanels, however, have no diagnostic significance.

Arnold Lea directed attention to the occasional presence of what he designated as the *sagittal fontanel,* which is a lozenge-shaped space found in the sagittal suture at a point about halfway between the greater and lesser fontanels. He considers that it results from faulty ossification of the parietal bones, and states that it occurred in 4.4 per cent of 500 fetal skulls which he examined. Adair and Scammon state that it occurs in a rudimentary form in about 30 per cent of all newborn children, but attains an area of one square centimeter or more in only 3.27 per cent. Whenever it is large enough to be confused with the large fontanel it may give rise to serious error in diagnosis.

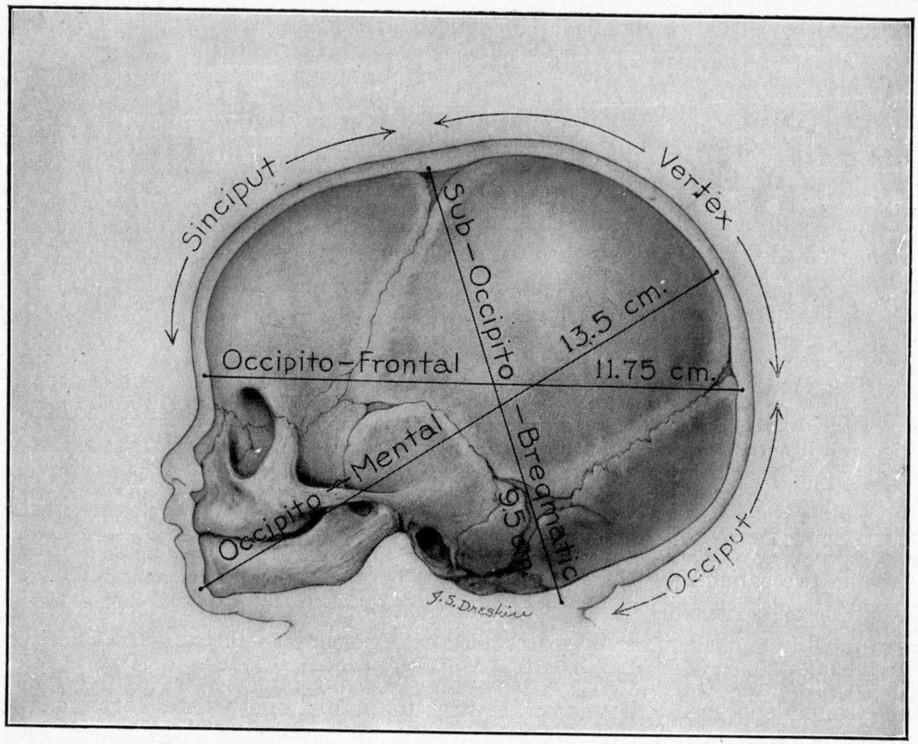

FIG. 134.—DESIGNATING AREAS AND DIAMETERS OF THE CHILD'S HEAD AT TERM.

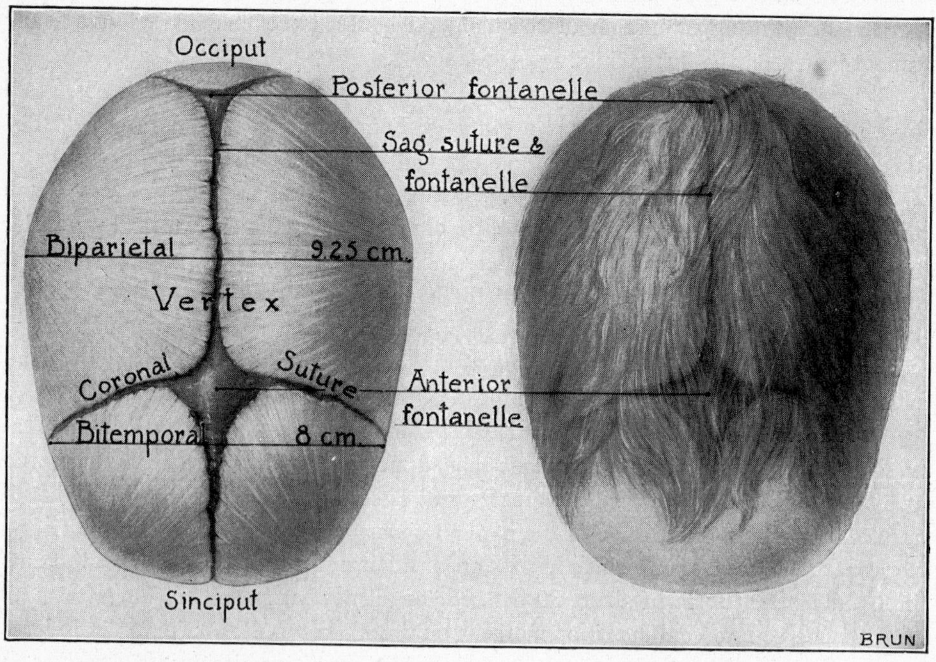

FIG. 135.—CHILD'S HEAD AT TERM SHOWING VARIOUS FONTANELS AND DIAMETERS.

To aid us in forming definite ideas concerning the shape and size of the fetal head, it is customary to measure certain *diameters* and *circumferences*. The diameters most frequently used are: (1) the occipitofrontal, which follows a line extending from the root of the nose to the most prominent portion of the occipital bone; (2) the biparietal, which represents the greatest transverse diameter of the head, and extends from one parietal boss to the other; (3) the bitemporal, which represents the greatest distance between the two temporal sutures; (4) the occipitomental, from the chin to the most prominent portion of the occiput; and (5) the suboccipitobregmatic, which follows a line drawn from the middle of the large fontanel to the under surface of the occipital bone, just where it joins the neck. For convenience the various diameters are frequently designated by initials, which, with their several average measurements, as well as Riggs' figures for the white and colored races, respectively, are given in Table 5.

	Initials	Average Length, Centimeters	Riggs' Figures, Centimeters	
			White	Black
Occipitofrontal	O. F.	11.75	11.71	11.26
Biparietal	B. P.	9.25	9.25	9.05
Bitemporal	B. T.	8.00	8.00	7.81
Occipitomental	O. M.	13.5	13.33	13.31
Suboccipitobregmatic	S. O. B.	9.5	9.70	9.29

TABLE 5. AVERAGE DIAMETERS OF THE FETAL HEAD. (Riggs.)

The greatest circumference of the head, which corresponds to the plane of the occipitofrontal diameter, is 34.5 cm., while the least circumference, corresponding to the plane of the suboccipitobregmatic diameter, is 32 cm. These figures just given are based upon the average measurements of a large number of heads just after birth, individual variations being frequently encountered. As a rule, boys have somewhat larger heads than girls, and the children of multiparae than those of primiparae. As indicated in the table, Riggs' figures show that all of the diameters are shorter in Negro children; but such measurements give no idea of the greater softness and compressibility of their heads. According to Calkins the various measurements of the head bear a constant relation to the standing height of the child. Consequently, he states that measurements of the head, when plotted as ordinates against the standing height as abscissae, result in a straight-line curve. This being the case, he concludes that the relationship between any two dimensions can be expressed by the straight line empirical formula: $y = ax \pm b$; where x and y are body dimensions and a and b are constants.

A certain amount of motility exists at the sutures between the various bones composing the skull. This may vary within relatively wide limits in different individuals, so that heads which afford the same diameters on actual measurement frequently differ markedly in the obstacle which they offer to labor; as the bones of one may be soft, compressible, and readily displaced, while those of another are firmly and densely ossified and admit of but little motility, the former being readily molded to the pelvic canal, while the latter are incapable of reduction in size.

PHYSIOLOGY OF THE FETUS

Nutrition of the Fetus. Owing to the small amount of yolk contained in the human ovum, the growth of the fetus is almost entirely dependent upon the amount of nutritive material which it obtains from its mother.

During the first few months of pregnancy, the embryo consists almost entirely of water, and it is during this period that it grows most rapidly. In the later months of pregnancy, when more solids are being added, the increase in size becomes gradually slower. Fehling analyzed the fetus at various periods with the results noted in Table 6, which indicates that, as the fetus increases in age, it contains relatively less water and a markedly increased quantity of albuminoid materials, salts and fats. Fehling showed that the total quantity of calcium contained in the fetus, estimated as CaO, increases from 0.045 gm. at the third month to 28 gm. at term, while the daily increment increases from 0.0015 to 0.399 gm. at corresponding periods.

	Water, Per Cent	Albuminoids, Per Cent	Salts, Per Cent	Fats, Per Cent
At 2½ months	93.82	4.49	Trace	Trace
Third to fourth month	89.95	7.05	1.729	0.0379
Seventh month	84.75	10.04	2.487	1.823
At term	69.16	13.96	3.373	11.75

TABLE 6. PROPORTIONS OF WATER AND SOLIDS IN THE FETUS AT VARIOUS STAGES OF PREGNANCY.

For the first few days after implantation, the nutrition of the ovum must be derived from the serum which accompanies the edematous condition of the decidua. Furthermore, the surrounding maternal tissue which has undergone necrosis as the result of the digestive action of the trophoblast, as well as the greatly augmented glandular secretion which characterizes this period, probably serves as a pabulum, to which is added glycogen which accumulates in the endometrium during the secretory phase. Within the next week, intervillous spaces which are filled with maternal blood begin to develop between the trophoblast and decidua. As the chorionic villi at this period are devoid of vessels, the only way in which nutritive material, which has been taken up by the trophoblast from the maternal blood, can be transmitted to the embryo is by means of direct osmosis. The relationship of decidua to the trophoblast is shown in Figs. 90, 104, 109 and 111.

In the third week of pregnancy the omphalomesenteric vessels make their appearance upon the surface of the umbilical vesicle, and convey to the embryo whatever nutritive materials the latter may contain. During the fourth week branches of the umbilical vessels appear in the chorionic villi, and from that time on make possible the direct transmission through the placental filter of nutritive material from the maternal to the fetal blood.

The Fetal Circulation. Owing to the fact that the lungs do not function and that the materials needed for the nutrition of the fetus are brought to it from the placenta by the umbilical vein, the fetal circulation differs materially from that of the adult (Figs. 136A and 136B). The blood is purified and laden with nutritive material in the placenta, and is then carried to the fetus through the umbilical vein, which, after penetrating the abdominal wall, divides into two branches. Of these the smaller

NOTE

The two following illustrations represent an attempt to show not only the shunts of the fetal circulation but also the resultant degrees of oxygen unsaturation of the fetal blood by gradations of color.

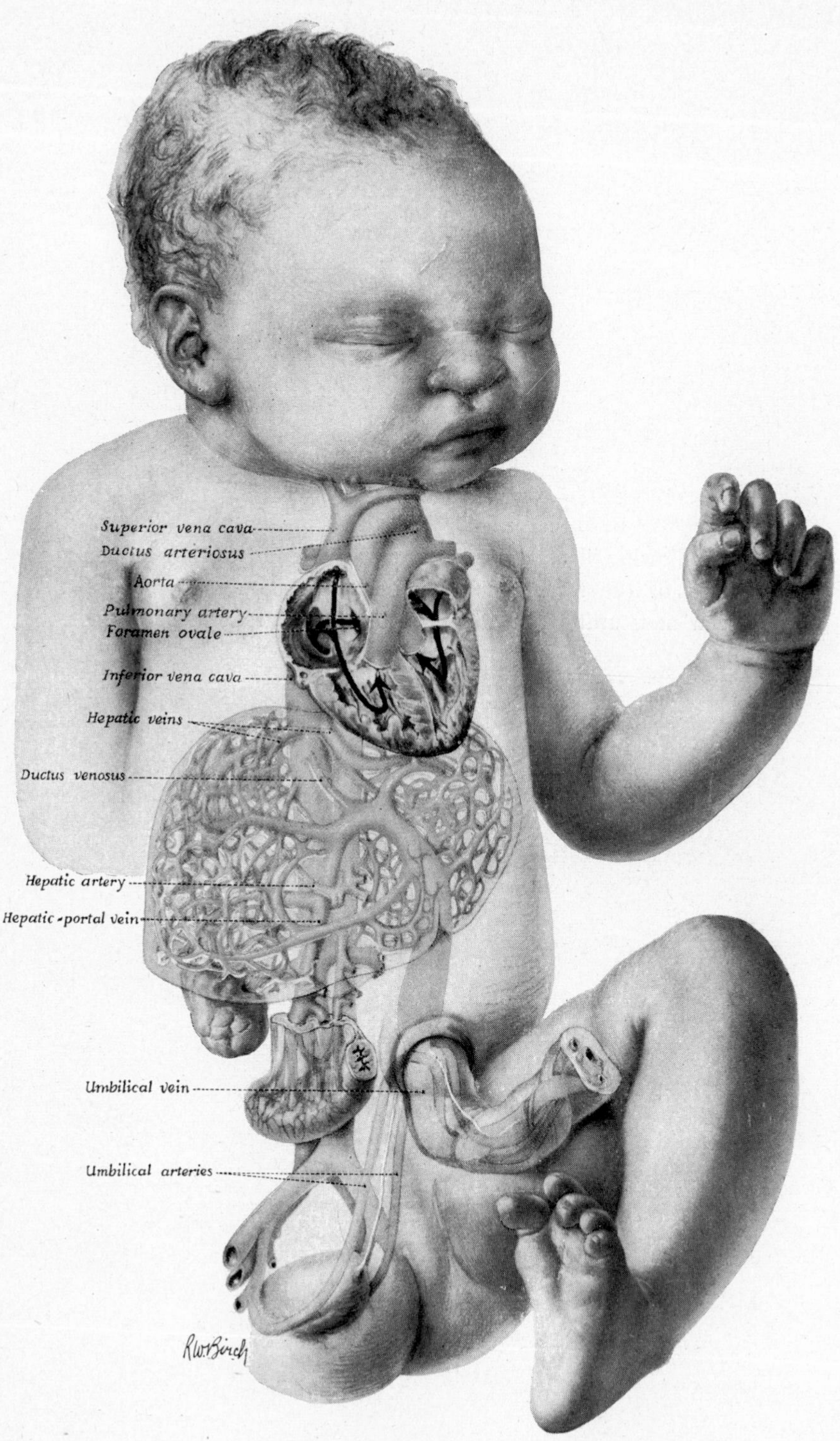

FIG. 136A.—CARDIOVASCULAR SYSTEM OF FETUS IN UTERO.

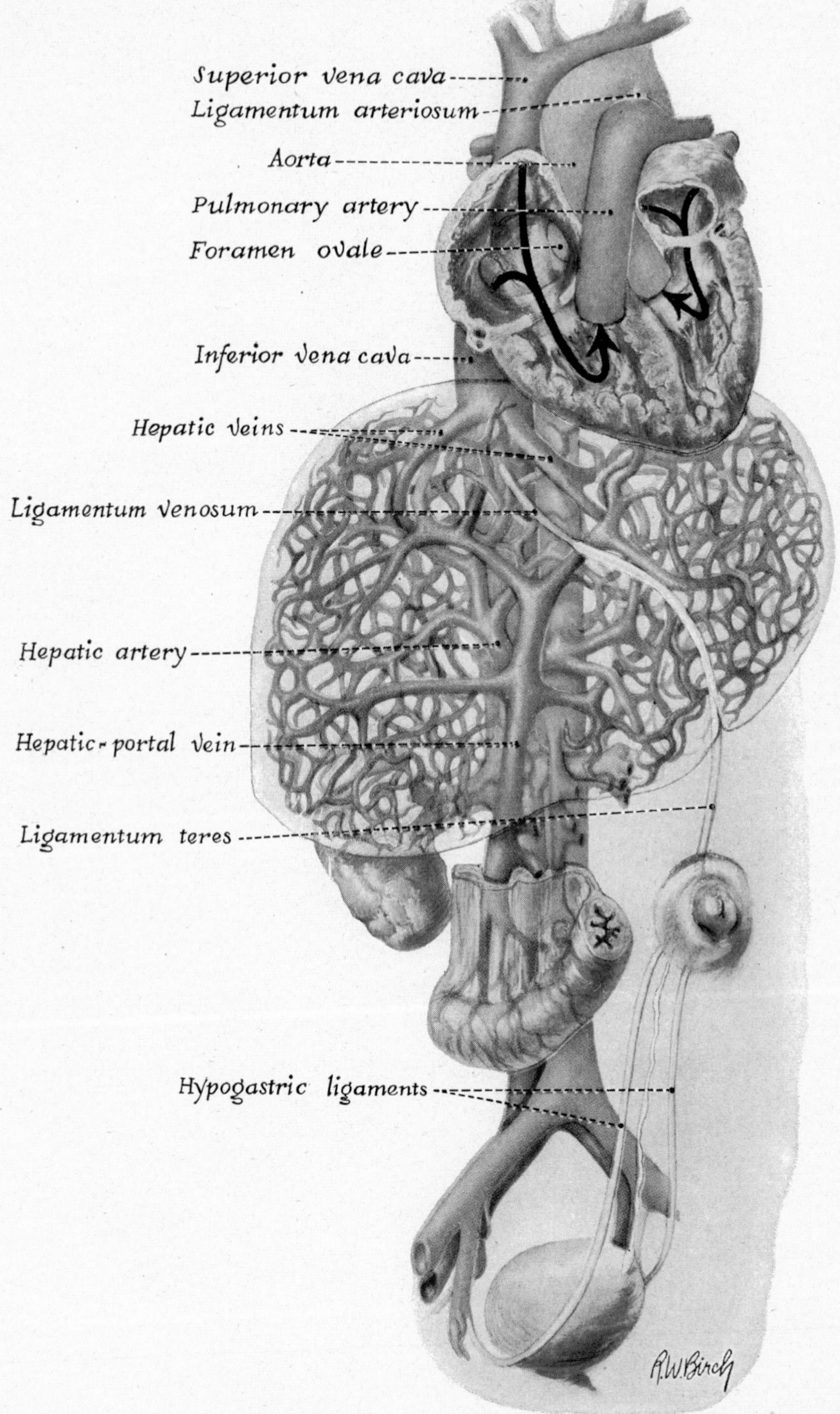

Fig. 136B.—Cardiovascular System of Infant after Birth.

unites with the portal vein, the blood from which circulates through the liver and then gains access to the inferior vena cava through the hepatic vein. The other larger branch, which is designated as the ductus venosus, empties directly into the vena cava. The contents of the vena cava above the hepatic vein, therefore, consist of a mixture of arterial blood from the placenta and venous blood returning from the lower extremities of the fetus. It has been generally taught that upon entering the right auricle the blood is deflected by the intervention of the eustachian valve in such a manner as to pass through the foramen ovale into the left auricle, whence it passes into the left ventricle which forces it into the aorta. On the other hand, the blood returning from the head and upper extremities by way of the superior vena cava is poured into the right auricle and, crossing the current from the inferior vena cava, passes into the right ventricle, whence it is forced into the pulmonary arteries. But so long as the lungs do not function, only a small portion of this blood gains access to them, the greater part of it passing through the ductus arteriosus to the arch of the aorta and being then carried to the rest of the body of the embryo.

According to this older view, the blood from the inferior and superior vena cava does not mix in the right auricle, but the two currents cross each other in such a way that the purer blood from the inferior cava passes directly to the left side of the heart through the foramen ovale and is supplied in great part to the head and neck, while the less pure blood from the superior cava passes through the right auriculoventricular opening and is forced by the right ventricle into the pulmonary arteries and the ductus arteriosus. The other theory supposes that thorough mixing of the blood takes place in the right auricle. The investigations made by Barcroft on oxygen content and of Barclay with radiopaque substances, as well as those of Windle and others, support, in a large measure, the earlier concept that the blood from the inferior vena cava, with its high oxygen content, passes to both the left and right auricles, while that from the superior vena cava, entering the right auricle, goes entirely to the right ventricle. These recent contributions on the subject are strong evidence against complete mixing of the two streams, occurring in the right auricle. Abel and Windle concluded from their experimental work on guinea pigs that, late in prenatal life, a circulation is present in the lungs, which is capable of caring for oxygenation pending assumption of active pulmonary respiration.

The blood which has gained access to the aorta directly from the left ventricle, as well as indirectly from the right ventricle through the ductus arteriosus, is propelled down the aorta and given off to the various organs according to their needs; but the bulk of it enters the internal iliac and hypogastric arteries—the latter after passing the umbilicus being designated as the umbilical arteries—and through them gains access to the placenta.

From the foregoing description, it is apparent that the blood circulating in the fetus is at no time strictly arterial or strictly venous but that the content of the inferior vena cava is purer than that of the aorta.

The distinctive features of the fetal circulation are the ductus venosus and arteriosus, the foramen ovale, the hypogastric arteries, and the umbilical cord. After birth these structures undergo marked changes. As soon as the child is born and begins to breathe, the pulmonary circulation becomes established. As a result, a much greater quantity of blood is pumped by the right ventricle into the pulmonary arteries, while a lessened amount passes through the ductus arteriosus. Moreover, as soon as the circulation in the cord is abolished, the umbilical vein becomes functionless, and a diminished quantity of blood is returned to the right auricle by the inferior vena cava. This change leads to a diminution in the tension in the right auricle, while that in the left side of the heart is increased, bringing about the sudden closure of the valve-like foramen ovale. The experiments of Barcroft and Barclay indicate that the functional closure of the foramen ovale occurs within a matter of minutes and not over a long period of time, as supposed by some writers.

As the circulation through the umbilical arteries ceases almost immediately after the pulmonary circulation is established, the function of the hypogastric arteries is in abeyance, and their distal ends rapidly undergo atrophy and obliteration within three or four days after birth and are then known as the hypogastric ligaments. The ductus venosus and umbilical veins also become occluded soon after birth, whereas the closure of the ductus arteriosus is supposed to be more gradual. However, studies by Barron and others strongly suggest that the ductus arteriosus as well as the ductus venosus are closed functionally within a few minutes after birth and that such closure is brought about by the action of sphincter muscles. The remnants of the umbilical veins form the ligamentum teres, those of the ductus venosus the ligamentum venosum, while the obliterated ductus arteriosus becomes the ligamentum arteriosum. Arey states that anatomic fusion of the two septa of the foramen ovale is not completed until about one year after birth, and that in 25 per cent of individuals perfect closure is never attained. Where the foramen ovale remains patent circulatory disturbances of greater or less gravity result from its persistence.

Oxygen Relationships of Fetal Blood. As shown in Fig. 137, the oxygen relationships of fetal blood in utero differ decidedly from those of maternal blood. The principal characteristics of fetal blood in its relation to oxygen are the high capacity, the low arterial content, the very low venous content, and as a result of these three factors, an extremely high degree of unsaturation of the capillary blood. This very high unsaturation of fetal blood in respect to oxygen indicates that the full-term fetus in utero exists normally in a state of cyanosis. The low oxygen content of the umbilical vein blood becomes more striking if, instead of referring to the quantity of oxygen present in volumes per cent (cubic centimeters of gas per hundred cubic centimeters of blood), we express it as a percentage of the total amount of oxygen with which the blood will combine; that is, in terms of percentage saturation. It will then be found that, while the arterial blood of the mother is usually 96 per cent or more saturated with oxygen and the maternal venous blood 71 per cent saturated, the arterial blood going to the fetus in utero is only 63 per cent saturated and falls at birth to approximately 50 per cent saturation. The low oxygen content of fetal arterial blood is the result of two circumstances: (1) the fact that the blood in the intervillous spaces is a mixture of arterial and venous blood and hence presents to the chorionic villi a lower oxygen tension than is presented by the pulmonary alveoli to the maternal blood and (2) the well-known physicochemical fact that oxygen diffuses through a wet membrane rather slowly.

In view of the low oxygen tension to which umbilical blood is exposed, the high hemoglobin content of this blood assumes particular significance, since there is general agreement that the usual response of adult blood to low oxygen tensions is a rapid increase in the number of erythrocytes and in the amount of hemoglobin. Thus, in individuals living in high altitudes, high figures for hemoglobin are constantly found, acclimated individuals showing a rise of 10 per cent in hemoglobin for every 100 mm. drop in barometric pressure. The increase in hemoglobin, moreover, seems to be associated with an increased hematopoietic activity of the bone marrow, and during the expedition of Barcroft to the Peruvian Andes, a marked increase in the number of reticulocytes was noted, which number fell to normal after the descent. Barcroft and other students of the subject believe that the purpose of the increase in hemoglobin is to provide a larger storehouse of oxygen in the blood, from which the necessary tension may be maintained in the plasma. Similarly, it seems altogether probable that the high hemoglobin content of fetal blood is essentially an adaptive or "acclimatization"

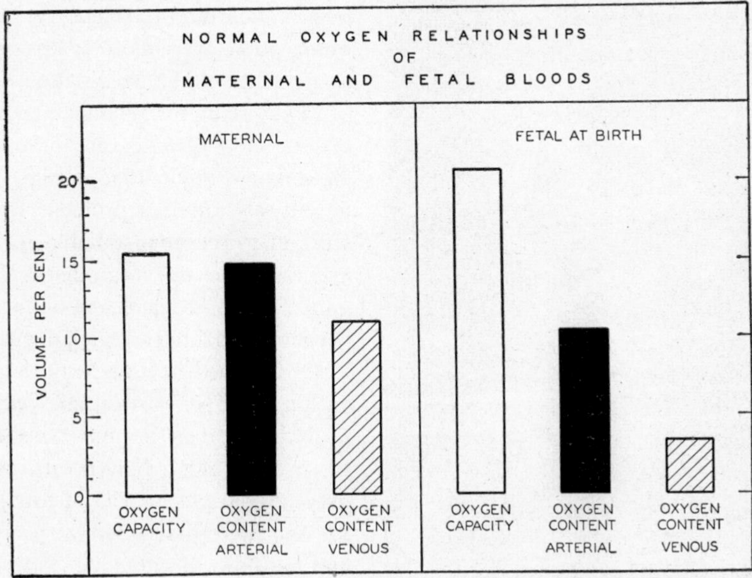

Fig. 137.—Oxygen Relationships of Fetal Blood.

mechanism resulting from constant exposure to low oxygen tensions. Plausibility is lent to such a view by the fact that as soon as a fetus is born and is subject to atmospheric conditions, the high hemoglobin and increased number of erythrocytes fall rapidly. Further support of this belief is found in the observation that fetal blood at birth shows evidence of increased bone marrow activity, with nucleated red cells, polychromatophilia, anisocytosis and poikilocytosis, changes which disappear in the first few weeks of extra-uterine life.

It must not be inferred from these findings, however, that the fetus in utero normally suffers from oxygen want, since the amount of oxygen lost by the umbilical vein blood in its passage through the fetus would seem to be plentiful for an organism resting in a dormant state in a medium at constant body temperature. Further confirmatory evidence that the fetus in utero does not normally experience oxygen want is supplied by figures on the lactic acid content of fetal blood, which are only slightly higher than those of the mother. Barcroft has aptly summarized these unique oxygen relationships of the fetus in utero in the phrase, "Everest in utero."

Intra-uterine Respiration. As far back as 1905 Ahlfeld thought he was able to see, on occasion, characteristic rhythmic movements of the abdomen in slender pregnant women. He interpreted these as excursions of the fetal thorax and even succeeded, by means of a tambour placed on the abdomen, in securing rather convincing tracings of these movements. Subsequent efforts by others, however, to confirm these observations on experimental animals—the mother animals having been anesthetized with ether—were completely unsuccessful. Of course, they did not know at that time, as we know now, that ether completely inhibits these movements and consequently, for well over a quarter of a century, Ahlfeld's observations were more or less dismissed as figments of the imagination.

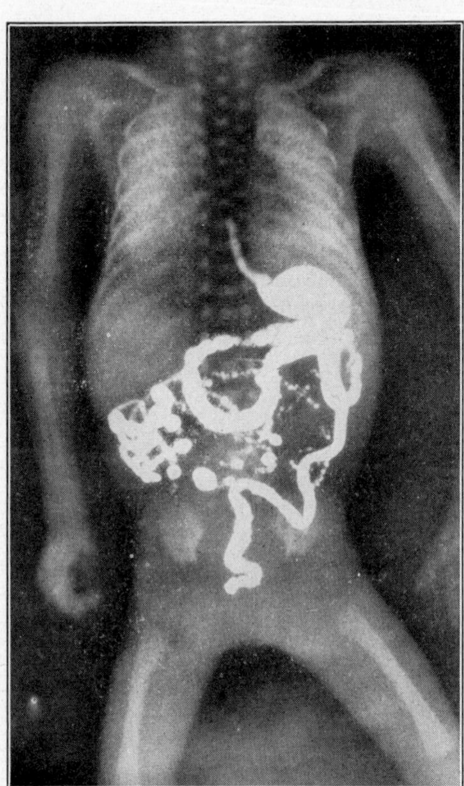

Fig. 138.—X-ray of 115 gm. Fetus in which Thorotrast Is Present in the Lungs. Esophagus, Stomach and Entire Intestinal Tract Following Injection of the Amniotic Cavity with Thorotrast 24 Hours before Delivery.

This demonstrates not only intra-uterine respiration of the fetus, but also that the fetus swallows amniotic fluid actively. (Courtesy of Dr. M. E. Davis and Dr. E. L. Potter.)

The credit for reviving the old idea of fetal respiration is due to Snyder and Rosenfeld. About 1935, while studying an entirely different problem, they were startled to see unmistakable respiratory excursions of the fetal thorax in pregnant rabbits in which the abdomen had been opened under regional anesthesia. They followed up this fortuitous observation by a series of studies which appeared to prove beyond question that these respiratory movements were not only normal phenomena of intra-uterine life but were associated with an inflow and outflow of amniotic fluid. Again, however, doubt was cast on the whole hypothesis, this time by Windle and his associates, who claimed that the findings of Snyder and Rosenfeld were due to the artificial stimulation produced by the experimental technic. The matter rested for some four or five years in this state of uncertainty until a seemingly decisive paper by Davis and Potter appeared. These authors studied intra-uterine respiration of the human fetus by injecting thorium hydroxide into the amniotic sac of pregnant women prior to therapeutic abortion and also prior to cesarean section. By x-ray examination of the fetal lungs after delivery they demonstrated that amniotic fluid and its contents are normally aspirated into the lungs as part of the intra-uterine respiratory activity and that this phenomenon is demonstrable as early as the twelfth week of gestation and continues throughout the intra-uterine life of the fetus (Fig. 138). At birth, air is substituted for fluid as a medium of exchange and the respirations become deeper, regular and continuous.

From a biological viewpoint, the occurrence of these fetal respiratory movements appears logical, since other important systems, such as the cardiac, renal and hepatic, function in utero, and it would be singular indeed if the important mechanism of pulmonary respiration, characterized by rhythmic muscular movements, should suddenly start functioning at birth without any preliminary activity. From a practical, clinical viewpoint the existence of fetal respiration has far-reaching implications, since we are no longer led to believe that respiration at birth is precipitated by some complicated chemical mechanism which we must try to imitate artificially. On the other hand, with this new viewpoint, we are inclined to regard this first breath as a continuation of a delicate, easily arrested mechanism which has been in action for some time.

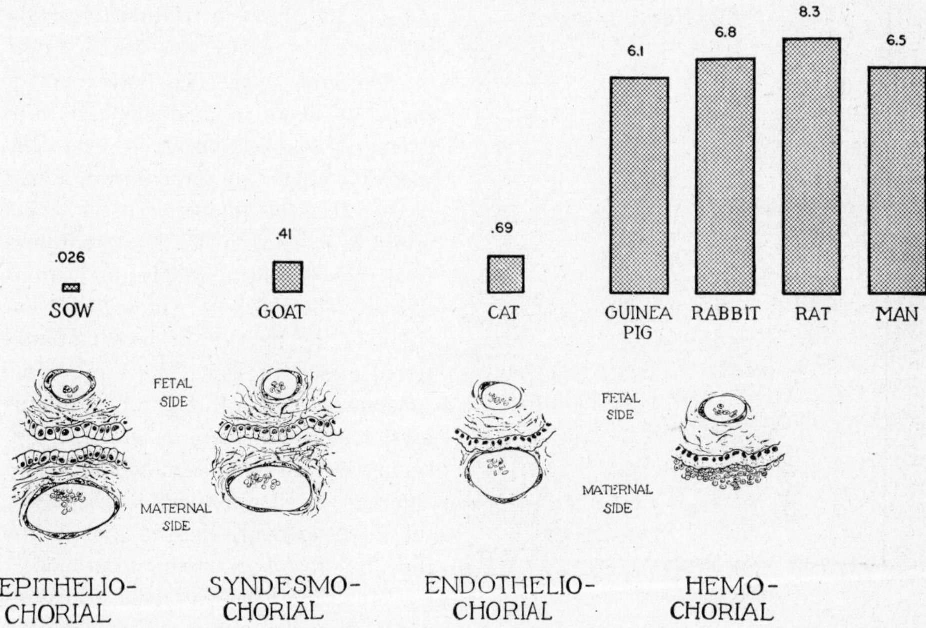

Fig. 139.—Variation of Transfer Rate per Unit Weight of Placenta with the Morphologic Type of Placenta.

The numerical values give the milligrams of sodium transferred across a unit weight of placenta per hour as observed in each instance at the middle of the ninth tenth of pregnancy. The relative magnitudes of the transfer rates are indicated by the relative areas of the dotted rectangles. The diagrams indicate the number and kind of tissue layers interposed between maternal and fetal circulations in each of Grosser's four groups (Flexner, Cowie, Hellman, Wilde and Vosburgh).

The Placenta as an Organ of Transfer

The placenta serves two main functions. As explained in Chapter 6, one of these is the production of the three hormones, chorionic gonadotrophin, estrogen and progesterone. The other is the transfer of oxygen and various nutritive materials from mother to fetus and, conversely, the conveyance of carbon dioxide and waste products from fetus to mother. As previously stated when the structure of the placenta was considered, there is no direct communication between the vessels of the chorionic villi and the intervillous spaces. The independence of the two circulations is most convincingly demonstrated, perhaps, during the first months of pregnancy by comparing the contents of the fetal vessels with that of the intervillous spaces. In the former, large numbers of nucleated red corpuscles are found, which are never present in the latter. At term, moreover, the red cell count of the fetus is regularly much higher than that of the mother, being roughly 5.5 million as against about 4 million in the mother.

Factors Concerned in Placental Permeability. Whether or not a given substance traverses the placental barrier and at what rate, depends upon a number of factors. These are: (1) the type of placenta concerned, a circumstance which varies with the species of the animal; (2) the stage of pregnancy; (3) the molecular weight of the substance in question; and (4) the selective activity which the placenta appears to exhibit in relation to certain substances.

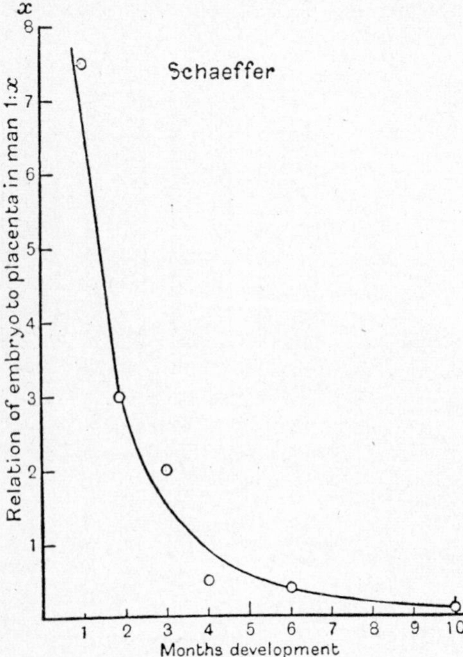

Fig. 140.—Ratio of Placental Weight to Fetal Weight in Man According to Duration of Pregnancy (From *Chemical Embryology,* by Joseph Needham. Cambridge University Press.)

Placental Type. The lower part of Fig. 139 shows in diagrammatic form Grosser's classification according to the species of animal concerned. Here it may be seen that the number of tissue layers interposed between the maternal and fetal blood differs widely in various species. The point of variance lies entirely in the number of layers of maternal tissue present. Thus, in swine, substances passing from mother to fetus must traverse the maternal endothelium, connective tissue and epithelium before entering the chorionic villus, whereas at the other extreme, in man and in the rodents, substances passing from mother to fetus enter the chorionic villus directly from the maternal blood without traversing any maternal tissues whatsoever. It will be seen from the upper half of Fig. 139 that these anatomical circumstances have a most important bearing upon the permeability of the placenta to simple substances such as the sodium ion. Thus, because of the greater intimacy of the two bloods, the human placenta is able to transfer approximately 250 times more sodium per gram of placenta per hour than is the sow placenta. These facts are important not only in showing how anatomical structure affects placental function, but serve also to recall that experimental work on placental permeability carried out on certain of the lower species is not necessarily applicable to placental behavior in man.

Stage of Pregnancy. The stage of pregnancy affects placental transfer through two factors: (1) the changing placental-fetal weight ratios as gestation progresses and (2) the structural alterations which the placenta undergoes as pregnancy advances.

If the weight of the placenta is divided by the weight of the fetus and the resultant figures be plotted for various stages of human pregnancy, a curve will be obtained such as is shown in Fig. 140. During the first trimester of pregnancy the trophoblastic tissue weighs decidedly more than the fetus, approximates its weight at three and one-half months, and thereafter shows a diminishing ratio in respect to fetal weight, so that at term the placenta weighs about one-sixth as much as the infant. This wide shift in relationship imposes upon the placenta the necessity of supplying a larger and larger mass of fetal tissue, per gram of placenta, as pregnancy progresses. In other words, the fetus increases in size very rapidly in comparison to placental growth. Indeed, between the twelfth week and term, the fetus grows 12 times more than the placenta. The placenta accommodates itself to this increasing demand, by structural alterations which parallel the increment in fetal requisites.

The alterations in placental architecture which make possible an increasing capacity for transfer in the course of pregnancy are of two sorts: (1) an increasing surface area which the villi present to the maternal blood and (2) a thinning of the villous coat. The relative size of the villus at 12, 19, 28 and 40 weeks of pregnancy, respectively, is shown in Fig. 141 where it may be seen that the size of an individual villus at term is only a small fraction of that of the same structure early in pregnancy. Paralleling this change, of course, is a great increase in the total area of the villous surfaces. Although microscopic examination of placentas gives clear evidence of an increase in the total surface area of the villi as pregnancy advances, no quantitative studies on the magnitude of this change are available. Several attempts have been made, however, to estimate the total surface area of chorionic villi in the human placenta at term. The first investigation of this kind was that of Dodds in 1922, who found that the total surface area of the villi in the normal human placenta at term was approximately 7 square meters. Rech found values ranging between 4.5 and 8 square meters with a mean of 6.3 square meters. More recent studies have indicated that these estimates are too small. Thus, Dees-Mattingly has found that the total absorptive area of the chorionic villi is 15 square meters, while Christoffersen, on the basis of a study of 61 human placentas at term, has placed the total villous surface from 10 to 20 square meters with an average of 14.5 square meters. In order better to visualize the area presented by the chorionic villi, it may be stated on the basis of the above figures that this area corresponds roughly to the size of a 9 by 12 living-room rug.

The other alteration in the placenta which makes for increasing permeability as pregnancy advances is to be found in alterations in those layers of the villus which interpose themselves between the maternal and the fetal bloods. As is well known, the layer of Langhans' cells disappears before the twentieth week with the result that the villus is then coated by merely one layer of syncytium instead of a double covering of cell layers. The walls of the villous capillaries likewise undergo alteration in the direction of thinning, showing a progressive decrease in the cellularity of their walls, until at term the endothelial nuclei are few, flattened and compact. Meanwhile, fetal vessels have become more numerous. As the result of these several changes the amount of sodium which the placenta is able to transfer per gram per hour increases as gestation advances until, near term, it transfers 12 times as much per gram per hour as at the third month. It will be noted that this figure corresponds exactly with that cited for the differential between fetal and placental growth.

Molecular Weight of Substance. Substances of a molecular weight under 1,000, with certain exceptions, appear to pass through the placenta by simple diffusion and tend to assume equal concentrations on both sides of the placental barrier. For instance, the following substances appear in equal concentrations in maternal and fetal bloods: sodium, chloride, magnesium, water, urea, uric acid, creatine, creatinine,

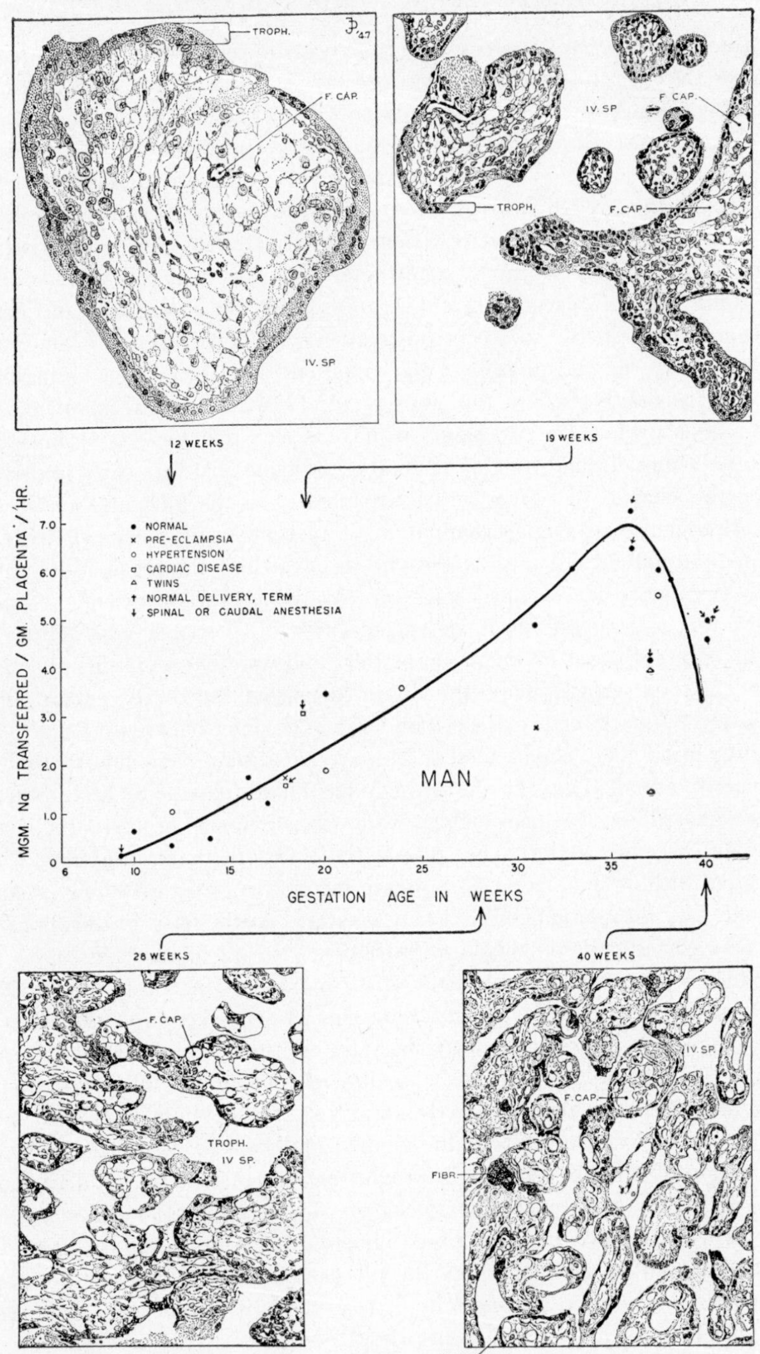

FIG. 141.—VARIATION IN THE RATE OF TRANSFER OF SODIUM WITH RESPECT TO GESTATION AGE.

The camera lucida drawings are from sections of normal human placentas at the indicated gestational ages and illustrate the histological changes which can be correlated with the change in permeability. Note, as the placenta ages, decrease in thickness of trophoblast (*Troph.*), increase in surface of villi exposed to intervillous space (*Iv. Sp.*) and increase in number of fetal capillaries (*F. Cap.*). *Fibr.*, fibrin (Flexner, Cowie, Hellman, Wilde and Vosburgh).

and total phosphorus. The concentrations of the following substances are slightly higher in fetal than in maternal blood: calcium, inorganic phosphorus, free amino nitrogen, and nucleic acid. Since these latter substances are essential architectural units for fetal growth, the concept has developed that the placenta possesses certain selective powers in regard to this special class of substances and transfers them in larger amounts. This hypothesis will be elaborated upon in the next section. The concentration of glucose, on the other hand, is slightly higher in the maternal circulation. From a practical standpoint it should be noted that almost all drugs, being of relatively low molecular weight, pass readily through the placenta and appear in the fetal blood and tissues within an hour or so after administration to the mother; included among these are all narcotic and sedative drugs (morphine, barbiturates, and such), all general anesthetic agents (ether, sodium pentothal, and such), the sulfonamides, penicillin, and streptomycin.

In general, substances of large molecular weight do not traverse the placenta, as evidenced by the fact that their concentrations in the two bloods show no regular relationships. This is true, for example, of the plasma proteins. It is believed that the fetus synthesizes its own proteins from the amino acids which, as indicated, do traverse the placenta and assume slightly higher concentrations on the fetal side of the placental barrier. The behavior of the placenta toward lipids is a moot question with present-day evidence suggesting that fetal fat may have a dual origin: first, placental transfer of fatty acids, cholesterol, and such; and second, synthesis of fat, by the fetus, from carbohydrate.

The earliest investigations on this question seemed to show that the fetus synthesized all its lipids from carbohydrates. Thus, Slemons and Stander reached the conclusion that the placenta in man is absolutely impermeable to fatty acids, and this attitude was taken by Slemons in his monograph on placental transmission. Slemons and Stander laid especial emphasis on the fact that there was no sort of parallelism between the variations in the level of fatty acids in the two bloods. The studies of Plass and Tompkins on the phosphatides agreed in showing that the several lipid fractions, like total lipids, were always higher in the maternal plasma than in the fetal, but that no constant ratio between the two bloods could be demonstrated.

Then, other evidence came to light which showed that some of the fetal lipids, at least, must be transmitted through the placenta. This evidence is of two types. In the first place, the feeding of certain fats to pregnant animals influences the iodine value of the fetal fats. Thus, if a fat with a low iodine number is given, the fat stores of the mother will have lower iodine values than when she is otherwise fed; the same effect is noted in the fetus but to a lesser degree. A similar relationship is found when fats of high iodine number are fed. The second type of evidence demonstrating placental transmission of fats is that contributed by Boyd and Wilson, who found a higher concentration of lipid substances in blood coming from the placenta than in that going to the placenta. This is plain evidence, of course, that fatty substances are given off to the fetal blood in transit through the placenta. The same investigators clamped the cord immediately after birth and took blood from the umbilical cord at that time and again when the placenta separated. The second specimen invariably showed a higher concentration of phospholipids and usually more free cholesterol, ester cholesterol, and neutral fat. This indicated that in the few minutes between clamping of the cord and placental separation the lipids mentioned passed from maternal to fetal bloods. In this connection it may be noted that Needham, on general biologic principles, has long been skeptical of the thesis that all fetal fat derives from synthesis. Thus, he remarks, "No oviparous animal requires its embryo to synthesize its fatty acids from carbohydrates and the idea that viviparous embryos should be asked to do so does not fit in with the biologically valuable properties of intra-uterine development."

Goldwater and Stetten have studied the transplacental passage of fatty acids and of cholesterol by the administration to pregnant rats of samples of these materials suitably labeled with deuterium, followed by the isolation of corresponding products from their fetuses. The feeding of deutero fatty acids and deutero cholesterol to pregnant rats in the latter part of gestation resulted in the appearance of the corresponding deutero compounds in the fetuses, proving that these compounds cross the rat placenta. On the other hand, enrichment of the body fluids of pregnant rats with deuterium oxide resulted in the rapid incorporation of deuterium into fetal glycogen, fatty acids, and cholesterol at rates indicating that these compounds are synthesized in the fetal organisms. From these observations the authors reached the conclusion that fetal fat is of dual origin, in part placental transfer of fatty acids, cholesterol, and such and in part synthesis by the fetus from carbohydrates.

Studies by Flexner, Vosburgh and their associates, who used radioactive isotopes for their investigations, indicate that the fetus obtains its iron from the plasma iron of the maternal blood and that the old idea that the trophoblast takes up iron from hemolyzed maternal blood corpuscles plays little if any role in the transport of this mineral.

Since the naturally occurring estrogens have a relatively small molecular weight (*e.g.*, estradiol, 272) this hormone might be expected to traverse the placenta, and it does so quite readily. Estrogen is present in the blood and urine of the infant at birth, but diminishes gradually to disappear entirely about the sixth day of life. Moreover, the effects of the intra-uterine action of estrogen on the fetus are clearly demonstrable. Thus, the vagina of the newborn is a multilayered membrane resembling that of the adult woman, but during the neonatal period it becomes thin and remains so until puberty. Other evidence of estrogen activity on the fetus is to be found in the slight bloody vaginal discharge which newborn girls occasionally exhibit during the first week of life and which is due to estrogen withdrawal. Similarly, the breast enlargement which the newborn sometimes shows is the result of estrogen action.

Since fetal urine is not present in sufficient amounts for pregnanediol determination, chemical proof that progesterone traverses the placenta is not available. The endometrium of the newborn shows no secretory activity, an observation indicating that progesterone does not pass through to the fetus in substantial quantity and in active form. However, the fact that the molecular weight of progesterone is about the same as that of estradiol suggests that progesterone may be transferred to some degree. Chorionic gonadotrophin does not traverse the placenta, a circumstance in keeping with the fact that it is a protein of large molecular weight.

Thyroxin, with a molecular weight of 777, appears to pass through the placenta, since, according to Döderlein, thyroxin given to pregnant guinea pigs causes an increase in the metabolism of the newborn offspring. On the other hand, parathyroid hormone, an albuminose, does not traverse the barrier. Snyder and Hoskins have shown that adrenalin, insulin, and posterior pituitary extract when injected into the fetus in utero do not appear in the maternal blood. However, the work of Cattaneo and of Schlossman raises some question about the behavior of adrenalin, as they found that following the injection of this hormone into either the fetal heart or umbilical artery, the maternal blood pressure rises almost directly in proportion to the dosage used.

Vitamin A shows no correlation between maternal and fetal blood levels. Moreover, the fetal concentration cannot be raised by increasing the maternal vitamin A or carotene levels. Only traces of carotene are present in the fetal plasma, often none at all. Thiamin, the only member of the vitamin B complex which has been studied in fetal circulation thus far, seems to pass rapidly from maternal to fetal bloods and is present in about the same concentration in each.

Selective Activity. As has been indicated, the molecular size of any given substance undoubtedly plays an important role in whether or not it will transgress the placenta; moreover, since most solutes of small molecular weight tend to assume equal concentrations on the two sides of the barrier, it can be assumed that they go back and forth across the placenta by a process of simple diffusion. Certain slight deviations from this general principle, as in the cases of amino acid nitrogen, calcium, and inorganic phosphorus, have been mentioned, but the degree of the deviation in these instances is scarcely enough to furnish proof that the basic mechanism involved is other than simple diffusion.

On the other hand, the behavior of a number of substances in relation to the placental barrier is such as to indicate clearly that the placenta possesses the power to exert selective activity in certain cases. Let us consider ascorbic acid for an example. This is a crystalline substance which resembles in its chemical configuration the pentose and hexose sugars and would be expected to pass through the placenta, like glucose, by simple osmosis. Nevertheless, studies by Braestrup, by Manahan and Eastman, by Teel, Burke and Draper, by Lund and Kimble, and by others, agree in showing that the amount of ascorbic acid in plasma from the umbilical cord blood of infants at birth is regularly from two to four times higher than that in the maternal plasma taken at the time of delivery. Teel, Burke and Draper have brought out the point especially that the greatest differences are found when the values for the maternal blood are lowest. They feel that the fetus in utero acts parasitically on the mother with respect to ascorbic acid, and as long as appreciable amounts of vitamin C are present in maternal plasma, the fetus tends to take what it needs irrespective of the maternal requirements. This is simply another way of saying, of course, that the placenta, in response to fetal needs, possesses the power of maintaining the ascorbic acid level of the fetal plasma at concentrations which are severalfold those of the maternal plasma. In vitro studies by Barnes on placental slices have revealed no evidence to indicate that the human placenta can synthesize ascorbic acid. By means of histochemical technics, moreover, Holzaepfel and Barnes have demonstrated that the placenta concentrates vitamin C in the syncytial layer of the chorionic villus. Both these observations are in keeping with the viewpoint that the placenta transfers vitamin C to the fetus through a process of selective activity.

In respect to antibodies, the placenta behaves in such an irregular manner as to controvert entirely the idea that large molecular size is necessarily a deterrent to placental transmission. Antibodies are believed to be gamma globulins or to be inseparably associated with that fraction of the plasma proteins. The molecular weight of the plasma globulins has been variously estimated between 103,000 and 175,000; even if it be assumed that the gamma globulins approach the serum albumins in molecular weight, we would be dealing with a weight of the general magnitude of 68,000. This is some 50 times the weight of polypeptides, which do not transgress the placenta. Yet the evidence is overwhelming that antibodies regularly traverse the placenta whether they be of foreign origin passively introduced into the mother, or whether they originate in the maternal organism as the result of active immunization.

Thus, as long ago as 1904 Polano reported a study of the passive transfer of diphtheria antitoxin from mother to child. That antibodies to diphtheria are transferred through the placenta was shown also by Park and Zingher who compared Schick tests on mothers and infants and showed that the newborn infant almost invariably gave the same reaction as the mother. These observations were confirmed by Kuttner and Ratner, who worked with the Schick test and made comparative titrations of the antitoxin content of the maternal and cord blood. Tetanus antitoxin is also transmitted through the placenta, as was first shown by Ten Broeck and Bauer in 1922. Leach, Zia and Lim have investigated the possibility of immunizing newborn infants to tetanus by administering tetanus toxoid to the mother. Seventy-one mothers were injected with tetanus formol toxoid, the number of injections varying from one to three. The tetanus antitoxin titer of the serum in 59 mothers taken at the time of delivery showed an average of 23.2 units. Cord blood from 70 newborn infants of mothers who had received tetanus toxoid injections showed an average titer of 11.2, whereas the amount present in infants of untreated mothers was negligible. Active immunization of mothers and passive immunization of the infants in utero to pertussis during the last third of pregnancy have been successfully effected by Cohen and Scadron, who feel that this procedure provides a most desirable protection for the young infants against pertussis. Similarly, isohemolysins, isoagglutinins and other agglutinins may readily traverse the placenta. The antibodies against influenza, lymphogranuloma venereum, and other virus diseases have been transmitted from mother to fetus. Antistreptolysins, staphylococcus antitoxin and antipneumococcic antibodies also pass through the placenta.

It is generally held that bacteria and viruses do not pass through the placenta, and whenever they do traverse it, it is a consequence of pathologic lesions produced in the placenta by these agents. Nevertheless, intra-uterine infection with viruses is occasionally seen, and until recent years it has been most frequently observed in smallpox. Intra-uterine infections with measles and chickenpox, though rare, are authentically reported.

Of great current interest is the probable passage of the virus of rubella through the placenta with resultant malformations in the fetus, provided the virus acts upon it during the early developmental stages. Because of these effects on the infant it has been generally assumed that the virus of rubella does pass through the placenta. However, in a recent study by Gillman, Gilbert and Gillman, it was considered not inconceivable that the type of metabolic disorder associated with rubella may mediate its effects through disturbances produced in the mother without actual passage of the virus into the fetal tissues. This subject is discussed further on page 707.

The Amniotic Fluid

From an extremely early period in embryologic development a clear fluid collects in the amniotic cavity and surrounds the fetus. The amount at term varies between 500 and 1,000 cc. as a rule, but quantities up to 2,500 cc. are not regarded as abnormal.

The amniotic fluid is alkaline in reaction, with a specific gravity of 1.007 to 1.025 and consists of 98 to 99 per cent water and 1 to 2 per cent solids, of which approximately half is organic and half inorganic. Cantarow, Stuckert and Davis have made extensive chemical studies of amniotic fluid and maternal blood obtained simultaneously from 36 women in the seventh to the ninth month of normal pregnancy. They reported average values for protein content of 0.53 gm.; for nonprotein nitrogen, 24.25 mg.; for uric acid, 4.54 mg.; for sugar, 19 mg.; for calcium, 5.46 mg.; and for phosphorus, 3.1 mg., per hundred cubic centimeters of amniotic fluid. Other recent studies on the chemical composition of the amniotic fluid in general confirm these findings. Many other organic substances have been reported as present in the amniotic fluid. These include fructose, lactic acid, carotene, adrenaline, glutathione, citric acid, and the enzymes erepsin, diastase, lipase, pepsin and rennin.

The source of the amniotic fluid has been a matter of much speculation, and from time to time four main views have been advanced as to its origin: (1) fetal urine; (2) transudation from maternal blood; (3) secretions through the amniotic epithelium; and (4) a mixed origin. It is known that the fetal kidneys excrete urine and small quantities doubtless escape into the amniotic fluid, but present-day opinion maintains that fetal urine constitutes only a very small fraction of the total amount of fluid present. Polano and other investigators have found that in normal pregnancy the amniotic epithelium frequently exhibits a very striking formation of vacuoles

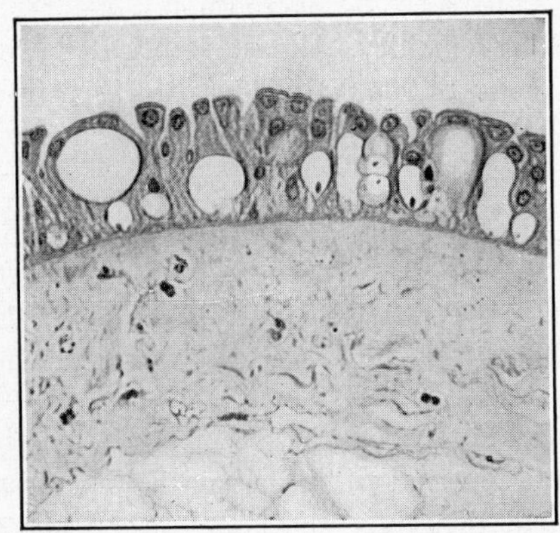

FIG. 142.—VACUOLES IN AMNIOTIC EPITHELIUM INDICATING SECRETORY ACTIVITY.

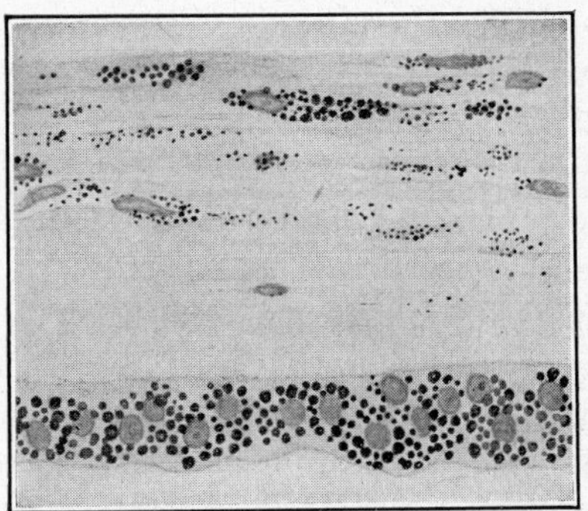

FIG. 143.—FAT IN AMNIOTIC EPITHELIUM. (Adapted from Polano.)

whose contents at times can be seen in the act of becoming extruded into the amniotic sac. Such changes occur so frequently that they must indicate some physiological function and thus lend support to the secretory theory. Moreover, by appropriate methods of staining, Polano was able to demonstrate the abundant presence of fat in the amniotic epithelium and associated it with secretory activity (Figs. 142 and 143). On the other hand, some authorities are skeptical about the secretory function of the amnion and regard the fluid as a pure dialysate. The question is hence an unsettled one, with opinion divided as to whether the amniotic fluid is a dialysate or a secretory product of the amniotic epithelium, or whether it comes from both these sources.

The amniotic fluid is by no means a static medium but is being continuously renewed at an amazingly rapid rate. Thus, Vosburgh, Flexner and their associates have shown by means of heavy water studies that, on the average, 35.4 per cent of the water of amniotic fluid is replaced per hour by water from the maternal plasma. This means that the average rate of renewal of the water of the amniotic fluid is once every 2.9 hours. At term a fetus weighing 3,400 gm. is surrounded by approximately 1,000 cc. of amniotic fluid which is exchanging water at the rate of 350 cc. per hour. The picture becomes all the more striking when it is recalled that while the molecules in this 350 cc. of water are migrating in one direction, an approximately equal number of molecules of water are passing in the other. It should be noted that this extremely active state of flux is in itself rather conclusive evidence against the urinary origin of the amniotic fluid.

The amniotic fluid serves a number of important functions. It keeps the fetus at an even temperature, cushions it against possible injury, and provides a medium in which it can move easily. Furthermore, as already indicated, the fetus continually drinks this fluid. However, any role the amniotic fluid may play in fetal nutrition is probably very slight.

SEX OF THE FETUS

More boys are born at full term than girls, the ratio being approximately 106 to 100. Thus, in a sample of 46,000,000 births registered in Western Europe from 1929 to 1937 the sex ratio was 105.5 males per 100 females for live-born infants, 126.7 for stillbirths, and 106.2 for all fetuses reaching viability. Almost identical figures have been found in the United States where, among 14,000,000 births registered from 1941 to 1945, the sex ratio was 105.6 for live births, 124.1 for stillbirths and 106.0 for the two groups combined (Tietze).

It has long been thought that the sex ratio at the time of conception, usually called the primary sex ratio, differs decidedly from that at term in the direction of a much higher proportion of males. Data recently collected by Tietze indicate that this old belief is incorrect and is attributable to erroneous diagnoses of the sex of young embryos. As shown by Karl M. Wilson, even trained experts cannot make a reliable diagnosis by inspection of the external genitalia if the embryo has not reached the crown-rump length of 50 mm., corresponding to the end of the eleventh week from the onset of the last menstruation. Even beyond this stage the large clitoris of the female will often be mistaken for a penis by less experienced observers. Pertinent information has been collected by Tietze from the main catalogue of the Carnegie Institution covering 5,667 fetuses of 50 to 249 mm., corresponding to the fourth to the seventh month of pregnancy. The sex of these embryos and younger fetuses was determined by microscopic examination of the gonads, most of these determinations having been made by the late Dr. George L. Streeter. Tietze's findings are shown in Table 7 and can leave little doubt that the sex ratio from the third to the seventh month of gestation is approximately the same as it is among viable infants.

Crown-Rump Length (mm.)	Month of Gestation	Number of Males	Number of Females	Percentage Males	Sex Ratio
20- 49	3rd	58	62	48.3 ± 4.6	93.5
50- 99	4th	598	555	51.9 ± 1.5	107.7
100-149	5th	771	667	53.6 ± 1.3	115.6
150-199	6th	801	730	52.3 ± 1.3	109.7
200-249	7th	775	770	50.2 ± 1.3	100.6
20-249	3rd to 7th	3003	2784	51.9 ± 0.7	107.9

TABLE 7. SEX RATIOS OF SPECIMENS IN THE CARNEGIE COLLECTION. (Tietze.)

The sex of the fetus is determined in the germ cells, either primarily or immediately after their union, so that it has become immutable by the time segmentation of the ovum begins. Support is lent to such a view by observations upon twin pregnancy in human beings. It has long been known that these result either from the fertilization of one or of two ova, and that a distinction can usually be made by the study of the fetal membranes. In the first case the children are always of the same sex, whereas in the latter the sex may or may not be the same. Furthermore, still more striking evidence is afforded by the armadillo. In this animal each litter consists of four young which are always of the same sex, and that they are derived from a single ovum is shown by the fact there is only one placenta and one chorion, but four amnions. While such observations show that the sex had been determined before segmentation had begun, they give no information as to the mechanism of its determination, and leave us doubtful whether it had been predetermined in the ovum or in the spermatozoon, or was due to changes taking place at the time of fertilization.

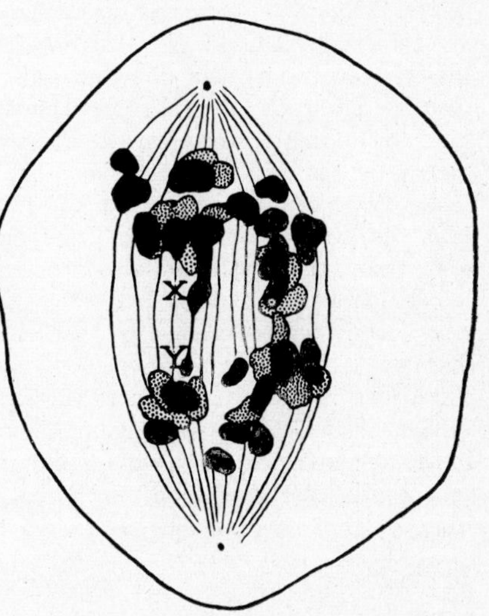

FIG. 144.—HUMAN PRIMARY SPERMATOCYTE SPINDLE WITH X-Y CHROMOSOME NOT YET DIVIDED. See Fig. 81.

(From Evans and Swezy, *The Chromosomes in Man*. Courtesy of University of California Press.)

Today, as a result of the investigations of Morgan, Painter, Evans and others, it is generally accepted that the determining factor must be attributed to a chromosome, called the *sex, x,* or *accessory* chromosome. The oogonia contain 46 ordinary and two x-chromosomes and after maturation the ovum, as well as the second polar body, will have 23 + x chromosomes. On the other hand, the spermatogonia, while having 46 ordinary chromosomes, contain only one x-chromosome and a mate to it, which is smaller, functionless and known as the y-chromosome. Thus the spermatozoon, after reduction of the chromosomes is completed, contains either 23 + x or 23 + y chromosomes, the former joining the ovum (23 + x) producing a female (46 + 2x) and the latter a male (46 + x + y). In other words, for practical purposes, spermatozoa containing the x-chromosome may be regarded as female and those containing the y-chromosome as male spermatozoa, giving rise to female and male offspring, respectively. More recent work by Evans and Swezy corroborates the earlier findings of Painter and of Evans and gives final proof of a true sex chromosome and two types of spermatids, which are different only insofar as the composition of one chromosome is concerned, one half carrying the x-chromosome and the other half the y-chromosome. The sex chromosomes are also shown in Figs. 81 and 82.

Prediction of Sex of Fetus in Utero. The number of tests, supernatural and otherwise, which have been proposed for this purpose are myriad. They appear in all centuries and emanate from all peoples: ancient Egyptian, Hippocratic Greek, Arabian, Indian, Chinese, Jewish, Russian, etc. The supernatural omens range from the prophetic interpretation of numerology, astrology and dreams, to the examination of entrails, the flight of birds, and "ordeals." As Blakely points out in his interesting survey of this subject, the use of strictly supernatural means to diagnose fetal sex has never been persistent or extensive, compared with what he calls "natural phenomena." These he divides into three broad groups:

Group 1. The supposed origin of the male from the right side of the uterus, the female from the left; and the changes in the right side of the pregnant woman's body ascribed to, or imagined to result from, such origin.

Group 2. The position, outlines, attitude and activities of the fetus during pregnancy and labor.

Group 3. The effects of a male fetus on the total maternal organism, that is, the reaction of the female body to the introduction therein of a male element. This is the largest and most important group.

In regard to the first of these ideas, the belief is widespread that boys develop from eggs coming from the right ovary and girls from the left. Various attempts have been made on the part of the gullible to control sex on this basis. Thus it has been recommended that the woman lie on the right side during coitus for a boy and on the left side for a girl, the idea being, of course, that gravity will direct the spermatozoa to the proper ovary. Another notion along the same lines was introduced by Rumley Dawson in a monograph which appeared in 1917 in which he attempted to prove that the two ovaries ovulate alternately, so that it is possible to control the sex, provided the woman had previously given birth to a child. To do so, it is only necessary to remember that, at the first ovulation following labor, the ovum would come from the ovary which had not functioned at the last conception. Accordingly, if the child were a boy, the next ovum would be from the left ovary, so that by making the necessary calculation, coitus could be had when the right or the left ovary was to function, according as a boy or girl was desired. That this whole concept is erroneous is demonstrated by the fact that women from whom one ovary has been removed continue to have children of either sex, and Murray conclusively showed the fallacy of such a belief. In 64 cases of cesarean section, Williams found the corpus luteum 36 times in the right ovary and 28 times in the left ovary. In the first instance, there were 23 boys and 13 girls, while in the second there were 16 boys and 12 girls, thereby demonstrating that children of either sex may develop from eggs coming from either ovary, and thus disproving the above theory.

By far the best known of the second group of signs is the fetal heart rate. In 1859, on the basis of a study of 100 cases, Frankenhaeuser suggested that fetal sex might be determined by the rate of the fetal heart in the last three months of pregnancy, a persistently slow rate (averaging 124 or less a minute) indicating a boy, and a persistently more rapid rate (averaging 144 or more a minute), a girl. All obstetricians are acquainted with this old sign and practically all hold no brief for it—if for no other reason, because the fetal heart rate usually falls between the figures given.

The last group of diagnostic methods is the most numerous and includes a wide variety of procedures from a modification of the Abderhalden test (the formation of protective ferments against living foreign protein) and vaginal pH to the more modern endocrine approach. All these tests, however, have been shown to be unreliable, and it must be concluded that there is at present no reliable method of predicting the sex of the unborn child. For complete literature on this topic up to 1937, Blakely should be consulted.

BIBLIOGRAPHY

Abel, S., and Windle, W. F. Relation of the Volume of Pulmonary Circulation to Respiration at Birth. Anat. Rec., 1939, 75:451.

Adair, F. L., and Scammon, R. E. A Study of the Ossification Centers of the Wrist, Knee and Ankle at Birth. Am. J. Obst. & Gynec., 1921, 2:35.

——— Observations on the Parietal Fontanelle in the Newborn and Young Infant. Am. J. Obst. & Gynec., 1927, 14:149.

Ahlfeld, F. Die intrauterine Tatigkeit der Thorax- und Zwerchfellmuskulatur Intrauterine Atmung. Monatschr. f. Geburtsh., 1905, 21:143.

Arey, L. B. Developmental Anatomy: A Textbook and Laboratory Manual of Embryology, 5th Ed. W. B. Saunders Co., Philadelphia, 1946.

Ballantyne, J. W., and Browne, F. J. The Problem of Fetal Postmaturity and Prolongation of Pregnancy. J. Obst. & Gynaec. Brit. Emp., 1922, 29:177.

Barclay, A. E., Barcroft, J., Barron, D. H., and Franklin, K. J. Radiographic Demonstration of Circulation through Heart in Adult and in Foetus, and Identification of Ductus Arteriosus. Brit. J. Radiol., 1939, 12:505.

——— X-ray Studies of Closing of Ductus Arteriosus. Brit. J. Radiol., 1938, 11:570.

Barcroft, J. Researches on Prenatal Life. Blackwell, Oxford, 1946.

Barnes, A. C. Placental Metabolism of Vitamin C. I. Normal Placental Content. Am. J. Obst. & Gynec., 1947, 53:645.

Barron, D. H. The Changes in the Fetal Circulation at Birth. Physiol. Rev., 1944, 24:277.

Becker, R. F., Windle, W. F., Barth, E. E., and Schultz, M. D. Fetal Swallowing, Gastrointestinal Activity and Defecation in Amnio. Surg., Gynec. & Obst., 1940, 70:603.

Belcher, D. P. A Child Weighing 25 Pounds at Birth. J.A.M.A., 1916, 67:950.

Blakely, S. B. The Diagnosis of the Sex of the Human Fetus in Utero. Am. J. Obst. & Gynec., 1937, 34:322.

Boyd, E. M., and Wilson, K. M. The Exchange of Lipids in the Umbilical Circulation at Birth. J. Clin. Investigation, 1935, 14:7.

Braestrup, P. W. Studies of Latent Scurvy in Infants. II. Content of Ascorbic (Cevitamic) Acid in the Blood Serum of Women in Labor and in Children at Birth. Acta Paediat., 1937, 19: Suppl. 1, 328.

Byrn, J. N., and Eastman, N. J. Vitamin A Levels in Maternal and Fetal Blood Plasma. Bull. Johns Hopkins Hosp., 1943, 73:132.

Calkins, L. A. Morphometry of the Human Fetus. Am. J. Obst. & Gynec., 1922, 4:109.

Cantarow, A., Stuckert, H., and Davis, R. C. Chemical Composition of Amniotic Fluid: A Comparative Study of Human Amniotic Fluid and Maternal Blood. Surg., Gynec. & Obst., 1933, 57:63.

Cattaneo, L. Contribution Experimentale à l'Étude du Passage des Hormones Foetales à travers le Placenta. Arch. Ital. de Biol., 1931, 86:1.

Christie, A. Prevalence and Distribution of Ossification Centers in the Newborn Infant. Am. J. Dis. Child., 1949, 77:335.

Christoffersen, A. K. La Superficie des Villosités Choriales du Placenta à la fin de la Grossesse (Étude d'Histologie Quantitative). Compt. rend. Soc. de biol., 1934, 117:641.

Cohen, P., and Scadron, S. J. Placental Transmission of Protective Antibodies against Whooping Cough by Inoculation of Pregnant Mother. J.A.M.A., 1943, 121:656.

Davis, M. E., and Potter, E. L. Intra-uterine Respiration of the Human Fetus. J.A.M.A., 1946, 131:1194.

Dawson, R. The Causation of Sex in Man. New York, 1917.

Dees-Mattingly, M. Absorptive Area of Chorionic Villi in Circumvallate Placenta. Am. J. Anat., 1936, 59:485.

Dodds, E. A. The Area of the Chorionic Villi in the Full Term Placenta. Anat. Rec., 1924, 24:285.

Döderlein, G. Experimenteller Hyperthyroidismus und seine Wirkung auf Fortpflanzung und Nachkommenschaft. Arch. f. Gynäk., 1928, 133:680.

Eastman, N. J. Fetal Blood Studies. I. The Oxygen Relationships of Umbilical Cord Blood at Birth. Bull. Johns Hopkins Hosp., 1930, 47:221.

——— Geiling, E. M. K., and DeLawder, A. M. Fetal Blood Studies. IV. The Oxygen and Carbon-Dioxide Dissociation Curves of Fetal Blood. Bull. Johns Hopkins Hosp., 1933, 53:246.

Evans, H. M., and Swezy, O. The Chromosomes in Man, Sex and Somatic. Mem. Univ. California, Berkeley, 1929, 9:1.

Flexner, L. B., and Gellhorn, A. Comparative Physiology of Placental Transfer. Am. J. Obst. & Gynec., 1942, 43:965.

Flexner, L. B., Cowie, D. B., Hellman, L. M., Wilde, W. S., and Vosburgh, G. J. The Permeability of the Human Placenta to Sodium in Normal and Abnormal Pregnancies and the Supply of Sodium to the Human Fetus as Determined with Radioactive Sodium. Am. J. Obst. & Gynec., 1948, 55:469.

Gillman, J., Gilbert, C., and Gillman, T. A Preliminary Report on Hydrocephalus, Spina Bifida and Other Congenital Anomalies in the Rat Produced by Trypan Blue. The Significance of These Results in the Interpretation of Congenital Malformations Following Maternal Rubella. South African J. M. Sc., 1948, 13:47.

Goldwater, W. H., and Stetten, DeW., Jr. Studies in Fetal Metabolism. J. Biol. Chem., 1947, 169:723.

Greene, R. R., et al. A Note on the Respiration-like Movements of the Human Fetus. Surg., Gynec. & Obst., 1938, 66:987.

Grosser. Frühentwicklung, Eihautbildung, und Plazentation des Menschen und der Säugetiere. München, 1927.

Grosser, O. Human and Comparative Placentation Including Early Stages of Human Development. Lancet, 1933, 1:999, 1053.

Hellman, L. M., Flexner, L. B., Wilde, W. S., Vosburgh, G. J., and Proctor, N. K. The Permeability of the Human Placenta to Water and the Supply of Water to the Human Fetus as Determined with Deuterium Oxide. Am. J. Obst. & Gynec., 1948, 56:861.

HOLZAEPFEL, J. H., and BARNES, A. C. Placental Metabolism of Vitamin C. II. Histochemical Analysis. Am. J. Obst. & Gynec., 1947, 53:864.

HOLZBACH, E. Uber den Wert der Merkmale zur Bestimmung des Reife des Neugeborenen. Monatschr. f. Geburtsh. u. Gynäk., 1906, 24:429.

HOSKINS, F. M., and SNYDER, F. F. Placental Transmission of Parathyroid Extract. Am. J. Physiol., 1933, 104:530.

JACKSON, C. M. On the Prenatal Growth of the Human Body. Am. J. Anat., 1909, 9:119.

KUTTNER, A. G., and RATNER, B. The Importance of Colostrum to the Newborn Infant. Am. J. Dis. Child., 1923, 25:413.

LEA, A. W. W. The Sagittal Fontanelle in the Heads of Infants at Birth. Tr. Obst. Soc. London, 1898, 40:263.

LEACH, C. N., ZIA, S. H., and LIM, K. T. An Attempt to Immunize Newborn Infants to Tetanus Neonatorum Through the Administration of Tetanus Toxoid to Pregnant Mothers. Am. J. Hyg., 1936, 24:439.

LUND, C. J., and KIMBLE, M. S. Some Determinants of Maternal and Fetal Vitamin C Levels. Am. J. Obst. & Gynec., 1943, 46:635.

MAKEPEACE, A. W., FREMONT-SMITH, F., DAILY, M. E., and CARROL, M. P. The Nature of the Amniotic Fluid. A Comparative Study of Human Amniotic Fluid and Maternal Serum. Surg., Gynec. & Obst., 1931, 53:635.

MANAHAN, C. P., and EASTMAN, N. J. The Cevitamic Acid Content of Fetal Blood. Bull. Johns Hopkins Hosp., 1938, 62:478.

NEEDHAM, J. Chemical Embryology. Cambridge University Press, 1931.

——— Biochemistry and Morphogenesis. Cambridge University Press, 1942.

PAINTER, T. S. The Spermatogenesis of Man. J. Exper. Zoöl., 1923, 37:291.

PLASS, E. D. Total Creatinine in Plasma, Whole Blood and Corpuscles of Mother and Fetus; Additional Analysis by a New Method. Bull. Johns Hopkins Hosp., 1917, 28:297.

PLASS, E. D., and MATTHEW, C. W. Placental Transmission. III. The Amino Acids, Nonprotein Nitrogen, Urea and Uric Acid in Fetal and Maternal Whole Blood, Plasma and Corpuscles. Bull. Johns Hopkins Hosp., 1925, 36:393.

PLASS, E. D., and TOMPKINS, E. H. Placental Transmission. II. The Various Phosphoric Acid Compounds in Maternal and Fetal Serum. J. Biol. Chem., 1923, 56:309.

POLANO, O. Exp. Beiträge zur Biologie der Schwangerschaft. Würzburg, 1904.

——— Der Antitoxinübergang von der Mutter auf das Kind. Ein Beitrag zur Physiologie der Plazenta. Ztschr. f. Geburtsh. u. Gynäk., 1904, 53:456.

RECH, W. Untersuchungen über die Grösse der Zottenoberfläche der Menschlichen Plazenta. Ztschr. Biol., 1924, 80:349.

REYNOLDS, S. R. M. Unpublished data on dynamics of circulation in umbilical cord, for which I am most indebted.

RIGGS. A Comparative Study of White and Negro Pelves, etc. Johns Hopkins Hospital Reports, 1904, 12:42.

SCHLOSSMAN, H. Beiträge zur Biologie der Plazenta. III. Die Durchlässigkeit der Plazenta für Adrenalin. Arch. f. Exper. Path. u. Pharmakol., 1932, 166:74.

SHREWSBURY, J. F. D. The Chemistry of the Liquor Amnii. Lancet, 1933, 1:415.

SHUMAN, H. H. Varicella in Newborn. Am. J. Dis. Child., 1939, 58:564.

SKINNER, H. H. A Baby Weighing Fifteen Pounds Two Ounces at Birth. Am. J. Obst. & Gynec., 1936, 32:511.

SLEMONS, J. M., and STANDER, H. J. The Lipoids of the Maternal and Foetal Blood at the Conclusion of Labor. Bull. Johns Hopkins Hosp., 1922, 34:7.

SMITH, C. A., and BARKER, R. H. Ether in the Blood of the Newborn Infant. Am. J. Obst. & Gynec., 1942, 43:763.

SMITH, C. A., and KAPLAN, E. Adjustment of Blood Oxygen Levels in Neonatal Life. Am. J. Dis. Child., 1942, 64:843.

SNYDER, F. F. The Rate of Entrance of Amniotic Fluid into the Pulmonary Alveoli during Fetal Respiration. Am. J. Obst. & Gynec., 1941, 41:224.

——— Obstetric Analgesia and Anesthesia. W. B. Saunders Co., Philadelphia, 1949.

SNYDER, F. F., and HOSKINS, F. M. Placental Transmission of Adrenalin, Insulin and Pituitrin. Anat. Rec., 1927, 35:33.

SNYDER, F. F., and ROSENFELD, M. Intra-uterine Respiratory Movements of the Human Fetus. J.A.M.A., 1937, 108, 1946.

SPEERT, H. Placental Transmission of Sulfathiazole and Sulfadiazine and Its Significance for Fetal Chemotherapy. Am. J. Obst. & Gynec., 1943, 45:200.

——— and BABBITT, D. The Passage of Sulfanilamide through the Human Placenta. Bull. Johns Hopkins Hosp., 1938, 63:337.

STANDER, H. J. The Respiratory Exchange of the Fetus. Am. J. Obst. & Gynec., 1927, 13:39.

——— and TYLER, M. The Moisture and Ash of Maternal and Fetal Blood, Surg., Gynec. & Obst., 1920, 31:276.

STREETER, G. L. Weight, Sitting Height, etc., and Menstrual Age of the Human Embryo. Carnegie Inst. of Wash., 1920, Publ. No. 274, Contrib. to Embryology, 2.

SWINGLE, W. W. The Determination of the Sex in Animals. Physiol. Rev., 1926, 6:28.

TEEL, H. M., BURKE, B. S., and DRAPER, R. Vitamin C in Human Pregnancy and Lactation; Studies during Pregnancy. Am. J. Dis. Child., 1938, 56:1004.

TEN BROECK, C., and BAUER, J. H. The Transmission of Tetanus Antitoxin through the Placenta. Proc. Soc. Exper. Biol. & Med., 1923, 20:399.

TIETZE, C. A Note on the Sex Ratio of Abortions. Human Biol., 1948, 20:156.

VOSBURGH, G. J., and FLEXNER, L. B. Maternal Plasma as a Source of Iron for the Fetal Guinea Pig. Am. J. Physiol., 1950, May.

VOSBURGH, G. J., FLEXNER, L. B., COWIE, D. B., HELLMAN, L. M., PROCTOR, N. K., and WILDE, W. S. The Rate of Renewal in Woman of the Water and Sodium of the Amniotic Fluid as Determined by Tracer Techniques. Am. J. Obst. & Gynec., 1948, 56:1156.

WILSON, K. M. Correlation of External Genitalia and Sex Glands in the Human Embryo. Carnegie Inst. of Wash., 1926, Contrib. to Embryology, 18:23.

WINDLE, W. F. Physiology of the Fetus. W. B. Saunders Co., Philadelphia, 1940.

——— Circulation of Blood through the Fetal Heart and Lungs and Changes Occurring with Respiration at Birth. Quart. Bull. Northwestern Univ. M. School, 1940, 14:31.

WINDLE, W. F., and BECKER, R. F. Relation of Anoxemia to Early Activity in the Fetal Nervous System. Arch. Neurol. & Psychiat., 1940, 43:90.

WINDLE, W. F., BECKER, R. F., BARTH, E. E., and SCHULZ, M. D. Aspiration of Amniotic Fluid by the Fetus. Surg., Gynec. & Obst., 1939, 69:705.

WOLTZ, J. H. E., and WILEY, M. M. Transmission of Streptomycin from Maternal Blood to Fetal Circulation and Amniotic Fluid. Proc. Soc. Exper. Biol. & Med., 1945, 60:106.

WOLTZ, J. H. E., and ZINTEL, H. A. Transmission of Penicillin to Amniotic Fluid and Fetal Blood in Human. Am. J. Obst. & Gynec., 1945, 50:338.

8

MATERNAL PHYSIOLOGY IN PREGNANCY

DURATION OF PREGNANCY

The average duration of human pregnancy, counting from the first day of the last menstrual period, is about 280 days or 10 lunar months (Fig. 145). Since the interval between the first day of menstruation and ovulation averages approximately 13 days, the mean duration of actual pregnancy, counting from the day of con-

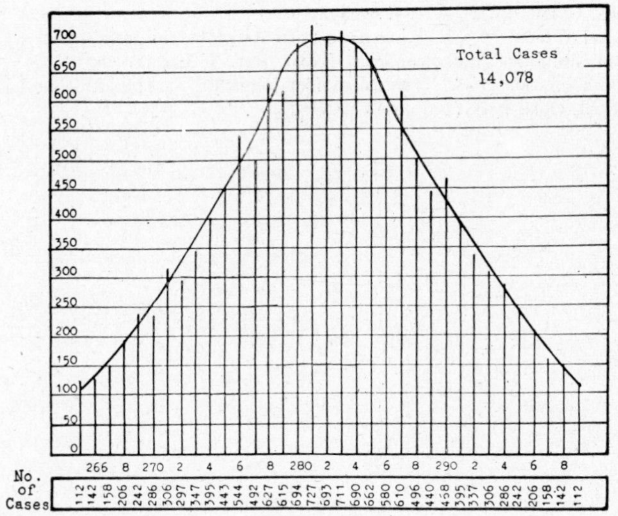

FIG. 145.—DISTRIBUTION CURVE OF DURATION OF PREGNANCY (FROM FIRST DAY OF LAST MENSTRUAL PERIOD) IN 14,078 CASES.

The infants were at least 48 cm. in length and 2,800 gm. in weight. In addition, to the 14,078 cases graphed above, there were in the author's series 961 cases (with infants showing same length and weight specifications) in which the duration of pregnancy was either less than 265 days or more than 299 days—that is, 6.4 per cent. In 624 of these, the pregnancy exceeded 299 days. It will be noted that the median duration of pregnancy in this series was 282 days (Speitkamp).

ception, must be close to 267 days. Ahlfeld analyzed 425 cases in which the date of fruitful coitus was supposed to have been known and found the average duration of gestation from the time of conception to be 269.91 days; but individual cases in the series ranged from 231 to 329 days. Cary has stated that in 15 cases of artificial insemination the duration of pregnancy ranged between 261 and 282 days, with an average of 272 days.

It is customary to estimate the expected date of delivery by counting back three months from the first day of the last menstrual period and adding seven days (Naegele's rule). For instance, if the patient's last menstrual period began on September 10, the expected date of confinement (often abbreviated E.D.C.) would be June 17. This method of calculation is made easier if the months are taken as numbers. Then, the above example becomes: 9/10 minus three months equals 6/10 plus 7 days equals 6/17. In view of the known variations in the duration of pregnancy this method of calculation must be regarded as the sheerest approximation. Thus, as shown in Table 8, less than 5 per cent of gravidae go into labor on the calculated date. In an additional 35 per cent of cases, a deviation of one to five days, before or after that date, may be expected; in the majority of cases, the deviation is still greater. In over three per cent of patients, labor does not ensue until three weeks or more after the calculated date.

Deviation in Days	Early Delivery	Delivery on Calculated Date	Late Delivery
0		189 (4.1)	
1 — 5	860 (18.5)		773 (16.6)
6 — 10	610 (13.1)		570 (12.2)
11 — 20	733 (15.7)		459 (9.9)
21 — 30	211 (4.5)		134 (2.9)
31 and over	75 (1.6)		42 (0.9)

Table 8. Deviation from Calculated Date of Confinement, According to Naegele's Rule, of 4,656 Births of Mature Infants.

The menstrual cycles of the mothers were 28 ± 5 days. The infants were at least 47 cm. in length and 2,600 gm. in weight. (Burger and Korompai.)

Since the interval between ovulation and the next menstrual period is more constant than the pre-ovulatory phase of the cycle, the duration of pregnancy, when calculated from the first day of the last period, is related to the length of the cycle. In other words, a patient with a long cycle will ovulate later in respect to the previous period than a woman with a short cycle, and hence any pregnancy will begin later in respect to the last menstrual period from which the calculation is made and therefore, on the average, it will end later.

The upper limit of the duration of pregnancy is of great medicolegal importance in cases in which the husband has been away for 10 months or more and the legitimacy of the child is in question. In the United States and England there is no law with respect to the duration of pregnancy, and individual cases are decided on their own merits. In 1921 an English court ruled in favor of the legitimacy of a child delivered 331 days after the departure of the husband. In a recent case reported by Wells the duration of pregnancy was presumably 334 days from the first day of the last period.

In not a few instances, especially in nursing women, conception may take place during a period of amenorrhea. Under such circumstances Naegele's rule is of no value and it is necessary to depend upon other means, which, unfortunately, are less satisfactory. In such cases the calculations are based upon the enlargement of the abdomen and the height to which the fundus of the uterus has risen. Generally speaking, with the patient on her back, the fundus is found at the fourth lunar month at a level about four finger-breadths above the symphysis pubis; at the fifth lunar month, just below the umbilicus; at the sixth lunar month, at the level of the umbilicus or slightly above; at the seventh lunar month, three finger-breadths above the umbilicus; at the eighth lunar month, three finger-breadths below the xiphoid process; at the ninth lunar month, just below the xiphoid; whereas in the last month, particularly in primigravidous women, it sinks downward and assumes almost the level it occupied at the eighth lunar month.

Precocious and Late Pregnancy. The youngest age at which childbirth has been authentically reported is probably four years and eight months—the famous case of Lina Medina who was delivered in Lima, Peru on May 15, 1939 of a 6½-pound male infant. Delivery was by cesarean section at the Maternity Hospital in Lima. It so happened that several American physicians were in Lima at the time and all attest the fact that this little girl, who appeared to be about five years old, was delivered by cesarean section as described. A careful investigation of the birth records of Lina Medina makes it possible that she was five years and eight months old instead of four years and eight months, but even then the case breaks all records.

Pregnancy after the age of 47 is very rare. In 65,000 deliveries at the Johns Hopkins Hospital, only one such case is recorded and that in a feeble-minded colored woman who stated she was 49 but may not have known her correct age.

UTERUS

The most apparent changes caused in the maternal organism by pregnancy are observed in the generative tract, and especially in the uterus which undergoes a very great increase in size. Thus, it is converted from a small, almost solid organ 6.5 cm. long, into a thin-walled, muscular sac capable of containing the fetus, placenta, and a large quantity of amniotic fluid. At the end of pregnancy it is about 32 cm. long, 24 cm. wide, and 22 cm. deep. It has been estimated that its capacity is increased 519 times. A corresponding increase in weight is also observed, the uterus at full term weighing in the neighborhood of 1,000 gm. (2.2 pounds), as compared with 30 gm. (1 ounce) in the virginal condition.

This enlargement is due principally to the hypertrophy of pre-existing muscle cells, but partly also to the formation of new ones during the earlier months of pregnancy. The fully developed muscle fibers are from two to seven times wider and from 7 to 11 times longer than those observed in the nonpregnant uterus, measuring 0.009 to 0.014 mm. by 0.2 to 0.52 mm. in the former, as compared with 0.005 by 0.05 to 0.07 mm. in the latter.

With the increase in the number and size of the muscle fibers is associated a marked development of mesenchymal tissue between the muscle bands, particularly in the external muscular layer, which resembles embryonic connective tissue. At the same time there is a considerable increase in the amount of elastic tissue. This forms a network about the various muscle bundles which hypertrophy with advancing pregnancy, and thus adds materially to the strength of the uterine walls. At the same time, there is a great increase in the size of the blood vessels, especially the veins, which, in the neighborhood of the placental site, become converted into large spaces, the so-called placental sinuses. Marked hypertrophy of the lymphatic and nervous supply of the uterus also takes place; this is well illustrated by the increase in size of Frankenhäuser's cervical ganglion from 2 by 2.5 cm. to 3.5 by 6 cm.

During the first few months, the hypertrophy of the uterus probably is brought about by a stimulus derived from the action of estrogen on the muscle fibers. That it is not directly due to the presence of the ovum in the uterine cavity is shown by the occurrence of precisely similar changes in extra-uterine pregnancy when the ovum is implanted in the tube or ovary. After the third month, however, the increase in size is in part mechanical, due to the pressure exerted by the growing product of conception.

During the first few months of pregnancy the uterine walls are considerably thicker than in the nonpregnant condition, but as gestation advances they gradually become thinner, so that at the end of the fifth month they are from 3 to 5 mm. in thickness. This measurement is retained throughout the succeeding months, so that at term the walls of the body of the uterus are rarely above 5 mm. thick, and occasionally

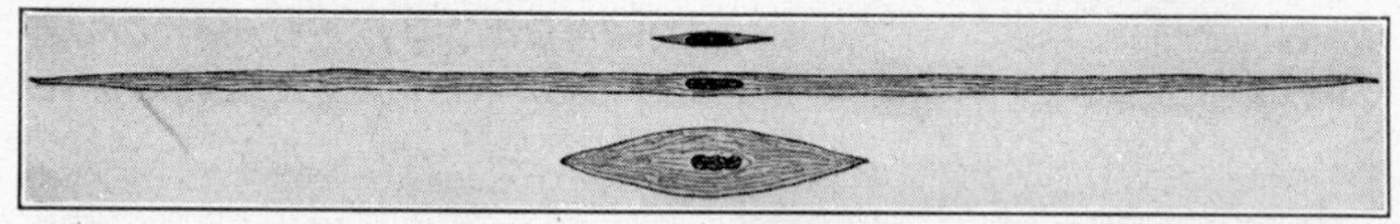

FIG. 146.—MUSCLE FIBERS FROM NORMAL NONPREGNANT, PREGNANT, AND PUERPERAL UTERUS (Stieve).

they measure considerably less. Consequently, the organ soon loses the firm, almost cartilaginous consistence which is characteristic of the nonpregnant condition, and in the later months becomes converted into a muscular sac having very thin, soft and readily compressible walls. This is well demonstrated by the ease with which the fetus can usually be palpated in the later months, and by the readiness with which the uterine walls yield to the movements of the fetal extremities.

The enlargement of the uterus is not symmetrical but is most marked in the fundal region. This can readily be appreciated by observing the relative positions of the insertions of the tubes and ovarian ligaments, which in the early months of pregnancy are only a little below the level of the fundus; whereas in the later months their attachments are found at points slightly above the middle of the organ.

The position of the placenta also exerts a determining influence upon the extent of the hypertrophy, the portion of the uterus to which it is attached enlarging more rapidly than elsewhere. This is clearly shown by the position of the uterine ends of the round ligaments; these are close together when the placenta is inserted upon the posterior and far apart when it is upon the anterior wall.

Arrangement of the Muscle Fibers. The musculature of the pregnant uterus is arranged in three strata: (1) an external hoodlike layer, which arches over the fundus and extends into the various ligaments; (2) an internal layer, consisting of sphincter-like fibers around the orifices of the tubes and the internal os; and lying between the two, (3) a dense network of muscle fibers perforated in all directions by blood vessels. The main portion of the uterine wall is formed by this middle layer, which consists of an interlacing network of muscle fibers, between which extend the blood vessels. Each fiber comprising this layer has a double curve so that the interlacement of any two gives approximately the form of the figure "8." As a result of such an arrangement, when the fibers contract after delivery they constrict the vessels and thus act as living ligatures. *From a clinical viewpoint, this is one of the most important facts in obstetrics.*

The muscle fibers composing the uterine wall in pregnancy, especially in its lower portion, overlap one another and are arranged like shingles on a roof, one end of each fiber arising beneath the peritoneal covering of the uterus, and extending obliquely downward and inward, to be inserted into the decidua, thus giving rise to a large number of muscular lamellae. The various lamellae are connected with one another by short muscular processes, so that when the tissue is slightly spread apart it presents a sievelike appearance which, on closer examination, is seen to be due to the presence of innumerable rhomboidal spaces.

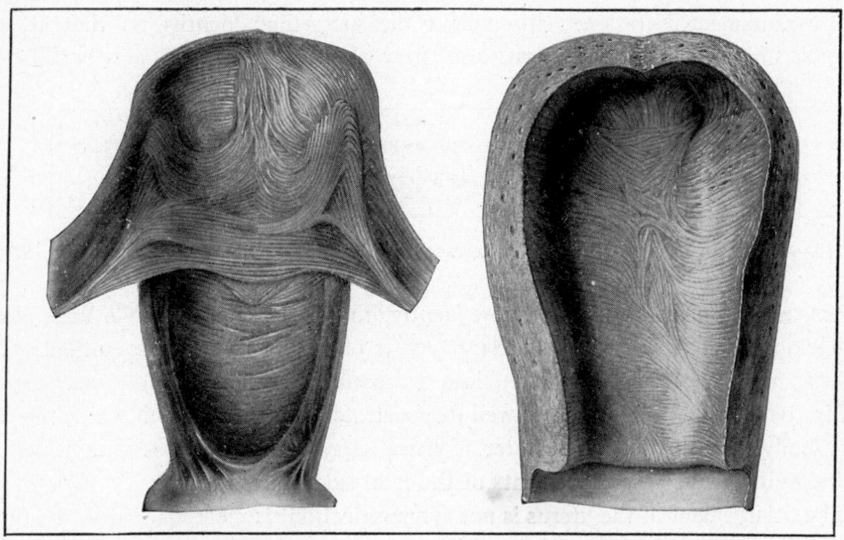

Fig. 147.—External and Internal Muscular Layers of Pregnant Uterus (Hélie).

The outermost layer of the uterine musculature can be especially well appreciated at the time of cesarean section. When the uterus contracts down after the delivery of the child and placenta, it is seen that the superficial margins of the incision retract some millimeters beyond the bulk of the muscular wall, and it is this layer which is brought together by the superficial suture. Upon microscopic examination it is in turn found to be made up of several thinner layers—an outermost layer consisting of muscle bundles running vertically, a median layer running circularly, and beneath the latter a thicker layer of loosely interlacing fibers, separated from one another by loose connective tissue and including many vessels. Indeed, the vessels are so abundant that this layer may appropriately be designated as the stratum vasculare.

Changes in Size and Shape of the Uterus. As the uterus increases in size, it also undergoes important modifications in shape. For the first few weeks its original pyriform outlines are retained, but the body and fundus soon assume a more globular form, which becomes almost spherical at the third month. After this period, however, the organ increases more rapidly in length than in width, and assumes an oval form, which persists until the end of pregnancy.

As the body of the uterus becomes larger the angle which it forms with the cervix becomes more acute—in other words, its physiological anteflexion is increased. By the fourth month the organ becomes too large to be contained in the pelvic cavity, and forms a tumor, the upper border of which reaches midway between the symphysis pubis and the umbilicus. As it becomes still larger it comes in contact with the anterior abdominal wall, displacing the intestines to the sides of the abdomen, and gradually rises up until it almost impinges upon the liver. As the uterus leaves the pelvis for the abdominal cavity considerable tension is exerted upon the broad ligaments, which then become more or less unfolded at their median and lower portion and thus contribute to the mobility of the pelvic peritoneum.

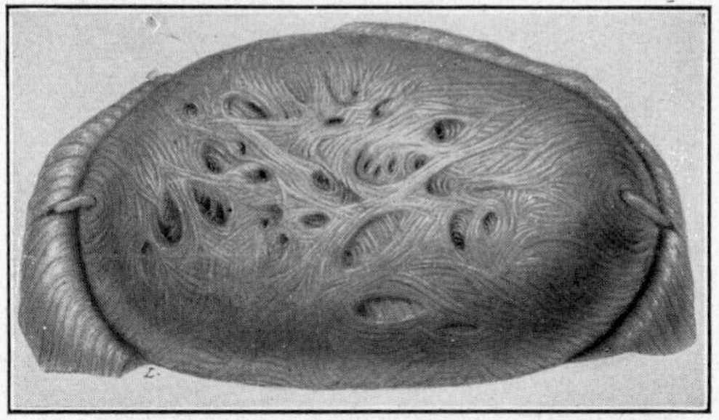

FIG. 148.—MEDIAN MUSCULAR LAYER OF PREGNANT UTERUS (Hélie).

The pregnant uterus possesses a considerable degree of mobility. Since its upper portion projects into and lies free in the abdominal cavity, and its lower portion is held in check by the cervical attachments, it readily changes its position. With the woman in a standing posture its longitudinal axis corresponds closely with that of the superior strait, the organ resting in great part upon the anterior abdominal wall; but, when she lies on her back, the uterus falls backward and rests upon the vertebral column.

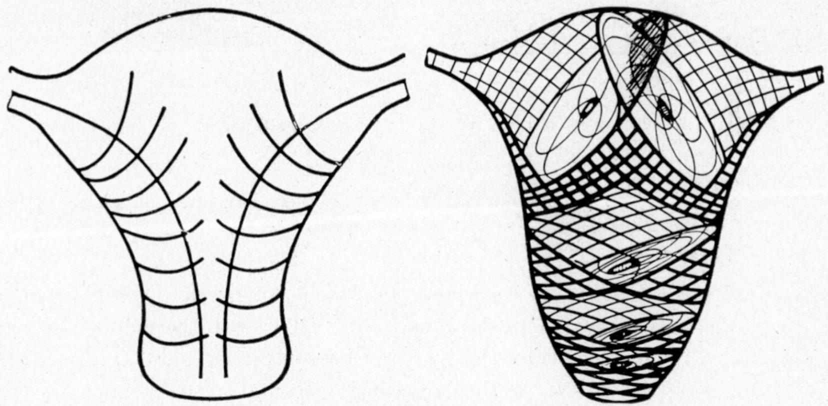

FIG. 149.—ARRANGEMENT OF THE TWO CHIEF SYSTEMS OF MUSCULAR FASCICULI IN THE NONPREGNANT UTERUS WHICH RESULTS FROM THE FUSION OF THE MULLERIAN DUCTS.
(From Ivy, *American Journal of Obstetrics and Gynecology.*)

As the uterus grows out of the pelvic cavity, it usually rotates slightly to the right, so that its left margin is directed more anteriorly than is the right. Occasionally the torsion may be in the opposite direction, statistics showing that it occurs to the right in 80 per cent and to the left in 20 per cent of the cases. The torsion is due in great part to the presence of the rectum which occupies the left side of the pelvis, though, occasionally, the condition may represent merely an exaggeration of the original position of the nonpregnant uterus which, as is well known, is not always perfectly symmetrical.

Changes in the Spiral Arteries. During the progestational stage of the cycle, the endometrial coiled arteries grow rapidly toward the uterine lumen, at the same time becoming increasingly coiled. Ramsey finds that when implantation occurs, the arterial tips still lie some millimeters below the surface epithelium, but a week or so later, slightly before the nineteenth day (ovulation age), the process of continued growth plus trophoblastic invasion effect an opening of the maternal arteries into the intervillous spaces of the fetal placenta. Beyond the fifty-third day the spiral arteries do not increase materially in length and there is no further significant alteration in their coils for another five to seven weeks. At the end of that time the vessels pass

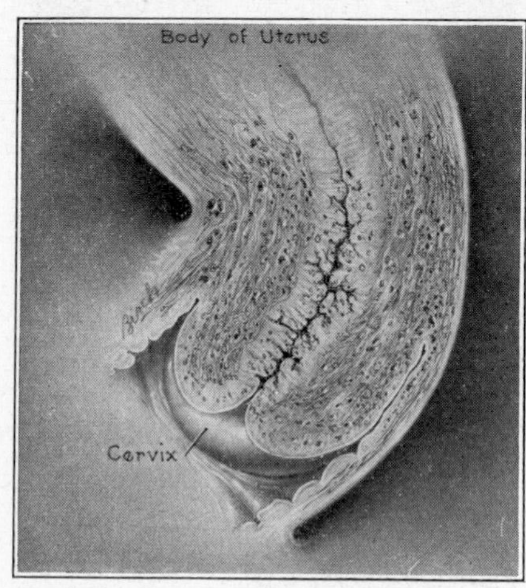

Fig. 150.

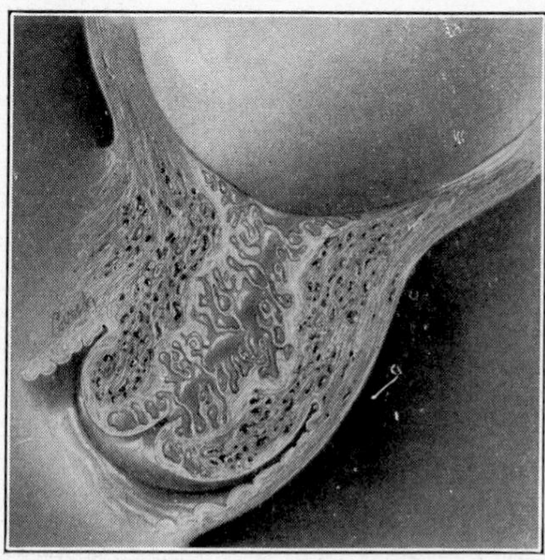

Fig. 151.

Fig. 150.—Cervix in the Nonpregnant Woman.

Fig. 151.—Cervix in Pregnancy.

Note the elaboration of the mucosa into a honeycomb-like structure, the meshes of which are filled with tenacious mucus—the so-called "mucous plug."

through an abrupt transition, in the course of which two major qualitative changes occur. First, the coils of the arteries are paid out, and second, the number of vessels communicating with the intervillous spaces is decreased. After these transformations have been effected, the course of the remaining placental arteries, now a smooth, straight, direct course interrupted only by an occasional right-angle bend, remains unchanged to term. It would thus appear that the coiling of the arteries is a mechanism which, when they become uncoiled, permits them to cover the greater distances presented by the enlarged pregnant uterus. As pregnancy advances another alteration occurs in these arteries, namely, intimal fibrosis, which makes its appearance around the fifty-third day and persists thereafter up to term. As described by Ramsey, the process is of variable extent, completely and permanently obliterating some stems and narrowing the lumen of others. It commences high up in the endometrium and, like the other two vascular changes, progresses towards the muscularis. At 154 days it is pronounced in the myometrial arcuate arteries. It is conceivable, in Ramsey's opinion, that this intimal fibrosis establishes a mechanism which may be of value in controlling hemorrhage at parturition.

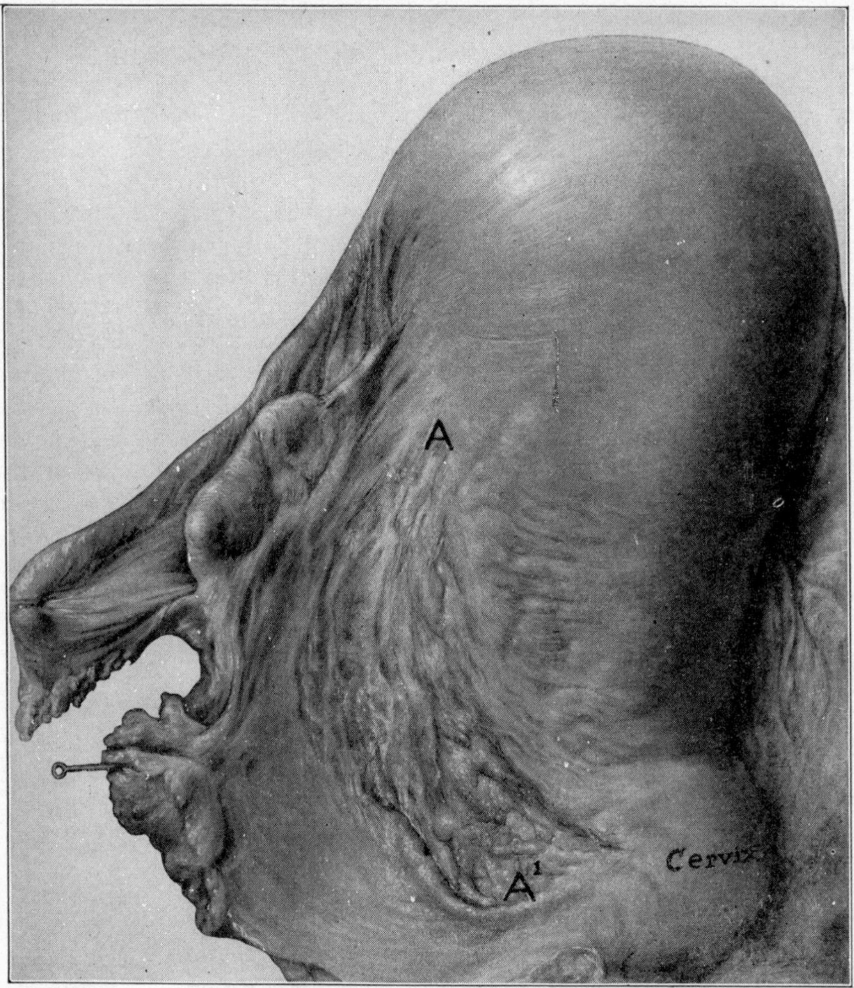

Fig. 152.—Ectopic Decidual Formation on Posterior Surface (A to A′) of Puerperal Uterus. × ⅔. (Hofbauer.)

Changes in the Cervix. Prior to 1927 it was generally stated that, apart from pronounced softening, slight changes occur in the cervix during the course of pregnancy and, until labor sets in, it appears as a mere appendage to the enlarged body of the uterus. Stieve, however, has shown that such views are erroneous and that most striking and important changes occur. In the first place, the cervical mucosa undergoes such marked proliferation that, at the end of pregnancy, it occupies approximately one half of the entire bulk of the cervix instead of only a small fraction of it as at other times. Moreover, the septa separating the glandular spaces become progressively thinner, resulting in the formation of a honeycomb-like structure whose meshes are filled with tenacious mucus, so that when the so-called "mucous plug" is expelled at the onset of labor practically the entire structure is carried away with it. Furthermore, the glands in the neighborhood of the external os proliferate beneath the stratified mucosa covering the vaginal portion and give the cervix the velvety consistence characteristic of pregnancy (Figs. 150 and 151).

In the second place the muscle fibers, instead of taking part in the hypertrophy of the body, actually diminish in number, although those which remain increase in size. At the same time, the connective tissue becomes looser and reverts to a younger stage, while in the third place, there is a great increase in the number of vessels, particularly veins, with the result that the cervical wall outside of its canal becomes converted into an almost erectile tissue.

Ectopic Decidua. Following the description by Schmorl and Kinoshita in 1897 of small decidual nodules on the posterior surface of the pregnant uterus and on the adjacent peritoneum, it has become generally recognized that decidual formation occasionally occurs in various portions of the body.

Geipel in 1928 described 40 personal observations of ectopic decidual formation, not only about the genitalia, but also in the pelvic lymph glands, omentum, diaphragm, appendix and spleen. In every fourth or fifth uterus removed at operation or autopsy at the end of pregnancy, one finds ectopic decidual formation. Usually this consists of small pale nodules, varying from 1 to 3 mm. in diameter, just beneath the peritoneum covering the lower portion of the posterior wall of the uterus. Occasionally, however, they present a pinkish color and suggest minute adhesions which have been torn through, while very exceptionally, the decidual formation involves large areas which are reddish in color and at first glance suggest an inflammatory change (Fig. 152).

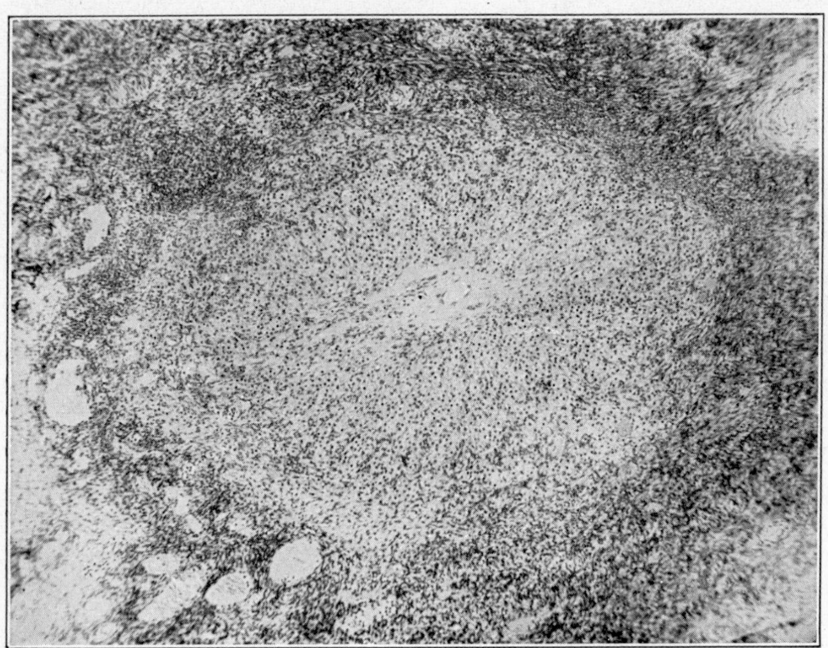

FIG. 153.—SECTION THROUGH OVARY OF PREGNANT WOMAN, SHOWING EXAGGERATED FOLLICULAR ATRESIA—THE SO-CALLED "INTERSTITIAL GLAND." × 60.

TUBES AND OVARIES

As has already been mentioned, the tubes and ovaries undergo marked changes in position with the advance of pregnancy, so that instead of extending outward almost at right angles from the cornua, their long axes become nearly vertical. Occasionally, as the result of the upward traction exerted by the enlarging uterus, the ovaries become greatly elongated. More important, however, is their increase in vascularity, to which the large size of the corpus luteum of pregnancy is in great part due. Ovulation ceases during pregnancy, so that new follicles do not ripen and, accordingly, only the single

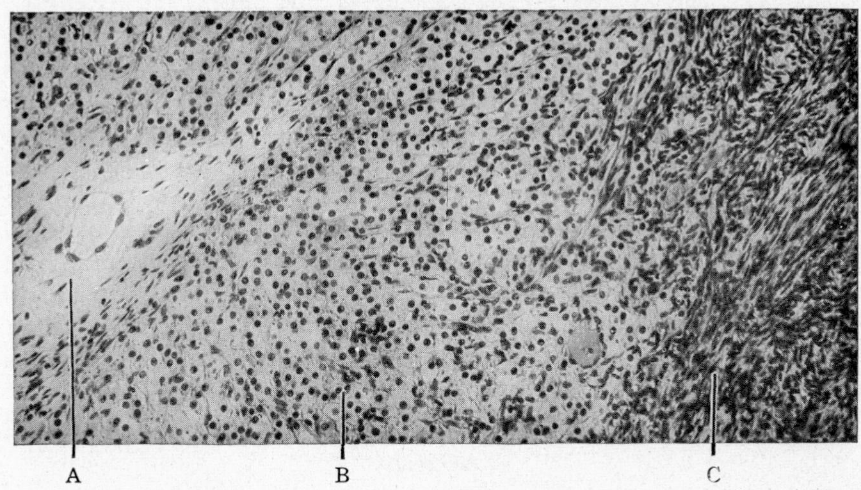

Fig. 154.—Portion of Figure 153, Magnified 200 Times.
A., connective tissue core; B., hypertrophied theca cells; C., normal ovarian stroma.

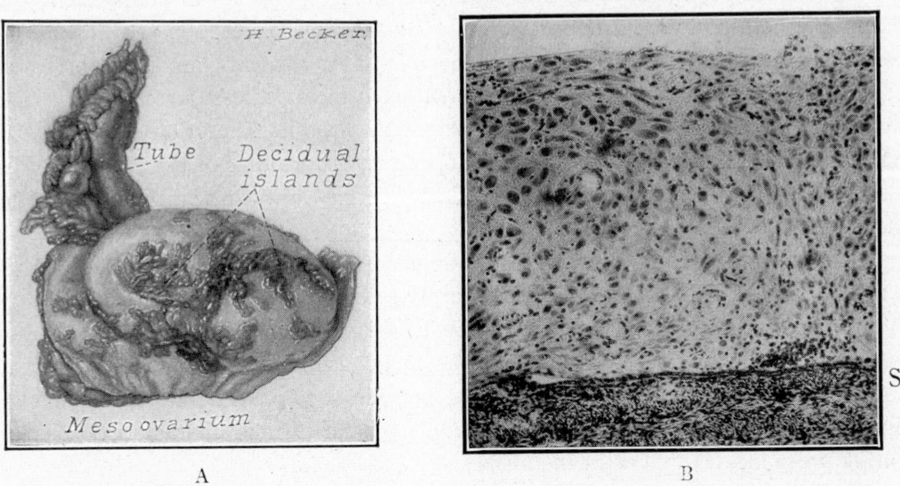

Fig. 155.—A, Gross Specimen; B, Microscopic Picture of Decidual Formation on Surface (S) of Ovary.

large corpus luteum of pregnancy can be found in one of the ovaries. While typical ovulation does not occur, many follicles begin to grow and, after reaching a certain stage of development, undergo atretic changes associated with a marked development of lutein-like cells in the theca folliculi. In many instances these cells come to occupy the greater part of the interior of the ovary and are designated by many writers as the "interstitial gland." In the early stages of atresia the interstitial cells form a layer surrounding the follicular cavity. Later this layer is broken up into separate clusters of cells and scattered in various directions so that their original relationship to the follicle rapidly becomes obscure. These formations present so characteristic an appearance as to permit the experienced observer to make a diagnosis of pregnancy (Figs. 153 and 154). They disappear within a few weeks after labor.

Inspection of the ovaries at cesarean section shows that in every third or fourth case a number of flattened pinkish elevations, rarely exceeding a few millimeters in diameter, project from their surface, and at first glance give the impression of being freshly torn adhesions. Closer examination, however, shows that they are not such, but that they consist of masses of decidual cells beneath the ovarian epithelium (Fig. 155). Their function is not known.

It is generally stated that the muscular fibers of the tubes undergo considerable hypertrophy during pregnancy, but if hypertrophy occurs at all, it is very slight in extent. Moreover, the epithelium of the tubal mucosa is flatter during pregnancy than it is in the nonpregnant state. Occasionally, in uterine pregnancy, decidual cells may develop in the stroma of the tubal mucosa, but they never lead to the formation of a continuous membrane as in the uterus.

VAGINA

Increased vascularity is the most marked change in the vagina, and to it are due the more copious secretion and the characteristic violet coloration of pregnancy. Stieve has shown that the vaginal wall undergoes very striking changes to prepare it for the distention incident to labor. He describes a considerable increase in the thickness of the mucosa, a great loosening of the connective-tissue elements, and an hypertrophy of the muscle cells to almost as great an extent as in the uterus. As a result, the vaginal walls may increase in length to such an extent that the lower portion of the anterior wall protrudes slightly through the vulval opening. The papillae of the vaginal mucosa also undergo considerable hypertrophy, whence results an increased roughness of the membrane.

The vaginal secretion is considerably augmented and normally is represented by a thick, white, crumbly substance. It is sharply acid, with a pH varying from 3.5 to 6, due to the presence of lactic acid which in turn is derived from the glycogen in the vaginal epithelium. It is believed that the lactic acid plays an important part in keeping the vagina relatively free from pathogenic bacteria. The cellular content of the vaginal secretion has been shown to undergo marked and characteristic changes during pregnancy as well as in the menstrual cycle.

The increased vascularity attending pregnancy is not confined to the genitalia, but extends to the various organs in their vicinity and in part may account for the slight relaxation of the pelvic joints, which is accompanied by an increase in their motility. As already noted (page 81), the relaxation of the pelvic joints occurring during gestation may be due to an ovarian hormone (relaxin). The tissues in the perineal region likewise undergo hypertrophic changes in anticipation of the strain of labor. The changes consist in increased vascularity and hypertrophy of the skin and muscles, combined with a general loosening up of the elements constituting the connective tissue.

With the enlargement of the uterus, the skin covering the anterior abdominal wall and the adjoining portions of the thighs is subjected to considerable tension which results in the rupture of the elastic fibers of the reticular stratum of the cutis, and in the formation of depressed areas which are known as the *striae of pregnancy*. In primigravidae these present a pinkish or slightly reddish appearance, as illustrated in Fig. 156, whereas in multiparae two varieties are observed: some resemble those of primigravidous women, while others present a glistening silvery appearance. The former result from the present pregnancy, and the latter represent cicatrices from previous pregnancies.

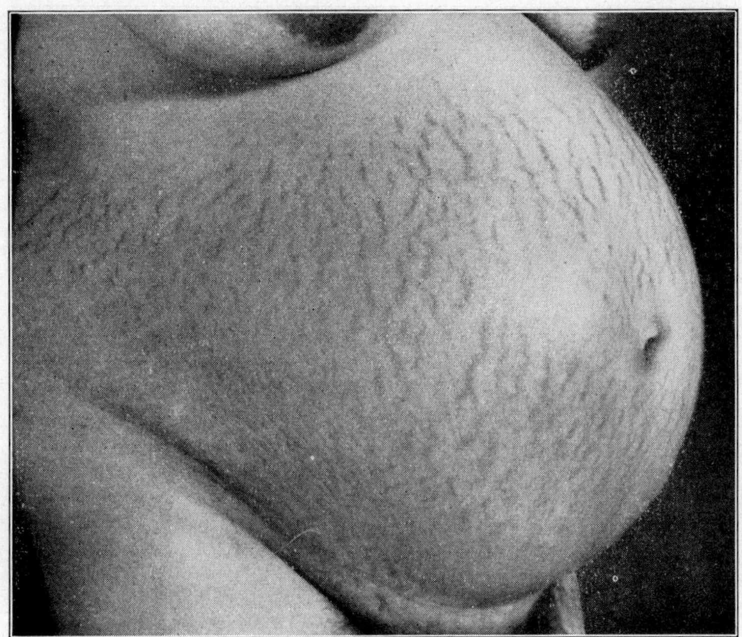

Fig. 156.—Primigravida at Term, Showing Striae of Abdomen.

Since 1923 considerable literature has accumulated in connection with the striae of pregnancy, and Sellheim and others claim that they are due less to passive stretching than to the fact that the skin cannot accommodate itself to the hypertrophic changes which occur in the abdominal walls under the influence of pregnancy. Certain force is lent to such contentions by the fact that striae do not usually follow passive distention of the abdominal walls as the result of ascites or tumor formation, and more particularly by the constitutional studies of Seynsche, which show that they occur more frequently in the robust pyknic types than in hypoplastic and asthenic women. They occur to some extent in about 75 per cent of all pregnant women.

Not infrequently the abdominal walls are unable to withstand the tension to which they are subjected, and the recti muscles become separated in the middle line, giving rise to a *diastasis* of greater or less extent. Where the process is exaggerated, a considerable portion of the anterior wall of the uterus is covered by nothing beyond a thin layer of tissue consisting only of skin, fascia, and peritoneum. In rare instances the separation is sufficiently extensive to admit a hernial protrusion of the gravid uterus.

BREASTS

During pregnancy marked changes occur in the breasts and, in the early weeks, the woman not infrequently complains of a sense of tenseness and tingling in these regions. After the second month the breasts begin to increase in size and offer a somewhat nodular sensation on palpation, which is due to the hypertrophy of the mammary alveoli; as they become still larger a delicate tracery of bluish veins appears just beneath the skin (Figs. 157 and 158). Even more characteristic, however, are the changes occurring in the nipples and the tissues in their vicinity. The nipples them-

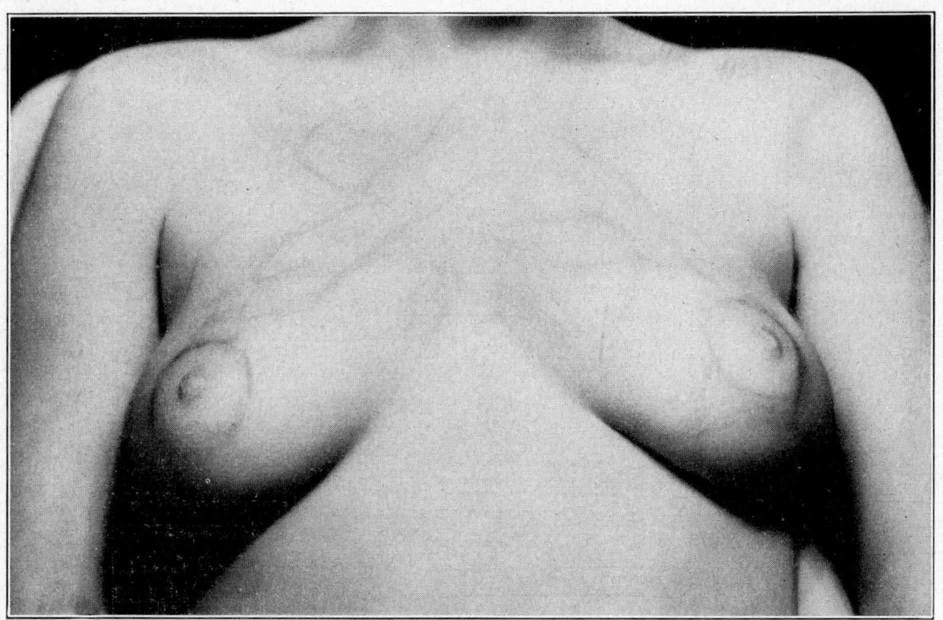

FIG. 157.—INFRA-RED PHOTOGRAPH OF A NONLACTATING BREAST IN A NONPREGNANT WOMAN.

selves soon become considerably larger, more deeply pigmented, and more erectile, and after the first few months a thin, yellowish fluid—*colostrum*—may be expressed from them by gentle massage. At this time the areola surrounding the nipple becomes considerably broader and much more deeply pigmented, the degree of pigmentation varying according to the complexion of the individual. In blondes the areolae and nipples assume a pinkish appearance, while in brunettes they become dark brown and occasionally almost black. Scattered through the areola are a number of small roundish elevations, the so-called *glands of Montgomery,* which result from the hypertrophy of the sebaceous glands. In a small number of cases similar structures make their appearance in a less deeply pigmented area outside of the periphery of the areola which is designated as the *secondary areola.* If the increase in the size of the breasts is very marked, the skin frequently presents striations similar to those observed in the abdomen.

Formerly it was believed that direct nervous connection existed between the uterus and the breasts, but the demonstration that lactation can be established after excluding the spinal nervous mechanism by severing all nerves supplying the breast, or even after transplanting the organ to other portions of the body, clearly indicates that some other factor must be invoked in explanation of the mammary changes in pregnancy. As previously indicated, it is evident that the stimulation to growth of the mammary gland is hormonal and not nervous in origin.

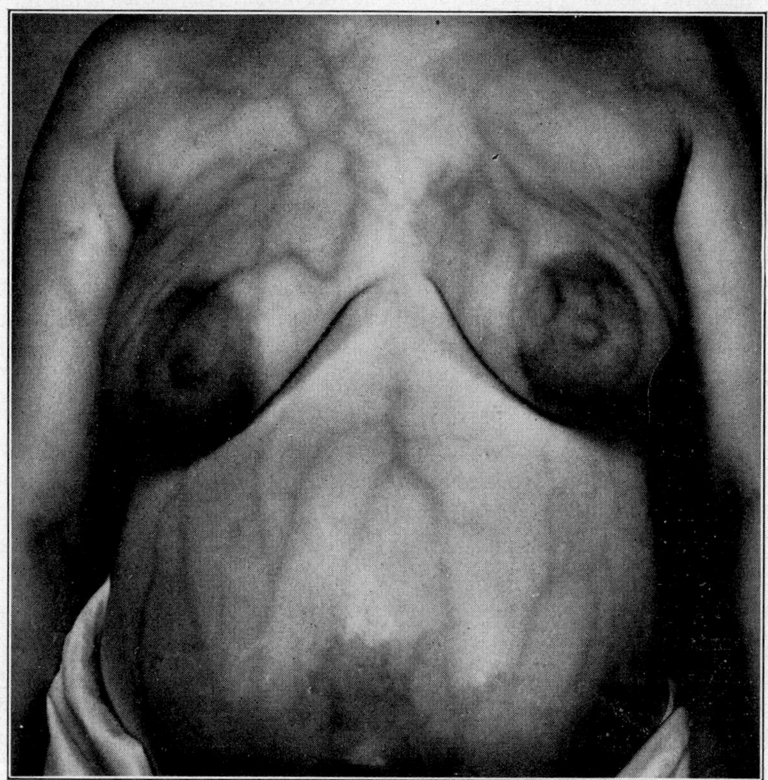

FIG. 158.—INFRA-RED PHOTOGRAPH OF GRAVIDA ONE MONTH BEFORE TERM, SHOWING ACCENTUATED VENOUS PATTERN OVER BREASTS AND ABDOMEN.

METABOLIC CHANGES

Weight Gain. One of the most notable alterations in pregnancy is weight gain. This is in part attributable to local changes, namely, the weight of the fetus, uterus, placenta and amniotic fluid, and in part to metabolic alterations, namely, water retention, acquisition of fat, and such. In an exhaustive survey of the literature, in which 19 publications and 11,960 cases were analyzed, Chesley found that the average total gain reported in pregnancy was 24.0 pounds. Of this increment, about one half, or 11.2 pounds, was gained in the last trimester; a similar amount, or 10.8 pounds, was added in the second trimester; while only a small fraction of the gain, or about 2 pounds, was made in the first trimester. The rate of gain in the last trimester was 0.86 pounds per week. However, the rate of increment for this period is not constant throughout but declines as term approaches. Chesley gives the following figures for the average number of pounds gained in the last four lunar months respectively: seventh month, 4.2; eighth month, 3.7; ninth month, 3.6; tenth month, 2.6. Wide individual variations, however, are noted even in completely normal patients. This is especially true in the last trimester, and as term approaches the variability tends to increase. Although many attempts have been made to correlate weight gain in pregnancy with initial weight, age and parity, the results have shown such disagreement that any conclusions about the roles played by these factors would seem to be unfounded.

What constitutes the maternal weight gain? Since in the average case at term, the infant weighs 7½ pounds, the placenta 1 pound, and the amniotic fluid about 1½ pounds, the weight represented by these products of conception, or the "reproductive weight gain," is approximately 10 pounds. Because of the growth of the mammary parenchyma, together with deposition of mammary fat, the breasts increase in weight to a variable degree, but the average is probably about 3 pounds. The weight of the uterus at term ranges from 1,000 to 1,400 gm., an increment of 2 to 3 pounds, with 2.5 pounds as an average figure. The augmentation in weight thus far accounted for is: "reproductive weight gain," 10 pounds; breasts, 3 pounds; and uterus, 2.5 pounds, a total of 15.5 pounds which might be regarded as tangible weight gain. This leaves 8.5 pounds still unaccounted for. The remaining increment is presumably due to protein storage (outside the uterus) and water retention (including blood water). The former factor (page 215) is of the order of 4 pounds of protein stored outside of the reproductive organs. Water retention, which will be discussed in detail in the next section, accounts for about 3 pounds gain in the form of increased blood water and an additional amount of extracellular water in the tissues. The latter increment has been variously estimated in normal pregnancy as between 1.4 and 5 pounds, depending upon a number of factors.

In about a quarter of gravidae the maximal weight gain is reached on about the third day antepartum, following which there is a weight loss of 2 pounds or so. Although it was once thought that this terminal loss was a phenomenon exhibited by almost all pregnant women and could even be utilized to predict the onset of labor, the bulk of evidence indicates that it occurs only in a minority of patients and that it is in general a very inconstant phenomenon.

Water Metabolism. An increased retention of water is one of the most characteristic biochemical alterations of later pregnancy. Since an exaggeration of this phenomenon may result in one of the gravest complications of gestation, eclampsia, its importance both from a theoretical and practical point of view is great.

The clearest evidence that water retention does occur regularly in normal pregnancy is the postpartum diuresis which almost all puerperae exhibit between the second and fifth day (page 456). The release of water which occurs at this time, moreover, is not only renal in origin but is augmented by the sweating, often profuse, which is so characteristic of this period. As a consequence, the weight loss during these early days of the puerperium averages about 5 pounds (Chesley). Further evidence of water retention in pregnancy is found in the augmented plasma volume which is a regular accompaniment of gestation (page 220). This is associated with an elevated water content of the blood, a reduction in red cell count, hemoglobin, hematocrit, and plasma proteins. Moreover, a substantial increase in available extracellular water is regularly seen in pregnancy. In women weighing less than 120 pounds, Chesley has found the available extracellular water to range from 33 to 37 per cent of the total body weight, whereas in nonpregnant women the average is between 20 to 26 per cent.

In considering the water retention in normal pregnancy it is necessary to differentiate the dependent edema of the ankles and legs from a generalized edema, latent or manifest. Clearly demonstrable pitting edema of the ankles and legs is seen in a substantial proportion of gravidae, especially in warm weather, and is due, as discussed on page 223, to an increase in the venous pressure of the blood in the extremities which is a regular accompaniment of gestation. Generalized retention of water, on the other hand, is usually not demonstrable clinically except by means of the scales. Occasionally, however, the patient's fingers will swell and her wedding ring will become tight.

The cause of generalized water retention in pregnancy is not definitely known, but the following factors bear upon it:

1. *The Effective Intracapillary Hydrostatic Pressure.* This impels filtration from the vascular bed. Because of the great technical difficulties involved, measurements of actual capillary pressure are not available, but it is known that the rate of filtration through normal capillaries is directly proportional to the increase in venous pressure and hence this factor in edema formation has been approached by determinations of venous pressure. As shown in Fig. 159 from McLennan's paper, antecubital venous pressure in normal pregnancy is not significantly different from that in the nonpregnant state and shows no particular trends during the course of pregnancy. Hence there is no evidence that increased capillary pressure is a cause of generalized edema in pregnancy.

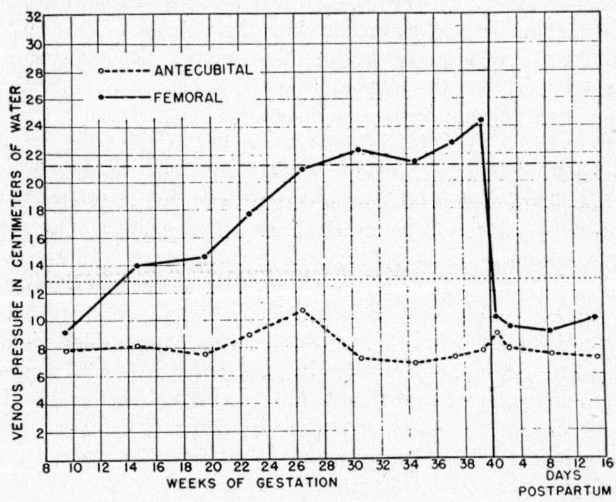

FIG 159.—THE AVERAGE COURSE OF ANTECUBITAL AND FEMORAL VENOUS BLOOD PRESSURE THROUGHOUT NORMAL PREGNANCY AND THE IMMEDIATE PUERPERIUM.

This series consisted of 173 antecubital and 227 femoral determinations in 160 pregnancies. The lower straight dotted line represents the upper limit of normal variation for antecubital venous pressure; and the upper line, the same for femoral venous pressure (McLennan).

2. *The Effective Colloidal Osmotic (Oncotic) Pressure of the Plasma.* This limits filtration and effects reabsorption of filtered water. Pregnancy is characterized by a diminution in serum proteins amounting to about 1 gm. per 100 cc. of plasma and as a consequence, the colloidal osmotic pressure of the plasma is diminished by about 20 per cent. As Chesley has noted, while the changes in proteins occurring in a normal pregnancy are not great enough to cause edema, they may well lead to some degree of water retention which would not show up as visible edema. In other words, the lowered serum proteins may conceivably be responsible for the latent generalized water retention of pregnancy, but it is the general consensus that the

degree of their diminution is not sufficient to explain any outright palpable edema in pregnancy. In this connection the findings of Weech, Snelling and Goettsch, who produced edema in dogs by plasmapheresis and by protein restriction, are pertinent. Their results ". . . suggest an equilibrium between plasma proteins and the volume of fluid in the interstitial spaces. The equilibrium seems to be maintained throughout the entire range of protein variation in such a way that very slight protein decline leads to a correspondingly slight increase in interstitial fluid." On the other hand, many observers such as Oberst and Plass, as well as Dexter and Weiss, believe that the hypoproteinemia of pregnancy is the result rather than the cause of the general hydration which the body undergoes. Dieckmann and Wegner share this view and recall furthermore that the diuresis of the puerperium begins when the plasma proteins are at their lowest level.

3. *Increased Capillary Permeability*. Capillary permeability may be ascertained either indirectly by determining the amount of protein in the edema fluid or directly by the pressure plethysmograph. Using the former method Dexter and Weiss found that the protein contents of the edema fluid in normal pregnancy is less than 0.40 gm. per cent and conclude that such very low protein concentrations in the edema fluid indicate conclusively that the permeability of the capillaries to protein is not increased either in the edema of pregnancy or in the hypertensive toxemias of pregnancy. Using the pressure plethysmograph, McLennan found in a small series of patients that the rate of filtration through the capillary wall is somewhat increased over the normal in the latter weeks of pregnancy. He points out that this may be the result of an increase in the permeability of the capillary wall or may possibly be attributable to other factors.

4. *Sodium Retention.* Several studies collected by Chesley show that the total retention of sodium in pregnancy ranges between 1.6 and 8.8 gm. per week with an average of about 3 gm. If all of the sodium is held extracellularly, the volume of extracellular water gained per week is even larger than is actually met in pregnancy. Rossenbeck found from direct analysis of various tissues that the sodium content is increased in normal pregnancy and markedly increased in eclampsia. In normal pregnancy, he calculates that excessive muscle sodium amounts to about 3 gm. This is only a fraction of the total amount stored during pregnancy. Taylor and his associates report that the total loss of sodium during the first 10 days postpartum is 4.89 gm. These same observers believe that the steroidal sex hormones are the main cause of the sodium and water retention in pregnancy. The evidence that these hormones do cause sodium and water retention is considerable. Thorn and Engel have injected estrone and estriol into dogs and have observed a decreased excretion of sodium. Likewise, Friedlander and his associates have found that estrogen administration was followed by sharp rises in the blood volume in both human subjects and in cats. The sodium-retaining effect of the estrogens and progesterones has already been given a clinical application by Thorn, Nelson and Thorn in an explanation of the so-called menstrual edema. If the hormones of the menstrual cycle are capable of causing retention of sodium and fluids, there is considerable reason to expect a more marked retention of these substances in pregnancy, when the hormones are present in much greater concentration and over a much longer period of time.

Basal Metabolism. A definite elevation of the basal metabolic rate occurs in the latter half of pregnancy when it ranges between + 5 and + 25 per cent. Plass and Yoakam found that the average increase in the basal metabolic rate is from + 1 per cent in the third lunar month (no change) to + 9 per cent in the tenth lunar month, with a return to + 1 per cent during the first week of the puerperium. It appears probable that most if not all of the increase in metabolic rate has its source in the products of conception. As shown by Sandiford and Wheeler, if the calculated theoretical body surface of the fetus is superimposed on that of the mother and if the sum of these two is employed for the calculation of calories per hour per square meter, it is found that the basal metabolic rate of the maternal tissues is not altered by pregnancy. Sontag and his associates support this viewpoint by showing that, in general, the larger the baby the greater is the increase in metabolic rate.

Type	Fluid ingested	Quantity of Urine	Nitrogen in Food	Nitrogen in Urine	Nitrogen in Feces	Nitrogen Balance
Primigravida	1780 cc.	1306 cc.	13.80. gms.	12.43 gms.	0.95 gm.	+ 0.42
Multigravida	1890 cc.	1007 cc.	16.77 gms.	13.26 gms.	0.53 gm.	+ 2.98
Twin pregnancy .	2354 cc.	1135 cc.	15.00 gms.	8.28 gms.	2.00 gms.	+ 4.72

Table 9. Daily Nitrogenous Exchange in Three Pregnant Women. (Slemons.)

Protein Metabolism. Substantial quantities of nitrogen are retained in pregnancy when adequate diets are allowed. This storage of nitrogen appears to begin very early in pregnancy. In a patient studied by Karl M. Wilson, daily observations upon the nitrogen exchange from the tenth to the fourteenth week of pregnancy revealed a considerable capacity for storing nitrogen. Even at that early period the total storage for the four weeks amounted to 60.0 gm. In a patient studied by Hoffström for the last 24 weeks of pregnancy, the storage of nitrogen was observed throughout the entire period. This averaged 1.84 gm. per day, the total amounting to 310 gm., the most marked storage occurring from the twenty-ninth week onward, when the needs of the growing fetus were at a maximum. Hoffström estimated that 101 gm. of this were needed for the development of the fetus, whereas the balance must have been added to the general maternal organism. He calculated that approximately 51 gm. of this balance were utilized in the development of the uterus and breasts, leaving 158 gm. to be added to the maternal nitrogen capital, although it was impossible to make a definite statement as to the exact manner in which it was stored. Similar results were obtained in two patients studied in 1915 by Wilson during the last 19 and 15 weeks of their respective pregnancies. In 1935 Hunscher, Hummel, Erickson and Macy reported the results of an extensive and well-controlled balance study which covered the last 21 weeks of pregnancy, parturition and the puerperium up to the eighth week postpartum. Their findings corroborate but are more striking than those of Hoffström. They reveal that the net gain to the mother amounts to 250 gm. of nitrogen after allowing for the nitrogen required by the fetus, for nitrogen lost at the time of delivery in placenta, amniotic fluid, blood and vomitus and, during the period of involution, in lochia and excreta, and for nitrogen required for the production of milk during 53 days of lactation.

Carbohydrate Metabolism. Abundant evidence attests the fact that pregnant women show an increased tendency to excrete glucose in the urine. This evidence is severalfold: (1) the relatively high frequency with which glycosuria is encountered in pregnant women, as reported in many series of cases; (2) the fact that the majority of pregnant women, following the ingestion of 100 gm. of glucose, will exhibit glycosuria while normal nonpregnant persons will usually not do so; and (3) the fact that some 90 per cent of gravidae, following the intramuscular injection of 2 mg. of phlorizin, will show glycosuria, whereas normal nonpregnant persons will seldom do so.

If we limit our consideration of glycosuria to cases showing 100 mg. per cent or more (that is, yielding a positive Benedict reaction), the frequency, as reported in the past two decades, ranges between 5 and 35 per cent. In 640 unselected pregnant women Williams and Wills found that 5.4 per cent of the cases were glycosuric. Rowe, Gallivan and Matthews, in a series of thoroughly studied and well-controlled patients seen at frequent intervals, found that 35 per cent showed sugar at some time during the antepartum period. Only 18 per cent showed repeated recurrence of glycosuria and in the majority of these there were aglycosuric intervals throughout the course of pregnancy.

The ingestion of glucose, levulose or galactose by pregnant women is so commonly followed by sugar in the urine that several tests for pregnancy have been based on this phenomenon. In 1920 Frank and Nothmann reported 30 cases in the first trimester of pregnancy in which glycosuria was produced by feeding 100 gm. of glucose; in 3 cases which were later found not to be pregnant no glycosuria could be produced. About the same time Long and Hirst concluded that ingestion glycosuria was a valuable aid in the diagnosis of pregnancy. Gottschalk and Strecker gave 100 gm. of levulose and regarded the presence of levulosuria as diagnostic of pregnancy, though a negative result was not thought to exclude it. Similarly, Rowe has shown that the pregnant woman has a lowered tolerance for galactose since she can tolerate only 20 gm. of this sugar without its excretion in the urine, whereas normal persons can ingest 40 gm. without galactosuria. In 1921 Kamnitzer and Joseph, wishing to utilize glycosuria as a diagnostic test for pregnancy and desirous of avoiding the uncertainties of alimentary absorption following the ingestion of glucose, endeavored to induce artificial glycosuria by the injection of phlorizin. This drug produces glycosuria through interfering with the reabsorption of sugar by the kidney tubules, the exact site of action being apparently the epithelial cells lining the proximal convoluted tubules. If the dosage is reduced to 2.0 or 2.5 mg., the great majority of gravidae will manifest glycosuria within an hour, whereas nonpregnant persons will seldom do so. Kamnitzer and Joseph reported 300 cases in which this method was used as a test for pregnancy with only six contradictory results. Subsequent studies by various authors showed an accuracy in the neighborhood of 90 per cent. Compared with the later Aschheim-Zondek test and its modifications, the phlorizin procedure is obviously less dependable, but the results obtained with it show clearly the decided tendency of pregnant women toward glycosuria.

Sugar tolerance curves on normal pregnant women indicate that this tendency toward glycosuria is the result of a reduced renal threshold for glucose upon which there may be superimposed a diminished tolerance for sugar. John found that the average renal threshold in pregnancy was but 117 mg. per cent, in contrast to an average of 149 mg. per cent in normal, nonpregnant persons. Richardson and Bitter carried out sugar tolerance tests on 247 antepartum patients at various stages of pregnancy. Sixty per cent of the women were normal both in respect to their blood sugar curve and in regard to the absence of sugar in the urine. The second largest group, 20 per cent, showed a normal blood sugar curve indicating a normal metabolism of carbohydrate, but the patients in this group excreted sugar into the urine, from a blood sugar definitely below the normal kidney threshold. A certain number with sugar in the urine had a maximal blood sugar, at some time during the two hours, of only 140 to 150 mg. per cent, and many were not above 120 mg. per cent. Williams and Wills believe that the renal threshold must be definitely lowered in the majority of gravidae, since 60 per cent of their cases showed sugar leaks after the ingestion of 100 gm. of glucose. Elias, Güdeman and Roubitschek have shown in a series of observations on pregnant women that in the earlier months, though the rise in the blood sugar curve after the intravenous injection of glucose is practically the same as in normal nonpregnant women, the leak point is definitely lowered. This was determined by a series of simultaneous sugar estimations in blood and urine, the latter obtained by continuous catheterization. Faber has reported two cases in which, during pregnancy, the sugar threshold was at a level of about 130 mg. per 100 cc. Some months after delivery the threshold in one patient had risen to 150 mg. and in the other to 200 mg. In keeping with this general viewpoint Rowe, Gallivan and Matthews have shown that the blood sugar is at low normal or slightly subnormal levels throughout pregnancy and returns to midnormal levels early in the postpartum period; their average figure for blood sugar in pregnancy is 83 mg. per cent and for several weeks postpartum is 94 mg. per cent.

While there is general agreement that pregnancy is frequently associated with a reduction in the renal threshold for sugar, most students of the subject believe that there is often also a lowered tolerance for sugar. In Richardson and Bitter's study eight per cent of the gravidae showed a blood sugar curve upon which a diagnosis of lowered carbohydrate tolerance would usually be made. In the opinion of Williams and Wills, the lowering of the renal threshold, though a factor in all the glycosuric cases, is not the major one in the causation of the glycosurias of pregnancy; the cause lies, rather, in the combination of a lowered renal threshold with an abnormally raised blood sugar curve. Only 4 of their 21 cases of glycosuria were simple renal leaks, the remaining 17 showing a glucose tolerance curve which, while not diabetic in type, approximated an exaggerated "lag" curve. The "lag" type of glucose tolerance curve so frequently met in gravid women suggests that there is active, even in normal pregnancy, some process which tends to reduce somewhat the sugar tolerance. In keeping with this viewpoint Hurwitz and Jensen, on the basis of serial glucose tolerance tests done on 25 normal pregnant women, believe that normal pregnancy exerts a "deleterious" effect on carbohydrate metabolism.

Fat Metabolism. Pregnancy is characterized by a hyperlipemia and a tendency to ketosis. Boyd reports an increase during pregnancy of 129 per cent in neutral blood fat and of 46 per cent in total lipids. He found the phospholipid-to-cholesterol ratio to be only slightly changed, as also the ratio of cholesterol esters to total cholesterol. He further noted that this lipemia of pregnancy is due to an elevated plasma lipid content, the change in the lipid content of the red cells being only an insignificant rise. The increase in neutral fat makes its appearance as early as the third month of gestation. In regard to the tendency toward ketosis Stander and Radelet found acetone bodies to be increased in the blood of normal pregnant women as did Bokelmann and Bock. More recently, Rossenbeck has found that the increase in plasma ketone bodies is particularly marked during the first trimester, after which the values gradually decrease. At term, however, the values are still above those for nonpregnant women. The reason for the increased lipemia of pregnancy is not known. It may be concerned with the fat requirements of the fetus or may represent a mechanism designed to assist the mammary apparatus in subsequent lactation.

Mineral Exchange. The calcium content of the fetus at term is about 25 gm. This calls for an average daily utilization of 0.08 gm. of calcium throughout pregnancy. However, almost two thirds of the total deposition takes place during the last month and it is then that drain of the maternal calcium to supply the osseous development of the fetus is greatest. Balance studies under optimal conditions show that the mother stores about 50 gm. of calcium and 35 to 40 gm. of phosphorus in the course of pregnancy. Only half of the calcium appears in the fetus, the remainder being stored in the maternal tissues. The studies of Bodansky, of Mull and Bill, of Newman and others indicate that there is a progressive decline of total serum calcium as pregnancy progresses, but this amounts to less than 10 per cent. The decrease in the maternal calcium occurs in the nondiffusible fraction, moreover, and hence there is no diminution in the concentration of the physiologic active, diffusible calcium ion. The serum phosphorus values in normal pregnancy fall within the usual nonpregnant range of 1.5 to 6.5 mg. per cent and tend to show a reciprocal relationship to the diffusible calcium concentration.

The average daily transfer of iron from mother to fetus amounts to about 0.4 mg. during the first two thirds of pregnancy, but during the last third the accretion becomes 10 times greater, or about 4.7 mg. of iron daily. A total iron content of 375 mg. in the mature human fetus may be accepted as a fair average from the various analyses reported. It must be recalled also that the maternal organism, in addition to fetal demands, has further need for iron in connection with the greatly hypertrophied uterus. This latter requirement is probably even greater than the fetal needs and has been estimated by Coons to be about 0.5 gm. of iron; this, together with the nearly 0.4 gm. for the fetus, makes a total of 0.9 gm. to be supplied from food or body reserves during pregnancy. An average daily storage of 3.2 mg. for the entire period of gestation would cover this need. In a recent study of 23 iron balances in 9 women at different periods of pregnancy, Coons has shown that iron was retained by the maternal body during the first six months of pregnancy in excess of the low fetal needs then existing. However, during the last three months, the daily iron retention rarely reached the 3.2 mg. calculated as necessary, and often fell far short of it. It will be noted that the total additional iron needed during pregnancy, namely 0.9 gm., is several times the 0.2 gm. of iron saved by nine months of amenorrhea (page 102).

The concentration of copper in the serum appears to be considerably raised in the terminal stages of pregnancy. Thus, Thompson and Watson report that the average value during the latter weeks of pregnancy is 230 micrograms per 100 ml. of serum in contrast to 106 micrograms per 100 ml. in nonpregnant women. The rise in serum copper seems to occur at an early stage in pregnancy, the level being significantly increased by the tenth to sixteenth weeks. The significance of this raised serum copper level in pregnancy is not known.

Acid-Base Equilibrium. The carbon dioxide combining power of the blood is decreased, and at term it is approximately 45 volumes per cent, as compared with about 65 volumes per cent in nonpregnant women. This reduction in alkali reserve has been confirmed by numerous investigators, and has led to the assumption that an "acidosis" exists during normal pregnancy. On the other hand, work on the total serum electrolytes by Oard and Peters, as well as by Stander, Eastman, Harrison and Cadden, has shown that the phrase is a misnomer, since normal pregnancy is not associated with an acidosis nor with an accumulation of abnormal acids. Stander and his associates found that normal gestation is accompanied by a decrease in alkali reserve as well as by a reduction in total base, amounting to 5 per cent, and regard such a finding as a remarkable departure from the normal. They further observed a reduction in the anions—serum protein and serum bicarbonate. Dieckmann and Wegner, in a more extensive study, have corroborated these findings, reporting a total base decrease of from 4 to 6 millimols below the normal, a decrease in the conductivity of the serum likewise corresponding to from 4 to 6 millimols (thus substantiating the diminution in total base), a reduction in carbon dioxide content of from 6 to 10 per cent, and no significant change in either the pH or serum chloride of the blood. They observed a decrease in the total amount of conductivity, expressed as percentage of sodium chloride and of total base, which in individual cases is of the same magnitude as the increase of the plasma volume. Oberst and Plass report higher values for total base and total acid, but confirm the earlier observations of a decrease of total base in pregnancy. These changes, however, do not affect the hydrogen ion concentration or pH of the blood, which remains unaltered at about 7.40. Consequently, with a normal blood pH, with no increase in organic acids nor with any accumulation of abnormal acids in the blood associated with the reduction in the bicarbonate or alkali reserve, it would appear that in normal pregnancy we have to deal with a compensated alkali deficit rather than with a true or definite acidosis.

The reason for this compensated alkali or carbon dioxide deficit is as yet not quite clear. Meyers, Muntwyler and Bill, as well as Plass and Oberst, are of the opinion that hyperventilation accompanying gestation is the cause of the carbon dioxide reduction. The latter writers suggest that the long period of pregnancy results in an equilibrium in which a potentially increased pH of the blood, due to hyperventilation, is returned to normal by a lowered plasma bicarbonate level and a proportionately lowered carbonic acid level.

Blood Chemical Constituents. Some of the most important blood chemical changes in pregnancy have already been noted, such as blood dilution, the lowering of the carbon dioxide combining power, the lipemia and the calcium and phosphorus trends. Another noteworthy alteration is an increase in blood fibrinogen from 0.3 gm. per cent in the nonpregnant to 0.4 gm. per cent or above at term. Since the other plasma protein fractions decrease in pregnancy as the result of the blood dilution, this augmentation in plasma fibrinogen is of a greater relative magnitude than the absolute figures would indicate. Closely paralleling the increase in plasma fibrinogen is a decided acceleration in the sedimentation rate which becomes five times more rapid as term approaches, but is demonstrable in the first trimester of gestation. From a clinical viewpoint, this increased sedimentation rate means that this phenomenon has no prognostic value when employed for the usual clinical purposes, such as the assessment of activity of tuberculous lesions and activity of rheumatic heart disease.

As the result of blood dilution, the serum proteins are diminished in pregnancy, from an average of about 7.25 gm. per cent in the nonpregnant state, to approximately 6.5 gm. per cent in gestation. There is wide variability, however, and values as low as 5.5 gm. per cent may be considered as within the normal range. Although many attempts have been made to demonstrate a shift in the albumin–globulin ratio in pregnancy, my own observations have indicated very little alteration, with the ratio in gestation averaging about 1.7. The importance of the A/G ratio in obstetrics has probably been overemphasized since, provided the chemical analyses have been done by a carefully standardized technic, little change is found either in normal pregnancy or in the toxemias (page 677). In this connection it is well to remember that this ratio in any given serum will vary widely with the minutiae of laboratory technic employed.

CHANGES IN VARIOUS SYSTEMS AND ORGANS

Blood. Except for the primary fetal and uterine development, an increase in blood volume is the greatest single alteration which the gravid organism undergoes. If the reports of several recent investigations are averaged, it will be found that the increase in total blood volume associated with gestation approximates 30 per cent, the increase in plasma volume about 40 per cent, and the increase in red cell volume about 20 per cent (Dieckmann and Wegner; Thomson et al.; Roscoe and Donaldson; McLennan and Thouin; Caton et al.). As can be surmised from the relative magnitude of the plasma and red blood cell volume changes, there is a concomitant decrease both in the hematocrit reading and in blood viscosity. Cohen and Thomson have placed the average decrease in hematocrit at 15 per cent, and in viscosity at 12 per cent. This remarkable increase in blood volume is presumably an adaptation designed to meet the demands of the enlarged uterus with its greatly hypertrophied vascular system.

The massive increase which occurs in plasma volume is attributable chiefly to hydremia. In 1924 Stander and Tyler showed that the moisture content of the blood increases gradually until the seventh month of pregnancy and then remains constant or diminishes very slightly. The constant diminution in serum proteins which occurs in the course of pregnancy is likewise evidence of plasma dilution. As already noted, Dieckmann and Wegner have demonstrated that the conductivity of the serum is decreased in pregnancy, reaching a minimum at term corresponding to from 4 to 6 millimols below normal. This represents, of course, a diminution in the electrolyte activity and predicates a decrease in the total base per unit volume of serum.

These alterations in the volume of the total blood, the plasma and the red cell mass in pregnancy are of the very greatest clinical importance for several reasons. In the first place, as will be discussed more in detail presently, the increase in total blood volume imposes on the heart the burden of pumping a proportionately greater quantity of blood per minute. This fact is of immense importance in cases of rheumatic heart disease in pregnancy (page 718). In the second place, the reduced hematocrit readings in pregnancy will frequently simulate an anemia, giving per cubic millimeter of blood examined in routine blood counts and hemoglobin determinations a lowered red cell count and a reduced hemoglobin level. The degree of diminution in red cell count is of the order of 750,000 and in the hemoglobin value is of the order of 2.0 gm. In other words, if the average red cell count of a group of normal nonpregnant women is, let us say, 4.5 million, the same group of women in pregnancy will show an average count of perhaps 3.75 million; similarly, the hemoglobin concentration will fall on the average from 13.0 gm. or so to 11.0 gm. or thereabout. This simulated anemia has been called the "pseudo-anemia" of pregnancy, but actually the total red cell volume is increased some 20 per cent. Hence, the blood picture is by no means that of a true anemia, but merely a natural result of the disproportionate increase in plasma volume as the result of blood hydration. For this reason, the diagnosis of anemia in pregnancy should not be made, as a rule, unless the red cell count falls below 3.25 million, the hemoglobin level below 10 gm., and the hematocrit reading below 30 per cent.

The changes in blood volume described, including the diminution in hematocrit, red cell count, and hemoglobin concentration, are progressive phenomena as pregnancy advances and usually reach the maximum about the seventh month. Roscoe and Donaldson find a mean decline in hemoglobin from 12.8 gm. to 10.8 gm. in normal pregnancy and believe that the magnitude of the fall is in proportion to the month of gestation. Despite these physiologic changes in the red cell count, cell size as well as the color index remains normal.

The white cell count in pregnancy is usually in the upper limit of normal, that is, between 8,000 and 10,000. On the basis of my own experience, the so-called "leukocytosis of pregnancy" is merely a slight tendency in that direction and only white counts in excess of 12,000 should be regarded as attributable to infection. This statement, however, does not apply to labor or the puerperium in which the white count may normally be twice or even three times the usual figure. Carey and Litzenberg, in a study of 134 normal pregnancies, found the average count for pregnancy, irrespective of the duration of gestation, to be between 10,000 and 11,000, and conclude that there may be a physiologic leukocytosis of pregnancy, but that it is not invariable.

The Heart. During the latter months of pregnancy the growing uterus pushes the diaphragm upward with the result that the heart is displaced to the left, upward and somewhat in the direction of the anterior chest wall; at the same time a certain degree

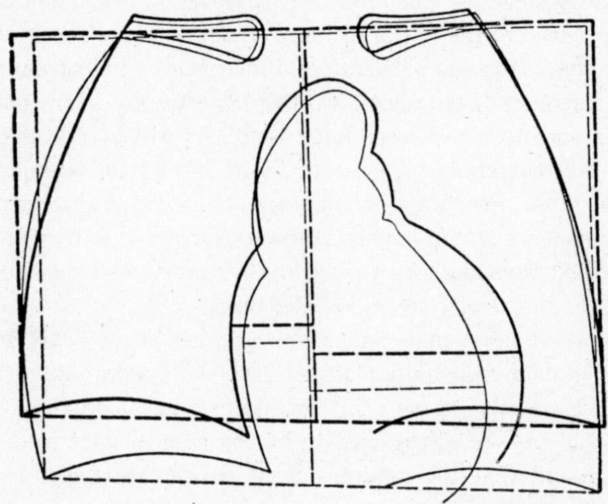

FIG. 160.—CHANGE IN CARDIAC OUTLINE WHICH OCCURS IN PREGNANCY.

The light lines show the relationships between the heart and thorax in the nonpregnant woman, while the heavy lines show the conditions existing in pregnancy. This diagram, which is based on teleoroentgenograms, shows the average findings in 33 women (Klaften and Palugyay).

of rotation of the heart is believed to take place. These changes are not constant either in degree or direction and vary according to the size and position of the child, the amount of amniotic fluid, the strength of the abdominal muscles and the constitutional type of the thorax. As the result of the same factor, namely, the upward pressure upon the diaphragm, the chest wall itself undergoes definite changes during pregnancy, its height being diminished and its circumference increased. This alteration is shown in Fig. 160 from Klaften and Palugyay, which represents the average change found in the chest wall and the heart of 33 pregnant women. These authors found that the distance from the midline of the sternum to the left margin of the heart was increased, on an average, 13 mm. and to the right margin of the heart 3 mm.; these changes were thought due in part to the shift of the position of the heart and in part to an increase in its apparent size owing to greater proximity to the anterior chest wall. Similar observations have been made by many other observers.

Inasmuch as the outline of the heart increases during gestation, the doctrine has been advanced that a certain degree of cardiac hypertrophy is a constant concomitant of pregnancy. This question has been long debated, some authors believing that a moderate hypertrophy of the heart takes place during gestation, others that a slight dilatation occurs, with the balance of evidence probably in favor of the latter if any actual change does take place in heart size. The suspicion that the change in cardiac outline associated with pregnancy is brought about by some factor other than, or in addition to, the upward pressure of the diaphragm, is based on the observation that alterations in cardiac outline may occur at an earlier stage in pregnancy than would be anticipated from abdominal pressure alone.

However, the conclusions to be reached from these investigations from a practical point of view are clear. During pregnancy, as the result of the upward pressure of the diaphragm or other factors, the positional relationships of the heart in the thoracic cavity are frequently changed. The apex beat is moved outward and upward. The left cardiac wall is displaced to the left, a distance which averages about one-half inch but which may reach almost one inch. Therefore, the attending physician must be cautious about making a diagnosis of pathologic cardiac hypertrophy in pregnancy unless it is evident that he is dealing with a very large heart. As will be discussed more fully in connection with the diagnosis of rheumatic heart disease in pregnancy, the normal heart in gestation often presents other manifestations simulating heart disease, such as an increased incidence of functional murmurs, of accentuation of the pulmonary second sound and extrasystoles. According to Hermann and King, normal pregnancy produces no changes in the electrocardiogram.

The most important functional change which occurs in the heart during pregnancy is a great increase in its minute output of blood which approximates 30 per cent in the last trimester. In view of the 40 per cent increase in total blood volume this alteration is an understandable one. It was proved to be the case in dogs by Stander, Duncan and Sisson, who found that the minute output of the heart was increased by one third to one half during the latter part of pregnancy. On the basis of repeated determinations on 13 pregnant women by means of Grollmann's acetylene method, Stander and Cadden reached the conclusion that the cardiac output begins to rise at the start of the fourth month and that at term it has increased to over 50 per cent of the normal nonpregnant value. Schmidt concluded that a significant increase occurs even in the first trimester. Recent studies by Hamilton and by Palmer and Walker have made use of cardiac catheterization in determining heart output in pregnancy. These two investigations, which are in remarkable agreement, indicate that the average output in midpregnancy is approximately 5.8 liters per minute in contrast to 4.6 liters per minute in the nonpregnant woman, an increase of about 26 per cent. In both series the cardiac output rose rapidly about the twelfth week and remained elevated until the last month when it fell rather sharply (especially in Hamilton's series) to reach pregravid levels during the last week or so of gestation. Wide individual variations, however, were encountered.

From a clinical viewpoint, the increase in the cardiac output which occurs in pregnancy is a change of the greatest importance. It allows us to dispense with such vague phrases as "the strain of pregnancy" and permits us to speak in quantitative physical terms as follows: As the result of pregnancy, the heart is obliged to perform at least 25 per cent more work than it did in the pregravid state.

Circulation. In normal pregnancy the arterial blood pressure shows little if any change. In Andros' study of 300 cases of normal pregnancy, the 661 pre-pregnancy readings averaged 114.6/72.6 mm. Hg (pulse pressure 42). In pregnancy the average systolic pressure for the group remained unchanged while the diastolic pressure tended to be only slightly (3 to 4 mm. Hg) below the pre-pregnancy figure. Other studies, notably those of Henry and of Burwell and his associates, indicate that in pregnancy there is a slight lowering of the systolic blood pressure and a somewhat greater lowering of the diastolic pressure, both values returning toward the nonpregnant levels during the last month. In the opinion of these authors there is an increase of about 10 mm. in the pulse pressure during the major part of pregnancy. Agreement is unanimous that normal pregnancy never causes an increase in systolic and diastolic blood pressures and any rise of 20 mm. or more above pre-existing levels, under basal conditions, is indicative of a pathologic process, usually preeclampsia (page 648).

As shown by McLennan, the antecubital venous pressure remains constant in pregnancy but the femoral venous pressure shows a steady rise from 8 to 24 cm. of water pressure at term (Fig. 159). Recently, by means of radioactive tracer substances, Wright, Osborn and Edmonds have shown that a retardation of blood flow occurs in the legs during pregnancy. This tendency toward a stagnation of blood in the extremities during the latter part of pregnancy is due entirely to the pressure of the enlarged uterus on the pelvic veins as shown by the fact that the elevated venous pressure returns to normal immediately after delivery of the infant at cesarean section (McLennan). From a clinical viewpoint the retarded blood flow and increased venous pressure in the legs which are demonstrable in the latter months of pregnancy are of great importance since they contribute to the ankle edema which gravidae frequently experience as they approach term, and play an important role in the development of varicose veins in the legs and vulva during gestation.

Burwell has observed the similarity between the changes in circulation in arteriovenous fistulae and certain circulatory alterations in pregnancy and believes that the latter are due mainly to the arteriovenous shunt constituted by the placenta and obstruction to venous return by the enlarged uterus. The circulatory changes in pregnancy, strikingly similar to those associated with an arteriovenous fistula, are the accelerated pulse rate, slightly decreased arterial blood pressure, elevated venous pressure in the pelvis and legs, increased blood volume and cardiac output and the placental murmur or bruit.

Respiratory Tract. It has long been known that pregnancy may exert a deleterious influence upon the voice of singers, and Hofbauer has shown that it is associated with changes in the larynx which occur in three quarters of all pregnant women. These consist in reddening and edema of the false vocal cords, as well as of the interarytenoid region. In addition to the usual histologic manifestations of inflammation, decidual-like cells may make their appearance in the submucosa. Owing to the upward displacement of the diaphragm in the later months of pregnancy, it would seem as though the capacity of the lungs would be decreased. Nevertheless, such is not the case, since the diminished height of the pleural cavities is compensated for by an increase in width. Furthermore, from the investigations on cardiac output referred to above, which are based on oxygen consumption per unit of time, it is evident that there must be a great increase in the amount of air inspired. Estimations of vital capacity reveal an actual increase during gestation. Plass and Oberst, in carefully controlled experiments, noted that the volume of tidal air and the minute volume of respired air increase progressively as term is approached, to return to normal during the second week of the puerperium.

Digestive Tract. The majority of pregnant women have a notable reduction in the free hydrochloric acid and total acidity of their gastric juice, accompanied by a parallel reduction in ferment content and hydrogen ion activity. While wide individual variations occur, there is, on an average, a 50 per cent decline in maximum free acidity from the third month to the sixth month of gestation with a rise in the last month to the level observed in the third month. According to Strauss and Castle, 75 per cent of women fail to secrete normal amounts of free hydrochloric acid or pepsin during the greater part of pregnancy and the gastric juice after delivery contains three times as much free acid as during the sixth month, and double the quantity secreted during the major portion of pregnancy. This hypochlorhydria of pregnancy has two important clinical relationships: (1) diminution in acid content of the stomach is usually paralleled by a decrease in gastric motility which, in turn, is believed to be the cause of heartburn and flatulence and may be an etiological factor in vomiting, all common complications of pregnancy; and (2) hypochlorhydria interferes with the ability of the stomach to absorb iron and so predisposes to anemia. The suspicion that gastric motility may be impaired in pregnancy has been confirmed by the x-ray studies of Hansen, and of Norman H. Williams. The former found that toward the end of pregnancy the stomach was pushed up into the left dome of the diaphragm and was rotated some 45 degrees until it lay as a flaccid bag more or less horizontally on the top of the fundus of the uterus. The tone of the stomach was so much diminished that the emptying time was definitely increased. Likewise, Norman H. Williams has found that the position and motility of the stomach in pregnancy delay the emptying time of this organ and favor the development of reverse currents that carry material cephalward. At least one half of all pregnant women suffer from constipation, a fact which suggests that the entire gastro-intestinal tract may be handicapped by diminished tone in gestation.

The status of the liver in normal pregnancy has long been the subject of debate with the evidence almost evenly balanced between those who claim that this organ shows no changes in normal gestation and those who maintain that it often manifests slight but significant diminution in function. The many studies which have been made on the liver in pregnancy by means of functional tests were reviewed in detail by Cantarow, Stuckert and Gartman. These investigators reported also observations of their own on serum bilirubin levels and bromsulfalein retention tests in normal and toxemic gravidae. They conclude that although serum bilirubin concentration remains within normal limits during normal pregnancy, some degree of hepatic functional impairment is present in a not inconsiderable proportion of cases. They make the further observation that the ability of the liver to eliminate bromsulfalein is more readily impaired by anesthetic agents in the pregnant than in the nonpregnant state. Ingerslev and Teilum have carried out liver biopsy studies on 17 pregnant women and find no particular deviation in the histological picture from that met in normal nonpregnant women, although vacuolar accumulation of fat in the central part of the lobules appears to be somewhat more pronounced during pregnancy. Their biochemical findings show that gestation is associated with certain changes in the intermediate metabolism of the liver, but they conclude with the statement that there is no basis, either on histological or biochemical grounds, to maintain the concept of "liver of pregnancy."

Spleen. In 1930 Barcroft made the interesting observation that in dogs during the second half of pregnancy the spleen becomes greatly diminished in size and regains its normal dimensions shortly after delivery. He was inclined to correlate this phenomenon with the normal increase in blood volume and thought that it probably occurs in women as well. It is barely possible that this splenic factor may play a role in the increased red cell mass characteristic of pregnancy and its return to normal values very early in the puerperium.

Urinary System. *Bladder.* There are few significant changes in the bladder previous to the fourth month of pregnancy. From this time onward, the increase in size of the uterus together with the hyperemia which affects all the pelvic organs, as well as a definite hyperplasia of the muscular and connective tissue elements, bring about an elevation of the trigone, with a thickening of its posterior or interureteric margin. This process continues to the end of pregnancy, producing a marked deepening and widening of the trigone. The bladder mucosa undergoes no change except for an increase in the size and tortuosity of the blood vessels supplying it. Toward the end of pregnancy, particularly in primigravidae in whom the presenting part usually engages deeply in the pelvis, there is a pushing forward and upward of the whole base of the bladder, converting the normal convex surface into one which is concave when viewed through the cystoscope. This development greatly increases the difficulty of diagnostic and therapeutic procedures. In addition, the pressure of the presenting part impairs the blood and lymph drainage of the base of the bladder so that this area is often edematous, easily traumatized and more susceptible to infection. Residual urine does not usually exist in primigravidae, but in multiparae with relaxed vaginal walls and cystocele, it is a frequent occurrence. It is thought by some that an incontinence of the ureterovesical valve frequently develops with the probability of vesico-ureteral reflux of urine, but the weight of evidence seems to indicate that this structure is no less competent in the gravid than in the nonpregnant individual.

Ureters. Since Sippel and Cruveilhier in 1843 demonstrated that women dying in pregnancy had dilated ureters, various theories have been propounded to explain this phenomenon. Formerly it was thought that the predominating factor consisted in compression of the ureter at the brim of the pelvis by the pregnant uterus with damming back of urine, although this did not account for the marked preponderance of dilatation on the right side as compared to the left, nor did it account for the fact that dilatation usually commences about the fourth month when the uterus could not exert very considerable pressure. Dextrorotation of the uterus with consequent torsion of the left ureter and angulation of the right, as well as the difference in relation between the left and right ureter to the large iliac and uterine vessels and to the sigmoid, have also been advanced as causative factors giving rise to a preponderance of right-sided dilatation. On the other hand, hyperplasia of the base of the bladder, the ureters, and broad ligaments, but particularly of the circular muscle fibers of the ureter with consequent narrowing of the intraligamentary portion of the ureter, was thought by Hofbauer to account for the ureteral dilatation. If this were true, then both ureters should be equally affected, but this is not borne out by the facts. These findings should be regarded only as contributory factors all of which may and probably do play some role; however, none of them alone seems particularly convincing. It now seems clear that in most pregnant women a condition of atonia develops which expresses itself not only in relaxation or loss of irritability of the musculature of the uterus, but also of the smooth musculature of the ureters, large bowel and bile ducts. The exact mechanism whereby this is brought about is not known but is thought by some to be hormonal, while others feel that it has its basis in the sympathetic nervous system. These smooth muscle structures have all been demonstrated to develop a marked atony during pregnancy.

Recent investigations by Jona, Fuchs and others have shown that the peristaltic activity of the urinary tract is dependent upon several factors. Systematic contrac-

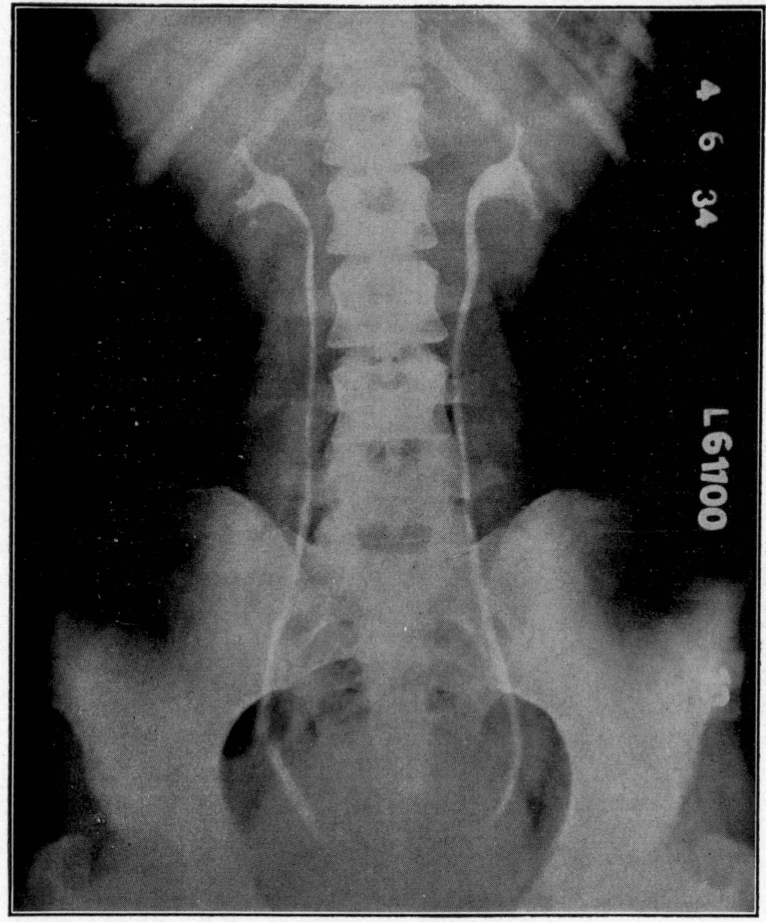

Fig. 161.—Pyeloureterogram Following Intravenous Injection of Neo-skiodan; Normal Nulligravida.

tions of the renal calices force urine into the kidney pelvis, where responsive contractions of the pelvic musculature propel it into the upper portion of the ureter. The ureter in like manner responds by means of a peristaltic wave, which, according to Fuchs, consists of a cystoid-detrusor type of activity. He describes three zones, two in the abdominal and one in the pelvic portion of the ureter, where such cystoids form to receive urine from above and then, by muscular contraction, to force it downward. Thus the systematic muscular contractions of calices, kidney pelvis and ureter are to force urine from kidneys to bladder, as a result of which the fluid pressure in the latter is uniformly higher than that in the kidney pelvis, as shown by Kreutzmann and others. It is, therefore, evident that drainage of the kidney is not dependent upon gravity but upon this peristaltic activity. The uretero-vesical valve, the obliquity of the course of the ureter through the wall of the bladder, as well as the ureteral peristaltic activity itself protect the kidneys against the resultant fluid pressure built upon the bladder. In addition there exists, according to Bloeninghaus, an autonomic bladder reflex, dependent upon intracystic tension, antagonistic to ureteral peristalsis.

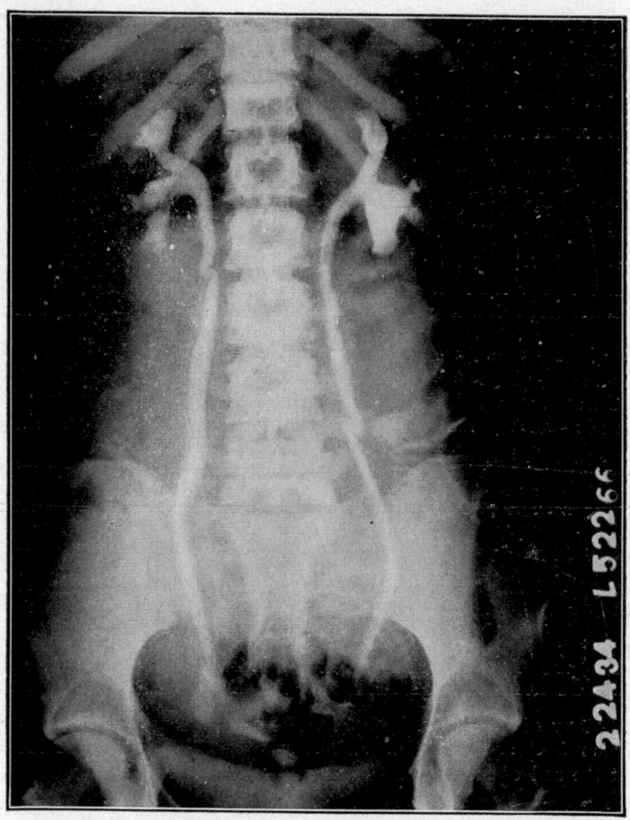

FIG. 162.—INTRAVENOUS PYELOGRAM ILLUSTRATING THE CHANGES IN THE URETER USUALLY ASSOCIATED WITH PREGNANCY.

The kidneys are normal. Both ureters are dilated and elongated, the right more than the left. They are also displaced laterally. These changes may be considered as normal.

That this mechanism of kidney drainage is fundamentally interfered with during gestation is evidenced by the findings of Kreutzmann and others that as pregnancy proceeds the pressure in the renal pelvis becomes greater than that obtained in the bladder. In 1937 Traut and McLane showed that during pregnancy the dilatation of the ureters is inversely proportional to the degree of atony as measured by kymographic tracings. Thus, this altered mechanism of kidney drainage seen in pregnancy undoubtedly is associated with varying degrees of ureteral atony.

It appears then that some dilatation of the ureters and renal pelvis is a natural concomitant of the pregnant state, and that this dilatation is associated with stasis of urine. The widening of the urinary tract is most marked on the right side and

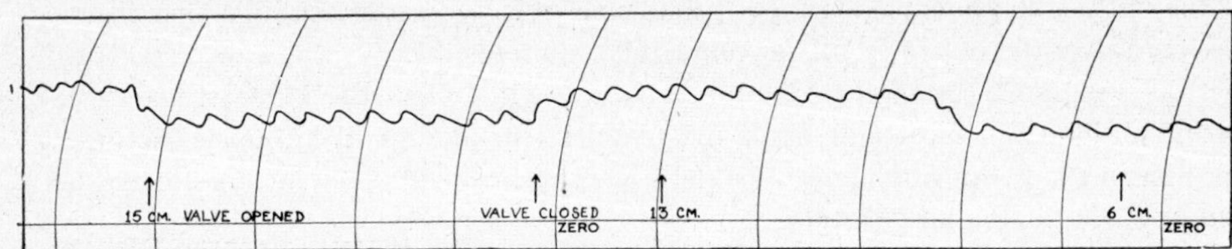

A. The curve made by the peristalsis of the normal ureter in a nonpregnant woman, acting upon a water manometer with tambour and writing lever. The musculature is competent to contract rhythmically at all levels of pressure, 15 cm. of water, 13 cm., and 6 cm.

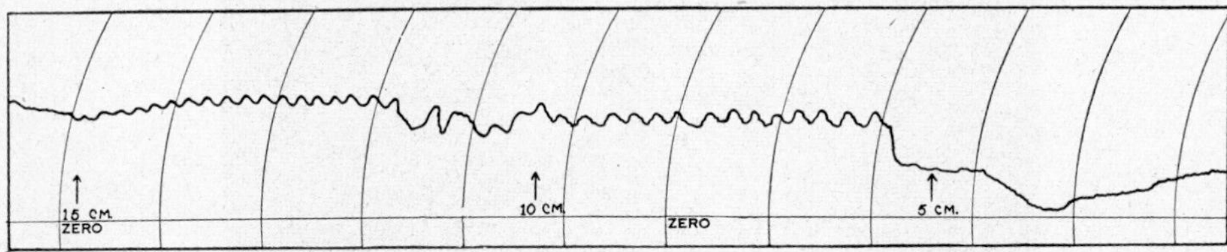

B. The effect of early pregnancy (fourth month) upon ureteral peristalsis. The amplitude is diminished at 15 cm. of water pressure, but is better though somewhat irregular at 10 cm., while at 5 cm. of pressure the contractions drop out completely. This is a frequent observation from the 3rd to the 6th months of pregnancy and seems to indicate a reduced irritability of the ureteral musculature.

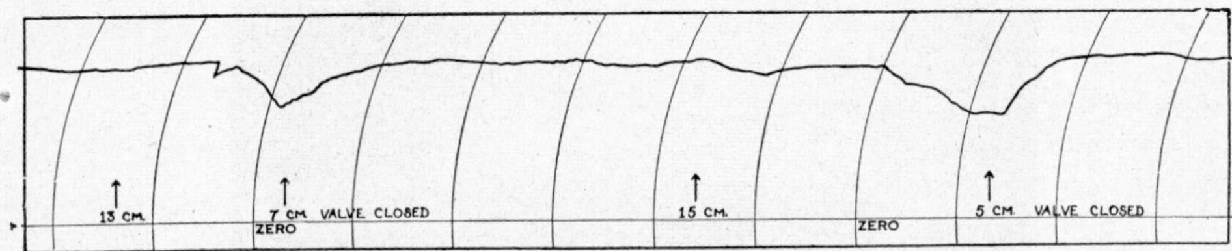

C. The ureteral atony of pregnancy. Peristalsis is completely absent at all levels of pressure. In addition the ureter is refractory to stimulation by injection of salt solution into the lumen. This is a frequent finding at the end of the second trimester of pregnancy.

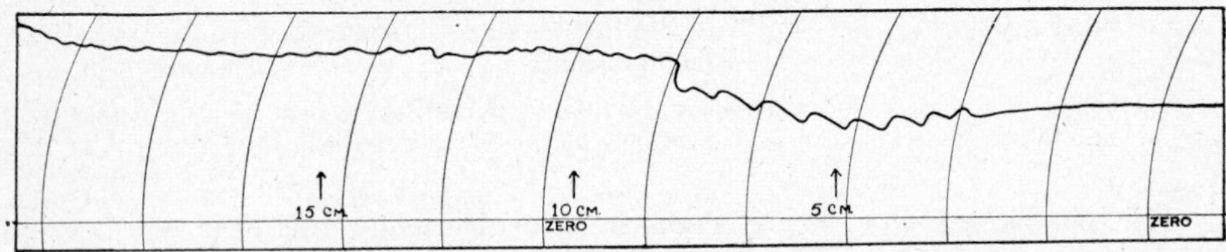

D. A return of irritability as indicated in this graph is common in the last month of pregnancy. This is usually seen in the lower pressure levels. Here it is definite at the 5 cm. level. Following delivery there is a tendency for the ureter to again become atonic. It usually has resumed its normal tone by the sixth week postpartum.

Fig. 163.—Normal Physiologic Variations of Ureteral Peristalsis in Pregnancy, B, C, D; with Tracing A from Nonpregnant Woman for Comparison.

usually involves that portion lying above the inlet of the true pelvis, although it is also occasionally seen in the pelvic ureter. The distention of the excretory duct is accompanied by elongation so that it is frequently thrown into curves of varying size, the smaller of which may approach sharp angulation producing, at least theoretically, partial or complete obstruction. These are the so-called "kinks," a most unfortunate term as it connotes obstruction. As a matter of fact these are, in a large majority of cases, merely single or double curves which, when viewed in the roentgenogram taken in the same plane as that occupied by the curve, appear as more or less acute angulations of the ureter. Another exposure made at right angles will nearly always reveal them as true curves with no kink. In addition to elongation, the ureter in both its abdominal and pelvic portions is frequently displaced laterally by the pressure of the enlarged uterus upon the bellies of the psoas muscles.

These changes in the urinary duct occur most commonly and in the greatest degree in primigravidae and in multiparae who have had pregnancies in rapid succession, while less frequently in those who have had long intervals between pregnancies. Approximately 80 per cent of all pregnant women have demonstrable dilatation of the ureter, or what has been termed "hydro-ureter of pregnancy." The right side is affected two or three times more frequently than the left, due undoubtedly to the fact that the dextrorotation of the uterus brings about more complete occlusion of the former than of the latter. As a result of this dilatation, the capacity of the kidney pelvis and ureter is increased from its normal limits of 6 to 15 cc. to values ranging from 20 to 60 cc., according to Crabtree. In the interpretation of kidney function tests done during pregnancy in which dependence is placed upon the clearance of a substance from the blood stream, this variation in the amount of urinary stasis in the upper tract may be the source of very misleading results. The tendency is, of course, to obtain lower values for the kidney function than actually exist, because of the dilution of the phenolsulfonephthalein or urea, and so forth, by the urine contained in the ureter and kidney pelvis.

The dilatation of the ureter and kidney pelvis is progressive from the fourth to the eighth month, after which time the ureter begins to show a return of irritability. Following delivery the resolution takes place rapidly in normal women so that in four to six weeks it has returned to pregestational dimensions. The stretching and dilatation do not continue long enough to impair permanently the elasticity of the ureter, unless infection has supervened, or the pregnancies are so rapidly repeated that involutional changes are not complete before the process is again initiated.

Bacteriuria in Pregnancy. There is evidence that the healthy kidney excretes bacteria. In 1913 Franke demonstrated the passage of *B. coli* from various portions of the bowel by way of the lymphatics to the capsule of the kidney, particularly on the right side. Falls, Dodds, and Crabtree have shown bacteria to be present in large numbers in the urine in from 11 to 14 per cent of normal pregnant women in the antepartum period. The invading organism in the majority of instances was *B. coli,* although streptococci and staphylococci were also found. On the other hand, Traut and McLane report an exceedingly low incidence of bacteriuria in 30 normal women studied at frequent intervals throughout pregnancy and the puerperium and were thus unable to substantiate the theory that the kidney excretes micro-organisms during gestation. Hundley and his co-workers likewise obtained positive cultures from the upper urinary tract in only 6 per cent of 500 normal pregnant women studied. From these investigations it would appear that bacteriuria, contrary to earlier views, is an infrequent occurrence during normal gestation.

Endocrine Glands. The most important endocrine changes in pregnancy have already been discussed; namely, the placental production of estrogen, progesterone, and chorionic gonadotrophin (pages 156-163).

A moderate degree of hypertrophy of the thyroid is a usual concomitant of normal pregnancy and may be recognized clinically in 65 to 90 per cent of all cases. Its significance is not clear, but that the thyroid plays an important part in pregnancy was shown by the experiments of Halsted and of Ukita. The former found that when the gland was partially removed from pregnant dogs, puppies were born whose thyroids were many times the normal size, thereby indicating that they had hypertrophied in order to supplement the deficient maternal secretion. The latter states that the removal of the gland from pregnant rabbits led to prolongation of the duration of pregnancy and to the birth of undersized and poorly developed offspring, whose thyroids were definitely hypertrophied and showed signs of increased secretory activity. The enlargement of the thyroid gland seen in pregnancy is due to a true hyperplasia of the adenomatous tissue, to an increased blood supply, and to the formation of new follicles according to the research of Falls, and of Mussey and Plummer. It seems clear that these changes are associated with an increased function of the gland evidenced by an increase in the basal metabolic rate of the woman and an actual increase of iodine content in the blood, as shown by Bokelmann and Scheringer, and more recently by Peters, Man and Heinemann.

The parathyroids undergo a considerable hypertrophy during pregnancy, and their secretion is essential to its normal progress. To a great extent they act through the calcium metabolism. Insufficiency of the parathyroid secretion occasionally manifests itself by the development of tetany in the mother, as is described in another section. Spingarn and Geist suggest that pregnancy may aggravate hyperparathyroidism, thus accounting for the increased incidence of this disease in the female.

As the thymus gland ordinarily atrophies with the approach of puberty, it would not appear to exert any influence upon pregnancy. Bompiani, however, has shown that when it persists abnormally, the organ undergoes diminution in size during pregnancy, to enlarge again after delivery. Anderson, in a review of the experimental work on the thymus and its relation to reproduction, states that thymectomy has no effect on the morphology or physiology of reproduction.

The anterior lobe of the pituitary gland undergoes hypertrophy during pregnancy and returns to the usual size after its completion. The hypertrophy, which may double the size of the lobe, is due in great part to an increase in the number and size of the "Hauptzellen." The so-called "pregnancy cells" are large ovoid cells, probably derived from the chromophobe cells, which are regarded by most workers as the reserve or undifferentiated foundation cells. Severinghaus, in a review of the literature, states that the "pregnancy cell" is an acidophile in high secretory activity, developing from the chromophobes and reverting to that state after termination of pregnancy. Furthermore, the basophiles show even more striking changes than the acidophiles, presenting large granular forms during the middle of pregnancy and, as term approaches, becoming depleted of granules with hypertrophied

Golgi apparatus and increased mitochondria. These changes observed in the acidophiles and basophiles are believed to be indicative of increased cellular activity.

On account of the known relation existing between abnormalities of the hypophysis and the development of acromegaly, a similar origin has been suggested for the nonedematous thickening of the features, as well as of the extremities, which is observed in so many pregnant women. The posterior or infundibular portion of the hypophysis does not hypertrophy during pregnancy but, in addition to its effect upon the blood pressure, it possesses the power of markedly stimulating uterine contractions, as has been shown by Dale, Bell, and others. Abel and his co-workers have isolated from the posterior lobe a crystalline product in the form of a tartrate, which possesses an almost miraculous power of stimulating nonstriated muscle. Whether this hormone is normally concerned in the regulation of the uterine contractions at the time of labor is not known, but the researches of Knaus show clearly that susceptibility to its action increases markedly as the end of pregnancy is approached. Extracts of the posterior lobe are extensively used in obstetrical practice to stimulate inefficient uterine contractions.

It is also definitely known that the cortex of the suprarenal bodies undergoes definite hypertrophy during pregnancy which, according to Kolde, is most marked in the zona fasciculata. Aschner, as a result of his studies, emphasizes the great increase in the lipid content of the gland. This increased activity of the adrenal glands appears to be more marked during the early and late phases of gestation.

Skeleton and Teeth. Rokitansky described the formation of irregularly shaped plaques of porous, newly formed bone, or osteoid tissue, upon the internal surface of the cranial bones during pregnancy. These he designated as puerperal osteophytes, but neither he nor the subsequent observers who have confirmed his findings are clear as to their significance. Dreyfuss states that their existence may be demonstrated in every third pregnant woman by the use of the x-ray and is inclined to believe that their production is in some way associated with the activity of the pituitary body. Hanau considers that they are most pronounced when an excessive formation of osteoid tissue occurs in other parts of the body. This he is inclined to attribute to a slight grade of osteomalacia, which he and Gelpke regard as physiological in all pregnancies and associated with the supply of calcium salts to the fetus.

According to Ziskin and his associates who have studied the teeth in pregnancy for many years, the process of gestation per se does not produce dental caries. Hence the old aphorism, "a tooth for every child," has no scientific basis. Already existing caries may occasionally extend very rapidly in pregnancy, however, from causes which are unknown. "Pregnancy gingivitis" is a rather rare condition characterized by swollen, spongy gums which bleed easily and which show in biopsies a loss of surface keratin with hypertrophic and inflammatory changes in the underlying tissues. According to Ziskin it is due to hormonal influences.

Nervous System. Mild degrees of disturbed mental equilibrium are frequently observed. In this category may be placed the longings and cravings for unusual or abnormal articles of diet. Many women also experience pronounced changes in disposition, and not a few multiparous patients recognize the occurrence of pregnancy by the appearance of these. In patients of neuropathic tendencies, the mental equilibrium may be overthrown to a greater or less degree, the patient becoming excitable, morbid, or morose, and in rare instances developing a true psychosis.

Skin. Reference has already been made to the formation of striae and to the pigmentation of the nipple and areola. In many cases the linea alba becomes markedly pigmented, assuming a brownish black color—the *linea nigra*. Occasionally irregularly shaped, brownish patches of varying size appear on the face and neck, the condition being known as *cloasma* or the "mask of pregnancy," which fortunately usually disappears after delivery. Very little is known concerning the nature of these pigmentary changes, but Wychgel has demonstrated that the pigment deposited in the papillary layer of the skin responds to the usual tests for iron. It is conceivable that these skin changes are associated with the hypertrophy of the cortex of the adrenals, or perhaps the changes noted in the hypophysis.

Vascular spiders develop in about two thirds of white women and some 10 per cent of colored women during pregnancy, as demonstrated by Bean, Cogswell, Dexter and Embick. These are minute, fiery red elevations of the skin with branching legs or radicles coming out from the central body and show a particular predilection for the face, neck, upper chest and arms. The condition is often designated as nevus, angioma or telangiectasis. Palmar erythema is also frequently encountered in pregnancy, having been observed by Bean and his associates in 62.5 per cent of white women and 35 per cent of Negresses. The two conditions frequently occur together. They are of no clinical significance and in most cases disappear shortly after the termination of pregnancy. It is the reserved opinion of the above authors that this high incidence of vascular spiders and palmar erythema in pregnancy may be due to the high saturation of the tissues with estrogen.

BIBLIOGRAPHY

Ahlfeld, F. Beobachtungen über die Dauer der Schwangerschaft. Monatschr. f. Geburtsh., 1869, 34:266.

Andersen, D. H. The Relationship between Thymus and Reproduction. Physiol. Rev., 1932, 12:1.

Andros, G. J. Blood Pressure in Normal Pregnancy. Am. J. Obst. & Gynec., 1945, 50:300.

Anthony, A. J., and Hansen, R. Beat Volume and Minute Volume of Heart at End of Pregnancy and Following Delivery. Ztschr. f. Geburtsh. u. Gynäk., 1935, 110:1.

Arnott, P. H. The Duration of Pregnancy. West. J. Surg., 1942, 50:115.

Balfour, W. M., and others. Radioactive Iron Absorption in Clinical Conditions: Normal Pregnancy, Anemia and Hemochromatosis. J. Exper. Med., 1942, 76:15.

Barcroft, J. Alterations in the Volume of the Normal Spleen and Their Significance. Am. J. M. Sc., 1930, 179:1.

Bean, W. B., Cogswell, R., Dexter, M., Embick, J. F. Vascular Changes of the Skin in Pregnancy —Vascular Spiders and Palmar Erythema. Surg., Gynec. & Obst., 1949, 88:739.

Bethell, F. H. The Blood Changes in Normal Pregnancy and Their Relation to the Iron and Protein Supplied by the Diet. J.A.M.A., 1936, 107:564.

Bland, P. B., Goldstein, L., and First, A. The "Physiological" Anaemia of Pregnancy. Surg., Gynec. & Obst., 1930, 50:954.

Bodansky, M. Changes in Serum Calcium, Inorganic Phosphate and Phosphatase Activity in the Pregnant Woman. Am. J. Clin. Path., 1939, 9:36.

——— and Duff, V. B. Regulation of the Level of Calcium in the Serum during Pregnancy. J.A.M.A., 1939, 112:223.

Boyd, E. M. The Lipemia of Pregnancy. J. Clin. Investigation, 1934, 13:347.

Burger, K., and Korompai, I. Die Bewertung der Berechnung des Geburtstermines nach Naegele auf Grund unserer heutigen Kenntnise. Zentralbl. f. Gynäk., 1939, 63:1290.

Burwell, C. S. The Placenta as a Modified Arteriovenous Fistula, Considered in Relation to the Circulatory Adjustments to Pregnancy. Am. J. M. Sc., 1938, 195:1.

——— and others. Circulation during Pregnancy. Arch. Int. Med., 1938, 62:979.

Cantarow, A., Stuckert, H., and Gartman, E. Studies of Hepatic Function. IV. Hepatic Function during Pregnancy. Am. J. Obst. & Gynec., 1935, 29:36.

CAREY, J. B., and LITZENBERG, J. C. Total Leucocyte Counts in Human Blood during Pregnancy. Ann. Int. Med., 1936, 10:25.

CATON, W. L., ROBY, C. C., REID, D. E., and GIBSON, J. G. Plasma Volume and Extravascular Fluid Volume during Pregnancy and the Puerperium. Am. J. Obst. & Gynec., 1949, 57:471.

CHESLEY, L. C. Weight Changes and Water Balance in Normal and Toxic Pregnancy. Am. J. Obst. & Gynec., 1944, 48:565.

——— A Study of Extracellular Water Changes in Pregnancy. Surg., Gynec. & Obst., 1943, 76:589.

——— and BOOG, J. M. Changes in Extracellular Water at Delivery and in the Puerperium. Surg., Gynec. & Obst., 1943, 77:261.

COHEN, M. E., and THOMSON, K. J. Studies on the Circulation in Pregnancy. J.A.M.A., 1939, 112:1556.

COONS, C. M. Iron Retention by Women during Pregnancy. J. Biol. Chem., 1932, 97:215.

COONS, C. M., and BLUNT, K. J. The Retention of Calcium, Phosphorus and Magnesium by Pregnant Women. J. Biol. Chem., 1930, 86:1.

COONS, C. M., and COONS, R. R. Some Effects of Cod Liver Oil and Wheat Germ on the Retention of Iron, Nitrogen, Phosphorus, Calcium and Magnesium during Human Pregnancy. J. Nutrition, 1935, 10:289.

COONS, C. M., COONS, R. R., and SCHIEFELBUSCH, A. T. The Acid-Base Balance of the Minerals Retained during Human Pregnancy. J. Biol. Chem., 1934, 104:757.

CRABTREE, E. G. Changes in the Urinary Tract in Women. The Result of Normal Pregnancy. New England J. Med., 1931, 205:1048.

DEXTER, L., and WEISS, S. Preeclamptic and Eclamptic Toxemia. Little, Brown & Co., Boston, 1941.

DIECKMANN, W. J., and WEGNER, C. R. Studies of the Blood in Normal Pregnancy. I. Blood and Plasma Volumes. Arch. Int. Med., 1934, 53:71.

——— Studies of the Blood in Normal Pregnancy. II. Hemoglobin, Hematocrit and Erythrocyte Determinations and Total Amount of Variations of Each. Arch. Int. Med., 1934, 53:188.

——— Studies of the Blood in Normal Pregnancy. III. Hemoglobin and Cell Volume Coefficients; Erythrocyte Volume, Hemoglobin Content and Concentration; Color, Volume and Saturation Indices. Arch. Int. Med., 1934, 53:345.

——— Studies of the Blood in Normal Pregnancy. IV. Percentages and Grams per Kilogram of Serum Protein and Fibrin and Variations in Total Amount of Each. Arch. Int. Med., 1934, 53:353.

——— Studies of the Blood in Normal Pregnancy. V. Conductivity, Total Base, Chloride and Acid Base Equilibrium. Arch. Int. Med., 1934, 53:527.

——— Studies of the Blood in Normal Pregnancy. VI. Plasma Cholesterol in Milligrams per Hundred Cubic Centimeters, Grams per Kilogram and Variations in Total Amount. Arch. Int. Med., 1934, 53:540.

DODDS, G. H. Immediate and Remote Prognosis of Pyelitis of Pregnancy and Puerperium. J. Obst. & Gynaec. Brit. Emp., 1932, 39:46.

EASTMAN, N. J. The Serum Proteins in the Toxemias of Pregnancy. Am. J. Obst. & Gynec., 1930, 19:343.

ELIAS, H., GÜDEMAN, J., and ROUBITSCHEK, R. Insulin and Pregnancy Glycosuria. Wien. Arch. f. inn. Med., 1925, 11:567.

ENGLISH COURT. Gestation of 331 Days Allowed. J.A.M.A. (Foreign letters—London), 1921, 77:716.

ENRIGHT, L., COLE, V. V., and HITCHCOCK, F. A. Basal Metabolism and Iodine Excretion during Pregnancy. Am. J. Physiol., 1935, 113:221.

FABER, K. Benign Glycosuria Due to Disturbances in the Blood Sugar Regulating Mechanism. J. Clin. Investigation, 1926-27, 3:203.

FALLS, F. H. A Contribution to the Study of Pyelitis in Pregnancy. J.A.M.A., 1923, 81:1590.

——— Hyperthyroidism Associated with Pregnancy. Am. J. Obst. & Gynec., 1929, 17:536.

FRANK, E., and NOTHMANN, M. Ueber die Verwertbarkeit der renalen Schwangerschaftsglykosurie zur Frühdiagnose der Schwangerschaft. München. med. Wchnschr., 1920, 67:1433.

GEIPEL, P. Weiterer Beitrag zur Kenntnis des decidualen Gewebes. Arch. f. Gynäk., 1927, 131:650.

GILLIGAN, D. R., and ERNSTENE, A. C. The Relationship Between the Erythrocyte Sedimentation Rate and the Fibrinogen Content of Plasma. Am. J. M. Sc., 1934, 187:552.

GOTTSCHALK, A., and STRECKER, J. Test Glycosuria in Pregnancy. Klin. Wchnschr., 1922, 1:2467.

GRIFFIN, R. J. The Sedimentation Rate and Schilling Index in Pregnancy. Am. J. Obst. & Gynec., 1934, 28:532.

HAMILTON, B., DASEF, L., HIGHMAN, W. J., Jr., and SCHWARTZ, C. Parathyroid Hormone in the Blood of Pregnant Women. J. Clin. Investigation, 1936, 15:323.

HAMILTON, H. F. H. The Cardiac Output in Normal Pregnancy: As Determined by the Cournand Right Heart Catheterization Technique. J. Obst. & Gynaec. Brit. Emp., 1949, 56:548.

HANNA, G. C., Jr. The Basal Metabolic Rate in Normal Pregnancy. Am. J. Obst. & Gynec., 1938, 35:155.

HANSEN, R. Zur Physiologie des Magens in der Schwangerschaft. Zentralbl. f. Gynäk., 1937, 61:2306.

HARDING, V. J. Metabolism in Pregnancy. Physiol. Rev., 1925, 5:279.

HARE, D. C., and KARN, M. N. An Investigation of Blood Pressure, Pulse Rate and the Response to Exercise during Normal Pregnancy and Some Observations after Confinement. Quart. J. Med., 1928-29, 22:381.

HENRY, J. S. The Effect of Pregnancy upon the Blood Pressure. J. Obst. & Gynaec. Brit. Emp., 1936, 43:908.

HOFBAUER, J. Maternal Changes Incident to Pregnancy. In Curtis, Obstetrics and Gynecology. W. B. Saunders Co., Philadelphia, 1934, 1:613.

——— Structure and Function of the Ureter during Pregnancy. J. Urol., 1928, 20:413.

——— Die Bedeutung der Generationsvorgänge für die Klinik der Tuberkulose. Ztschr. f. Geburtsh. u. Gynäk., 1910, 67:572.

——— Larynx und Schwangerschaft. Monatschr. f. Geburtsh. u. Gynäk., 1908, 28:45.

HOTELLING, H., and HOTELLING, F. A New Analysis of Duration of Pregnancy Data. Am. J. Obst. & Gynec., 1932, 23:643.

HUGGETT, A. S. Foetal Blood-gas Tensions and Gas Transfusion through the Placenta of the Goat. J. Physiol., 1927, 62:373.

HUGHES, E. C. A Study of 1,250 Basal Metabolisms during Pregnancy. New York State J. Med., 1934, 34:873.

HUMMEL, F. C., and others. A Consideration of the Nutritive State in the Metabolism of Women during Pregnancy. J. Nutrition, 1937, 13:263.

HUMMEL, F. C., STERNBERGER, H. R., HUNSCHER, H. A., and MACY, I. G. Metabolism of Women during the Reproductive Cycle. VII. Utilization of Inorganic Elements (a Continuous Study of a Multipara). J. Nutrition, 1936, 11:235.

HUNSCHER, H. A., HUMMEL, F. C., ERICKSON, B. N., and MACY, I. G. Metabolism of Women during the Reproductive Cycle. VI. A Case of the Continuous Nitrogen Utilization of a Multipara during Pregnancy, Parturition, Puerperium and Lactation. J. Nutrition, 1935, 10:579.

HUNTER, W. The Anatomy of the Gravid Uterus, 1774.

INGERSLEV, M., and TEILUM, G. Biopsy Studies on the Liver in Pregnancy. II. Liver Biopsy on Normal Pregnant Women. Acta obst. et gynec. Scandinav., 1946, 25:352.

JENSEN, J. The Heart in Pregnancy. C. V. Mosby Co., St. Louis, 1938.

JOHN, H. J. Therapy of Non-Diabetic Glycosuria. Ohio State M. J., 1941, 37:136.

JOHNSTON, J. A., and others. The Basal Metabolism in Pregnancy. J. Nutrition, 1938, 15:513.

JONA, J. L. A Further Contribution to the Physiology and Pathology of the Kidney Pelvis. Surg., Gynec. & Obst., 1934, 59:713.

KAMNITZER and JOSEPH. Glycosuria Test for Beginning Pregnancy. Med. Klin., 1922, 18:396.

KLAFTEN, E., and PALUGYAY, J. Vergleichende Untersuchungen über Lage und Ausdehnung von Herz und Lunge in der Schwangerschaft und im Wochenbett. Arch. f. Gynäk., 1927, 131:347.

KRAUL, L. Zur Berechnung des Geburtstermines nach Naegele. Wien. klin. Wchnschr., 1935, 48:305.

KRETSCHMER, H. L., and HEANEY, N. S. Dilatation of the Kidney Pelvis and Ureter during Pregnancy and the Puerperium. A Pyelographic Study. J.A.M.A., 1925, 85:406.

KRETSCHMER, H. L., HEANEY, N. S., and OCKULY, E. A. Dilatation of the Kidney Pelvis and Ureter during Pregnancy and the Puerperium. A Pyelographic Study in Normal Women. J.A.M.A., 1933, 101:2025.

KREUTZMANN, H. R. Studies in Normal Ureteral and Vesical Pressure. J. Urol., 1928, 19:4; 517.

LONG, C. F., and HIRST, J. C., Jr. Ingestion Glycosuria, an Aid to Early Diagnosis of Pregnancy. New York M. J., 1923, 118:543.

MCLENNAN, C. E. Antecubital and Femoral Venous Pressure in Normal and Toxemic Pregnancy. Am. J. Obst. & Gynec., 1943, 45:568.

——— Rate of Filtration through Capillary Walls in Pregnancy. Am. J. Obst. & Gynec., 1943, 46:63.

——— and THOUIN, L. G. Blood Volume in Pregnancy. Am. J. Obst. & Gynec., 1948, 55:189.

MACY, I. G., and HUNSCHER, H. A. An Evaluation of Maternal Nitrogen and Mineral Needs during Embryonic and Infant Development. Am. J. Obst. & Gynec., 1934, 27:878.

MENGERT, W. F. The Relation of Maternal Metabolism to Infant Birth Weight. Surg., Gynec. & Obst., 1933, 56:1009.

MULL, J. W., and BILL, A. H. Variations in Serum Calcium and Phosphorus during Pregnancy. I. Normal Variations. Am. J. Obst. & Gynec., 1934, 27:510.

MUSSEY, R. D., and PLUMMER, W. A. Treatment of Goiter Complicating Pregnancy. J.A.M.A., 1931, 97:602.

MYERS, V. C., MUNTWYLER, E., and BILL, A. H. The Acid-Base Balance Disturbance of Pregnancy. J. Biol. Chem., 1932, 98:253.

NEWMAN, R. L. Blood Calcium: Normal Curve for Pregnancy. Am. J. Obst. & Gynec., 1947, 53:817.

NICE, M., MULL, J. W., MUNTWYLER, E., and MYERS, V. C. The Acid-Base Balance of the Blood during Normal Pregnancy and Puerperium. Am. J. Obst. & Gynec., 1936, 32:375.

OARD, H. C., and PETERS, J. P. The Concentration of Acid and Base in the Serum in Normal Pregnancy. J. Biol. Chem., 1929, 81:9.

OBERST, F. W., and PLASS, E. D. Water Concentration of the Blood during Pregnancy, Labor and the Puerperium. Am. J. Obst. & Gynec., 1936, 31:61.

——— The Acid-Base Balance in the Plasma and Blood Cells of Normal Nonpregnant, Pregnant and Puerperal Women. J. Lab. & Clin. Med., 1940, 26:513.

PALMER, A. J., and WALKER, A. H. C. The Maternal Circulation in Normal Pregnancy. J. Obst. & Gynaec. Brit. Emp., 1949, 56:537.

PETERS, J. P., MAN, E. B., and HEINEMANN, M. Pregnancy and the Thyroid Gland. Obst. & Gynec. Surv., 1948, 3:647.

PLASS, E. D., and BOGERT, L. J. The Calcium and Magnesium Content of the Blood Serum during Pregnancy, Labor and the Puerperium. Am. J. Obst. & Gynec., 1923, 6:427.

PLASS, E. D., and MATTHEW, C. W. Plasma Protein Fractions in Normal Pregnancy, Labor and the Puerperium. Am. J. Obst. & Gynec., 1926, 12:346.

PLASS, E. D., and OBERST, F. W. Respiration and Pulmonary Ventilation in Normal Nonpregnant, Pregnant and Puerperal Women. Am. J. Obst. & Gynec., 1938, 35:441.

PLASS, E. D., and YOAKAM, W. A. Basal Metabolism Studies in Normal Pregnant Women with Normal and Pathologic Thyroid Glands. Am. J. Obst. & Gynec., 1929, 18:556.

PYLE, S. I., POTGIETER, M., and COMSTOCK, G. On Certain Relationships of Calcium in the Blood Serum to Calcium Balance and Basal Metabolism during Pregnancy. Am. J. Obst. & Gynec., 1938, 35:283.

RAMSAY, J., THIERENS, V. T., and MAGEE, H. E. The Composition of the Blood in Pregnancy. Brit. M. J., 1938, 1:1199.

RAMSEY, J. The Vascular Pattern of the Endometrium of the Pregnant Rhesus Monkey (Macaca Mulatta). Carnegie Inst. of Wash., 1949, Publ. 583, Contrib. to Embryology, 33:113.

RICHARDSON, R., and BITTER, R. S. Glycosuria in Pregnancy. Am. J. Obst. & Gynec., 1932, 24:362.

ROSCOE, M. H., and DONALDSON, G. M. M. The Blood in Pregnancy. I. The Haemoglobin Level. J. Obst. & Gynaec. Brit. Emp., 1946, 53:430.

——— The Blood in Pregnancy. Blood Volume, Cell Volume and Hemoglobin Mass. J. Obst. & Gynaec. Brit. Emp., 1946, 53:527.

ROSSENBECK, H. Behavior of Ketone Bodies, Residual Nitrogen, Lactic Acid, Chlorides and Alkali Reserve in Healthy Pregnant Women. Arch. f. Gynäk., 1939, 168:709.

——— Eklampsie und Ionenhaushalt. Blut- und organ-analytische Untersuchungen als Beitrag zur Patho-Biologie der Eklampsie. Arch. f. Gynäk., 1931, 145:331.

ROWE, A. W. Sugar Tolerance as an Aid to Diagnosis. J.A.M.A., 1927, 89:1403.

ROWE, A. W., ALCOTT, M. D., and MORTIMER, E. The Metabolism in Pregnancy. II. Changes in the Basal Metabolic Rate. Am. J. Physiol., 1925, 71:667.

ROWE, A. W., and BOYD, W. C. The Metabolism in Pregnancy. IX. The Foetal Influence on the Basal Rate. J. Nutrition, 1932, 5:551.

ROWE, A. W., GALLIVAN, D. E., and MATTHEWS, H. The Metabolism in Pregnancy. V. The Carbohydrate Metabolism. Am. J. Physiol., 1931, 96:94.

——— The Metabolism in Pregnancy. VI. The Respiratory Metabolism and Acid Elimination. Am. J. Physiol., 1931, 96:101.

SANDIFORD, I., and WHEELER, T. Basal Metabolism before, during and after Pregnancy. J. Biol. Chem., 1924, 62:329.

SCHMIDT, H. R., BICKENBACK, W., and JONEN, P. Stoffwechselphysiologische Untersuchungen an trächtigen Hündinnen, mit besonderer Berücksichtigung der chemischen Zusammensetzung der Organe. Ztschr. f. Geburtsh. u. Gynäk., 1927, 91:527.

SCHMORL. Ueber grosszellige (decidua-ähnliche) Wucherungen auf dem Peritoneum und den Ovarien bei intrauteriner Schwangerschaft. Monatschr. f. Geburtsh. u. Gynäk., 1897, 5:46.

SEEGERS, W. H. The Nitrogen Balance of a Young Primipara. Am. J. Obst. & Gynec., 1937, 34:1019.

SELLHEIM, H. Weiterstellung des Bauches, Fasiendehnung und Dehnungsstreifen der Haut. Monatschr. f. Geburtsh. u. Gynäk., 1923, 63:185.

SEYNSCHE, K. Schwangerschaftsstreifen und Konstitution. Zentralbl. f. Gynäk., 1926, 50:1749.

SLEMONS, J. M., and STANDER, H. J. The Lipoids of the Maternal and Fetal Blood at the Conclusion of Labor. Bull. Johns Hopkins Hosp., 1923, 34:7.

SONTAG, L. W., REYNOLDS, E. L., and TORBET, V. Relation of Basal Metabolic Gain during Pregnancy to Nonpregnant Basal Metabolism. Am. J. Obst. & Gynec., 1944, 48:315.

SPEITKAMP, L. Uber die Länge der Schwangerschaft beim Menschen. Ztschr. f. Geburtsh. u. Gynäk., 1937, 116:10.

SPINGARN, C. L., and GEIST, S. H. Hyperparathyroidism and Pregnancy. J.A.M.A., 1939, 113:2387.

Stander, H. J., and Cadden, J. F. The Cardiac Output in Pregnant Women. Am. J. Obst. & Gynec., 1932, 24:13.

Stander, H. J., and Creadick, A. N. Blood Volume in Pregnancy. Bull. Johns Hopkins Hosp., 1924, 35:1.

Stander, H. J., Duncan, E. E., and Sisson, W. E. Heart Output during Pregnancy. Am. J. Obst. & Gynec., 1926, 11:44.

Stieve, H. Der Halsteil der menschlichen Gebärmutter, etc. Leipzig, 1927.

——— Die regelmässigen Veränderungen der Musculatur u. des Bindegewebes in der menschlichen Gebärmutter, etc. Ztschr. f. mikr.-anat. Forschung, 1926, 6:351.

——— Das Schwangerschaftswachstum und die Geburts-Erweiterung der menschlichen Scheide. Ztschr. f. mikr.-anat. Forsch., 1925, 3:307.

——— Muskulatur u. Bindegewebe in der Wand der menschlichen Gebärmutter, etc. Ztschr. f. mikr.-anat. Forsch., 1929, 17:371.

——— Ueber die Neubildung von Muskelzellen in der Wand der schwangeren menschlichen Gebärmutter. Zentralbl. f. Gynäk., 1932, 56:1442.

Strauss, M. B., and Castle, W. B. Studies of Anemia in Pregnancy. Am. J. M. Sc., 1932, 184:655; 1933, 185:539.

Taylor, H. C., Jr., Warner, R. C., and Welsh, C. A. Relationship of Estrogens and other Placental Hormones to Sodium and Potassium Balance at the End of Pregnancy and in the Puerperium. Am. J. Obst. & Gynec., 1939, 38:748.

——— Relationship of Estrogens and Progesterone to Edema of Normal and Toxemic Pregnancy. Am. J. Obst. & Gynec., 1943, 45:547.

Thompson, R. H. S., and Watson, D. Serum Copper Levels in Pregnancy and in Preeclampsia. J. Clin. Path., 1949, 2:193.

Thomson, K. J., Hirsheimer, A., Gibson, J. G., and Evans, W. A., Jr. Studies on the Circulation in Pregnancy. III. Blood Volume Changes in Normal Pregnant Women. Am. J. Obst. & Gynec., 1938, 36:48.

Thomson, K. J., and Cohen, M. E. Studies on the Circulation in Pregnancy. II. Vital Capacity Observations in Normal Pregnant Women. Surg., Gynec. & Obst., 1938, 66:591.

Thomson, K. J., Reid, D. E., and Cohen, M. E. Studies on Circulation in Pregnancy. IV. Venous Pressure Observations in Normal Pregnant Women, in Pregnant Women with Compensated and Decompensated Heart Disease and in the Pregnancy "Toxemias." Am. J. M. Sc., 1939, 198:665.

Thorn, G. W., and Engel, L. L. Effect of Sex Hormones on Renal Excretion of Electrolytes. J. Exper. Med., 1938, 68:299.

Thorn, G. W., Nelson, K. R., and Thorn, D. W. Study of Mechanism of Edema Associated with Menstruation. Endocrinol., 1938, 22:155.

Traut, H. F., and McLane, C. M. Physiological Changes in the Ureter Associated with Pregnancy. Surg., Gynec. & Obst., 1936, 62:65.

Van Liere, E. J., and Sleeth, C. K. The Question of Cardiac Hypertrophy during Pregnancy. Am. J. Physiol., 1938, 122:34.

Wallis, R. L. M., and Bose, J. P. Glycosuria in Pregnancy. J. Obst. & Gynaec. Brit. Emp., 1922, 29:274.

Way, S. Relation Between Gastric Acidity and the Anterior-Pituitary-Like Hormone Content of Urine in Pregnant Women. Brit. M. J., 1945, 2:182.

Weech, A. A., Snelling, C. E., and Goettsch, E. The Relation between Plasma Protein Content, Plasma Specific Gravity and Edema in Dogs Maintained on a Protein Inadequate Diet and in Dogs Rendered Edematous by Plasmapheresis. J. Clin. Investigation, 1933, 12:193.

Wells, S. M. A Case of Prolonged Pregnancy. Guy's Hosp. Gaz., 1948, 62:299. Abstracted in Obst. & Gynec. Surv., 1949, 4:378.

Williams, J. W. Decidual Formation throughout the Uterine Muscularis. Tr. South. Surg. & Gynec. Ass., 1905, 17:119.

Williams, E. C. P., and Wills, L. Studies in Blood and Urinary Chemistry during Pregnancy. Quart. J. Med., 1928-29, 22:493.

Williams, N. H. Variable Significance of Heartburn. Am. J. Obst. & Gynec., 1941, 42:814.

Wilson, K. M. Nitrogen Metabolism in Pregnancy. Bull. Johns Hopkins Hosp., 1916, 27:121.

Wright, H. P., Osborn, S. B., and Edmonds, D. G. Measurement of the Rate of Venous Blood Flow in the Legs of Women at Term and in the Puerperium, Using Radioactive Sodium. J. Obst. & Gynaec. Brit. Emp., 1949, 56:36. Abstracted in Obst. & Gynec. Surv., 1949, 4:476.

Ziskin, D. E. The Incidence of Dental Caries in Pregnant Women. Am. J. Obst. & Gynec., 1926, 12:710.

Section Three: MANAGEMENT OF NORMAL PREGNANCY

9

DIAGNOSIS OF PREGNANCY

Ordinarily, the diagnosis of pregnancy offers little or no difficulty, and the patient is usually aware of the true condition before she consults a physician. In a small minority of cases, however, the task is by no means easy, and despite every known method at our command we are occasionally unable to decide with certainty.

Mistakes in diagnosis are most frequently made in the first few months, while the uterus is still a pelvic organ, although it is by no means impossible to confound a pregnancy, even at full term, with a tumor of some other nature. Such errors are usually the result of hasty or imperfect examination, but a false conclusion may sometimes be arrived at even after the most conscientious exploration of the patient. Some idea of the frequency of such mistakes may be realized when it is stated that there is hardly a gynecologist of experience who has not opened the abdomen on one or more occasions, with the expectation of removing a tumor of the uterus or its appendages, and has been surprised to find himself in the presence of a normal pregnancy.

It is often a matter of considerable importance that a diagnosis be made in the early months of pregnancy, but, unfortunately, it is just at this period that our diagnostic ability is most restricted, as the absolutely positive signs do not, as a rule, become available until the fifth month. Hence, it follows that in cases in which the existence of such a condition might affect the reputation or interests of the patient a positive expression of opinion should be deferred until the diagnosis is beyond all doubt.

The diagnosis is based upon the presence of certain symptoms and signs. The former are chiefly subjective and are appreciated by the patient; while the latter are made out by the physician after a careful physical examination, in which the senses of sight, hearing, and touch, as well as certain laboratory procedures, are employed.

The signs and symptoms are usually classified into three groups: the positive signs, which cannot usually be detected until after the fourth month; the probable signs, which can be appreciated at an earlier period; and the presumptive evidences, which are usually subjective in character, and may be experienced at varying periods.

Positive Signs of Pregnancy. These are three in number and consist in: (1) hearing and counting the fetal heart beat; (2) perception of active fetal movements by the examiner; and (3) recognition of the fetal skeleton by means of the x-ray. When any one of these signs is obtained, the diagnosis is established beyond all doubt.

1. *The Fetal Heart Beat.* Whenever one can hear and count the pulsations of the fetal heart, the diagnosis of pregnancy is assured beyond peradventure. Unfortunately, however, this sign cannot usually be appreciated until the eighteenth or

twentieth week, though not a few writers claim that it may be possible as early as the twelfth or fourteenth week.

The fetal heart beat, after the eighteenth or twentieth week of pregnancy, should be detected without difficulty. Ordinarily it varies in frequency from 120 to 140 beats to the minute and is a double sound, closely resembling the tick of a watch under a pillow. In order to hear it, the abdomen should be bared, or at most covered by a thin cloth. In the earlier months it is best detected by means of a head stethoscope. One should not be content with merely hearing the fetal heart but should always attempt to count its rate and compare it with that of the maternal pulse.

In the early months the heart should be sought just over the symphysis pubis; but in the later months the situation at which it is best heard varies according to the position and presentation of the fetus, details concerning which will be given when we consider the methods of obstetrical examination.

Other Sounds Which May Be Heard on Auscultation. In addition to hearing the fetal heart, auscultation of the abdomen in the later months of pregnancy often reveals other sounds, the most important of which are the funic souffle, the uterine or placental souffle, sounds due to movements of the fetus, the maternal pulse, and the gurgling of gas in the intestines of the mother.

The *funic,* or *fetal,* or *umbilical souffle* is a sharp, whistling sound, synchronous with the fetal pulse, which can be heard in about 15 per cent of all cases. It is very inconstant in its appearance, as it may be recognized distinctly at one examination and be absent on succeeding occasions. It is due to the rush of blood through the umbilical arteries under circumstances in which they are subject to torsion, tension or pressure, as, for example, when the cord is coiled around the neck of the fetus. This is not, however, a sign of very great importance, although, when heard, it is distinctly characteristic of pregnancy and is of some value.

The *uterine souffle* is a soft, blowing sound, synchronous with the maternal pulse, and is usually most distinctly heard upon auscultating the lower portion of the uterus. It is due to the passage of blood through the dilated uterine vessels. This sign is not characteristic only of pregnancy, as it may be present in any condition in which the blood supply to the genitalia becomes markedly increased, and accordingly may be heard in nonpregnant women presenting large myomatous tumors of the uterus or enlarged ovaries.

Certain *movements of the fetus* may likewise be recognized on auscultation. Also, the *maternal pulse* can frequently be distinctly heard on auscultating the abdomen, and in some instances the pulsation of the aorta is unusually loud. Occasionally the pulse may become so rapid during examination as to simulate the fetal heart sounds. In addition to the sounds just mentioned, it is not unusual to hear certain others produced by the passage of gases or fluids through the intestines of the mother.

2. *Movements of the Fetus.* The second positive sign of pregnancy is present whenever the physician is able to feel the spontaneous movements of the fetus.

After the fifth month the *active movements* may be felt at intervals on placing the hand over the abdomen. These vary from a faint flutter in the early months to quite violent motions at a later period, which are sometimes visible as well. Occasionally, somewhat similar sensations may be produced by contractions of the intestines or the muscles of the abdominal wall, though these should not deceive an experienced observer.

3. *The X-Ray.* Whenever the outlines of the fetal skeleton can be distinguished by means of the roentgen ray, the existence of pregnancy is assured. Unfortunately, like the other positive signs, this method of diagnosis is usually not available until after the fourth month. By this means Bartholomew, Sale and Calloway were able to make a positive diagnosis in one third of their patients at the fifth month, in one half at the sixth month, and almost constantly later. Just how early the fetal skeleton

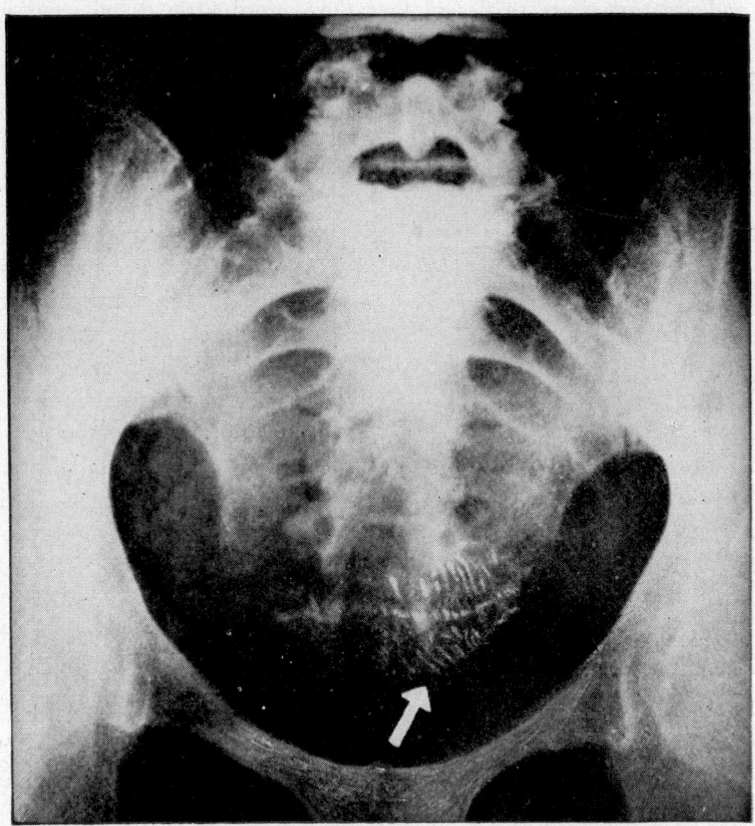

FIG. 164.—X-RAY OF EARLY PREGNANCY. DURATION OF PREGNANCY, 95 DAYS OR LESS. (Courtesy, the late Dr. Joseph F. Elward and Dr. Joseph F. Belair, *Radiology*, 31:678, 1938.)

will show in the roentgenogram depends upon the thickness of the abdominal wall, the x-ray equipment and other factors. It has been demonstrated as early as the fourteenth week by Elward and Belair. The method is of especial value in differentiating the pregnant uterus from abdominal tumors, particularly when the child is dead.

Probable Signs of Pregnancy. These consist of (1) enlargement of the abdomen; (2) changes in the shape, size and consistence of the uterus; (3) changes in the cervix; (4) the detection of intermittent contractions of the uterus; (5) ballottement; (6) mapping the outlines of the fetus; and (7) positive hormonal test for pregnancy.

1. *Enlargement of the Abdomen.* From the third month onward the uterus can be felt through the abdominal walls as a tumor, which gradually increases in size up to the end of pregnancy. Generally speaking, any enlargement of the abdomen during the childbearing period should be regarded as prima facie evidence of the existence of pregnancy.

The abdominal enlargement is less pronounced in primigravidae than in multiparae, for the reason that in the latter the abdominal walls have lost a great part of their tonicity and are sometimes so flaccid that they afford little or no support to the uterus, which then sags forward and downward, giving rise to a *pendulous abdomen.* This difference is so apparent that it is not unusual for women in the latter part of a second pregnancy to suspect the existence of twins from the increased size of the abdomen, as compared with that noted in the corresponding month of the previous pregnancy. It should also be borne in mind that the abdomen changes its shape materially according as the woman is in the upright or horizontal position, being much less prominent when she is lying down.

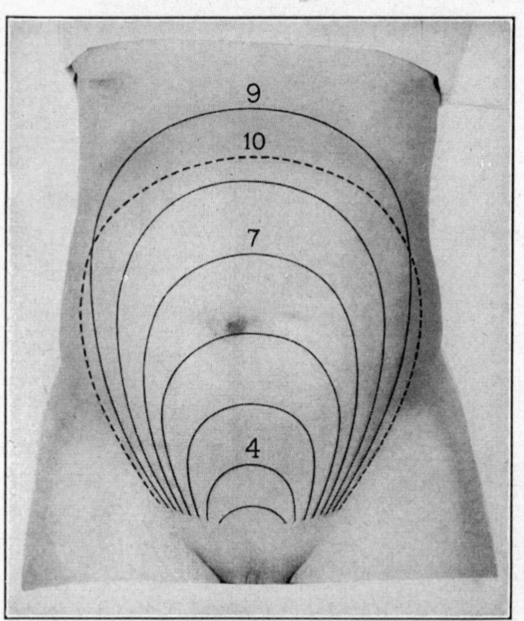

Fig. 165.—Relative Height of the Fundus at the Various Lunar Months of Pregnancy.

2. *Changes in Size, Shape and Consistence of Uterus.* In the first three months these are the only physical signs available.

During the first few weeks the increase in size is limited almost entirely to the anteroposterior diameter, but at a little later period the body of the uterus becomes almost globular in shape, and at the third month attains the size of an orange. During the first two months the pregnant uterus still continues to be entirely a pelvic organ, whereas during the third month it begins to rise above the symphysis. At the same time the angle between the body and cervix becomes accentuated—in other words, the physiological anteflexion is increased.

More characteristic than the changes in shape are those affecting its consistence. On bimanual examination the uterine body offers a doughy or elastic sensation and in some instances becomes so soft as to be hardly distinguishable. At about the sixth week another sign of very considerable value—the so-called *Hegar's sign*—becomes available. On careful examination with one hand upon the abdomen and two fingers of the other hand in the vagina, the firm, hard cervix is felt, and above it the elastic body of the uterus, while between the two the isthmus is felt as a soft compressible area. Occasionally the change in consistence in this location is so marked that no connection between the cervix and body appears to exist, so that inexperienced observers may mistake the cervix for a small uterus, and the softened body for a tumor of the tubes or ovaries.

The value of this sign is universally admitted, and we consider it the most valuable physical sign of early pregnancy. Its production probably depends upon forcing the portion of the ovum occupying the lower uterine segment into the upper part of the body of the uterus, so that the empty and softened isthmus can then be readily

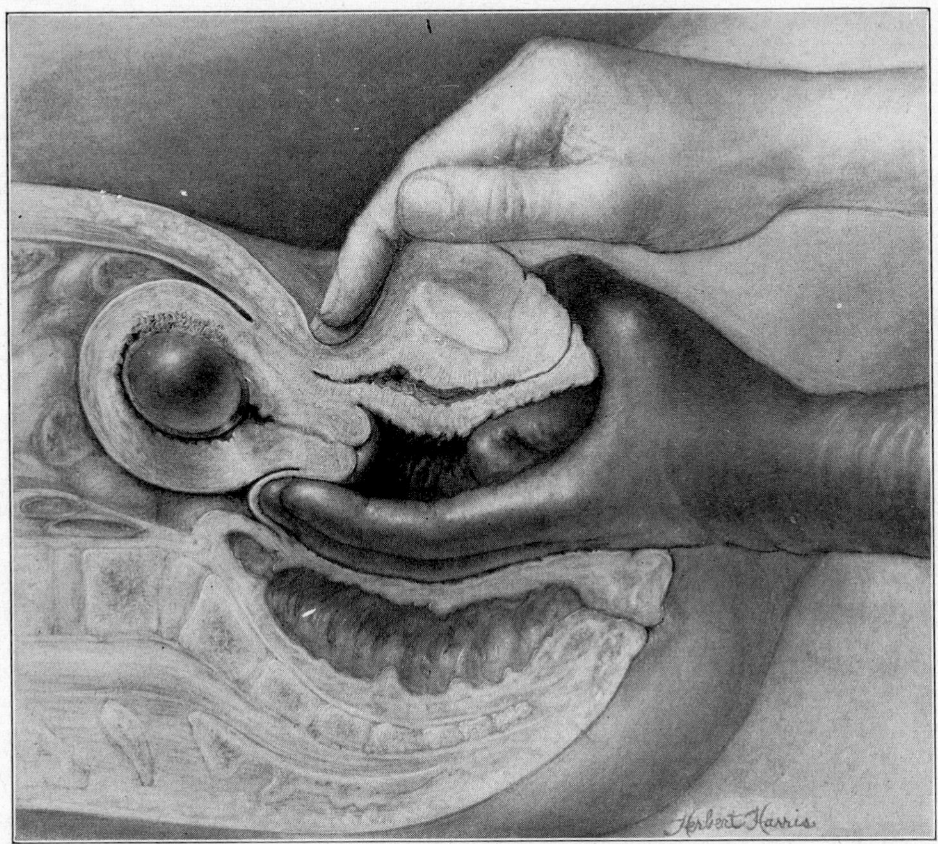

FIG. 166.—METHOD OF DETECTING HEGAR'S SIGN.

compressed between the fingers. Figures 166 and 167 give a good idea of how the sensation is to be obtained on bimanual examination. This sign is not, however, absolutely characteristic or dependable, as it may occasionally be elicited when the walls of the nonpregnant uterus are unduly soft.

3. *Cervix.* Beginning with the second month of pregnancy, the cervix becomes considerably softened, and in primiparous women the os externum offers to the finger a sensation similar to that obtained by pressing upon the more yielding lips instead of the harder cartilage of the nose, as at other times. Occasionally, however, the softening does not occur until much later in pregnancy, and in certain inflammatory conditions, as well as in carcinoma, the cervix may remain firm and hard until the onset of labor. Moreover, as pregnancy advances, the cervical canal becomes so patulous

that it frequently admits the tip of the finger, which in extreme cases can be introduced through the internal os.

4. *Intermittent Contractions of the Uterus.* From the first weeks on, at intervals of from three to ten minutes, the pregnant uterus undergoes painless contractions, which in the second trimester can be appreciated by bimanual examination, and later by the hand upon the abdomen, when the previously relaxed organ is felt to become firm and hard, remaining so for a few moments, and then returning to its original condition. Attention was first called to this phenomenon by Braxton Hicks, and the sign has since

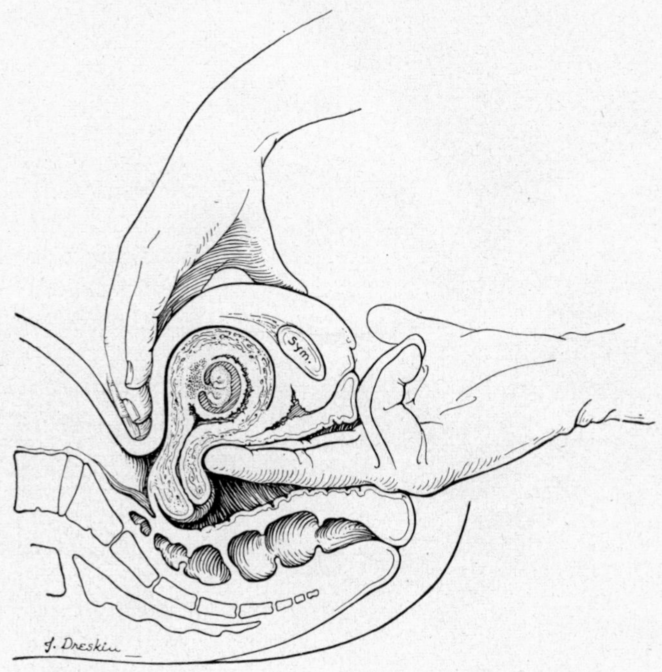

FIG. 167.—ALTERNATE METHOD OF DETECTING HEGAR'S SIGN.

been known by his name. It is not infallible, however, since Braxton Hicks contractions are sometimes observed in hematometra, and occasionally in cases of soft myomata.

5. *Ballottement.* This term is derived from the French "ballotter," to toss up like a ball. During the fourth and fifth months of pregnancy, the fetus is small in relation to the amount of amniotic fluid present, and a sudden tap on the uterus makes the fetus rise in the amniotic fluid and then rebound to its original position and in turn tap the examining finger. When elicited by an experienced examiner, this is one of the most certain of the probable signs of pregnancy, and many authorities even regard it as a positive sign. It is not, however, absolute evidence of pregnancy, since it can be simulated by a pedunculated tumor surrounded by ascitic fluid. The sign may be obtained through either the vagina or the abdominal walls. To obtain vaginal ballottement the patient should be on her back; the physician then introduces two fingers into the vagina and carries them up to the anterior fornix to which he imparts a sudden motion with his fingertips, afterward retaining them in the same position. After a

moment the part of the fetus which occupies the lower segment of the uterus drops down upon them again. External ballottement can be obtained by imparting a sudden motion to the portion of the abdominal wall covering the uterus; in a few seconds the rebound of the fetus can be felt.

6. *Mapping the Outlines of the Fetus.* In the second half of pregnancy it is possible to distinguish the outlines of the fetus by palpation through the abdominal walls, and this becomes easier the nearer term is approached. However, some serous myomata occasionally simulate the head or small parts, or both, and may give rise to serious diagnostic errors and hence a diagnosis of pregnancy should not be made on this sign alone. Furthermore, in the late stages of pregnancy when it becomes demonstrable, x-ray is the easiest and most certain answer to the question.

7. *Endocrine Tests.* As explained in Chapter 6, a hormone, chorionic gonadotrophin, is produced by the trophoblast shortly after implantation, is excreted in the urine and may readily be detected there because of its action on the rodent ovary and on the gonads of various amphibia. Upon this fact a large number of tests for pregnancy have been based, of which the most widely used are the following: (1) the Aschheim-Zondek test; (2) the Friedman test; (3) the Xenopus or Hogben test; and (4) the American male frog or *Rana pipiens* test.

The great advantage of all these endocrine tests over other methods of diagnosticating pregnancy is that they become positive extremely early in gestation and make it possible to establish a diagnosis with 95 to 98 per cent accuracy about three weeks after implantation of the ovum, or about two weeks after the first missed period. Under carefully controlled research conditions, the accuracy between the fiftieth and the one hundred and twentieth day after the last menstrual period approaches 100 per cent, but in actual routine use errors occasionally occur due to various causes such as mixing of specimens, mixing of animals, sickness of animals so that they do not respond, and so on. Moreover, before the fiftieth day and after the one hundred and twentieth day, if the patient does not follow instructions about withholding fluid the night before the morning specimen is obtained and happens to have a diuresis, the concentration of the hormone may be too dilute to give a reaction. For these reasons the hormone tests are not listed under the positive signs of pregnancy, but with reasonable care they approximate 98 per cent in accuracy and are by far the most dependable of the probable signs of pregnancy.

During the first week after the first missed period, the hormone, although present in the urine, may or may not be in sufficient concentration to give a positive reaction, and hence negative tests at that time carry little significance. It is therefore desirable to postpone the test until two weeks after the first missed period when either a positive or a negative reaction becomes of diagnostic value. The patient is asked to withhold all fluid after 7 P.M., to void at bedtime, discarding the specimen, and then to void in the morning, in a clean container, the specimen to be examined. The technics of the four most commonly employed endocrine tests for pregnancy are outlined below.

Aschheim-Zondek Test.

1. Collect first morning specimen of urine.
2. Filter if necessary. Always keep in refrigerator when not being used.
3. Warm just enough to remove chill by allowing to stand at room temperature just before injecting into mice.

4. Inject subcutaneously into each of five immature female white mice (6 to 8 gm. in weight) 0.4 cc. of the urine specimen on six different occasions over a period of two days, each mouse receiving a total of 2.4 cc.

5. One hundred hours after the first injection, kill the mice and examine the ovaries for the presence of hemorrhagic follicles or corpora lutea. The presence of either or both of these structures in at least one mouse indicates a positive reaction. In case of doubt, serial sections of the ovaries stained with hematoxylin and eosin may be examined microscopically.

6. In cases of suspected hydatidiform mole and chorionepithelioma, dilutions of the urine with distilled water from 1:10, 1:100 and so on, are injected in the same way.

The Aschheim-Zondek test is the original endocrine test from which all others have stemmed. It is not used extensively in the United States at the present time, however, because of the multiple injections required, the long time interval before an answer can be obtained and also because of the difficulty of having on hand at all times the immature mice of the weight specified.

Friedman Test.

1. Collect first morning specimen of urine and proceed as described for the Aschheim-Zondek test.

2. Inject slowly into the ear vein of a mature female rabbit, previously isolated for four weeks, 10 cc. of the urine specimen.

3. Twenty-four hours or longer after the injection, the rabbit is anesthetized, its abdomen is opened and the ovaries examined for the presence of hemorrhagic ruptured follicles, which indicate a positive reaction. Care must be taken to differentiate between hemorrhagic ruptured and unruptured follicles. The latter do not indicate a positive reaction. If the reaction is negative, the ovaries are explored again 24 hours later to make certain that a delayed positive reaction has not occurred. The animal can be used again after four weeks. Because of adhesions, it is undesirable to employ a single rabbit for more than three tests.

Since the Friedman test does away with the three objections of the Aschheim-Zondek test mentioned above, it has been the most extensively employed diagnostic procedure for pregnancy in this country. Recently, however, many clinics and laboratories are giving it up in favor of one or the other of the two tests listed below.

Xenopus or Hogben Test. This procedure is based upon egg extrusion in the South African clawed toad (*Xenopus laevis*) and has been extensively used, especially in the British Empire ever since the reaction was described by Hogben in 1930. Of some 5,300 tests reported by six different observers, the percentage of accuracy is stated to be between 96 and 100. In a study carried out in our clinic by Foote and Jones, it was found that, from the fortieth day after the last menstrual period onward, the Hogben test gave an accuracy which approximated 96 per cent. They point out that an important clinical advantage of the Hogben over the Friedman test is that it gives no false positive results.

The method used by Foote and Jones was that described by Weisman and, briefly, involves concentration of 40 cc. of the first morning urine by acetone precipitation, and the injection of 1 cc. of the aqueous concentrate into the dorsal lymph sac of the toad. If the urine specimen contains a sufficient concentration of chorionic gonadotrophin, ovulation occurs and myriads of eggs are extruded in from 8 to 16 hours following the injection. These eggs can be readily seen on the floor of the aquarium, especially if a black background is placed underneath it. The injections are usually given to the toad in the evening, and observations made the following morning. This is in order to allow the animal to remain in darkness overnight, as it has been found that light sometimes inhibits egg extrusion. A month is allowed as a resting period for each animal after a positive test, and two weeks following a negative. Landgrebe and Samson, who have had a vast experience with these toads, have used the same animals over a period of 12 years and find no loss of sensitivity to stimulation. Their records also show that each animal in their colony is used approximately 10 times a year.

The advantages of the Xenopus or Hogben test over the two procedures described above are several: (1) the reaction is an all or none affair, and no experience or skill is required to read it; (2) as mentioned, it rarely gives a false positive; (3) the time required for completion is short; and (4) the toads are much cleaner and easier to keep than either rabbits, rats, or mice. The only objection to the test is that at the present writing the toads are somewhat expensive and occasionally difficult to procure.

Male Frog Test. This test employs the American male frog, *Rana pipiens,* as the test animal and is based on the fact that the injection of a pregnant woman's urine into the lateral lymphatic sinus of the male frog leads to the appearance of spermatozoa in the urine of the latter which can be readily detected microscopically. The technic of the test as described by Wiltberger and Miller is simple and is as follows: A first morning (overnight) specimen of urine is obtained and 5 cc. carefully injected subcutaneously into the dorsal or lateral lymph sac of the frog. Each frog is placed in a separate, clean, dry glass jar with a perforated lid and set aside for two to four hours at room temperature. At the end of this time any urine that has been voided by the frogs is examined microscopically. If spermatozoa are not present, the urine is carefully drained from the jar without disturbing the frog. The frog is then seized in the hand while still in the jar. This pressure usually induces another urination. The new specimen of urine is then examined for spermatozoa. The frog sperms are easily identifiable. When spermatozoa are present, the test is positive; when they are not present, the test is negative. The fact that there are no intergrades eliminates all subjective interpretations. The test animals are not killed and may be used for another test after four or five days.

Although this test has not had the extensive trial which the three procedures described above have had, reports by Wiltberger and Miller on 200 cases and by Robbins and Parker on 122, indicate that it is just as reliable as the older tests. In our own clinic, Job has employed it in 244 cases and found it to be 95.6 per cent accurate and entirely satisfactory in other respects. One of the important advantages of this test is that the male frogs are easily obtainable in the United States and are quite inexpensive. Moreover, positive reactions make themselves known within two to four hours.

Other Diagnostic Tests. Excretion of chorionic gonadotrophin varies widely from individual to individual and from specimen to specimen in the same individual. As pointed out by Foote and Jones, although it roughly parallels the blood serum gonadotrophin, it does not do so exactly. For this reason no pregnancy test based upon urinary excretion of chorionic gonadotrophin approaches in accuracy or sensitivity those based upon the concentration of this hormone in the blood serum. Therefore, in cases which present an especial diagnostic problem and particularly in those in which the quantitative assay of chorionic gonadotrophin is desired as it exists in the body, it is advisable to use a serum technic. One of the most delicate and dependable of these has been described by Delfs and has been employed in our clinic with great satisfaction for a number of years. It is based on the principle that chorionic gonadotrophin, when injected into immature rats, produces, through its ovarian action, an increase in uterine weight proportionate to the amount injected. Although rather time-consuming for routine use as a test for pregnancy, we have found it a welcome addition to our armamentarium whenever certainty and precision are essential.

Presumptive Signs of Pregnancy. The presumptive evidences of pregnancy are afforded in great part by subjective symptoms which may be appreciated by the patient herself. These consist of (1) cessation of the menses, (2) changes in the breasts, (3) morning sickness, (4) quickening, (5) discoloration of the mucous membranes, (6) abnormalities in pigmentation, and (7) disturbances in urination.

1. *Cessation of the Menses.* In a healthy, married woman who has previously menstruated regularly, cessation of menstruation strongly suggests that impregnation has occurred. Not until the date of the expected period has been passed by 10 days or more, however, can any reliance be put on this symptom. But when the expected period has been passed by more than 10 days, the likelihood of pregnancy is indicated. When the second period is also missed, the probability naturally becomes stronger.

Although cessation of menstruation is the earliest and one of the most important symptoms of pregnancy, it should be noted that pregnancy may occur without prior menstruation and that menstruation may occasionally continue after conception. An example of the former circumstance is noted in certain Oriental countries where girls marry at a very early age; here pregnancy frequently occurs before the menstrual periods are established. Again, nursing mothers, who usually do not menstruate during the period of lactation, often conceive at this time; more rarely, women who think they have passed the menopause are startled to find themselves pregnant. Conversely, it is not uncommon for a woman to have one or two periods after conception. But almost without exception, these are brief in duration and scant in amount. In such cases the first period ordinarily lasts two days instead of the usual five, and the next only a few hours. Although there are instances in which women are said to have menstruated every month throughout pregnancy, these are of questionable authenticity and are probably ascribable to some abnormality of the reproductive organs. Indeed, vaginal bleeding at any time during pregnancy should be regarded as abnormal and investigated at once.

Absence of menstruation may result from a number of conditions other than pregnancy. Probably one of the most common causes of delay in the onset of the period is psychic influence, particularly fear of pregnancy. Change of climate, exposure to cold, as well as certain chronic diseases such as anemia, may likewise suppress the menstrual flow.

2. *Changes in the Breasts.* In the section on Maternal Physiology in Pregnancy, reference was made to the changes which occur in the breasts. Generally speaking, these changes are quite characteristic in primigravidae, but are of less value in multiparae, since the breasts of the latter not infrequently contain a small amount of milk or colostrum for months or even for years following the last labor. Occasionally, changes in the breasts similar to those produced by pregnancy may be observed in women suffering with ovarian or uterine tumors. Instances have also been reported of such breast changes occurring in cases of spurious or imaginary pregnancy.

3. *Nausea and Vomiting.* The establishment of pregnancy is frequently manifested by disturbances of the digestive system and even more particularly by nausea and vomiting. The so-called "morning sickness" of pregnancy, as the name implies, usually comes on in the earlier part of the day and passes off in a few hours, although it occasionally persists longer or may occur at other times. It usually appears about the end of the first month and disappears spontaneously six or eight weeks later, although some patients suffer from it for a longer period.

4. *Quickening.* From about the eighteenth to the twentieth week the pregnant woman becomes conscious of slight, fluttering movements in her abdomen, which gradually increase in intensity. These are usually due to movements of the fetus, and their first appearance is designated as "quickening," or the perception of life. Occasionally fetal movements may be perceived as early as the tenth week, while in rare instances they are not experienced at all.

This sign offers only corroborative evidence of pregnancy, and is of no value unless confirmed by the hand of the physician, as in many nervous women similar sensations are experienced in its absence.

5. *Discoloration of the Mucous Membrane of Vagina and Vulva.* Under the influence of pregnancy the mucosa about the vaginal opening and the lower portion of the anterior vaginal wall frequently takes on a dark bluish or purplish, congested ap-

pearance. Attention was first called to this condition by Jacquemier and Kluge, but particular stress was laid upon its significance by Chadwick, of Boston, so that in America it is known as *Chadwick's sign*. Its presence supplies valuable presumptive evidence, but is not conclusive, as it may likewise be observed in any condition leading to intense congestion of the pelvic organs.

6. *Pigmentation of the Skin and Abdominal Striae.* These manifestations, which have already been referred to in the section on the physiology of pregnancy, are often observed in pregnant women, but are not characteristic, as they are sometimes lacking, and, on the other hand, may be associated with tumors of other origin.

7. *Urinary Disturbances.* In the early weeks of pregnancy the enlarging uterus, by exerting pressure on the bladder, may cause a desire for frequent micturition. This continues for the first few months, and gradually passes off as the uterus rises up into the abdomen, to reappear when the head descends into the pelvis a few weeks before term.

Differential Diagnosis of Pregnancy. The pregnant uterus is often mistaken for other tumors occupying the pelvic or abdominal cavities, and vice versa, though, as a rule, the former mistake is more frequently made. The early periods of pregnancy may be simulated by enlargement of the uterus due to interstitial or submucous myomata, sarcoma, hematometra, and conditions resulting from inflammatory disturbances. As a rule, the uterus in these circumstances is harder and firmer than in pregnancy, and does not present its characteristic elastic or boggy consistency. Moreover, except in hematometra, such conditions are not attended by cessation of the menses. If, however, there is any possibility of a mistake, a delay of a few weeks will usually clear up the diagnosis.

The pregnant uterus is occasionally mistaken for a small ovarian or tubal tumor, though this error should rarely occur if the patient be carefully examined bimanually and the pelvic contents palpated, if necessary under an anesthetic. As the tumor becomes larger and rises up into the abdomen, other points become available, for differential diagnosis, notably the positive signs of pregnancy and the intermittent contractions of Braxton Hicks.

The diagnosis of pregnancy in a myomatous uterus often presents serious difficulties, and for a time may be impossible. But a short delay will show a more rapid increase in the size of the tumor than is consistent with the existence of an uncomplicated myoma, and variations in the consistency of its different parts should also serve to direct one's attention to the pregnant condition.

Occasionally, an ovarian cystoma may be complicated by pregnancy. In the early stages the diagnosis, as a rule, can be easily made, as careful bimanual examination should enable one to differentiate between the two tumors; but in the later months it may become extremely difficult and sometimes impossible, owing to the increased distention of the abdomen. Furthermore, if the positive signs cannot be elicited, the existence of pregnancy is usually overlooked and a simple cystoma diagnosticated, whereas, if the heart sounds are heard and the x-ray findings are positive, the cystoma may escape recognition and the excessive abdominal enlargement be attributed to hydramnios.

In the early months, hypertrophy of the supravaginal portion of the cervix may seriously increase the difficulties of diagnosis, as the enlarged cervix may be mistaken for the entire uterus, the soft and elastic body being either overlooked or regarded as a tumor of the uterine appendages. Careful bimanual examination under anesthesia usually does away with the possibility of this error.

Irregular development of the pregnant uterus, associated with a sacculation of its anterior or posterior wall, may seriously complicate the diagnosis, especially if the fetus is dead, as even after the most careful examination, the existence of pregnancy may remain unrecognized and the sacculation be mistaken for an ovarian cyst. This is especially apt to occur when the sacculation occupies the posterior wall, as in such cases the anterior wall may remain practically unchanged, and when, under anesthesia, one can feel the fundus with both tubes extending from it, it is a pardonable error to conclude that the fluctuant tumor lying posterior to it is an ovarian cyst.

Spurious Pregnancy. Imaginary pregnancy, or *pseudocyesis,* is a condition with which almost every practitioner, sooner or later, will meet. It is usually observed in patients nearing the menopause, or in younger women who intensely desire offspring. Such patients may present all the subjective symptoms of pregnancy, associated with a considerable increase in the size of the abdomen, which is due either to an abnormal and rapid deposition of fat or to the existence of tympanites and occasionally of ascites. When it occurs in the earlier years of life the menses do not, as a rule, disappear, but they may present certain abnormalities which the patient may consider are due to her supposed condition.

In many instances the woman may imagine that she detects fetal movements, which are sometimes so violent as to make her fearful that they may be visible to onlookers. Paddock finds that such "movements" are more common among older women and are possibly associated with such disorders as gas in the intestines, excessive fat deposits and tumors.

Changes in the breasts, such as enlargement, the appearance of a secretion, and increased pigmentation, are sometimes observed. These are probably due to endocrine disturbance, involving the ovary, anterior pituitary and possibly the adrenal glands. In a majority of these cases, there is actual "morning sickness," due perhaps to a psychic cause.

Pseudopregnancy has been produced experimentally in lower animals. It is known that the rabbit, the ferret and the cat do not ovulate unless sexually excited and may thus stay in a state of estrus when there are no corpora lutea but only follicles in the ovary. In these animals, pseudopregnancy may be induced by sterile mating with vasectomized males, resulting in corpora lutea formation, changes in the uterine mucosa and mammary gland hypertrophy. Long and Evans have produced similar changes in the rat and mouse by sterile mating. Hisaw states that from the present data one may conclude, for the rabbit at least, that copulation stimulates the anterior pituitary (perhaps nervously) to secrete sufficient hormone to cause ovulation and beginning of lutein development.

The supposed fetal movements usually result from contractions of the intestines or the muscles of the abdominal wall, and occasionally are so marked as to deceive even physicians. Careful examination of the patient usually enables one to arrive at a correct diagnosis without great difficulty, as the small uterus can be demonstrated on bimanual examination, made, if necessary, under anesthesia. The greatest difficulty in these cases is to persuade the patient as to the correctness of the diagnosis. Bichebois has pointed out that insane women frequently suffer from the delusion that they are pregnant, and persist in such a belief for years.

Distinction between First and Subsequent Pregnancies. Occasionally, it is a matter of practical importance to decide whether a patient is pregnant for the first time or has previously borne children. Ordinarily, child-bearing leaves indelible traces behind it, which are readily appreciated, but very exceptionally such signs are lacking. Again, in very rare instances, all the signs indicating a previous labor may follow the delivery of a large tumor through the vagina.

In a pregnant woman who has never borne children the abdomen is usually tense and firm, and the uterus is felt through it only with difficulty. The characteristic old striae and the distinctive changes in the breasts are naturally absent. The labia majora are usually in close apposition, the frenulum is intact, and the hymen torn in several places. The vagina is usually narrow and marked by well-developed rugae. The cervix is softened, but does not usually admit the tip of the finger until the very end of pregnancy, and during the last four to six weeks of pregnancy, the presenting part is usually found engaged in the superior strait, unless some disproportion exists.

In multiparous women, on the other hand, the abdominal walls are usually lax, flabby, and frequently pendulous, and the uterus is readily palpated through them. In addition to the pinkish striae due to the present condition, the silvery cicatrices of past pregnancies may also be noted. The breasts are usually not as firm as in the first pregnancy, and frequently present striae similar to those observed on the abdomen. The vulva is usually more or less gaping, the frenulum has disappeared and the hymen is replaced by the *carunculae myrtiformes*. The external os, even in the early months of pregnancy, usually shows signs of laceration and at a little later period readily admits the tip of the finger which can be carried up to the internal os. Furthermore, in the majority of cases the presenting part does not engage in the superior strait until the onset of labor.

Diagnosis of the Life or Death of the Fetus. Generally speaking, the fetus should be considered to be alive unless definite evidence to the contrary can be adduced. In the early months of pregnancy the diagnosis of fetal death offers considerable difficulty and can be made only after repeated examinations have demonstrated that the uterus has remained stationary in size for a number of weeks. Since the placenta may occasionally live and continue to manufacture chorionic gonadotrophin for as long as four weeks after fetal death, a positive endocrine test for pregnancy is not necessarily an indication that the fetus is alive (Zondek). On the other hand, a negative test points to fetal death, especially if further tests continue negative.

In the later months of pregnancy, the disappearance of fetal movements usually directs the attention of the patient to this possibility. Careful investigation shows that the uterus does not correspond in size with the estimated duration of pregnancy, or even has become smaller than previously, while at the same time retrogressive changes have occurred in the breasts which have become soft and flabby. The diagnosis cannot usually be made at a single examination; it is permissible only after repeated examinations, when in addition to the signs just mentioned one has failed to hear the fetal heart or perceive the movements of the child.

Occasionally, a positive diagnosis can be made at once by palpating the macerated skull through the partially dilated cervix; in this event one feels that the bones of the head are loose and present a sensation as if they were contained in a flabby bag. Spalding showed that a positive diagnosis of fetal death can sometimes be made by the employment of the roentgen ray. In such cases the plate will show overlapping of the bones of the skull at the several sutures, associated with distinct signs of shrinkage of the skull contents.

BIBLIOGRAPHY

ARNOT, Philip H. The Duration of Pregnancy. West. J. Surg., Obst. & Gynec., 1942, 50:115.

ASCHHEIM, S. Die Schwangerschaftsdiagnose aus dem Harn durch Nachweis des Hypophysenvorderlappenhormons, etc. Zentralbl. f. Gynäk., 1929, 53:15.

——— Die Schwangerschaftsdiagnose aus dem Harn. Berlin, 1930, p. 62.

——— and ZONDEK, B. Die Schwangerschaftsdiagnose aus dem Harn durch Nachweis des Hypophysenvorderlappenhormons. Klin. Wchnschr., 1928, 7:1404.

BARTHOLOMEW, R. A., SALE, B. E., and CALLOWAY, J. T. Diagnosis of Pregnancy by the Roentgen Ray. J.A.M.A., 1921, 76:912.

CHADWICK, J. R. Value of the Bluish Coloration of the Vaginal Entrance as a Sign of Pregnancy. Tr. Am. Gynec. Soc., 1886, 11:399.

COWIE. Pregnancy Diagnosis Tests: A Review. Commonwealth Agricultural Bureaux Joint Publication No. 13, 1948.

CREW, F. A. E. Biologic Pregnancy Diagnosis Tests: Comparison of the Rabbit, the Mouse and the "Clawed Toad" (Xenopus Laevis) as the Experimental Animal. Brit. M. J., 1939, 1:766.

DELFS, E. An Assay Method for Human Chorionic Gonadotropin. Endocrinology, 1941, 28:196.

DICKINSON, R. L. The Diagnosis of Pregnancy between the Second and Seventh Weeks by Bimanual Examination. N. York J. Gynaec. & Obst., 1892, 2:544.

DOUGLAS, H. S. Simple Amenorrhea or Pregnancy? Use of Prostigmin in Differentiation and Treatment. West. J. Surg., 1943, 51:245.

ELKAN, E. Xenopus Pregnancy Test. Presse Méd., Paris, 1939, 47:308.

ELWARD, J. F., and BELAIR, J. F. Roentgen Diagnosis of Pregnancy. Radiology, 1938, 31:678.

ENGLE, E. T., in Allen, Danforth and Doisy, Sex and Internal Secretions, 2nd Ed. The Williams & Wilkins Company, Baltimore, 1939.

FOOTE, E. C., and JONES, G. E. S. An Evaluation of the Hogben Pregnancy Test. Am. J. Obst. & Gynec., 1946, 51:672.

FRENCH, H. C. A Modification of the Visscher-Bowman Pregnancy Test, with a Report on 513 Observations. Am. J. Obst. & Gynec., 1937, 33:854.

FRIEDMAN, M. H. Mechanism of Ovulation in the Rabbit. II. Ovulation Produced by the Injection of Urine from Pregnant Women. Am. J. Physiol., 1929, 90:617.

GOODYER, Allan V. N., GEIGER, Arthur J., and MONROE, Willys M. Clinical Fetal Electrocardiography. Yale J. Biol. & Med., 1942, 15:1.

GREENHILL, J. P. Editorial note, in Year Book of Obstetrics and Gynecology. The Year Book Publishers, Chicago, 1948, p. 27.

HAINES, M. The Male Toad Test for Pregnancy. Lancet, 1948, 2:923.

HICKS, J. B. On the Contraction of the Uterus throughout Pregnancy. Tr. Obst. Soc., London, 1872, 13:216.

HISAW, F. L., in Allen, Danforth and Doisy, Sex and Internal Secretions, 2nd Ed. The Williams & Wilkins Company, Baltimore, 1939.

HOTELLING, H., and HOTELLING, F. A New Analysis of Duration of Pregnancy Data. Am. J. Obst. & Gynec., 1932, 23:643.

HURWITT, E., ABRAMSON, D., and LESNICK, G. Relaxin in Human Serum as a Test of Pregnancy. Surg., Gynec., & Obst., 1937, 65:335.

JOB, B. K. Unpublished Data.

KIKUGAWA, M. The Influence of the Urine of Pregnant Women on Sweet Water Fish. Ztschr. f. Geburtsh. u. Gynäk., 1938, 116:103.

LANDGREBE, F. W., and SAMSON, L. The Hogben Pregnancy Test with a Note on the Breeding of Xenopus for the Test. J. Obst. & Gynaec. Brit. Emp., 1944, 51:133.

LONG, J. A., and EVANS, H. M. The Oestrous Cycle in the Rat and Its Associated Phenomena. Memoirs Univ. Calif., 1922, 6:1.

LÖWENHARDT, P. Die Berechnung und die Dauer der Schwangerschaft. Arch. f. Gynaek., 1872, 3:456.

MAININI. Diagnostic Test for Pregnancy Utilizing the Male Frog as the Reactive Animal. Sem. Med. 1947, 54:337.

MAZER, C., and HOFFMAN, J. Three Hormone Tests for Early Pregnancy; Their Clinical Evaluation: Comparative Study. J.A.M.A., 1931, 96:19.

MONTGOMERY, W. F. H. An Exposition of the Signs and Symptoms of Pregnancy, 2nd Ed. London, 1863.

PADDOCK, R. Spurious Pregnancy. Am. J. Obst. & Gynec., 1928, 16:845.

PETERSON, R. Value of Pneumo-peritoneal Roentgenography in Obstetrics and Gynecology. J.A.M.A., 1922, 78:397.

RATHBUN, L. S. Analysis of 250 Cases of Postmaturity. Am. J. Obst. & Gynec., 1943, 46:278.

ROBBINS, S. L., and PARKER, F., JR. The Rana Pipiens Test for Pregnancy. Endocrinol., 1948, 42:237.

SIEGEL, P. W. Beitrag zur menschlichen Schwangerschaftsdauer. Zentralbl. f. Gynäk., Leipzig, 1921, 45:984.

SPALDING, A. B. A Pathognomonic Sign of Intra-uterine Death. Surg., Gynec. & Obst., 1922, 34:754.

STRASSMAN, E. O. Development of Fetal Electrocardiography. Tri-State Med. J., 1943, 15:2880.

WAHL, F. A. Are Children Larger and Does Pregnancy Last Longer than Formerly? Deutsche med. Wchnschr., 1937, 63:769.

WEISMAN, A. I., and COATES, C. W. A New Experimental Laboratory Animal, the South African Clawed Frog (Xenopus Laevis); Its Use in Pregnancy Diagnoses, Hormone Assays, and Endocrine Evaluation. Bull. N. Y. Acad. Med., 1943, 19:660.

——— The Frog Test (Xenopus Laevis) for Pregnancy. A Report of One Thousand Tests Over a Period of Four Years of Study. West. J. Surg., 1944, 52:171.

WILTBERGER and MILLER. The Rana Pipiens Test for Pregnancy. Science, 1948, 107:198.

ZONDEK, B. Zur Methodik der Schwangerschaftsreaktion aus dem Harn durch Nachweis des Hypophysenvorderlappenhormons; Fällungsschnelbreaktion; Entgiftung des Harns. Verbesserung der Schwangerschaftsreaktion. Klin. Wchnschr., 1930, 9:964.

——— and ASCHHEIM, S. Das Hormon des Hypophysenvorderlappens. Klin. Wchnschr., 1927, 6:248.

10

THE NORMAL PELVIS

As the mechanism of labor is essentially a process of accommodation between the fetus and the bony passage through which it must pass, it is apparent that the size and shape of the pelvis is of transcendent importance in obstetrics. In both sexes the pelvis forms the bony ring through which the body weight is transmitted to the lower extremities, but in the female it assumes a special form which adapts it to the purposes of childbearing.

It is composed of four bones: the sacrum, the coccyx, and two innominate bones, the last two being united by strong articulations with the sacrum at the sacro-iliac synchondroses, and with one another at the symphysis pubis. The purely anatomical characteristics of the pelvis are dealt with at length in the standard works on anatomy, so that we shall limit our considerations to the peculiarities of the female pelvis which are of importance in childbearing.

PELVIC ANATOMY FROM AN OBSTETRICAL POINT OF VIEW

General Considerations. The linea terminalis forms the boundary between the false and the true pelvis, the former lying above and the latter below it. The *false pelvis* is bounded posteriorly by the lumbar vertebrae and laterally by the iliac fossae, while in front the boundary is formed by the lower portion of the anterior abdominal wall. It possesses no particular obstetrical significance, but serves to support the intestines in the nonpregnant woman, and the enlarged uterus in the pregnant condition. It varies considerably in size in different individuals, according to the flare of the iliac bones; but ordinarily in dried specimens the distances between the anterior superior spines of the ilium and between the most widely separated portions of the iliac crests measure 23 and 26 cm., respectively.

The *true pelvis* lies beneath the linea terminalis and is the portion concerned in childbearing. It is bounded above by the promontory and alae of the sacrum, the linea terminalis, and the upper margins of the pubic bones, and below by the pelvic outlet. Its cavity, roughly speaking, may be compared to an obliquely truncated cylinder with its greatest height posteriorly, since its anterior wall at the symphysis pubis measures 4.5 to 5 cm., and its posterior wall 10 cm. With the woman in the upright position, the upper portion of the pelvic canal is directed downward and backward, while in its lower course it curves and becomes directed downward and forward.

The walls of the true pelvis are partly bony and partly ligamentous. Its posterior boundary is furnished by the anterior surface of the sacrum; its lateral limits are formed by the inner surface of the ischial bones and by the sacrosciatic notches and ligaments, while in front it is bounded by the obturator foramina, the pubic bones, and the ascending rami of the ischial bones.

If the planes of the ischial bones were extended downward they would meet somewhere about the region of the knee. Extending from the middle of the posterior margin of each ischium are the ischial spines which are of great obstetrical importance, inasmuch as a line drawn between them represents the shortest diameter of the pelvic cavity. Moreover, since they can be readily felt on vaginal or rectal examination, they serve as valuable landmarks in determining the extent to which the presenting part has descended into the pelvis.

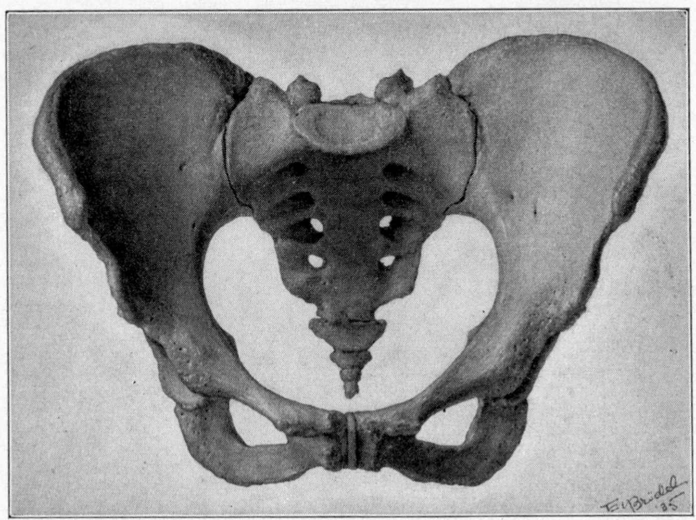

Fig. 168.—Normal Female Pelvis. × ⅓.

The sacrum forms the posterior wall of the pelvic cavity. Its upper anterior margin, corresponding to the body of the first sacral vertebra and designated as the promontory, can be felt on vaginal examination and offers a landmark which serves as the basis of internal pelvimetry. Normally, the sacrum presents a marked vertical and a less pronounced lateral concavity, which, in abnormal pelves, may undergo important variations. A straight line drawn from the promontory to the tip of the sacrum usually measures 10 cm., whereas if the concavity be followed the distance averages 12 cm.

In the female the pubic arch presents a characteristic appearance. The descending rami of the pubic bones unite at an angle of 90 to 100 degrees and form a rounded arch through which the head can readily pass. Its margins are more delicate than in the male, and are considerably everted.

Planes and Diameters of the Pelvis. Owing to the peculiar shape of the pelvic cavity and the difficulty experienced in rendering clear the exact location of a body occupying it, for greater convenience in description it is customary to construct certain imaginary planes through it. Those most frequently employed are designated as (1) the superior strait, (2) the inferior strait, (3) the plane of greatest, and (4) the plane of least, pelvic dimensions (Figs. 169 and 171).

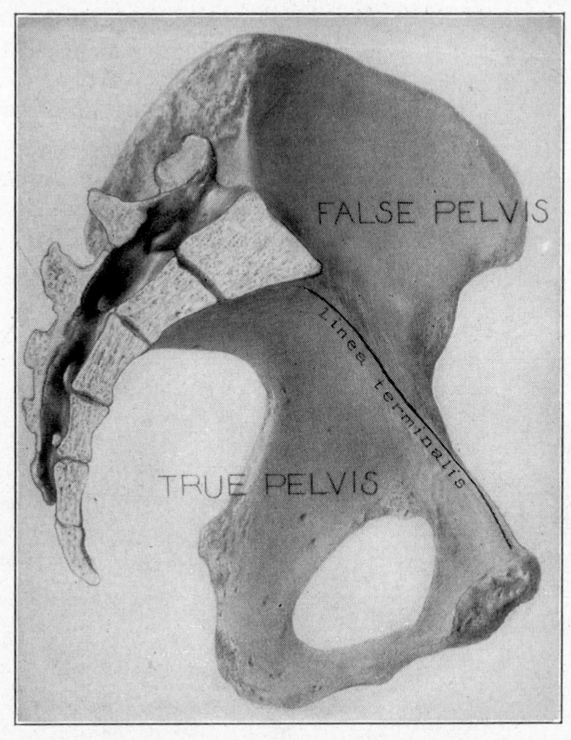

FIG. 169.—SAGITTAL SECTION OF PELVIS, SHOWING FALSE AND TRUE PELVIS.

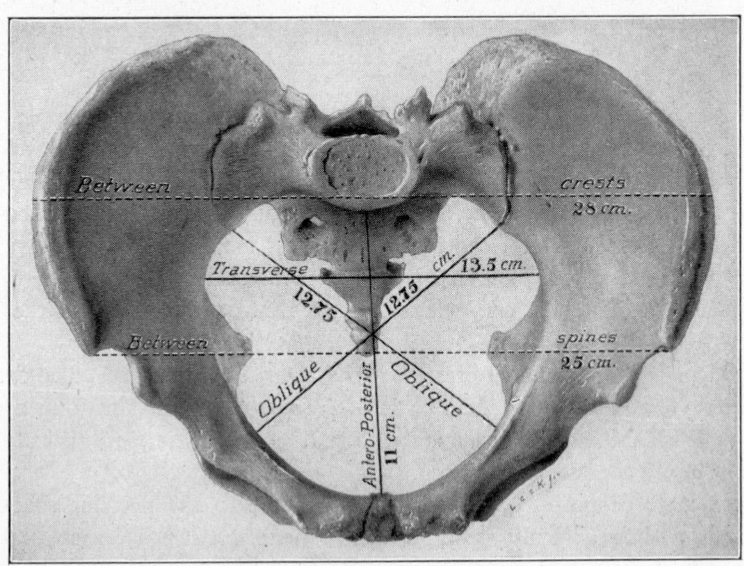

FIG. 170.—NORMAL FEMALE PELVIS SHOWING DIAMETERS OF THE SUPERIOR STRAIT. × ⅓.

The superior strait represents the upper boundary of the true pelvis, and is frequently spoken of as the pelvic inlet. In the past it has been regarded as somewhat oval in shape, with a depression on its posterior border corresponding to the promontory of the sacrum. Thoms, however, found that the oval type occurred in only 34 per cent of a series of 800 white women, while the round type is more frequently encountered, its incidence being 45.8 per cent. Caldwell and Moloy have likewise described the typical female or "gynecoid" pelvis as one in which the inlet is more rounded than oval or heart-shaped. Their incidence of 50.6 per cent for the round or gynecoid pelvis compares closely with the above figure of Thoms. From these investigations, based upon roentgenological studies of large series of cases, we must conclude that the typical female pelvis, as representing the predominant type observed in women, has a superior strait which is more nearly round than oval in shape. Thoms has described "round inlet" as one in which the transverse is equal to, or slightly greater (not more than 1 cm.) than, the anteroposterior diameter.

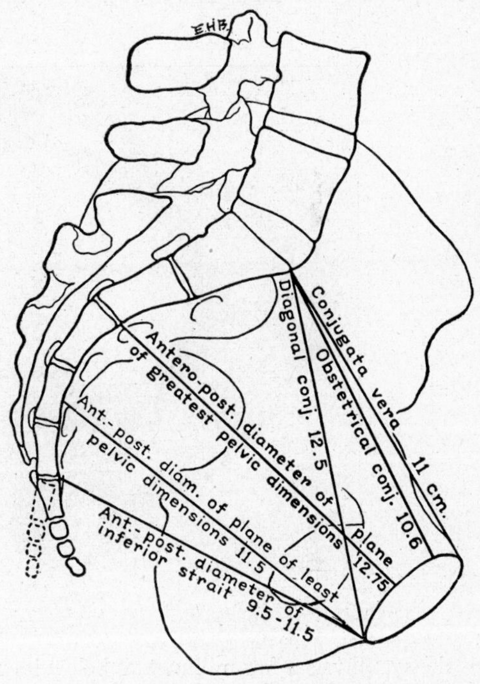

FIG. 171.—DIAGRAM SHOWING VARIOUS PELVIC PLANES AND DIAMETERS.

The superior strait is bounded posteriorly by the promontory and alae of the sacrum, laterally by the linea terminalis, and anteriorly by the horizontal rami of the pubic bones and the upper margin of the symphysis pubis. Strictly speaking, it is not a mathematical plane, since its lateral margins, as represented by the linea terminalis, are at a lower level than its central portion between the promontory and the upper border of the symphysis, as is clearly seen in the sagittal section through a normal pelvis (Fig. 169).

Four diameters are usually described as traversing the superior strait: the anteroposterior, the transverse, and two oblique diameters. The anteroposterior diameter extends from the middle of the promontory of the sacrum to the upper margin of the symphysis pubis, and is designated as the *conjugata vera* or *true conjugate*. This term was first employed by Roederer, who likened the superior strait to an ellipse whose shorter diameter ran anteroposteriorly. Normally the conjugata vera measures 11 cm. or more, but it may become markedly shortened in abnormal pelves. From a practical point of view it is the most important diameter, inasmuch as, in actual practice, it is the point of departure for all attempts to estimate the size of the pelvis. The transverse diameter is constructed at right angles to the conjugata vera and represents the greatest distance between the linea terminalis on either side; it usually intersects the conjugata vera at a point about 5 cm. in front of the promontory.

In the oval or brachypellic type of pelvis it measures about 13 cm., Thoms' average being 12.67 cm., while in the round or mesatipellic type it is somewhat shorter. Each of the oblique diameters extends from one of the sacro-iliac synchondroses to the iliopectineal eminence on the opposite side of the pelvis. They measure 12.75 cm., and are designated as right and left, respectively, according as the starting-point is the right or left sacro-iliac synchondrosis.

The anteroposterior diameter of the superior strait, or conjugata vera, does not represent the shortest distance between the promontory of the sacrum and symphysis pubis, which is along a line drawn from the former to a point on the inner surface

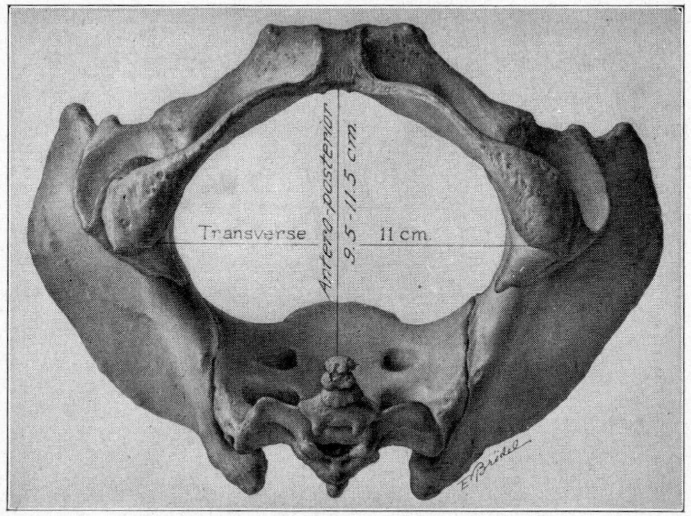

Fig. 172.—Pelvic Outlet. × 1/3

of the symphysis a few millimeters below its upper margin. The latter line is the shortest diameter through which the head must pass in descending into the superior strait, and was designated by Michaelis as the *obstetrical conjugate*. It is a few millimeters shorter than the anatomical or true conjugate, but for practical purposes the distinction is rarely made, except in x-ray pelvimetry.

Unfortunately, in the living woman, the conjugata vera cannot be measured directly with the examining finger, and various more or less complicated instruments have been devised for its determination, none of which gives perfectly satisfactory results. For clinical purposes, therefore, we are content to estimate its length indirectly, by measuring the distance from the lower margin of the symphysis to the promontory of the sacrum and subtracting from the result 1.5 to 2 cm., according to the height and inclination of the symphysis pubis. This diameter is the *conjugata diagonalis,* the importance of which was first emphasized by Smellie.

The outlet of the pelvis is designated as the inferior strait. It is not a plane in a mathematical sense, but consists of two triangular planes whose bases would meet on a line drawn between the two ischial tuberosities. It is bounded posteriorly by the tip of the coccyx, laterally by the greater sacrosciatic ligaments and the ischial tuberosities, and anteriorly by the lower margin of the pubic arch (Fig. 172). For the pelvic outlet two diameters are described: the anteroposterior and the transverse. The former extends from the lower margin of the symphysis pubis to the tip of the sacrum, and the latter between the inner margins of the ischial tuberosities. The anteroposterior diameter measures 11.5 cm., while the transverse diameter measures 10.0 to 11 cm.

The plane of greatest pelvic dimensions, as its name implies, represents the roomiest portion of the pelvic cavity. It extends from the middle of the posterior surface of the symphysis pubis to the junction of the second and third sacral vertebrae, and laterally passes through the ischial bones over the middle of the acetabulum. Its anteroposterior and transverse diameters measure 12.75 and 12.5 cm., respectively. Since its oblique diameters terminate in the obturator foramina and the sacrosciatic notches, their length is indeterminate.

The plane of least pelvic dimensions extends through the lower margin of the symphysis pubis and the ischial spines. Its anteroposterior diameter measures 11.5 cm. Its transverse diameter extends between the ischial spines and measures 10.5 cm., being the shortest diameter in the normal pelvic cavity.

In order to facilitate the study of the pelvic cavity, Hodge constructed four parallel planes, the first of which is the superior strait, while the other three are parallel to it and pass through the lower margin of the symphysis pubis, the ischial spines, and the tip of the coccyx, respectively. Caldwell and Moloy divided the pelvis into the upper pelvis (inlet), the midpelvis (level of the ischial spines), the lower posterior pelvis (the space above the sacrococcygeal platform) and the lower anterior pelvis (outlet) and pointed out that these levels, parallel to the inlet, are somewhat similar to the four parallel planes of Hodge. On the other hand, Thoms has defined the midpelvic plane as the plane which passes through the lower border of the symphysis, the ischial spines, and intersects the lower region of the sacrum. This area, the plane of the least pelvic dimensions, is of great practical importance in some pelves.

Pelvic Inclination. The normal position of the pelvis, with the woman in the erect position, can be reproduced by holding the specimen in such a way that the incisions of the acetabula look directly downward. The same result is obtained when the anterior superior spines of the ilium and the pubic spines are placed in the same vertical plane. Under these conditions the promontory of the sacrum is 9.5 to 10 cm. higher than the upper margin of the symphysis pubis.

By the term *pelvic inclination* is understood the angle which the plane of the superior strait forms with the horizon (see Fig. 169). With the woman in the upright position, the pelvic inclination is usually about 55 degrees. Except when markedly abnormal, the pelvic inclination possesses no practical obstetrical significance and is of value only in the study of atypical pelves and in anthropology.

Much more important, however, is the angle which is formed between the posterior surface of the symphysis pubis and the conjugata vera. This is usually estimated at 90 to 100 degrees, but varies considerably according to the shape, height, and inclination of the symphysis. This must always be taken into consideration in estimating the length of the conjugata vera from that of the conjugata diagonalis, since it is evident that the amount to be subtracted from the diagonal conjugate will vary with the size of the angle in question.

The Pelvic Axis. At the end of pregnancy the axis of the superior strait, if extended directly upward, would pass through the abdominal wall at about the region of the umbilicus, while the axis of the inferior strait would impinge upon the promontory of the sacrum. As the pelvic canal is practically cylindrical in shape down to the plane of greatest pelvic dimensions, it is apparent that the head must descend along the downward prolongation of the axis of the superior strait until it has nearly reached the level of the ischial spines, and only begins to curve forward in the region of the inferior strait. Therefore, the obstetrical pelvic axis should be represented as straight in its upper and curved only in its lower portion (see Fig. 173).

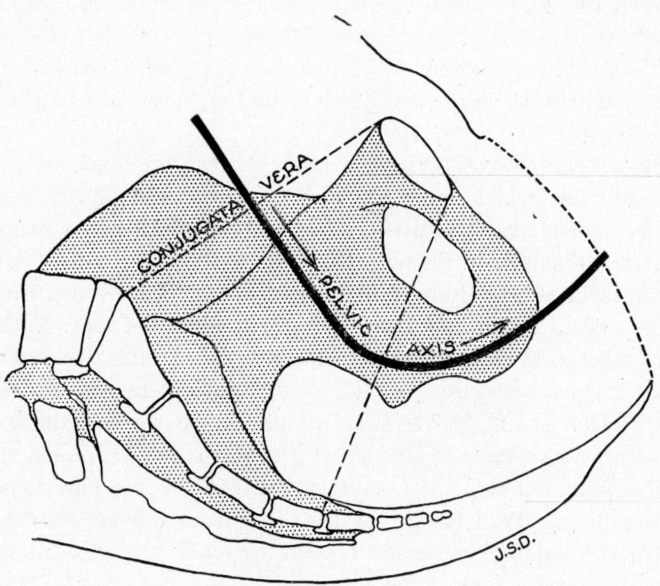

FIG. 173.—DIAGRAM SHOWING THE PELVIC AXIS. × ⅓.

The Pelvic Joints. Anteriorly, the pelvic bones are held together by the symphysis pubis, which consists of a mass of fibrocartilage, and by the superior and inferior pubic ligaments, the latter being frequently designated as the ligamentum arcuatum pubis. The symphysis admits of a certain amount of mobility, which becomes more marked during pregnancy, particularly in multiparous women. This fact was demonstrated by Budin, who showed that if the finger were inserted into the vagina of a pregnant woman, and she were made to walk, one could distinctly feel the ends of the pubic bones move up and down with each step. Likewise, the articulations between the sacrum and innominate bones possess a certain amount of mobility.

Relaxation of the pelvic joints is a normal accompaniment of pregnancy and is probably the result of hormonal activity, as stated in a previous section dealing with the hormones during pregnancy. Abramson, Roberts and Wilson observed relaxation of the symphysis pubis in the human, beginning in the first half of pregnancy and increasing during the last three months. These authors noted that retrogression begins immediately following parturition, being complete within three to five months. The roentgen-ray studies of Roberts confirm these observations and show that the symphysis pubis increases in width during pregnancy, being more in multiparae than in primigravidae, and returning to normal soon after delivery, no further appreciable widening occurring during parturition.

Because of the elasticity which the pelvic joints exhibit in pregnancy, it used to be thought that positioning the patient in extreme hyperextension increased the obstetrical conjugate. To obtain this objective the patient was placed on her back with her buttocks extending slightly over the edge of the delivery table and with her legs hanging down by their own weight,—the so-called "Walcher position." The x-ray studies of Young, and of Brill and Danelius, show clearly that this old concept is erroneous and that no appreciable increase in pelvic size results from the Walcher position. This posture is very distressing to the patient, besides being futile, and is no longer employed.

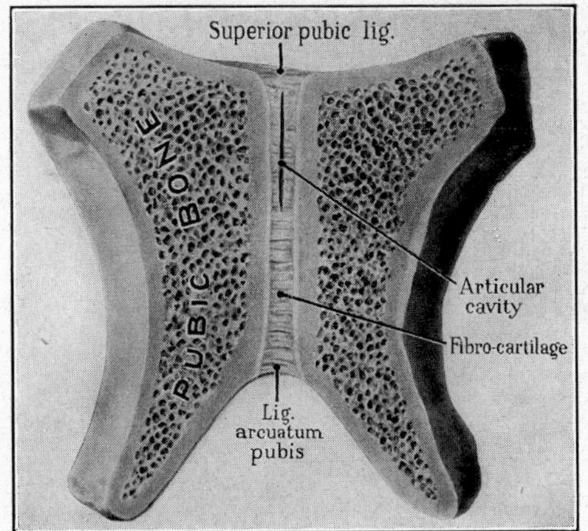

FIG. 174.—FRONTAL SECTION SYMPHYSIS PUBIS (Spalteholz). × 1.

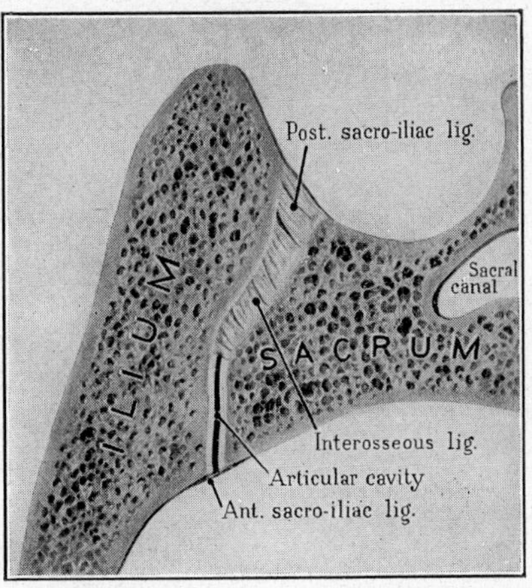

FIG. 175.—SACRO-ILIAC SYNCHONDROSIS (Spalteholz). × 1.

Sexual Differences in the Adult Pelvis. The pelvis presents marked sexual differences. Speaking generally, we may say that in the male the pelvis is heavier, higher, less graceful, and presents a more conical appearance than in the female. In the male the muscular attachments are much more strongly marked, and the iliac bones are less flared than in the female. The pubic arch is more angular in shape, and presents an aperture of 70 to 75 degrees, as compared to 90 to 100 degrees in the female. This difference is so marked that one usually speaks of the pubic angle in the male and the pubic arch in the female. In the male pelvis the superior strait is smaller and more triangular in outline, while the pelvic cavity is deeper and more conical in shape; the sacrosciatic notch is narrower and the distance between the lower border of the sacrum and the ischial spine smaller than in the female pelvis. These differences are readily noted in Figs. 176 to 178 and may be especially emphasized by a comparison of the various measurements in the two sexes.

Broadly speaking, the external measurements are practically alike in both sexes, though the distance between the anterior superior spines of the ilium is somewhat less in the male, while all the diameters of the pelvic cavity are shorter. Indeed, the outlet of the male type of pelvis is contracted to such a degree as to render difficult the passage of a living child under the pubic angle. Occasionally the female pelvis may approach the male type, and such funnel pelves may offer insuperable obstacles to the birth of the child and necessitate radical operative procedures to effect delivery.

Numerous, although not very satisfactory, attempts have been made to explain the cause of the differences between the male and female pelvis. According to Fehling and others, sexual differences make their appearance as early as the fourth or fifth month of intra-uterine life, so that the sex can be ascertained long before term by examination of the pelvis. On the other hand, Morton in a recent study of 27 fetal pelves of various ages was unable to note any significant sexual differences.

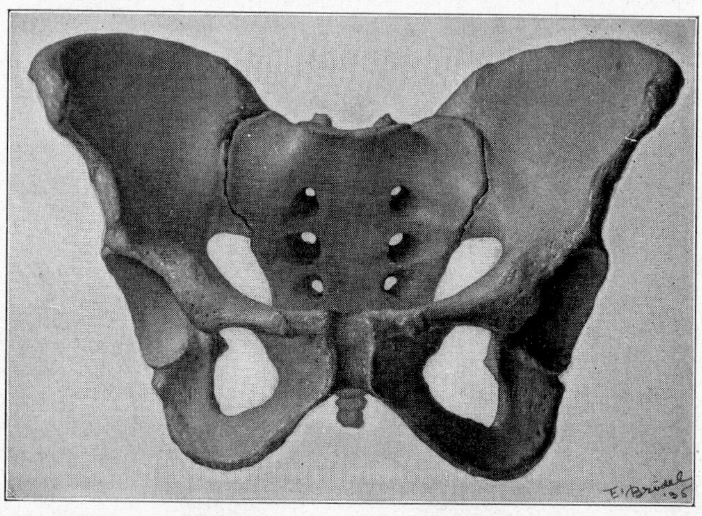

FIG. 176.—FRONT VIEW FEMALE PELVIS. × ⅓.

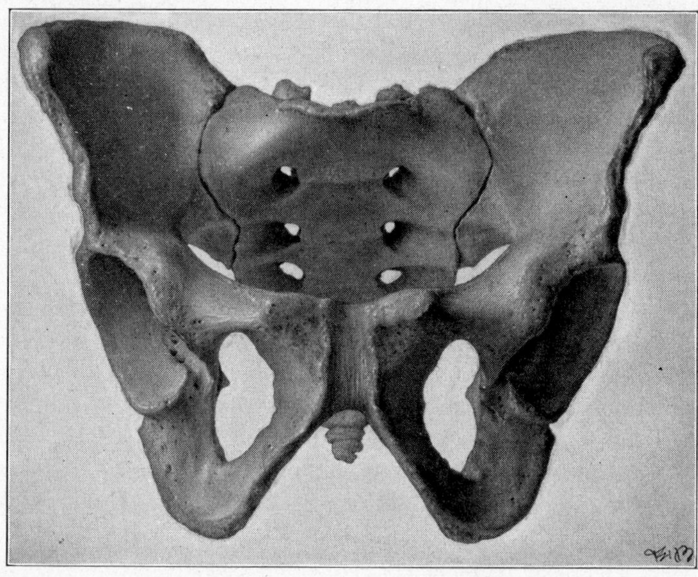

FIG. 177.—FRONT VIEW MALE PELVIS. × ⅓.

Pelvis of the Newborn Child. The mechanism by which the pelvis of the fetus is converted into the adult form is of interest, not only from a scientific, but also from a practical point of view, as it affords important information concerning the mode of production of certain varieties of deformed pelves.

The pelvis of the child at birth is partly bony and partly cartilaginous. The innominate bone does not exist as such, its place being taken by the ilium, ischium, and pubis, which are united by a large Y-shaped cartilage, the three bones meeting in the acetabulum. The iliac crests and the acetabula, as well as the greater part of the ischiopubic rami, are entirely cartilaginous in structure.

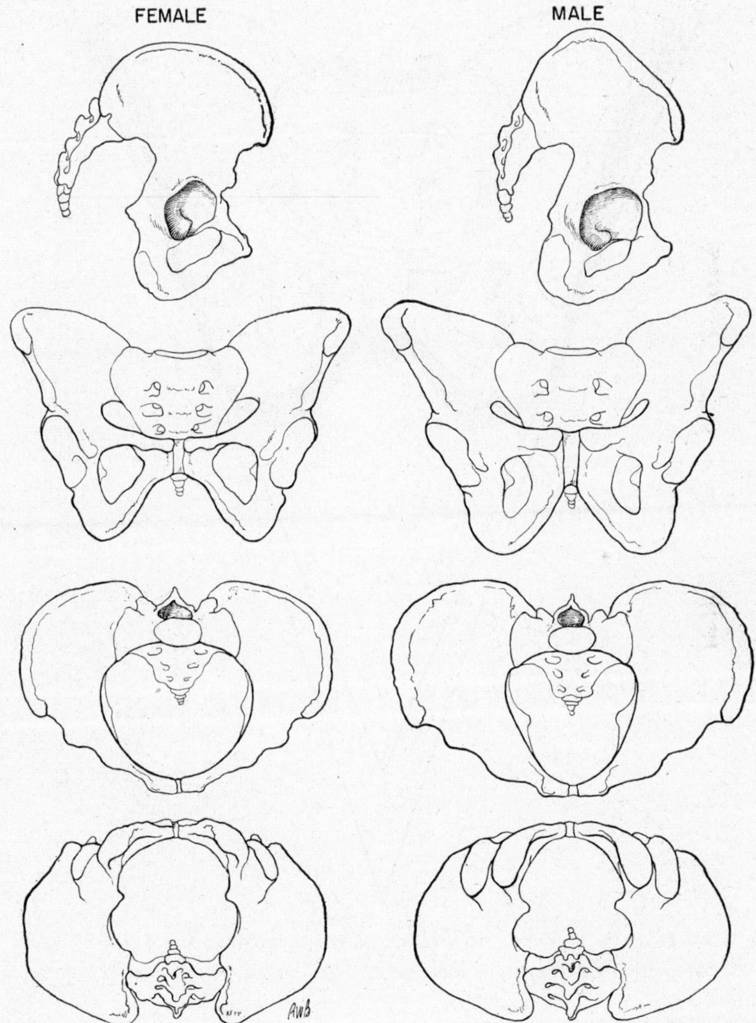

Fig. 178.—Lateral, Anterior, Superior and Inferior Views of Female and Male Pelvis, Respectively.

The cartilaginous portions of the pelvis gradually give place to bone, but complete union in the neighborhood of the acetabulum does not occur until about the age of puberty, and occasionally even at a later period. Indeed, we may say that the innominate bones do not become completely ossified and fully developed until between the twentieth and twenty-fifth years.

Each innominate bone is developed from 12 centers of ossification. Three of these are primary and give rise to the ilium, ischium, and pubis. According to Adair, they appear in the order named and are all present by the nineteenth week of pregnancy. The remaining nine centers—the so-called epiphyseal centers—are secondary, and do not develop until a considerably later period, some of them not until after the age of puberty.

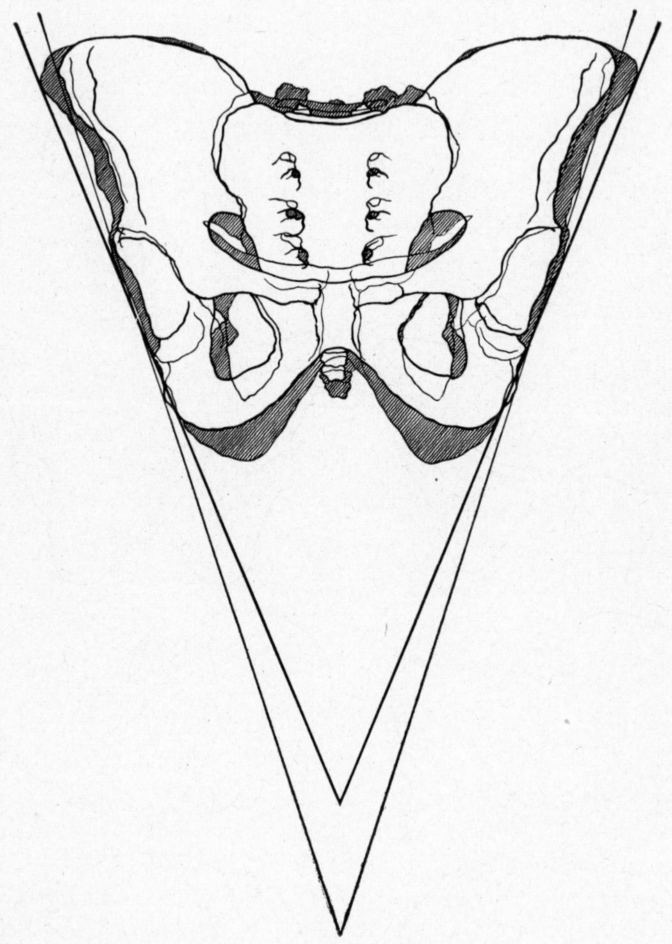

Fig. 179.—Diagram Showing Difference in Shape of Male and Female Pelves. The shaded portion represents the male pelvis; the outline portion, the female pelvis.

The sacrum at birth is likewise partly bony and partly cartilaginous. It is made up of 21 distinct bones, each of which is derived from a single center of ossification. The 21 centers are arranged as follows: one for each vertebral body (five), three for the alae on either side (six), and two for the arches of each vertebra (10). To these must be added the various epiphyseal centers which appear later. The cartilage gradually becomes ossified, and the various component parts of the sacrum fuse together. The alae are the first portions to become united, after which the vertebral bodies gradually become welded together, the fusion extending from below upward. According to Litzmann, the bodies of the sacral vertebrae are not entirely united until the seventh year, and complete ossification of the sacrum is not effected until the twenty-fifth year. Figure 180 represents the disarticulated pelvis of a child three years old, and clearly shows the extent to which ossification has progressed at that age.

The pelvis of the newborn child differs from that of the adult not only in being made up of a large number of bones, which are united by cartilage, but more particularly in its characteristic shape. In the newborn child, the vertebral column is almost vertical, and its lumbar curvature practically absent. The promontory is very slightly marked, and is situated at a much higher level than in the adult. The sacrum is almost straight from above downward, but presents a more marked transverse concavity

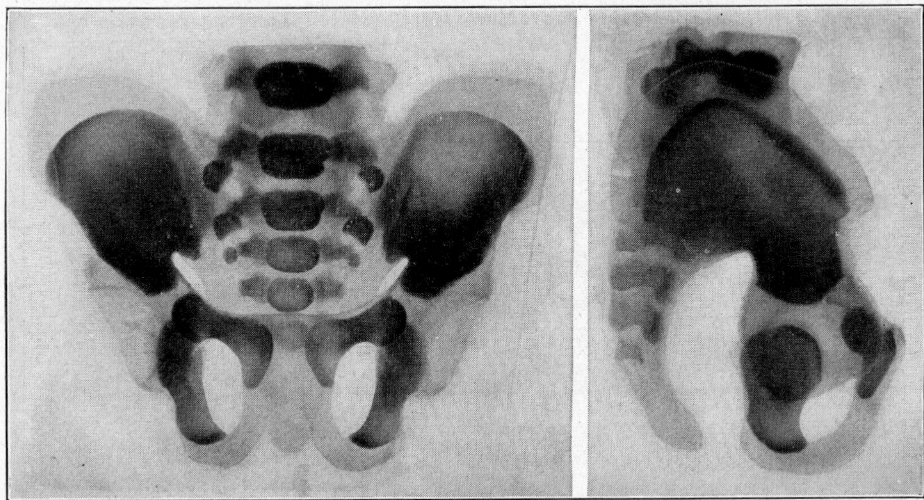

Fig. 180.—Fetal Pelvis Near Term.
Frontal and lateral views showing extent of ossification.

than in the adult. Its alae are only slightly developed, and as a consequence the pelvis is relatively narrower. The iliac fossae are almost vertical, and the horizontal rami of the pubis are far shorter than in the adult. The pubic arch is much more angular, while the pelvic inclination is decidedly greater. The superior strait is narrower and more angular in shape, the relation between the conjugata vera and the transverse diameter being 100 to 105, instead of 100 to 122.5 as in the adult. The cavity of the pelvis is relatively much smaller, and is distinctly funnel-shaped. The antero-posterior and transverse diameters of the pelvic outlet, when expressed in terms of the conjugata vera, are respectively 93 and 73, instead of 104.5 and 100 as in the adult.

Transformation of Fetal into Adult Pelvis. At present it is generally believed that in the evolution of the form of the pelvis two sets of factors—developmental and inherent tendencies, and mechanical influences—are concerned. That the process is not entirely the result of the action of mechanical forces is manifested by the existence of sexual and racial differences in the adult pelvis. On the other hand, the mechanical influences which come into play after birth are identical in both sexes, but despite this fact the sexual differences become established as puberty is approached.

The part played by developmental and hereditary influences was clearly demonstrated by Litzmann, who showed that the female sacrum is characterized by a marked increase in width as compared with that of the male. At birth, in both sexes, the body of the first sacral vertebra is twice as broad as the alae (100 to 50), but in the adult the relation becomes 100 to 76 in the female, and 100 to 56 in the male, indicating a much more rapid growth of the alae in the female. Falk, in 1908, held that all the changes in the developing pelvis are due to similar causes, and that the influence of the various mechanical factors is merely accessory. The growth and development of that portion of the ilium forming the upper boundary of the great sacrosciatic notch, as shown later, profoundly effects the shape and size of the pelvic inlet.

Three mechanical forces take part in bringing about the final shape of the pelvis: the body weight, the upward and inward pressure exerted by the heads of the femora, and the cohesive force exerted by the symphysis pubis. So long as the child remains constantly in the recumbent position these forces are in abeyance, but as soon as it sits

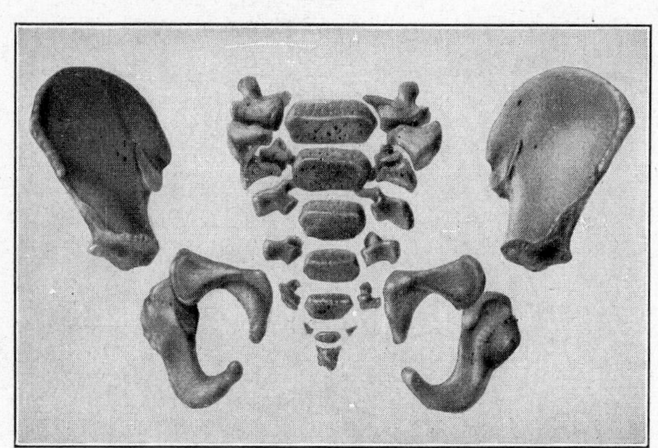

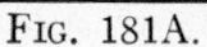

Fig. 181A.

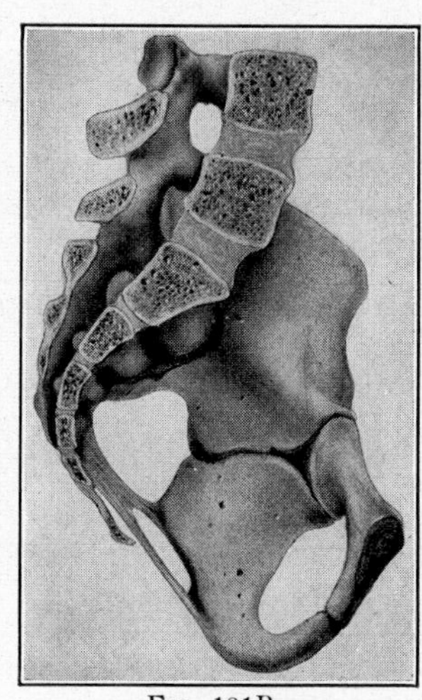

Fig. 181B.

Fig. 181A.—Disarticulated Pelvis of Three-year-old Girl. × ¼.

Fig. 181B.—Sagittal Section through Pelvis of Five-year-old Girl. × ¼.

up or walks the body weight is transmitted through the vertebral column to the sacrum, and, as the center of gravity is anterior to its promontory, the force transmitted is resolved into two components, one of which is directed downward and the other forward. Accordingly, the two together tend to force the promontory of the sacrum downward and forward toward the symphysis pubis, a process which can only be accomplished by the sacrum rotating about its transverse axis so that its tip tends to become displaced both upward and backward. This displacement, however, is resisted by the strong sacrosciatic ligaments, which therefore permit of only slight extension, with the result that the partly cartilaginous sacrum becomes bent upon itself just in front of its axis—*i.e.*, about the middle of its third vertebrae—so that its anterior surface becomes markedly concave from above downward, instead of flat as it was previously. At the same time, the body weight forces the bodies of the sacral vertebrae forward, so that they project slightly beyond the alae, thereby diminishing the transverse concavity of the sacrum.

As the anterior surface of the sacrum is wider than its posterior, the bone tends to sink down into the pelvic cavity under the influence of the body weight, and would prolapse completely into it were it not held in place by the strong posterior iliosacral ligaments, which suspend it, so to speak, from the posterior superior spines of the ilium. Accordingly, as the sacrum is pushed downward into the pelvic cavity it exerts traction upon these ligaments, which in turn drag the posterior superior spines inward toward the middle line, and consequently tend to rotate the anterior portions of the innominate bones outward. Excessive outward rotation is prevented, however, by the cohesive force exerted at the symphysis, but particularly by the upward and inward pressure exerted by the heads of the femurs. Practically, then, the iliac bone becomes converted into a two-armed lever, with the articular surface of the sacrum as a fulcrum; as a consequence, it bends at its point of least resistance, which is just anterior to the articulation, and thus gives the pelvis a greater transverse and a lesser anteroposterior diameter. At the same time, it must be remembered that a considerable part of the transverse widening is more apparent than real, and is due to the relative shortening of the conjugata vera by the downward and forward displacement of the promontory of the sacrum.

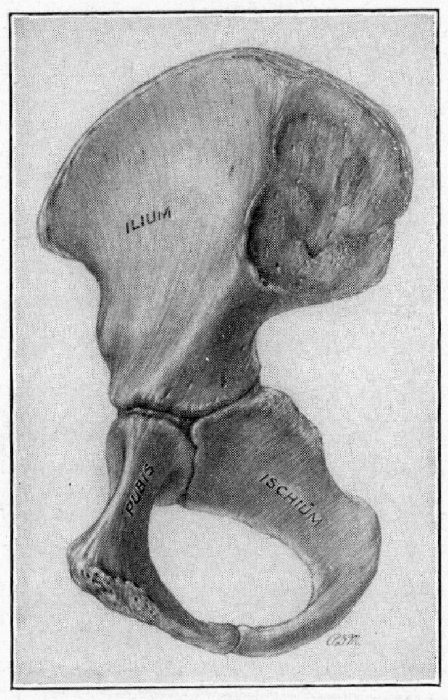

Fig. 182.—Innominate Bone in Three-year-old Child Showing Its Component Parts.

It is apparent that the forces just mentioned must act in identically the same manner in the two sexes, so that, while they may serve to explain many points in the transformation of the fetal into the adult pelvis, they fail to give a satisfactory explanation of its sexual differences, which probably are due to the sex hormones as well as to hereditary and other factors.

Breus and Kolisko insist that too great stress has been laid upon the action of mechanical forces in the production of the ultimate shape of the pelvis, and hold that the relative flattening of the superior strait is due not so much to the downward and forward displacement of the base of the sacrum as to the unequal rate of growth before puberty of the sacrum and the several component parts of the innominate bones. In making this contention, they lay great stress upon the so-called terminal length of the latter. This includes not only the linea terminalis, but also its imaginary continuation which extends from the ventral margin of the sacro-iliac articulation to the iliac crest just above the superior posterior spine. In the normal adult pelvis, the terminal length measures from 19.5 to 21 cm., and is divided into three parts—the sacral, iliac, and pubic portions. The first extends from the posterior margin of the iliac crest to the ventral margin of the articular surface, the second from the latter to the line upon the linea terminalis which indicates the union of the iliac and pubic bones, and the third from that point to the anterior end of the pubic bone. These portions measure 6.5 to 7, 6 to 6.5, and 7 to 7.5 cm., respectively, and therefore are of practically equal length. During the period of development, the sacral portion grows from the cartilage covering the iliac crest, the iliac portion from the upper limb of the Y-shaped cartilage of the acetabulum, and the pubic portion from the latter as well as from the symphyseal cartilage.

Up to the seventh or eighth year the sacrum increases steadily in width, and then ceases to grow until just before puberty, when it rapidly attains its full development. During the earlier period the superior strait grows relatively more rapidly in its transverse diameter, and therefore assumes a flattened shape. Normally, the iliac portion of the innominate bone increases steadily in length, until it has attained its full development just before puberty, while the sacral and pubic portions grow much more slowly. Accordingly, as a result of these variations, combined with the arrested growth of the sacrum, the anteroposterior diameter of the superior strait will at some time equal or exceed the transverse diameter in length, so that between the eighth and twelfth years the pelvic inlet tends to become round

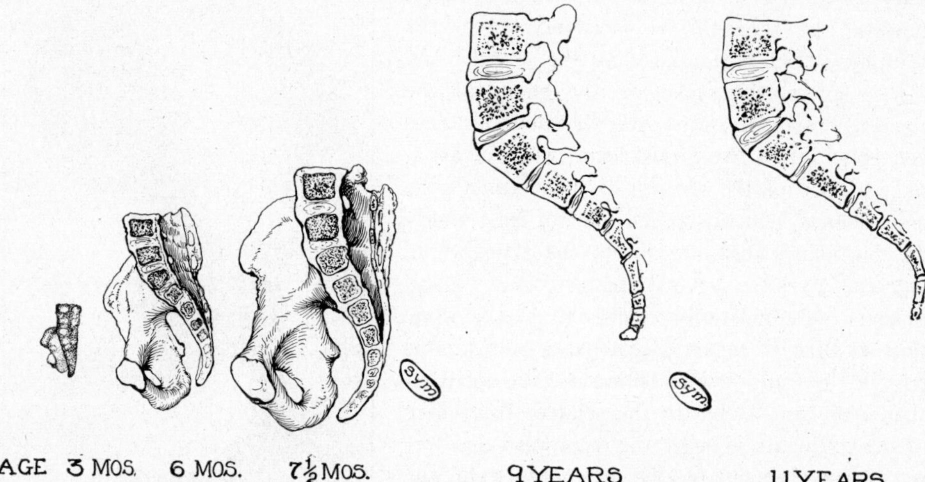

Fig. 183.—Progressive Changes in the Sacral Curvature.

(From Morton and Hayden, *American Journal of Obstetrics and Gynecology.*)

or even oval in shape, with its long diameter extending anteroposteriorly. This, however, is only a transient phenomenon, as shortly before puberty the sacrum suddenly begins to increase rapidly in width, and the pubic bones in length, so that the superior strait reassumes its typical flattened shape with the long diameter extending transversely.

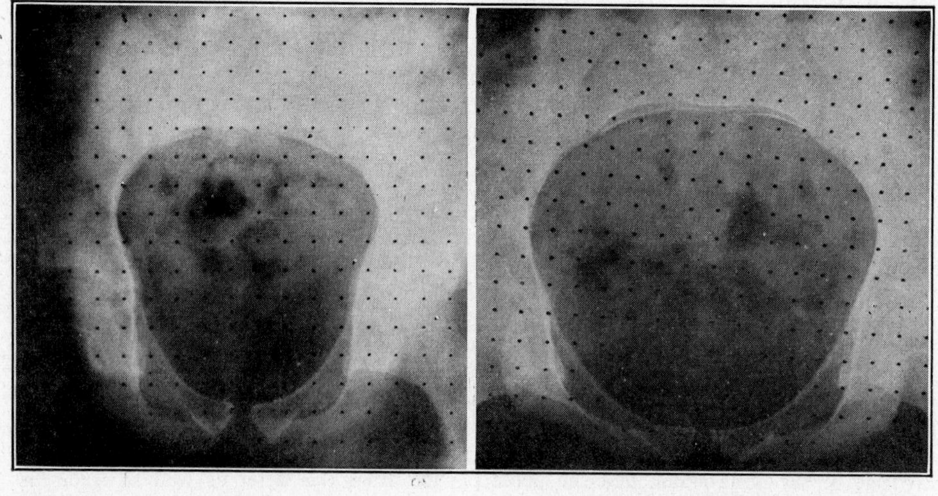

A B

Fig. 184.—Changes in the Inlet of the Female Pelvis During Adolescence.

A, at 12 years and B, at 16 years of age. (From Morton and Hayden, *American Journal of Obstetrics and Gynecology.*)

Breus and Kolisko, therefore, contend that these variations indicate that the changes in shape of the pelvis must be attributed to something more than mere mechanical influences, since the latter come into play in infancy and continue as long as the individual is able to sit up or walk. Were they the only factors concerned, the pelvis would necessarily continue to become more and more flattened, until it had attained its ultimate form, whereas the occurrence of a rounded superior strait between the eighth and twelfth year clearly indicates that some other factor must be concerned. As yet they have advanced no explanation for the variable rate of growth of the sacrum and the component parts of the innominate bone, but they nevertheless hold that its occurrence precludes the acceptance of the mechanical theory to the exclusion of all others, while at the same time they admit that the latter may also play an important part in the development of the pelvis.

The effect of the mechanical factors is particularly emphasized in the production of certain varieties of contracted pelvis, which have been studied by Meyer and Schroeder. In rare instances, as in one recorded by Gurlt, none of the mechanical forces had come into play, and then one has an opportunity of studying the development of the pelvis in their absence. In Gurlt's case, autopsy upon a 31-year-old hydrocephalic woman who had been bedridden since infancy and had never sat or walked showed that the pelvis had retained its fetal characteristics.

The cohesive force exerted at the symphysis pubis cannot act by itself, as it is manifested only when the force exerted by the body weight causes a tendency toward gaping of the pubic bones. Likewise, the effect of the upward and inward force exerted by the femurs cannot be observed by itself, as this force comes into play only when it has to react against that resulting from the body weight. Nor has the action of the body weight alone ever been observed, though theoretically it might be noted in an individual presenting a split pelvis (congenital lack of union at the symphysis pubis) who has never walked. Its action, however, has been studied experimentally by Freund, who suspended a cadaver by the iliac crests after cutting through the symphysis; he found that the innominate bones gaped widely.

The effect of the combined action of the body weight and the force exerted by the femurs has been studied by Litzmann in cases of congenital absence of the symphysis pubis. In such circumstances there is a marked transverse widening of the posterior portion of the pelvis, while the force exerted by the femurs causes the anterior portions of the innominate bones to become almost parallel.

The action of the body weight and the cohesive force exerted at the symphysis, without the upward and inward pressure exerted by the femurs, can be studied in individuals whose lower extremities are absent, and occasionally in cases of congenital dislocation of the hips. Holst has described a case in which the lower extremities were congenitally absent, the pelvis being characterized by a marked increase in width and a marked decrease in its anteroposterior diameter. Owing to the excessive pressure exerted upon the tubera ischii in the absence of the counteracting force exerted by the femora, the innominate bones are rotated in such a manner as to turn their crests inward and the tubera ischii outward, thus producing a considerable transverse widening of the inferior strait. More or less similar changes may be observed in cases of congenital dislocation of the hip if the patients have never walked.

The effect of the various mechanical influences is particularly emphasized when they are exerted upon pelves whose bones are softened by disease, as in rachitis and osteomalacia. Consideration of the changes so produced will be deferred until the study of deformed pelves is taken up.

PELVIC SIZE AND ITS ESTIMATION

It is essential that the obstetrician be able to determine the existence and extent of any pelvic contraction before the onset of labor in order that he may, as far as possible, decide in advance upon the proper treatment to be instituted in each case. With this in view, accurate pelvic mensuration should constitute an integral part of the examination of every pregnant woman.

Clinical Pelvimetry

The Diagonal Conjugate Measurement. In the majority of abnormal pelves the most marked deformity affects the anteroposterior diameter of the inlet, or superior strait, and as a consequence we are especially anxious to ascertain the length of the obstetrical conjugate. As already explained, however, this measurement cannot be obtained in living women without the aid of x-ray technic and, therefore, it is customary

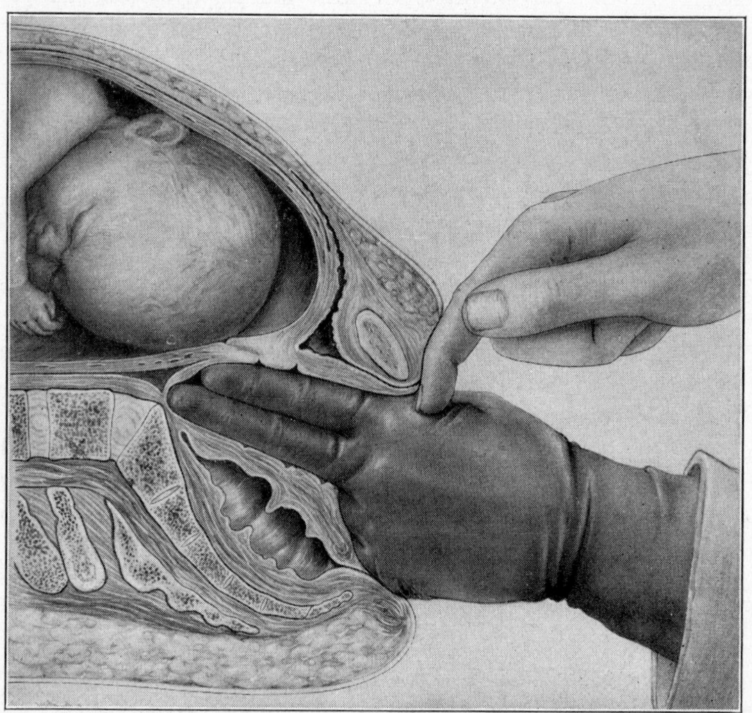

Fig. 185.—Measuring the Diagonal Conjugate.

in routine practice to estimate the anteroposterior dimension of the inlet by measuring the distance from the promontory of the sacrum to the lower margin of the symphysis pubis. **This distance, the diagonal conjugate dimension, is the most important clinical measurement of the pelvis and every practitioner of obstetrics should be intimately familiar with its technic and interpretation.**

For this purpose the patient should be placed upon an examining table with her knees drawn up, and her feet supported by suitable stirrups. If this cannot be conveniently arranged, she should be brought to the edge of the bed and a firm pillow placed beneath her buttocks. Two fingers are introduced into the vagina, and, before measuring the diagonal conjugate, the motility of the coccyx is determined and the anterior surface of the sacrum is palpated. The first is ascertained by seizing the coccyx between the fingers in the vagina and the thumb externally and attempting to move it to and fro. The anterior surface of the sacrum is then methodically palpated from below upward and its vertical and lateral curvature noted. In normal pelves only the last three sacral vertebrae can be felt without pushing up the perineum, whereas in markedly contracted varieties the entire anterior surface of the sacrum is usually readily accessible.

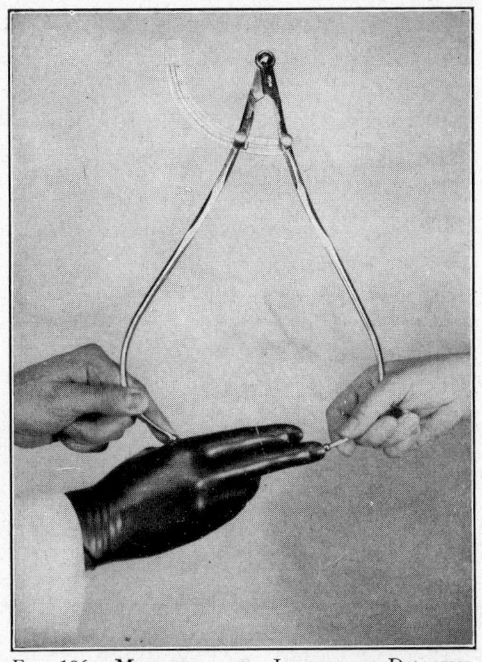

Fig. 186.—Measuring the Length of Diagonal Conjugate with Pelvimeter.

Except in extreme degrees of contraction, in order to reach the promontory of the sacrum, the elbow must be depressed and the perineum forcibly pushed upward by the knuckles of the third and fourth fingers. In order to effect this, it is customary for the examiner to place one foot upon a stool and to rest against the knee the elbow corresponding to the examining hand. Then, by moving the knee, strong pressure can be exerted without interfering with the motility of the wrist or of the examining fingers. The index and second fingers, firmly held together, are carried up over the anterior surface of the sacrum when by sharply depressing the wrist the promontory is felt by the tip of the second finger as

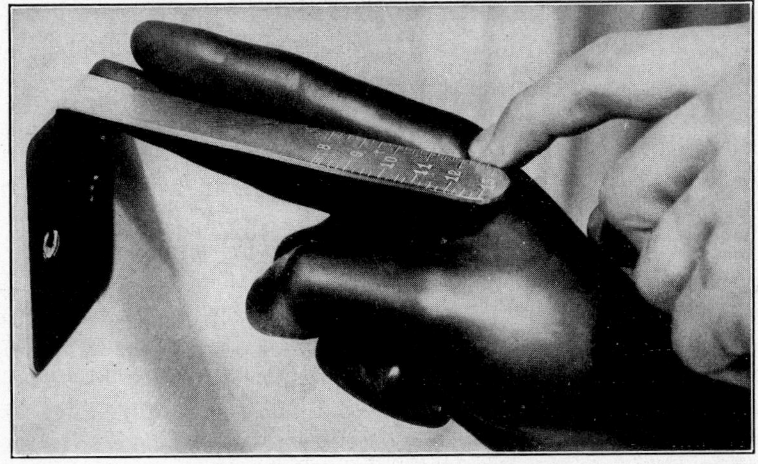

Fig. 187.—Metal Scale, Fastened to Wall, for Measuring the Diagonal Conjugate Diameter as Determined Manually. (Douglas.)

a projecting bony margin at the base of the sacrum. With the finger closely applied to its most prominent portion, the hand is elevated until the radial surface of the index finger is brought into close contact with the pubic arch. This point is then marked by the nail of the index finger of the other hand, after which the fingers are withdrawn from the vagina and the distance between the mark and the tip of the second finger is measured (Figs. 185 and 186). This represents the diagonal conjugate, from which the true conjugate is estimated by deducting 1.5 to 2 cm., according to the height and inclination of the symphysis pubis. Due to the fact that the pelvimeter often registers an error of one half to one centimeter, we now employ a rigid measuring scale, attached to the wall, as shown in Fig. 187.

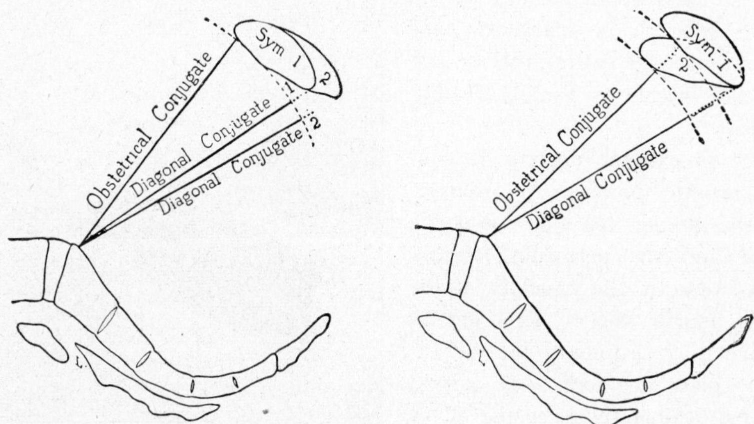

FIG. 188.—DIAGRAMS SHOWING VARIATIONS IN LENGTH OF DIAGONAL CONJUGATE DEPENDENT ON THE HEIGHT AND INCLINATION OF THE SYMPHYSIS PUBIS.

In this method the problem consists in estimating the length of one side of a triangle, the conjugata vera; the other two—diagonal conjugate and the height of the symphysis pubis—being known. Were we able to measure satisfactorily the angle formed between the symphysis and conjugata diagonalis, the exact length of the true conjugata could readily be ascertained by the ordinary rules of trigonometry. Unfortunately, this cannot be done accurately in the living woman, but for practical purposes it suffices to estimate the length of the diagonal conjugate as just described, deducting 1.5 cm. from it if the pubis is low and slightly inclined, and 2 cm. if it is high and has a marked inclination. The length of the diagonal conjugate also varies according to the position of the promontory, being longer when it is elevated, and vice versa (Fig. 188).

If this measurement is greater than 11.5 cm. or if the promontory of the sacrum cannot be reached at all, it is justifiable to assume that the pelvic inlet is of adequate size for childbirth. Thus, as shown in Fig. 189, in 61 consecutive cases in which the diagonal conjugate measurement exceeded 11.5 cm. in our clinic, there was not a single instance in which the obstetrical conjugate fell below 10.0 cm. But the question may be raised about the possibility of transverse contraction of the inlet. It is true that this is occasionally seen, but in our experience it is unusual for it to occur in sufficient degree to cause dystocia, provided the anteroposterior dimension of the inlet is adequate.

The objection to the diagonal conjugate measurement is sometimes made that it is painful to the patient. It doubtless does cause some momentary discomfort of mild degree, but having carried this measurement out personally in several thousand patients, including a large number of private patients, I cannot be much impressed by this criticism. If properly done and deferred to the middle part of pregnancy when the distensibility of the vagina is greater, patients do not object to it any more than they do to a venipuncture.

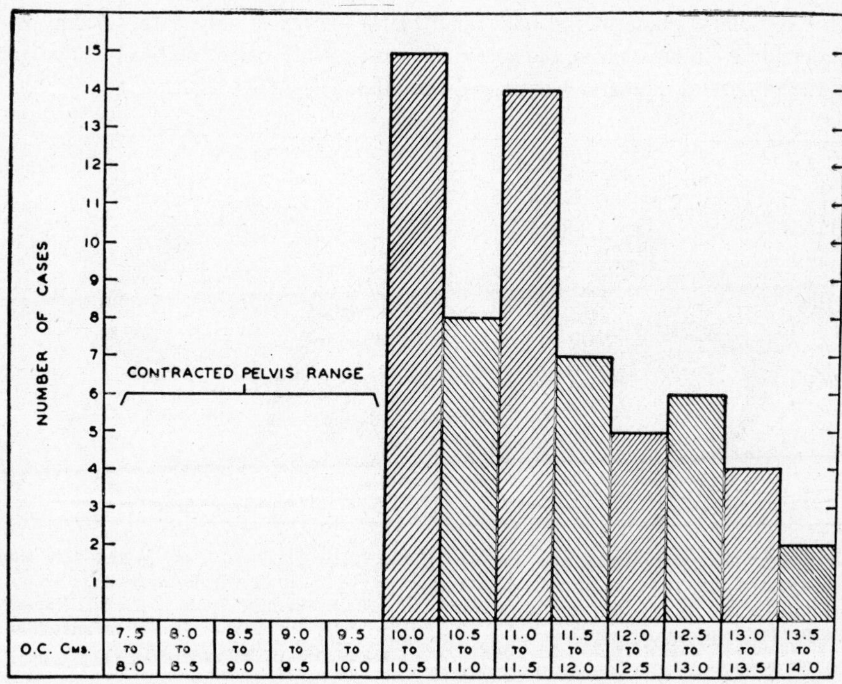

FIG. 189.—THE DISTRIBUTION OF THE OBSTETRICAL CONJUGATE MEASUREMENT (X-RAY) IN 61 CASES IN WHICH THE DIAGONAL CONJUGATE WAS GREATER THAN 11.5 CM.

Mean length of obstetrical conjugate was 11.4 cm.; shortest length, 10.0 cm.; greatest length, 13.7 cm. (Dippel).

Any diagonal conjugate measurement in excess of 11.5 cm. is considered to be normal.

Engagement. By engagement is meant the descent of the biparietal plane of the fetal head to a level below that of the pelvic inlet. In other words, when the biparietal or largest diameter of the head has passed through the inlet, it is said that engagement has taken place, or, that the head is engaged. Although engagement is usually regarded as a phenomenon of labor (and will be discussed later in that connection), it is important to note here that in primigravidae it frequently occurs during the last few weeks of pregnancy, and when it does so, is an all-important confirmatory evidence that the pelvic inlet is adequate for that particular head. Accordingly, when this phenomenon has occurred, it may be considered that the fetal head has served as a sort of internal pelvimeter to demonstrate beyond all question that the inlet is ample for that particular infant.

Whether or not the head is engaged may be determined either by rectal examination or by abdominal palpation. After a little experience with rectal (or vaginal) examination, it becomes relatively easy to determine the station of the lowermost part of the head in relation to the level of the ischial spines. Is it above, at, or below an imaginary line drawn between the ischial spines? **If the lowest part of the occiput is at or below the level of the spines, the head, as a rule, must be engaged for the following reason:** The distance from the plane of the pelvic inlet to the level of the ischial spines approximates 5 cm. in most pelves, whereas the distance from the biparietal plane of the fetal head to the vertex is only 3 to 4.5 cm. or so, and under these circumstances, the vertex cannot possibly reach the level of the spines unless the biparietal diameter has passed the inlet. (See Figs. 190-191.)

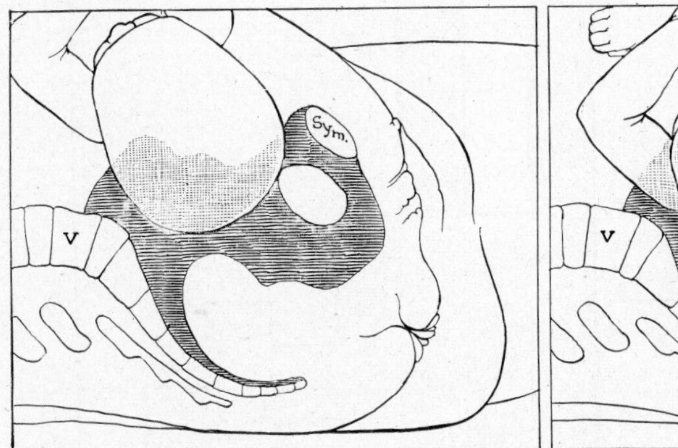

Fig. 190.—Showing that When the Lowermost Level of the Head Is Several Centimeters above the Ischial Spines, It Is Not Engaged.

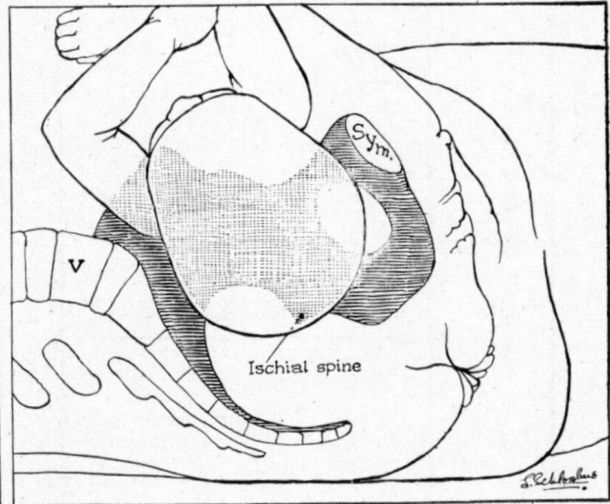

Fig. 191.—Showing that When the Lowermost Level of the Head Is at or below the Ischial Spines, It Is Engaged. Exceptions to this Rule May Occur if there Is Extreme Caput Formation.

Engagement may also be determined by abdominal examination. If, in a mature infant, the biparietal plane has descended through the inlet, that plane so completely fills the inlet that the examining fingers (as shown in Fig. 192) cannot reach that part of the head which is lowermost. Hence, the examining fingers when pushed downward over the lower abdomen, as shown, will slide over that portion of the head which is proximal to the biparietal plane (nape of the neck) and hence will diverge. Conversely, if the head is not engaged, the examining fingers can easily palpate the lower part of the head and will hence converge as shown in Fig. 193. Fixation of the fetal head, it should be noted, is not necessarily synonymous with engagement. It is true that a head which is freely movable on abdominal examination cannot be engaged, but, contrariwise, fixation of the head is sometimes seen when the biparietal plane is a centimeter or more above the inlet. In my experience, the maneuver just described, based on divergence or convergence of the examining fingers, is a much more reliable method of determining engagement of the fetal head than its fixation.

Engagement occurs at or prior to the onset of labor in over 90 per cent of primigravidae. Thus, in Bäder's study of 7,898 primigravidae, there were 499 instances of an unengaged head at the onset of labor, or 6.3 per cent. Similarly, in an investigation of 3,828 primigravidae, Farkas found 305 unengaged heads at the onset of labor, or 8 per cent. In close agreement with these statistics are the more recent observations of Auer and Simmons who found in 773 primigravidae that the head was engaged in 91.3 per cent prior to the onset of labor. Data on the frequency of engagement in primigravidae 10 days to 2 weeks before the expected date of confinement are meager but on the basis of my own experience it is probably of the order of 75 per cent. In multiparae, on the other hand (in whom there is usually less concern about pelvic contraction because of previous childbearing record), engagement is present at the onset of labor in only a minority of cases.

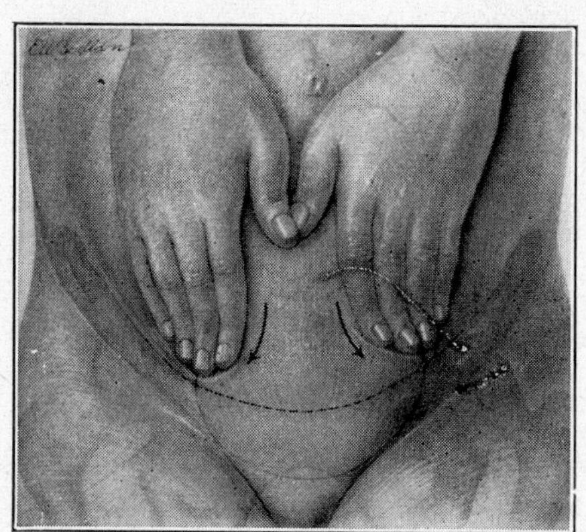

Fig. 192.—If the Fingers Diverge When Palpating the Lateral Aspects of the Fetal Head, the Head Is Engaged.

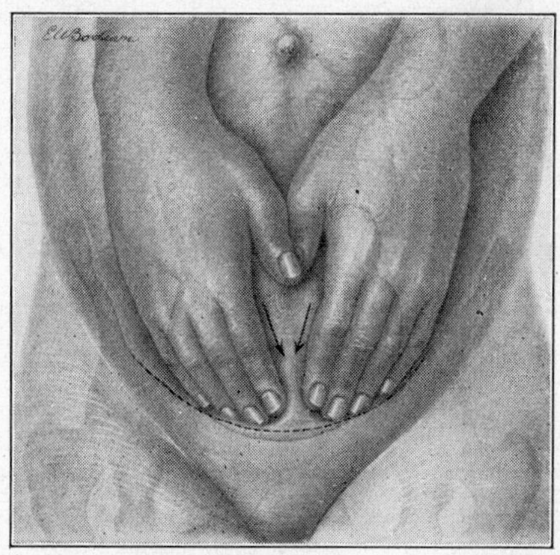

Fig. 193.—If the Fingers Converge When Palpating the Lateral Aspects of the Fetal Head, the Head Is Not Engaged.

Although the presence of engagement is conclusive evidence of an adequate pelvic inlet for the baby concerned, its absence is by no means indicative of pelvic contraction. For instance, in Bäder's study cited above, labor was entirely normal in 87 per cent of the 499 primigravidae with unengaged heads at the onset of labor. Nevertheless, the incidence of contraction of the inlet is decidedly higher in this group than in the female population at large. Hence, an unengaged head in a primigravida at the onset of labor always calls for careful revaluation of the whole cephalopelvic picture.

Outlet Measurements. Next to the diagonal conjugate measurement the most important clinical dimension of the pelvis is the diameter between the ischial tuberosities. This is variously called the tuberischii diameter (often abbreviated T.I.), the bisischial diameter, the intertuberous diameter and the transverse diameter of the outlet. With the patient in lithotomy position the measurement is taken from the inner and lowermost aspect of the ischial tuberosities, as shown in Fig. 194. A measurement in excess of 8 cm. is considered to be normal. For measuring the tuberischii diameter we have used almost exclusively the pelvimeter devised by Thoms. This possesses the additional advantage that it also makes possible the measurement of the anterior and posterior sagittal diameters of the outlet. The posterior sagittal diameter of the pelvis extends from the midpoint of a line between

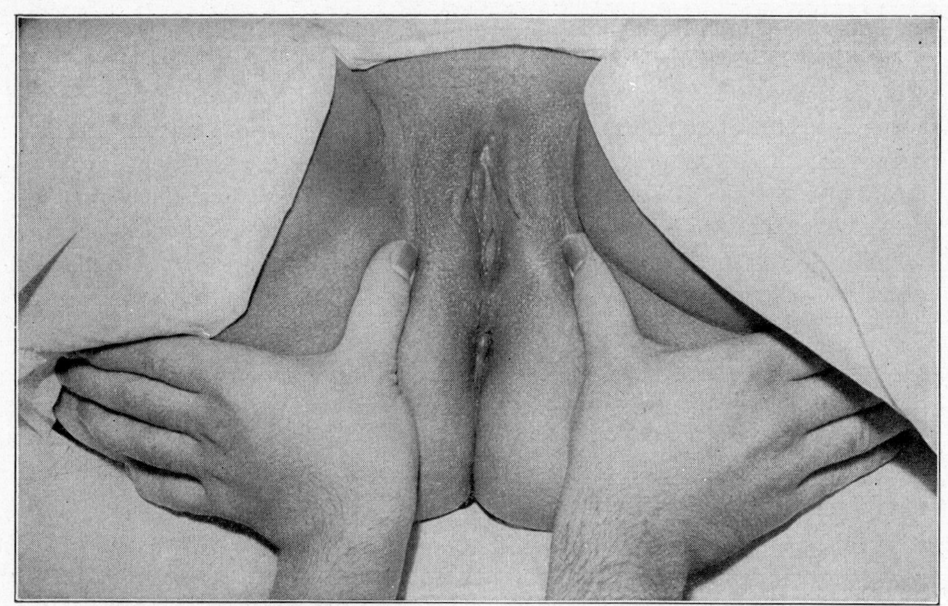

Fig. 194A.—Palpation of Pubic Arch.

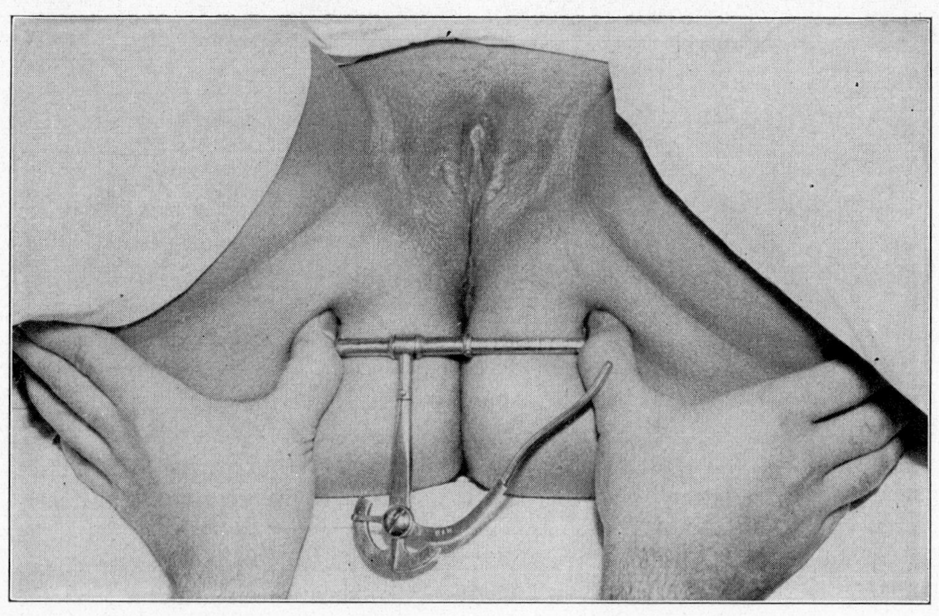

Fig. 194B.—Showing Mensuration of Transverse Diameter of Outlet by Means of Thoms' Pelvimeter.

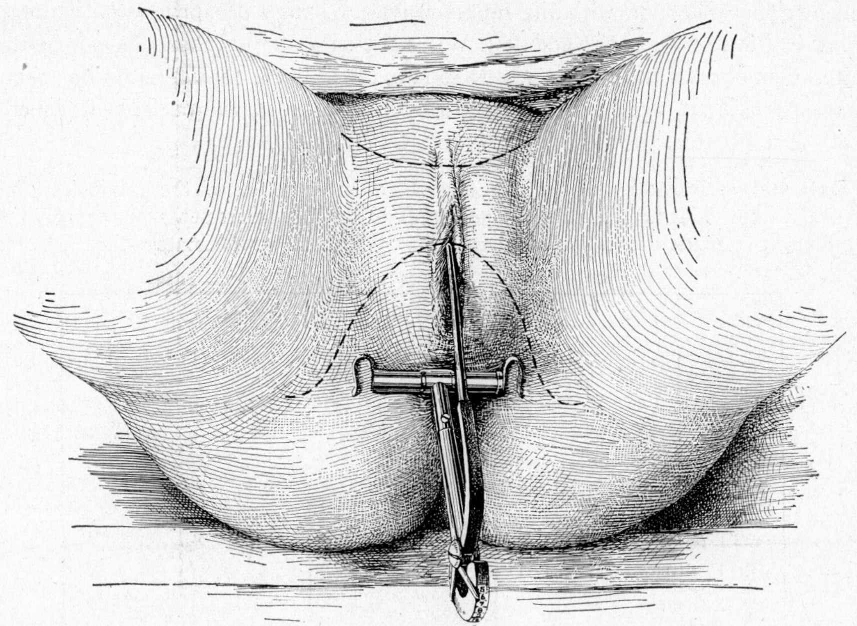

FIG. 195.—SHOWING MENSURATION OF ANTERIOR SAGITTAL DIAMETER OF OUTLET BY MEANS OF THOMS' PELVIMETER. × ⅓.

the ischial tuberosities to the tip of the sacrum. For this measurement the transverse bar of the Thoms pelvimeter is held by the fingers of one hand in relation to the transverse diameter of the outlet and its long arm is rotated posteriorly in such a way that its tip rests on the lowermost part of the sacrum with skin and subcutaneous fat interposed. The measurement can then be read off on the pelvimeter. The clinical measurement of the anterior and posterior sagittal diameters of the outlet by means of Thoms' pelvimeter is shown in Figs. 195 and 196. The importance of the posterior sagittal measurement in relation to the tuberischii diameter will be discussed sub-

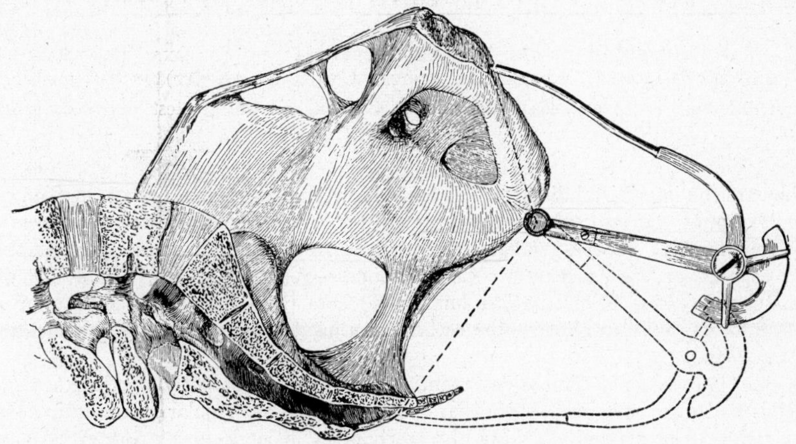

FIG. 196.—DIAGRAM ILLUSTRATING MENSURATION OF THE ANTERIOR AND POSTERIOR SAGITTAL DIAMETERS OF OUTLET BY MEANS OF THOMS' PELVIMETER. × ⅓.

sequently in connection with the funnel pelvis and may be appreciated at once by a consideration of Figs. 452 and 454. When the sum of the tuberischii and posterior sagittal diameters of the outlet exceeds 15 cm., the outlet is considered to be adequate, whereas if it is appreciably less than 15 cm., dystocia at the outlet will sometimes occur—Thoms' rule.

External Pelvimetry of Inlet. Since direct mensuration of the pelvic inlet is impractical except by x-ray technics, a number of external measurements of the pelvis have long been in common use in the belief that they permit an approximate estimation of inlet

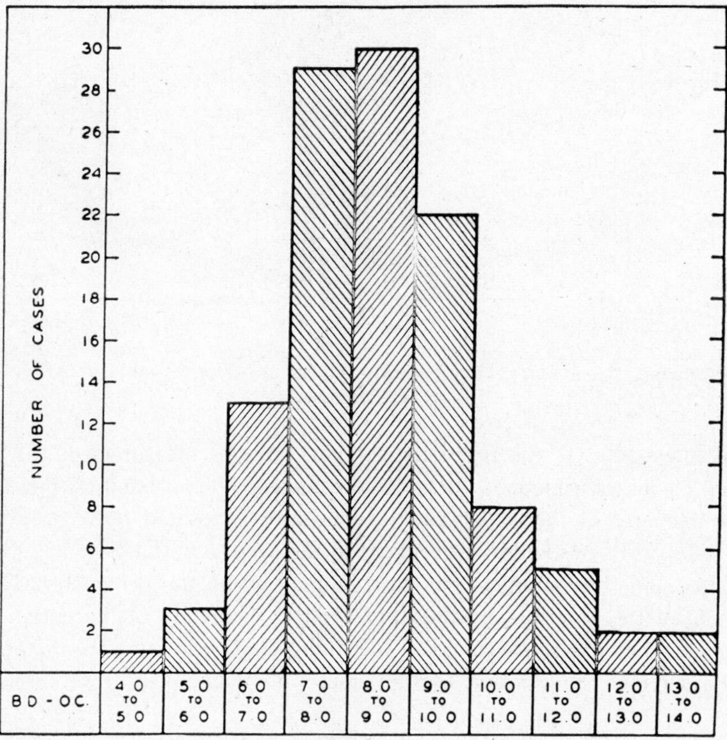

Fig. 197.—The Distribution of the Difference between the External Conjugate (Baudelocque's Diameter) and the Obstetrical Conjugate (X-ray) in 115 Cases.

Mean difference is 8.5 cm., least difference is 4.9 cm. and the greatest difference is 13.5 cm. (Dippel).

size. They are the intercristal diameter (distance between the external lips of the iliac crests—average, 28 cm.); the interspinous diameter (distance between the external aspects of the anterior superior iliac spines—average, 25 cm.); intertrochanteric diameter (distance between external aspects of the trochanteric protuberances—average, 31 cm.); and the distance between the depression below the last lumbar vertebra posteriorly and the anterior surface of the symphysis pubis anteriorly—the external conjugate or Baudelocque's diameter—average, 18 to 20 cm.

The first two external dimensions mentioned above are patently measurements of the false pelvis and experience has shown that their size bears no regular relationship to that of the true pelvis. The distance between the trochanters depends to a great extent upon the angle which the neck of the femur forms with its shaft; and as a consequence its shortening does not indicate a corresponding decrease in the transverse diameters of the pelvic cavity.

As methods of measuring the true pelvis, therefore, these procedures are of no value. It has been claimed, however, that a flaring outward of the ilium, so that the anterosuperior spinous diameter approximates or equals the intercristal, is indicative of rachitic changes in the true pelvis. In a large experience with rickets in Negresses in Baltimore, we have ample evidence that rachitic changes in the pelvic inlet, even though extreme, are not frequently associated with the changes described. Hence we agree with Thoms and others that these transverse external measurements serve no useful obstetrical purpose and we abandoned them a good many years ago.

Of all the pelvic measurements which have been recommended, the external conjugate has probably been more widely employed and, until very recently, more universally depended upon than any other index of pelvic contraction. In the opinion of Baudelocque, who first recommended this measurement in 1775, this dimension was regularly about 7.5 cm. greater than the conjugata vera and hence, through simple subtraction, yielded the conjugata vera. It is true that Baudelocque's contention does contain an element of validity because, in most cases, it does bear the approximate relationship to the conjugata vera which Baudelocque claimed; however, as shown in Fig. 197, the difference between this dimension and the conjugata vera may vary, even in a series of 115 cases, between 5 and 13 cm. This means that it is not unusual for a woman to have an external conjugate diameter of 19 or 20 cm. with contracted internal measurements and, contrariwise, a measurement of 16 or 17 cm. with a normal inlet. This criticism of the external conjugate is not new since it was made by contemporaries of Baudelocque, was emphasized in the nineteenth century by Michaelis and in the present era by Thoms. The number of unnecessary cesarean sections which have been performed solely because of a reduced external conjugate diameter and contrariwise, the number of women who have been allowed to suffer hours of hopelessly obstructed labor because this dimension was normal, are legion.

At the present writing external pelvimetry of the inlet is in a state of transition, the trend being toward elimination of these procedures. Nevertheless, many experienced obstetricians still use them in the belief that they do possess some value and they are still routine in a large number of clinics. Medical students might note, moreover, that they constitute a favorite question on State Board Examinations. For the reasons stated, however, it may be confidently predicted that external pelvimetry of the inlet will be abandoned universally before long.

Clinical Estimation of Midpelvic Size. Clinical estimation of midpelvic capacity is not satisfactory. It is true that both DeLee and Hanson have devised pelvimeters for measuring the interischial spinous diameter and that the latter has made valuable observations by means of his instrument but, in the main, adequate recognition of contraction in this region demands roentgenologic mensuration.

X-ray Pelvimetry

Status of X-ray Pelvimetry. Although x-ray pelvimetry was described in 1900, its development and popularity are phenomena of the past two decades. Even today, however, the greatest divergency of opinion exists about its value. Some feel that it is superfluous and may even be misleading. Others regard x-ray pelvimetry as the panacea for all perplexities in the management of pelvic contraction. As is usually true under such circumstances, the truth lies somewhere between these two extremes.

Let it be emphasized in the first place that the prognosis for successful labor in any given case cannot be established on the basis of x-ray pelvimetry alone, since the pelvic factor is but one of several circumstances which will determine the outcome. As enumerated by Mengert, the factors concerned are at least five in number as follows: (1) size and shape of the bony pelvis, (2) size of the fetal head, (3) force exerted by the uterine contractions, (4) moldability of the head and (5) presentation and position. Of these, only the first is susceptible to precise measurement and it is simply the objective of x-ray pelvimetry to eliminate this one factor from the category of the unknown. X-ray pelvimetry must hence be regarded merely as a valuable adjunct in the management of patients with contracted pelvis, just as the electrocardiogram is a helpful aid to the cardiologist in the management of patients with heart disease.

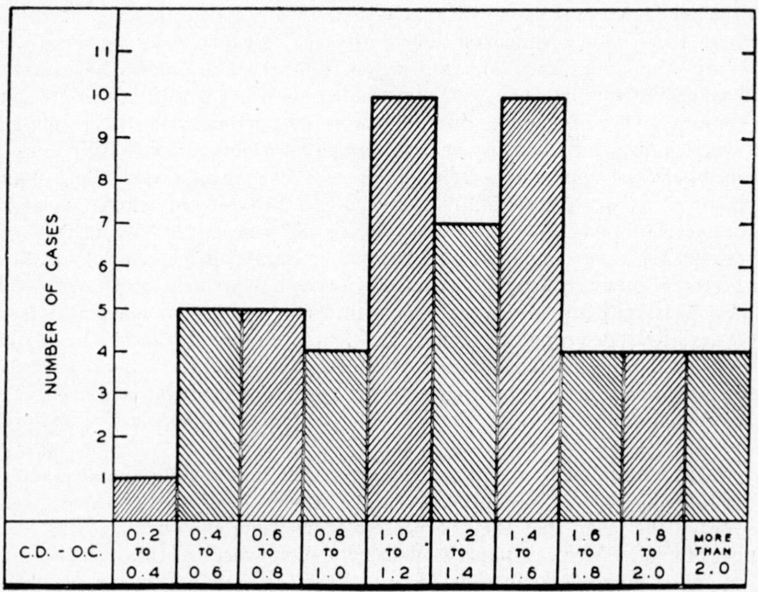

Fig. 198.—The Distribution of the Difference between the Diagonal Conjugate and the Obstetrical Conjugate (X-ray) in 54 Cases in which the Diagonal Conjugate Measured 11.5 cm. or Less.

Mean difference is 1.3 cm., greatest difference is 3.1 cm. and least difference is 0.1 cm. (Dippel).

X-ray pelvimetry possesses numerous advantages over manual estimation of pelvic size, such as the following:

1. It provides precision of mensuration to a degree which is possible in no other way. The clinical importance of such precision will become apparent when the shortcomings of the diagonal conjugate measurement are considered. As stated, it has been our experience that when this exceeds 11.5 cm., the anteroposterior dimension of the inlet is very rarely contracted (Fig. 189). On the other hand, when the diagonal conjugate is under 11.5, this dimension is not always a reliable index of the obstetrical conjugate, since the difference between these two diameters (usually said to be about 1.5 cm.) may range between 0.1 and 3.1 cm. as shown in Fig. 198. For instance, two primigravidae may have diagonal conjugates of 10.5 cm. But in one the obstetrical conjugate may be 10.2 cm. and vaginal delivery be easy; whereas in the other it may be 8.2 cm. and cesarean section become obligatory.

2. It provides mensuration of certain diameters which were previously not easily obtainable, such as the transverse diameter of the inlet and the interischial spinous dimensions. The latter measurement is receiving increasing recognition as an important cause of midpelvic arrest and of difficult forceps operations.

3. By the stereoscopic technic, x-ray pelvimetry permits visualization of the general architecture of the pelvis and, in experienced hands, this type of information is almost as valuable as actual mensuration.

4. When standing films are taken from time to time in the course of labor, very precise information is obtainable concerning the descent or lack of descent of the biparietal plane of the head. This information is sometimes difficult to obtain by palpating the presenting part because elongation of the head in labor may make such digital findings misleading.

Special Indications for X-ray Pelvimetry. Because of the expenses involved and other reasons, radiographic pelvic measurement is not feasible for all pregnant women, nor is it necessary in the great majority of cases. There are, however, certain clinical circumstances which point to the probability of pelvic contraction or potential dystocia and make x-ray pelvimetry highly desirable. These are as follows:

A. History
  1. Difficult forceps delivery
  2. Unexplained stillbirth or neonatal death
  3. Previous cesarean section
B. Palpation
  1. Prominent ischial spines
  2. Narrow, pointed pubic arch
C. Manual mensuration
  1. Inlet
    a. Ability to touch sacral promontory easily on vaginal examination
    b. Diagonal conjugate measurement below 11.5 cm.
  2. Outlet
    a. Intertuberous diameter of 8.0 cm. or less
    b. Sum of tuberischii and posterior sagittal diameters 15 cm. or less
D. Nonengagement of fetal head at term in a primigravida
E. Failure to make progress in labor
F. Breech, face and other abnormal presentations
G. Elderly primigravidae
H. Very young primigravidae

Technics of X-ray Pelvimetry. The essential problem in x-ray pelvimetry is that of correcting for distortion of the image produced by divergence of the x-rays. The amount of distortion depends upon (1) the distance of an object (or a pelvic diameter) from the x-ray film, and (2) the distance from the x-ray tube to the film (Fig. 199). The latter can be eliminated as an unknown by establishing a standard tube-film distance. The farther above the film an object is, the greater will be the distortion of its image. Unfortunately, in some diameters of the pelvis the exact distance above the x-ray film is an unknown. A great variety of mechanical and mathematical methods have been devised to correct for this variable image distortion of the different pelvic diameters.

Thoms' Method. This is an example of position type of pelvimetry which is widely used and is given below in detail. It is reasonably simple and gives accuracy adequate for clinical purposes in most pelvic diameters of interest to the obstetrician.

LATERAL (ISOMETRIC) FILM—TECHNIC FOR ANTEROPOSTERIOR MEASUREMENTS. The problem of correction for distortion here is a simple one. The measurements that are desired from this view, such as the obstetrical conjugate, anteroposterior diameter of the midpelvis, and the posterior sagittal of the outlet, are all located in the same midline plane which is easily located by anatomical landmarks. A metal ruler placed in this plane will be subject to the same distortion as the pelvic diameters and its image may be used to measure these diameters directly (isometric scale).

TAKING THE LATERAL FILM. The patient stands with one side against a vertical Bucky diaphragm in symmetrical profile position. A canvas binder is helpful in preventing motion (Fig. 200). The tube is centered just above the trochanter at a tube-film distance of 36 inches. A metallic ruler with centimeter notches supported on a standard is placed close to the sacrum in the midline and parallel to the film. The exposure varies with the thickness of the patient.

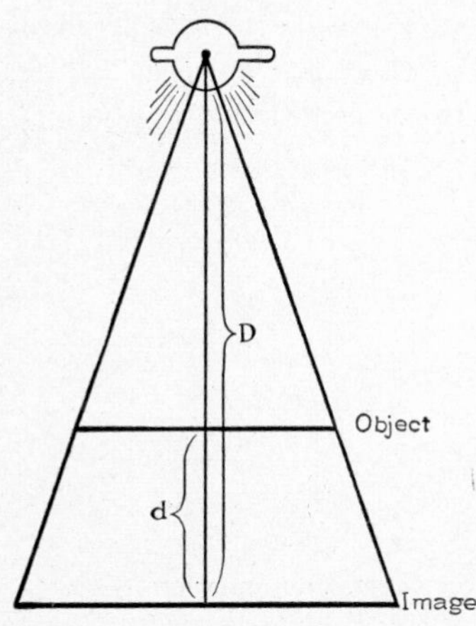

FIG. 199.—PRINCIPLE OF DIVERGENT DISTORTION.

Size of the image depends on object-film distance (d) and tube-film distance (D).

If a standing film is inconvenient, the patient may be positioned lying on the side with the table horizontal. A head pillow, lateral lumbar pad and pads between knees and ankles are necessary to good positioning (Fig. 201). The marker is positioned between the buttocks and parallel to the table top. Other factors are the same as for the standing film.

MEASURING THE LATERAL FILM. The end points of each diameter are located. Each diameter is then spanned by a caliper and this distance is transferred directly to the image of the centimeter scale on the film which gives the corrected diameter. Diameters which may be measured are the obstetrical conjugate, posterior sagittal at the inlet, midpelvis and outlet, and anteroposterior diameter at midpelvis and outlet. Observation should be made of the curvature and inclination of the sacrum and of the appearance of the sacrosciatic notch.

The lateral isometric film with its exact measurement of the important obstetrical conjugate is the most valuable single tool in the commonest type of serious pelvic contraction, *i.e.*, of the inlet. Let it be stressed that such a film can be taken by any physician with access to a standard x-ray machine. The only special equipment needed is a metal ruler with centimeter notches or perforations. A review of the contours and bony anatomy of the lateral view of the pelvis will facilitate location of the symphysis, sacrum, and ischial spines; this can be accomplished with a little practice by anyone.

ANTEROPOSTERIOR FILM—TECHNIC FOR TRANSVERSE MEASUREMENTS. Correction for divergent distortion in this view is more complicated because the diameters of interest (the transverse of the inlet, interspinous and intertuberal diameters) are at somewhat different levels. Moreover, the locations of these levels are not clearly marked anatomically as is the midline. Hence the use of isometric scales is more difficult.

TAKING THE ANTEROPOSTERIOR FILM. The patient is placed on the table in semi-recumbent position supported by a back-rest. The pelvic inlet should be horizontal. This is accomplished by measuring (1) the perpendicular distance from the interspace between the fourth and fifth lumbar vertebrae to the table top and (2) the distance from a point on the symphysis 1 cm. below its superior border to the table top. The patient's position is adjusted until these measurements are equal. (Note is made of this height of the inlet plane for use later in positioning the grid.) The tube is centered about 6 cm. above the symphysis at a tube-film distance of 36 inches. The exposure is varied with the thickness of the patient.

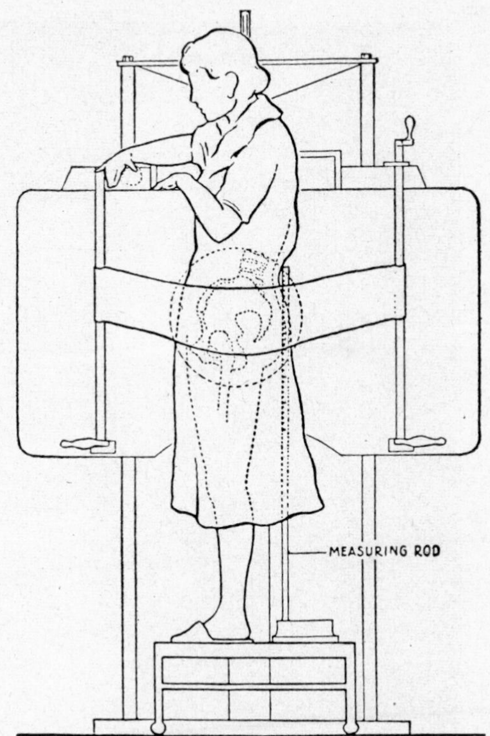

FIG. 200.—POSITIONING OF THE PATIENT, STANDING, FOR LATERAL X-RAY OF PELVIS TO OBTAIN ANTEROPOSTERIOR DIAMETERS BY THOMS' TECHNIC. (Courtesy of Dr. Herbert Thoms.)

The patient is removed from the table, leaving the tube and exposed film in place. The centimeter grid, a special lead plate with perforations along one edge, is placed in the same plane as that previously occupied by the pelvic inlet as determined by the measurements (Fig. 203). A second (flash) exposure is made on the edge of the previously exposed film; for this the tube is positioned over the perforated region in the grid, at a distance of 36 inches.

MEASURING THE ANTEROPOSTERIOR FILM. The transverse diameter of the inlet is spanned by a caliper and measured on the top row of centimeter perforations which is the correction for the level of the pelvic inlet. Below this are correction scales for levels 5, 6, 7, 8 and 9 cm. below the inlet. On the lateral film the corrected distance from the inlet to the ischial spines is determined. This distance below the inlet is then used to choose the appropriate scale on the anteroposterior film to use in correcting the interspinous image. A similar procedure is used in correcting the transverse diameter of the outlet.

Colcher and Sussman have introduced a simplified single-scale anteroposterior

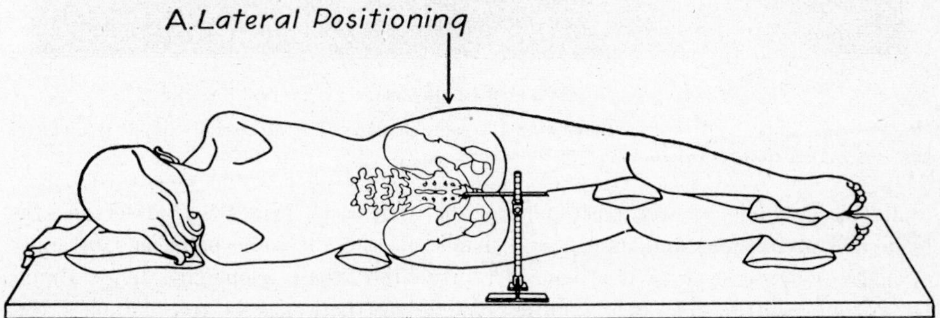

FIG. 201.—POSITIONING OF THE PATIENT, RECLINING, FOR LATERAL X-RAY OF PELVIS TO OBTAIN ANTEROPOSTERIOR DIAMETERS BY THOMS' TECHNIC.
(Courtesy of Dr. Herbert Thoms.)

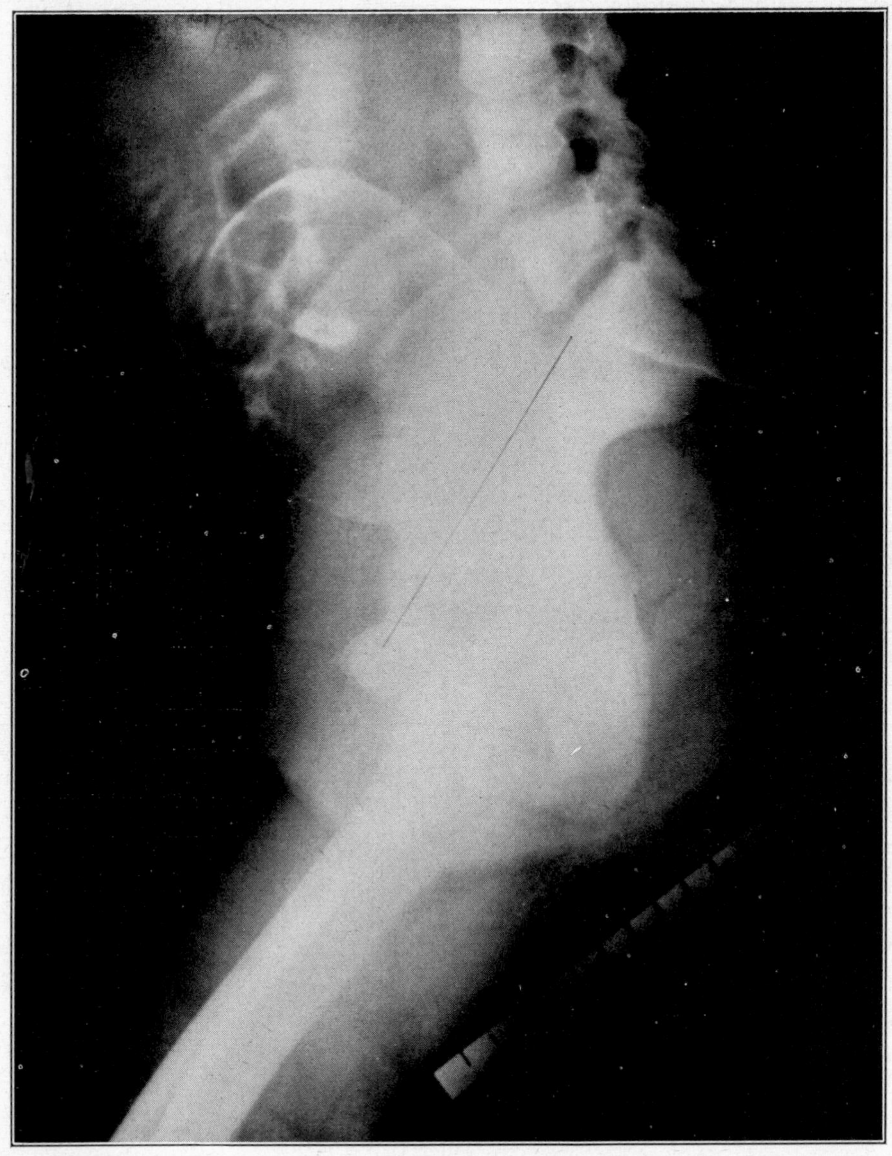

FIG. 202.—LATERAL ROENTGENOGRAM OF PELVIS BY THOMS' TECHNIC.

The scale shows corrected centimeters in the sagittal plane. The obstetrical conjugate diameter has been drawn on the pelvis.

film. This method seeks, by positioning of the patient, to bring the transverse of the inlet, the interspinous and intertuberal diameters into the same plane and to apply a single isometric scale to this plane. Unfortunately, these diameters cannot always be brought into the same plane and in some pelves there may be considerable error, especially in the interspinous diameter.

Alternate Anteroposterior Method—Stereoscopic Films. This technic illustrates the parallax type of pelvimetry. It depends upon two films taken under standard

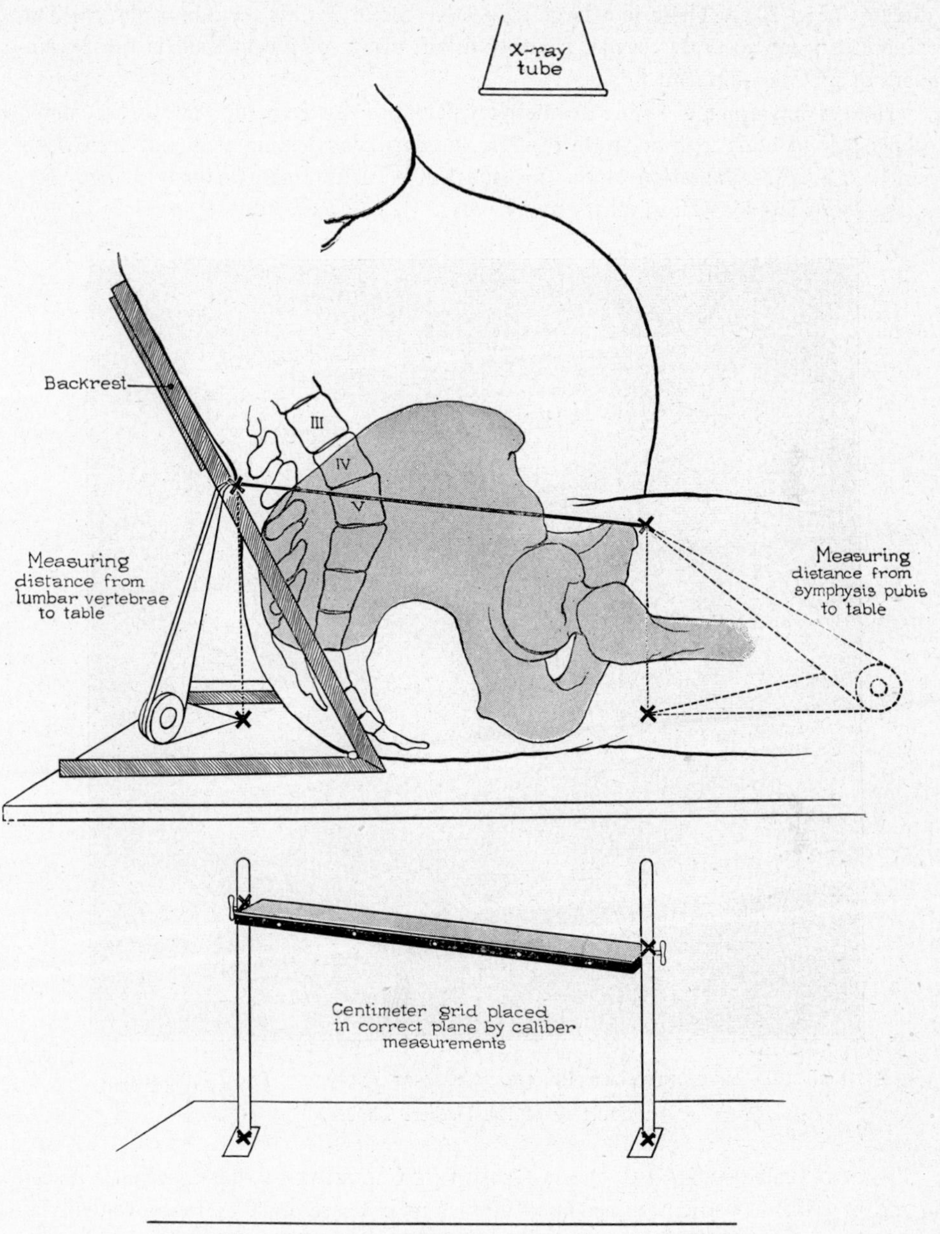

FIG. 203.—POSITIONING OF PATIENT AND MARKERS FOR THE THOMS' ANTEROPOSTERIOR PELVIC X-RAYS.

conditions, the x-ray tube being shifted a known distance between exposures. Correction for distortion can be accomplished either with a precision stereoscope or by geometric calculation or construction.

Caldwell and Moloy developed a precision stereoscope in which the factors used in taking the films are duplicated in the optical system. When the system is properly adjusted, a centimeter ruler is applied to the image in space and it is measured directly (Fig. 205). There is a large subjective factor in this method and experience is necessary for accurate results. Another disadvantage of the method is the requirement of special equipment.

Hodges has applied simple geometric calculation by triangulation to the stereoscopic pair of films with accurate results. Standard x-ray equipment and stereoscope can be used. An adaptation of this method has been used satisfactorily in our clinic at the Johns Hopkins Hospital for many years.

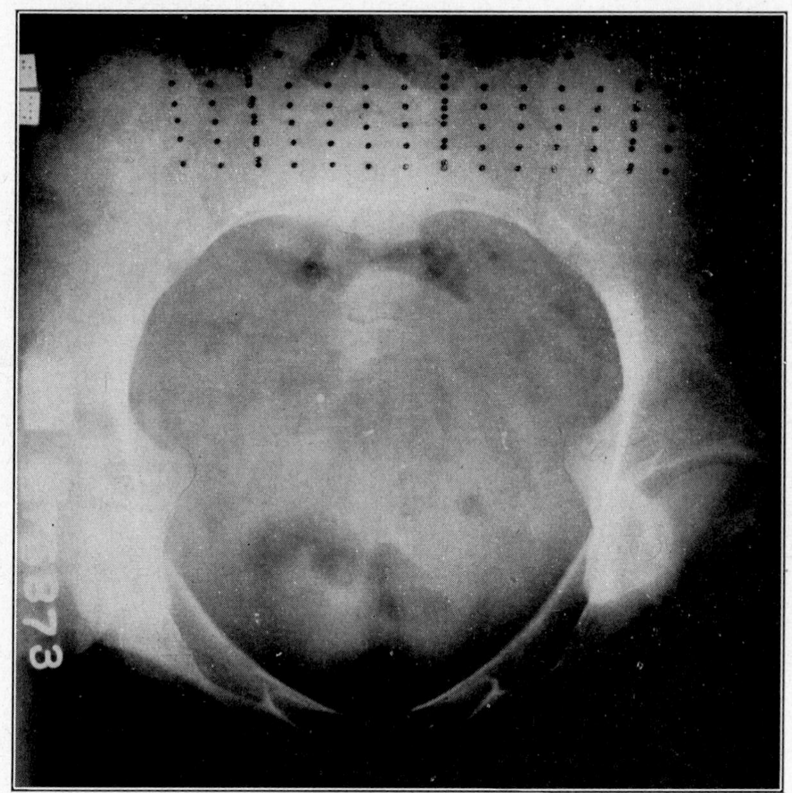

FIG. 204.—ANTEROPOSTERIOR ROENTGENOGRAM OF PELVIS BY THOMS' TECHNIC. (Courtesy of Dr. Herbert Thoms.)

TAKING STEREOSCOPIC FILMS FOR GEOMETRIC CALCULATION. The patient is placed in the recumbent position with a small lumbar pad. There must be no movement between the two exposures. Centering is at the level of the anterior iliac spines. Tube-film distance is constant at 36 inches, and tube shift between exposures is *exactly* 10 cm. The tray and cassettes must occupy a fixed position for the two exposures. A perforated lead marker is centered over one side of the cassette to register on each film and allow accurate superimposition of the two films.

MEASURING THE FILMS. End points of the diameters to be measured (the transverse of the inlet, interspinous and intertuberal diameters) are perforated with a stylet and each distance measured. The two films are then superimposed over a view-box using the register markers for alignment. The parallax shift (P) of each end point is measured. A correction factor for *each* diameter is calculated using the parallax shift for that diameter:

$$\text{Factor} = \frac{\text{tube shift}}{\text{parallax} + \text{tube shift}} = \frac{10}{\text{P} + 10}$$

This factor is derived from the geometric setup used in taking the films. Each diameter measured on the film is multiplied by its own correction factor.

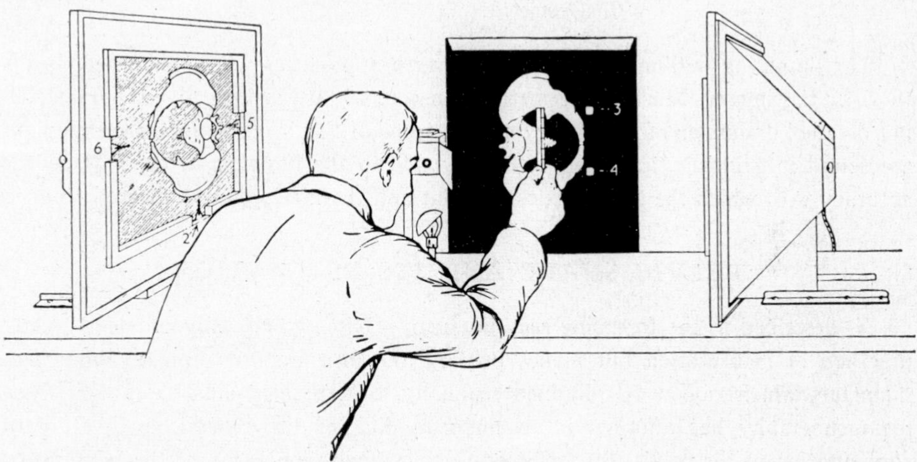

FIG. 205.—X-RAY PELVIMETRY EMPLOYING STEREOSCOPIC TECHNIC OF CALDWELL AND MOLOY.

The stereoscopic anteroposterior films are augmented by an isometric lateral film of the Thoms type. This combined isometric and stereoscopic work-up has the advantage of both complete mensuration and morphological study of the pelvis in three dimensions. Steele and Javert also have developed and stressed the advantages of a combined isometric and stereoscopic method.

In an excellent review of the many technics of x-ray pelvimetry that have been developed during the recent years, Hodges and Dippel state that most of these fall into four general types, as follows:

- I. Position methods
  - A. Isometric scales
  - B. Proportional scales
  - C. Triangular proportion
    - 1. Direct application of equations
    - 2. Graphs of equations
    - 3. Slide rules
- II. Parallax methods
  - A. Stereoscopic
    - 1. Direct parallax
    - 2. Measurement of virtual image
    - 3. Geometric construction
      - a. Plane
      - b. Solid
  - B. Non-stereoscopic
    - 1. Single film
    - 2. Multiple films (Cartesian co-ordinate)

III. Ninety-degree triangulation
   A. Empirical
   B. Geometrical construction
      1. Plane
      2. Cartesian co-ordinate
IV. Orthometric reproduction
   A. Pantographic
   B. Orthoscopic
   C. Geometric

This imposing outline illustrates the diverse approaches which have been made to x-ray pelvimetry. Most of the methods in common use belong to types I and II, but detailed discussion of each is beyond the scope of this book. A number of methods are sound in principle, and their ultimate value to the obstetrician depends on the accuracy with which the technic is carried out and the interpretation derived from it.

PELVIC SHAPE AND ITS ESTIMATION

As described in the foregoing section, x-ray pelvimetry not only provides greater precision of mensuration but makes possible the measurement of many important diameters which cannot be obtained manually. Still a third advance which pelvic roentgenography has afforded is an understanding of the general architecture or configuration of the pelvis. By architecture or configuration is meant the relationship of certain dimensions of the pelvis to one another, that is, its shape quite apart from its size. As a result of the classical studies of Caldwell and Moloy, a classification of the pelvis according to shape—known as the Caldwell-Moloy classification—is now in wide use. Likewise, Thoms has evolved a valuable classification of pelves according to their configuration. Familiarity with one or another of these classifications is a necessary prerequisite to a full understanding of the mechanism of labor as it is also to the intelligent management of labor in pelvic contraction. In the latter connection, pelvic shape has introduced the important concept of the pelvic space actually available to the fetal head in contradistinction to the total space as indicated by absolute dimensions. For example, consider the space presented by a square opening in comparison with that of a circular opening which happens to be slightly smaller in square centimeters than the former. It is understandable that a ball a bit smaller than the circle could pass through it easily since all the space is usable, whereas it might not be able to get through the square opening because part of the measured space, the corners, are not available to a globular object.

The Caldwell-Moloy classification is based on the type of the posterior and anterior segments of the inlet (Figs. 206 and 207). A line drawn through the greatest transverse diameter of the inlet divides the inlet into anterior and posterior segments. The posterior segment determines the type, while the anterior segment may show variations. Many pelves are not pure types. Thus in mixed types we may speak of a gynecoid pelvis with android "tendency," meaning that the hindpelvis is gynecoid in characteristics and the forepelvis is android. Before taking up the specific Caldwell-Moloy classification and its various pelvic types, it is necessary to survey those relationships which are taken into consideration in assigning a pelvis to this or that category. The particular pelvic characteristics which must be known before the Caldwell-Moloy classification can be employed are as follows:

The Inlet. The pelvic inlet is divided into an anterior and posterior segment by the widest transverse diameter. The posterior sagittal diameter of the inlet is represented by that portion of the anteroposterior diameter which lies posterior to the

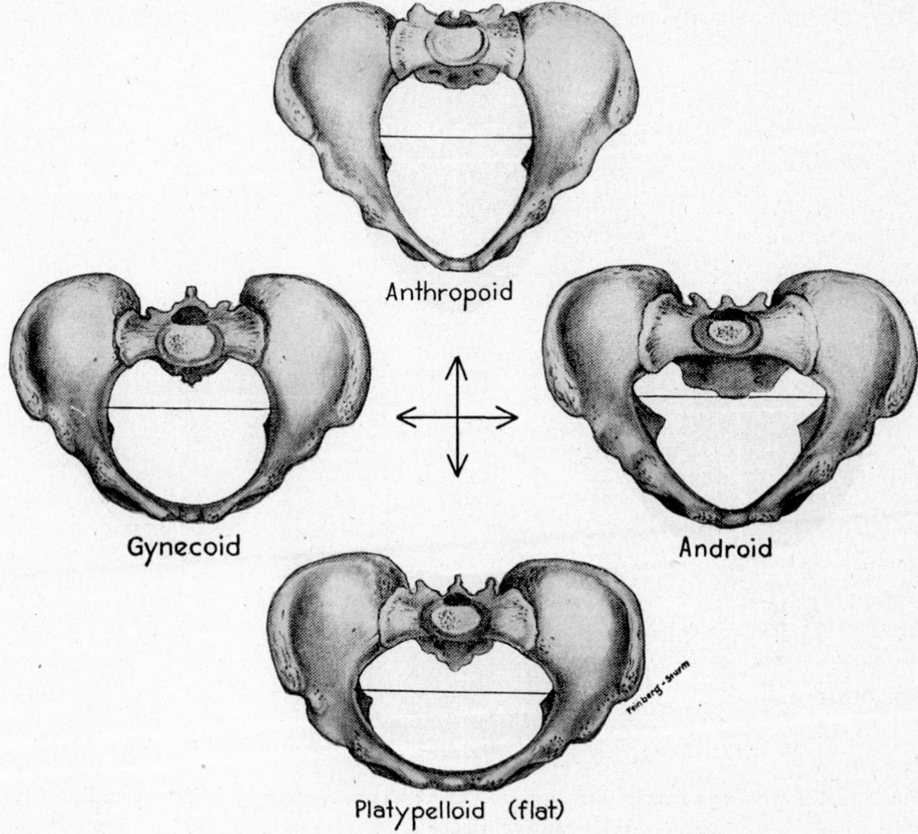

Fig. 206.—The Four Parent Pelvic Types.

A line passing through the widest transverse diameter divides the inlet into an anterior and posterior segment. (From Moloy and Swenson, *Diagnostic Roentgenology*. Courtesy of Thos. Nelson & Sons, New York.)

point of intersection by the transverse diameter. The first question to be answered concerns itself with this posterior sagittal diameter. Is it unduly short? Is it unduly long? In other words, is the transverse diameter of the pelvis very close to the promontory of the sacrum or some distance removed? Expressed in different words, does the posterior segment tend to be flattened anteroposteriorly or elongated? Furthermore, are the sides of the posterior segment well rounded or wedge shaped? Turning now to the anterior segment, does it appear to be a fairly good semicircle or is it wedge-shaped or triangular, or does it present the shape more or less of a flattened semicircle? Moreover, is the anterior sagittal diameter unusually long or unusually short? Finally, looking at the inlet as a whole, is its transverse diameter greater than, equal to or less than the anteroposterior diameter? If the transverse diameter is greater than the posterior, the appearance of the inlet will naturally be that of an ovoid transversely; if the reverse is true, the ovoid will be anteroposterior, while if the measurements are approximately equal the inlet will of course present the shape of a circle.

The Sacrosciatic Notch. Is the sacrosciatic notch wide, average or narrow? Posterior inlet capacity, as has just been discussed, is controlled largely by the size

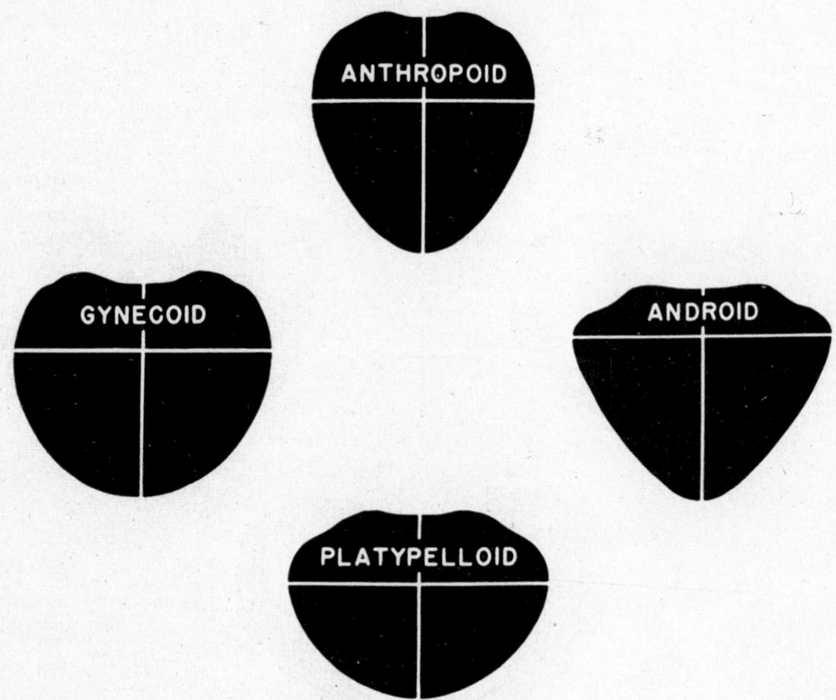

Fig. 207.—Showing the Pelvic Inlet of the Parent Types, Anterior and Posterior Segments. (Steele.) (See Fig. 206.)

of the sacrosciatic notch. If the notch is large, the posterior sagittal diameter of the inlet will be large, whereas if it is small, that diameter will be short. This relationship exists because the width or narrowness of the sacrosciatic notch is transmitted through the ilium to affect the length of the posterior iliac portion of the inlet behind the widest transverse diameter.

Splay of Side Walls. Are the side walls divergent, straight or convergent? The answer to this question is of clinical importance since the obstetrician desires to know whether the width present at the inlet is preserved through the pelvis. The splay may be actually divergent and these forms are always associated with a very wide subpubic arch, although the angle of the forepelvis may be wide or narrow. The convergent side walls are usually found in conjunction with a narrow subpubic arch but here again the angle of the forepelvis may be wide or narrow.

Character of the Ischial Spines. Do the ischial spines jut into the pelvic cavity or are they barely visible or not visible at all as one looks at the inlet from above? Prominent ischial spines, since they are located in the plane of least pelvic dimensions, may be a source of great difficulty in labor and they imply also the possibility of definite convergence of the side walls of the pelvis which is also an unfavorable prognostic sign.

The Sacrum. The inclination of the sacrum concerns the sacrum as a whole and may be defined as the fixed position of the anterior sacral surface in relation to the true pelvis. It determines the anteroposterior diameter of the bony pelvis—symphysis to sacrum—at the level of any pelvic plane. Is the sacrum forward in the pelvis? Or is it parallel to the symphysis or does it slope backward and approach an almost horizontal position? What is the length and width of the sacrum and what is its curvature? How many segments are there? An increase in length of the sacrum is usually due to partial or complete fusion of the fifth lumbar vertebra with the first sacral segment above or by bony union of the last sacral segment with the first coccygeal vertebra below. Complete fusion results in the sacrum with six segments, sometimes termed "assimilation." Assimilation is very common and occurs often in normal pelves, as well as in the more abnormal types.

Subpubic Arch. Is the subpubic arch wide, moderate or narrow? Roentgenograms of the subpubic arch afford an opportunity of judging the character of the bones. Three types are recognized: delicate, average and heavy.

Caldwell, Moloy and Swenson consider it most advisable for the obstetrician to acquire the habit of dividing the pelvis into the component parts described above and noting the characteristics of the inlet, the sacrum, the ischial spines and the pubic arch, while viewing the stereoroentgenograms, or even when estimating pelvic shape and size by vaginal examination. It then becomes easier to judge the obstetrical capacity of any individual pelvis, even if it may be difficult to classify it.

In the Caldwell-Moloy classification, four parent categories are recognized. However, it should be emphasized that these four so-called parent types are largely for purposes of classification only; they are hypothetical except in the very rare instance when one finds a pelvis which confirms to one of these pure types in every detail. The four parent groups of Caldwell-Moloy are as follows:

Gynecoid Pelvis. The term as used refers to the average female pelvis which displays the anatomic characteristics ordinarily attributable to the human female. The posterior sagittal diameter at the inlet is only slightly shorter than the anterior sagittal. The sides of the posterior segment are well rounded and the forepelvis is also well rounded and wide. Accordingly, since the transverse diameter of the inlet is either slightly greater or about the same as the anteroposterior diameter, the inlet as a whole presents either a slightly oval or round shape. The side walls of the pelvis are straight, the spines not prominent, the pubic arch is wide with a transverse diameter of above 10 cm. The sacrum is inclined neither anteriorly nor posteriorly. The sacrosciatic notch is well rounded and never narrow. Caldwell, Moloy and Swenson established the frequency of occurrence of the four parent types in skeletal material from inspecting T. Wingate Todd's collection of pelves of known sex at Western Reserve University. They found that among pure types of pelves in white women the gynecoid is the most frequently encountered, comprising 41.4 per cent. The corresponding figure for Negresses was 42.1 per cent.

Android Type. The posterior sagittal diameter at the inlet is much shorter than the anterior sagittal, making it impossible for the fetal head to avail itself of this posterior space. The sides of the posterior segment are not rounded but tend to form with the corresponding sides of the anterior segment a sharp wedge at their point of junction. The forepelvis is narrowed and triangular. The side walls are usually convergent, the ischial spines prominent, and the subpubic arch narrowed. Further study of the latter will usually indicate that the bone structure is characteristically heavy. The sacrosciatic notch is narrow and high arched. The sacrum is set forward in the pelvis and the posterior sagittal diameter is decreased from inlet to outlet by the forward inclination. The android type of pelvis in its more extreme examples presages a

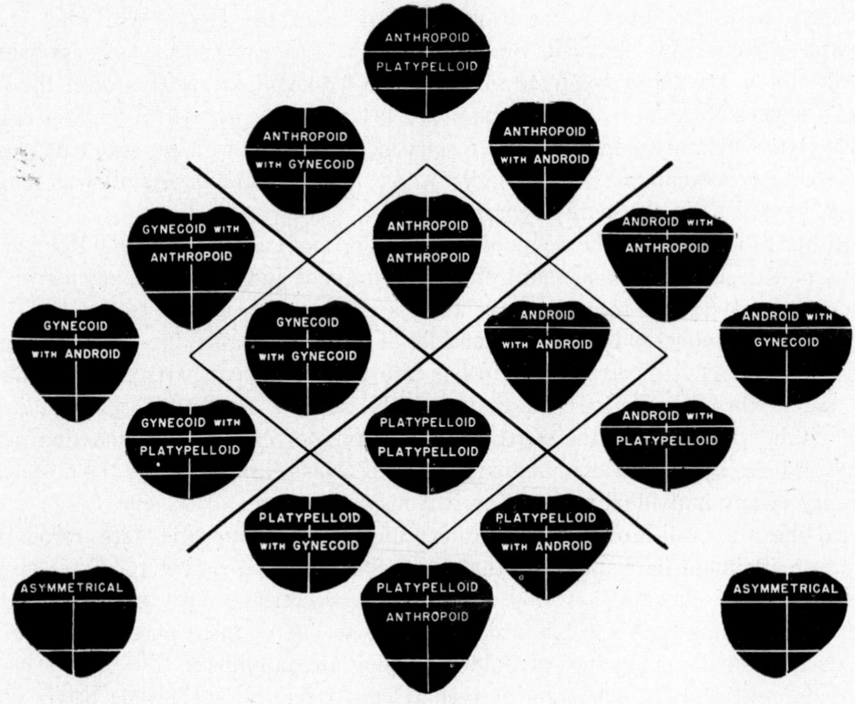

Fig. 208.—Pelvic Inlet Types.
(From Javert, *North Carolina Medical Journal.*)

very poor prognosis by the vaginal route, and the frequency of difficult forceps operations and stillbirths increases substantially in this type when combined with small size. The android type of pelvis makes up 32.5 per cent of pure-type pelves encountered in white females and 15.7 per cent in Negresses in the Todd collection.

Anthropoid Pelvis. This pelvis is characterized essentially by the fact that the anteroposterior diameter of the inlet is greater than the transverse so that the inlet appears more or less like an oval anteroposteriorly, but an oval with the anterior segment somewhat narrowed and pointed. The sacrosciatic notch is large. The side walls are often somewhat convergent and the sacrum is inclined posteriorly, thus increasing the posterior space at all levels. The ischial spines are not likely to be prominent. The subpubic arch is frequently somewhat narrow but well shaped. The anthropoid type of pelvis is said to be more commonly found in the Negro race, whereas the android form is more frequently met in the white race. Thus anthropoid types make up 23.5

per cent of pure-type pelves in white females in comparison to 40.5 per cent in Negresses.

Platypelloid Type. This pelvis is in actuality simply a flat gynecoid pelvis, being characterized by a short anteroposterior and a wide transverse diameter. The latter is set well in front of the sacrum as in the typical gynecoid form. The angle of the forepelvis is very wide and the anterior pubo-iliac and posterior iliac portions of the

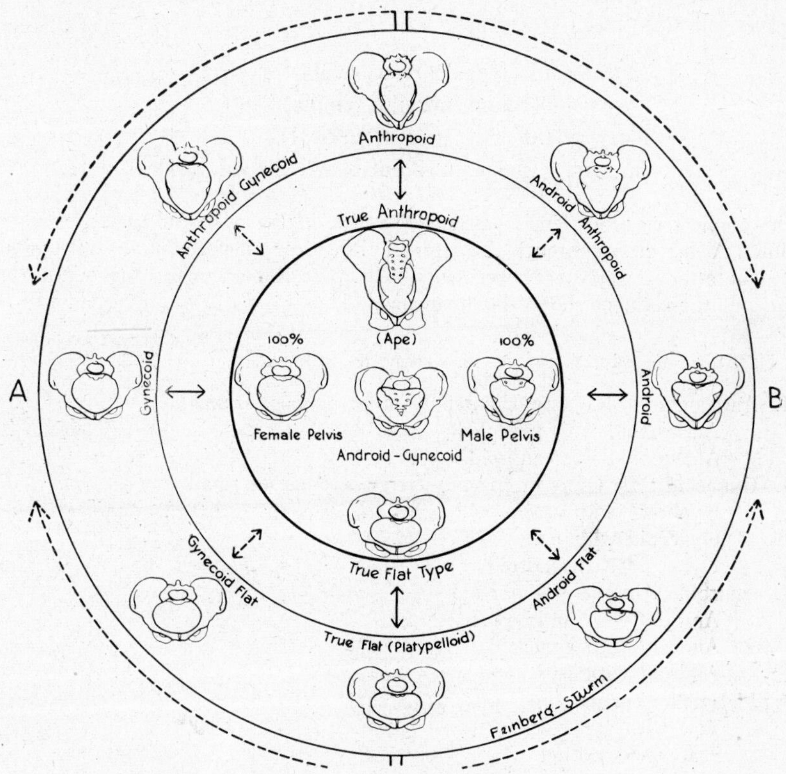

FIG. 209.—INTERMEDIATE FORMS OF THE PARENT TYPES WITH EVOLUTIONARY AND SEXUAL MODIFICATIONS.

(From Caldwell, Moloy and D'Esopo, *American Journal Obstetrics and Gynecology.*)

iliopectineal lines are well curved. The platypelloid type of pelvis is the rarest of the pure varieties, having been encountered in but 2.6 of white females and in 1.7 per cent of Negresses.

Intermediate Types. As already indicated, intermediate or mixed types of pelves are much more frequent than the pure types which have just been reviewed. The many varieties of these mixed types are clearly shown in Fig. 208. It may be recalled again that the character of the posterior segment determines the type and that of the anterior segment the tendency.

The influences which bring about such diversity in shape in female pelves are illustrated in Fig. 209. Two major forces are recognized, *i.e.,* evolutionary and sexual. Within the inner circle two axes may be noted. The vertical axis begins with a diagram of a gorilla pelvis and terminates with a flat or platypelloid human form.

These transmitted influences are thought to produce the cycle of change in pelvic form shown to the left in the outer circle referred to as the "evolutionary" cycle. In the horizontal axis a typical gynecoid, or 100 per cent female, pelvis is illustrated to the left with a typical 100 per cent male pelvis to the right. This "sexual" cycle is supposed to produce the adult android forms and their intermediate types shown to the right in the outer circle.

To summarize, the classification of pelvic shape of Caldwell and Moloy may be outlined as follows:

Anthropoid (long, narrow, oval)
Gynecoid (round, normal, female)
Platypelloid (flat, transverse oval)
Android (wedge or blunt-heart shaped, male)

Their complete classification is based on the type of the posterior and anterior segments of the inlet. A line drawn through the greatest transverse diameter of the inlet divides the inlet into anterior and posterior segments. The posterior segment determines the type, while the anterior segment shows the "tendency." Thus we speak of "gynecoid with android tendency."

The classification may, therefore, be written as follows:

I. Anthropoid type (pure or parent)—large, average or small
  Anthropoid with gynecoid
  Anthropoid with android
II. Gynecoid type (pure or parent)—large, average or small
  Gynecoid with anthropoid
  Gynecoid with flat
  Gynecoid with android
III. Android type (pure or parent)
  Android with anthropoid
  Android with gynecoid
  Android with flat
IV. Platypelloid or flat type (pure or parent)
  Flat with gynecoid
  Flat with android
V. Asymmetrical pelves
VI. In each individual pelvis, the following regions of the lower pelvis must be described in detail:
  a. Subpubic arch—wide, moderate, narrow
  b. Pubic rami—straight or curved
  c. Splay or side walls—divergent, straight or convergent
  d. Shape of forepelvis—well-formed or funnel
  e. Character of the ischial spines
  f. The sacrosciatic notch—wide, average, or narrow masculine type
  g. The sacrum—a general concept of length, width, curvature and number of segments
  h. Sacral inclination—forward, average, backward
  i. Lateral bore—straight, convergent or divergent
  j. Posterior pelvic capacity at the inlet and at the level of the spines and the relationship of the sacrococcygeal platform to the latter
  k. Shape of the outlet in front of the sacral tip

Finally, the pelvis should be studied as a whole to determine whether it is well formed or angular, irrespective of the gynecoid, android, anthropoid, or flat character of the pelvic inlet.

In 1922 Thoms described his original method of outlining the superior strait of the pelvis by means of the x-ray. Since that time he has made many important contributions to the field of roentgen-ray pelvimetry and has evolved a simple classification along the lines of the one proposed by Turner in 1886. His classification, based on the ratio of the anteroposterior to the transverse diameter of the pelvic inlet, is as follows:

1. Dolichopellic or anthropoid type pelvis. The transverse is less than the anteroposterior diameter.
2. Mesatipellic or round type pelvis. The transverse is equal to, or slightly greater (not more than 1 cm.) than, the anteroposterior diameter.
3. Brachypellic or oval type pelvis. The transverse diameter is more than 1 and less than 3 cm. greater than the anteroposterior diameter.
4. Platypellic or flat type pelvis. The transverse diameter is 3 cm. or more greater than the anteroposterior diameter.

Thoms considers the following diameters of the bony pelvis significant:

Pelvic inlet	Anteroposterior Transverse Posterior sagittal
Midpelvic plane	Anteroposterior Transverse or bispinous Posterior sagittal
Pelvic outlet	Transverse or bituberal Posterior sagittal

The posterior sagittal diameter of the inlet is represented by that portion of the anteroposterior diameter which lies posterior to the point of intersection by the transverse diameter. Similarly the posterior sagittal diameter of the midpelvic plane is that part of the anteroposterior diameter which lies posterior to the point of intersection by the transverse or bispinous diameter. The midpelvic plane, or plane of least dimensions, as previously defined, is bounded anteriorly by the lower border of the symphysis pubis, laterally by the ischial spines, and posteriorly, as emphasized by Hanson and Thoms, usually by the lower border of the fourth sacral segment.

BIBLIOGRAPHY

Abramson, D., Roberts, S. M., and Wilson, P. D. Relaxation of the Pelvic Joints in Pregnancy. Surg., Gynec. & Obst., 1934, 58:595.

Auer, E. S., and Simmons, J. M. The Floating Fetal Head in the Primipara at Term. Am. J. Obst. & Gynec., 1949, 58:291.

Bäder, A. Die Bedeutung des uber dem Eingange beweglichen Kopfes bei de Geburt von Primiparen. Orvoskepzes, 25, Toth-Sonderh., 315-321, 1935. (Abstracted in Berichte, 1936, 31:395.)

Ball, R. P. Roentgen Pelvimetry and Fetal Cephalometry. Surg., Gynec. & Obst., 1936, 62:798.

——— and Marchbanks, S. S. Roentgen Pelvimetry and Fetal Cephalometry; A New Technic. Radiology, 1935, 24:77.

Brakemann, O. Weiterer Beitrag zur röntgenologischer Diagnose des intrauterinen Fruchttodes. Arch. f. Gynäk., 1934, 157:197.

——— Haltung und Konfiguration des kindlichen Kopfes bei der Beckenendlage. Ztschr. f. Geburtsh. u. Gynäk., 1936, 112:154.

Breus, C., and Kolisko, A. Die pathologischen Beckenformen. F. Deuticke, Leipzig & Wien, 1902-1912.

——— Die Pathologische Beckenformen. Leipzig u. Wien, 1900.

Brill, H. M., and Danelius, G. Roentgen Pelvimetric Analysis of Walcher's Position. Am. J. Obst. & Gynec., 1941, 42:821.

Caldwell, W. E., and Moloy, H. C. Anatomical Variations in the Female Pelvis and Their Effect in Labor with a Suggested Classification. Am. J. Obst. & Gynec., 1933, 26:479.

CALDWELL, W. E., MOLOY, H. C., and D'ESOPO, D. A. Studies on Pelvic Arrests. Am. J. Obst. & Gynec., 1938, 36:928.

——— A Roentgenologic Study of the Mechanism of Engagement of the Fetal Head. Am. J. Obst. & Gynec., 1934, 28:824.

CALDWELL, W. E., MOLOY, H. C., and SWENSON, P. C. The Use of the Roentgen Ray in Obstetrics. Part I. Roentgen Pelvimetry and Cephalometry; Technic of Pelvioroentgenography. Am. J. Roentgenol., 1939, 41:305.

——— The Use of the Roentgen Ray in Obstetrics. Part II. Anatomical Variations in the Female Pelvis and Their Classification According to Morphology. Am. J. Roentgenol., 1939, 41:505.

——— The Use of the Roentgen Ray in Obstetrics. Part III. The Mechanism of Labor. Am. J. Roentgenol., 1939, 41:719.

CHAMBERLAIN, W. E., and NEWELL, R. R. Pelvimetry by Means of the Roentgen Ray. Am. J. Roentgenol., 1921, 8:272.

CLIFFORD, S. H. I. The X-ray Measurement of the Fetal Head Diameter in Utero. Surg., Gynec. & Obst., 1934, 58:727.

——— The Stereoroentgenometric Method of Fetometry and Pelvimetry with Its Obstetrical Application. West Virginia M. J., 1935, 31:401.

COLCHER, A. E., and SUSSMAN, W. A Practical Technique for Roentgen Pelvimetry with New Positioning. Am. J. Roentgenol., 1944, 51:207.

DICKINSON, K., and PROCTER, I. Comparative Measurements of the Female Pelvis. Am. J. Obst. & Gynec., 1942, 44:585.

DIPPEL, A. L. The Diagonal Conjugate versus X-ray Pelvimetry. Surg., Gynec. & Obst., 1939, 68:642.

EASTMAN, N. J. Pelvic Mensuration: a Study in the Perpetuation of Error. Obst. & Gynec. Surv., 1948, 3:301.

ELLER, W. C., and MENGERT, W. Recognition of Midpelvic Contraction. Am. J. Obst. & Gynec., 1947, 53:252.

FARKAS, J. Zur Frage des über dem Beckeneingang beweglich stehender Kopfes bei Erstgebärenden. Monatschr. f. Geburtsh. u. Gynak., 1935, 100:138.

FRAY, W. W., and POMMERENKE, W. T. Roentgenographic Pelvimetry and Fetalometry. Elimination of Error Due to Movements Between X-ray Exposures. Radiology, 1939, 32:261.

GRANZOW, J. Eine einfache Methode zur röntgenographischen Messung der Conjugata vera. Arch. f. Gynaek., 1930, 141:155.

GREULICH, W. W., and THOMS, H. The Dimensions of the Pelvic Inlet of 789 White Females. Anat. Rec., 1938, 72:45.

HANSON, S. Internal Pelvimetry as a Basis for the Morphological Classification of Pelves. Am. J. Obst. & Gynec., 1938, 35:228.

——— A New Pelvimeter for the Measurement of the Bispinous Diameter. Am. J. Obst. & Gynec., 1930, 19:124.

HARRIS, J. W. Some Practical Considerations of Labor Complicated by Contracted Pelvis. West. J. Surg., Obst. & Gynec., 1940, 48:23.

HAYDEN, Charles T. Roentgen-ray Pelvimetry, A Study of Three-Hundred-Twenty Labors. Calif. & West. Med., 1938, 49:25.

HEATON, C. E. Pelvioradiography. A Clinical Evaluation. N. Y. State J. Med., 1938, 38:83.

HODGES, P. C. An Epiphyseal Chart. Am. J. Roentgenol., 1933, 30:809.

——— Roentgen Pelvimetry and Fetometry. Am. J. Roentgenol., 1937, 37:644.

——— The Role of X-ray Pelvimetry in Obstetrics. Minnesota Med., 1949, 32:33.

HODGES, P. C., and DIPPEL, A. L. Collective Review. The Use of X-rays in Obstetrical Diagnosis, with Particular Reference to Pelvimetry and Fetometry. Internat. Abstr. Surg., 1940, 70:421.

HODGES, P. C., and HAMILTON, J. E. Pelvic Roentgenography in Pregnancy. Further Experiments with 90° Triangulation Methods. Radiology, 1938, 30:157.

HODGES, P. C., HAMILTON, J. E., and PEARSON, J. W. Roentgen Measurement of the Obstetrical Conjugate of the Pelvic Inlet. Am. J. Roentgenol., 1940, 43:127.

HODGES, P. C., and LEDOUX, A. C. Roentgen Ray Pelvimetry—A Simplified Stereoroentgenographic Method. Am. J. Roentgenol., 1932, 27:83.

HOLST. Beschreibung des Beckens u. der Geburtstheil eines 40 Jahre alten weiblichen Amelus. Holst's Beiträge, 1869, Heft 2, ff. 145-148.

INCE, J. G. H., and YOUNG, M. The Bony Pelvis and Its Influence on Labour: A Radiological and Clinical Study of 500 Women. J. Obst. & Gynaec. Brit. Emp., 1940, 47:130.

JACOBS, J. B. Further Improvement in Pelvimetric Roentgenography. Am. J. Obst. & Gynec., 1936, 32:76.

——— Management and Outcome of Labor in 742 Women with Borderline Pelves. Am. J. Obst. & Gynec., 1942, 43:267.

JAVERT, C. T. A Combined Isometric and Stereoscopic Technic for Radiographic Examination of the Obstetrical Patient. North Carolina Med. J., 1943, 4:465.

JAVERT, C. T., and STEELE, K. B. The Transverse Position and the Mechanism of Labor. Int. Abst. Surg., 1942, 75:507.

JAVERT, C. T., STEELE, K. B., and POWLITIS, M. E. Clinical Pelvimetry and Pelvic Palpation as a Basis for Morphologic Classification of the Obstetric Pelvis. Am. J. Obst. & Gynec., 1943, 45:216.

JOHNSON, C. R. Roentgen Mensuration by Stereoroentgenometry. Radiology, 1935, 25:492.

——— Pelvimetry by Stereoroentgenometry. Am. J. Roentgenol., 1937, 38:607.

——— A Method for Mensuration by Means of the Roentgen Ray. Am. J. Surg., 1930, 8:151.

KAUFMAN, Julius. The Planeogram. Analysis and Practical Application, with Especial Reference to Mensuration of the Pelvic Inlet. Radiology, 1936, 27:732.

KELLOGG, F. S. Has X-ray Pelvimetry Reduced the Incidence of Caesarean Section for Cephalopelvic Disproportion? M. Rec. & Ann., 1942, 36:399.

LITWER, H. Roentgen Pelvimetry. J. Obst. & Gynaec. Brit. Emp., 1936, 43:1158.

LITZMANN. Die Formen des Beckens. Berlin, 1861.

MARTIUS, H. Welchen Wert hat die Röntgendiagnostik bei den Geburt beim engen Becken. Monatschr. f. Geburtsh. u. Gynäk., 1937, 106:257.

MENGERT, W. Estimation of Pelvic Capacity. J.A.M.A., 1948, 138:169.

——— and ELLER, W. C. Graphic Portrayal of Relative Pelvic Size. Am. J. Obst. & Gynec., 1946, 52:1032.

MICHAELIS, G. A. Das Enge Becken. Leipzig, 2nd Ed., 1865.

MOIR, J. C. The Use of Radiology in Predicting Difficult Labour. J. Obst. & Gynaec. Brit. Emp., 1946, 53:487; 54:20.

MOORE, G. E. Roentgen Measurements in Pregnancy. A Few Practical Methods and a Simplified Procedure Used by the Author. Surg., Gynec. & Obst., 1933, 56:101.

MORTON, D. G., and HAYDEN, C. T. A Comparative Study of Male and Female Pelves in Children with a Consideration of the Etiology of Pelvic Conformation. Am. J. Obst. & Gynec., 1941, 41:485.

PETTIT, A. V., GARLAND, L. H., DUNN, R. D., and SHUMAKER, P. Correlation between Shape of Female Pelvis and Clinical Course of Labor. West. J. Surg., 1936, 44:1.

PLASS, E. D. Contracted Pelvis and Delayed Labor. Texas State J. Med., 1941, 37:363.

PORTES, MAYER, and MATHIEU. Application de la Sériescopie aux Études Radiopelvimétriques. Bull. Soc. gynéc. et d'obst. de Paris, 1938, 27:60.

RAPPAPORT, E. M., and SCADRON, S. J. Pelviradiography and Clinical Pelvimetry. Comparative Values in the Prognosis of the Outcome of Labor. J.A.M.A., 1939, 112:2492.

REUTER, E. G., and REEVES, R. J. Roentgen Pelvimetry, a Simplified Method. Am. J. Roentgenol., 1939, 42:847.

ROBBINS, O. F. Method of Roentgen Pelvimetry; Preliminary Report. Lancet, 1937, 57:418.

SCHAFER, G. Die röntgenologische Untersuchung geburtshilflicher Fragen durch die Seitenaufnahme. Ztschr. f. Geburtsh. u. Gynäk., 1937, 115:195, 331.

SCHUMAN, W. A New Measurement (Clinical) for Estimating the Depth of the True Pelvis. Am. J. Obst. & Gynec., 1934, 28:497.

SCHUMANN, E. A. The Size and Shape of the Pelvic Inlet as Determined by Direct Measurement. Am. J. Obst. & Gynec., 1936, 32:832.

SNOW, William. Late Extrauterine Pregnancy Diagnosed by Soft Tissue Roentgenography. Am. J. Roentgenol., 1939, 41:537.

——— and ROSENSOHN, M. Roentgenologic Visualization of the Soft Tissues in Pregnancy. Am. J. Roentgenol., 1939, 42:709.

STEELE, K. B., and JAVERT, C. T. The Mechanism of Labor for Transverse Positions of the Vertex. Surg., Gynec. & Obst., 1942, 75:477.

——— Roentgenography of the Obstetric Pelvis. Am. J. Obst. & Gynec., 1942, 43:600.

——— Classification of the Obstetric Pelvis Based on Size, Mensuration and Morphology. Am. J. Obst. & Gynec., 1942, 44:783.

STEELE, Kyle B., WING, Lucius A., and MCLANE, Chas. M. A Clinical Evaluation of Stereoroentgenography of the Female Pelvis. Am. J. Obst. & Gynec., 1938, 35:938.

TENGBERGEN, J. Die Beckenmessung mittels der Redressionsmethode mit Vorführung eines dazu konstruierten Apparates. Acta radiol., 1928, Supp. 3, p. 57.

THOMS, H. Outlining the Superior Strait of the Pelvis by Means of the X-ray. Am. J. Obst. & Gynec., 1922, 4:257.

——— The Uses and Limitations of Roentgen Pelvimetry. Am. J. Obst. & Gynec., 1937, 34:150

THOMS, H. Routine Roentgen Pelvimetry in 600 Primiparous White Women Consecutively Delivered at Term. Am. J. Obst. & Gynec., 1939, 37:101.

——— The Estimation of Pelvic Capacity. Am. J. Surg., 1940, 47:691.

——— The Obstetric Pelvis. Baltimore, 1935.

——— Roentgen Pelvimetry as a Routine Prenatal Procedure. Am. J. Obst. & Gynec., 1940, 40:891.

——— The Clinical Application of Roentgen Pelvimetry and a Study of the Results in 1,100 White Women. Am. J. Obst. & Gynec., 1941, 42:957.

——— The Relation of the Sacral Promontory to the Pelvic Inlet. Am. J. Obst. & Gynec., 1943, 46:110.

——— Precision Methods in Cephalometry and Pelvimetry. Am. J. Obst. & Gynec., 1943, 46:753.

THOMS, H., and GODFRIED, M. S. The Suboccipitobregmatic Circumference. Am. J. Obst. & Gynec., 1940, 39:841.

THOMS, H., and GREULICH, W. W. A Comparative Study of Male and Female Pelves. Am. J. Obst. & Gynec., 1940, 39:56.

THOMS, H., and WILSON, H. M. Lateral Roentgenometry of the Pelvis. A Newly Modified Technic. Yale J. Biol. & Med., 1937, 9:305.

——— Practical Application of Modern Pelvimetric Methods. Yale J. Biol. & Med., 1939, 11:179.

——— Roentgen Methods for Routine Obstetrical Pelvimetry. Yale J. Biol. & Med., 1938, 10:437.

——— The Roentgenological Survey of the Pelvis. Yale J. Biol. & Med., 1941, 13:831.

THOMS, H., FOOTE, W. R., and FRIEDMAN, I. The Clinical Significance of Pelvic Variations. Am. J. Obst. & Gynec., 1939, 38:634.

TORPIN, R. Description of a New Method of Studying Placentation by Amniotic Sac Distention. Am. J. Obst. & Gynec., 1938, 35:683.

——— HOLMES, L. P., and HAMILTON, W. F. A Roentgen Pelvimeter Simplifying Thoms' Method. Radiology, 1938, 31:584.

TURNER, W. The Index of the Pelvic Brim as a Basis of Classification. J. Anat. & Physiol., London, 1885-1886, 20:125.

——— The Sachral Index in Various Races of Mankind. J. Anat. & Physiol., London, 1886, 20:317.

WAHL, F. A. Wesentliche Messpehler bie der mittels der röntgenologischen Beckenprofilaufnahme durchgefuhrten Grossenbestimmung der Conjugata vera. Arch. f. Gynäk., 1932, 151:587.

——— Spezialraster für die praktische anwendung der Segmentarstereometrie. Arch. f. Gynäk., 1939, 168:1.

WEINBERG, A., and SCADRON, S. J. The Value of Pelvioradiography in the Management of Dystocia. Am. J. Obst. & Gynec., 1943, 46:245.

WEINTRAUB, S., and SNOW, W. Roentgenologic Visualization of the Soft Structures of Pregnancy. Am. J. Roentgenol., 1939, 42:718.

WEITZNER, S. F. A Simple Roentgenographic Method for Accurately Determining the True Conjugate Diameter of the Pelvis. Am. J. Obst. & Gynec., 1935, 30:126.

WESTERGAARD, B. Stereoscopic Measurement of Distances in the Female Pelvis and on the Foetal Skull. Acta radiol., 1939, 20:33.

YOUNG, J. Relaxation of Pelvic Joints in Pregnancy: Pelvic Arthropathy of Pregnancy. J. Obst. & Gynaec. Brit. Emp., 1940, 47:493.

11

PRESENTATION AND POSITION OF THE FETUS —METHODS OF DIAGNOSIS

Irrespective of the relation which it may bear to the mother, the fetus in the later months of pregnancy assumes a characteristic posture, which is described as its *attitude* or *habitus;* and, as a general rule, it may be said to form an ovoid mass, which roughly corresponds with the shape of the uterine cavity. It is usually taught that the fetus is folded or bent upon itself in such a way that the back becomes markedly convex, the head is sharply flexed so that the chin is almost in contact with the chest, the thighs are flexed over the abdomen, the legs are bent at the knee joints, and the arches of the feet rest upon the anterior surfaces of the legs. The arms are usually crossed over the thorax or are parallel to the sides, while the umbilical cord lies in the space between them and the lower extremities. Warnekros, on the other hand, contends that the normal habitus is much less constrained, and that the contrary view is due to the fact that our conclusions have been based upon the study of frozen or hardened specimens in which the uterus has become so retracted as to exert an abnormal pressure upon its contents. In his valuable x-ray atlas, he shows that before the onset of labor the head normally occupies a position midway between flexion and extension, the back is but slightly flexed, and the extremities are relatively freely movable—in other words, the fetus, when at rest, is in an unconstrained position, analogous to that which it maintains outside of the uterus.

The attitude is frequently modified by changes in the consistency of the abdominal and uterine walls, by the abundance or lack of liquor amnii, as well as by movements of the extremities. Occasionally the head may become deflected, and a totally different posture is assumed. The characteristic attitude results partly from the mode of growth of the fetus, and partly from a process of accommodation between it and the outlines of the uterine cavity.

PRESENTATION AND POSITION OF FETUS

Presentation. By this term is understood the relation which the long axis of the fetus bears to that of the mother, and we accordingly distinguish between longitudinal and transverse presentations. Occasionally during pregnancy the fetal axis may cross the maternal axis at an angle, and thus give rise to oblique presentations; but, as these always become longitudinal or transverse during the course of labor, they need not be considered. Longitudinal presentations are noted in over 99 per cent of all labors at full term.

Considerable confusion has resulted from confounding the terms *presentation* and

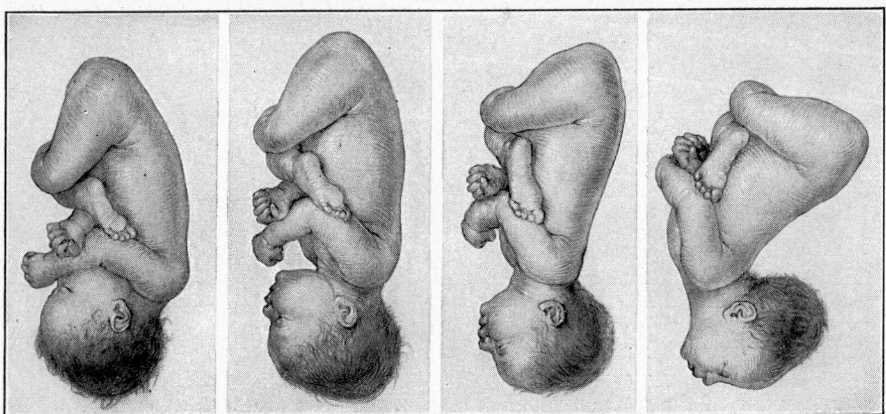

Fig. 210.—Showing Difference in Attitude of Fetus in Vertex, Sinciput, Brow and Face Presentations.

presenting part. By the latter we understand the portion of the fetus which engages at the superior strait and is felt through the cervix on vaginal examination. Accordingly, in longitudinal presentations the presenting part may be either the head or the breech, and we speak of *cephalic* or *breech presentations*, respectively. When the fetus lies with its long axis transversely, the shoulder is the presenting part, and we speak of a *transverse presentation* with the *shoulder presenting*.

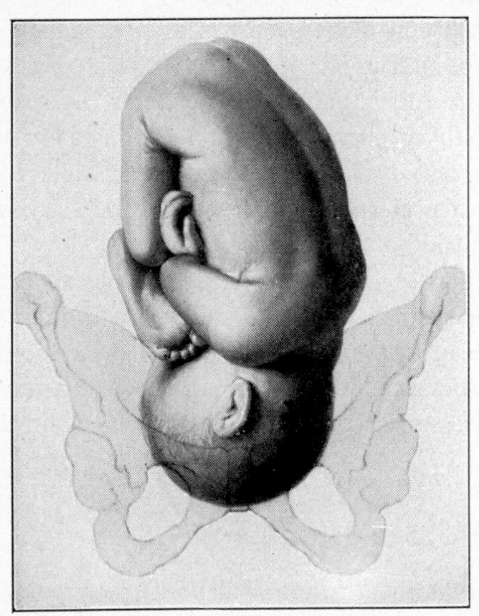

Fig. 211.—Left Occiput Anterior Position. (L. O. A.)

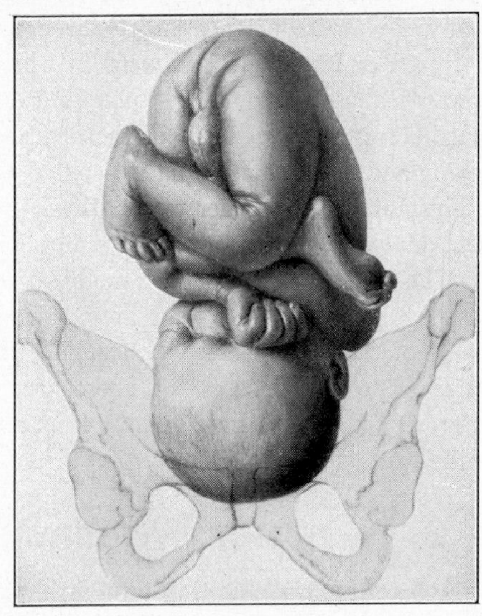

Fig. 212.—Left Occiput Posterior Position. (L. O. P.)

Cephalic presentations are divided into several groups, according to the relation which the head bears to the body of the child. Usually the head is sharply flexed, so that the chin is in contact with the thorax. In these circumstances the vertex is the presenting part—*vertex presentation*. More rarely the neck may be sharply extended, so that the occiput and back come in contact and the face engages in the superior strait—*face presentation*. Again, the head may assume a position intermediate between these extremes, being partially flexed in some cases, when the large fontanel presents—*sincipital presentation;* or partially extended in other cases, so that the brow becomes the presenting part—*brow presentation*. The last two are not usually classified as distinct varieties, as they are usually transient, and as labor progresses become converted into vertex or face presentations, by flexion or extension, respectively.

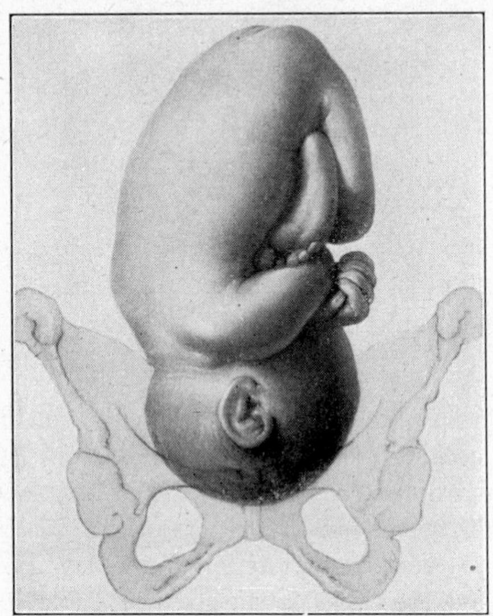

FIG. 213.—RIGHT OCCIPUT ANTERIOR POSITION. (R. O. A.)

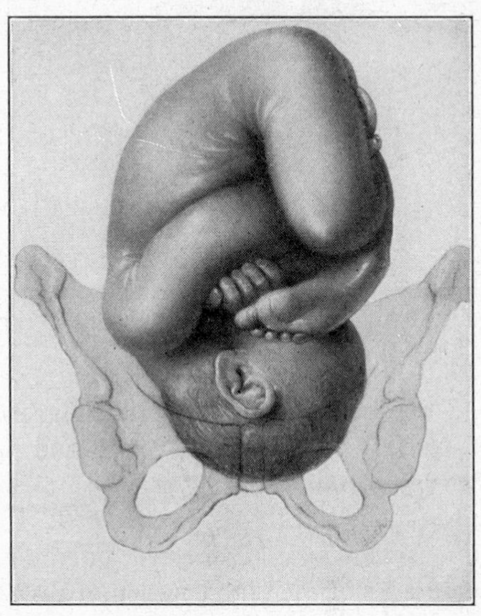

FIG. 214.—RIGHT OCCIPUT TRANSVERSE POSITION. (R. O. T.)

When the child presents by its pelvic extremity, the thighs may be flexed and the legs extended over the anterior surfaces of the body—*frank breech presentation;* again, the thighs may be flexed on the abdomen and the legs upon the thighs—*full breech presentation;* or the feet may be the lowest part—*foot* or *footling presentation*. Occasionally one leg may retain the position which is typical of one of the above-mentioned presentations, while the other foot or knee may present—*incomplete foot* or *knee presentation*. As the mechanism of labor, however, is essentially the same in all modifications of breech presentations, the several varieties need not be considered separately.

Position. By this term we designate the relation of some arbitrarily chosen portion of the child to the right or left side of the mother. Accordingly, with each presentation we have one or other of two positions—right or left. With us and in France, the occiput, chin, and sacrum are the determining points in vertex, face, and breech presentations, respectively; in Germany the child's back is the orienting portion.

Variety. Furthermore, for the purpose of still more accurate orientation, we take into consideration the relationship of some given portion of the presenting part to the anterior, transverse, or posterior portion of the mother's pelvis. Thus, as there are two positions, there will be in all six varieties for each presentation.

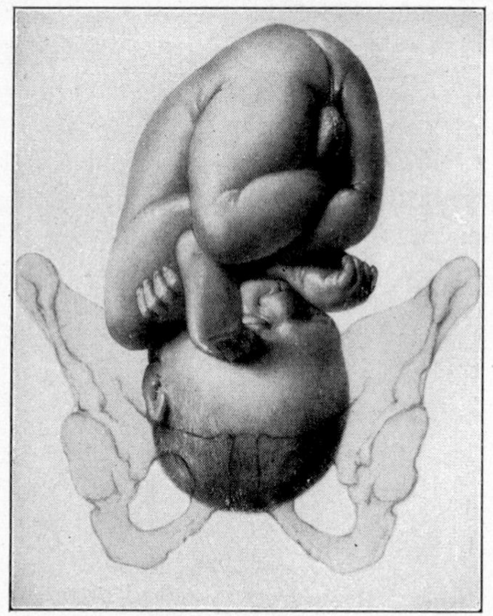

Fig. 215.—Right Occiput Posterior Position. (R. O. P.)

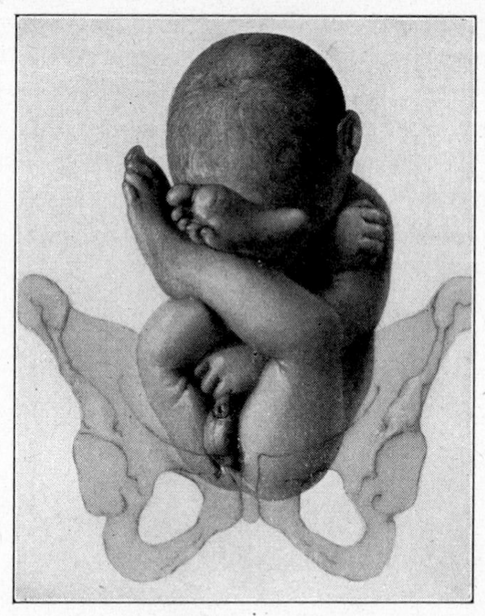

Fig. 216.—Left Sacrum Posterior Position. (L. S. P.)

Nomenclature. As the presenting part in any presentation may be either in the left or right position, we have left and right occipital, left and right mental, and left and right sacral presentations, which in an abbreviated form may be written L. O. and R. O., L. M. and R. M., L. S. and R. S. Again, as the presenting part in each of the two positions may be directed anteriorly, transversely, or posteriorly, we may have six varieties of each presentation. Thus, we have the classification given in Table 10.

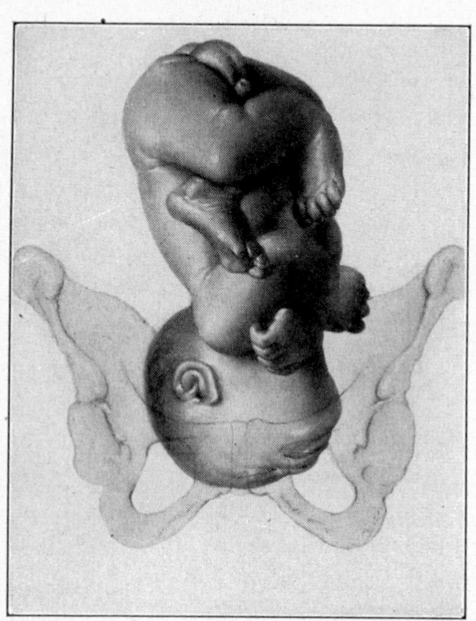

Fig. 217.—Left Mentum Anterior Position. (L. M. A.)

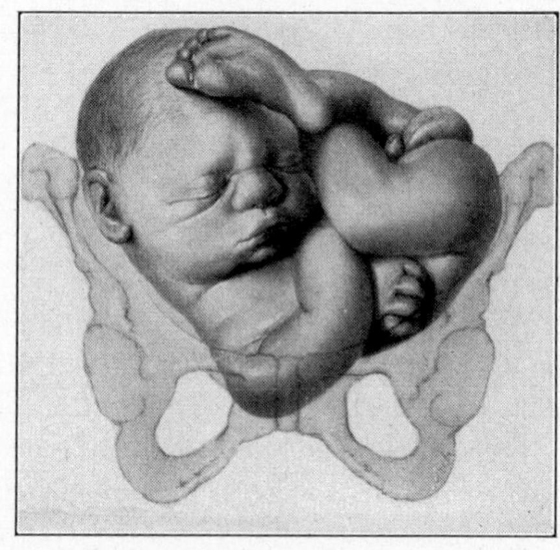

Fig. 218.—Right Acromiodorso Posterior Position. (R. A. D. P.)

This means that the acromium is to the mother's right and the back is posterior.

	Position	Presentation	Variety	Abbreviation
Vertex presentations	Left	Occiput	Anterior	L.O.A.
	"	"	Transverse	L.O.T.
	"	"	Posterior	L.O.P.
	Right	"	Anterior	R.O.A.
	"	"	Transverse	R.O.T.
	"	"	Posterior	R.O.P.
Face presentations	Left	Mentum	Anterior	L.M.A.
	"	"	Transverse	L.M.T.
	"	"	Posterior	L.M.P.
	Right	"	Anterior	R.M.A.
	"	"	Transverse	R.M.T.
	"	"	Posterior	R.M.P.
Breech presentations	Left	Sacrum	Anterior	L.S.A.
	"	"	Transverse	L.S.T.
	"	"	Posterior	L.S.P.
	Right	"	Anterior	R.S.A.
	"	"	Transverse	R.S.T.
	"	"	Posterior	R.S.P.

TABLE 10. CLASSIFICATION OF VERTEX, FACE AND BREECH PRESENTATIONS.

Frequency of the Various Presentations and Positions. According to the statistics collected by Schroeder, based upon several hundred thousand cases, the vertex presents in 95 per cent, the face in 0.6 per cent, and the breech in 3.11 per cent, transverse presentations occurring in only 0.56 per cent of all cases. Markoe, in fifty-one thousand deliveries occurring in the New York Lying-In Hospital, noted 94.2, 0.48, 3.9 and 0.9 per cent, respectively, while in the first seventy-five hundred admissions to the obstetrical service of the Johns Hopkins Hospital the incidence of the several presentations was 94.6, 0.34, 3.9, and 0.96 per cent, respectively. These figures apply to the conditions observed at or near full term, but prior to the seventh month breech and transverse presentations occur more frequently.

It is usually stated that about 70 per cent of all vertex presentations occur in the left, and only 30 per cent in the right position, and we have found 64 and 36 per cent, respectively. The former becomes more and the latter less frequent the nearer pregnancy approaches term. Naegele first pointed out that the occiput was usually directed anteriorly in left, and posteriorly in right positions, so that it is usually found at one or other extremity of the right oblique diameter of the pelvis, owing to the fact that the left oblique diameter is materially encroached upon at its posterior extremity by the rectum.

Although the incidence of breech presentation is only three per cent or slightly more at term, its frequency is much greater earlier in pregnancy. Thus, at the thirtieth week, Vartan states, one gravida in every four has a breech presentation whereas Ryder's comparable figure is one in six. The great majority of these breech cases at the thirtieth week undergo spontaneous version to a vertex presentation, usually about the thirty-second week.

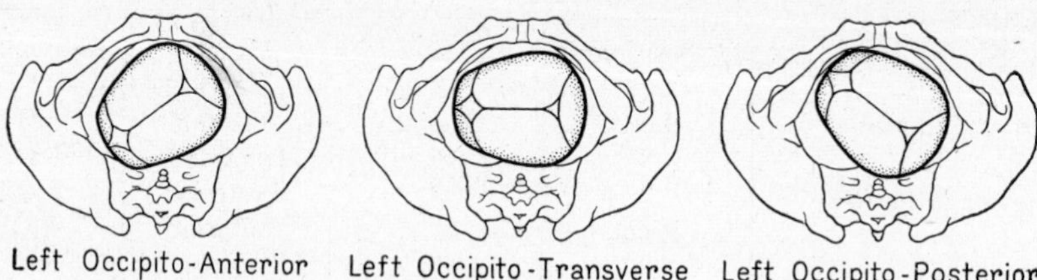

Fig. 219.—Various Left Positions in Occiput Presentations.

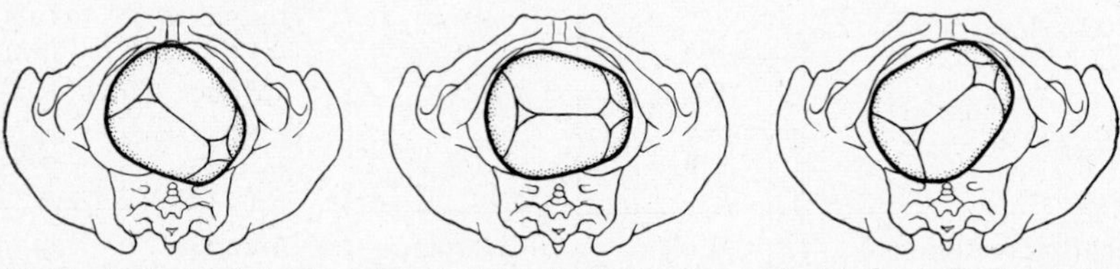

Fig. 220.—Various Right Positions in Occiput Presentations.

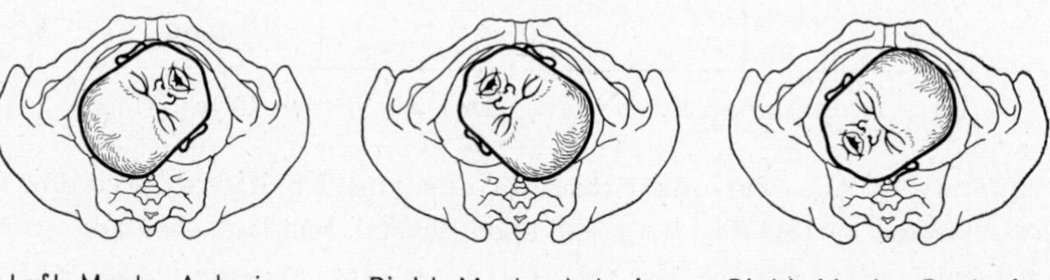

Fig. 221.—Left and Right Positions in Face Presentations.

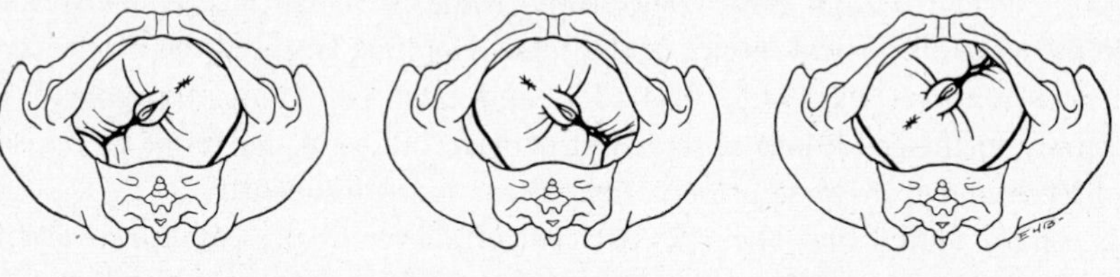

Fig. 222.—Left and Right Positions in Breech Presentations.

Reasons for the Predominance of Head Presentations. Of the several reasons which have been advanced to explain why the baby at term usually presents by the vertex, about the only tenable one seems to be the pyriform shape of the uterus. Although the measurement of the fetal head at term is slightly larger than the breech, the entire podalic pole of the fetus—that is, the breech plus its flexed extremities—is bulkier than the cephalic pole and more motile; the cephalic pole is represented by the head only, since the upper extremities are some distance removed, small and less protruding. Until about the thirty-second week the mass of amniotic fluid is large in relation to fetal mass and there is no crowding of the fetus by the uterine walls. At approximately this time, however, the ratio between amniotic fluid mass and fetal mass alters in the direction of a relative diminution in amniotic fluid. This brings the uterine walls in closer apposition to the fetal parts and it is only then that the pyriform shape of the uterus exerts its effect. The fetus, if it has been presenting by the breech, changes its polarity in order to make use of the roomier fundus for its bulkier and more motile podalic pole. The high incidence of breech presentation in hydrocephalic fetuses is in keeping with this theory, since here the cephalic pole is definitely larger than the podalic. Nor is the high frequency of breech presentations in anencephalic monsters an argument against it since such fetuses are usually premature at delivery and hydramnios is the rule.

As Vartan points out, the cause of breech presentation must be some circumstance which prevents the physiological mechanism described above from taking place. Obviously, abnormal uterine shape can play a role in rare cases only, for instance, in cases in which a septum bulges into the upper segment; otherwise, breech presentations would repeat themselves much more often than they do. Vartan believes that some peculiarity of fetal attitude, particularly extension of the vertebral column in frank breeches, may prevent the fetus from turning itself, and his series of roentgenograms of cases in which the baby did not turn and could not be turned affords convincing evidence of this contention. Another important factor, he points out, is a diminished amount of amniotic fluid.

DIAGNOSIS OF PRESENTATION AND POSITION OF FETUS

The diagnostic methods at our disposal are fourfold: abdominal palpation, vaginal and rectal touch, combined examination and auscultation, and in certain doubtful cases, the x-ray.

Obstetrical Palpation. In order to obtain satisfactory results, the examination should be made systematically by following the four maneuvers suggested by Leopold. The patient should be on a firm bed or examining table, with the abdomen bared. During the first three maneuvers the examiner stands at the side of the bed which is most convenient to him, and faces the patient, but reverses his position and faces her feet for the last maneuver (see Figs. 223 and 224).

First Maneuver. After outlining the contour of the uterus, and determining how nearly its fundus approaches the xiphoid cartilage, the fundus is gently palpated with the tips of the fingers of two hands, and the fetal pole occupying it differentiated, the breech giving the sensation of a large, irregularly shaped, nodular body, and the head that of a hard, round object which is freely movable and ballottable.

Second Maneuver. Having determined which pole of the fetus lies at the fundus, the examiner places the palmar surface of his hands on either side of the abdomen and makes gentle but deep pressure. On one side he feels a hard resistant plane—the back—and on the other numerous nodulations—the small parts. In women with thin abdominal walls the fetal extremities can readily be differentiated, but in fat persons only irregular nodulations can be felt. In the latter case, or when a considerable quantity of amniotic fluid is present, the appreciation of the back can be facilitated by making deep pressure with one hand while palpating with the other. After determining upon which side the back is situated, we next note whether it is directed anteriorly, transversely, or posteriorly, and thereby gain an exact idea of the orientation of the body.

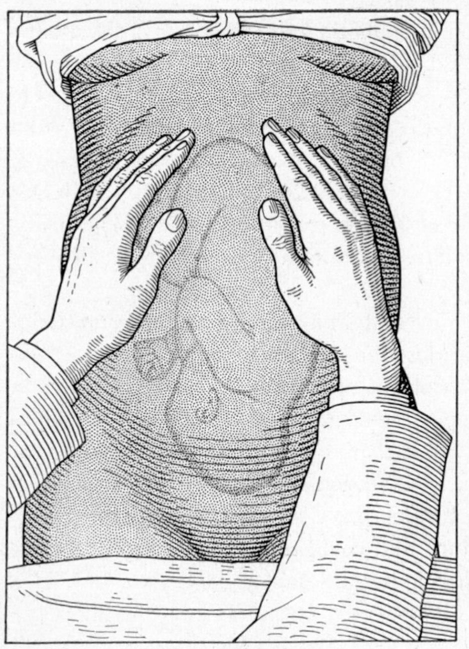

First Maneuver.

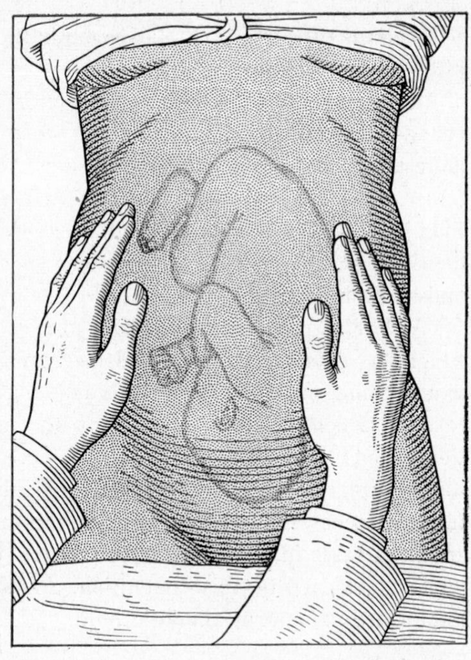

Second Maneuver.

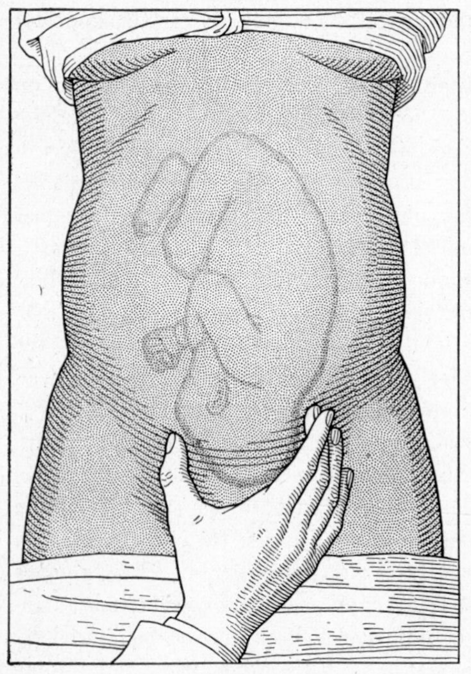

Third Maneuver.

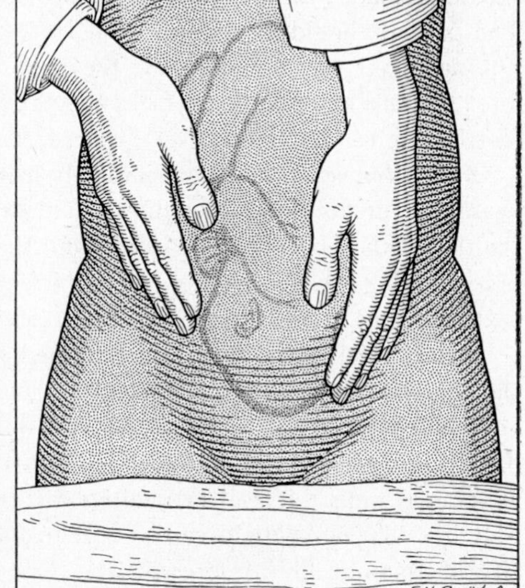

Fourth Maneuver.

Fig. 223.—Palpation in Left Occiput Anterior Position.

Third Maneuver. The examiner grasps the lower portion of the abdomen, just above the symphysis pubis, between the thumb and fingers of one hand. If the presenting part be not engaged, a movable body will be felt, which is usually the head. The differentiation between it and the breech is made as at the fundus, the former being appreciated as a hard, round, ballottable body. If the presenting part be not engaged, this practically completes the examination, as we now know the situation of the head, breech, back, and extremities, and all that remains is to determine the attitude of the head. If careful palpation shows that the greatest cephalic prominence is on the same side as the small parts, we know that the head is flexed and that the vertex is the presenting part; but when the reverse is the case we know that the head is extended and that we have a face presentation. On the other hand, if the presenting part is deeply engaged, this maneuver simply shows that the lower pole of the fetus is fixed in the pelvis, and the details concerning it are ascertained by carrying out the following instructions:

Fourth Maneuver. The examiner faces the patient's feet, and with the tips of the first three fingers of each hand, makes deep pressure in the direction of the axis of the superior strait. If the head presents, he finds that one hand is arrested sooner than the other by a rounded body, the cephalic prominence, while the other hand descends deeper into the pelvis. In vertex presentations the prominence is on the same side as the small parts, and in face presentations on the same side as the back. Again, the degree of ease with which the prominence is felt indicates the extent to which descent has occurred. In many instances, when the head has descended into the pelvis, the anterior shoulder of the child can be readily differentiated by the third maneuver. In breech presentations the information obtained from this maneuver is not so definite.

Abdominal palpation is available throughout the later months of pregnancy, and in the intervals between the pains at the time of labor. By its use we can not only determine the presentation and position of the child, but also obtain important information as to the extent to which the presenting part has descended into the pelvis. For example, we know so long as the cephalic prominence is readily palpable that the vertex has not descended to the level of the ischial spines; whereas, when it can no longer be palpated from above, the head has descended so deeply that its most dependent part can be palpated through the pelvic floor. Moreover, when there is disproportion between the size of the head and the pelvis, its seriousness can be gauged by determining the extent to which the anterior portion of the head overrides the symphysis pubis. Likewise, with practice, it is possible to estimate roughly the size of the child, while in twin pregnancy the second fetus can be mapped out and its presentation determined.

During uterine contractions, on carefully palpating in the region of the internal abdominal ring, one can often distinguish a rounded cord on either side—the *round ligaments*—from which important information may be obtained. In the first place, the intensity of their contraction gives some idea of the manner in which the uterus is acting; second, by noting their course, it is possible to diagnose the situation of the placenta in about 80 per cent of all cases. Leopold and Palm showed that when the round ligaments converge toward the fundus of the uterus, the placenta is usually situated upon the posterior wall, whereas it is upon the anterior wall when they are parallel or diverging.

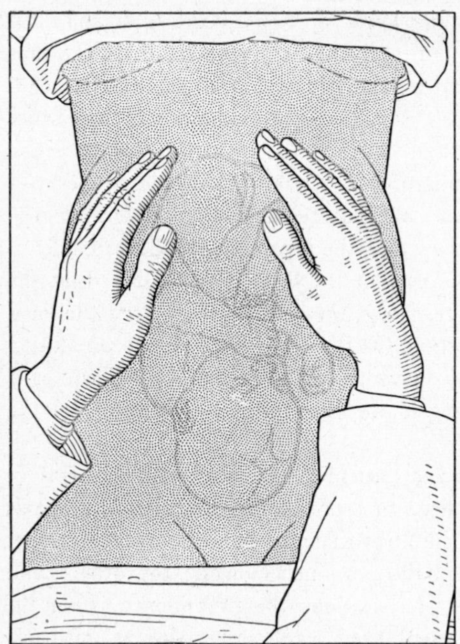

First Maneuver.

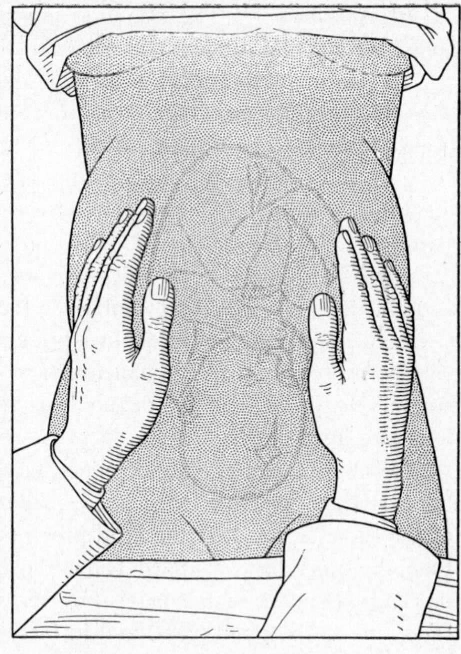

Second Maneuver.

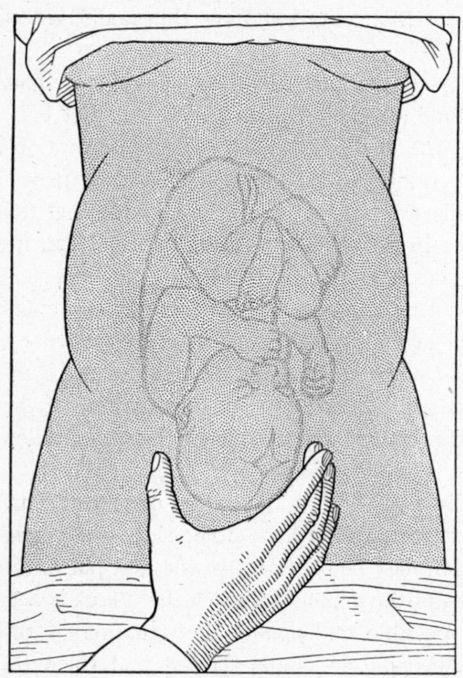

Third Maneuver.

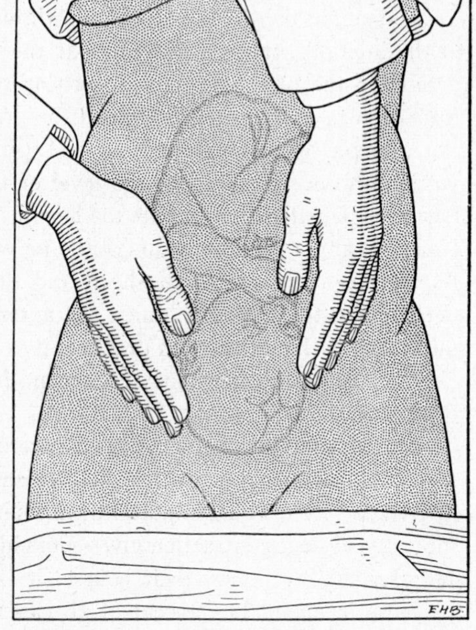

Fourth Maneuver.

Fig. 224.—Palpation in Right Occiput Posterior Position.

During labor, palpation also gives us valuable information concerning the *lower uterine segment;* when there exists some obstruction to the passage of the child, the *contraction ring* may be felt as a transverse or oblique ridge extending across the lower portion of the uterus. Moreover, even in normal cases, we can differentiate, by palpation, between the contracting body of the uterus and the passive lower uterine segment; for during a pain the former presents a firm, hard sensation, while the latter appears elastic and almost fluctuant.

Vaginal Examination. During pregnancy the results arrived at by vaginal examination, concerning the presentation and position of the child, are necessarily somewhat inconclusive, for, as the cervix is still closed, one is obliged to palpate the presenting part through the lower uterine segment. During labor, on the other hand, after more or less complete dilatation of the cervix, important information may be obtained. In vertex presentations the position and variety are determined by the differentiation of the various sutures and fontanels; in face presentations, by the differentiation of the various portions of the face; and in breech presentations, by the palpation of the sacrum and ischial tuberosities.

Under the most favorable circumstances the information to be derived from vaginal touch alone is not more accurate than that obtained by abdominal palpation, and in vertex presentations the fontanels are frequently mistaken for one another, and occasionally face and breech presentations escape differentiation. Moreover, later in labor, after the formation of the *caput succedaneum,* detection of the various diagnostic points often becomes impossible.

A much more serious objection, however, is the danger of puerperal infection, no matter how careful one's technic may be; for it is now generally admitted that absolute hand disinfection cannot be effected, and, even granting that the use of sterile rubber gloves overcomes this difficulty, the gloved fingers may still carry up into the vagina pathogenic micro-organisms from the margins of the vulva, and thus give rise to infection.

Accordingly, it is advisable to limit vaginal examination during labor, and in normal cases to do away with it altogether. For, if the preliminary examination has shown that the patient has a normal pelvis and presents no other abnormality, and we find by the fourth maneuver that the head is deeply engaged, all that we gain by vaginal examination is information as to the degree of dilatation of the cervix and the condition of the membranes, and this can usually be ascertained equally well by rectal examination. As a result, vaginal examination becomes absolutely necessary only in the few cases in which palpation and rectal examination do not give satisfactory results, or in patients presenting some abnormality, or in whom the course of labor is unduly delayed.

In attempting to determine the presentation and position by vaginal examination, it is advisable to pursue a definite routine, which is readily accomplished by three maneuvers (Figs. 225 and 226).

First Maneuver. After appropriate preparation of the patient, two fingers of either the right or left gloved hand, as best suits the examiner, are introduced into the vagina and carried up to the presenting part. A few moments suffice to determine whether it is a vertex, face or breech.

Second Maneuver. If the vertex be presenting, the fingers are carried up behind the symphysis pubis, and are then swept backward over the head toward the sacrum.

During this movement they necessarily cross the sagittal suture. When it is felt, its course is outlined, and we know that the small fontanel must lie at one end and the large fontanel at the other end of it.

Third Maneuver. We then attempt to determine the position of the two fontanels. For this purpose the fingers are passed to the anterior extremity of the sagittal suture, and the fontanel there encountered is carefully examined and identified; then, by a cir-

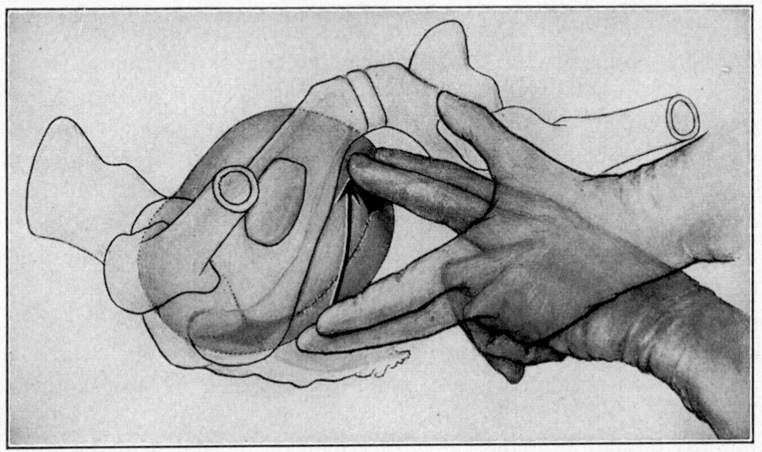

FIG. 225.—LOCATING THE SAGITTAL SUTURE ON VAGINAL EXAMINATION.

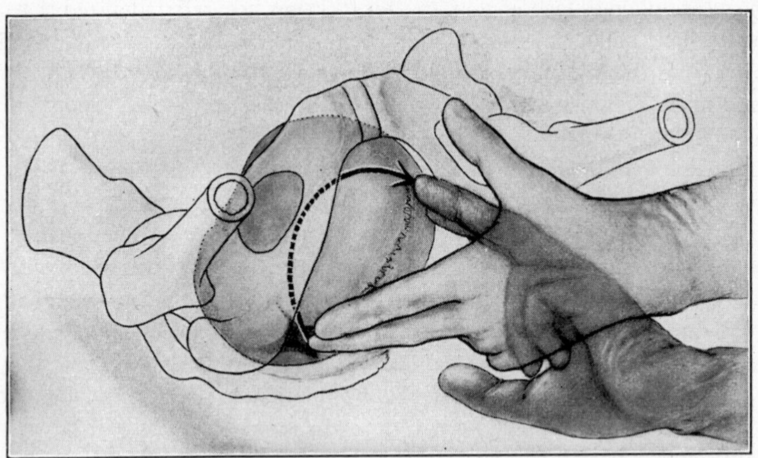

FIG. 226.—DIFFERENTIATING THE FONTANELS ON VAGINAL EXAMINATION.

cular motion, the fingers are passed around the side of the head until the other fontanel is felt and differentiated. By this means the various sutures and fontanels are readily located, and the possibility of error is considerably lessened. In face and breech presentations it is still further minimized, as the various parts are more readily distinguished.

Combined Examination. By combined examination we understand the introduction of two fingers of one hand into the vagina, and the application of the other hand over the lower portion of the abdomen. This method is rarely employed except when the presenting part is not engaged, and the external hand is used to fix it so as to permit the internal fingers to explore it satisfactorily, as well as to determine the existence of disproportion between the size of the head and the superior strait and its degree.

Auscultation. By itself, auscultation does not give very important information as to the presentation and position of the child, but it sometimes reinforces the results obtained by palpation. Ordinarily, the heart sounds are transmitted through the convex portion of the fetus, which lies in intimate contact with the uterine wall. Accordingly they are best heard through the back in vertex and breech, and through the thorax in face presentations. The region of the abdomen in which the fetal heart is heard most plainly varies according to the presentation and the extent to which the presenting part has descended. In head presentations the point of maximum intensity is usually midway between the umbilicus and the anterior superior spine of the ilium, while in breech presentations it is usually about on a level with the umbilicus.

Auscultation frequently gives us not a little supplementary aid in determining the position of the child. Thus, in occipito-anterior positions the heart is usually best heard a short distance from the middle line; in the transverse varieties it is heard more laterally, and in the posterior varieties well back in the patient's flank. Occasionally, however, in obliquely posterior positions, the information gained from the location of the fetal heart is misleading, and may give rise to serious diagnostic errors; for if the flexion of the head be imperfect, the thorax may become convex, in which event the heart sounds may be transmitted through it and lead one to suppose that one has to deal with an obliquely anterior position.

X-ray. With the increasing perfection of x-ray apparatus, we have gained another diagnostic aid which is of particular value in doubtful cases. In fat women, or those with abdominal walls so rigid as to make palpation difficult, a well-taken plate may clear up many diagnostic difficulties and enable us to recognize the existence of a breech or transverse presentation, which otherwise might have escaped detection until late in labor.

BIBLIOGRAPHY

Barnum, C. G. The Effect of Gravitation on the Presentation and Position of the Foetus. J.A.M.A., 1915, 64:498.

Duncan, J. M. The Position of the Foetus. Researches in Obstetrics. Edinburgh, 1868, pp. 14-37; also Edinb. M. & S. J., 1855.

Griffith, W. S. A. An Investigation of the Causes which Determine the Lie of the Foetus in Utero. J. Obst. & Gynaec. Brit. Emp., 1915, 27:105.

Hecker, C. Statistisches aus der Gebäranstalt München. Arch. f. Gynaek., 1882, 20:378.

International Medical Congress. Uniformity in Obstetrical Nomenclature. Am. J. Obst., 1887, 20:1084.

La Chapelle. Pratique des Accouchements. Paris, 1821, T. 1, pp. 17.

Leopold and Spörlin. Die Leitung der regelmässigen Geburten nur durch äussere Untersuchung. Arch. f. Gynaek., 1894, 45:337.

Markoe, J. W. Observations and Statistics on Sixty Thousand Labors, etc. Bull. N. Y. Lying-in Hosp., 1909, 6:101-115.

Müller, A. Ueber die Ursachen der Ungleichheit und Unklarheit in der Benennung und Einteilung der Kindeslagen. Monatsch. f. Geburtsh. u. Gynaek., 1900, 12:161, 266.

Naegele, H. F. J. Die Lehre vom Mechanismus der Geburt Nebst Beitragen zur Geschichte Derselben. Mainz, 1838.

Palm, R. Ueber die Diagnose des Placentarsitzes in der Schwangerschaft, etc. Ztschr. f. Geburtsh. u. Gynäk., 1893, 25:317.

Ryder, G. H. External Cephalic Version in Treatment of Breech Presentations. M. Rec., 1944, 157:601.

Schatz, F. Ueber den Schwerpunkt der Frucht. Zentralbl. f. Gynäk., 1900, 24:1033.

——— Die Ursachen der Kindeslagen. Arch. f. Gynaek., 1904, 71:541.

Schultze, B. S. Untersuchungen über den Wechsel der Lage und Stellung des Kindes in den letzten Wochen der Schwangerschaft, Leipzig, 1868.

Seitz, L. Ueber den Einfluss der Schwerkraft auf die Entstehung der Schädellagen. Arch. f. Gynaek., 1908, 86:114.

Sellheim, H. Exp. und vergleichend physiologische Untersuchungen über die Entwicklung der typischen Fruchtlage. Arch. f. Gynaek., 1917, 106:1.

Simpson, J. W. Attitude and Position of the Foetus *in utero*. Month. J. Med. Sc., 1848-1849, 9:423, 639, 863.

Tompkins, P. An Inquiry into the Causes of Breech Presentation. Am. J. Obst. & Gynec., 1946, 51:595.

Vartan, C. K. The Behavior of the Fetus in utero with Special Reference to the Incidence of Breech Presentation at Term. J. Obst. & Gynaec. Brit. Emp., 1945, 52:417.

Warnekros, K. Schwerkraft und Kopflage. Arch. f. Gynaek., 1919, 111:21.

——— Schwangerschaft und Geburt in Roentgenbilde. München, 1921.

12

PRENATAL CARE

From a biological point of view, pregnancy and labor represent the highest function of the female reproductive system, and a priori should be considered as a normal process. But when we recall the manifold changes which occur in the maternal organism, it is apparent that the borderline between health and disease is less distinctly marked during gestation than at other times, and derangements, so slight as to be of but little consequence under ordinary circumstances, may readily be the precursors of pathological conditions which may seriously threaten the life of the mother or the child, or both.

It accordingly becomes necessary to keep pregnant patients under strict supervision, and to be constantly on the alert for the appearance of untoward symptoms. In all cases the services of an obstetrician should be engaged early in pregnancy, as upon him devolves the duty of advising the patient as to her mode of life during the months preceding labor.

Unless it be found upon inquiry that the patient has been leading an ill-ordered existence, very little change should be made in her mode of living, and she should be encouraged to go on much as usual, care being taken that she receives the proper amount of exercise, amusement and diversion. It is the duty of the physician to gain the confidence of his patient and encourage her to come to him whenever anything occurs to worry her, instead of taking advice from her women friends. A woman in her first pregnancy generally stands in need of a certain amount of reassurance with regard to the dangers of parturition, and the knowledge that she is in the hands of a competent and careful physician will contribute largely to her peace of mind as well as to her physical well-being.

One of the creditable achievements of American obstetrics consists in the development of so-called "prenatal care." The term has a wider application than the words imply, and may be defined as such supervision and care of the pregnant, parturient and puerperal woman as will enable her to pass through the dangers of pregnancy and labor with the least possible risk, to give birth to a living child, and to be discharged in such condition that she may be able to suckle it and thus afford it the greatest prospect of attaining maturity, as well as to fulfill her duties as mother and housewife with a minimal amount of invalidism.

Prior to the rise of present-day obstetrics, the physician usually had but one interview with his patient before he saw her in labor, and often at this interview merely sought to compute the expected date of confinement. When he next saw her, she might be in the throes of an eclamptic convulsion or striving vainly to overcome the resistance offered by a contracted pelvis. It is in the prevention of such calamities as these that care and supervision of the pregnant woman has been found to be of such value. Indeed, prenatal care is an absolute necessity if a substantial number of women are to avoid disaster; and it is helpful to all. The patient should be seen as early in pregnancy as possible and every four weeks thereafter until the seventh month; she should then make visits every two weeks until the last month during which it is most important that she be seen every week.

GENERAL PROCEDURE

Definitions. Certain terms are routinely employed to indicate the childbearing experience of any given patient and these must be clearly delineated.

A *gravida* is a pregnant woman. A *primigravida* is one pregnant for the first time. A *secundigravida* is one who is pregnant for the second time. A *multigravida* is a woman who has been pregnant several times.

A *primipara* is a woman who has delivered one viable child. Usage of this term, however, is not entirely uniform and in a loose way it is sometimes employed interchangeably with primigravida.

A *multipara* is a woman who has had two or more children. The word *pluripara* is a synonym for *multipara*. The word *gravida* refers to a pregnancy regardless of its duration. The word *para* refers to past pregnancies that have gone to the period of viability. A patient is a primigravida, or gravida I, and para O during her first pregnancy. She becomes a primipara when she delivers a fetus which has been viable whether or not the child is dead or alive at birth. During her second pregnancy she is a secundigravida, or gravida II, and at the same time she is a primipara, or para I. If a patient after two abortions then becomes pregnant, she is gravida III, para O. When she delivers a viable baby she is a gravida III, para I, and so on. The terms *gravida* and *para* refer to pregnancies and not to fetuses. Hence, a woman who delivers twins at the end of her first pregnancy is still para I.

In certain clinics it is customary to summarize the past obstetrical history of a patient by a series of digits connected by dashes, thus: 6-1-2-6. The first digit refers to the number of full-term infants the patient has delivered, the second digit to the number of premature infants, the third digit to the number of abortions the patient has had, and the fourth to the number of children now alive. Thus, the above example would indicate that the patient has had six full-term deliveries, one premature delivery, two abortions, and has six children at the present time. This gives a more complete picture than the mere statement that she is para VII.

A *parturient* is a woman in labor.

A *puerpera* is a woman who has just given birth.

The History. The name and address of the patient, her age and parity, and the date of the last menstrual period are recorded and the date of delivery estimated. Inquiries are made regarding the family history, with special reference to any condition likely to affect childbearing, such as hereditary disease, tuberculosis or multiple pregnancy. The personal history of the patient is then reviewed not only in regard to previous diseases and operations, but particularly in relation to any difficulties experienced in previous pregnancies and labors, such as miscarriages, prolonged labor, death of infant, hemorrhage and other complications. Inquiry is then made into the history of the present pregnancy, especially in relation to nausea, edema of the feet or face, headache, disturbances of sight, vaginal bleeding, constipation, breathlessness, sleeplessness, cramps, heartburn, lower abdominal pain, vaginal discharge and varicose veins. A suitable form for recording these particulars is usually employed. Obstetricians, hospital clinics, and organizations usually have their own forms for recording these details.

The General Medical Examination. This includes weighing the patient, taking the blood pressure, inspecting the teeth and throat and making an examination by auscultation and percussion of the heart and lungs. Opportunity is taken at this time to inspect the breasts and nipples, particularly in relation to their suitability for subsequent nursing. From an obstetric viewpoint, the most important part of the general medical examination is the taking of the blood pressure, both systolic and diastolic. This is usually carried out first, and should always be done whenever the patient is seen on subsequent visits. As will be explained subsequently, any substantial increase in blood pressure indicates one of the most serious complications in pregnancy—toxemia.

The Obstetric Examination. The obstetric examination is comprised of three parts: (1) palpation and auscultation of the abdomen; (2) estimation of pelvic measurements; and (3) vaginal examination. Palpation and auscultation of the abdomen yield valuable information concerning the size and position of the fetus. The great importance of careful pelvic mensuration has already been emphasized, while the purpose of the vaginal examination (aside from its use in the diagnosis of pregnancy) is to rule out abnormalities of the birth canal (particularly those which might impede labor), and to take the diagonal conjugate measurement.

Laboratory Tests. The most important laboratory tests carried out in prenatal care are the urine examination, the blood test for syphilis, the estimation of the hemoglobin and the Rh determination. At the first and second examinations the urine is tested for albumin and sugar and at all subsequent examinations for albumin. If the patient brings the specimen from home she should be instructed to collect a part of the first urine voided in the morning. The blood for the Wassermann or other syphilis test is obtained by venipuncture, and a portion of this same blood may be employed for Rh and hemoglobin estimation. Since many pregnant women develop anemia, the latter examination is highly important. A metabolism test is routine in the practice of some obstetricians.

Return Visits. At return visits careful inquiry is made into the general well-being of the patient, and questions are asked concerning any untoward signs and symptoms such as edema of the fingers or face, bleeding, constipation and headache. The patient is then weighed, her blood pressure is taken and the urine is analyzed for albumin. While an abdominal examination is usually carried out at this time, some physicians limit their abdominal examinations, insofar as return visits are concerned, to the later months.

Instructions to Patients. After the routine examination, the patient is instructed regarding diet, rest and sleep, daily intestinal elimination, proper exercise, fresh air and sunshine, bathing, clothing, recreation and dental care. It is usually possible, and always desirable, to assure the patient that the findings on examination were normal, and that she may anticipate an uneventful pregnancy followed by an uncomplicated delivery. At the same time, however, she is tactfully instructed regarding certain danger signals which demand immediate report to the doctor. These symptoms are as follows:

1. Vaginal bleeding, no matter how slight
2. Swelling of the face or fingers
3. Severe continuous headache
4. Dimness or blurring of vision
5. Pain in the abdomen
6. Persistent vomiting
7. Chills and fever
8. Sudden escape of fluid from the vagina

DIET IN PREGNANCY

Total Caloric Intake. In normal pregnancy the diet should be no more or less than that to which the patient has been accustomed unless weight gain is excessive. As shown in Table 11, the Food and Nutrition Board of the National Research Council recommends no increase in caloric intake, which should be in the neighborhood of 2,500 calories a day. It is true that the increased metabolic rate of later pregnancy would ordinarily call for augmentation of caloric intake, but this is counterbalanced, or more than counterbalanced in many cases, by diminished activity.

Nutrients	Nonpregnant	Pregnant (Latter Period)	Lactating
Calories	2500	2500	3000
Protein (Gm.)	60	85	100
Calcium (mg.)	0.8	1.5	2.0
Iron (mg.)	12	15	15
Vitamin A (I. U.)	5000	6000	8000
Thiamin (mg.)	1.5	1.8	2.3
Ascorbic acid (mg.)	70	100	150
Riboflavin (mg.)	2.2	2.5	3.0
Nicotinic acid (mg.)	15	18	23
Vitamin D (I. U.)	+	400-800	400-800

TABLE 11. DAILY ALLOWANCES OF SPECIFIC NUTRIENTS FOR THE NONPREGNANT, PREGNANT AND LACTATING WOMAN.

Recommendations of the Food and Nutrition Board of the National Research Council (1941).

Curtailment of Weight Gain. Excessive weight gain in pregnancy is highly undesirable from a number of viewpoints, and increasing emphasis is being laid on the importance of curtailing weight increment to 25 pounds at the most, or better, to 20 pounds. In Dieckmann's opinion, weight gain should be limited to 8 kg., or about 18 pounds; and to this end he employs, with the aid of dietitians, an 1,800 calorie diet. The more one practices obstetrics, the more one is convinced that an excessive weight gain in pregnancy is the cause of no end of complications, both major and minor. However, to keep weight gain down to 20 pounds may be difficult in many cases and will require careful dietary control and not a little discipline. It is an end, however, much to be desired.

General Character of Diet. If the patient is already eating a well-balanced variety of foods including an ample amount of meat, green vegetables, fruits, brown cereals and milk, there is no need for change. In general, however, the diet of the pregnant woman should include as a minimum daily intake one quart of milk, one serving of meat, fish or chicken, with liver once a week, one egg, three to four slices of a dark, whole grain or enriched bread, two to three servings of vegetables, of which one should be raw and one green or yellow, one or two servings of fruit, one of which should be a citrus fruit, and one to two tablespoons of butter or fortified margarine, with sufficient additional foods to make up her total caloric needs.

Protein. As pointed out by P. F. Williams and many other authors, the pregnant woman differs from other persons in her protein requirements. To the basic need of the nonpregnant woman for material building and repair there is added during pregnancy the demand of an increased metabolism, fetal growth and repair, the growth of the uterus, the increased blood volume and the development of mammary tissue. The increased protein requirements of the pregnant woman are emphasized by the increased allowance recommended by the Food and Nutrition Board of the National Research Council, namely, 85 gm. for the average pregnant woman and 100 gm. for the average lactating woman as compared with 60 gm. for the nonpregnant woman of equal weight. At least two thirds of the protein requirement in gestation should be supplied by animal protein such as meat, milk, eggs, cheese, poultry and fish, since these furnish all the essential amino acids in highly beneficial form. The remaining one third of the protein requirements may be made up of vegetable proteins, such as occur in beans, peas and cereals of whole grain, especially wheat.

Many surveys have been made of the protein intakes of various groups and indicate that inadequate protein consumption is a common dietary lapse throughout the country. They indicate, moreover, that it is a common cause of anemia and may possibly have some bearing also on the development of certain other complications such as toxemia, edema and prematurity. As already pointed out, the iron lost in nine menstrual periods is less than the additional iron required by tissue growth in pregnancy, and in the last three months the demands are especially great. On the basis of extensive studies Coons has concluded that under fairly ideal conditions of diet and well-being it seems possible for the maternal organism to assimilate during the period of pregnancy enough iron from food to supply the newborn infant with the needed reserves but that the margin of safety is very small. She feels that only the best diets are capable of supplying the iron demands of pregnancy, while poor diets, particularly when associated with gastro-intestinal disturbances such as hyperemesis, are inadequate. In this connection Bethell, Gardiner and McKinnon found that when the daily intake of animal protein fell below 50 gm., the incidence of anemia rose rapidly with increasing deficiency of animal protein and reached 40 per cent of the patients studied when the daily animal protein intake was below 30 gm.

The role which inadequate protein consumption may play in causing the toxemias of pregnancy is much less clear-cut and, indeed, is doubted by many authorities including Dieckmann. Strauss has long contended that a diet low in protein may be a cause of toxemia of pregnancy. He feels that with a dietary protein deficiency the fetus draws on the maternal organism for its dietary factors, including its protein precursors. If the mother's protein intake has been barely sufficient for her own economy, the depletion of her protein in the last trimester of pregnancy would be pronounced, using up the various protein reserves and finally the plasma protein. When the plasma protein becomes depleted, of course, the balance between the intracapillary hydrostatic pressure and the colloid osmotic pressure of the blood becomes disturbed; as a result, an excess of extracellular tissue fluid, or edema, presents itself, with a consequent disturbance in the electrolyte balance and a resulting inefficiency in the liver and kidney function, elevation of blood pressure and other signs of specific toxemia of pregnancy.

As will be explained when the toxemias of pregnancy are considered, decided hypoproteinemia can rarely be demonstrated in these disorders and when present probably plays only an auxiliary role in augmenting the degree of edema. Dieckmann states that he did not find any correlation between the serum protein concentration and the amount of edema. Only 16 per cent of preeclamptic and 12 per cent of the eclamptic women whom he studied showed a serum protein concentration at the edema level or lower, indicating that the edema in the majority of toxemic women was not occasioned by hypoproteinemia. Kooser found a median protein intake of 45 gm. daily in one group of women among 4,000 obstetric patients of the Frontier Nursing Services in Kentucky. This must be regarded as a very low dietary intake of protein, and yet but 3 per cent incidence of all types of toxemia and 0.2 per cent incidence of eclampsia were observed.

Minerals. Experimental evidence indicates that 13 or more mineral elements are essential for human nutrition. Calcium, phosphorus, iron and iodine have been studied the most extensively, and it is believed that if these are provided in sufficient amounts the other nine or so will also be present in sufficient quantities. Actually, since phosphorus is an almost invariable constituent of protein, a sufficiency of the latter is a guarantee of an adequacy of the former. Except in regions of endemic goitre, iodine need receive no special consideration. In such areas the use of iodized salt is usually recommended.

The calcium content of the fetus at term is about 25 gm. This requires an average utilization of 0.08 gm. daily throughout pregnancy. However, almost two thirds of the fetal calcium is deposited during the last month and, as a consequence, considerable storage of calcium must take place in the early months of gestation if the drain of the last month is to be withstood without depletion of maternal stores. Authorities agree that the normal nonpregnant adult requires 0.68 gm. of calcium a day. To avoid robbing the tissues of the mother and to assure storage, an ample excess over these combined requirements should be provided, and the amount recommended is 1.5 gm. daily. The calcium in one quart of milk (1.2 gm.), together with the quantity consumed in other foods, meets this need.

There is some evidence that the calcium and phosphorus in milk are more valuable than that from other foods and that it is difficult, if not practically impossible, to supply in other foods or in medicinal form amounts comparable to those which can be supplied readily in milk. The calcium of milk, moreover, is more effectively utilized than that ingested in other forms and, in addition, the milk provides proteins of especial nutritive value.

The increased iron requirements of the pregnant woman have been emphasized on page 218. To meet these, the National Research Council recommends a daily intake of 15 mg. daily. If at all possible, this quantity of iron should be provided by natural foods, because absorbability of iron derived from animal protein and certain green vegetables is much greater than is true of medicinal iron. For instance, only about 15 per cent of the iron in ferrous sulfate is absorbed, whereas the iron in liver is utilized to the extent of 45 per cent (Goodman and Gilman). The foods which contribute mainly to the iron content of the diet are red meats (especially liver), green vegetables, whole wheat, egg yolk, carrots and fruits, and the importance of these should be stressed in any diet list given to gravidae.

Vitamins. The importance of the relationship of the vitamins to reproduction is becoming more apparent. Unfortunately the problem is still largely in the animal experimentation stage. Most of the knowledge regarding the relation of vitamins to pregnancy we have obtained from laboratory investigations on animals.

All investigators seem to be agreed that vitamin A is essential to the individual for the maintenance of body resistance to infection. In pregnancy this is of the utmost importance when we consider the incidence of intercurrent diseases such as pneumonia and pyelitis, as well as the danger of infection during labor and the puerperium. Although, according to Burton and Balmain, this vitamin may have no prophylactic value with regard to puerperal infection, we must conclude that a marked deficiency in vitamin A will result in lowered body resistance to such an infection. Lund and Kimble observed that with the advancement of pregnancy there occurred a decrease in the plasma vitamin A values, the appearance of which may be delayed by the amount of the vitamin in the diet. They noted less complications of gestation and parturition, and a decreased puerperal morbidity, with adequate plasma vitamin A levels than when a deficiency exists, although they are careful not to attribute definitely the unfavorable effects to a vitamin A deficiency, as many other factors may be involved. Byrn and Eastman, on the other hand, found the incidence of obstetrical complications unaffected by levels of vitamin A below 50 International Units (I.U.) per 100 ml. of maternal plasma. Bodansky and his associates suggest that the decrease in the maternal plasma vitamin A level during pregnancy may be due to storage in the fetal liver and utilization by the fetus. Dieckmann and co-workers, likewise, report no marked differences in the complications of pregnancy and labor following addition of calcium, phosphorus, iron and vitamins A and D to the diet. However, they point out that a large enough number of patients to permit definite conclusions has not been studied and that unquestionably an adequate diet predisposes to a normal pregnancy and healthy offspring.

Milk and dairy products containing butter fat are good sources of vitamin A and provitamin A (carotene), while the latter is found abundantly in green leafy and yellow vegetables and yellow fruits. According to Lund and Kimble, an adequate diet, based on accepted standards, provides the necessary amount of vitamin A required during the first third of pregnancy, but should be supplemented with 5,000 to 10,000 I.U. of this vitamin daily during the later months.

Vitamin B complex includes various fractions essential to proper nutrition: vitamin B_1 or thiamin, riboflavin, nicotinic acid, pantothenic acid, and B_6 or pyridoxine. Thiamin (B_1) is the antineuritic vitamin, while riboflavin and nicotinic acid are antipellagric factors, referred to sometimes as B_2 complex. It has been shown that an abundant supply of B_1 is essential to the pregnant woman, as the offspring readily depletes her reserve of this all-important dietary factor. A deficiency in B_1 may lead to a polyneuritis with fatal outcome. As the modern American diet is often lacking in this vitamin, due to the method of preparation of such articles of food as cereals, as well as to the fact that the meat and milk used by the patient are obtained from animals on feeds low in B_1, it is often necessary to supply the vitamin separately. It is also to be borne in mind that lack of vitamins A and B, predisposes to infections.

Riboflavin appears to be essential to the formation of an enzyme necessary for tissue oxidation, while nicotinic acid definitely prevents pellagra. As riboflavin and nicotinic acid are absolute essentials in the diet, the pregnant patient should take plenty of the natural foods containing them, such as meat, milk, eggs and green vegetables.

Such conditions as pyloric obstruction and bleeding in the babies, an increased incidence of postpartum hemorrhage in the mothers and a tendency toward anemia and atrophy of the ovaries, have been ascribed to deficiencies in the B complex. These observations then may be further reasons for ensuring an adequate supply of these vitamins for the pregnant woman. During lactation from three to five times more of vitamin B complex is required, according to Sure, and Evans and Burr.

The water-soluble vitamin C, or ascorbic acid, the absence of which results in scurvy, appears necessary for the proper development of the offspring. Ingier observed that in guinea pigs a deficiency of vitamin C was followed by stillborn offspring, often premature or underdeveloped. Even on slight deficiencies in vitamin C, pregnant guinea pigs will show an anemia and lowered calcium content of the tooth pulp according to Reyher, Walkhoff and Walkhoff. The quantitative estimation of ascorbic acid in the urine, following a tolerance test with vitamin C, furnishes an index of vitamin C deficiency. Such estimations, as well as plasma vitamin C determinations, conducted on women at various stages of gestation indicate the tendency toward a reserve deficiency and emphasize the need of an abundant supply of this vitamin throughout pregnancy. Lund and Kimble noted that the plasma vitamin C level reflects the amount in the diet and that an adequate level can be maintained throughout pregnancy by a daily diet containing fresh citrus fruits or tomatoes or berries.

Vitamin D, the antirachitic vitamin, is also essential during pregnancy. Hess is of the opinion that vitamin D, given during the pregnant period, has only slight value in preventing subsequent rickets in the children. However, from our knowledge of its relation to calcium and phosphorus metabolism, we cannot doubt that vitamin D is of great importance in safeguarding the mother and her offspring during the gestation period. This is to be borne in mind particularly where exposure to sunshine is limited, in which event vitamin D, in the form of cod-liver oil or some other product, may be administered. It must be pointed out, however, that there is some evidence indicating that too much calcium and vitamin D may result in early calcification in the fetal bones (osteosclerosis). Thus, should it become necessary because of lack of sunshine or inability to obtain an adequate diet (including milk) to supply vitamin D and calcium and phosphorus compounds, one should exercise care in their administration. It should be borne in mind that the ordinary diet does not supply sufficient vitamin D to comply with the requirements for the latter half of pregnancy and lactation (400 to 800 I.U.), as stipulated by the National Research Council.

Vitamin E (a-tocopherol) is essential to reproduction, as the development of the embryo depends upon it. It is also essential to the nutrition of the suckling offspring. The important role of this vitamin will be discussed in greater detail in the section on abortion.

From a consideration of these vitamins it must be apparent that a well-balanced diet, containing all the vitamins, is of first importance during pregnancy and lactation. Such a diet should have generous amounts of calcium-containing and iron-containing foods, green vegetables and legumes, fresh citrus fruits as well as one quart of milk daily. It is to be noted that a quart of milk, taken daily, supplies the calcium requirement in pregnancy, as well as furnishing other minerals, vitamins, particularly A, and protein, carbohydrate and fats. It is apparent, as brought out by the investigations of Williams, Hark and Fralin, and others, that the food habits of the average woman lead to marked deficiencies in many of these dietary essentials. The obstetrician must not only find out the food habits of his patient but must give her specific instructions as to her essential dietary needs as they pertain to vitamins, minerals, fluid and carbohydrate, protein and fats.

There can be no doubt that a certain number of pregnant and lactating women suffer from symptoms due to calcium deficiency as shown by Mendenhall and Drake, Reed and others. These symptoms may be relieved by a proper balanced diet containing sufficient calcium and vitamins.

GENERAL HYGIENE

Exercise. During normal pregnancy the woman should be encouraged to take an average amount of light outdoor exercise, though in individual cases it is often difficult to specify the exact amount—a safe rule being to instruct her to desist while still feeling that she could do more without tiring herself. Exercise should consist mainly of walking, and a good rule is half an hour's walk each morning and afternoon, unless this proves to be tiring, in which event it should be curtailed. The more strenuous forms of exercise such as tennis and horseback riding should be interdicted. Swimming is allowed in mild form early in pregnancy, but not diving. Patients in whom there is a history of or tendency to abortion should be particularly careful as to exercise. When for various reasons outdoor exercise cannot be taken, massage in the hands of a skilful person is to be recommended. In the later months long journeys should not be undertaken unless absolutely necessary, and driving over rough roads should be avoided. When possible, the pregnant woman should lie down for an hour or two after the midday meal.

Bath. The patient should be advised to take a shower or sponge bath during the last month of pregnancy. While a daily warm tub bath is very desirable during the first eight months, it should be avoided the month preceding the expected date of confinement, because of the danger of slipping on the floor of the tub, with consequent injury to the uterus and placenta. Prolonged hot baths are to be avoided because of their fatiguing effect.

The Bowels. During pregnancy the enlarged uterus sometimes interferes with the normal intestinal peristalsis and gives rise to more or less marked constipation. The more sedentary mode of living is undoubtedly a further factor in the causation of this very frequent complication of pregnancy. As will be discussed later, constipation may play an important role in the production of pyelitis and for this and other reasons care should be taken that the bowels are moved daily. To ensure this it is necessary for the patient to have regular habits with regard to bowel movements, to avoid indigestible foods, to select those foods inducive to bowel movement and to obtain fairly regular exercise, such as walking. If with these precautionary methods constipation still prevails, a daily movement is best accomplished by the administration of light petrolatum or mineral oil. However, it must be borne in mind that the constant use of mineral oil may lead to a vitamin deficiency, in which event protective measures should be employed. Some patients may require a mild laxative, such as milk of magnesia, in addition to the oil, while the occasional woman may do better on small doses of phenolphthalein. The use of active cathartics or purgatives is inadvisable, as they may sometimes stimulate the smooth muscle of the uterus and so bring about labor.

Clothing. The physician is frequently asked concerning the clothing which is best adapted to the pregnant state. Generally speaking, the clothing should be loose and so arranged as to exert as little pressure upon the waist as possible; and in the later months of pregnancy, if the patient is accustomed to the use of a corset, the ordinary type should be replaced by a loosely fitting low girdle or by one of the specially designed "maternity" corsets. In multiparous women, when the abdomen is markedly relaxed from previous childbearing, the wearing of an abdominal support of elastic material, or an ordinary scultetus bandage, adds materially to their comfort. When varicose veins of the extremities are present the legs should be bandaged or encased in elastic stockings, and when large varices exist about the vulva the patient should be cautioned concerning the possibility of their rupture.

Sexual Intercourse. In healthy persons sexual intercourse in moderation usually does no harm, as long as the abdominal enlargement is not too great to make it inconvenient for the patient. But where there is a tendency to abortion or premature labor it should be interdicted. It should be strictly forbidden in the last month of pregnancy, as in numerous instances severe puerperal infection has followed sexual intercourse just before the onset of labor.

The Breasts. In the last months of pregnancy attention should be devoted to the condition of the breasts, and more particularly to the nipples, as by appropriate preliminary treatment nursing may sometimes be rendered easier, and the occurrence of fissures and the consequent danger of mammary infection in part prevented. For this purpose the patient, during the last two months, may anoint her nipples night and morning with lanolin or cocoa butter, which tends to render them more elastic. Some obstetricians believe it advisable to do as little as possible to the breasts and nipples during pregnancy, an opinion with which we are largely in agreement. Certainly, any attempts to lengthen the small nipples by making traction upon them night and morning must be carried out with great care and with no undue optimism that this procedure will cure the condition. We know of no means, however, by which retracted or inverted nipples can be made serviceable.

In the New York Hospital each patient is given a printed booklet which contains all the necessary instructions and advice. This form includes the following:

Directions for Patients during Pregnancy

Food: The following foods should be included in your diet every day. These foods will protect your health and will provide for the growth of your baby:

Milk—One quart—either as a drink or in cooking. Evaporated milk may be substituted for bottle milk.

Vegetables—Two servings other than potato—one of which should be raw.

Fruit—Two servings—one of which should be raw.

Breads and Cereals—Dark breads and dark cereals should be used.
Eggs—One a day if possible; at least three or four eggs every week.
Meat, Fish or Liver—One serving.
Prepare three regular meals, eat slowly, and chew your food well.

Fluids: Drink at least eight glasses of fluids daily.

Sleep and Rest: The old saying "Early to bed and early to rise" is good advice for the expectant mother. Sleep at least eight hours every night in a well-ventilated room. Rest several times a day, if only for a few minutes. Lie down for at least an hour sometime during the day.

Exercise: If possible walk or rest out of doors every day. Housework is good exercise, but it does not take the place of that taken in the sunshine and fresh air. Heavy lifting and stretching may be harmful.

Recreation—Mothers' Club: Some pleasure is necessary for health. Carry on your usual diversions except the more active ones. You will find the Mothers' Clubs enjoyable, and the nurse will give you the address of the one nearest your home.

Dental Care during Pregnancy: The teeth should be put in good condition at the beginning of pregnancy and kept so. The health in general is dependent upon a clean mouth and sound teeth.

Care of the Skin: Bathe all over every day with warm water. After the seventh month take a sponge bath or shower only; tub baths should be taken only with your doctor's consent.

To Insure Good Elimination: Special attention must be paid to the diet, to the regularity of meals, and to the formation of the habit of going to the toilet at the same time every day, preferably after breakfast. Be sure that you are taking as much as eight glasses of fluids daily.

Constipation is seldom caused by one thing. Rest, relaxation, or exercise may be equally important for a satisfactory bowel movement daily. If you are unable to have a good elimination every day add more fruits and vegetables to the diet as outlined. Be sure that dark breads and dark cereals are being used. If necessary ask the nurse how to prepare prunes and senna. Cathartics should be taken only when ordered by the doctor. If you have hemorrhoids (piles) let your doctor know.

Clothing for the Mother: At least one becoming dress is an excellent investment and if made early in pregnancy can serve for the entire period. All clothing during this time should be light, loose, and hang from the shoulders. Ask the nurse for information regarding patterns and styles. Discuss your abdominal support with the nurse also. A good supporting corset or binder will make you more comfortable, will help to prevent fatigue, and will eliminate the necessity of wearing tight bands around the waist or legs.

BIBLIOGRAPHY

Aring, C. D., Evans, J. P., and Spies, T. D. Some Clinical Neurologic Aspects of Vitamin B Deficiencies. J.A.M.A., 1939, 113:2105.

Bethell, F. H., Gardiner, S. H., and MacKinnon, F. Influence of Iron and Diet on Blood in Pregnancy. Ann. Int. Med., 1939, 13:91.

Bodansky, O., Lewis, J. M., and Lillienfeld, M. C. C. The Concentration of Vitamin A in the Blood Plasma during Pregnancy. J. Clin. Invest., 1943, 22:643.

Burke, B. S., Beal, V. A., Kirkwood, S. B., and Stuart, H. C. Nutrition Studies during Pregnancy. Am. J. Obst. & Gynec., 1943, 46:38.

——— Nutritional Needs in Pregnancy in Relation to Nutritional Intakes as Shown by Dietary Histories. Obst. & Gynec. Surv., 1948, 3:716.

Burton, A. H. G., and Balmain, A. R. Vitamin A and Streptococcal Immunity. Lancet, 1930, 1:1063.

Byrn, J. N., and Eastman, N. J. Vitamin A Levels in Maternal and Fetal Blood Plasma. Bull., Johns Hopkins Hosp., 1943, 73:132.

Coons, C. M. Iron Retention by Women during Pregnancy. J. Biol. Chem., 1932, 97:215.

Cowgill, G. R. The Need for the Addition of Vitamin B_1 to Staple American Foods. J.A.M.A., 1939, 113:2146.

Darby, W. G., Cannon, R. O., and Kaser, M. A. The Biochemical Assessment of Nutritional Status during Pregnancy. Obst. & Gynec. Surv., 1948, 3:704.

Dieckmann, W. J., Adair, F. L., Michel, H., Kramer, S., Dunkle, F., Costin, M., Campbell, A., Wensley, A. C., and Lorang, E. Calcium, Phosphorus, Iron and Nitrogen Balances in Pregnant Women. Am. J. Obst. & Gynec., 1944, 47:357.

Dieckmann, W. J., Turner, D. F., and Ruby, B. A. Diet Regulation and Controlled Weight in Pregnancy. Am. J. Obst. & Gynec., 1945, 50:701.

Dieckmann, W. J., and others. Diet in Pregnant Patients. Obst. & Gynec. Surv., 1948, 3:731.

Eastman, N. J. Expectant Motherhood, 2nd Ed. Little, Brown & Co., Boston, 1947.

——— Editorial note. Obst. & Gynec. Surv., 1946, 1:811.

Ebbs, J. H. Nutritive Requirements in Pregnancy and Lactation. J.A.M.A., 1943, 121:339.

Evans, H. M., and Bishop, K. S. On the Relation between Fertility and Nutrition. I. The Ovulation Rhythm in the Rat on a Standard Nutritional Regimen. II. The Ovulation Rhythm in the Rat on Inadequate Nutritional Regimen. J. Metab. Research, 1922, 319, 335.

Evans, H. M., and Burr, G. O. The Antisterility Vitamin Fat-Soluble E. Memoirs University of California, 1927, Vol. 8.

Fitzgerald, J. E., and Webster, A. Effect of Vitamin K Administered to Patients in Labor. Am. J. Obst. & Gynec., 1940, 40:413.

Friedman, G. J., Sherry, S., and Ralli, E. P. The Mechanism of the Excretion of Vitamin C by the Human Kidney at Low and Normal Plasma Levels of Ascorbic Acid. J. Clin. Invest., 1940, 19:685.

Garry, R. C., and Wood, H. O. Dietary Requirements in Human Pregnancy and Lactation. A Review of Recent Work. Nutrition. Abstr. & Rev., 1946, 15:591.

Goodman, L., and Gilman, A. The Pharmacological Basis of Therapeutics. The Macmillan Co., New York, 1941, pages 1106 and 1113.

Hess, A. F., and Weinstock, M. Rickets as Influenced by Diet of the Mother during Pregnancy and Lactation. J.A.M.A., 1924, 83:1558.

Hirst, J. C., and Shoemaker, R. E. Vitamin A in Pregnancy. Average Capacity According to the Feldman Adaptometer. Am. J. Obst. & Gynec., 1940, 40:12.

Horwitz, O., and Farley, D. L. Vitamin B_1 Deficiency in Pregnancy as Indicated by a Test for OBT Principle. Surg., Gynec. & Obst., 1940, 71:313.

Kooser, J. H. Observations on the Possible Relationship of Diet to Late Toxemia of Pregnancy. Am. J. Obst. & Gynec., 1941, 41:288.

Lund, C. J., and Kimble, M. S. Plasma Vitamin A and Carotene of the Newborn Infant. With Consideration of Fetal-Maternal Relationships. Am. J. Obst. & Gynec., 1943, 46:207.

——— Vitamin A during Pregnancy, Labor and the Puerperium. Am. J. Obst. & Gynec., 1943, 46:486.

——— Some Determinants of Maternal and Plasma Vitamin C Levels. Am. J. Obst. & Gynec., 1943, 46:635.

Mackie, Thomas T. Diet and Deficiency Disease in Clinical Medicine. New York State J. Med., 1940, 40:475.

Mendenhall, A. M., and Drake, J. C. Calcium Deficiency in Pregnancy and Lactation. Am. J. Obst. & Gynec., 1934, 27:800.

Moore, C. U., and Brodie, J. L. The Relation of Maternal Diet to Hemorrhage in the Newborn. Am. J. Dis. Child., 1927, 34: 53.

Müller, Carl. Das Fruchtbarkeitsvitamin E. Arch. f. Gynäk., 1939, 169:483.

Nixon, W. C. W. Diet in Pregnancy. J. Obst. & Gynaec. Brit. Emp., 1942, 49:614.

Oberst, F. W., and Plass, E. D. Calcium, Phosphorus, and Nitrogen Metabolism in Women during the Second Half of Pregnancy and in Early Lactation. Am. J. Obst. & Gynec., 1940, 40:399.

People's League of Health (Interim Report): Nutrition of Expectant and Lactating Mothers. Lancet, 1942, 2:10.

Reed, C. B. The Calcium Problem in Pregnancy. Am. J. Obst. & Gynec., 1933, 26:814.

Reyher, W., Walkhoff, E., and Walkhoff, O. Studien über die Wirkung C-hypovitaminotischer Nahrung auf Schwangere, Feten and Neuegeborene. München med. Wchnschr., 1928, 75, 2087-2090.

Reynolds, E., and Macomber, D. Certain Dietary Factors in the Causation of Sterility in Rats. Am. J. Obst. & Gynec., 1921, 2:379.

Sadovsky, A., Weber, D., and Wertheimer, E. Concentration of Vitamin C in Blood during and after Pregnancy. J. Lab. and Clin. Med., 1939, 25:120.

Sherman, H. C., and MacLeod, F. L. The Relation of Vitamin A to Growth, Reproduction and Longevity. J. Am. Chem. Soc., 1925, 47:1658.

Shute, E. Vitamin E in Habitual Abortion and Habitual Miscarriage. J. Obst. & Gynaec. Brit. Emp., 1942, 49:534.

Stander, H. J. Calcium Needs during Pregnancy. Am. J. Obst. & Gynec., 1938, 35:530.

Straumfjord, J. V. Vernix Caseosa. A Manifestation of Vitamin A Deficiency. West. J. Surg., 1940, 48:341.

Strauss, M. B. Observations on the Etiology of the Toxemias of Pregnancy. The Relationship of Nutritional Deficiency, Hypoproteinemia, and Elevated Venous Pressure to Water Retention in Pregnancy. Am. J. M. Sc., 1935, 190:811.

Sure, B. Dietary Requirements for Fertility and Lactation: A Dietary Sterility Associated with Vitamin A Deficiency. J. Agr. Research, 1928, 37:87.

——— Dietary Requirements for Reproduction. Vitamin B Requirements for Normal Lactation. J. Biol. Chem., 1927, 74:55.

Vogt, E. Ueber Reformen der Schwangerschaftsdiät mit Rücksicht auf das Vitaminbedürfnis des Fetus. München med. Wchnschr., 1929, 76:1959.

Vogt-Moller, P. The Therapeutic Application of Vitamin E in Human Clinical Medicine. Acta obst. et gynec. Scandinav., 1940, 20:85.

Vorhaus, M. G. Evaluation of Vitamin B_1 (Thiamin Chloride) in the Treatment of Polyneuritis. Am. J. M. Sc., 1939, 198:837.

Warkany, J. Experimental Studies on Nutrition in Pregnancy. Obst. & Gynec. Surv., 1948, 3:693.

Williams, P. F. Importance of Adequate Protein Nutrition in Pregnancy. J.A.M.A., 1945, 127:1052.

Williams, P. F., Hark, B., and Fralin, F. G. Nutrition Study in Pregnancy; Correlation between Dietary Survey of Vitamin A Content and Dark Adaption Time. Am. J. Obst. & Gynec., 1940, 40:1.

Williams, P. F., and Fralin, F. G. Nutrition Study in Pregnancy. Food Habits of 514 Pregnant Women. Am. J. Obst. & Gynec., 1942, 44:647.

Section Four: PHYSIOLOGY AND CONDUCT OF LABOR

13

THE FORCES CONCERNED IN LABOR

By labor is meant the series of processes by which the mature, or almost mature, products of conception are expelled from the mother's body. Childbirth, travail, accouchement, confinement and parturition are all synonyms. The word "delivery" refers to the actual birth of the baby.

CAUSE OF THE ONSET OF LABOR

Regardless of species, whether the fetus weighs 2 gm. at the end of a 21-day pregnancy, as in the mouse, or whether it weighs 200 pounds at the end of a 640-day pregnancy, as in the elephant, labor regularly begins at just the right time; namely, when the fetus is mature enough to cope with extra-uterine conditions but not yet large enough to cause mechanical difficulties in labor. The process responsible for this beautifully synchronized and salutary achievement is obscure. Indeed, despite much research, about all we know definitely concerning the cause of the onset of labor may be epitomized in the old adage, "When the fruit is ripe it will fall."

The crux of the question is not what initiates uterine contractility, because Braxton Hicks contractions occur throughout pregnancy and similar contractions are demonstrable even in the nonpregnant uterus. The question is how these painless and seemingly futile contractions are converted into the painful, exquisitely coordinated and efficient contractions which dilate the cervix and expedite expulsion of the child. Of the main theories which attempt to explain the onset of labor, no single one is adequate. Nevertheless each seems to contain a grain of truth and, in all probability, the mechanism proposed by each does play some role. In other words, it appears likely that the onset of labor is not due to a single cause, but to a number of factors all converging toward the same end, and all playing some part in the specialized pattern of uterine contractions characteristic of labor.

1. **Estrogen Theory.** This theory rests on the belief that a nice balance exists throughout pregnancy between the uterine-stimulating action of estrogen and the uterine-relaxing effect of progesterone a balance which is finally upset, as progesterone production regresses. The data bearing on this theory are contradictory. As indicated on page 80, the supposed relaxing effect of progesterone on uterine muscle is itself open to question. Moreover, as indicated, estrogen is not an oxytocic, and huge quantities can be given to gravidae near term without inducing labor. Venning has failed to discover any regular decline in pregnanediol excretion prior to labor and, on the contrary, has observed that labor may begin on a rising pregnanediol output. On the other hand, Lyon has found in 68 cases that there is a steady decline in the excretion of pregnanediol from about 30 mg. of sodium pregnanediol glucuronidate four days before labor to an average of about 19.5 mg. 48 hours preceding labor and 14 mg. one day prior to the onset of labor. In further support of this theory Snyder has

shown that the administration of chorionic gonadotrophin to pregnant rabbits near term causes prolongation of pregnancy through the resultant formation of new corpora lutea and the continued manufacture of progesterone. More recently Heckel and Allen have found that 1.5 mg. of progesterone per day, injected subcutaneously into rabbits, not only delays but may even prevent parturition.

2. **Posterior Pituitary Theory.** This theory supplements the estrogen theory by postulating that estrogen makes the uterine muscle increasingly sensitive to posterior pituitary hormones, whose oxytocic powers are well known. (Chief objection: pregnant rats, rabbits and cats in which the pars posterior and pars intermedia of the hypophysis have been removed, experience normal labor.)

3. **Estrogen and Progesterone Withdrawal Theory.** On the basis of extensive endocrine studies, Smith, Smith and Schiller suggest that the onset of labor may resemble the onset of menstruation in its mechanism. They find that during the week or two before the onset of labor a progressive change in steroid metabolism takes place, characterized by progesterone and estrogen withdrawal. Since the changes in steroid metabolism before and at the time of menstruation are similar to those before and at the onset of labor, and since vasoconstriction in the endometrium is the most striking premenstrual phenomenon, they are inclined to think of vascular spasm as an incitant to labor contractions.

4. **Distention Theory.** Any hollow viscus, whether bladder, bowel or uterus, tends to contract and empty itself when distended to a certain point. In the case of the uterus, Reynolds has shown that as pregnancy nears term, uterine growth slackens, whereas the rate of fetal growth increases. The result is a rapid increment in intra-uterine pressure. The resultant tension imposed on the uterine muscle fibers may itself initiate labor. Reynolds, however, believes that the resultant pressure on the placental site with consequent decrease in the flow of blood through the placenta is the determining factor. This general hypothesis is supported by a number of considerations: in rabbits, the greater the number of fetuses in a litter, the shorter (within limits) will be the duration of pregnancy. Conversely, the smaller the litter size, the longer pregnancy lasts (Wishart and Hammond). Since it has been demonstrated that the larger the litter size, the greater is the total mass of conceptus tissue and fluids, it follows that distention mass determines the duration of pregnancy in the rabbit, other things being equal. In the human, the average duration of twin pregnancies is about twenty-one days shorter than single gestations (Guttmacher).

Smith, Smith and Schiller have pointed out that the distention theory is not incompatible with the estrogen and progesterone withdrawal theory and may be interrelated. Thus, withdrawal of estrogen may be responsible for cessation of uterine growth; and compression of the placental site may be responsible for a diminished production of estrogen and progesterone by the placenta.

5. **Mechanical Irritation Theory.** The stretching of the lower uterine segment by the fetal head and, more particularly, the pressure exerted by it on the retrocervical nervous ganglia, are probably important factors in the onset of labor. This theory finds its chief support in the efficacy of the several methods of artificial induction of labor. Thus, the regularity with which artificial puncture of the membranes near term induces labor is best explained by the resultant descent of the fetal head, which stretches the lower uterine segment and makes pressure on the surrounding ganglia. Also, a bag introduced in the lower uterine segment has a similar effect.

THE THREE STAGES OF LABOR

The process of labor is divided, for convenience of description, into three distinct stages:

The First Stage of Labor, or the dilating stage, begins with the first true labor pain and ends with the complete dilatation of the cervix.

The Second Stage of Labor, or the stage of expulsion, begins with the complete dilatation of the cervix and ends with the delivery of the baby.

The Third Stage of Labor, or the placental stage, begins with the delivery of the baby and ends with the birth of the placenta.

THE CHARACTERISTICS OF UTERINE CONTRACTIONS IN LABOR

Alone among physiologic muscular contractions, those of labor are painful. Thus, the common designation in all languages for such a contraction is "pain." The cause of the pain is not definitely known, but the following hypotheses have been suggested: (1) anoxia of the compressed muscle cells (as in angina pectoris); (2) compression of nervous ganglia in the cervix and lower uterine segment by the tightly interlocking muscle bundles; (3) stretching of the cervix during dilatation; and (4) stretching and displacement of the peritoneum due to direct pull and to shifting of the underlying muscle fibers. Uterine contractions are *involuntary*. Their action is not only independent of the mother's will, but of extra-uterine nervous control. Patients with paraplegia have normal, though painless, contractions, as do women who have had bilateral lumbar sympathectomy; the uterus, moreover, can contract after removal from the body, and in Locke's solution, strips of uterine muscle contract for hours. Stimulation of the hypogastric plexus and the nervus erigens in the dog, Rudolph and Ivy find, yields results which lack uniformity and they conclude that the extrinsic nerves of the uterus play a subordinate role in parturition. In other words, uterine action in labor, like that of the heart, is *under intrinsic nervous control* which must reside either in the muscle cell itself or in the ganglia present in the uterine wall. The observations of Ivy, Hartman and Koff indicate that the uterus, again like the heart, possesses "pacemakers" which initiate uterine contractions and control their rhythmicity. In the monkey these are located near the insertion of each fallopian tube; from these two sites contractions pass in ever widening concentric waves, elliptical in form, forward and medially until the waves meet in the midline, whence they travel caudally.

The contractions of the uterus during labor are *intermittent,* with periods of relaxation between, resembling in this respect the systole and diastole of the heart. The *interval between contractions* diminishes gradually from about ten minutes early in labor, to one or two minutes in the second stage. These periods of relaxation not only provide rest to the uterine muscle and to the mother, but are essential for the welfare of the baby, since unremitting contractions may so interfere with placental function as to produce fetal anoxemia. The *duration of each contraction* ranges from 45 seconds to a minute and a quarter, averaging about one minute. Each contraction presents three phases—increment, acme and decrement, the increment or crescendo phase being longer than the other two combined. Ever since Uncle Toby in *Tristram Shandy* first estimated that the force exerted by each labor pain amounted to some 470 pounds, this question has been the object of much speculation and some study, but precise information is still lacking. Certain it is, however, that Uncle Toby's estimate was a gross exaggeration, modern studies placing the force exerted in the neighborhood of 25 pounds.

Local Characteristics of Uterine Behavior in the Two Uterine Segments. During labor and under the influence of uterine contractions, the uterus gradually becomes differentiated into two distinct portions. The upper is the active contrac-

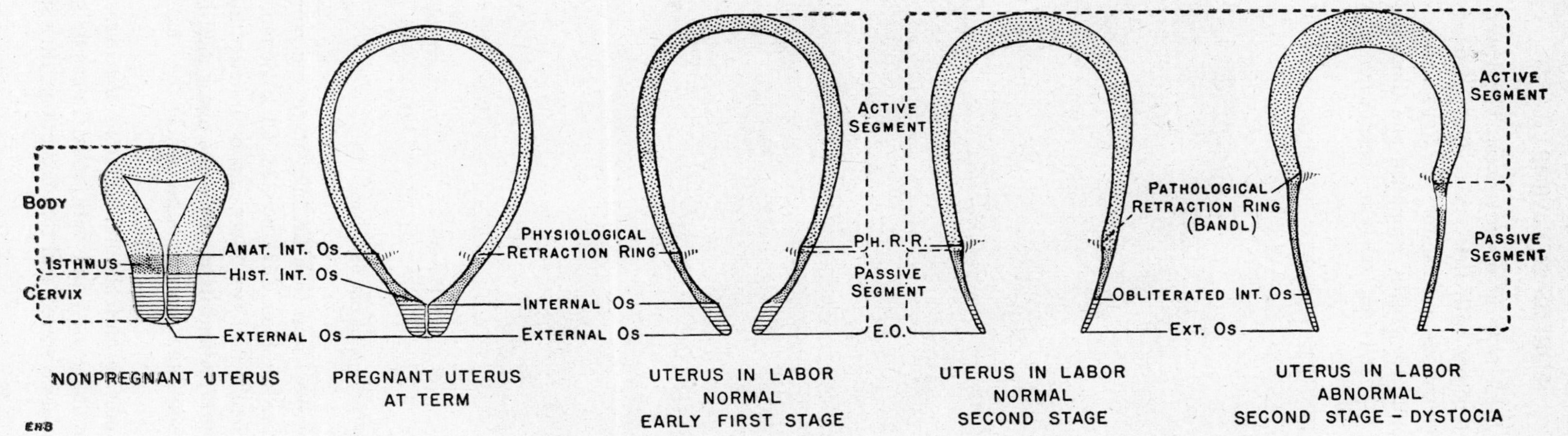

Fig. 227.—Progressive Development of the Segments and Rings of the Uterus at Term.

Note comparison between the nonpregnant uterus, uterus at term, and uterus in labor. The passive segment is derived from the lower uterine segment (isthmus) and cervix; the physiological retraction ring, from the anatomical internal os. The pathological retraction ring which forms under abnormal conditions develops from the physiological ring.

tile portion and becomes thicker as labor advances. The lower portion—that is, the lower uterine segment together with the cervix—plays a passive part, becoming developed into a thin-walled muscular tube for the transmission of the fetus. The lower uterine segment is simply the greatly expanded and thinned-out isthmus of the nonpregnant uterus (page 31). It is not solely a phenomenon of labor but expands

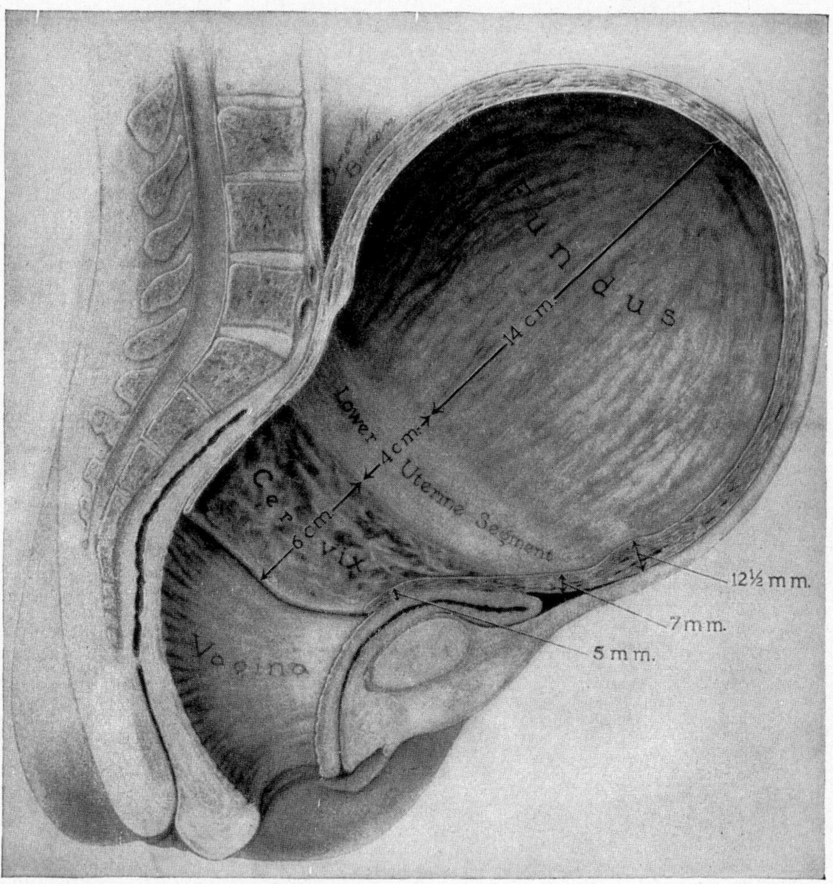

Fig. 228.—The Relationships of the Upper Portion of the Uterus, the Lower Uterine Segment and the Cervix as Found in a Patient Dying in the Second Stage of Labor of Poliomyelencephalitis.

The twin pregnancy was about 28 weeks in duration.

gradually as pregnancy progresses and then becomes more and more thinned out as labor advances. It is illustrated in Figs. 227 and 228. On abdominal palpation, even before the rupture of the membranes, two zones can be differentiated during a contraction, the upper one being firm and hard, while the lower affords a semifluctuant sensation. The former represents the contractile portion of the uterus; the latter, the distended, passive portion.

Were the entire sac of uterine musculature, including the lower uterine segment and cervix, to contract simultaneously and with equal intensity in all parts, it is obvious that no purpose would be served and that conditions after such a contraction would be the same as before. Herein lies the importance of the division of the uterus into an upper and lower segment, because these two segments differ not only anatomically but also in the physiologic properties of their musculature. Briefly, the upper segment contracts, thickens and expels the fetus, while the lower segment and cervix relax, dilate and come to constitute a greatly expanded, thinned out muscular tube through which the baby can pass.

The musculature of the upper uterine segment undergoes a type of contraction in which the muscle after contracting does not relax to its original length, but becomes relatively fixed at a shorter length, the tension, however, remaining the same

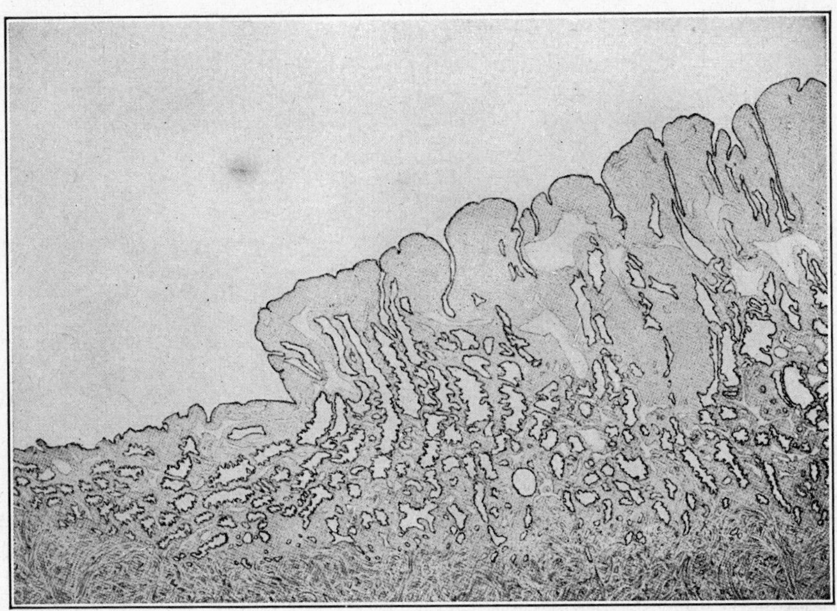

FIG. 229.—SECTION SHOWING DIFFERENCE BETWEEN MUCOSA OF BODY AND OF LOWER SEGMENT OF 2 MONTHS' PREGNANT UTERUS (Stieve). × 10.

Thick part—body. Thin part—lower uterine segment.

as before the contraction. This ability of the musculature of a viscus to contract down on its diminishing contents, with tension remaining constant, is known as *retraction*. It is designed to take up "slack," to hold the advantage gained and to maintain the uterine musculature in firm contract with the intra-uterine contents. If there were no retraction, each individual contraction would start at the same point (in relation to uterine size) at which its predecessor started. When retraction is present, however, each successive contraction starts at the point where its predecessor left off, the uterine cavity becoming permanently smaller as the result of each successive contraction, thus preventing the child's slipping back. As a result of this successive shortening of its muscle fibers with each contraction, the upper segment becomes progressively thickened throughout the first and second stages of labor, and tremendously thickened immediately after the birth of the baby. It is apparent that this phenomenon of retraction manifested by the upper uterine segment must be contingent upon a decrease in the volume of its contents. But how is it possible for its contents to be diminished, particularly early in labor, when the entire uterus is virtually a closed sac, with only a minute opening at the cervix? There can be only one answer, namely, that the musculature of the lower segment relaxes, or gives way, permitting a greater and greater bulk of the intra-uterine contents to distend its walls. This is exactly what happens, the upper segment retracting only to the extent that the lower segment and cervix relax.

It is important to note that this relaxation of the lower uterine segment is by no means complete relaxation, but is rather just the reverse of retraction. The muscle fibers of the lower segment become stretched with each contraction of the upper

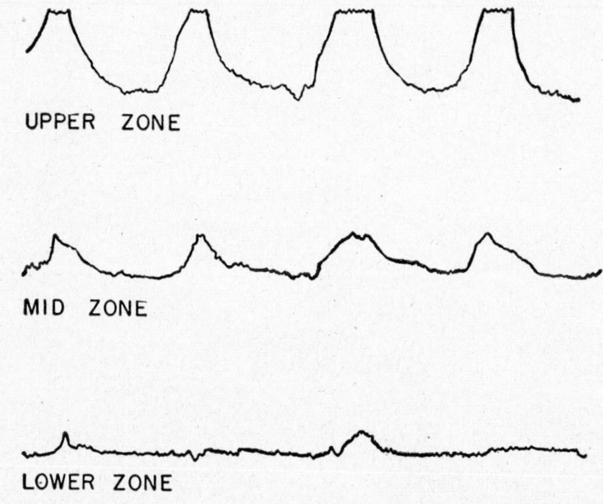

FIG. 230A.—TRACINGS OF UTERINE CONTRACTIONS IN VARIOUS PARTS OF THE UTERUS MADE BY REYNOLDS' TOKODYNAMOMETER.

The lower zone probably corresponds roughly with the lower uterine segment. The patient was a primigravida in active labor, 5 cm. dilated, with pains about three minutes apart. The original tracings have been inked over for clearer reproduction. (Courtesy of Dr. S. R. M. Reynolds, Dr. L. M. Hellman and Dr. P. Bruns.)

segment and at the end of such a contraction do not contract to their previous length, but remain relatively fixed at the longer length, the tension, however, remaining the same as before. In relaxation of this type the musculature still manifests tone, still resists stretch and will contract on stimulation. This phenomenon has been called "receptive" or "postural" relaxation; it might even be thought of as "tonal relaxation," however contradictory the term. The retraction of the upper uterine segment and the sustained relaxation of the lower have both been compared to a ratchet mechanism in which the advantage gained, as the result of a given force exerted, is held.

The successive lengthening of the muscle fibers in the lower uterine segment as labor progresses, naturally produces a thinning out of this structure, so that it may normally measure as little as 2.4 mm. in its thickest place (Stieve). At the same time its area increases so that it comes to constitute a larger and larger part of the muscular envelope encasing the fetus. As a result of this thinning of the lower uterine segment and the concomitant thickening of the upper, the boundary line between them becomes abrupt and is marked by a ridge on the inner uterine surface called the *physiologic retraction ring*. When the thinning of the lower uterine segment becomes extreme, as in obstructed labor, this ring becomes very pronounced and is then known as the *pathologic retraction ring,* or *Bandl's ring.* This is a pathologic condition and is discussed on page 786.

The different behavior of the upper and lower parts of the uterus in labor, as described above, has recently been studied from a quantitative viewpoint and new evidence adduced that there is a gradient of diminishing physiologic activity from the fundus to the lower uterine segment. The quantitative demonstration of this fact has been made possible by two ingenious devices: (1) the tokodynamometer of Reynolds and (2) the intra-uterine receptors of Karlson of Stockholm.

The former apparatus employs three resistance strain gauges set in heavy brass ring mountings which may be placed anywhere on the abdomen. When the uterus

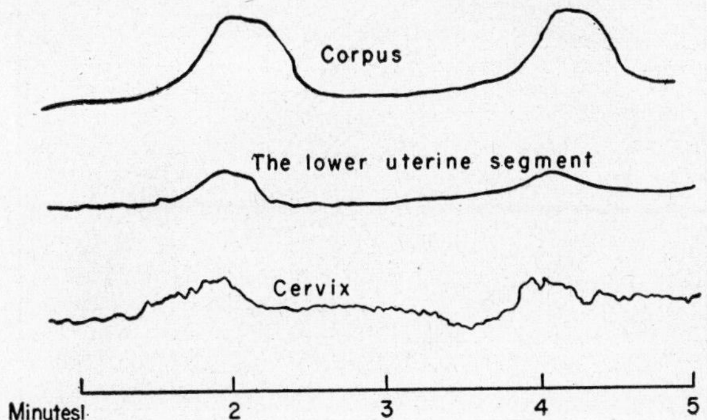

Fig. 230B.—Tracings of Uterine Contractions in Various Parts of the Uterus Recorded by Karlson by Means of Intra-uterine Receptors.

The patient was in early labor but from the time this tracing was made, progress was rapid. To permit clearer reproduction the background of the original record has been eliminated and the tracings inked over. (Courtesy of Dr. Stig Karlson.)

contracts, the increased convexity of the local arc of uterus underlying the ring pushes upward on the gauge and applies a strain to its elements proportional to the local force of the uterine contraction. A record is obtained electrometrically, an example of which is shown in Fig. 230A. It is at once apparent from these tracings that the intensity of each contraction is greater in the upper zone than in the midzone and, again, greater in the midzone than lower down. Equally noteworthy is the differential in the duration of the contractions, those in the midzone being much briefer than those above and the contractions in the lower zone being extremely brief and sometimes entirely absent. This subsidence of contraction in the midzone while the upper zone is still contracting can only mean that the upper part of the corpus, throughout a substantial portion of each contraction, is exerting pressure caudalward on the more relaxed parts of the uterus. In false labor, or when labor is not making progress, this gradient does not exist and both the intensity and the duration of the contractions are likely to be the same in the three zones.

The findings of Reynolds as described here have been observed in our clinic in several hundred labors, and have been reduplicated, quite independently and by means of an altogether different type of apparatus, by Karlson. This technic measures the internal pressure in the uterus at any point by means of so-called receptors. These are metal capsules with lengths of about 12 mm. and a diameter of 4.5 mm. in the middle of which is a small aperture or window. On the inner side of this aperture is a membrane sensitive to pressure. The receptors are soldered to a stiff steel tube with a lumen of 1 mm. and a length of about 37 cm. through which any pressure exerted against the window is carried through the tube and registered electrometrically. An example of one of Karlson's tracings is shown in Fig. 230B. Here again a gradient of diminishing activity is observed between the corpus and the lower uterine segment. Karlson's other tracings, like Reynolds', indicate that when this gradient is absent—that is, when the contraction of the lower segment equals or exceeds that of the corpus—the patient is either in false labor or stationary in respect to cervical dilatation.

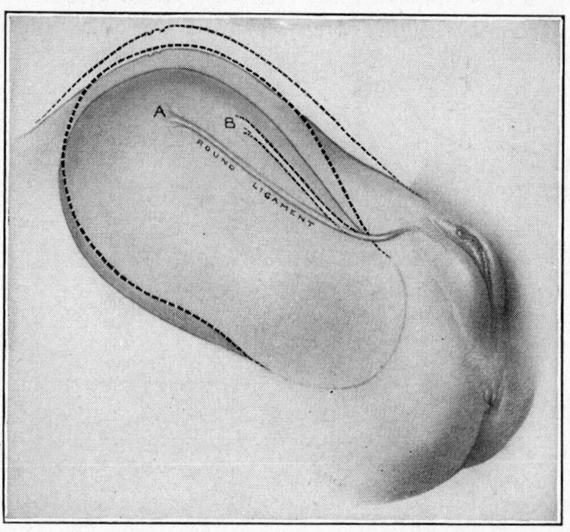

Fig. 231.—Action of Round Ligaments in Drawing Uterus Forward during a Contraction.
The halftone outlines show the round ligament, the uterus and the abdominal wall in the resting state, while the broken lines show the same structures during a contraction.

Ligamentous Action. The round ligaments are not mere reduplications of the peritoneum, but are composed principally of smooth muscle fibers prolonged from that organ. Accordingly, whenever the uterine musculature contracts, they contract also. Being anchored, like guy ropes, to the lowermost part of the anterior abdominal wall, they pull the parturient uterus forcibly forward with each contraction. The uterosacral ligaments posteriorly, being merely folds of peritoneum reinforced with small amounts of fibrous and muscular tissue, offer little resistance. With each contraction, therefore, the uterus rises from its resting place upon the vertebral column, and pushes the anterior abdominal wall forward. This positional change of the uterus is an important factor in labor, since it aligns the long axis of the uterus with the axis of the birth canal (Figs. 231 and 232).

Change in Uterine Shape. Each contraction produces an elongation of the uterine ovoid, with a concomitant decrease in the transverse and anteroposterior diameters, the result apparently of a preponderance of circular muscle fibers in the uterine wall. This change in shape has two important effects on the process of labor: (1) The decrease in lateral diameter produces a straightening out of the vertebral column of the fetus, causing its upper pole to be pressed firmly against the fundus of the uterus while the lower pole is thrust further downward into the pelvis. The amount of lengthening of the fetal ovoid produced in this manner has been estimated to range between 5 and 10 cm. The pressure so exerted is known as *fetal axis pressure.* (2) With the lengthening of the uterus, the longitudinal fibers are drawn taut and,

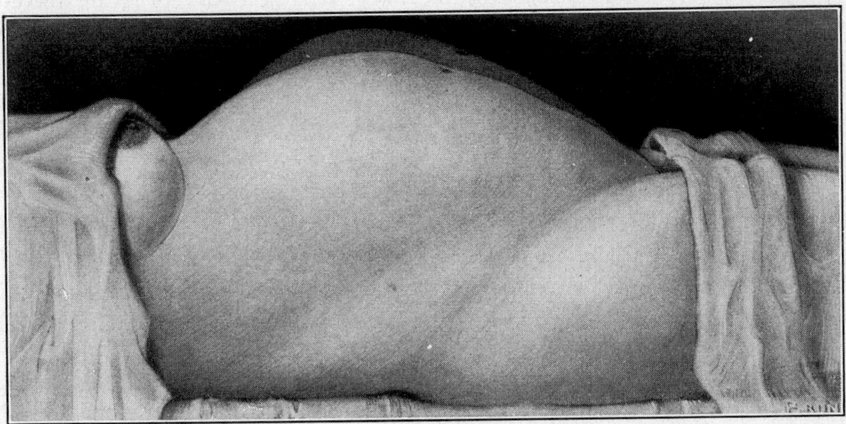

Fig. 232.—Composite Picture, Showing Shape of Abdomen Before and During a Uterine Contraction, the Shadowy Outline Indicating Contraction.

since the lower segment and cervix are the only parts of the uterus which will give, these structures are pulled upward over the lower pole of the fetus. This effect on the musculature of the lower segment and cervix is an important factor in cervical dilatation.

OTHER FORCES CONCERNED IN LABOR

Intra-abdominal Pressure. After the cervix is fully dilated, particularly after the bag of waters has ruptured, the chief driving force which expels the baby is contraction of the abdominal muscles, with consequent increase in intra-abdominal pressure. The nature of the force is similar to that involved in defecation, but greatly intensified. As the head reaches the perineal floor the character of the pain appears to produce a reflex stimulation which causes the patient to close her mouth firmly, contract her abdominal muscles and force her diaphragm downward. The important role played by intra-abdominal pressure in fetal expulsion is most plainly attested by the labors of paraplegic women. Such patients suffer no pain, although the uterus may contract violently. In these patients cervical dilatation (which is solely the result of uterine contractions) proceeds normally, but expulsion of the infant is rarely possible except under one circumstance: namely, when the attendant ascertains by palpation the onset of each contraction, informs the woman and instructs her about the use of her abdominal muscles, or "bearing down." Although intra-abdominal pressure, then, is a necessary force for the spontaneous completion of labor, it should be noted that it is futile unless acting on a contracted uterus. In other words, it is a necessary auxiliary to uterine contractions in the second stage of labor, both forces being essential. In the first stage of labor, it plays no role whatsoever.

Intra-abdominal pressure plays an important role not only in the second stage but also in the third stage of labor. After the placenta has become separated from its uterine attachment, it lies free in the lower uterine segment or upper vagina. In completely spontaneous labor its expulsion from this site is effected by the mother's bearing down, that is, by an increase in intra-abdominal pressure.

The Resisting Forces. Labor is work; and work, in the language of mechanics, is the causing of motion against a resisting force. It is necessary to recall, therefore, that the forces involved in labor are not limited to those uterine and abdominal powers which bring about the egress of the infant, but entail also certain resisting forces. These are the resistance offered by the cervix to dilatation, the frictional force presented by the birth canal to the presenting part and the forces exerted by the muscles of the pelvic floor and perineum.

Very little is known about the nature of the resistance which the cervix offers to dilatation, but the many hours required to bring it about, and especially the fact that almost all cervices suffer at least minor lacerations in labor, make plain the fact that substantial resistance has to be overcome. The frictional resistance of the birth canal is so great that the baby's head is molded to conform with it. The troughlike structure of the pelvic floor so resists the descent of the head that rotation of the latter is effected from a position in which its occipitofrontal diameter lies transverse to the maternal pelvis to one in which it is anteroposterior (page 359); while the resistance of the perineum is sometimes such an obstructing force that surgical incision of that structure becomes necessary.

In a sense, then, the process of a labor may be looked upon as a contest between the forces of expulsion and those of resistance.

CHANGES IN THE UTERUS DURING THE FIRST STAGE OF LABOR

The forces concerned in the first stage of labor are (1) the uterine contractions and (2) the resultant hydrostatic pressure of the bag of waters against the cervix and lower uterine segment or, in the absence of the bag of waters, the pressure of the presenting part against the cervix and lower uterine segment. As the result of the action of these forces, two all-important changes are wrought in the cervix: *effacement* and *dilatation*.

The Mechanism of Cervical Effacement. By "effacement" is meant the shortening of the cervical canal from a structure one or two centimeters in length to one in which no canal at all exists, but merely a circular orifice with almost paper-thin edges. The process takes place from above downward and is due to the fact that the muscle fibers in the region of the internal os are pulled upward, or "taken up," into the lower uterine segment, while the condition of the external os remains for the time being unchanged. As may be seen in Figs. 233 through 236, the edges of the internal os are drawn several centimeters upward, so that the former cervical mucosa becomes part of the lower uterine segment, and lies parallel and contiguous to the chorion. Accordingly, effacement may be compared to a funneling process in which the whole length of a moldable tube is converted into a very obtuse, flaring funnel, with only a small circular orifice for an outlet. Although cervical effacement is chiefly the result of muscular action, the process is greatly facilitated by the expulsion of the cervical plug of mucus (page 205). With the very first labor pains, the bag of waters burrows into the cervix in pouchlike fashion to expel this plug and with it the entire

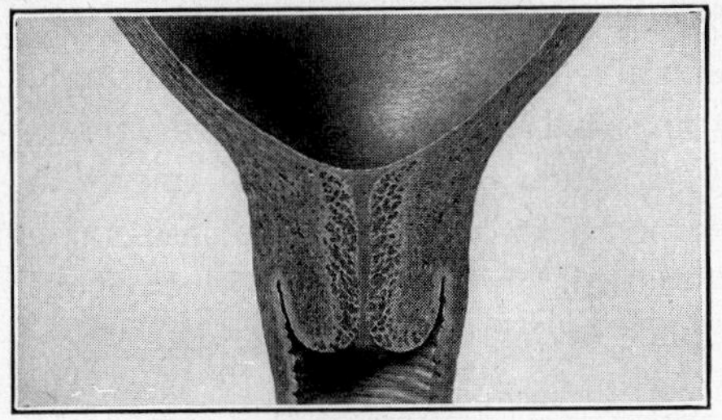

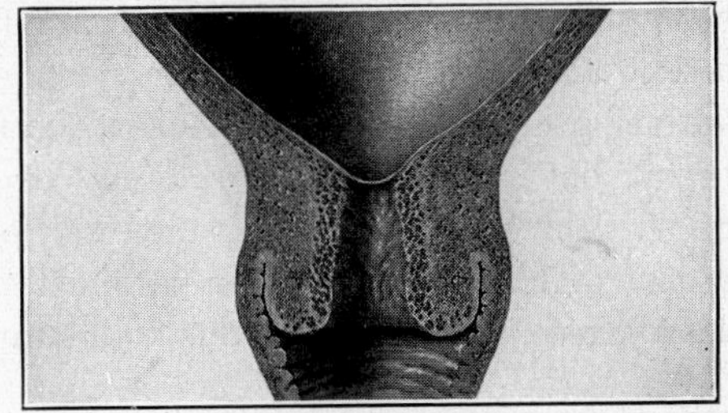

FIG. 233.—CERVIX AT END OF PREGNANCY.

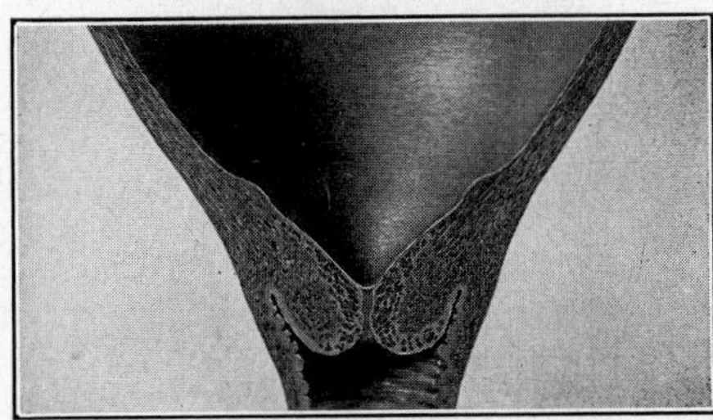

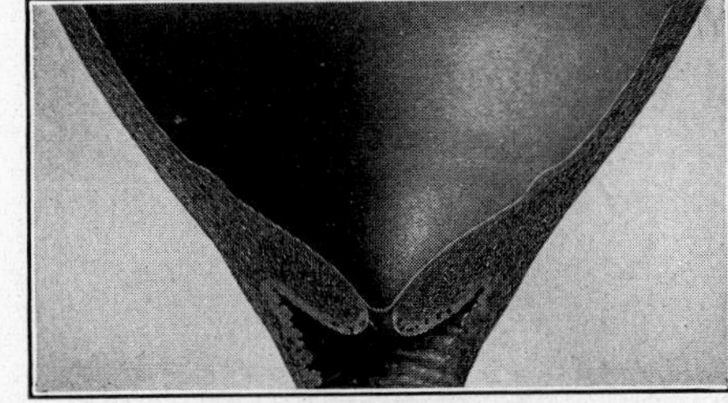

FIG. 234.—BEGINNING EFFACEMENT OF CERVIX. NOTE DILATATION OF INTERNAL OS AND FUNNEL SHAPED CERVICAL CANAL.

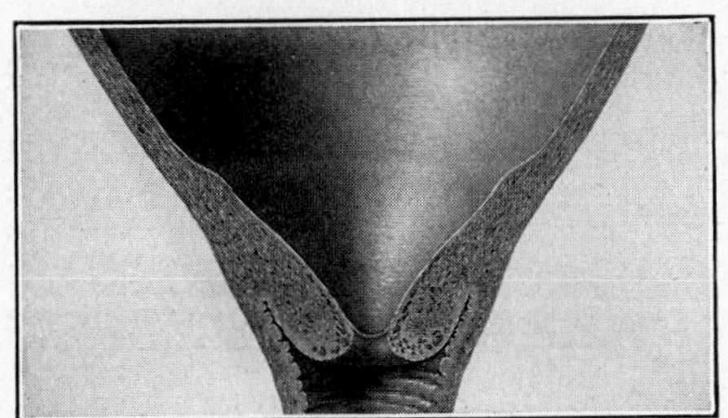

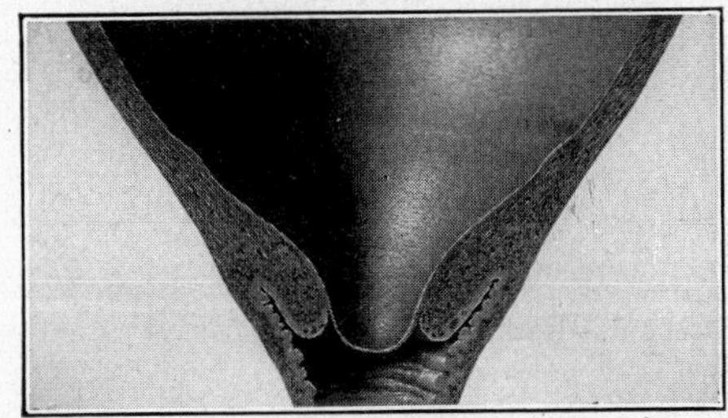

FIG. 235.—FURTHER EFFACEMENT OF CERVIX. NOTE HIGHER POSITION OF INTERNAL OS AND BULGING OF MEMBRANES.

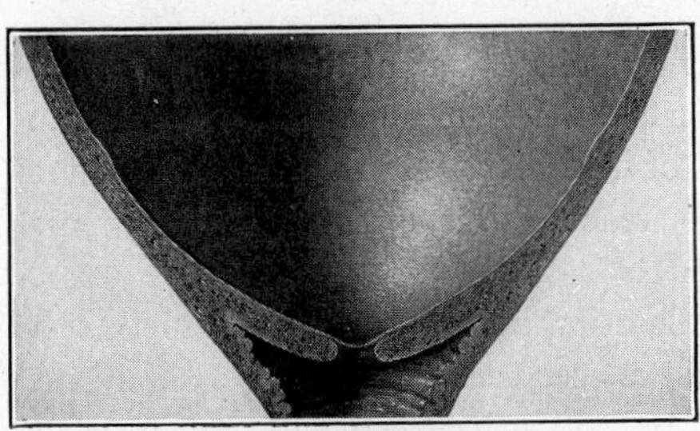

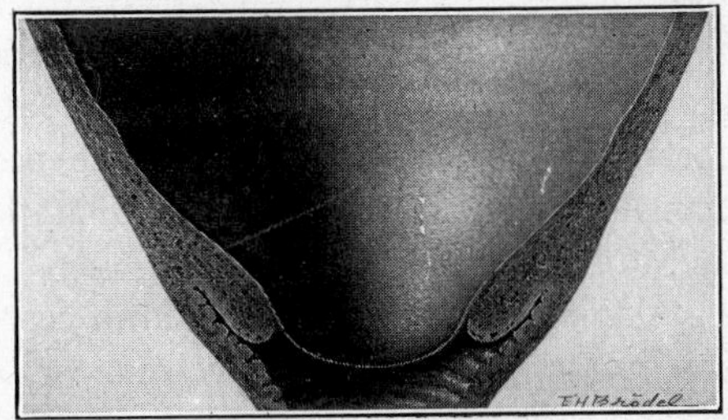

FIG. 236.—CERVICAL CANAL OBLITERATED.

Left, primigravida; right, multigravida.

honeycomb-like cervical mucosa. This not only canalizes the cervix but expresses a certain amount of blood from the erectile outer walls of the organ, thus producing a flattening effect. In primigravidae effacement is usually complete before dilatation begins, but in multiparae it is rarely complete, dilatation proceeding, as a rule, with rather thick cervical edges. As the result of Braxton Hicks contractions a considerable degree of effacement is often attained before actual labor starts in. Synonymous with "effacement" are the terms "obliteration" and "taking up" of the cervix.

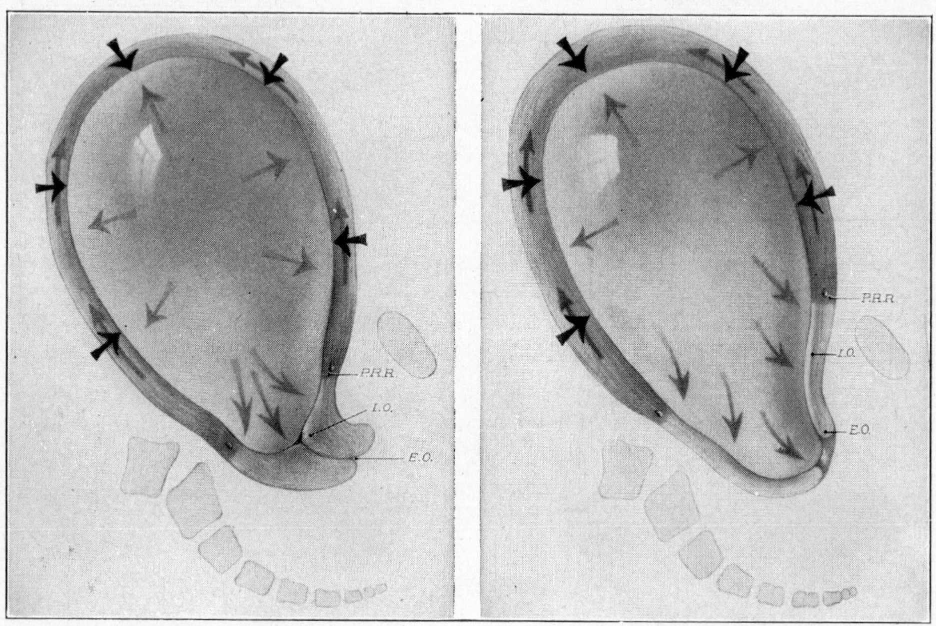

FIG. 237. FIG. 238.

FIG. 237.—HYDROSTATIC ACTION OF BAG OF WATERS IN EFFECTING CERVICAL EFFACEMENT AND DILATATION.

In absence of bag of waters, the presenting part acts similarly. In this and the next two illustrations note changing relationships of external os (*E.O.*), internal os (*I.O.*) and physiologic retraction ring (*P.R.R.*).

FIG. 238.—HYDROSTATIC ACTION OF BAG OF WATERS AT COMPLETION OF EFFACEMENT.

The Mechanism of Cervical Dilatation. By "dilatation" of the cervix is meant the enlargement of the external os from an orifice a few millimeters in size to an aperture large enough to permit the passage of the baby, that is, to one with a diameter of about 10 cm. When dilatation has reached this figure, it is commonly said to be "complete," or "full."

Although the forces concerned in cervical dilatation are not well understood, several factors appear to be involved. In the first place, the muscle fibers about the cervix are believed to be so arranged that they pull upon its edges and tend to draw it open through a mechanism similar to that by which the diaphragm of a microscope functions. Any proof, however, that the muscle fibers are so arranged is lacking. In the second place, with the onset of labor pains, the fluid contents of the uterus are subjected to pressure, and the force exerted on the liquor amnii is transmitted equally in all directions. As the lower uterine segment and cervix will naturally constitute a point of least resistance, they are consequently subjected to increased tension and distention in the course of which a centrifugal pull is exerted on the cervix. Moreover, as the uterine contractions make pressure on the bag of waters, the latter, in turn, burrows into the cervical canal in pouchlike fashion and exerts a dilating action in the manner of a wedge. This is usually referred to as the hydrostatic action of the bag of waters. In the absence of the bag of waters, the pressure of the presenting part against the cervix and lower uterine segment has a similar effect, as shown by the fact that rupture of the bag of waters, whether spontaneous or artificial, does not retard cervical dilatation. Furthermore, as previously explained, when the so-called "mucous plug" is expelled early in labor, it carries with it practically the entire honeycomb-like cervical mucosa, with the result that a relatively wide canal is exposed to the action of the dilating forces. Dilatation is facilitated also by the expression of blood from the erectile-like tissue of the outer walls of the cervix.

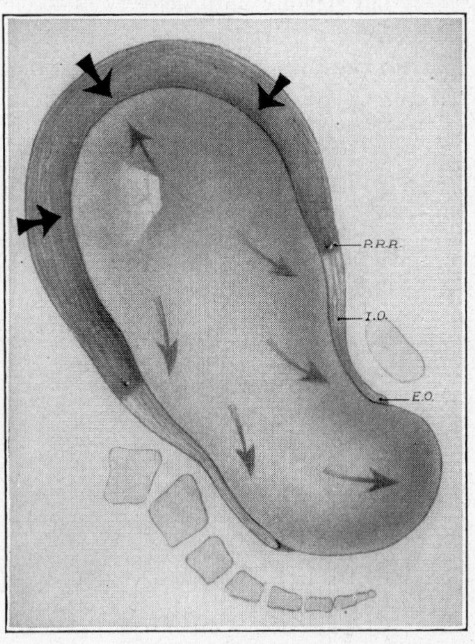

Fig. 239.—Hydrostatic Action of Bag of Waters at Full Cervical Dilatation.

As shown in Fig. 229, the decidua covering the lower uterine segment is thin and poorly differentiated. Toward the end of pregnancy the spongiosa layer in this area consists only of a few filaments representing thinned-out gland walls and it is readily conceivable that the slightest movement of the underlying musculature might sever them and allow the fetal membranes to slip back and forth over the mucosa. In a series of convincing studies, Stieve has shown that this loosening of the membranes in the lower segment is a regular accompaniment of early labor and, moreover, is prerequisite to successful cervical dilatation. A moment's visualization of the relationships will make it plain that a bag of waters which slides readily over the lower segment and partly through the cervix is a much more efficacious dilating agent than one attached to the surface. As all obstetricians know, digital stripping of the membranes in the region of the cervix sometimes suffices to initiate labor in gravidae at term, a fact in keeping with Stieve's observations.

CHANGES IN THE UTERUS DURING THE SECOND STAGE OF LABOR

By the end of the first stage of labor the uterine contractions have resulted in the differentiation of the organ into two parts, which are separated from one another by the physiologic retraction ring. Above is the active, contractile portion, which becomes thicker as labor advances, and below, the thin-walled, passive, lower uterine segment and cervix (see Fig. 240).

While these changes are being effected, often there has been no descent on the part of the fetus, and, as a rule, the position of the presenting part remains unchanged until after the cervix has become completely dilated. With the commencement of the second stage, however, descent begins, and under normal conditions continues slowly but steadily until delivery is accomplished. Naturally, the differentiation into stages is more or less arbitrary, so that, in a certain proportion of cases, it happens that the presenting part begins to descend during the latter part of the first stage of labor.

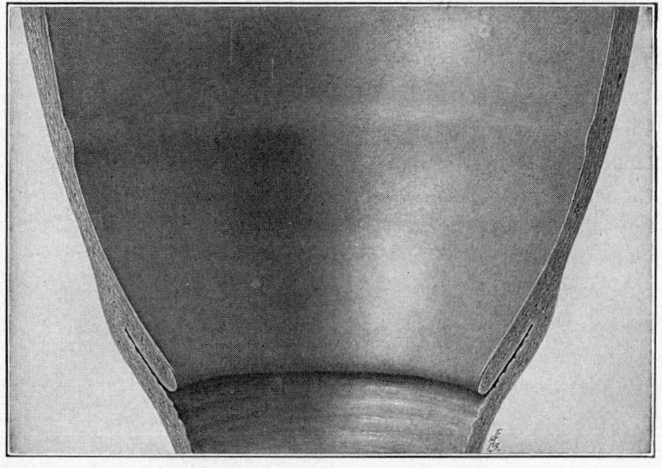

FIG. 240.—COMPLETE EFFACEMENT AND FULL DILATATION OF CERVIX.

After complete dilatation of the cervix, rupture of the membranes usually occurs, which is manifested by a sudden rush of a variable quantity of a quite clear fluid from the vagina. On the other hand, the membranes may give way some time before complete dilatation of the cervix has been brought about; while, on rare occasions, they may retain their integrity until the completion of labor, so that the fetus is born surrounded by them, the portion covering its head being designated as a *caul.*

Attention has already been directed to the changes in shape which the uterus presents during contraction. These may be noticed in the first, but more especially in the second stage, when the organ increases considerably in length, and at the same time diminishes in its transverse and anteroposterior diameter with each contraction. The increase in length is due partly to the stretching of the lower uterine segment, and partly to a straightening out of the fetus, but we are unable to make definite statements as to the part played by each factor. With the formation of the lower uterine segment, the upper portion of the uterus increases greatly in thickness, and, as labor proceeds, covers a progressively decreasing portion of the child. Thus, when the head is upon the perineum, less than one half of the fetus is in the upper segment. In obstructed labors, in which definite disproportion exists between the size of the presenting part and the pelvic canal, the lower uterine segment is subjected to excessive stretching, and consequently the retraction ring assumes a much higher level, when it can be palpated as a distinct transverse or oblique ridge at a variable level between the symphysis pubis and umbilicus. In such circumstances, its recognition indicates that rupture of the uterus is imminent and will occur if the labor is not promptly ended.

In addition to these factors, the contractions of the abdominal muscles of the woman also play no small part in effecting the extrusion of the child; indeed, according to some authorities, they alone bring it about. It is apparent that their action is usually essential for when it is absent, or only partially comes into play, labor is frequently so delayed that resort to forceps becomes necessary.

When the head has descended through the pelvis and is resting on the pelvic floor, more than half of the entire length of the child lies beneath the retraction ring; moreover, as the upper portion of the uterus becomes thicker and thicker, it necessarily exerts a diminished effect, so that, in the majority of cases, it becomes essential that the abdominal contractions should participate in the work.

Immediately after the birth of the child a striking change occurs in the position and size of the uterus, and on palpation it can be distinguished as a firm, rounded body which does not reach to the umbilicus. At this time its contracted and retracted body is freely movable above the collapsed lower uterine segment and cervix, and can readily be displaced in any desired direction.

CHANGES IN THE VAGINA AND PELVIC FLOOR DURING LABOR

The outlet of the pelvis is closed by a number of layers of tissue, which together constitute what is known as the pelvic floor. Beginning from within outward one meets successively with the peritoneum, the subperitoneal connective tissue, the internal pelvic fascia, the levator ani and coccygeus muscles, the external pelvic and perineal fascia, and, included between the latter, the superficial muscles of the perineum, external to which are the subcutaneous tissue and the cutaneous covering of the perineal and vulvar regions.

Of these structures the most important are the levator ani muscle and the fascia covering its upper and lower surfaces, which for practical purposes may be considered as constituting the pelvic floor. This muscle closes the lower end of the pelvic cavity as a diaphragm, and presents a concave upper and a convex lower surface. On either side it consists of a pubic and iliac portion. The former is a band 2 to 2.5 cm. in width, which arises from the horizontal ramus of the pubis 3 to 4 cm. below its upper margin, and 1 to 1.5 cm. from the symphysis pubis. Its fibers pass backward and encircle the rectum, and possibly give off a few fibers which pass behind the vagina. The greater or iliac portion of the muscle arises on either side from the white line—the tendinous arch of the pelvic fascia—and from the ischial spine, at a distance of about 5 cm. below the margin of the superior strait. Its fibers do not possess a uniform arrangement, but, according to Dickinson, the following portions can be distinguished: passing from before backward, there is a narrow band which crosses the pubic portion and descends to the rectovaginal septum. The greater part of the muscle passes backward and unites with that from the other side of the rectum, while the posterior portions meet together in a tendinous raphé in front of the coccyx, the most posterior fibers being attached to the bone itself. The posterior and lateral portions of the pelvic floor, which are not filled out by the levator ani muscle, are occupied by the pyriformis and coccygeus muscles on either side.

The levator ani muscle varies from 3 to 5 mm. in thickness, though its margins, which encircle the rectum and vagina, are somewhat thicker. It undergoes considerable hypertrophy during pregnancy, and on vaginal examination its internal

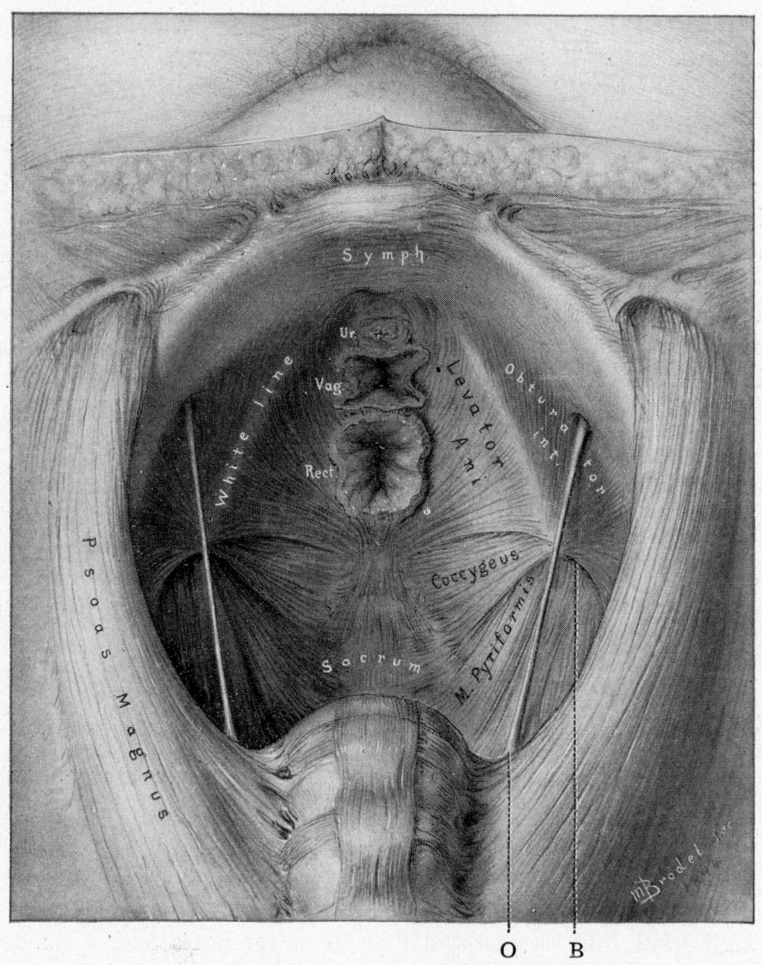

FIG. 241.—THE PELVIC FLOOR SEEN FROM ABOVE (Kelly).
O., obturator nerve; B., border of great sciatic foramen.

margin can be felt as a thick band extending backward from the pubis and encircling the vagina, about 2 cm. above the hymen. On contraction it serves to draw both the rectum and vagina forward and upward in the direction of the symphysis pubis, and is to be regarded as the real closer of the vagina, since the constrictor cunni, one of the superficial muscles of the perineum, is too delicate in structure to have more than an accessory function.

The internal pelvic fascia, which forms the upper covering of the levator ani, is attached to the margin of the superior strait, where it is joined by the fascia lining the iliac fossa, as well as by the transverse fascia of the abdominal walls. It passes down over the pyriformis and the upper half of the obturator internus muscle and is firmly attached to the periosteum covering the lateral wall of the pelvis, the white line indicating its point of deflection from the latter, whence it spreads out over the upper surface of the levator ani and coccygeus muscles.

The inferior fascial covering of the pelvic diaphragm is divided into two parts at a line drawn between the ischial tuberosities. Its posterior portion consists of a single layer which, taking its origin from the sacrosciatic ligament and the ischial tuberosity,

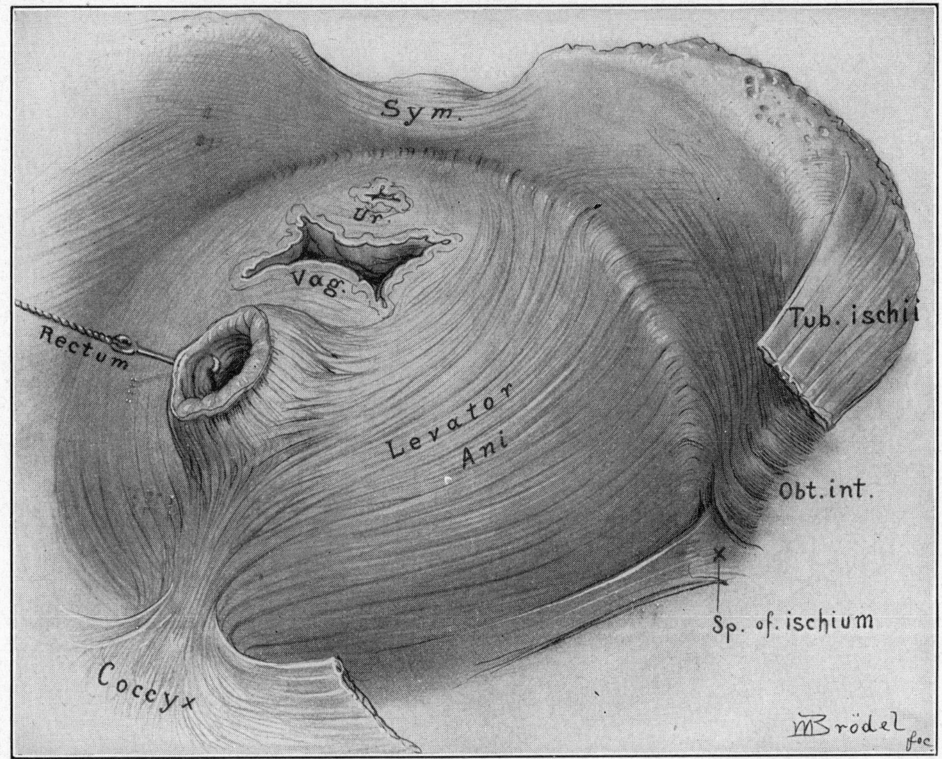

FIG. 242.—THE PELVIC FLOOR SEEN FROM BELOW (Kelly).

passes up over the inner surface of the ischial bones and the obturator internus muscles to the white line, in whose formation it takes part. From this tendinous structure it is reflected at an acute angle over upon the inferior surface of the levator ani, the space included between the latter and the lateral pelvic wall being designated as the *ischiorectal fossa.* The structure filling out the triangular space between the pubic arch and a line joining the ischial tuberosities is known as the *urogenital diaphragm,* which, exclusive of skin and subcutaneous fat, consists principally of three layers of fascia: (1) the deep perineal fascia which covers the anterior portion of the inferior surface of the levator ani muscle and is continuous with the fascia just described; (2) the middle perineal fascia which is separated from the former by a narrow space in which are situated the pudic vessels and nerves; (3) the superficial perineal fascia, which, together with the layer just described, forms a compartment in which lie the

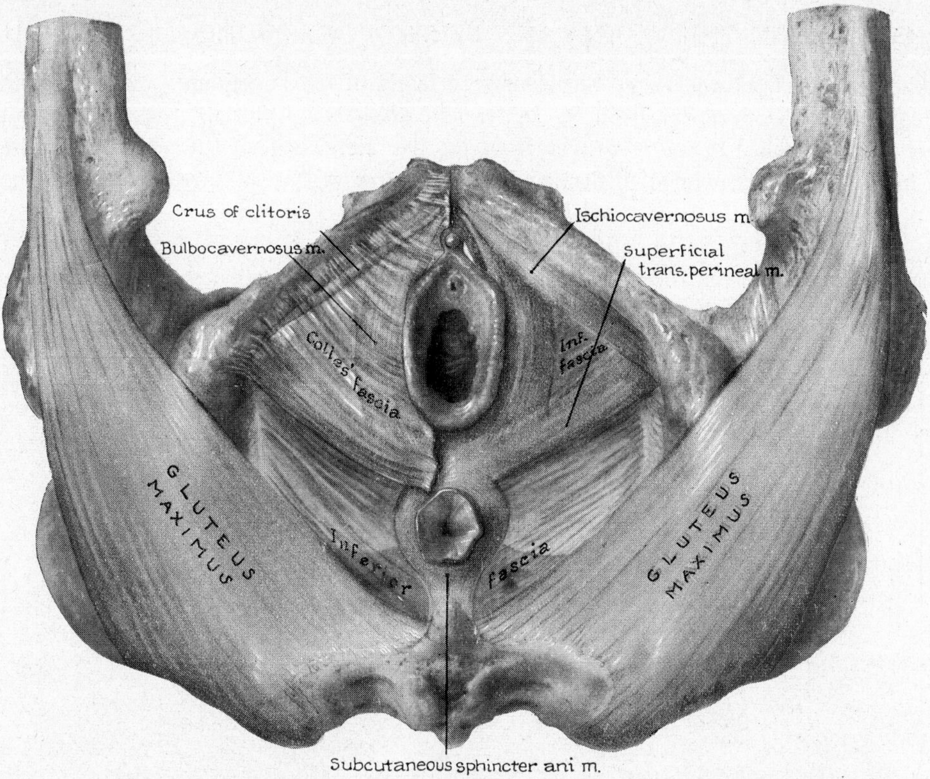

FIG. 243.—SUPERFICIAL MUSCLES AND FASCIA OF PELVIC FLOOR.

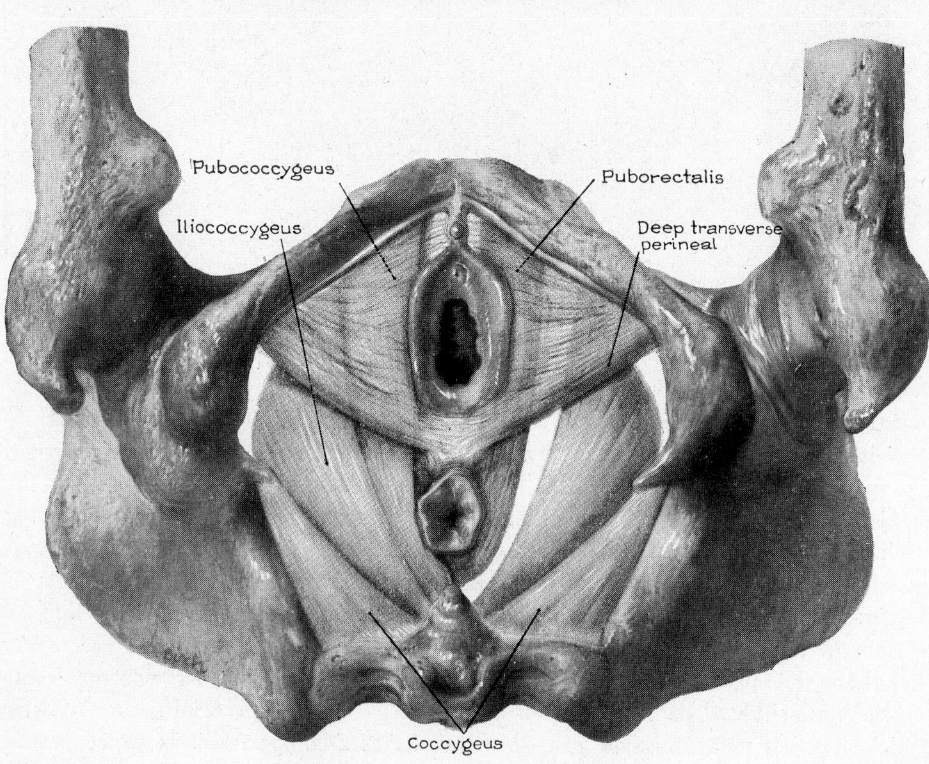

FIG. 244.—DEEP MUSCLES OF PELVIC FLOOR.

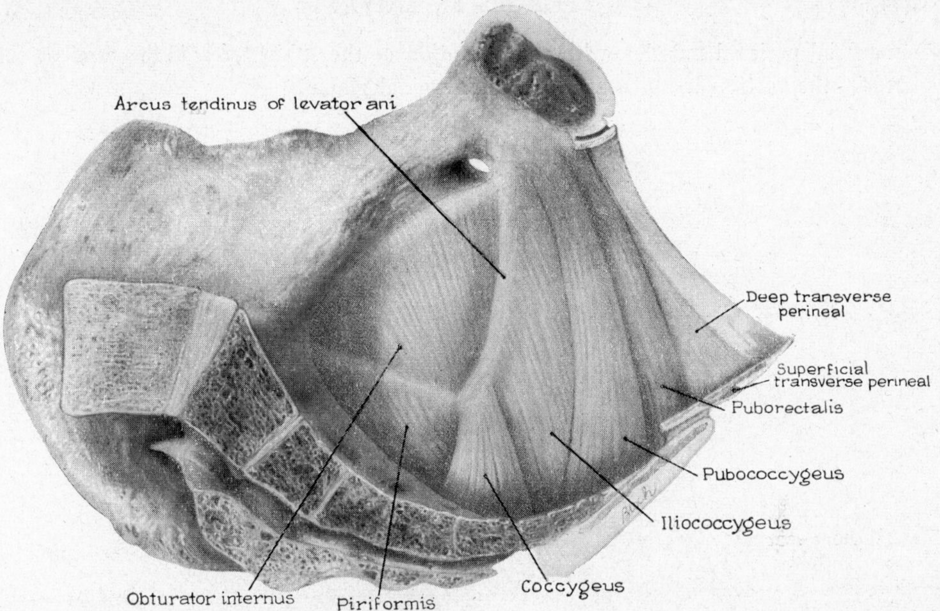

FIG. 245.—LATERAL VIEW OF MUSCLES OF PELVIC FLOOR.

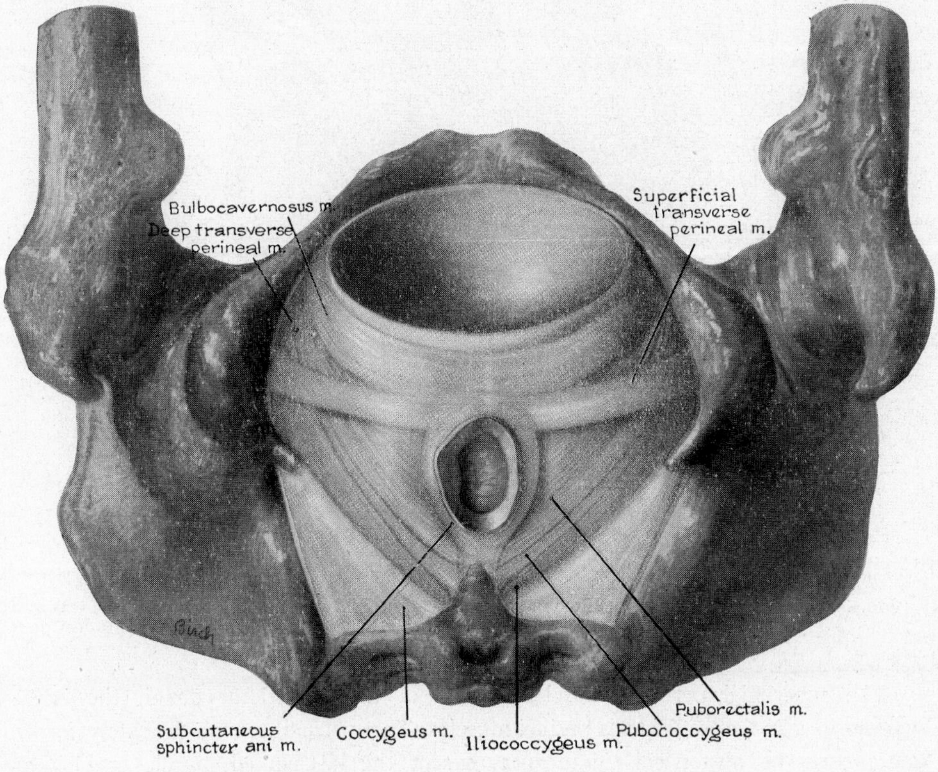

FIG. 246.—MUSCLES OF PELVIC FLOOR WHEN HEAD IS "CROWNING."

superficial perineal muscles, with the exception of the sphincter ani, the rami of the clitoris, the vestibular bulbs and the vulvovaginal glands (see Fig. 20).

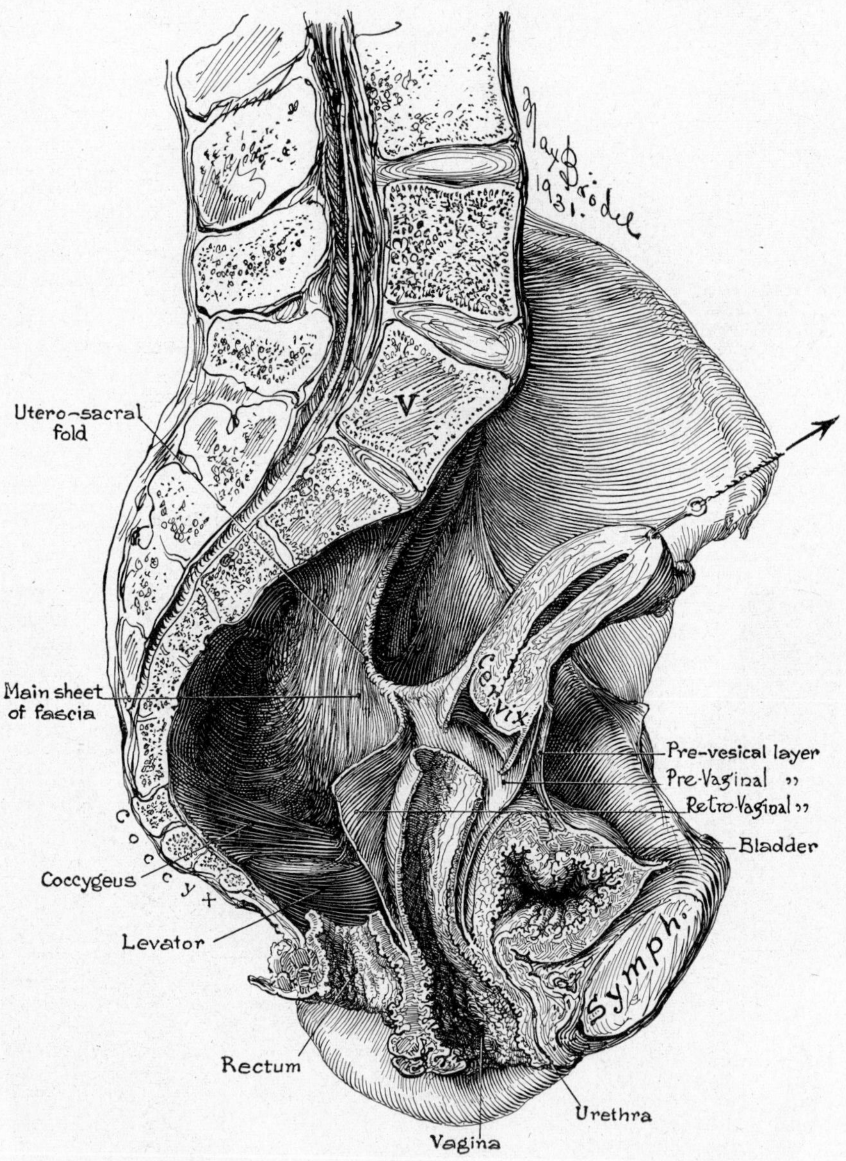

FIG. 247.—SAGITTAL SECTION OF PELVIC STRUCTURES TO SHOW FASCIA SURROUNDING VAGINA. (From Sears, *American Journal of Obstetrics and Gynecology.*)

The superficial perineal muscles consist of the constrictor cunni, the ischiocavernosus and the transversus perinei muscles. These structures are delicately formed and possess no obstetrical significance, except the last-named muscles, which are always torn through in perineal lacerations, when they serve in great part to bring about gaping of the wound. Studdiford held that the perineal body, anterior and interior to the sphincter ani, contains numerous strands of nonstriated muscle, which also plays an important part in perineal tears.

In the first stage of labor the bag of waters takes part in the dilatation and distention of the upper portion of the vagina which has been prepared for the process by important changes in its mucosa and connective tissue, while Stieve has shown that its unstriped muscular fibers undergo almost as great hypertrophy as those of

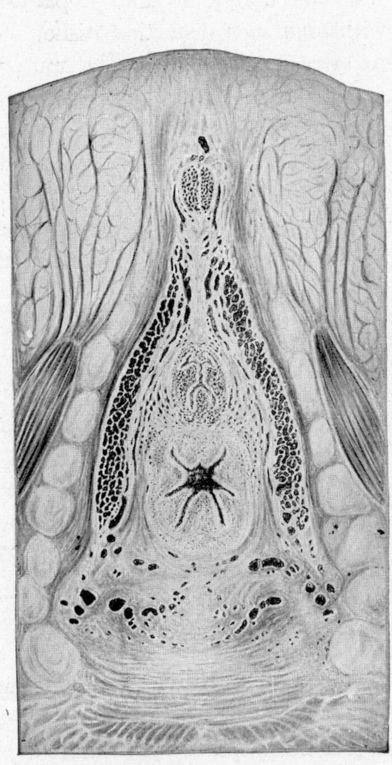

FIG. 248.—CROSS SECTION OF THE OUTLET OF A 27-YEAR-OLD BIPARA, EIGHT MONTHS AFTER DELIVERY.

The contents of the blood vessels are shown in black (Stieve).

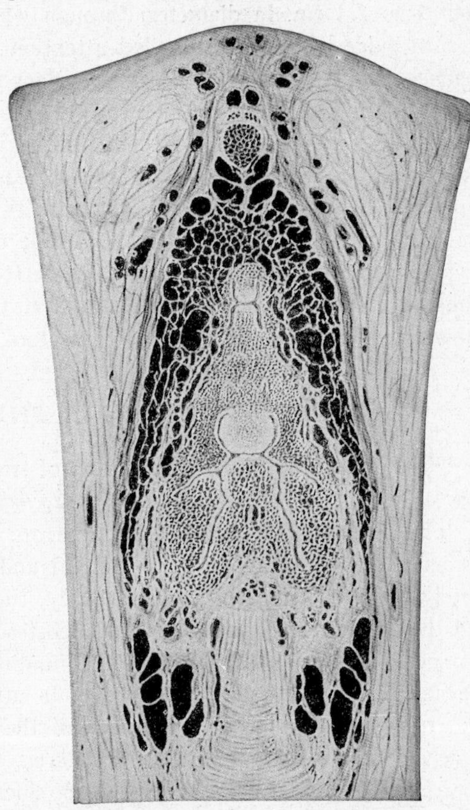

FIG. 249.—CROSS SECTION OF OUTLET OF 26-YEAR-OLD QUADRIPARA WHO DIED TWO DAYS AFTER DELIVERY.

The extreme vascularity of parts is shown (Stieve).

the uterus itself. Furthermore, Runge contends that radical chemical changes occur in the colloids of the vaginal wall, by which they become more hydrophilic, and thus better able to undergo the necessary plastic changes. But after the membranes have ruptured the changes occurring in the pelvic floor are due entirely to the pressure exerted by the presenting part. As this descends, the anterior portion of the pelvic floor becomes forced against the inferior and posterior portions of the symphysis. On the other hand, the posterior portion undergoes marked changes, becoming pushed downward and forward, and subjected to great stretching, eventually being converted into a thin-walled, tubular structure—the perineal gutter. When the head distends the vulva, the vulvar opening looks upward and forward, and the course of the birth canal along the pelvic floor follows the curve indicated in Fig. 245.

The most marked change consists in the stretching of the fibers of the levator ani muscle and the thinning of the central portion of the perineum, which becomes transformed from a wedge-shaped mass of tissue 5 cm. in thickness to a thin, almost transparent membranous structure 2 to 4 mm. thick. At the same time it is pushed down about 2.5 cm. from its original position. When the perineum is distended to the utmost, the anus becomes markedly dilated, and presents an opening which varies from 2 to 2.5 cm. in diameter, through which the anterior wall of the rectum is seen to bulge. Küstner has called attention to the fact that important preparatory changes make it possible for the pelvic floor to withstand such distortion without too much damage, and has adduced histological evidence to prove that the muscles, connective tissue and skin all undergo very considerable hypertrophy. Stieve has likewise emphasized the extraordinary increase in the number and size of the vessels supplying the vagina and pelvic floor, so that by the end of pregnancy practically the entire area between the anterior half of the vagina and the pubic arch has become converted into an erectile tissue. It is apparent that such an arrangement makes great compression possible, but at the same time it greatly increases the danger of hemorrhage if the tissues are torn through.

PHYSIOLOGY OF THE THIRD STAGE OF LABOR

The third stage of labor is made up of two phases, namely, *the phase of placental separation* and *the phase of placental expulsion.*

The Phase of Placental Separation. As the baby is being born, the uterus retracts down on its diminishing content and by the time the infant has been completely extruded from the mother's body, the uterine cavity has become obliterated and the organ is represented by an almost solid mass of muscle, the walls of which are several centimeters thick and the fundus of which lies just below the level of the umbilicus. This sudden diminution in uterine size is inevitably accompanied by a corresponding decrease in the area of the placental site. By way of an attempt to accommodate itself to this reduced area, the placenta becomes twice as thick as it was at the onset of labor. However, since its elastic properties are limited, the placenta is unable to follow this change very far and buckles on itself in folds. This places tension on the placental-uterine union and, as a consequence, the weakest layer of the decidua, the spongiosa, gives way and cleavage takes place in this layer. Separation of the placenta, therefore, is due primarily to a disproportion between the static size of the placenta and the reduced size of the placental site, this disproportion being the natural result of the uterine retraction associated with the birth of the baby.

The process of cleavage is greatly facilitated by the filamentous character of the spongiosa layer of the decidua. Indeed, to employ a crude analogy, this layer serves in this connection the same purpose as the row of perforations between postage stamps. As separation proceeds, more or less blood insinuates itself between the separating placenta and the remaining decidua basalis with the formation of a hematoma. But the formation of this hematoma is to be regarded as the result of the separation rather than the cause since in some cases there is no hematoma and bleeding is negligible. The hematoma may, however, accelerate the process.

In the majority of cases placental separation takes place within a few minutes after the birth of the baby. Thus, in a series of 30 cases, Brandt injected the umbilical

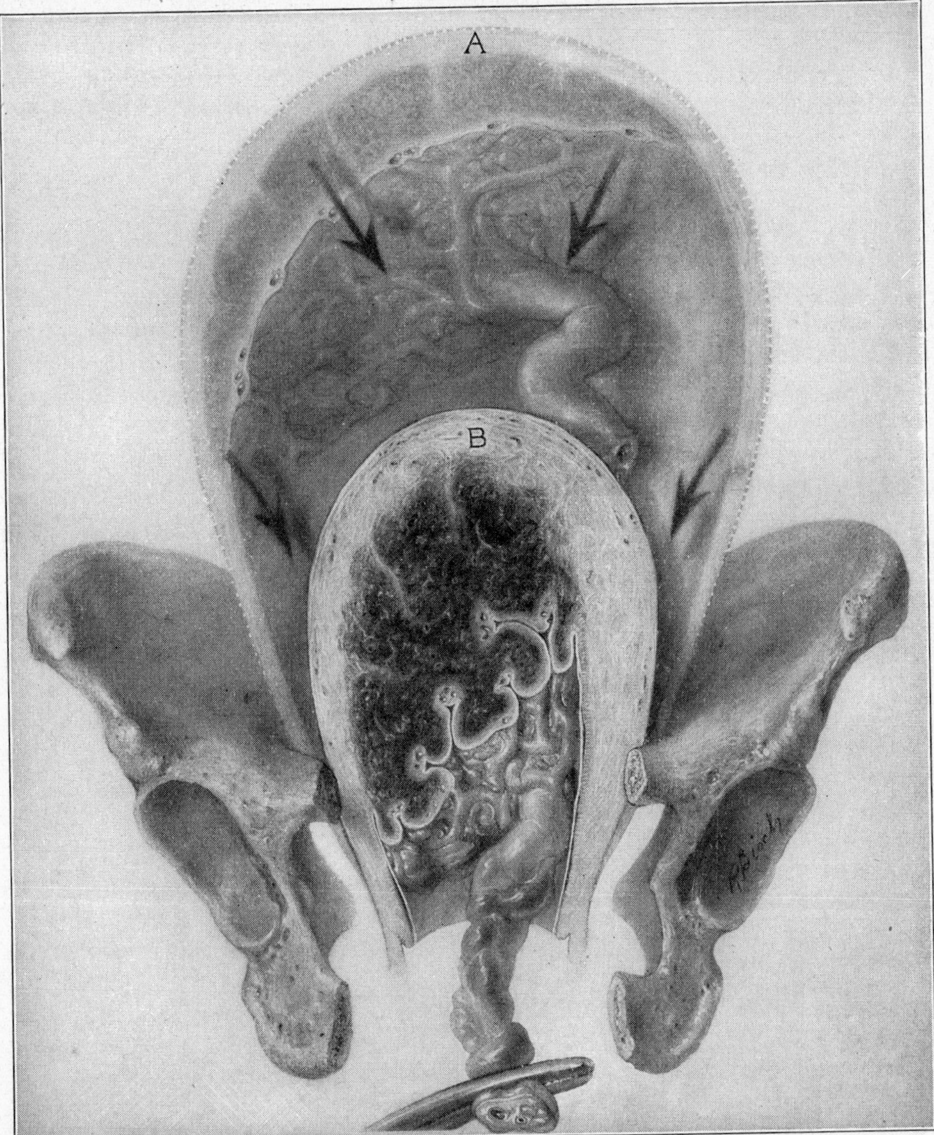

FIG. 250.—DIMINUTION IN SIZE OF PLACENTAL SITE AFTER BIRTH OF BABY.

A, placental relationships before delivery of infant; *B*, placental relationships after delivery of infant.

cord with a solution of sodium iodide and, three minutes later, was able to demonstrate, by means of x-rays, that the placenta in every instance had separated and lay folded on itself in the lower uterine segment. Calkins and also Pastore are likewise convinced that the detachment occurs very quickly, often in a few seconds.

Freeland demonstrated that the periphery of the placenta is the most adherent portion and as a result separation usually begins elsewhere. Brandt and others in recent clinical and roentgenologic studies have substantiated this conclusion, as well as the fact that some separation occurs even before the third stage of labor. This undoubtedly accounts for some of the fetal distress noted just before expulsion of the child.

As a result of the great decrease in the superficies of the rest of the interior of the uterus, the fetal membranes and the decidua vera are obliged to accommodate

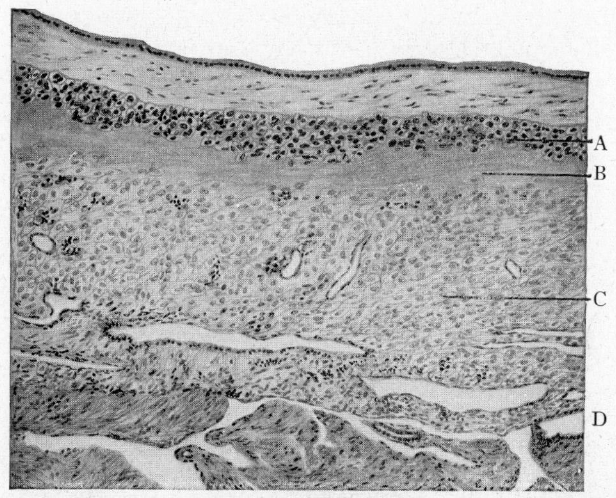

FIG. 251.—SECTION THROUGH WALL OF PREGNANT UTERUS OUTSIDE OF PLACENTAL SITE. × 66. A, amnion and chorion laeve; B, fibrin layer; C, decidua vera; D, muscularis.

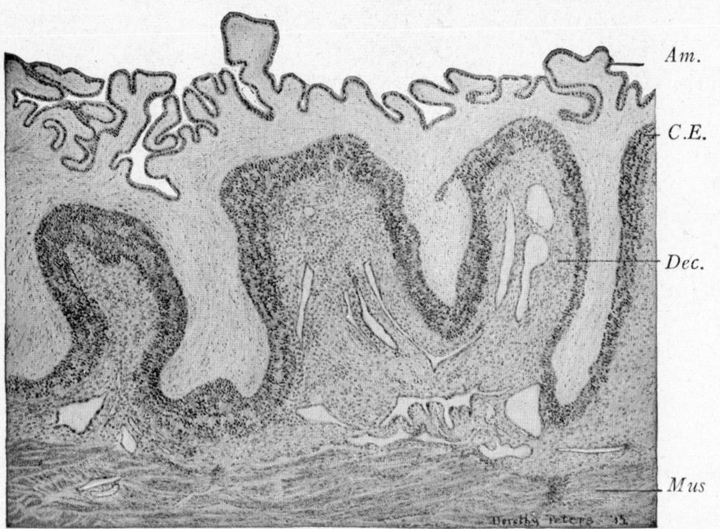

FIG. 252.—SECTION THROUGH UTERINE WALL OUTSIDE OF PLACENTAL SITE DURING THIRD STAGE, SHOWING FESTOONING OF MEMBRANES. × 25.
Am., amnion; *C.E.* epithelium of chorion; *Dec.*, decidua vera; *Mus.*, muscularis.

themselves to the changed conditions, and, as they are not contractile or elastic, they are thrown into innumerable small festoons or folds, so that the layer increases from a fraction of a millimeter to 3 or 4 mm. in thickness.

Figures 251 and 252, which represent the lining membrane of the uterus at the end of pregnancy and early in the third stage, respectively, give a good idea of the condition of affairs, and make it apparent that a very considerable proportion of the decidua vera has become included between the folds of the festooned amnion and chorion laeve.

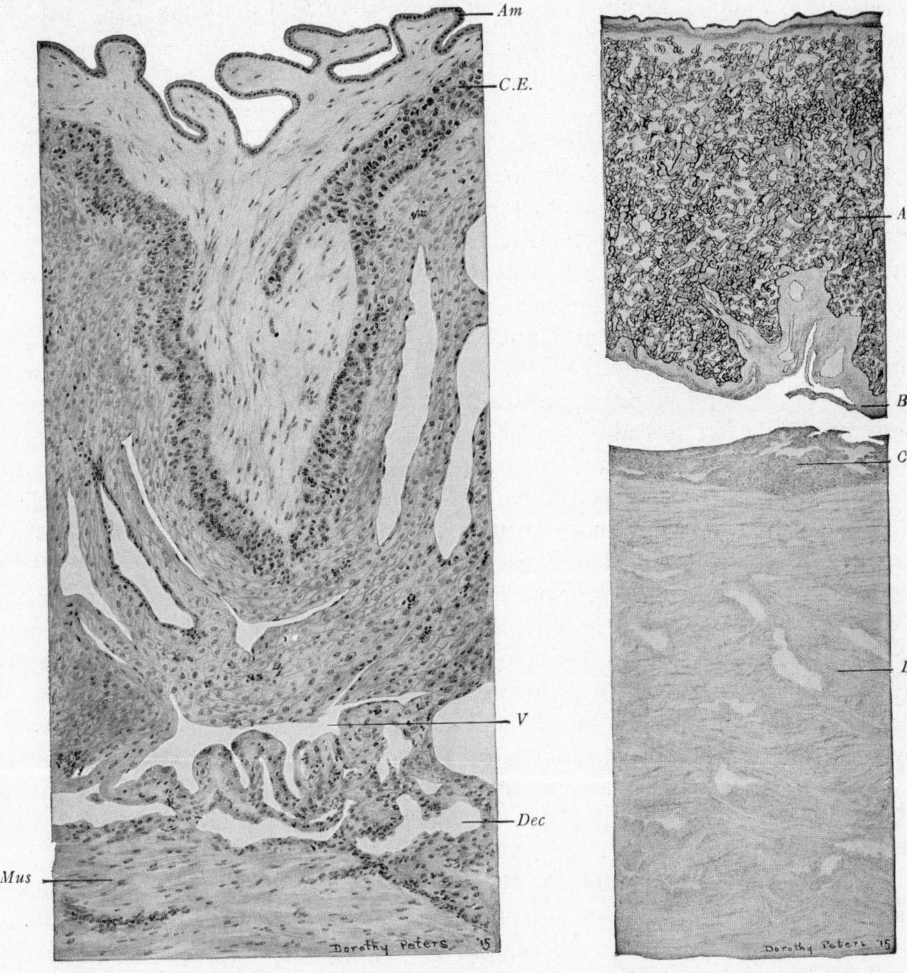

FIG. 253.—PORTION OF FIG. 252. MORE HIGHLY MAGNIFIED. × 66.

Am., amnion; *C.E.*, epithelium of chorion laeve; *Dec.*, decidua vera, gland spaces; *Mus.*, muscularis; *V.*, vascular spaces in decidua.

FIG. 254.—DIAGRAM SHOWING SEPARATION OF PLACENTA, AND APPROXIMATE AMOUNT OF DECIDUA BASALIS USUALLY CAST OFF WITH IT, AND RETAINED IN UTERO. × 3.

A, placenta; *B*, *C*, decidua basalis; *D*, muscularis.

As stated, the separation of the placenta takes place in the spongy layer of the decidua basalis, so that a portion is cast off with the placenta, while the balance remains attached to the muscularis (Fig. 253). The amount of decidual tissue which is retained at the placental site is dependent upon the original thickness of the decidua basalis, and varies within wide limits.

The membranes usually remain in situ until the separation of the placenta is practically completed, and are then peeled off from the uterine wall partly by the further contraction and retraction of the muscularis, and partly by traction exerted by the separated placenta, which now lies in the flabby lower uterine segment or the upper portion of the vagina. At this time the body of the uterus has become converted into an almost solid mass of muscle, whose anterior and posterior walls each measure 4 to 5 cm. in thickness and lie in such close apposition that the uterine cavity is practically obliterated.

Reference to Fig. 252 makes it clear that the greater portion of the decidua vera has been included between the festooned folds of the amnion and chorion laeve, and must be cast off when separation occurs. Consequently the portion which remains attached to the uterine wall is relatively thin, and, were it not for the great decrease in the size of the uterine cavity, it would represent only a fraction of the thickness noted during the last days of pregnancy.

The Phase of Placental Expulsion. After the placenta has separated, the pressure exerted upon it by the retracted uterine walls causes it to slide downward into the flaccid lower uterine segment or into the upper part of the vagina, where it then rests like a foreign body. In some cases it may be expelled from this location by increase in abdominal pressure, that is, by the same force which normally expels the infant. Modern woman, however, in the recumbent position cannot be expected to expel the placenta spontaneously in more than 15 to 20 per cent of cases. As long ago as 1884, Campe showed that the average duration of the third stage exceeded eight hours if women were left entirely to their own devices at that time. Among 500 women under a similar regime, Ahlfeld found that only 20 per cent were able to expel the placenta within one hour. In this day of anesthesia and analgesia the figure would doubtless be even lower and consequently some artificial means of terminating the third stage is usually necessary. The usual means employed is pressure over the fundus by the hand of an attendant in such a way that the uterus is used as a piston to shove the placenta out. In brief, then, the forces concerned in the expulsion of the placenta are either abdominal pressure or manual pressure, with the uterus used in either case as a sort of intermediary piston.

Schultze and Duncan Mechanisms of Placental Extrusion. As previously indicated, placental detachment usually occurs in the center of the placenta rather than at the periphery. When this central type of separation takes place, the retroplacental hematoma is believed to push the placenta toward the uterine cavity, first the central portion and then the rest. The placenta, inverted in this manner and weighted with the hematoma, now descends downward, but since the surrounding membranes are still attached to the decidua, it can only do so by dragging after it the membranes which peel off from the periphery of the placenta outward. As a consequence, the sac formed by the membranes is turned inside out, the placenta appearing at the vulva with the glistening fetal surface presenting. The retroplacental hematoma either follows the placenta or is demonstrable within the inverted sac. Because of the mechanism described, any bleeding from the placental site pours into the inverted sac and no blood escapes externally until after extrusion of the placenta. This is known as Schultze's mechanism of placental extrusion.

The other mechanism by which the placenta gains egress from the uterus and the vagina is known as the Duncan mechanism. In this, separation is believed to

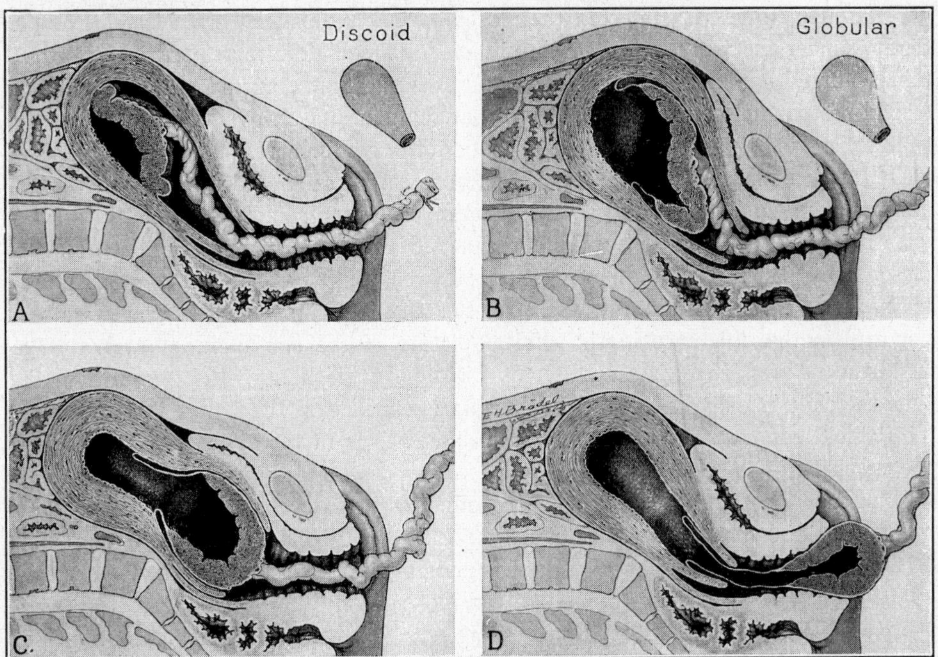

Fig. 255.—Schultze Mechanism.

A. Beginning central separation of placenta and collection of retroplacental blood. Uterus is changing from discoid to globular shape.

B. Complete separation. Placenta entering lower uterine segment. Uterus now globular.

C. Placenta entering vagina. Musculature of fundus is thicker.

D. Expression of placenta and completion of third stage of labor.

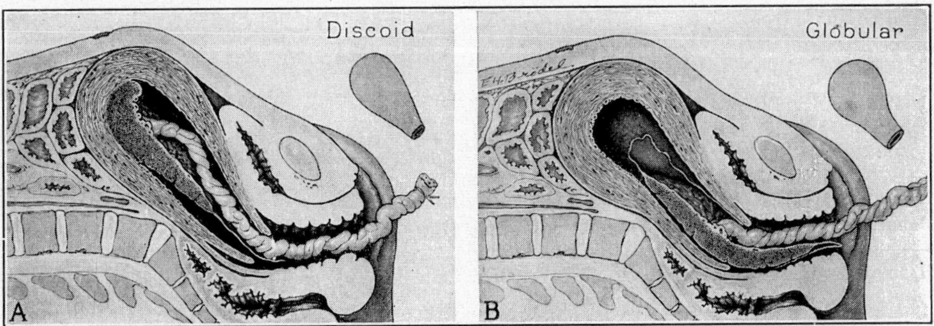

Fig. 256.—Duncan Mechanism.

A. Separation of placenta at one margin. Discoid uterus. Active bleeding.

B. Expulsion of placenta from lower uterine segment to vagina. Globular uterus.

occur first at the periphery with the result that blood insinuates itself between the membranes and the uterine wall and escapes out the vagina. In this event, the placenta descends to the vagina sideways and the maternal surface appears first at the vulva.

Interesting roentgen information about these two mechanisms has been contributed by Warnekros, who immediately after the birth of the child cut the cord, and, through its vessels, injected the placenta with a substance which would cast a shadow under the x-ray. Roentgenograms made immediately thereafter showed three things—first, that in two thirds of the cases separation occurred with the first or second postpartum contraction; second, that the placenta always passed through the contraction ring by its margin, and that the formation of a retroplacental hematoma played very little part in bringing about its separation; and third, that the mechanisms described by Duncan and Schultze developed only in the vagina and consequently applied only as the placenta emerged from the vaginal outlet. For this reason they contend that differentiation between the two methods is a matter of indifference, as the placenta always leaves the uterus in one way. This, however, does not explain the difference in the clinical picture of the two types of presentation. As already stated, there is a continuous trickling of blood from the uterus from the time the child is delivered until the placenta is expelled in the Duncan presentation. This would confirm the opinion that the difference is in the separation rather than the expulsion of the placenta.

Our experience is that the placenta usually escapes from the vulva by the Schultze mechanism, and similar views are held by Tucker and Freeland. The former, in 2,700 labors occurring at the Sloane Hospital, noted Schultze's mechanism in 64.8 per cent of the cases, as compared with 82.5 per cent observed by the latter in 2,600 labors at the Rotunda Hospital, Dublin. Freeland believes that a more frequent occurrence of Duncan's mechanism is due to the fact that the uterus had been kneaded during the third stage, and his belief is confirmed by the fact that in Tucker's series expression by Credé's method was routinely employed. In a series of 1,870 cases studied by Pastore, the Schultze presentation occurred in 71.1 per cent of the cases, while the Duncan mechanism was noted in only 28.9 per cent. In general, the total blood lost during the third stage of labor is greater with the Duncan presentation probably because of the partial peripheral separation of the placenta. (See Fig. 256A.)

BIBLIOGRAPHY

Ahlfeld, F. Die Blutung bei der Geburt und ihre Folgen für die Frau. Ztschr. f. Geburtsh. u. Gynäk., 1904, 51:341.

Aschoff, L. Das untere Uterinsegment. Ztschr. f. Geburtsh. u. Gynäk., 1906, 58:328.

——— Ueber die Berechtigung, etc., des Begriffes Isthmus uteri. Verhandl. d. deutsch. path. Gesellsch., 1908, 12:314.

Bandl, L. Ueber Ruptur der Gebärmutter. Wien, 1875.

——— Ueber das Verhalten des Uterus und Cervix, etc. Stuttgart, 1876.

Barbour, A. H. F. Atlas of the Anatomy of Labour Exhibited in Frozen Sections, 3rd Ed. Edinburgh, 1896.

——— Is There a Lower Uterine Segment? J. Obst. & Gynaec. Brit. Emp., 1908, 13:237.

Brandt, L. M. Mechanism and Management of the Third Stage of Labor. Am. J. Obst. & Gynec., 1933, 25:662.

Calkins, L. A. Management of the Third Stage of Labor. J. A. M. A., 1933, 101:1128.

Campe. Die Behandlung der Nachgeburtsperiode. Ztschr. f. Geburtsh. u. Gynäk., 1884, 10:416.

Corner, G. W. From Ourselves Unborn. An Embryologist's Essay on Man. Yale University Press, New Haven, 1944.

Danforth, D. N., Graham, R. J., and Ivy, A. C. Functional Anatomy of Labor as Revealed by Frozen Sagittal Sections in Macacus Rhesus Monkey. Surg., Gynec. & Obst., 1942, 74:188.

Danforth, D. N., and Ivy, A. C. Consideration of the Cause of Onset of Labor: Collective Review. Internat. Abstr. Surg., 1939, 69:351; in Surg., Gynec. & Obst., October, 1939.

Dickinson, R. L. Studies of the Levator Ani Muscle. Am. J. Obst., 1889, 22:897.

Duncan, J. M. The Expulsion of the Placenta. (Read to the Edinburgh Obstetrical Society, March 22, 1871.) Mechanism of Natural and Morbid Parturition. Edinburgh, 1875, pp. 246-256.

FREELAND, J. R. The Relationship Existing between the Mechanism and Management of the Third Stage of Labor. Am. J. Obst., 1914, 69:302.

HECKEL, G. P., and ALLEN, W. M. Prolongation of Pregnancy in the Rabbit by the Injection of Progesterone. Am. J. Obst. & Gynec., 1938, 35:131.

IVY, A. C. Functional Anatomy of Labor with Special Reference to Human Being. Am. J. Obst. & Gynec., 1942, 44:952.

——— and HARTMAN, C. G., and KOFF, A. The Contractions of the Monkey Uterus at Term. Am. J. Obst. & Gynec., 1931, 22:388.

KARLSON, S. On the Motility of the Uterus during Labour and the Influence of the Motility Pattern on the Duration of the Labour. Acta obst. et gynec. Scandinav., 1949, 28:209.

KOFF, A. K., and DAVIS, M. E. Mechanism of Prolongation of Pregnancy in the Rabbit. Am. J. Obst. & Gynec., 1937, 34:26.

LYON, R. Pregnanediol Excretion at the Onset of Labor. Am. J. Obst. & Gynec., 1946, 51:403.

MURPHY, D. P. The Tonus of the Uterus during Pregnancy and Its Relation to Labor. Surg., Gynec. & Obst., 1942, 74:182.

——— The Role of Intermittent Contractions of the Uterus in the Process of Labor; Observations Made with Lorand Tocograph. Am. J. Obst. & Gynec., 1945, 49:186.

PASTORE, J. B. A Study of the Blood Loss during the Third Stage of Labor and the Factors involved. Am. J. Obst. & Gynec., 1936, 31:78.

REYNOLDS, S. R. M. Physiology of the Uterus with Clinical Correlations. 2nd Ed. Paul H. Hoeber, New York, 1949.

——— and HEARD, O. O., BRUNS, P., and HELLMAN, L. M. A Multi-channel Strain-Gage Tokodynamometer: an Instrument for Studying Patterns of Uterine Contractions in Pregnant Women. Bull. Johns Hopkins Hosp., 1948, 82:446.

——— and HELLMAN, L. M., and BRUNS, P. Patterns of Uterine Contractility in Women during Pregnancy. Obst. & Gynec. Surv., 1948, 3:629.

RUDOLPH, L., and IVY, A. C. The Coordination of the Uterus in Labor. Am. J. Obst. & Gynec., 1931, 21:65.

SCHULTZ. Ueber den Mechanismus der Spontanen Ausscheidung der Nachgeburt, etc. Deutsche med. Wchnschr., Berlin, 1880, 6:252.

SMITH, P. E. Nonessentiality of Posterior Hypophysis in Parturition. Am. J. Physiol., 1932, 99:345.

SNYDER, F. F. The Prolongation of Pregnancy and Complications of Parturition in the Rabbit following Induction of Ovulation near Term. Bull. Johns Hopkins Hosp., 1934, 54:1.

STIEVE, H. Der Halsteil der menschlichen Gebärmutter, etc. Leipzig, 1927.

——— Die Enge der menschlichen Gebärmutter, ihre Veränderungen während der Schwangerschaft, der Geburt und des Wochenbettes, und ihre Bedeutung. Ztschr. f. mikr.-anat. Forsch., 1928, 14:549.

——— Schiedenwand und Scheidenmund während und nach der Geburt. Ztschr. f. mikr.-anat. Forsch., 1928, 13:441.

TORPIN, R. Physiology of Labor. Am. J. Obst. & Gynec., 1947, 53:78.

WARNEKROS. Die Nachgeburtsperiode in Röntgenbilde. Arch. f. Gynäk., 1918, 109:266.

WOODBURY, R. A., HAMILTON, W. F., and TORPIN, R. The Relationship between Abdominal, Uterine and Arterial Pressure during Labor. Am. J. Physiol., 1938, 121:640.

(For literature on the cause of the onset of labor, see the first Reynolds reference.)

14

THE MECHANISM OF LABOR IN VERTEX PRESENTATIONS

Vertex presentations occur in from 94 to 97 per cent of all cases—94.8 per cent in 31,000 consecutive cases in the obstetrical service of the New York Lying-In Hospital. Naegele and most subsequent observers believed that in vertex presentations the sagittal suture nearly always engages in the right oblique diameter of the pelvis. In other words, one usually has to deal with a left occipito-anterior or a right occipitoposterior position. Roentgenological studies, however, of Caldwell, Moloy, Thoms, Steele, Wing, McLane, and Javert show that this is not so, but that in the majority of instances the head enters the pelvic inlet in the transverse rather than in one or other of the oblique diameters.

Upon analyzing the incidence of the several varieties in the 28,494 consecutive vertex presentations occurring in the New York Lying-In Hospital, Stander found the occiput to the left in 63.90 per cent and to the right in 35.23 per cent. The occiput was located directly anteriorly or posteriorly in 0.87 per cent. Caldwell and his associates in a roentgenologic study of a series of 200 patients found the occiput directed to the left in 59 per cent, to the right in 35.5 per cent, and directly anterior in 5.5 per cent. Moreover, these studies indicate that transverse positions far exceed those of the oblique positions, 60 per cent engaging in the transverse diameter, two thirds with the occiput directed toward the left, and one third toward the right. The right oblique diameter accommodated 19 per cent, equally divided between L. O. A. and R. O. P., while in the left oblique, R. O. A. and L. O. P. occurred in 6.5 per cent and 9 per cent, respectively.

In the New York Lying-In Hospital Steele and his associates corroborated the findings of Caldwell and Moloy. They studied three series of cases, the first comprising patients not in labor and with the fetal head not fixed, the second, a similar group but with the head fixed, and the last, patients in labor and with the head fixed, in whom they made x-ray observations early in labor, as well as at the beginning of the second stage. Over half of the patients had an initial transverse position as revealed by the stereoscope, while about one quarter showed presentations between transverse and oblique. Slightly less than one quarter of the initial presentations were definitely oblique. These earlier observations have been corroborated by their later and more extended studies. The following table gives the incidence of the different positions, in percentage, as determined by the combined stereoscopic and isometric lateral technic, which is described in the section on x-ray pelvimetry.

Descent of Head	L.O.T.	R.O.T.	L.O.A.	R.O.A.	O.A.	R.O.P.	L.O.P.	O.P.	Number of Cases
Above or at inlet	39.9	23.5	13.2	9.6	1.8	7.3	3.0	.6	763
At, above or below spines	33.7	28.8	11.9	5.7	2.8	11.5	3.2	1.8	277

These findings show a transverse position of the head in over 60 per cent of the 1,040 patients studied, irrespective of whether the head is unengaged or in the mid-pelvis.

Mechanism in Left and Right Occipito-Anterior Positions. We shall consider in the first place the mechanism of labor in the anterior varieties of vertex presentation—namely, the left and right occipito-anterior (Fig. 257).

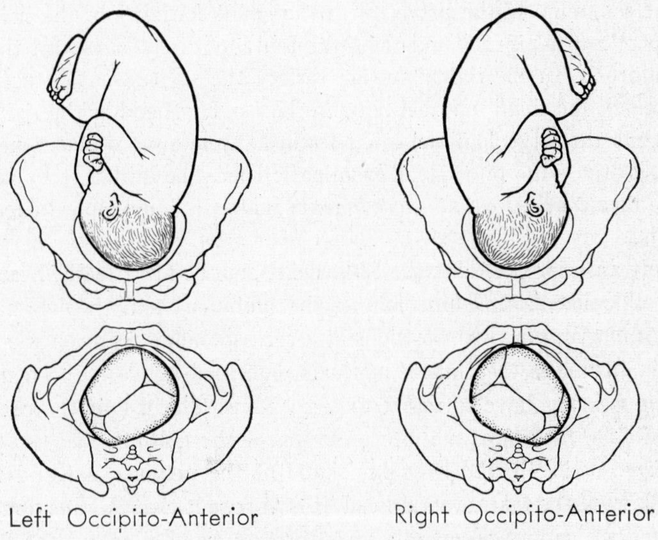

FIG. 257.—SHOWING CHILD IN L. O. A. AND IN R. O. A.

Diagnosis. The mode of presentation of the fetus is most reliably determined by abdominal palpation, which can be utilized not only during pregnancy but also at the time of labor, provided it be practiced in the intervals between the pains. Its accuracy, however, is greatly impaired in patients with very fat abdominal walls, or in whom the uterus is unduly distended by an excessive amount of amniotic fluid, or deformed by subperitoneal or intramural myomata; the latter may occasionally be mistaken for portions of the child.

For the purpose of diagnosis we employ the four maneuvers already described and, with the fetus in the left occipito-anterior position, obtain the following:

First maneuver: Irregular breech at fundus.

Second maneuver: Resistant plane of back on the left and anterior portion of the abdomen, with the small parts on the right side.

Third maneuver: If the head be not engaged, it is felt as a freely movable body over the superior strait; but if it be fixed, the anterior shoulder may be detected.

Fourth maneuver: Negative if the head is not engaged; otherwise the cephalic prominence is felt on the right side (Fig. 223).

For the right occipito-anterior position the findings are as follows:

First maneuver:	Irregular breech at fundus.
Second maneuver:	Resistant plane of back on the right and anterior portion of the abdomen, with the small parts on the left side.
Third maneuver:	As in L. O. A.
Fourth maneuver:	Cephalic prominence on the left side.

Until the head has become engaged the information obtained by vaginal or rectal examination is relatively meager, and even after engagement satisfactory results cannot usually be obtained until the cervix has become sufficiently dilated to permit the differentiation of the various sutures and fontanels. When this is possible and the child lies in the left anterior position the sagittal suture will be found to occupy the right oblique diameter of the pelvis, with the small fontanel in the neighborhood of the left iliopectineal eminence and the large fontanel directed toward the right sacro-iliac synchondrosis. In the right anterior variety the sagittal suture occupies the left oblique diameter, the small fontanel lying in the neighborhood of the right iliopectineal eminence, while the large fontanel looks toward the left sacro-iliac synchondrosis.

The diagnostic value of vaginal examination may be still further impaired when the presence of a marked *caput succedaneum* makes it impossible to feel the sutures and fontanels.

In the left anterior positions the fetal heart sounds are usually heard on the left side of the abdomen along a line joining the umbilicus and the left antero-superior spine of the ilium, and in right positions at a corresponding point on the right side.

In certain instances the clinical methods described above may be unsatisfactory, in which case we may have to resort to x-ray films. The use of the precision stereoscope, if available, facilitates the interpretation of the findings.

Mechanism. Owing to the irregular shape of the pelvic canal and the relatively large dimensions of the mature fetal head, it is apparent that any portion of the latter, chosen at random, cannot necessarily pass through every plane of the former. It follows that some process of adaptation or accommodation of suitable portions of the head to the various pelvic planes is necessary to insure the completion of childbirth. This is brought about by certain very definite movements of the presenting part, which constitute what is usually termed the mechanism of labor (see Fig. 263).

For purposes of instruction, one is obliged to describe the various movements as if they occurred separately and independently of one another, whereas, in reality, the mechanism of labor consists of a combination of movements, several of which may be going on at the same time as it is manifestly impossible for any one of them to occur unless the presenting part descends simultaneously. These movements are divided into two classes, depending upon whether they are essential to the completion of labor, or merely facilitate its progress. To the first group belong the so-called cardinal movements—*descent, internal rotation* and *extension;* to the second, the accessory movements—*flexion* and *external rotation.* As a preliminary to these movements, the uterine contractions bring about important modifications in the attitude or habitus of the fetus, which greatly facilitate the act of labor. These consist principally in a straightening out of the fetus, so that its back loses its convexity while the extremities and small parts are more closely applied against the body, with the result that the fetal ovoid becomes transformed into a cylindrical body with the smallest possible cross section for passage through the birth canal.

Engagement. As already stated, the mechanism by which the presenting part enters the superior strait is designated as engagement. This is best studied in women who have borne one or more children, for the reason that some weeks before the onset of labor in primigravidae the head normally descends so deeply into the pelvic canal that its most dependent portion lies just above a line joining the ischial spines, whereas in multiparous women this usually does not take place until after the commencement of labor.

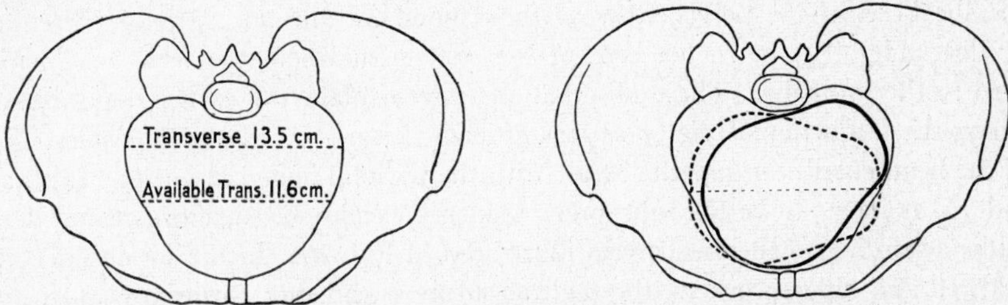

FIG. 258.—DIAGRAMS SHOWING HOW ENCROACHMENT OF THE SACRUM MAY PREVENT ENGAGEMENT IN THE TRANSVERSE DIAMETER, UNLESS HEAD IS ASYNCLITIC.

In most multiparae at the end of pregnancy the head, which occupies a position midway between flexion and extension, is freely movable above the superior strait, or rests upon one or other iliac fossa. Accordingly, when the uterine contractions set in and force it toward the pelvic opening, the cephalic circumference which first engages is the one that passes through the extremities of the fronto-occipital diameter. This normally measures 11.5 cm., and, as the conjugata vera is only 11 cm. in length in the bony pelvis and is encroached upon by various tissues in the living woman, it is apparent that a normal-size head usually does not engage with its sagittal suture directed anteroposteriorly. Accordingly, it must enter the superior strait either in the transverse or in one of its oblique diameters (12.75 cm.). As has already been said, this usually occurs in the transverse or, less frequently, in the right oblique diameter, so that one end of the sagittal suture is directed toward the left iliopectineal eminence and the other toward the right sacro-iliac synchondrosis. This is attributable to two factors. In the first place, the fetus, in the later months of pregnancy, tends to assume this position spontaneously; secondly, the posterior end of the left oblique diameter is encroached upon by the rectum, so that, for practical purposes, it is shorter than the right. Calkins is of the opinion that an additional and more adequate explanation lies in the fact that the urinary bladder occupies the right anterior quadrant.

Naegele, in 1838, held that engagement took place in such a way that the sagittal suture assumed an eccentric position, being nearer the promontory of the sacrum than the symphysis, and that therefore the anterior parietal bone of the fetus was first felt on vaginal examination—*Naegele's obliquity.* Others contend that the reverse is the case, and that the head enters the pelvis with its sagittal suture nearer the symphysis pubis—*Litzmann's obliquity*—so that the posterior parietal bone of the fetal head, instead of the anterior, is first felt on vaginal examination. (See Fig. 443.)

Until the recent studies of Caldwell and his associates, it has been generally believed that the head usually engages in such a manner that its sagittal suture lies either in the middle of the pelvis or approaches the promontory of the sacrum only slightly, but not to the extent that Naegele had supposed. In an extensive roentgenologic investigation of the mechanism of labor, Caldwell, Moloy and Swenson observed that with engagement the fetal head is usually in a posterior parietal presentation, or Litzmann's (Varnier's) obliquity, a presentation which we have commonly associated with considerable cephalopelvic disproportion. In corroboration of this observation, Javert and Steele noted Litzmann's obliquity in 75 per cent of their cases in which the fetal head was at the brim of the pelvis, whereas they found an anterior parietal presentation (Naegele's obliquity) in 76 per cent of the women in whom the fetal head had descended to the midpelvis. These observations may explain the earlier opposing views regarding the frequency of the two types of asynclitism—anterior and posterior.

If the head enters the superior strait with the parietal bone presenting (Litzmann's obliquity), as seems to be the rule rather than the exception, engagement and descent would be according to the mechanism illustrated in Fig. 266. In the former, according to Caldwell and his co-workers, the sagittal suture is directed downward and forward toward the symphysis, and as the head descends, the anterior parietal bone sinks behind the symphysis in a downward and backward direction until the head fits in the pelvic canal. Caldwell and his co-workers further state that when the fetal head has descended to fill the fully dilated cervix its long axis is usually almost parallel with the sacrum, and they believe that the lower uterine segment and cervix guide and direct the head to follow this curved axis of descent. Their stereoroentgenograms of normal labor show that the mechanism of engagement and descent usually takes place along an axis in the posterior pelvis, the most ample segment of the pelvic cavity. These authors have directed attention to several significant factors which come into play in different types of abnormal pelves.

Descent. The first requisite for the birth of the child is descent, the extent varying materially according as the patient is a primigravida or a multipara. In the former, when there is no disproportion between the size of the head and the pelvis, engagement is frequently so deep at the onset of labor that the most dependent part of the head is at, or only slightly above, the level of the ischial spines, so that further descent does not necessarily begin until the second stage of labor sets in. In multiparae, on the other hand, descent begins with engagement. It should, however, be remembered that in either event, once having been inaugurated, descent is inevitably associated with the various movements to which reference will be made. Descent is brought about by one or more of four forces: (1) intra-uterine fluid pressure; (2) direct pressure of the fundus upon the breech; (3) contraction of the abdominal muscles; and (4) extension and straightening of the child's body.

As the anterior surface of the sacrum and the posterior surface of the symphysis measure 12 and 5 cm., respectively, it is apparent that, if all parts of a body passing through the pelvic cavity are to reach the inferior strait at the same time, the portion lying posteriorly must descend more rapidly than the anterior portion. This compensatory difference in the rate of descent of the portions of the presenting part occupying the anterior and posterior segments of the pelvis is known as *synclitism.* In synclitism the sagittal suture of the head upon entering the pelvic inlet is midway between the symphysis and the promontory of the sacrum, and as the head descends the biparietal diameter successively assumes positions parallel to the various planes of the pelvis from above downward. As stated above, Caldwell and his associates in their roentgenological studies of engagement contend that early in the process the posterior parietal bone is actually presenting, the sagittal suture being close to the anterior border of the symphysis. With engagement there is a gradual slipping of the anterior parietal bone behind the symphysis pubis, necessitating varying degrees of lateral flexion of the fetal head. This method of descent is known as *asynclitism*.

Flexion. As soon as the descending head meets with resistance, whether it be from the margins of the superior strait or the cervix, the walls of the pelvis, or the pelvic floor, flexion results. In this movement the head rotates about its transverse axis in such a manner as to bring the chin into more intimate contact with the thorax, thereby substituting the suboccipitobregmatic for the fronto-occipital diameter.

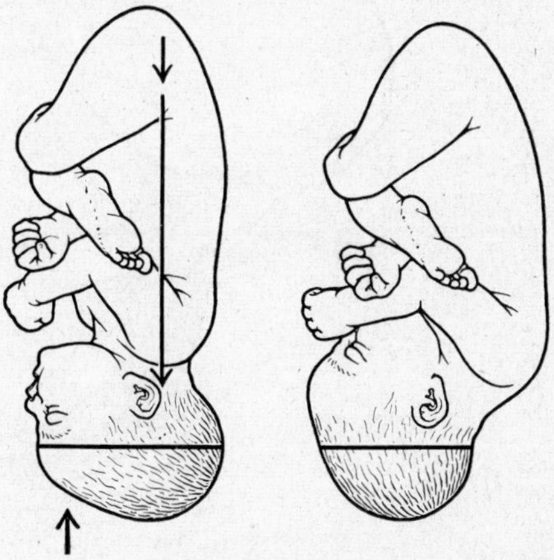

This purely mechanical phenomenon, by which a diameter of 9.5 replaces one of 11.75 cm., may be due to the manner in which the head is articulated with the vertebral column, whereby the head represents a two-armed lever, the short arm extending from the occipital condyles to the occipital protuberance, and the long arm from the condyles to the chin. When resistance is encountered the long arm of the lever, following the ordinary laws of mechanics, ascends while the short arm descends; thus flexion is brought about.

FIG. 259.—DIAGRAMS SHOWING LEVER ACTION PRODUCING FLEXION OF HEAD; CONVERSION OF OCCIPITOFRONTAL INTO SUBOCCIPITOBREGMATIC DIAMETER.

According to D'Esopo, flexion of the head depends upon the relationship between the line of force, transmitted in the direction of the fetal spine and foramen magnum, and the occipitofrontal plane rather than upon the lever action as outlined above.

The point of the birth canal at which this movement occurs varies greatly. When there is no disproportion between the presenting part and the pelvic canal, pronounced flexion does not occur until the resistance of the pelvic floor is encountered, but if descent begins before the external os is fully dilated, especially if its margins are resistant, flexion may be completed before the head has left the uterus; in generally contracted pelves the movement occurs in an exaggerated manner while engagement is being effected.

Internal Rotation. By this is understood a turning of the head about its vertical axis in such a manner that the occiput gradually moves from the position which it originally occupied, toward the symphysis pubis or the hollow of the sacrum as the case may be.

Internal rotation is absolutely essential for the completion of labor, except when the child is abnormally small, and in the anterior varieties always occurs from left to right in left positions, and in the reverse direction in right positions. (Figs. 261 and 262.) Indeed, no matter what the original position of the head may be, the occiput usually rotates to the front, although exceptionally, in occipitoposterior positions, it may turn toward the hollow of the sacrum.

It should be remembered that internal rotation does not occur by itself, but is always associated with the descent of the presenting part, and is usually not effected until the head has reached the level of the spines and therefore becomes engaged, as

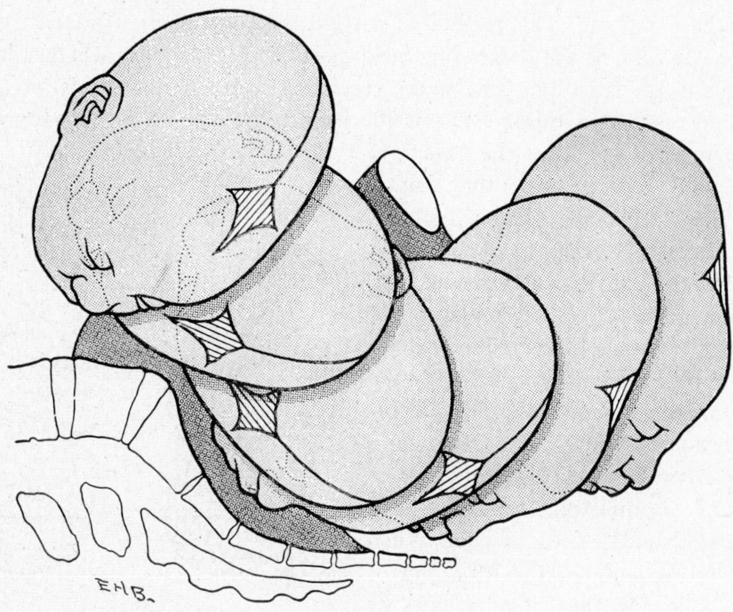

FIG. 260.—MECHANISM OF LABOR FOR LEFT OCCIPUT ANTERIOR POSITION.

shown by Steele's x-ray studies. Calkins has reported examinations during labor on some 2,900 primigravidae and some 2,500 multiparae to ascertain when internal rotation occurs. As a result, he believes that in approximately two thirds of all patients internal rotation is complete at the time the head reaches the pelvic floor. In somewhat less than 30 per cent, internal rotation is completed very shortly after the head reaches

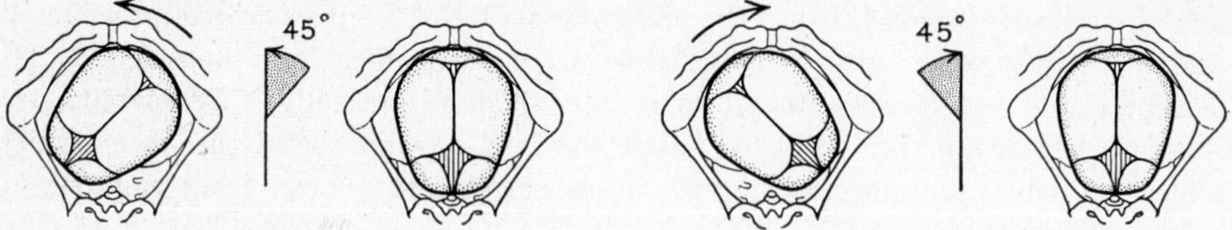

FIG. 261.—ANTERIOR ROTATION FROM L. O. A. FIG. 262.—ANTERIOR ROTATION FROM R. O. A.

the pelvic floor. In somewhat over four per cent of all patients, rotation to the anterior does not take place. When rotation does not occur until the head reaches the pelvic floor, it takes place in multiparae during the next one or two contractions, and in primigravidae during the next three to five contractions. Rotation before the head reaches the pelvic floor is definitely more frequent in multiparae than in primigravidae, according to Calkins; it is also frequent in women with good pains.

The factors responsible for internal rotation are to be found in the structures of the pelvic floor, in the oval shape of the vaginal outlet, and particularly in the levator ani muscle, which, yielding before the impact of the head, nevertheless exerts sufficient force upon it to compel it to adjust itself to its curvatures. Furthermore, the walls of the perineal gutter offer a concave inclined plane over which the rounded head readily glides in its downward course.

This explanation, although fairly satisfactory when the occiput is originally directed obliquely anteriorly in the pelvis, would not necessarily seem to apply with equal force to those cases in which it occupies an obliquely posterior position. But the following account of Dubois' experiment clearly demonstrates that even in such circumstances the pelvic floor exerts a predominating influence in the production of this movement: "In a woman who had died a short time previously in childbirth, the uterus, which had remained flaccid and of large size, was opened up as far as the cervical orifice and held by assistants in a suitable position above the superior strait. The fetus of the woman was then placed in the soft and dilated uterus in the right occipitoposterior position. Several pupil-midwives, pushing the fetus from above, readily caused it to enter the cavity of the pelvis. Much greater force was needed to make the head travel over the perineum and clear the vulva, and it was not without astonishment that we saw, in three successive attempts, that, when the head had traversed the external genital organs, the occiput had turned to the right anterior position, while the face was turned to the left and to the rear. In a word, rotation had taken place as in natural labor. We repeated the experiment a fourth time, but as the head cleared the vulva the occiput remained posterior. We then took a deadborn fetus of the previous night, but of much larger size than the preceding, and placed it in the same position as the first, and twice in succession witnessed the head clear the vulva after having executed the movement of rotation. Upon the third and following essays delivery was accomplished without the occurrence of rotation. Thus the movement only ceased after the perineum and vulva had lost the resistance which had made it necessary, or at least had been the inciting cause of its accomplishment."

Extension. When, after internal rotation, the sharply flexed head reaches the vulva, it undergoes another movement which is absolutely essential to its birth—namely, it becomes so extended that the base of the occiput comes in direct contact with the inferior margin of the symphysis pubis. This movement is brought about by two factors. In the first place, as the vulvar outlet looks upward and forward, extension must occur before the head can pass through it. If the sharply flexed head, on reaching the pelvic floor, continued to be driven downward in the same direction as heretofore—in the axis of the superior strait—it would impinge upon the end of the sacrum and the posterior portion of the perineum, and, if the *vis a tergo* was sufficiently strong, would eventually carry away the lowermost portion of the former, and be forced through the tissues of the latter. But when the head presses upon the pelvic gutter two forces come into play, the first acting downward, exerted by the uterus, and the second upward, supplied by the resistant pelvic floor, the resultant force being one directed forward and somewhat upward in the direction of the vulvar opening, thereby giving rise to extension.

After the suboccipital region has come in contact with the inferior margin of the symphysis pubis, the head is no longer to be regarded as a two-armed lever. It is simply a one-armed lever, the occiput being the fulcrum with the arm extending from it to the chin; any force exerted upon the head must necessarily lead to further extension. As this becomes marked, the vulvar opening gradually dilates and the scalp of the child becomes apparent through it. Now, if we mark the point which first appears, and carefully examine the child after its birth, we find in left occipito-anterior positions

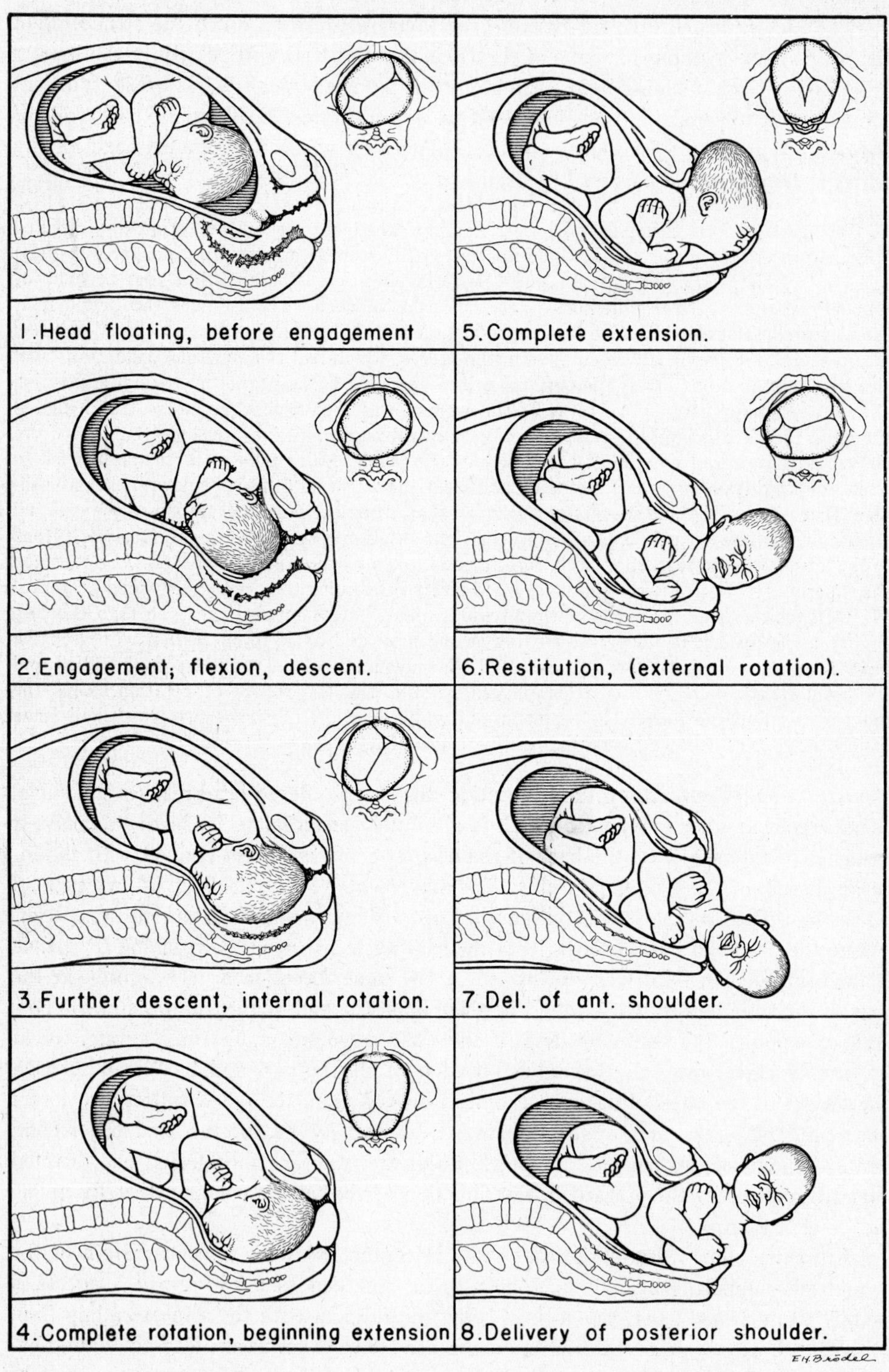

FIG. 263.—PRINCIPAL MOVEMENTS IN THE MECHANISM OF LABOR AND DELIVERY; L. O. A. POSITION.

that it was the upper and posterior margin of the right parietal bone that first came into view, while the reverse holds good in right occipito-anterior positions.

With increasing distention of the perineum and vaginal opening, a larger and larger portion of the occiput gradually appears, and the head is born by further extension, the occiput, bregma, forehead, nose, mouth, and finally the chin successively passing over the anterior margin of the perineum. Immediately after its birth the head falls downward and the chin comes in contact with the region of the anus (see Fig. 263).

External Rotation. A few moments after its birth the head undergoes another movement, and, when the occiput has been originally directed toward the left, it rotates toward the left tuber ischii, and in the opposite direction when it has been originally toward the right. This is known as external rotation or restitution, and is simply the index of a corresponding rotation of the body of the child, which serves to bring its bisacromial diameter into relation with the anteroposterior diameter of the pelvic outlet. This movement is brought about by essentially the same factors which produce the internal rotation of the head.

Expulsion. Almost immediately after the occurrence of external rotation, the anterior shoulder appears under the symphysis pubis, and in a short time the anterior margin of the perineum becomes distended by the posterior shoulder, which is first born, being rapidly followed by the other. Finally, the body of the child is quickly extruded along a curved line corresponding to the axis of the lower part of the birth canal—that is, with its upper side markedly concave and its lower convex.

Mechanism in Occipitoposterior Positions. In 28,494 cases of labor at the New York Lying-In Hospital in which the vertex presented, Stander observed 2,308 occipitoposterior positions (8.1 per cent), the incidence of R. O. P. being 5.2 per cent, of L. O. P. 2.7 per cent, and of O. P. 0.19 per cent. The number of primary occipitoposterior positions was probably twice as great as is here indicated, but, owing to the fact that many of the patients were not examined until well advanced in the second stage of labor, it happened in many cases that anterior rotation had already occurred. Danforth studied 1,565 private patients who were examined early in labor, and found the incidence of posterior positions 27.1 per cent, the right occiput posterior position being observed 6.7 times more frequently than the left occiput posterior.

Recent evidence gained from radiographic studies indicates that a narrow fore pelvis is often associated with posterior positions. D'Esopo found two different pelvic forms frequently encountered in these positions—one in which the transverse diameter is contracted at the brim, or midpelvis, or both, with compensating ampleness in the anteroposterior diameter; and the other, the converse, in which the anteroposterior diameter is short because of a flat posterior segment at the inlet or a forward sacrum at the midpelvis with ample length in the transverse diameter.

Torpin and Holmes believe that the placenta located on the anterior wall of the uterus has a tendency to produce posterior positions. They observed an increased incidence of posterior positions of the fetus with the placenta attached anteriorly as compared with the placenta on the posterior wall of the uterus.

Whenever the back of the child is felt on the right side of the mother, the possibility of a right posterior position should always be borne in mind; it occurs much more frequently than the right anterior variety. It should also be remembered, whenever the small parts are distinctly felt in the anterior portion of the abdomen, that one has in all probability to deal with a posterior position, more especially in the rare instances in which the occiput has rotated into the hollow of the sacrum. In the less frequent left posterior positions palpation gives similar results, except that the back is felt in the left flank, and the small parts and cephalic prominence are found on the right side of the abdomen.

Diagnosis. Palpation in a right occipitoposterior position gives the following data:

First maneuver:	The fundus is occupied by the breech.
Second maneuver:	The resistant plane of the back is felt well back in the right flank, the small parts being on the left side and in front and much more readily palpable than in anterior positions.
Third maneuver:	Negative if the head is engaged; otherwise the movable head is detected above the superior strait.
Fourth maneuver:	Cephalic prominence on the left side.

On vaginal or rectal touch in the right posterior position, the sagittal suture occupies the right oblique diameter; the small fontanel is felt opposite the right sacro-iliac synchondrosis, the large fontanel being directed toward the left iliopectineal eminence; in the left position the reverse obtains. In many cases, particularly in the early part of labor, owing to imperfect flexion of the head, the large fontanel lies at a lower level than in anterior positions, and is more readily felt.

On auscultation the heart is heard in the right or left flank of the mother, according as one has to deal with a right or left position. It should be remembered that in these positions the heart sounds are sometimes transmitted through the thorax of the child and are best heard either in the middle line or slightly to one side of it. This is due to a partial extension of the head and the altered relation of the body of the child, whereby the thorax comes in contact with the anterior uterine wall. Failure to realize this possibility sometimes results in serious diagnostic error.

Mechanism. In the great majority of occipitoposterior positions the mechanism of labor is identical with that observed in the anterior varieties, except that the occiput has to rotate from the region of the sacro-iliac synchondrosis to the symphysis pubis, instead of from the iliopectineal eminence—through 135 degrees instead of 45 degrees (Fig. 264).

In many instances internal rotation does not take place until the perineum begins to bulge, but occasionally it occurs only partially, or sometimes not at all, so that the occiput rotates only to a transverse or an obliquely anterior position, or remains obliquely posterior. In such circumstances spontaneous delivery is made less likely, unless the child is very small. Even in favorable cases considerable time is usually required for the completion of anterior rotation, so that there results a definite prolongation of labor. Varnier, upon comparing the histories in 400 cases of occiput posterior and in 660 cases of occiput anterior positions, found that, in the former, labor averaged 3 hours and 16 minutes to 1 hour and 50 minutes longer, according as the patient was a primiparous or multiparous woman; in our experience the prolongation is not so great.

In a small percentage of cases, particularly in women with funnel pelves, the occiput, instead of rotating anteriorly or retaining its original position, turns spontaneously toward the sacrum, and eventually occupies its concavity. According to West and Varnier this occurs in two or three per cent of the cases, while we have noted a somewhat higher incidence of *persistent occipitoposterior position* in our obliquely posterior cases (see Fig. 265).

In many instances it is difficult to explain why anterior rotation fails to occur, but it may be stated as a general rule that it is much more likely to take place when the head is well flexed than when it is imperfectly flexed or partially extended. In the latter event the large fontanel occupies a lower level than the small, whence it would appear that it is usually the most dependent part of the head which rotates anteriorly.

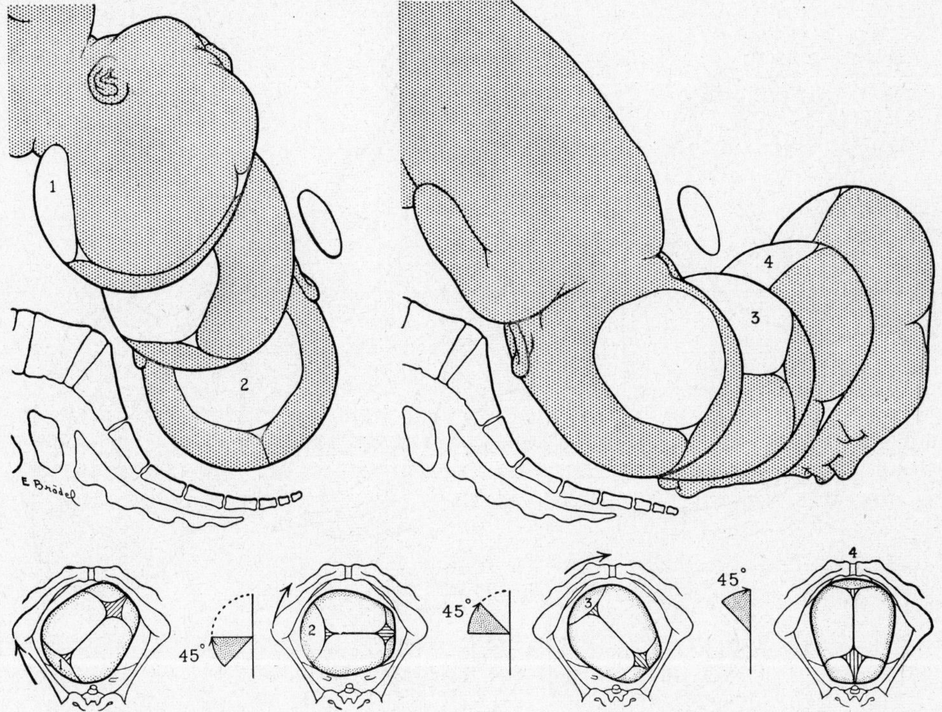

Fig. 264.—Mechanism of Labor for Right Occiput Posterior Position, Anterior Rotation.

After the occiput has rotated into the hollow of the sacrum, the child may be born in one of two ways. Ordinarily the head becomes markedly flexed and lengthened in its mento-occipital diameter so that eventually the region just anterior to the large fontanel impinges upon the lower margin of the symphysis pubis, after which the occiput is slowly pushed over the anterior margin of the perineum by a movement of flexion. Then, by a movement of extension, the occiput falls backward, and the brow, nose, mouth and chin appear successively under the symphysis. After the birth of the head, external rotation and expulsion of the body occur in the usual manner.

According to Sentex, Winckel, Weiss, and Müller, the head is occasionally born by another mechanism, which comes into play in those cases in which partial extension persists. In such circumstances the brow appears at the vulva, and, while the root of the nose impinges upon the symphysis, by a movement of flexion the brow, bregma and occiput successively pass over the perineum, until finally the face slips out from under the symphysis pubis. This mechanism approaches closely to that observed in brow presentations and is much more difficult than the one just described. It is more likely to lead to tears of the maternal soft parts, since it is evident that in the first instance the vulva is distended by the suboccipitofrontal circumference of the head, and in the second by the occipitofrontal, which measure 34 and 37 cm., respectively.

It is generally believed that occipitoposteriors offer a less favorable prognosis than occipito-anterior positions. This is probably due to the fact that Mauriceau, Smellie and all the early authorities taught that in such cases the occiput always

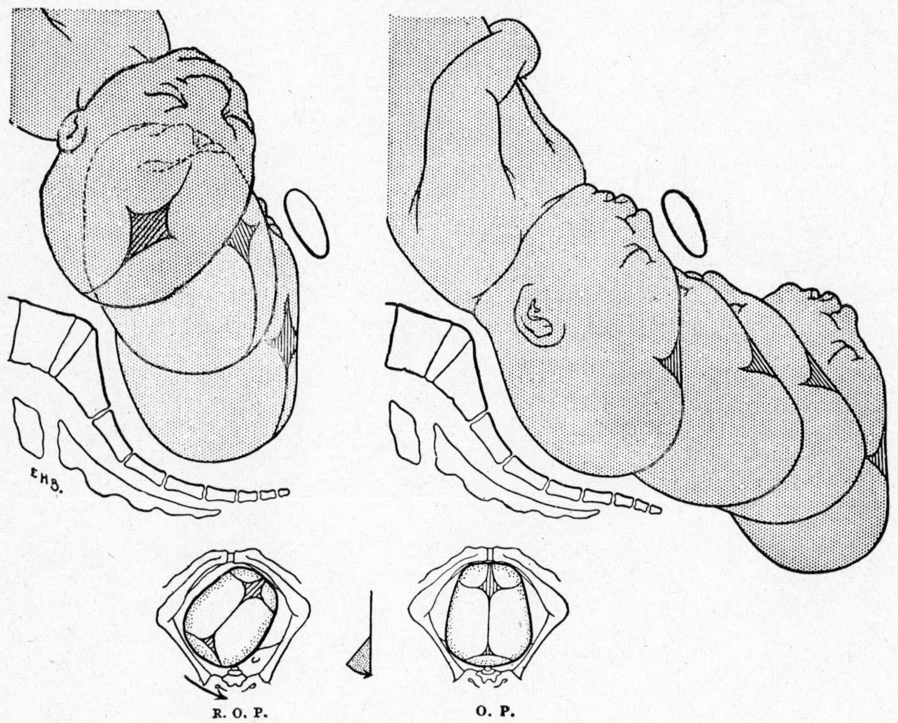

FIG. 265.—MECHANISM OF LABOR FOR RIGHT OCCIPUT POSTERIOR POSITION, POSTERIOR ROTATION.

rotated into the hollow of the sacrum, and that later many American writers, being led astray by their fears, have failed to realize what nature can accomplish. It is true that Naegele showed that in the vast majority of cases the occiput rotated anteriorly, but in spite of his teachings, the older views still prevail. Thus Capuron, in 1833, taught that spontaneous delivery could not take place; and Tarnier, while admitting the correctness of Naegele's conclusions, nevertheless held that the prognosis was always serious, for, even when anterior rotation occurred, the duration of labor was greatly increased and the maternal and fetal mortality augmented.

A comparatively large experience has led us to discount these gloomy views, and to regard the occurrence of obliquely posterior positions with equanimity, provided the pelvis and child are normal in size. Moreover, in view of our uniformly good results, we do not consider it advisable to attempt to convert them into other positions during the course of labor, except when the forceps is to be applied. It is true that labor is somewhat prolonged and instrumental interference is required more frequently—in 10 per cent of the cases, according to Varnier, as compared with 3.6 per cent in anterior positions. Even when only partial rotation occurs, so that one has to deal with the so-called "deep transverse arrest," the progress is excellent provided the head is rotated, usually manually, at the proper level and the forceps application

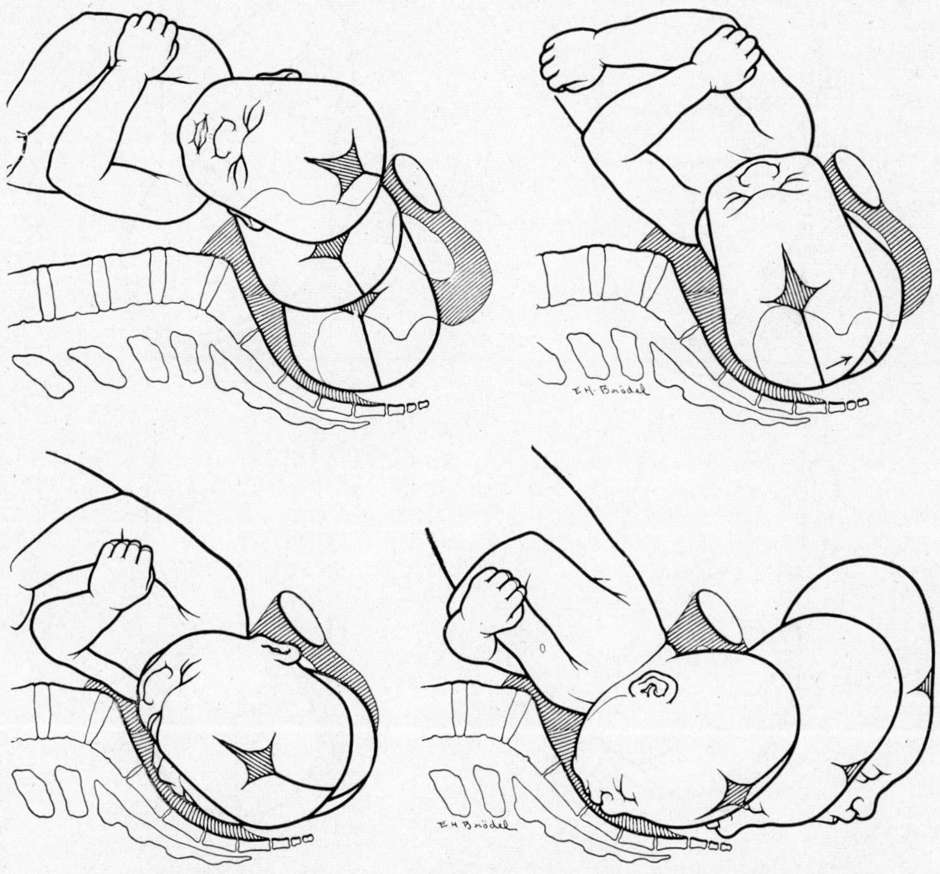

FIG. 266A.—MECHANISM OF LABOR FOR LEFT OCCIPUT TRANSVERSE POSITION, LATERAL VIEW.

Posterior parietal presentation at the brim (Litzmann's obliquity), followed by lateral flexion resulting in anterior parietal presentation after engagement, further descent, rotation and extension. (From Steele and Javert, by permission of Surgery, Gynecology and Obstetrics.)

and extraction correctly performed. In 635 cases reported by Plass in 1916, in which delivery occurred spontaneously or was aided by forceps, no maternal mortality was attributable to the posterior position, and the fetal mortality was not appreciably increased over that occurring in obliquely anterior positions.

Even in the comparatively rare instances in which posterior rotation occurs so that the occiput comes to lie in the hollow of the sacrum, the prognosis is not bad, as in the majority of cases spontaneous delivery occurs, being noted by Varnier in 30 out of 35 cases. No doubt in such cases there is an increased tendency toward perineal tears which is particularly marked when the head is born by the less frequent mechanism. But we feel tbe main cause of the dread in which posterior positions are held is the fact that they frequently escape recognition, with the result that the large number which rotate anteriorly and end spontaneously are overlooked, and only those cases are recognized in which rotation either fails to occur, deep transverse arrest results, or the occiput rotates into the hollow of the sacrum.

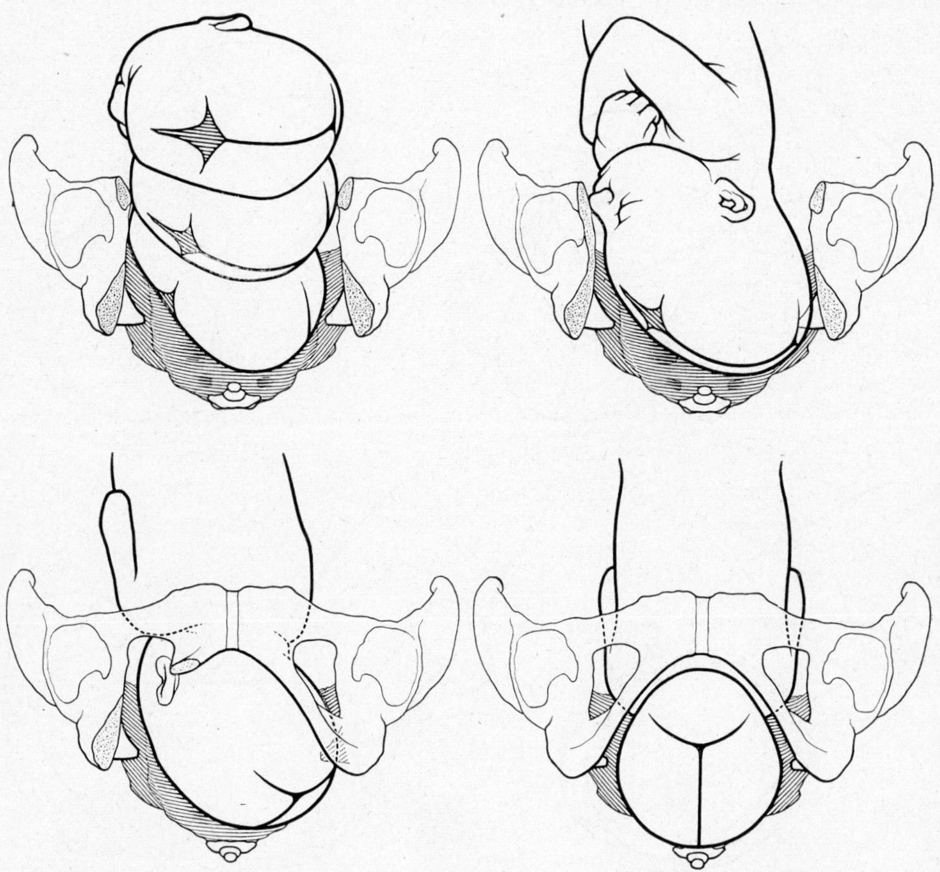

FIG. 266B.—MECHANISM OF LABOR FOR LEFT OCCIPUT TRANSVERSE POSITION, FRONTAL VIEW. (From Steele and Javert, by permission of Surgery, Gynecology and Obstetrics.)

Mechanism in Occipitotransverse Positions. As previously stated, transverse positions of the occiput occur most commonly, accounting for well over half of all positions. Caldwell, from his roentgenologic studies, concluded that 60 per cent of his series had transverse positions of the occiput. Steele and his associates found a comparable figure in cases studied in the New York Lying-In Hospital.

Diagnosis. Palpation in a left occipitotransverse gives the following data:

First maneuver: The fundus is occupied by the breech.

Second maneuver: The resistant plane of the back is felt directly to the left in the flank, the small parts being on the right side and readily palpated through the flank.

Third maneuver: Negative if the head is engaged; otherwise the movable head is detected above the superior strait.

Fourth maneuver: Cephalic prominence on the right side.

The left occipitotransverse position is seen somewhat more frequently than the right occipitotransverse position; in the latter event palpation reveals similar results, except the back is in the right flank and the small parts and cephalic prominence are found on the left side.

On vaginal or rectal examination the sagittal suture occupies the transverse diameter of the pelvis, more or less midway between the sacrum and the symphysis. In the case of left transverse positions the small fontanel is directed toward a point midway between the iliopectineal eminence and the sacro-iliac synchondrosis on that side,

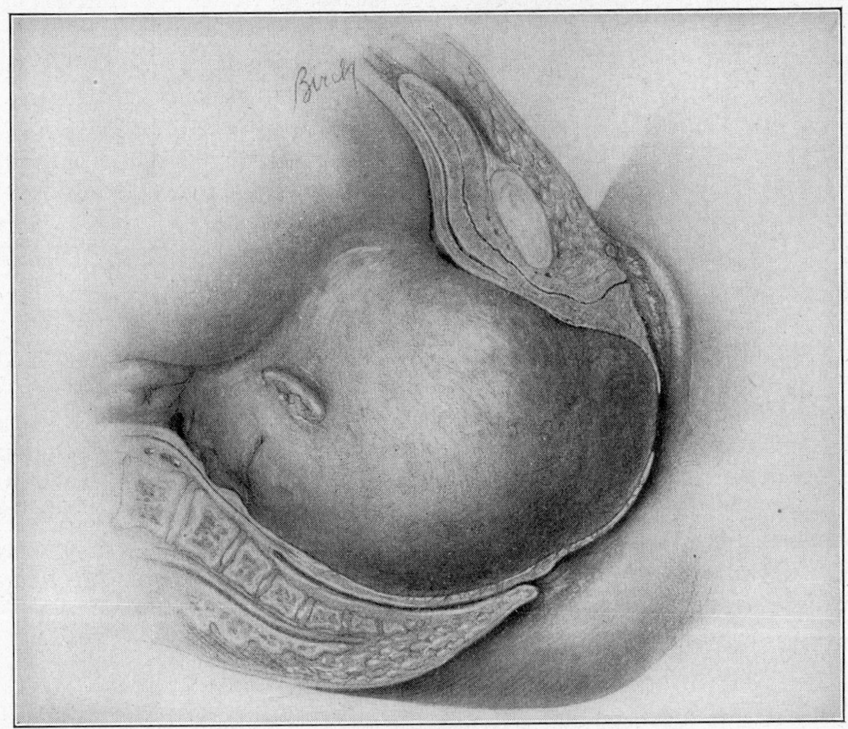

Fig. 267.—Formation of Caput Succedaneum.

the large fontanel being directed toward the same point on the right side of the pelvis. In right transverse positions the reverse of the above findings in left transverse holds true. On auscultation the fetal heart is usually heard in the right or left flank of the mother at or slightly below the level of the umbilicus, according as one has to deal with a right or left position. Less audible heart tones can sometimes be also heard on the side opposite the fetal back when for various reasons the sound is also transmitted through the thorax.

Mechanism. In the majority of instances of transverse positions the mechanism of labor is identical to that of the anterior positions, except that the occiput has to rotate from its transverse position to the symphysis pubis, a 90 degree rotation instead of 45 degrees as in anterior positions. The occiput does not often rotate posteriorly into the hollow of the sacrum as is occasionally seen in posterior positions. At the same time it must be borne in mind that anterior rotation does not always occur, in which event we have a "deep transverse arrest." The mechanism involved and the management will, of course, depend upon the type of pelvis but, in general, they are identical to this same complication that arises in posterior positions.

Stereoscopic views of the fetal head at different levels of descent through the pelvis indicate that in transverse positions of the occiput as it enters the superior strait the head lies in posterior asynclitism (Litzmann's obliquity) with the posterior parietal bone presenting and the anterior parietal bone slightly over the symphysis. As labor progresses, lateral flexion backward and descent bring the posterior parietal bone more into the posterior segment thus enabling the anterior parietal bone to come into the forepelvis. In the midpelvis, lateral flexion forward facilitates further descent and internal rotation can now take place to be followed by extension and expulsion as in the anterior varieties.

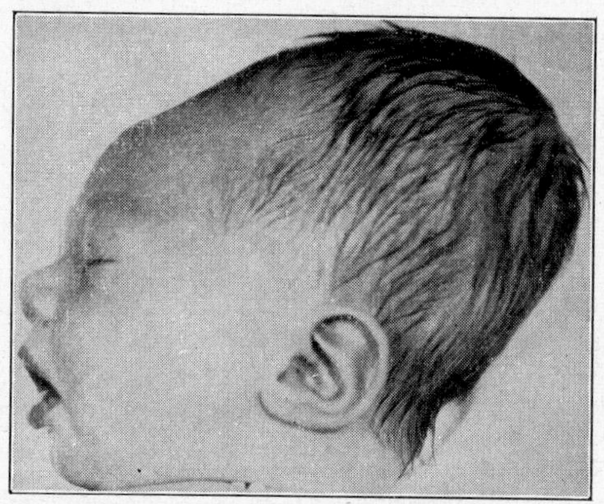

Fig. 268.—Molding of Head at Birth.

Changes in the Shape of the Head. In vertex presentations the child's head undergoes important and characteristic changes in shape, as the result of the pressure to which it is subjected during labor. In prolonged labors in which the membranes have ruptured before complete dilatation of the cervix, the portion of the head immediately over the os is relieved from the general pressure existing in the uterus, and, as a consequence, a serous exudate occurs under the scalp at this point, causing a soft swelling, known as the *caput succedaneum*. Usually this attains a thickness of only a few millimeters, but in prolonged labors it may become so considerable as to prevent

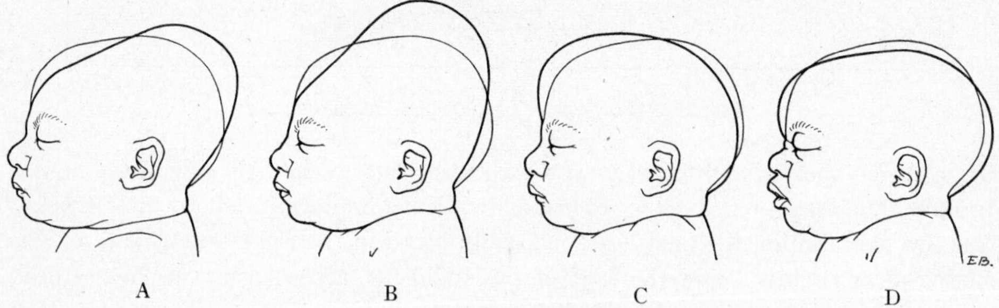

Fig. 269.—Molding of Head in Cephalic Presentations.
A, occiput anterior; B, occiput posterior; C, brow; D, face.

the examining finger from distinguishing the various sutures and fontanels. More usually the caput is formed when the head is in the lower portion of the birth canal, and frequently only after the resistance of a rigid vaginal outlet is encountered. It occurs upon the most dependent portion of the head and, therefore, in left occipito-iliac positions is found over the upper and posterior extremity of the right parietal bone, and in right positions over the corresponding area of the left parietal bone. Hence it follows that, in many instances, after labor we are enabled to diagnose the original position by the situation of the caput succedaneum.

More important, however, are the plastic changes which the head undergoes. Owing to the fact that the various bones of the skull are not firmly united, movement may occur at the various sutures. Ordinarily the margins of the occipital bone, and more rarely those of the frontal bone, are pushed under those of the parietal bones; in many cases one parietal bone may overlap the other, the rule being that the one occupying the posterior position is overlapped by the anterior. These changes are of great importance, especially in contracted pelves, when the ability of the child's head to become molded may make the difference between a spontaneous labor and a major obstetrical operation (see Fig. 268).

As a result of pressure the head also undergoes a marked change in shape, which consists in a diminution of its suboccipitofrontal and occipitofrontal diameters. In other words, it becomes lengthened from chin to occiput and compressed in other directions.

In occipitoposterior positions, when the occiput has rotated into the hollow of the sacrum, the frontal bone is sometimes markedly overlapped by the anterior margins of the parietal bones. This leads to a distinct depression on that part of the head and gives some idea of the force with which the region of the large fontanel has been pressed against the lower margin of the symphysis.

Such pressure changes are of much more serious import than was formerly believed, and it is now known that they may play an important part in the production of fatal subdural hemorrhage. Holland, in his important work upon cranial stress during labor, has shown that they subject the tentorium cerebelli or the falx to excessive tension, which may result in actual lesions associated with hemorrhage, and which readily account for many fetal deaths which were formerly considered inexplicable.

BIBLIOGRAPHY

Caldwell, W. E., Moloy, H. C., and D'Esopo, D. A. A Roentgenologic Study of the Mechanism of Engagement of the Fetal Head. Am. J. Obst. & Gynec., 1934, 28:824.

——— The Rôle of the Lower Uterine Soft Parts in Labor. Am. J. Obst. & Gynec., 1936, 32:727.

Caldwell, W. E., Moloy, H. C., and Swenson, P. C. The Use of the Roentgen Ray in Obstetrics. Part I. Roentgen Pelvimetry and Cephalometry; Technic of Pelvio-roentgenography. Am. J. Roentgenol., 1939, 41:305.

——— The Use of the Roentgen Ray in Obstetrics. Part II. Anatomical Variations in the Female Pelvis and Their Classification According to Morphology. Am. J. Roentgenol. & Radium Therapy, 1939, 41:505.

——— The Use of the Roentgen Ray in Obstetrics. Part III. The Mechanism of Labor Am. J. Roentgenol. & Radium Therapy, 1939, 41:719.

Calkins, L. A. The Etiology of Occiput Presentations. Am. J. Obst. & Gynec., 1939, 37:618.

Danforth, W. C. The Management of Occiput Posterior. Am. J. Obst. & Gynec., 1934, 28:756.

D'Esopo, D. A. The Occipitoposterior Position. Its Mechanism and Treatment. Am. J. Obst. & Gynec., 1941, 42:937.

Holland, E. Cranial Stress in the Foetus during Labor. J. Obst. & Gynaec. Brit. Emp., 1922, 29:549.

Javert, C. T., and Steele, K. B. The Transverse Position and the Mechanism of Labor. A Historical Collective Review. Internat. Abstr. Surg., 1942, 75:507.

Jones, J. Some Causes of Delay in Labor, with Special Reference to the Function of the Cervical Spine of the Foetus. J. Obst. & Gynaec. Brit. Emp., 1906, 10:407.

Klingensmith, P. Posterior Rotation of the Occiput during Labor. Am. J. Obst. & Gynec., 1942, 44:623.

Litzmann, C. C. T. Die Geburt bei Engem Becken. Leipzig, Breilkopfund Härtel, 1884.

Martius, H. Die Aetiologie des hohen Gradstandes. Ztschr. f. Geburtsh. u. Gynäk., 1915, 76:763.

——— Die regelwidrige Geburt. Halban-Seitz, Die Biologie und Pathologie des Weibes, Bd. VII, Teil 2, ff. 143.

MOIR, C. The Cause of Internal Rotation of the Foetus with Special Reference to the Occipito-Posterior Position. J. Obst. & Gynaec. Brit. Emp., 1932, 39:84.

MÜLLER, A. Ueber Hinterhauptslagen und Scheitellagen. Monatschr. f. Geburtsh. u. Gynaek., 1898, 7:382, 534.

NAEGELE, H. F. J. Die Lehre vom Mechanismus der Geburt Nebst Beiträgen zur Geschichte Derselben. Mainz, 1838.

PARAMORE, R. A Critical Inquiry into the Causes of Internal Rotation of the Foetal Head. J. Obst. & Gynaec. Brit. Emp., 1909, 16:213.

PLASS, E. D. A Statistical Study of 635 Labors with the Occiput Posterior. Bull. Johns Hopkins Hosp., 1916, 27:164.

PROCTOR, I. M., and DICKINSON, K. A Study of the Occipito-Posterior Positions of the Vertex. Analysis, Management and Results in 106 Consecutive Cases. J.A.M.A., 1940, 114:381.

RUDOLPH, L., and IVY, A. C. Internal Rotation of the Fetal Head from the Viewpoint of Comparative Obstetrics. Am. J. Obst. & Gynec., 1933, 25:74.

SENTEX. Étude Statistique et Clinique sur les Positions Occipitopostérieures. Paris, 1872.

STEELE, K. B., and JAVERT, C. T. Mechanism of Labor for Transverse Positions of the Vertex. Surg., Gynec. & Obst., 1942, 75:477.

THOMS, H., and GODFRIED, M. S. Suboccipitobregmatic Circumference. Am. J. Obst. & Gynec., 1940, 39:841.

TORPIN, R., and HOLMES, L. P. The Influence of the Placental Site upon Fetal Presentation. Am. J. Obst. & Gynec., 1943, 46:268.

VARNIER, H. Les Occipito-postérieures. Obstétrique journalière, 1900, p. 181.

WEISS. Zur Behandlung der Vorderscheitellagen. Samml. klin. Vortr., n. F., Leipzig, 1892, Nr. 60.

WINCKEL. Lehrbuch der Geburtshulfe, II. Aufl., 1893, ff. 147.

15

THE CLINICAL COURSE OF LABOR

Lightening. Several weeks before the onset of labor the abdomen undergoes a marked change in shape, its lower portion becoming more pendulous, whereas in the neighborhood of the costal margin it looks decidedly flatter. This change is perceived by the woman herself, who feels that her waist has become lower; and occasionally it occurs so suddenly as to cause her to fear that something has given way inside the abdomen. Abdominal palpation shows that the change is due to the fact that the fundus of the uterus has descended from the position which it occupied at the ninth month, and resumed that of the eighth, and that the head, which was previously freely movable, has descended and become fixed in the superior strait. These changes are most pronounced in primigravidae, and frequently do not occur in multiparae until the onset of labor. This descent of the uterus, due to the sinking of the fetal head into the pelvic inlet, is termed "lightening."

After this the patient experiences considerable relief from the respiratory disturbances from which she may have suffered; but at the same time locomotion may become more difficult, and she may suffer from cramplike pains in the lower extremities and a more frequent desire to urinate. During the last few weeks of pregnancy, the vaginal secretion is increased in amount, the labia become more swollen and succulent and, in multiparae, gape more or less widely.

False Labor Pains. For a varying period before the establishment of true labor pains, gravidae often suffer from so-called "false pains," and it is necessary to be able to distinguish between them and effective uterine contractions. False pains may begin as early as three or four weeks before the termination of pregnancy. They are merely an exaggeration of the intermittent uterine contractions which occur throughout the entire period of gestation but which are now painful. They occur at decidedly irregular intervals, are confined chiefly to the lower part of the abdomen and groin and rarely extend from the back girdlewise around to the front of the abdomen, as do true labor pains. The duration of false labor pains is short, and unlike true labor contractions they are rarely intensified by walking about and may even be relieved by being on the feet. As the hours go by, furthermore, false labor pains do not increase in intensity, duration and frequency as is characteristic of true labor contractions. However, observations such as the above may occasionally be inconclusive, and the only certain way to distinguish between false and true labor pains is to ascertain the effects which they exert on the cervix. True labor pains, in the course of a few hours, produce a demonstrable degree of effacement and possibly also some dilatation of the cervix, whereas the effect of false labor pains on the cervix is nil.

"Show." A rather dependable sign of impending labor (provided no rectal or vaginal examination has been done in the previous 48 hours) is "show." By this is meant the discharge from the vagina of a small amount of blood-tinged mucus which represents the extrusion of the mucous plug which has filled the cervical canal during pregnancy. This is a late sign, and labor usually ensues within the next 24 hours. It must be emphasized, however, that the quantity of blood which escapes with the

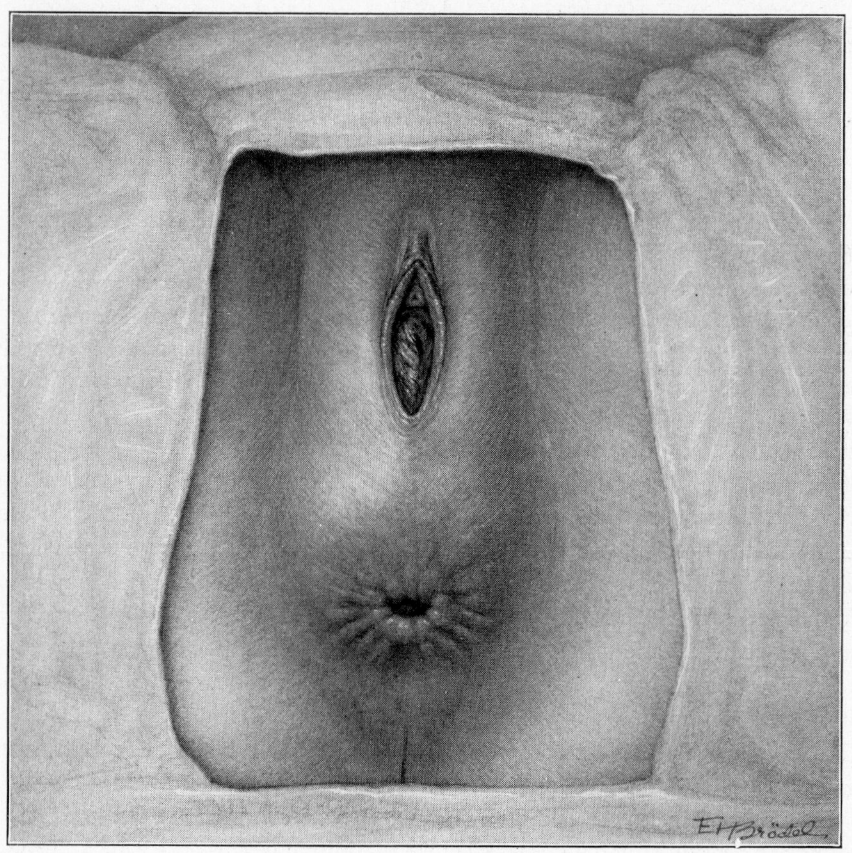

Fig. 270.—Birth of Head, Scalp Appearing at Vulva.

mucous plug amounts only to a few drops, or at the most a few cubic centimeters, and that any substantial escape of blood at this time should be regarded as suggestive of a pathologic condition.

First Stage of Labor. In the beginning of the first stage, the pains are short, slight in intensity, separated by long intervals of 10 or 15 minutes, and do not cause the patient any particular discomfort. She may be walking about, and between pains she is generally quite comfortable. Early in the first stage, the pain is usually located in the small of the back, but as time goes on it sweeps around girdle-like to the anterior part of the abdomen. The pains recur at shortening intervals, every three to five minutes, and become stronger, and last longer. Indeed, the pains which precede and accompany full dilatation are often of excruciating severity. At this time, furthermore, there is usually a marked increase in the amount of show due to rupture of capillary vessels in the cervix and lower uterine segment. The average duration of the first stage of labor in primigravidae is usually stated to be 16 hours; in multiparae, 11 hours.

Second Stage of Labor. The pains are now severe and long, lasting 50 to 100 seconds, and occurring at intervals of 2 or 3 minutes. Rupture of the membranes usually occurs during the early part of this stage of labor and is accompanied by a gush of amniotic fluid from the vagina. Sometimes, however, the membranes rupture during

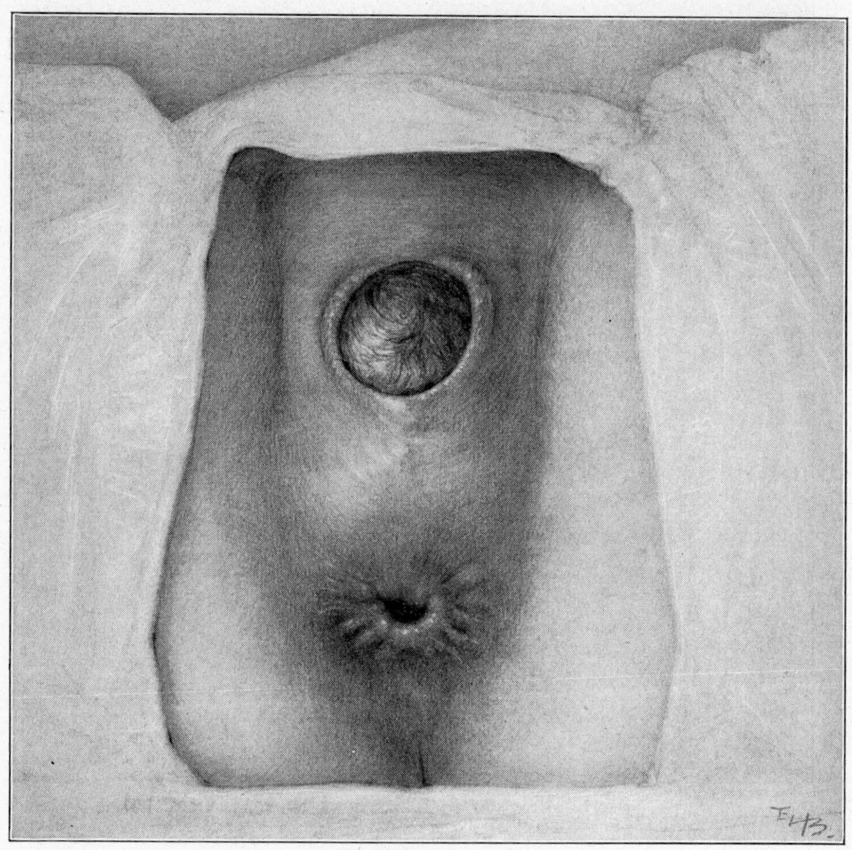

FIG. 271.—BIRTH OF HEAD, VULVA PARTIALLY DISTENDED.

the first stage and occasionally before labor starts. When rupture occurs before the onset of labor, pains ordinarily set in within 24 hours, but exceptionally, several days or even a week or longer may elapse, so that in such cases one should be cautious in expressing an opinion as to when labor will begin.

During this stage, as if by reflex action, the muscles of the abdomen are brought into play; and when the pains are in progress the patient will strain, or "bear down," with all her strength, so that her face becomes flushed and the large vessels in her neck are distended. At the onset of a pain the patient begins the grunt or groan so characteristic of this stage of labor and directs all her energy toward expelling the contents of the uterus. As a result of this exertion she may perspire profusely.

Toward the end of the second stage, when the head is well down in the vagina, its pressure often causes small particles of fecal material to be expelled from the rectum in association with each pain. As the head descends still farther, the perineal region begins to bulge and the skin over it becomes tense and glistening. At this time the scalp of the fetus may be detected through the slitlike vulvar opening. With each subsequent pain the perineum bulges more and more, and the vulva becomes more and more dilated and distended by the head, being gradually converted into an ovoid, and

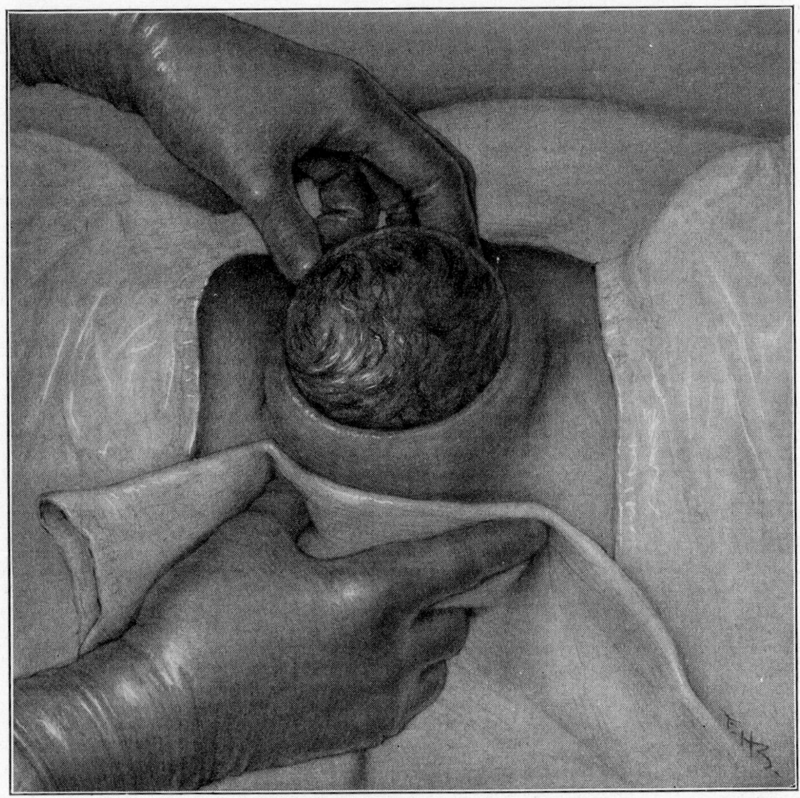

Fig. 272.—Birth of Head, Vulva Completely Distended.

at last into an almost circular opening. With the cessation of each contraction, the opening becomes smaller and the head recedes from it, to advance again with the next pain. As the head becomes increasingly visible, the vulva is stretched further, and finally it encircles the largest diameter of the baby's head. This encirclement of the largest diameter of the baby's head by the vulvar ring is known as "crowning." The perineum is now extremely thin so that its frenulum does not exceed a piece of paper in thickness and looks as if it would rupture with each pain. At the same time, the anus becomes greatly stretched and protuberant, and the anterior wall of the rectum may be easily seen through it. By now the perineum has become converted into a deep gutter 5 to 6 cm. long, at the end of which is the vulvar opening, which looks almost directly upward and is distended by the head of the child, whose occiput is firmly present against the symphysis pubis. The distention of the vulva is most marked at its perineal margin, and less so at its upper and lateral portions.

The head advances a little with each pain and recedes in intervals between them. This continues until the parietal bosses become engaged in the vulva, when further recession becomes impossible, and with the next two or three pains the head is rapidly expelled by a movement of extension, the base of the occiput rotating around the lower margin of the symphysis pubis as a fulcrum, while the bregma, brow and face

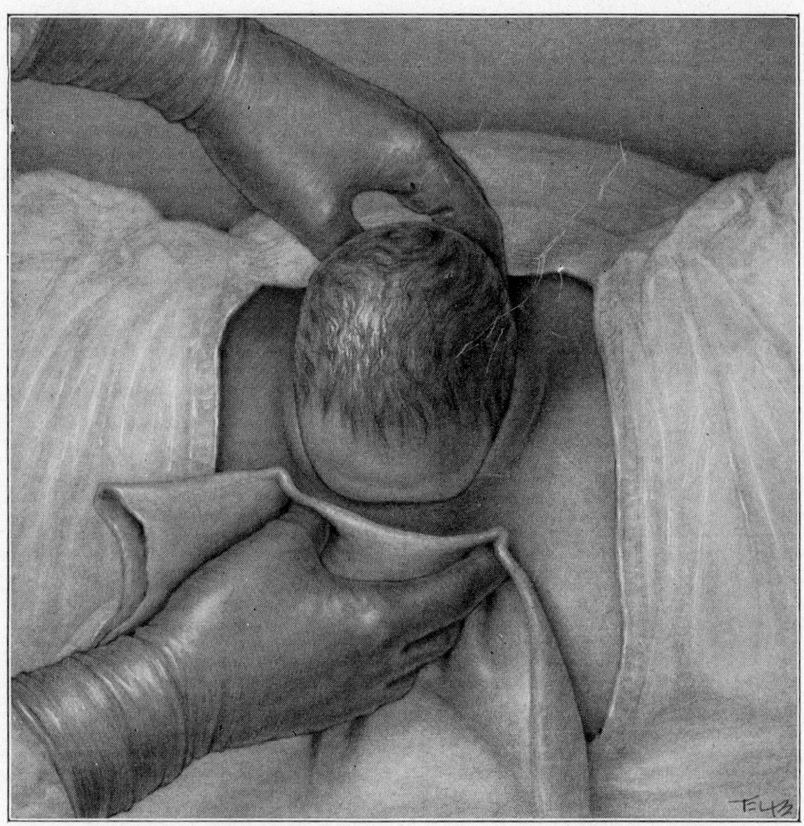

FIG. 273.—BIRTH OF HEAD, SHOWING DELIVERY BY EXTENSION.

successively pass over the fourchet. In the majority of primigravidae the perineum is unable to withstand the strain to which it is subjected, and tears in its anterior portion.

Immediately after its birth the head falls posteriorly, so that the face comes almost in contact with the anus. In a few moments the occiput turns toward the one or other thigh, and eventually the entire head assumes a transverse position. This is known as external rotation or restitution, and indicates that the bisacromial diameter of the child has rotated into the anteroposterior diameter of the pelvic outlet.

At this time the perineum is quite retracted around the neck of the infant, whose face in consequence may become so congested that the inexperienced obstetrician is often seized by an almost uncontrollable desire to complete delivery by traction upon the head. This, however, is usually unnecessary, for the next pain forces the anterior shoulder down under the symphysis pubis, where it becomes fixed; while the posterior shoulder emerges over the anterior margin of the perineum, after which the body of the child is rapidly expelled by a movement of lateral flexion, following a curve corresponding to the axis of the birth canal.

Immediately after extrusion of the child comes a gush of amniotic fluid, which represents the portion which did not escape when the membranes ruptured, and which may be more or less tinged with blood.

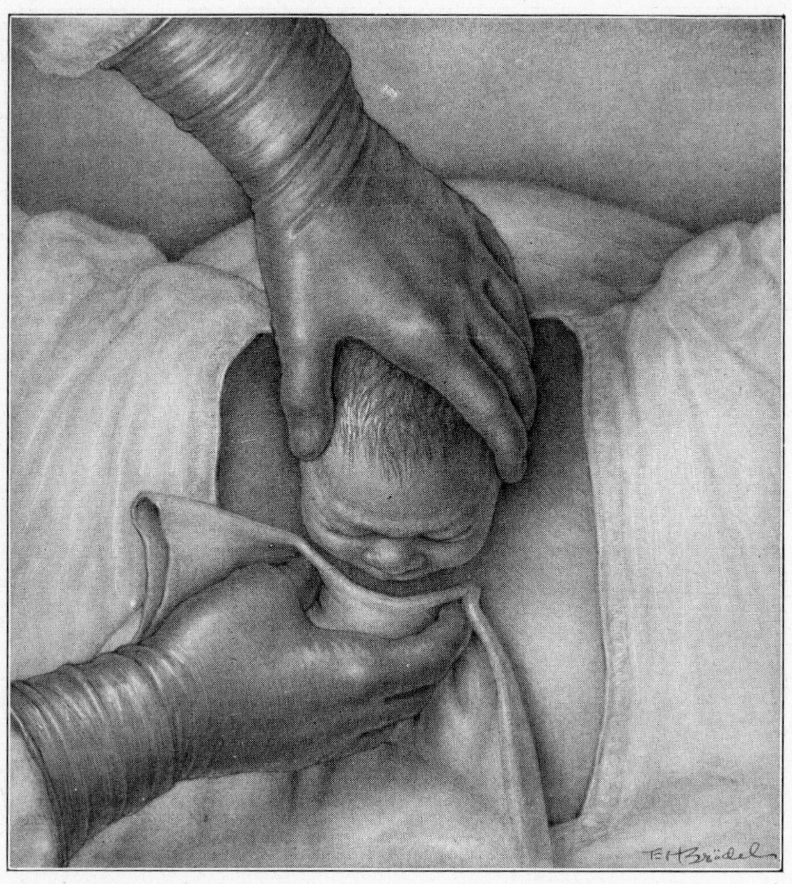

FIG. 274.—BIRTH OF HEAD, MOUTH APPEARING OVER PERINEUM.

In primiparous women the second stage of labor usually lasts from about one to two hours, but is much shorter in multiparous women, in whom two or three pains sometimes suffice for the completion of the period of expulsion.

Third Stage of Labor. Immediately following the birth of the child the remainder of the amniotic fluid escapes, after which there is usually a slight flow of blood. For a short time the patient experiences no pain, but after a few minutes uterine contractions begin again and recur at regular intervals, until the placenta becomes separated and is expelled into the lower uterine segment.

Immediately following delivery, the uterus can be felt as a firm globular mass just below the level of the umbilicus. Shortly thereafter the uterus relaxes and assumes a discoid shape. With each subsequent contraction and relaxation the uterus changes from a globular to a discoid shape. However, when the placenta is separated the globular shape persists even during relaxation of the fundus. Calkins has described this as the early sign of separation, although the placenta is still in the uterine cavity. He found this a good indication to express the placenta from the uterus. In his cases the duration of the third stage of labor was only four minutes and the blood loss was definitely reduced. Stander used this method for ten years in the New York Lying-In Hospital and confirmed Calkin's findings.

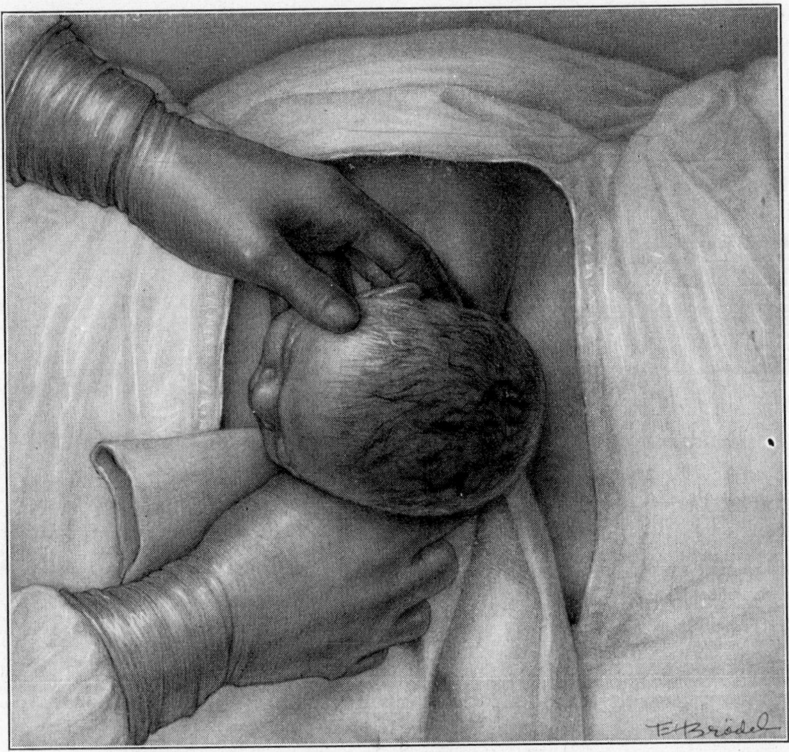

FIG. 275.—BIRTH OF HEAD, EXTERNAL ROTATION.

If the placenta is allowed to remain in the uterus following its separation, further clinical changes occur. At some time, varying between 5 and 30 minutes after the birth of the child, palpation shows that the fundus of the uterus has risen up to or above the umbilicus, or 3 to 7 cm. above its original position, while simultaneously a slight prominence has appeared immediately above the symphysis pubis. At the same time the portion of umbilical cord protruding from the vulva has increased by 10 or 12 cm. in length. These changes indicate that the placenta has been extruded from the uterine cavity proper into the lower uterine segment, or even into the upper part of the vagina. The rising of the fundus is due to the fact that the lower uterine segment, which immediately after the birth of the child had collapsed upon itself, is now distended by the placenta, and mechanically lifts the tightly contracted body of the uterus to a higher level.

In rare cases the placenta is born almost immediately after the child; in about one quarter of the cases it is delivered spontaneously 15 to 30 minutes later, while occasionally hours may pass before it appears at the vulva. The possibility of wide divergence in this respect can readily be appreciated when we remember that the action of the uterus ceases after the placenta has been extruded from its cavity, so that its further descent depends upon the contraction of the abdominal muscles, or upon the action of gravity. But owing to the great distention to which they have been subjected, the tonicity of the abdominal muscles is frequently so impaired that they can no longer exert sufficient force to expel the after-birth from the vagina, so that in many cases it will not be born for hours unless the patient assumes a sitting position or assistance is rendered by the physician.

It is important to differentiate between separation of the placenta and its expulsion from the uterus. The two cardinal signs of separation are the change in shape of the fundus from a discoid to a globular mass during relaxation, and the beginning of bleeding. This latter sign, however, is important in only the Schultze mechanism since there is a continuous trickling of blood with the Duncan mechanism. The signs of descent of the placenta occur later and formerly were considered as indicative of separation. These are the lengthening of the cord and the rise of the fundus. For that reason it had been thought that the average duration of the third stage of labor was from 14 to 17 minutes. With the earlier recognition of separation the phase of separation of the third stage will be found to average from four to seven minutes.

Blood Loss in Third Stage. In 348 consecutive vaginal deliveries in our clinic in which the blood loss was carefully measured with the Carroll plate (Fig. 291) and 10 per cent added in the calculation to allow for blood on sponges, towels and drapes, the average blood loss was 245 cc. Since any such series will inevitably include a few cases of excessive blood loss which distorts the average figure (in this series one of 1,500 cc.; 2 of 1,200 cc.; and 3 of 1,100 cc.), a better idea of the amount of blood most commonly lost is to be had from the median figure, that is, the figure above and below which half the figures fall. In this series the median blood loss was 192 cc. The blood loss was less than 200 cc. in 52.3 per cent and less than 300 cc. in 70.6 per cent. The most commendable statistics for low blood loss are those of Calkins whose figures for the two groups are 71 and 89 per cent respectively. His average blood loss in 800 cases was only 179 cc. Pastore found an average blood loss of 230 cc. in 2,394 cases.

While the figures cited in the above paragraph are representative of the total blood loss that may be expected in the third stage, it must be understood that this is made up, in most cases, of two components: blood loss from the uterus (mostly placental site) and blood loss from episiotomy and/or perineal lacerations. Especially in cases in which the total blood loss is less than 200 cc., episiotomy bleeding may constitute from a quarter to almost all the total blood loss.

Bleeding from the uterus in the third stage of labor varies with certain known factors, the most important of which is the size of the intra-uterine mass. Thus, Reich has shown that with a small baby of 5 pounds or less, the probability of hemorrhage in excess of 500 cc. is less than 1 in 21, whereas with a large baby of 9 pounds or more, the chance of such an amount of blood loss is 1 in 4. Multiple pregnancy is likewise associated with an increased frequency of postpartum hemorrhage. For instance, Guttmacher, in a series of 234 twin pregnancies at the Johns Hopkins Hospital, found that the incidence of postpartum hemorrhage (600 cc. +) was 14.5 per cent, whereas in the clinic population at large it was 6.3 per cent. In this connection it is well known of course that hydramnios also is frequently followed by postpartum hemorrhage. The fact that the amount of postpartum bleeding is related to the size of the fetal mass is not surprising since the larger the fetal mass the larger the placenta, and the larger the placenta the larger is the placental site, the usual source of blood loss at this time. Certain pathological conditions are also associated with an increased probability of postpartum hemorrhage, notably premature separation of the placenta (about 1 in 4 cases) and placenta previa (possibly as often as 1 in 2 cases).

Still another important cause of postpartum hemorrhage is operative delivery. The statistics of Pastore, Reich and others indicate that excessive bleeding is about three times more common after operative delivery than after spontaneous termination of labor. Both lacerations and anesthesia, especially ether anesthesia, contribute to this end. Internal podalic version (page 1091) is followed by serious postpartum hemorrhage in a high percentage of cases. According to Peckham and Kuder, lacerations are responsible for about six per cent of all postpartum hemorrhages, a figure with which Pastore's statistics are in close agreement. With the exception of rectal ether, perhaps, which Irving, Berman and Nelson have shown causes an increased incidence of postpartum atony, modern analgesia per se cannot be incriminated in this respect. Insofar, however, as it increases the frequency of operative delivery, it may well be a factor, Colvin and Bartholomew, on the other hand, report a very low incidence of hemorrhage in their paraldehyde series and are inclined to attribute the gratifying results to the greater amount of rest obtained during labor and the smaller quantity of ether used.

Duration of Labor. The duration of labor represents considerable individual variations, and is usually about six hours longer in primigravidae than in multiparae. Generally speaking, the average for the former is about 18 hours, of which 16 are occupied by the first, one and three quarters to two by the second, and a quarter to a half hour by the third stage of labor; for the latter it is about 12 hours, 11 of which are occupied by the first, and 1 by the second stage. Föderl gives slightly shorter average periods, 14 hours and 5 minutes for primigravidae, 8 hours and 8 minutes for secundiparae and 8 hours and 41 minutes for all other multiparae. His figures, however, are confined to normal labors in women with normal pelves and with babies weighing between 2,500 and 3,500 gm. and delivering in an occiput anterior position. Peckham, on the other hand, studied 13,658 consecutive deliveries at or near term and found the average primiparous labor to be 16.57 hours in the white and 17.66 hours in the black race, as contrasted with 10.91 and 12.49 hours, respectively, for the two races among the multiparae. The slower course of labor in the primiparous woman is due to the greater resistance offered by the soft parts. Occasionally labor may be extremely rapid, and even in primigravidae the entire process is sometimes completed within a few hours; while, on the other hand, a duration of 24 to 36 hours or even longer is not unusual.

In a review of 14,775 parturitions at the Johns Hopkins Hospital, Busby found that the median and modal durations of labor are more statistically significant than mean or average figures and certainly are more in keeping with general experience. In his series of white primigravidae, the mean duration of total labor was 13.04 hours, the median 10.59 and the mode, 7. Contrary to the general belief, labor is exceptionally rapid and easy in very young primigravidae. Harris, after analyzing the histories of 500 such cases, reached the conclusion that, from a purely obstetrical point of view, 16 years or less represents the optimum age for the birth of the first child—a view which is shared by several authors. In a more recent study Peckham places the optimum age somewhat higher, as he found a lower incidence of spontaneous labor in the very young woman than in the age group of 17 to 19 years. On the other hand, labor is usually definitely prolonged in primigravidae after the thirty-fifth year.

It is generally stated that delivery occurs most frequently between the hours of 2 and 4 A.M. Observations by Lynch, as well as the statistics of Knapp, which are based upon 39,000 cases, show that this is not correct, and that more children are born between 9 and 12 P.M. than in any other three hours of the day. Furthermore, if the day be divided, according as delivery occurs in the twelve hours preceding or following 6 P.M., respectively, it will be found that only four or five per cent more children are born in the latter than in the former period. Guthmann recently analyzed 121,794 labors, which included 26,707 from his own clinic, and found the incidence of day and that of night deliveries to be practically identical, being 49.1 and 50.9 per cent, respectively. The general belief that most births occur at night is due to the fact that labor usually lasts more than twelve hours, and accordingly either its beginning or end must necessarily fall between 6 P.M. and 6 A.M.

BIBLIOGRAPHY

Busby, T. The Duration of Labor: Mean, Median and Mode. Am. J. Obst. & Gynec., 1948, 55:846.

Calkins, L. A. The Second Stage of Labor—The Descent Phase. Am. J. Obst. & Gynec., 1944, 48:798.

——— The Second Stage of Labor. III. Number of Pains. Am. J. Obst. & Gynec., 1949, 57:106.

——— Management of the Third Stage of Labor. J.A.M.A., 1933, 101:1128.

Carroll, B. H., Meier, H. H., and Stone, O. H. Immediate Postpartum Hemorrhage Due to Retained Secundines. Am. J. Obst. & Gynec., 1948, 55:620.

Colvin, E. D., and Bartholomew, R. A. Improvements in the Paraldehyde Method of Relief of Pain in Labor. Am. J. Obst. & Gynec., 1938, 35:589.

Föderl, V. Investigation of the Average Duration of Labor in Primiparae, Secundiparae and Multiparae and Its Relation to the Age of the Woman in Labor. Monatschr. f. Geburtsh. u. Gynäk., 1936, 102:65.

Guthmann, H. The Onset of Labor Pains, the Duration and the Time of Day. Monatschr. f. Geburtsh. u. Gynäk., 1936, 103:337.

Guttmacher, A. G. An Analysis of 573 Cases of Twin Pregnancy. II. The Hazards of Pregnancy Itself. Am. J. Obst. & Gynec., 1939, 38:277.

Harris, J. Pregnancy and Labor in Young Primiparae. Bull. Johns Hopkins Hosp., 1922, 33:12.

Irving, F. C., Berman, S., and Nelson, H. B. The Barbiturates and Other Hypnotics in Labor. Surg., Gynec. and Obst., 1934, 58:1.

Knapp, C. B. The Hour of Birth. Bull. N. Y. Lying-In Hosp., 1909-10, 6:69.

Lynch, F. The Hour of Birth. Surg., Gynec. & Obst., 1907, 5:677.

Moir, C. The Nature of the Pain of Labor. J. Obst. & Gynaec. Brit. Emp., 1939, 46:409.

Pardee, H. E. B., and Mendelson, C. L. Pulse and Respiratory Variations in Normal Women during Labor. Am. J. Obst. & Gynec., 1941, 41:36.

Pastore, J. B. A New Method for Measuring the Blood Loss during the Third Stage of Labor. Am. J. Obst. & Gynec., 1935, 29:866.

——— A Study of the Blood Loss during the Third Stage of Labor and the Factors Involved. Am. J. Obst. & Gynec., 1936, 31:78.

Peckham, C. H. The Age Distribution of 15,370 Obstetric Patients and Its Effect upon the Type of Delivery. Am. J. Obst. & Gynec., 1932, 23:635.

——— and Kuder, K. Some Statistics of Postpartum Hemorrhage. Am. J. Obst. & Gynec., 1933, 26:361.

Reich, A. M. A Critical Analysis of Blood Loss following Delivery. Am. J. Obst. & Gynec., 1939, 37:224.

Robertson, E. M. The Effects of Emotional Stress on the Contractions of the Human Uterus. J. Obst. & Gynaec. Brit. Emp., 1939, 46:741.

16

THE CONDUCT OF NORMAL LABOR

Since most deliveries in this country are now conducted in hospitals, the first and larger portion of this chapter will deal with the institutional management of normal labor. This will be followed by a section describing the alterations in hospital technics which are required for home delivery. Actually the principles and the methods of examinations involved in the conduct of labor in the hospital and in the home are identical, the only modifications necessary for home delivery being in such matters as equipment, instructions to nurse, positioning of patient in bed, and anesthesia. Once a physician has been thoroughly drilled in the aseptic management of labor in a hospital, only a little ingenuity is required to adapt it to the circumstances encountered in most homes.

Psychological Approach to Patients. The pains of childbirth have been the stock and store of intimate conversation among women since time immemorial, and many young women approach childbirth in dread of the ordeal. It is no easy task to dispel this age-old fear, but from the first prenatal visit the obstetrician must make a conscious effort to give his patient a wholesome point of view. He must instill in her not only confidence, but also the feeling that he is her friend, a medically wise friend who is sincerely desirous of sparing her all the pain possible provided that this is compatible with her safety and that of the child. The very presence of such a friendly doctor and the realization that he is competent to handle any emergency is in itself a potent, basic analgesic. But all this involves qualities which cannot be put into a code of instructions. The attitude I have in mind comes only as the result of long nights in the labor room, and then only to those of understanding heart. It is the very stuff of which good doctors are made and is at once the safest and most welcome of obstetric anodynes.

During the past decade increasing emphasis has been placed on the fact that there is an "emotional labor" which is as definite and important as its physical counterpart. There can be no doubt that the attitude of a woman toward her confinement has a considerable influence on the ease of her labor. This fact has been stressed for many years by the British obstetrician, Grantly Dick Read, and has been endorsed by various groups in this country, notably by the Maternity Center Association of New York, by Thoms and Goodrich of New Haven and others. Read has attempted to find an answer to the following question: "Is labor easy because a woman is calm, or is she calm because her labor is easy?" And conversely: "Is a woman pained and frightened because her labor is difficult, or is her labor difficult and painful because she is frightened?" As the result of a scrutiny of many cases, the following hypothesis took shape in Read's mind: "Fear is in some way the chief pain-producing agent in otherwise normal labor." In succinct form, Read's main theme is that a tense woman means a tense cervix. Although the neuromuscular mechanism by which fear exerts a deleterious effect on uterine motility is obscure, the general validity of Read's contention is in keeping with common clinical experience.

In order to remove this harmful influence of fear in labor, a whole new school of thought in regard to childbirth has developed which emphasizes the advantages to be gained from what is called "natural childbirth" or "physiologic childbirth." As Thoms points out, natural childbirth is a broad concept and represents an attempt on the part of those who care for pregnant and parturient women to understand the physiology of pregnancy and labor, especially in its emotional aspects, so that these important functions may be viewed with less apprehension and better understanding by patients, and that greater skill in caring for them may be developed. Natural childbirth entails prenatal education designed to eliminate fear, exercises in relaxation, muscle control and breathing, adroit management in labor (the patient being attended throughout by a nurse or physician skilled in reassurance of the patient) and, at delivery, encouragement of properly co-ordinated muscular effort. The gaining of the confidence of the patient is all important. Thus, Read writes: "Women demand of all things complete confidence in the dependability, personal strength and skill of the man who is with them during labor. They do not want soft words or sob stuff but explanation, instruction, and encouragement. They want to hear that all is going well, that the baby is well and that they are conducting their job in an admirable manner."

It should be emphasized that the proponents of natural childbirth have never claimed that labor should be conducted without anesthetic aids or that it can be made devoid of pain (Thoms). Under the regime of natural childbirth most patients do experience pain to a greater or lesser degree and analgesics and anesthetics are not withheld when they are indicated. Nevertheless, the more these principles can be inculcated in the management of labor, the easier in general childbirth will be; moreover, the quantity and duration of medicinal analgesia and anesthesia required will be diminished to the benefit of both mother and infant.

Medical students, internes and nurses should note especially that the morale of women in labor is sometimes hopelessly shattered by careless remarks. Thus, comments outside the room of patients are often overheard to their discomposure. Laughter in the environs of the patient (about some entirely different matter) is inevitably interpreted by the patient in the light that it is she who is being laughed at. For some 15 years the famous lines of Oliver Wendell Holmes have had a prominent place on the wall of the doctors' office on our delivery floor. Medical students and internes would do well to memorize these words and take them to heart:

"The woman about to become a mother, or with her newborn infant upon her bosom, should be the object of trembling care and sympathy wherever she bears her tender burden or stretches her aching limbs . . . God forbid that any member of the profession to which she trust her life, doubly precious at that eventful period, should hazard it negligently, unadvisedly, or selfishly!"

ADMISSION PROCEDURES

Since every hospital has its own admission procedures, the minutiae of preparing a patient for hospital delivery will of necessity vary from institution to institution. In this connection it may be recalled that many things may be accomplished equally well in a number of ways. Although it may appear that the procedures employed in various hospitals differ greatly, actually the differences are in details only, the objectives being the same everywhere, namely, asepsis and antisepsis, together with a careful check on the patient for abnormalities. If this is the patient's first hospital experience, it will be much easier for her if she has been told about the necessary preliminary procedures, such as the vulvar and the perineal clean-up, and the methods of examinations which are employed. She should also be advised to come to the hospital at the onset of labor, for after labor progresses these activities are more difficult to carry out and much more distressing to the patient.

After greeting the patient the physician ascertains her general condition, including the frequency of her pains, their intensity, their duration, the amount of show if any, and whether the bag of waters has ruptured or is intact. The temperature, pulse and respiration are then taken by the nurse followed by a blood pressure reading either by the physician or nurse. Unless the patient is progressing very rapidly in labor, the physician orders the collection of a urine specimen, a soap and water enema, shaving and cleansing of the pubic area, vulva, and inner thighs and, depending upon circumstances, a shower or slab bath. Patients in labor are never allowed to use the toilet because it is important that the physician should have available for examination not only the urine specimen, but whatever material may be passed *per vaginam*.

Vulvar and Perineal Clean-up. The aim in shaving and washing the vulva should be to cleanse and disinfect the immediate neighborhood of the vagina, but to allow nothing to get into it. First, the patient is placed on a bedpan or douche pan with legs widely separated. A sponge soaked with an antiseptic solution, or simply a dry sponge, is usually placed just within the introitus prior to any lathering and shaving of the parts. This prevents contaminated fluids from entering the vagina. In some hospitals, the pubic and vulvar hair are lathered prior to shaving, but in others a dry shave is employed. An ordinary safety razor is used, the direction of the stroke being from above downward, care being taken not to get any hair and soap into the introitus.

Since a tub bath might permit infected bath water to gain access to the vagina, a tub bath is never given at this time, just as it is forbidden in the last months of pregnancy. The type of bath used, when it is deemed desirable, will depend to some extent upon the set-up of the hospital. The types usually given are the spray, the shower and the sponge bath.

While washing the genitals, the nurse again holds a sponge in the introitus to prevent wash water from running into the vagina; a dry towel pressed against the vulva serves the same purpose. The strokes must be from above downward and away from the introitus. Special attention should be paid to separating the vulvar folds and to the removal of such smegma as may have accumulated around the base of the clitoris and in the folds of the labia minora. In washing the region around the anus, it must be remembered that a sponge which has passed over that region must not be returned near the vulvar orifice, but must be thrown away immediately. The solutions used in cleansing the genitals vary in different hospitals, but sterile water with soap, followed by a wash with bichloride of mercury solution (1:1000) is possibly the most commonly employed technic. After the vulva has been cleansed, the labia are gently separated and the introitus flushed out with some antiseptic solution, usually a bichloride of mercury solution. The patient is now instructed not to handle her genitals (lest she infect herself), is put in a hospital gown and is taken to the labor room.

Is the Patient in Labor? As already indicated, false labor pains frequently simulate true labor and the question often arises as to whether we are dealing with the former or the latter type of contractions. While this is occasionally a difficult problem to settle, a decision usually can be reached on the grounds of the following differential points between true and false labor, especially the last mentioned one:

TRUE LABOR	FALSE LABOR
Pains	Pains
Occur at regular intervals	Occur at irregular intervals
Intervals gradually shorten	Intervals remain long
Intensity gradually increases	Intensity remains same
Located chiefly in back	Located chiefly in abdomen
Intensified by walking	Walking has no effect; often relieves
Show is usually present	No show
Cervix becomes effaced and dilated	*Cervix usually uneffaced and closed and remains so*

EXAMINATIONS IN LABOR

General. As soon as possible after admission a complete examination of the heart and lungs is carried out to make certain that there are no conditions present which might contraindicate a general anesthetic. As already indicated, the pulse, respiration and temperature are taken by the nurse and repeated every four hours. In cases in which there is fever or in which labor has lasted more than 24 hours, it is desirable to repeat these observations every two hours. The blood pressure reading which is made on admission should be repeated every six hours or so; but in cases of toxemia of pregnancy this is done more frequently. The general condition of the patient throughout labor is naturally of the utmost importance and the physician should develop the habit of making, on every visit, a survey of her general status which should include observations on the pulse rate, blood pressure, character of respirations, facies and mental attitude.

Abdominal. The abdominal examination is similar to that carried out in the prenatal course, comprising estimating the fetal size and position and listening to the fetal heart sounds.

The behavior of the fetal heart sounds in labor is of great importance and this examination is carried out at least every 3 hours during the first stage, while during the second stage it should be done every 5 or 10 minutes. It will be recalled that the rate of the fetal heart ranges between 120 and 150, averaging about 140. After a contraction, it normally becomes much slower than usual and may fall to the neighborhood of 90 or 100. Provided the baby is in good condition, however, it will return rapidly to its previous rate, usually within 15 or 20 seconds. On the other hand, if the baby is in distress, either because of the lack of oxygen or due to an abnormal degree of pressure exerted on its head, the fetal heart rate is constantly slow, often in the neighborhood of 80 per minute or below. This slow rate is occasionally accompanied by irregularity and sometimes by the passage of meconium which are other signs indicative of fetal distress. Repeated auscultation of the fetal heart sounds constitutes one of the most important parts of the conduct of the first and second stages of labor.

Rectal. The majority of the examinations carried out during labor are abdominal and rectal; vaginal examinations are performed only for special reasons. Rectal examinations are much safer than vaginal, since they avoid the risk of carrying pathogenic bacteria from the introitus and lower vagina to the region of the cervix and

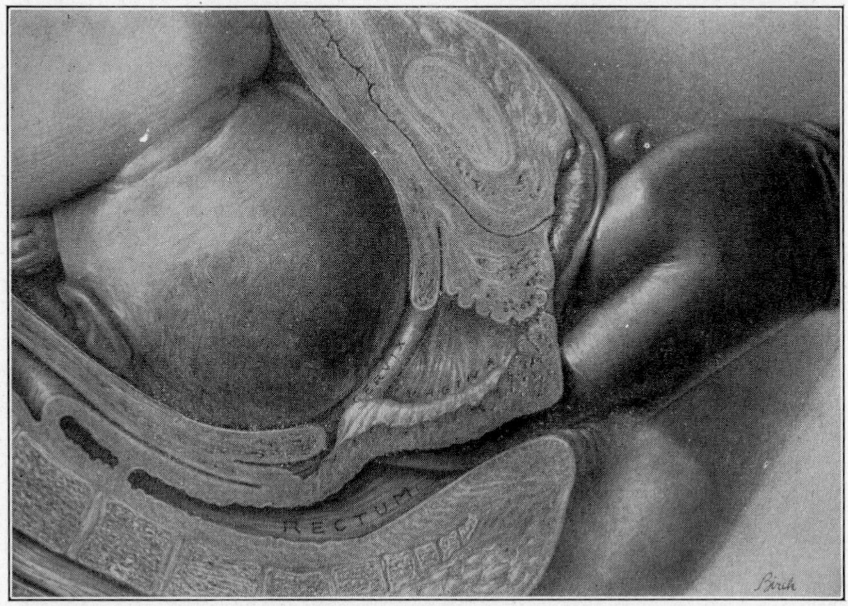

FIG. 276.—RECTAL EXAMINATION.

Note that the thumb is flexed into the palm of the hand so that it will not enter the vagina.

lower uterine segment. Furthermore, they have the advantage of not requiring disinfection on the part of the physician or the patient, as the nonsterile glove is drawn directly over the unwashed hand, the glove being boiled and the hand washed after the completion of the examination. In making a rectal examination the index finger is used, the hand being covered by a clean but not necessarily sterile rubber glove. As shown in Fig. 276 the thumb should be flexed into the palm of the hand, because otherwise it may enter the vagina and predispose to infection. The finger is now literally anointed with a lubricating jelly and introduced slowly into the rectum. The cervical opening can usually be felt as a depression surrounded by a circular ridge. The degree of dilatation and the amount of effacement are noted. Very often the membranes can be felt bulging into the cervix, particularly during a pain. The level of the fetal head is now ascertained and correlated with the level of the head as being a number of centimeters above or below the ischial spines.

The frequency with which rectal examinations are required during labor depends on the individual case. Not infrequently one or two such examinations are all that are necessary, while in some instances many more are required. In the normal patient with adequate pelvic measurements and a normal sized fetus, the progress of labor can be followed to a great extent by careful evaluation of the subjective and objective symptoms of the patient, accurate interpretation of the findings on abdominal examination and by palpation of the perineum, if necessary.

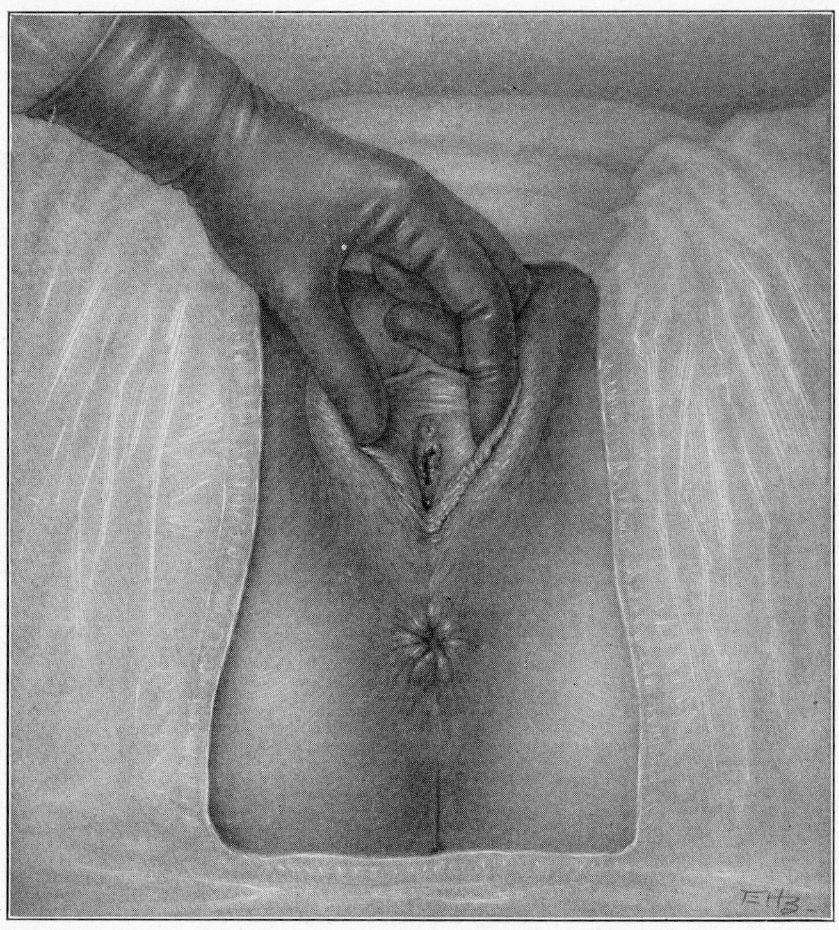

FIG. 277.—ILLUSTRATING SPREADING APART THE LABIA BEFORE MAKING A VAGINAL EXAMINATION.

Vaginal. Although rectal examinations possess the advantages stated, they suffer from the disadvantage that the findings are sometimes inconclusive and in that event, or if labor is not progressing satisfactorily, vaginal examination is indicated. In general, 9 labors out of 10 can be conducted by rectal and abdominal examinations only. Vaginal examination is naturally more reliable than rectal, since the cervix and fontanels can be palpated directly with no intervening rectovaginal septum to interfere with tactile sense.

After the patient has been properly prepared, the vulvar and perineal region scrubbed and draped, and the examiner has scrubbed and donned sterile gloves, the thumb and forefinger of one hand distend the labia widely, so as to expose the vaginal opening and prevent the examining fingers from coming in contact with the inner surfaces of the labia and the margins of the hymen, while the index and second fingers of the other hand are introduced into the vagina (Fig. 277).

In making the examination a definite routine should be followed: (1) A very important consideration in the technic of the examination is the fact that once the fingers are inserted in the vagina, they should not be withdrawn until the examination is entirely completed. The fingers should be introduced along the anterior surface of the vaginal wall, and the shape and size of the pubic arch and the height of the symphysis noted. (2) The cervix should then be examined to determine whether its canal is obliterated, the degree to which the external os is dilated, and the character of its margins. Next observe whether the membranes are intact or not, great care being taken to avoid rupturing them if the patient is in the first stage of labor. (3) If the os be dilated, the presentation and position of the child should be made out, and the relation of the presenting part to the superior strait and to the line connecting the ischial spines determined. (4) After having decided these points the palmar surface of the fingers should be directed posteriorly, and the perineum palpated between the two fingers in the vagina and the thumb outside, with special reference to its consistency, thickness and resistance. (5) The mobility of the coccyx should then be tested, after which the fingers should be passed upward over the anterior surface of the sacrum and its vertical and lateral curvature noted. If the presenting part is not low down, the three lower sacral vertebrae are readily palpable in normal women, whereas the first and second can be felt only in contracted pelves. (6) If the presenting part is not deeply engaged, and the diagonal conjugate has not been measured, its length should now be determined.

After completing the examination, the physician is usually expected to express an opinion as to the probable course of events. If everything is normal, he should assure the patient that all is well, but he should guard against making any precise statement as to the probable duration of labor, and be content with saying that, under the circumstances present, the average time is a certain number of hours, and that her labor will probably be ended within that period. The obstetrician who ventures to make more precise statements will speedily find that his predictions are often very faulty, even when the head is on the perineum. If some abnormality be present it is not always wise to inform the patient of the fact, but the physician should be careful to impart his knowledge to some responsible member of the family for his own protection.

Methods of Detecting Rupture of the Membranes. The clinical diagnosis of ruptured membranes may sometimes be surprisingly uncertain and a number of tests to decide the question have been recommended.

Perhaps the most widely employed procedure is one or another method of testing the acidity or alkalinity of the vaginal fluid. These tests are based on the fundamental fact that normally the pH of the vaginal secretion ranges between 4.5 and 5.5, whereas the pH of the amniotic fluid is usually 7.0 to 7.5.

Nitrazine Test. The use of the indicator substance, nitrazine, for the diagnosis of ruptured membranes was first suggested by Baptisti in 1938 and is a simple and fairly reliable method. Baptisti used indicator test papers impregnated with the dye. With these papers is furnished a color chart comprising a pH range from 4.5 to 7.5 (made by E. R. Squibb and Company). The papers are set at pH of 6.0. The pH of the vaginal secretion is determined by inserting a sterile cotton tipped applicator deeply into the vagina, and after withdrawal,

the cotton tip is touched to a strip of the nitrazine paper and the paper then compared with the color chart. Color changes are interpreted as follows:

Yellow	pH	5.0	Intact membranes
Olive yellow	pH	5.5	
Olive green	pH	6.0	
Blue green	pH	6.5	Ruptured membranes
Blue gray	pH	7.0	
Deep blue	pH	7.5	

Baptisti points out that a false reading is likely to be encountered in patients with intact membranes but who have an unusually large amount of bloody show since the blood, like amniotic fluid, will tend to turn the indicator to the alkaline side. His results in 50 consecutive cases were generally satisfactory.

A more extended study of the nitrazine test by a slightly different technic was made by Abe in 1940. He reported 176 cases in which the nitrazine test was used and found it correct in 98.9 per cent of patients with known rupture of membranes and in 96.2 per cent in patients with intact membranes. Abe, as well as Kushner, found that nitrazine is the most accurate indicator for the purpose.

We have employed nitrazine papers for the diagnosis of ruptured membranes ever since they were first suggested by Baptisti and have found the test easy to carry out and reasonably dependable. It must not be thought, however, that the ordinary clinical use of these pH tests will yield as good results as those reported above, because the practical employment which is usually made of the procedure is to test borderline cases in which the amount of fluid present is small and, since it is small, may sometimes be affected by the pH of blood and vaginal secretions.

Fat Globules. The demonstration of fat globules microscopically in the vaginal fluid is another fairly dependable test but is somewhat more troublesome to carry out than the nitrazine technics. It was first recommended by Numers in 1936 and is used in a number of clinics. The technic is as follows: a speculum is inserted 1 or 2 cm. above the introitus; one drop of secretion is taken and spread out on a clean slide. The preparation is air-dried and, without previous fixation, stained at room temperature in a dye solution, obtained by dissolving 0.2-0.3 gm. sudan III in 100 cc. 70 per cent hot alcohol. The slide is washed in water, dried by blotting paper and examined immediately after the staining under low magnifying power. The fat-substances are stained a distinct orange-red; particles of mucus are sometimes stained weakly yellowish-red. These, as well as small, faintly tinted drops of fat occurring in expelled cells of the vaginal epithelium, may be easily distinguished from the fetal fat-substances. In all, 280 cases were examined by Numers, 141 of them before the rupture of membranes and 139 afterward. Only four of the former cases gave a slight positive sudan reaction, the rest yielding a negative result (97.2 per cent). The samples taken after the rupture of membranes gave a positive outcome in 99.3 per cent; one negative case only was observed. Slight sudan reactions seem to be relatively more frequent in premature cases. The faulty reactions amount to about two per cent of the entire material.

Fetal Epithelium. Still another test is based on the demonstration of disintegrating squamous cells from fetal epithelium as proposed first by Bourgeois. Either the Shorr differential stain or some modification of it is used. The morphologic differentiation of fetal squamas from sheets of cells recently desquamated from the maternal vagina, vestibule, or urethra, is made on the fact that cells from the latter locations generally possess well-developed nuclei and granular cytoplasm which lacks the translucence of fetal cells. Bourgeois reported an overall accuracy of 97.1 per cent in 344 specimens of vaginal fluid from 275 patients. It should be noted, nevertheless, that characteristic fetal squamas are not consistently found in liquor amnii prior to the beginning of the ninth lunar month.

The fact that these several technics for the diagnosis of ruptured membranes have been recommended is indication enough that no one of them is without its weaknesses. Thus, the pH methods may be vitiated by admixture of blood and are less dependable when only minute quantities of amniotic fluids have escaped. The identification of fetal epithelium becomes of little value prior to the thirty-second week. This test, moreover, demands some little training in cytology since degenerating squamous epithelium, both from fetal and vaginal sources, may be encountered and they tend to converge in their morphology. The demonstration of fat globules, like that of fetal squamas, is more uncertain prior to the thirty-second week since the amount of vernix is much less. In other words, both these microscopic tests are of little value before the ninth lunar month.

In summary, the nitrazine test is certainly the simplest of the various procedures and, if allowances are made for the sources of error mentioned, is as accurate as any of the others. If, in a given case, there is reason to question it, the fat globule test is probably the next most practical.

OTHER ASPECTS OF FIRST STAGE MANAGEMENT

During the first stage of labor the patient usually prefers to move about her room and frequently is more comfortable when occupying a sitting position. This is permitted provided the membranes are intact and analgesia is not being administered. During this period, therefore, she should not be compelled to take to her bed unless she feels so inclined, and when she does so she should be cautioned against attempting to hasten labor by voluntarily bringing her abdominal muscles into play, for they have no effect upon the dilatation of the cervix, and the effort will only serve to exhaust her strength.

A perineal pad should not be worn during labor because of the nature of the vaginal discharge. The tenacious mucoid discharge frequently comes in contact with the anus and could easily be smeared about the external genitalia and vaginal orifice when changing or adjusting the pads. No antiseptic is applied to the external genitalia during labor prior to the time of preparation for delivery, unless it is necessary to prepare the patient for vaginal examination.

Careful watching of the bladder is an important part of the management of labor since a full bladder may be a serious impediment, especially in the second and third stages. Accordingly, the patient should be asked to void every three or four hours; if she is unable to do so and if the distended bladder can be palpated above the symphysis, catheterization should be carried out. Figure 495 illustrates a case in which failure to follow this injunction resulted in extreme delay in the progress of labor.

Since the median duration of labor is less than 10 hours and since ingestion of food may create anesthesia difficulties at delivery, it is customary to withhold solid food in parturient women. In fact, patients in labor rarely desire food, are prone to vomit it and show evidence that their powers of digestion are impaired at this time. Patients may take fluids early in labor when delivery is not imminent. If vomiting or dehydration occurs, or if labor is longer than 12 hours, administration of intravenous glucose is often desirable.

MANAGEMENT OF SECOND STAGE

There are certain signs which herald the onset of the second stage of labor and which should be watched for carefully. These are: (*a*) the patient begins to bear down of her own accord; this is caused by a reflex when the head begins to press on the perineal floor. (*b*) There is a sudden increase in show; sometimes there may be slight actual bleeding. (*c*) Patient thinks that she needs to evacuate; this symptom is also due to pressure of the head on the perineal floor and consequently against the rectum. (*d*) Membranes rupture with discharge of amniotic fluid. This, of course, may take place at any time but occurs most frequently at the beginning of the second stage. (*e*) Perineum begins to bulge and anal orifice to dilate. This is a late sign, but if *a, b, c,* and *d* occur, it should be watched for with every pain. Only rectal or vaginal examination (or the appearance of the head) can definitely confirm the suspicion.

If the above signs are overlooked, the delivery may occur without benefit of proper attention (colloquially called B.O.A., "born on arrival"). In general, primigravidae

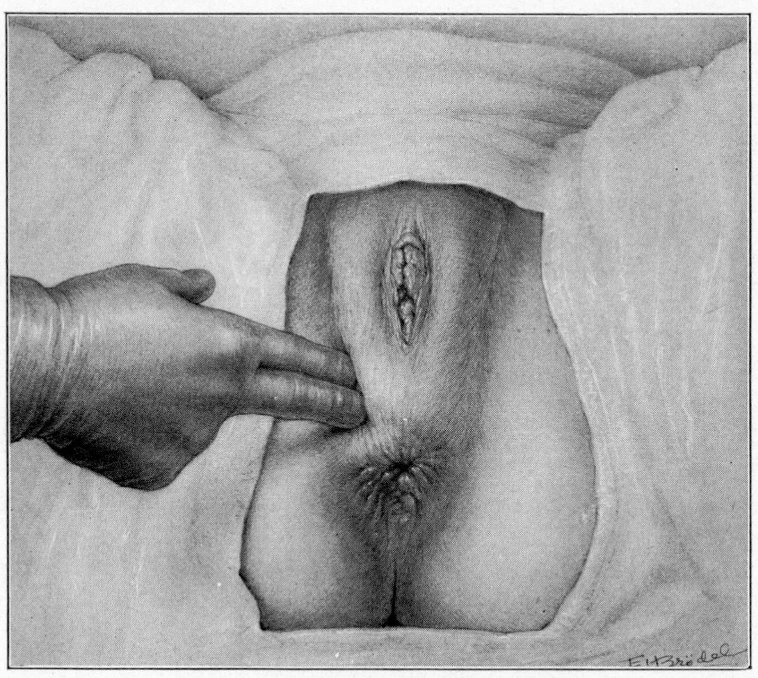

FIG. 278.—PALPATING HEAD THROUGH PERINEUM.

should be taken to the delivery room when fully dilated and multiparae when 7 or 8 cm. dilated.

Ordinarily, in the second stage of labor the necessary information can be obtained by rectal exploration, but when vaginal examination becomes necessary the most rigid aseptic technic should be observed. Furthermore, it should be remembered that after the head has become engaged, its descent can be followed readily by the increasing difficulty with which the cephalic prominence can be palpated on employment of the fourth maneuver. As long as the latter can be palpated, one knows that the most dependent portion of the vertex lies above the level of the ischial spines. Moreover, when the cephalic prominence can no longer be felt from above, if the legs are widely separated and the tips of the fingers applied to the perineum, to the side of and in front of the anus, and pressed firmly inward and upward, the presenting part can be felt as a firm, rounded body. Generally speaking, this maneuver becomes available as soon as the biparietal plane of the head has passed below the level of the ischial spines (Fig. 278).

In most cases, bearing-down efforts are reflex and spontaneous in the second stage of labor but occasionally the patient does not employ her expulsive forces to good advantage and coaching is desirable. In some hospitals straps are placed in the patient's hands. The straps are firmly attached to the delivery table and so adjusted in length that she can reach them comfortably. Her legs should be half flexed so that she can push with them against the floor of the table. Instructions should then be given the patient to take a deep breath just as soon as her next pain begins and, with her breath held, to exert downward pressure exactly as if she were straining at stool. Pulling on the straps at this time is a helpful adjunct. The effort should be as long and sustained as possible, since short "grunty" endeavors are of little avail. Usually these bearing-down efforts are rewarded by increasing bulging of the perineum, that is, by further descent of the head. The patient should be informed of such progress, for encouragement now is all important. During this period of active bearing down the fetal heart sounds should be auscultated after each pain. The maternal pulse must be counted frequently also, since any substantial increase in pulse rate indicates exhaustion and calls for some other means of meeting the situation than the continuation of bearing-down efforts.

As the head passes down into the pelvis small particles of feces are frequently expelled, and as they appear at the anus, they should be sponged off with large fresh pledgets soaked in antiseptic solution. *Asepsis* and *antisepsis* are all important in the second stage of labor and no one should be permitted in the delivery room unless he or she wears a sterile gown, as well as a mask covering both nose and mouth, and a cap which completely covers the hair of the head. Preparation for actual delivery entails a repetition of the vulvar and perineal clean-up previously described, plus the placing of suitable towels and draping over the patient so that only the immediate region about the vulva is exposed.

In putting the legs of the anesthetized patient up into stirrups, care should be used not to separate the legs too widely or to have one leg higher than the other. Both legs should be raised and lowered at the same time, with a nurse holding each. Failure to observe these instructions may result in straining the ligaments of the pelvis, with consequent discomfort in the puerperium.

Procedure in Hand Disinfection. It is now generally admitted that it is impossible to render one's hands absolutely sterile, no matter what method of disinfection may be employed. Even after the most rigorous directions have been scrupulously followed, there still remains a not inconsiderable danger of infection.

With the view of still further minimizing these risks, the use of rubber gloves has been introduced. These can be rendered absolutely sterile by boiling and, when drawn over the carefully disinfected hands, afford the greatest safety possible. Since they are likely to tear occasionally, the necessity for disinfecting the hands before putting them on is apparent. But their employment, even in conjunction with all our other precautions, does not entirely do away with the possibility of introducing pyogenic bacteria into the genital tract, since Williams has shown that they may be carried up from the vaginal outlet by the sterile gloved finger. As early as 1898, he demonstrated that pathogenic organisms are present upon the inner surfaces of the labia and the margins of the hymen in at least 60 per cent of pregnant women, and that the mere introduction of a sterile glass speculum 2 cm. in diameter, which is no larger than the two fingers employed for examination, carries micro-organisms into the vagina in one half of such cases. Inasmuch as the delicate structure of the parts renders their thorough disinfection out of the question and as the examining fingers necessarily come in contact with them, it must be admitted that vaginal examinations during labor can never be entirely devoid of danger, and they should therefore be avoided so far as is consistent with the welfare of the patient. While these considerations should not deter us from making as many examinations as may be necessary in abnormal cases, it should always be borne in mind that the best results are obtained by the least possible employment of the vaginal examination and the widest possible utilization of other methods of examination.

In all cases the hands should be disinfected as carefully as for a major surgical operation. The following technic is recommended:

1. The fingernails are cut and cleaned before starting to scrub.
2. Using a sterile brush, scrub the hands and forearms up to the elbows vigorously with green soap and hot water, for five minutes or as much longer as may be necessary to render them macroscopically clean, paying particular attention to the nails and palmar surface of the fingers. If running water is not available, the water must be changed at least once. After changing it, remove dirt from beneath the finger nails with nail cleaner, and renew the washing.
3. A sterile orangewood stick is now employed to clean thoroughly the fingernails.
4. A new sterile brush is employed to scrub the hands and arms for another period of five minutes as described under 2, above.
5. The hands and arms are immersed in an arm-tank 24 inches deep containing an antiseptic solution, for three minutes.

The amount of time required for the entire disinfection is approximately 18 minutes. Where the birth of the baby becomes imminent or in any case of hurry, the time is shortened accordingly. However, emphasis is placed on the immersion of the hands and arms in antiseptic solution and alcohol, and an attempt to soak the full three minutes in each solution is made whenever possible.

Following scrubbing and disinfection of the hands, a sterile gown is put on in such a manner that the hands do not touch the outer surface of the gown. This is most easily done if a nurse holds the gown full length by the collar tips with the armholes toward the operator. Likewise, the gloves are put on in such a manner that the skin of the hands never touches the outer sides of the gloves. This is shown in Fig. 279.

After the patient has been prepared for delivery, catheterization, if done, is carried out by the physician, but prior to that time is performed by the nurse at the physician's request. It is sometimes difficult to catheterize a patient in the second stage of labor since the baby's head may compress the urethra. If the catheter does not pass easily it is best to push the head up slightly, insinuate one's finger between the head and region of the urethra and in this manner make a space for the catheter; force should never be employed.

Cramps in the leg are common in the second stage of labor because of pressure exerted by the baby's head on certain nerves in the pelvis. These are readily relieved by changing the position of the leg, passive motion and massage for a few seconds. These should never be ignored since they sometimes appear to cause excruciating pain.

As soon as the head distends the perineum to a diameter of 6 or 8 cm., that is, when crowning is about to occur, it is desirable to place a towel over the rectum and exert forward pressure on the chin of the baby's head while the other hand exerts downward pressure on the occiput. This is called *Ritgen's maneuver,* and allows the physician to control the egress of the head; it also favors extension so that the head is born with the smallest diameter presenting. The head is usually delivered between pains, and as slowly as possible. All these measures (control of head by Ritgen's maneuver, extension and slow delivery between pains) help to prevent lacerations. As shown in Fig. 283, the posterior shoulder is usually delivered first and then the remainder of the body follows without particular mechanism.

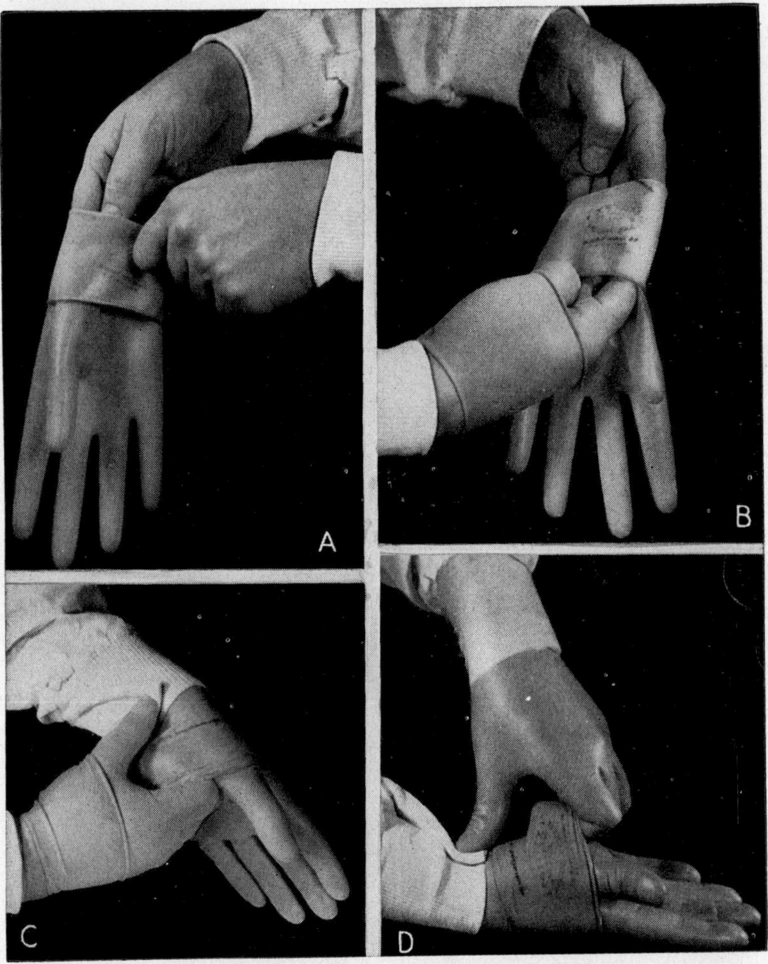

Fig. 279A, B, C and D.—Method of Putting on Sterile Gloves so that the Exteriors of the Gloves Are Never Touched by the Ungloved Hand.

In the majority of cases the shoulders appear at the vulva just after the occurrence of external rotation, and are born spontaneously. Occasionally a delay occurs and immediate extraction may appear advisable. To accomplish this the head should be held between two hands (Fig. 284), and downward traction made until the anterior shoulder appears under the pubic arch; next, by an upward movement, the posterior shoulder should be delivered, after which the anterior shoulder will usually drop down from beneath the symphysis (Fig. 285).

The body almost always follows the shoulders without difficulty, but in case of prolonged delay its birth may be hastened by traction upon the head, or by pressure upon the abdomen, but not by hooking the fingers in the axillae, since by the latter procedure the nerves of the arm may be injured and transient or permanent paralysis result. Indeed, even when the former method of extraction is employed, traction should

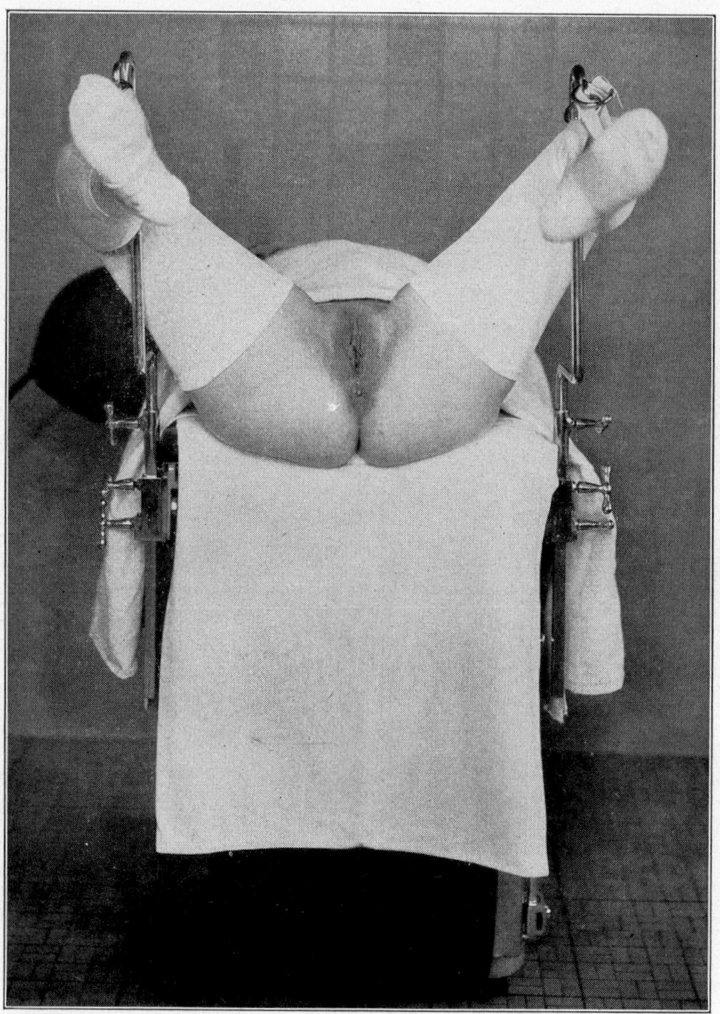

Fig. 280.—Showing Patient at Edge of Table, with Legs Held in Position with Stirrups.

be exerted only in the direction of the long axis of the child, for if it be made obliquely the neck will be bent upon the body, when excessive stretching of the brachial plexus on its convex side may occur, with subsequent paralysis.

Immediately after the birth of the head, the finger should be passed to the neck of the child in order to ascertain whether it is encircled by one or more coils of the umbilical cord. This complication occurs in about every fourth case and ordinarily does no harm but occasionally the coil is drawn so taut that the vessels are constricted and asphyxiation results. If such a coil be felt it should be drawn down between the fingers and, if loose enough, slipped over the child's head; but if it be too tightly applied to permit of this procedure, the cord should be seized and cut between two artery clamps, and the child immediately extracted before asphyxiation results.

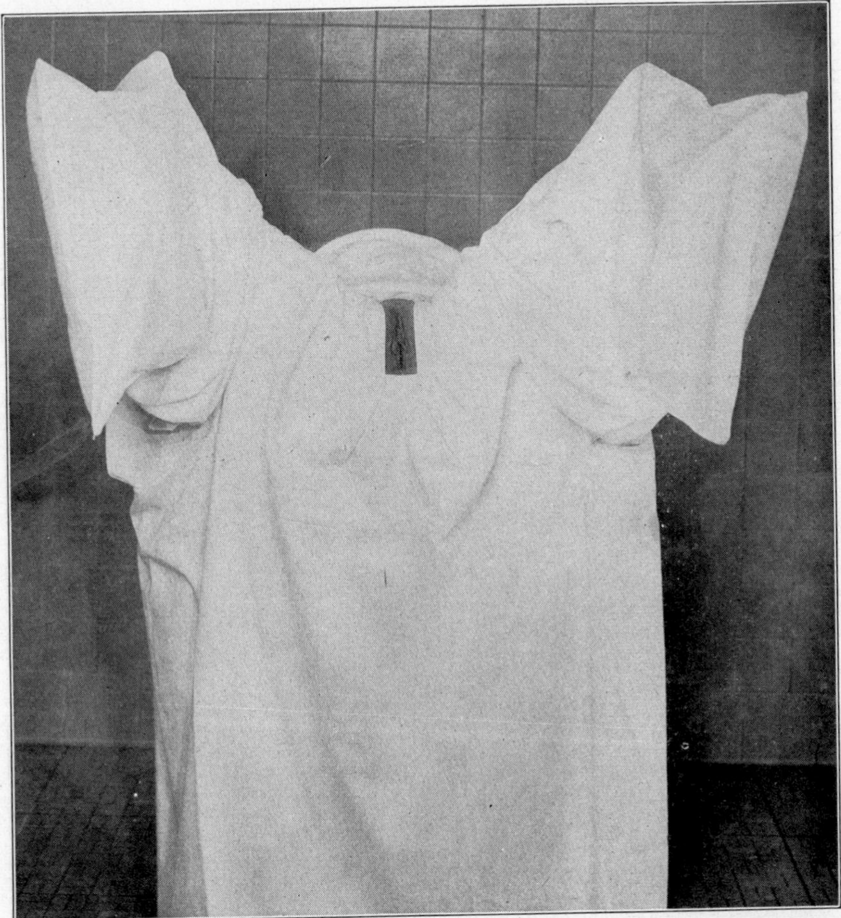

Fig. 281.—Showing Patient Covered with Sterile Draping Preparatory to Operation.

Tying the Cord. It is our practice to cut the cord between two Kelly clamps placed a few inches from the abdomen, and subsequently to apply a sterilized linen tape ligature tightly tied about 2 cm. from the abdomen. From time to time various types of clamps or other devices have been recommended to replace the ligature. Such a device is shown in Fig. 286 and this and other such clamps are used extensively in many institutions. Whenever possible clamping or ligating the umbilical cord should be deferred until its pulsations wane or, at least, for one or two minutes.

There has been a tendency of late, for a number of reasons, to ignore this precept. In the first place the widespread use of analgesic drugs in labor has resulted in a number of infants whose respiratory efforts are sluggish at birth and whom the obstetrician wishes to turn over immediately to an assistant for aspiration of mucus and, if necessary, resuscitation. This readily leads to the habit of clamping all cords promptly. Secondly, there is the episiotomy wound to suture; and the quicker the repair is started, the shorter will be the duration of anesthesia, and the less the blood loss from the wound. Finally, modern management of the third stage, especially if ergonovine has been given with the birth of the anterior shoulder, calls for immediate attention to the uterus and furnishes another reason for handing the

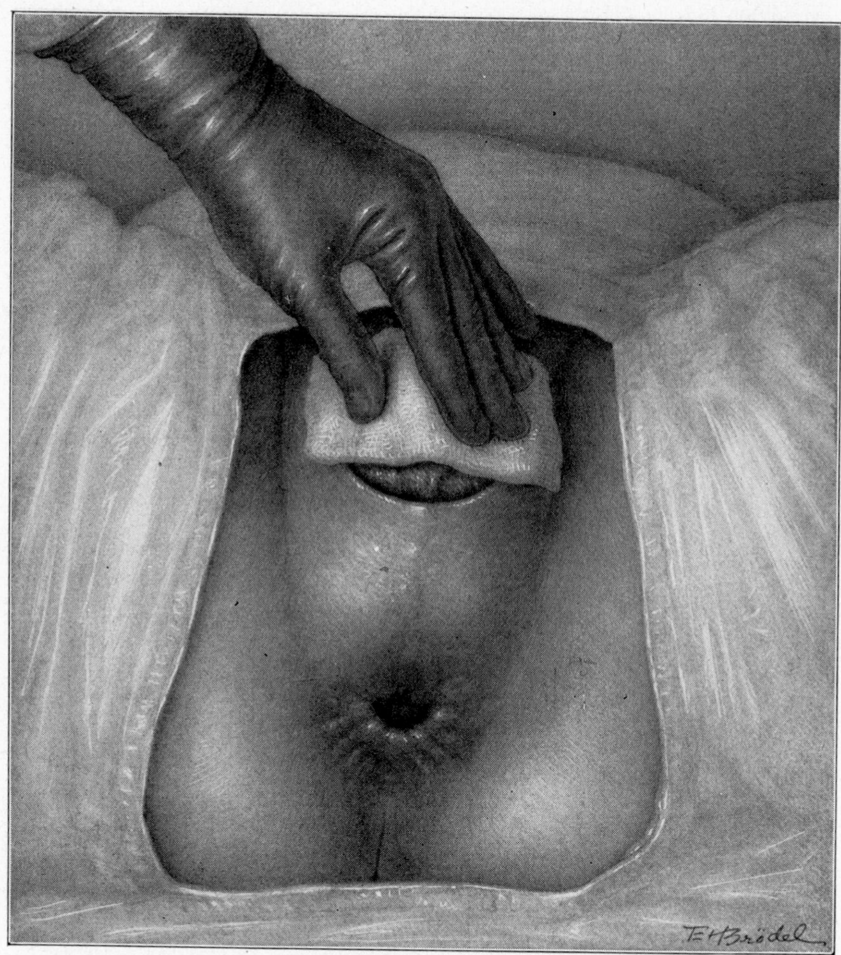

Fig. 282.—Method of Restraining Head to Increase Flexion and Protect Perineum.

baby to an assistant or nurse as promptly as possible. These three tendencies of modern obstetrics, then, notwithstanding their several merits, do militate against delayed clamping of the cord. As a result, two questions arise: How important is this additional blood to the infant? How can the possible advantages to the baby of late clamping be secured in the presence of these interfering technics?

The benefits which accrue to the baby from delayed ligature of the cord probably contribute more to his welfare during the neonatal period than has been realized. This fact has been stressed by many authors but most cogently perhaps by the well documented studies of DeMarsh, Alt, Windle and Hillis, working at the Cook County Hospital. Their first study dealt with the effect that depriving the infant of its placental blood had on the hematological picture during the first week of life Their findings may be summarized by stating that

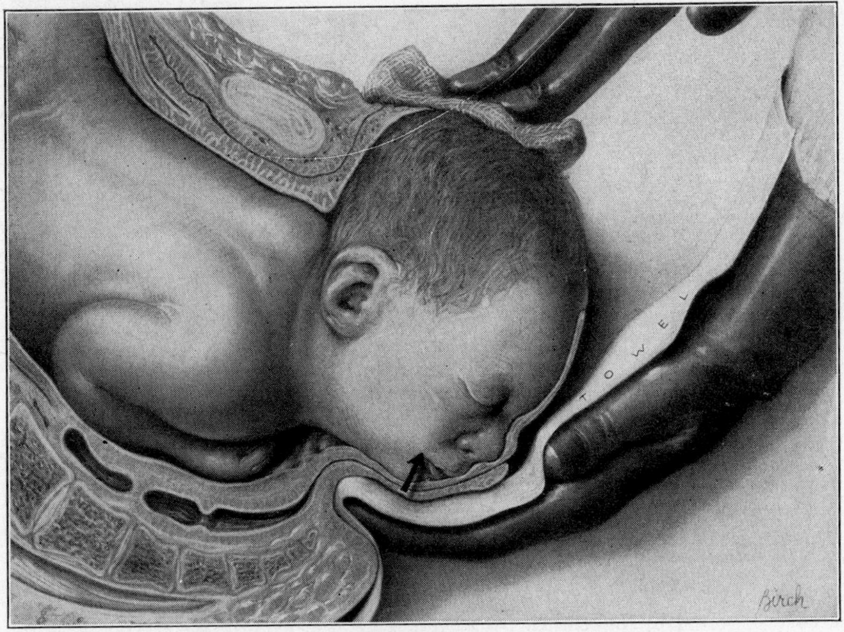

FIG. 283.—DELIVERY BY THE MODIFIED RITGEN'S MANEUVER.

the hemoglobin concentration, the red cell count and the body weight were, on the average, decidedly higher in infants whose cords were clamped late rather than immediately. These authors found also higher reticulocyte counts in infants whose cords were clamped immediately, a circumstance suggesting a greater demand for blood in this group than in the group whose cords were not clamped until placental separation. A subsequent paper had to do with the blood volume of the newborn infant in relation to early and late clamping of the umbilical cord. Here it was found that the deprivation of blood which the newborn suffers from immediate cord clamping averages 107 cc. This figure is in good agreement with the 96

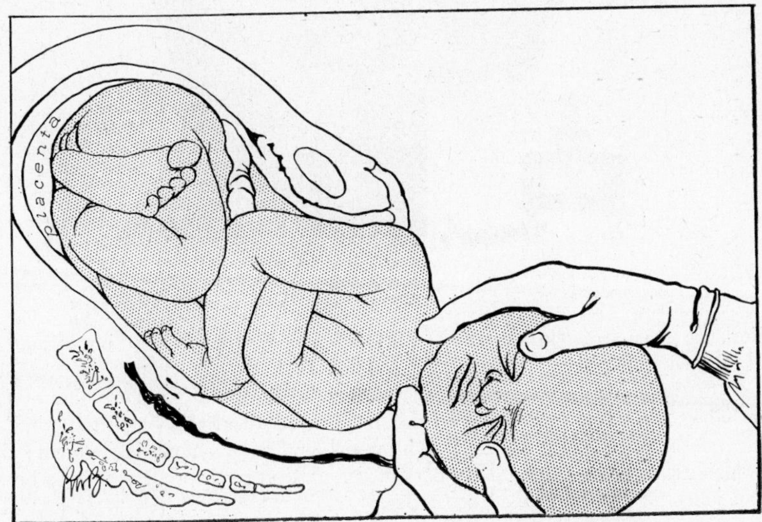

FIG. 284.—GENTLE TRACTION TO BRING ABOUT DESCENT OF ANTERIOR SHOULDER.

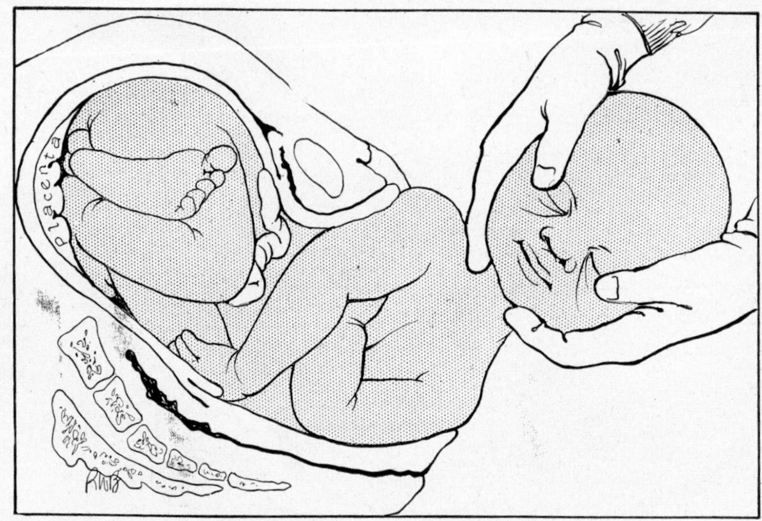

FIG. 285.—DELIVERY OF ANTERIOR SHOULDER COMPLETED; GENTLE TRACTION TO DELIVER THE POSTERIOR SHOULDER.

cc. recently reported by Ballentine. Moreover, while the average blood volume of infants allowed to retrieve this placental blood (delayed clamping) was 361 cc., it was only 301 when immediate clamping of the cord had been practiced, a difference equal to one sixth of the total blood volume of the newborn infant.

As shown by the figures cited above the quantity of blood received by the newborn infant from the placenta (96-107 cc.) looms tremendously large in relation to its total blood volume (about 360 cc.) and must have an important bearing on bodily economy during the neonatal

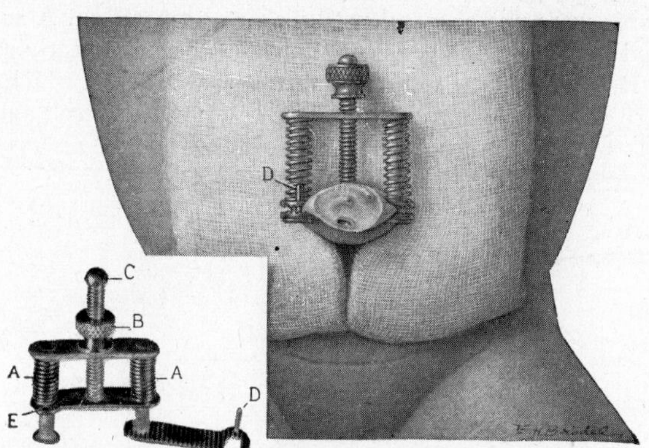

FIG. 286.—EXAMPLE OF A CORD CLAMP (Pastore).

period. For the premature infant this additional blood is especially important for two reasons: (1) since the placenta is larger in relation to body size than in the mature baby, the quantity of the transfusion is greater in relation to the infant's blood volume; (2) since premature babies are prone to develop anemia, they need all of this blood that they can get. The need of the mature infant for this additional blood is of course less urgent; but since this physiologic transfusion is inherently part of the natural birth process, it is to be regarded as desirable unless it can be proved otherwise.

The practical difficulties associated with delayed clamping of the cord, as mentioned above, disappear in large measure if consideration is given to the rate at which blood is transfused from placenta to infant after birth. This question was carefully studied in 1930 by two German investigators, Haselhorst and Allmeling. These workers placed 120 newborn infants on special spring scales immediately after delivery and observed their weight gain from minute to minute. The results were very informative. The total weight gain, about 90 gm., is in good agreement with the figures cited above. Most important, however, from a practical viewpoint is the fact that over half this weight of blood is transferred the first minute and about three-quarters within the first two minutes. After about three minutes the strong pulsations cease and thereafter the amount of blood transferred is a rather small fraction of the whole. From the viewpoint of the objective to be attained, therefore, delayed clamping or ligature of the cord might be defined very sensibly as postponement of this procedure for two to three minutes. Even a delay of one minute will give the infant over half of the blood it is supposed to receive. A delay of one minute should not interfere appreciably with the technics discussed above, but here, as always, common sense has to be employed and ironclad rules are undesirable.

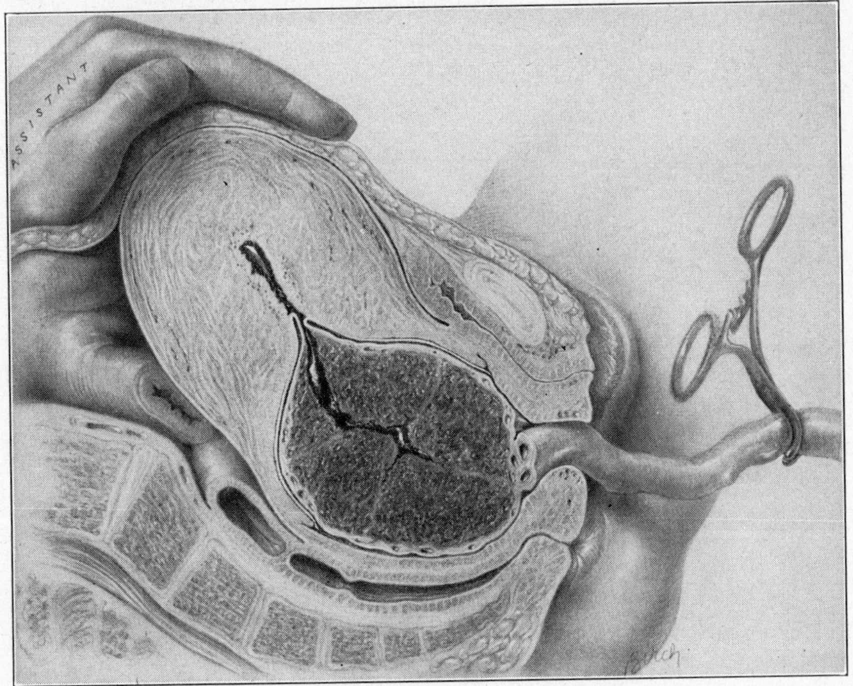

Fig. 287.—Expression of Placenta.

The fundus should be massaged before carrying out this procedure to make certain that the uterus is firmly contracted and hard. However, it is not squeezed.

MANAGEMENT OF THIRD STAGE

Immediately after delivery of the infant, the height of the uterine fundus and its consistency are ascertained. The physician may do this by palpating the uterus through a sterile towel placed on the lower abdomen, but it is a duty which is often delegated to an assistant or nurse, at least while the physician is engaged in clamping and cutting the umbilical cord. As long as the uterus remains hard and there is no bleeding, the policy is ordinarily one of watchful waiting until the placenta is separated; no massage whatsoever is practiced, the hand simply resting on the fundus to make certain that the organ does not balloon out with blood. Since attempts to deliver the placenta prior to its separation from the uterine wall are not only futile but may be dangerous, it is most important that the signs of placental separation be well understood. The signs which suggest that the placenta has separated are as follows:

1. The uterus rises upward in the abdomen; this is due to the fact that the placenta, having been separated, passes downward into the lower uterine segment and vagina where its bulk pushes the uterus upward.

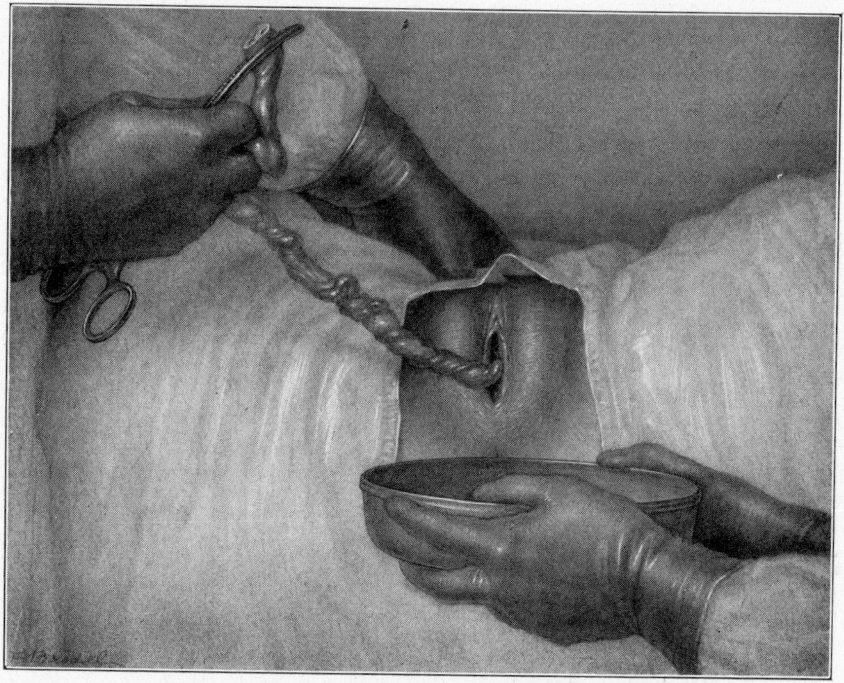

Fig. 288.—Expression of Placenta.

2. The umbilical cord protrudes three or more inches farther out of the vagina, indicating that the placenta also has descended.

3. The uterus assumes a globular shape and becomes, as a rule, firmer. This is the earliest sign to appear.

4. A sudden gush of blood often occurs.

These signs are sometimes apparent within a minute or so after delivery of the infant, usually within five minutes. When the placenta has certainly separated, the physician first ascertains that the uterus is firmly contracted. He may then ask the patient, if not anesthetized, to bear down, and the intra-abdominal pressure so produced may be adequate to expel the placenta. If this fails or if it is not practicable because of anesthesia the physician, again having made certain that the uterus is hard, exerts downward pressure with his hand on the fundus and, employing the placenta as a piston, simply shoves the placenta out of the vagina. This procedure, known as placental "expression," must be done gently and without squeezing. It should never be attempted unless the uterus is hard, otherwise the organ may be turned inside-out. This is one of the gravest complications of obstetrics and is known as "inversion" of the uterus (page 923).

The methods of expressing the placenta as described above should be sharply differentiated from the so-called "Credé expression" in which the body of the uterus is vigorously squeezed in order to produce placental separation. This latter procedure is usually futile, is likely to traumatize the placental site and is not recommended.

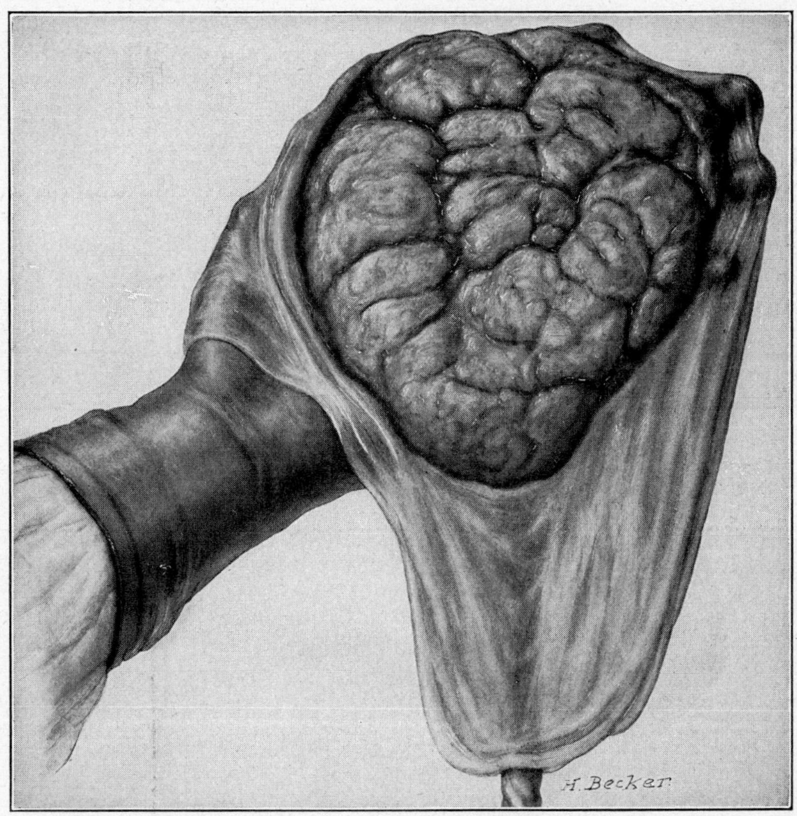

Fig. 289.—Inspection of Placenta Immediately after Its Delivery.

In the belief that much unnecessary blood loss occurs between the moment of separation and of expulsion, as the result of the growing retroplacental hematoma, Calkins has recommended a technic for the conduct of the third stage which aims at earlier recognition of placental separation and earlier expulsion. His procedure embraces two departures from the standard method quoted above: (1) Constant application of the hand to the uterine fundus after birth of the child in order to detect the first signs of placental detachment; (2) vigorous massage of the uterus immediately after separation, followed at once by efforts at expulsion. He describes his method as follows:

Directly after the delivery of the baby, the hand is placed on the abdomen; the uterus is held very gently with the fingers behind and the thumb in front and with no attempt to massage the organ unless it shows signs of relaxation and flaccidity. As soon as it changes *from a discoid to a globular shape* and a trickle of blood appears from the vagina, the organ is vigorously massaged until it becomes firmly contracted and then, by squeezing and gentle downward pressure, an attempt is made to express the placenta. Should the placenta not come out readily, no further attempt is made to express it and no further massage is instituted until some sign of enlargement or flaccidity appears or there is an increase of bleeding from the vagina.

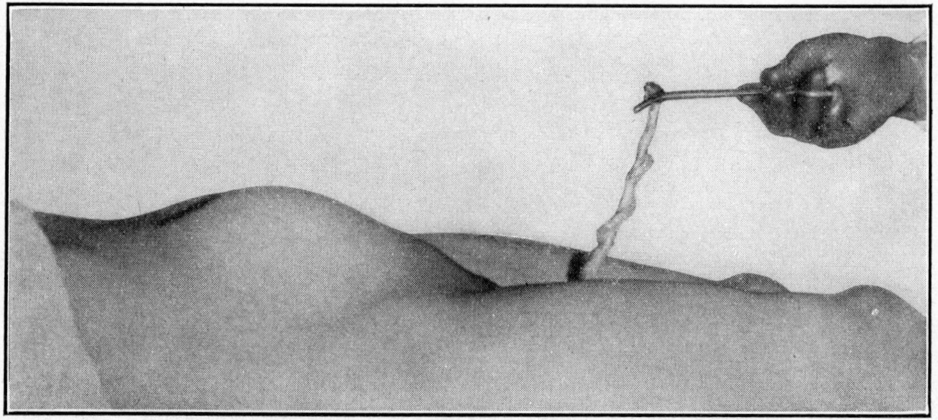

Fig. 290A.—Abdominal Contour after Completion of Second Stage.

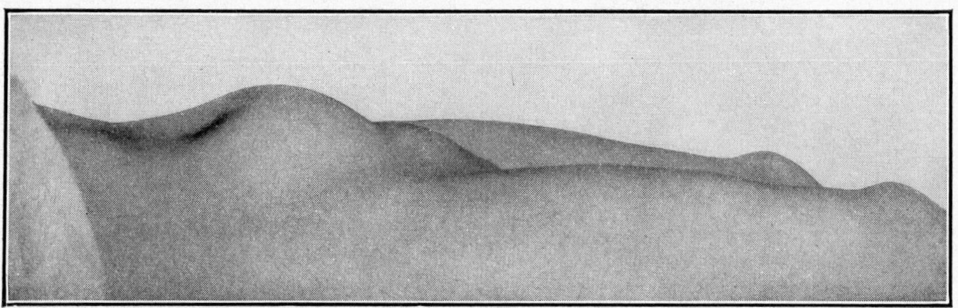

Fig. 290B.—Abdominal Contour after Completion of Third Stage.

Calkins believes that this technic not only will minimize excessive bleeding but also will reduce moderate losses such as would otherwise range between 200 and 600 cc. In this connection emphasis should be laid on the desirability of measuring blood loss with some degree of accuracy for only by so doing can the obstetrician be apprised at all times of the amount of blood which is being lost. Estimates of blood loss based on the general impression received of the amount of bleeding, are notoriously inaccurate and tend to be underestimates. We have found the Carroll plate, as shown in Fig. 291, a practical and reasonably simple device for this purpose.

Finally, it should be emphasized, that the hour following the delivery of the placenta is a most critical one. It is so critical that it has even been suggested that this hour be designated as the fourth stage of labor. It is at this time that postpartum hemorrhage is most likely to occur as the result of uterine relaxation and it is mandatory that the uterus be watched constantly throughout this period by a competent nurse who keeps her hand more or less constantly on the fundus and massages it at the slightest sign of diminishing retraction.

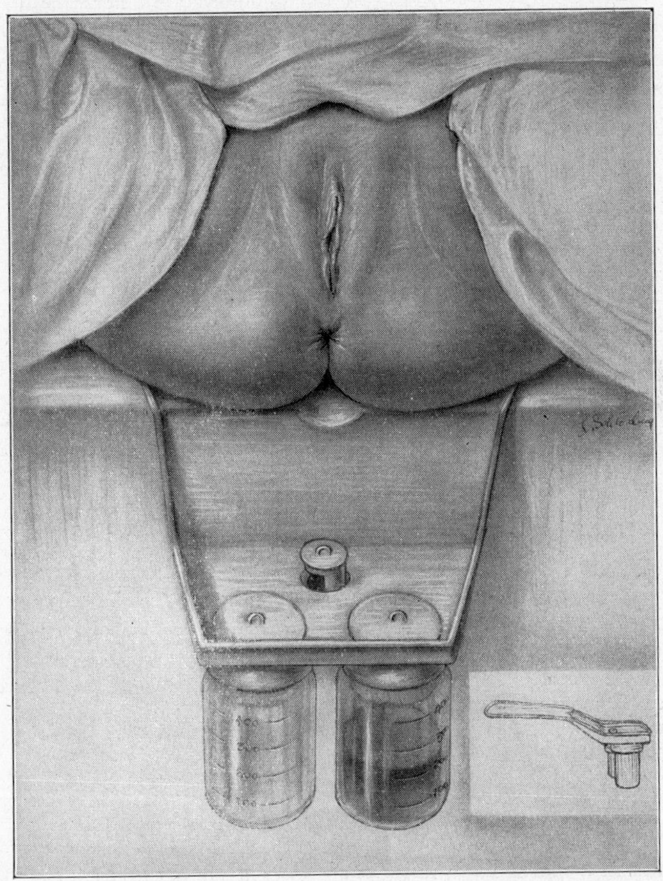

Fig. 291.—Carroll Plate for Measurement of Blood Loss at Delivery.

The small valve, shown open, permits amniotic fluid to be drained away separately from blood. With this closed, one of the larger valves is opened to collect blood in one of the attached glass jars. If desired, one jar may be used to measure episiotomy blood loss and the other, uterine hemorrhage. Ordinary pint fruit jars fit the threads of the plate. (Courtesy of Dr. B. H. Carroll.)

ERGONOVINE, PITUITARY EXTRACT AND PITOCIN

Ergot, which has been termed a "veritable treasure house of pharmacological constituents," is a fungus which grows upon rye and other grain. It has been the object of intensive chemical investigation for many years and as the result a large number of alkaloids of ergot have been isolated of which the most important from an obstetrical viewpoint is *ergonovine*. Since a number of investigators isolated this alkaloid almost simultaneously and each gave it a name, various synonyms exist. Of these the most important is ergometrine, the original name given to the alkaloid by Dudley and Moir of England, where it is so designated. Although the term "ergotrate" is a trade name for ergonovine, it was introduced very early in the history of this alkaloid and, in hospital parlance, is perhaps used more extensively than the name ergonovine which was given to the substance by the Council on Pharmacy and Chemistry of the American Medical Association in 1937.

Whether given by mouth, intramuscularly or intravenously, ergonovine is a powerful stimulant to myometrial contraction and exerts an effect, moreover, which may persist for several hours. One of its most valuable features from a clinical viewpoint is the rapidity with which it acts. The uterine response occurs almost immediately after intravenous injection of the drug and within a few minutes after intramuscular or oral administration. The sensitivity of the uterus to ergonovine is very great and in pregnant women an intravenous dose of as little as 0.1 mg. or an oral dose of only

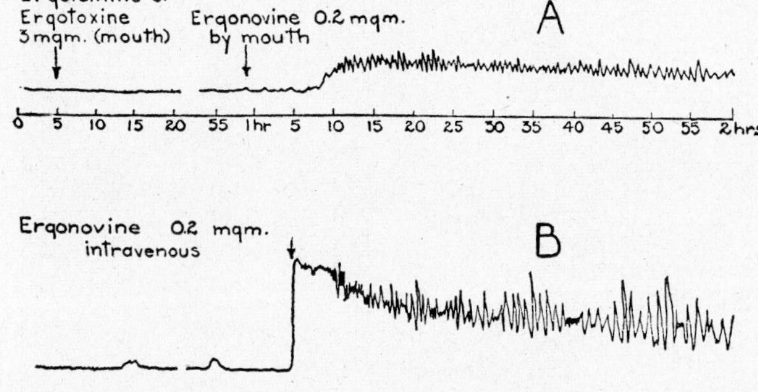

FIG. 292.—EFFECTS ON THE HUMAN UTERUS OF VARIOUS ALKALOIDS OF ERGOT.

A. Oral administration of 3 mg. of ergotamine or ergotoxin as compared with 0.2 mg. of ergonovine (B). This record is that of the uterine motility of a woman (para 4) seven days postpartum, obtained by means of a balloon and manometer.

B. Intravenous administration of 0.2 mg. of ergonovine. This record is that of a woman (para 2) seven days postpartum.

(After Davis, Adair and Pearl. From Goodman and Gilman, *The Pharmacological Basis of Therapeutics,* The Macmillan Co., New York.)

0.25 mg. results in a marked response. Moreover, as shown in Fig. 292, the response is sustained in character with no tendency toward relaxation. This tetanic effect makes it ideal for the prevention and control of postpartum hemorrhage.

Another agent frequently used in obstetrics is *extract of posterior pituitary* which, like ergonovine, causes a marked stimulation of the myometrium. The response of the uterus to a solution of posterior pituitary resembles that produced by ergonovine for the first 5 or 10 minutes, but then normal rhythmic contractions of amplified degree return, with intermittent periods of relaxation. This fundamental difference between the action of ergonovine and that of pituitary extract may be seen by comparing Figs. 292 and 293, and has most important clinical implications. Ergonovine administered before the delivery of the placenta may cause incarceration of that organ through tetanic uterine contraction, whereas pituitary extract given prior to placental expulsion produces a response which is characterized within a few minutes by periods of relaxation during which the placenta can escape from the uterus.

In 1928 Kamm and his associates separated two fractions from posterior pituitary extract. One possesses marked oxytocic activity and is usually referred to by the trade name "*pitocin.*" The other is strongly vasopressor and antidiuretic, and is usually referred to by the trade name *"pitressin."* Since one of the most common and serious complications of pregnancy and labor is a condition characterized by hypertension and water retention (toxemias of pregnancy, page 644-705), the vasopressor and anti-diuretic fraction of whole pituitary extract is undesirable for obstetric use and hence pitocin is preferable to the mother substance.

Ergonovine, pituitary extract and pitocin, are all employed widely in the conduct of the normal third stage of labor, but the timing of their administration differs greatly in various clinics. It should be noted in the first place that these agents are by no means necessary in most cases and that the third stage can usually be conducted with reasonably low blood loss without their aid. The most commonly employed program, perhaps, is the intramuscular administration of ergonovine, 0.2 mg., immediately after the delivery of the placenta. Having employed that program in past

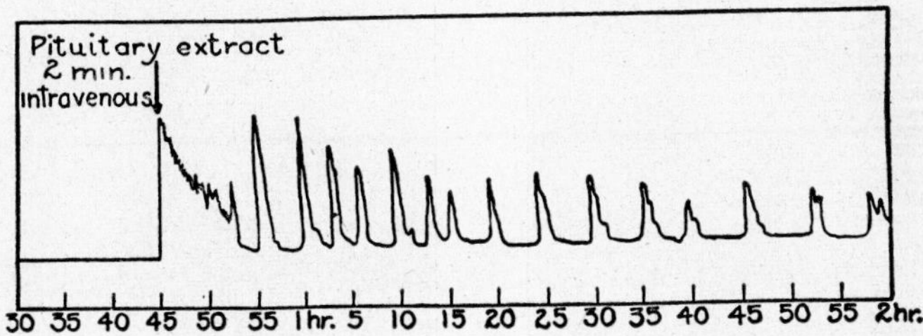

Fig. 293.—Effect on the Human Uterus of 0.15 cc. of Solution of Posterior Pituitary Given Intravenously to a Woman (para 3) on the Sixth Day Postpartum. (After Davis, Adair and Pearl. From Goodman and Gilman, *The Pharmacological Basis of Therapeutics,* The Macmillan Co., New York.)

Compare with Fig. 292.

years ourselves, it is our feeling that it can be improved upon in respect to control of blood loss by combining the ergonovine with the administration of pitocin intramuscularly immediately after the birth of the baby. To repeat and be more explicit, the drug technic which we consider ideal for the management of the third stage, both from the viewpoint of minimizing blood loss and general safety, is as follows: pitocin, 1 cc. or 10 units intramuscularly immediately after the birth of the baby, followed by ergonovine, 0.2 mg. intramuscularly immediately after the delivery of the placenta.

Still another ergonovine technic which is extensively employed by obstetrical specialists is the administration intravenously of ergonovine 0.2 mg. just as the anterior shoulder of the baby is being born. This violates the general rule that ergonovine should never be given before the delivery of the placenta for the reason stated above. However, when given at just this particular moment, the uterus, which is already retracting down rapidly on its diminishing contents, contracts very forcefully as the result of the oxytocic drug, and thereby produces immediate placental separation. If now, pressure is made on the fundus, the placenta can be expressed from the uterus before it has time to attain a tetanic state since its lower portion has been so recently dilated by the passage of the baby. When this method is meticulously carried out the third stage is greatly abbreviated and blood loss reduced to a very minimum. However, even in expert hands, the incidence of placental retention is higher than with other technics and it should be used only by experienced obstetricians.

LACERATIONS OF THE BIRTH CANAL

According to their extent, lacerations of the perineum are classified as of the first, second and third degree.

First degree lacerations are those which involve the fourchet, the perineal skin and vaginal mucous membrane without involving any of the muscles.

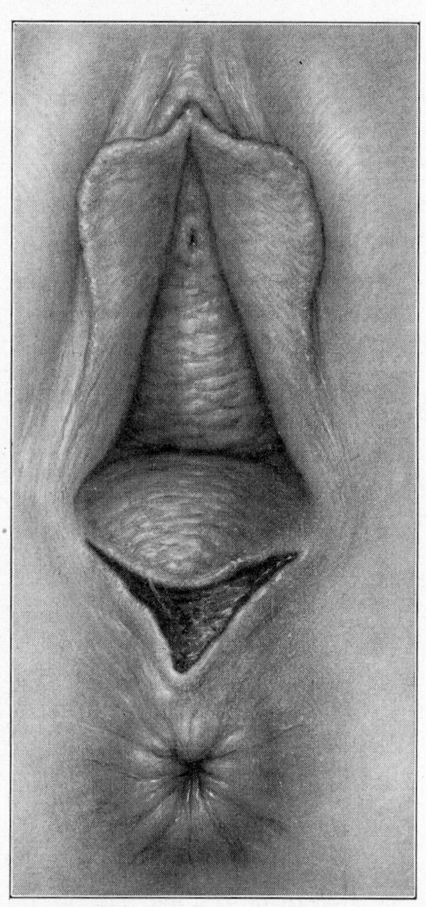

Fig. 294A.—First-Degree Perineal Tear.

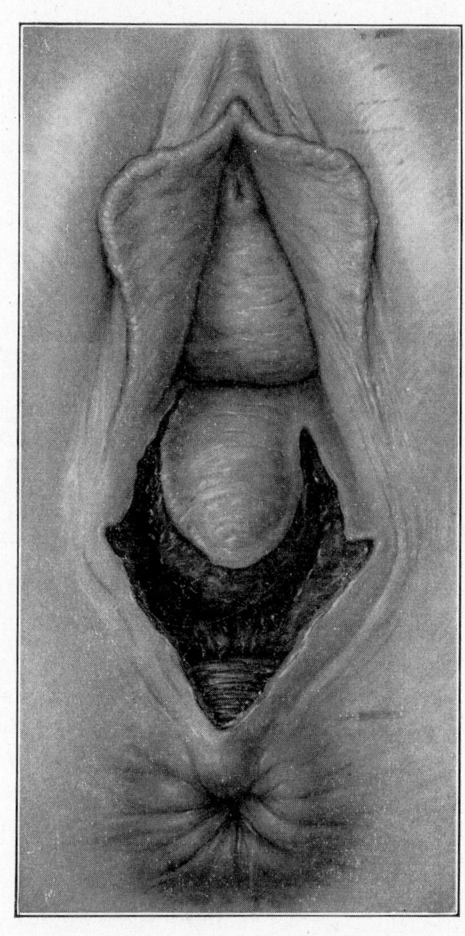

Fig. 294B.—Deep Second-Degree Perineal Tear.

Second degree lacerations are those which involve (in addition to skin and mucous membrane) the muscles of the perineal body but not the rectal sphincter. These tears usually extend upward on one or both sides of the vagina, making a triangular injury.

Third degree lacerations are those which extend completely through the skin, mucous membrane, perineal body *and* the rectal sphincter. This type is often referred to as a complete tear. Not infrequently, these third degree lacerations extend a certain distance up the anterior wall of the rectum.

In some clinics, including our own, a so-called "fourth degree laceration" is distinguished, this designation being applied to those third degree tears which extend a certain distance up the anterior wall of the rectum. For the sake of clarity the term "fourth degree laceration" will not be used in the ensuing discussion and when third degree lacerations with rectal wall extension are mentioned, they will be so designated.

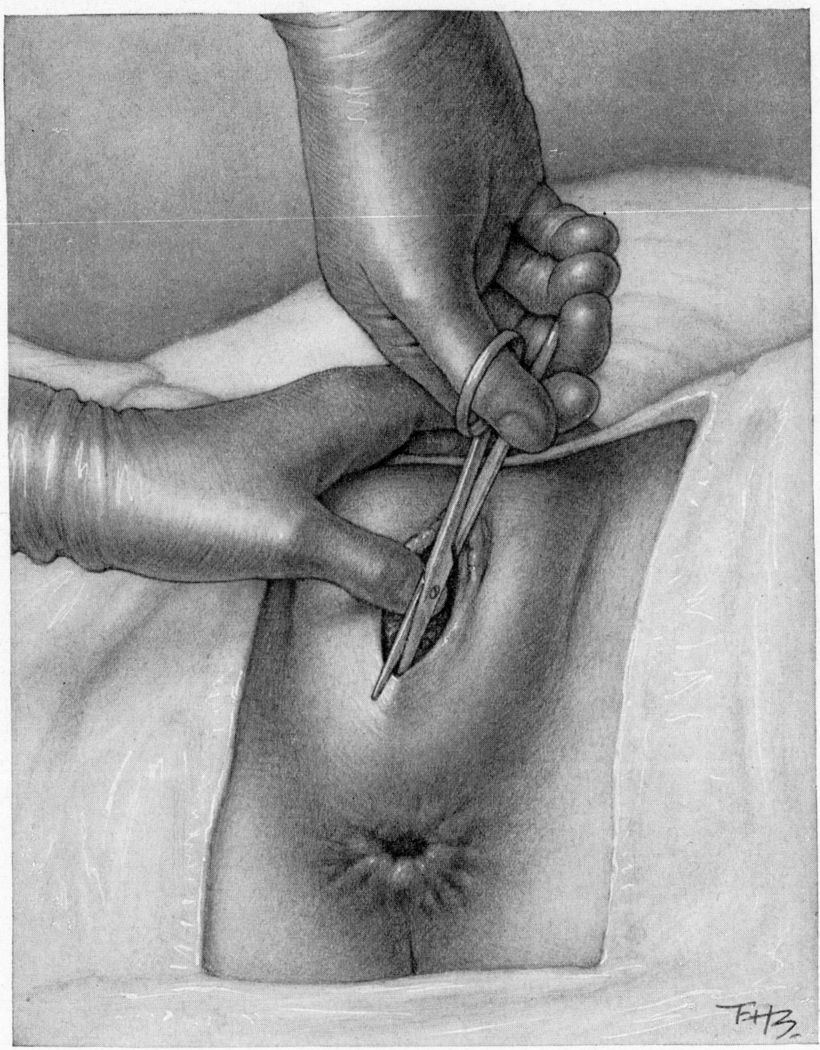

FIG. 295A.—SCISSORS PLACED FOR MEDIOLATERAL EPISIOTOMY.

The causes of perineal lacerations are rapid and sudden expulsion of the head (particularly when it "pops" out); excessive size of the infant; difficult forceps deliveries and breech extractions; outlet contraction of the pelvis, forcing the head posteriorly; exaggerated lithotomy position; and very friable maternal tissues. Some tears are unavoidable even in the most skilled hands. First and second degree lacerations are extremely common in primigravidae and it is for this reason, among others, that episiotomy is widely employed.

In addition to the types of perineal injury mentioned above, lacerations of the vagina at higher levels occasionally occur and may be responsible for extensive hemorrhage. Tears in the region of the urethra are especially prone to bleed profusely.

Since the repair of perineal tears is virtually the same as that of episiotomy incisions (albeit often more difficult because of irregular lines of tissue cleavage), the technic of suturing them will be discussed in the following section.

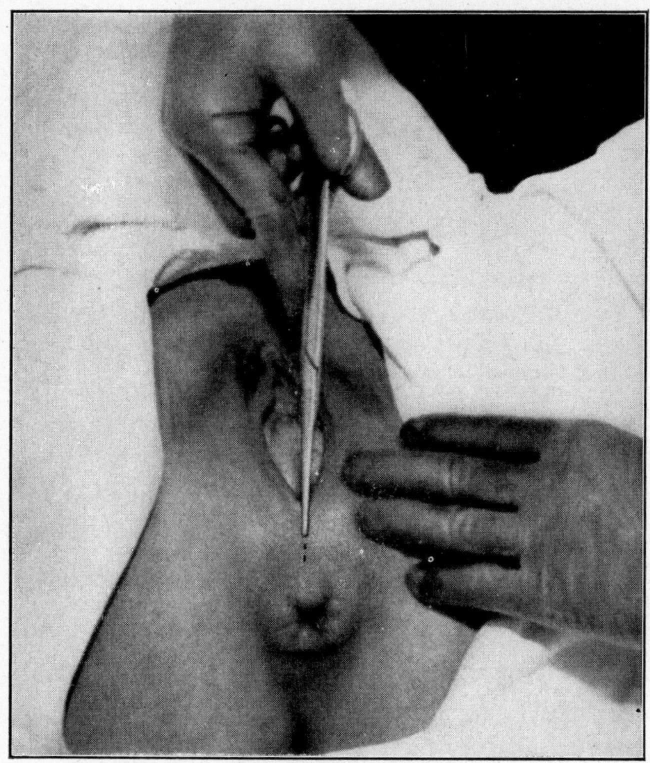

Fig. 295B.—Scissors Placed for Median Episiotomy.

EPISIOTOMY AND REPAIR

By episiotomy is meant incision of the perineum to facilitate delivery. The incision may be made in the midline, a *median episiotomy;* or it may be begun in the midline and directed laterally and downward away from the rectum, a *mediolateral episiotomy.*

Purposes of Episiotomy. Except for cutting and tying the umbilical cord, episiotomy is the most common operation in obstetrics. The reason for its popularity is not far to seek. In the first place, it substitutes a straight, clean-cut surgical incision for the ragged, contused laceration which is otherwise likely to ensue; such an incision is easier to repair and heals better than a tear. In the second place, it spares the baby's head the necessity of serving as a battering ram against perineal obstruction. If prolonged, this "pounding" of the infant's head against the perineum may cause brain injury. In the third place, the operation shortens the duration of the second stage of labor; and finally mediolateral episiotomy reduces the likelihood of third degree lacerations.

In regard to the carrying out of episiotomy, several important questions arise: (1) How soon before delivery should it be done? (2) Which type of operation is preferable, median or mediolateral? (3) When should the incision be repaired, before or after placental expulsion? (4) What suture material and technic are the best?

How Soon before Delivery Should Episiotomy Be Done? If episiotomy is done unnecessarily early, bleeding from the gaping wound may be substantial during the interim between the incision and the birth of the baby. As shown by Odell and Seski, blood loss from the episiotomy wound during this period is not inconsequential, far more indeed than occurs from this source during or following delivery. If episiotomy is done too late, the muscles of the perineal floor have already undergone undue stretching and one of the objectives of the operation is defeated. It is my practice, as a compromise, to perform episiotomy when the head is visible to a diameter of 2 to 3 cm., that is, slightly sooner than shown in Figs 295 A and B.

In this connection, the question arises as to whether episiotomy should be performed before or after the application of forceps. The usual practice is to perform the operation before the blades are applied. Having tried both plans, we lean somewhat to making the incision after the forceps are in place. Although it is slightly more awkward to perform episiotomy with the forceps in place, blood loss from the episiotomy wound is less with this technic since immediate traction on the forceps can be exerted and the resultant tamponade of the perineal floor by the baby's head is effected earlier than could otherwise be achieved.

Median versus Mediolateral Episiotomy. The advantages and disadvantages of the two types of episiotomy may be enumerated as follows:

MEDIAN EPISIOTOMY	MEDIOLATERAL EPISIOTOMY
1. Easy to repair	1. More difficult to repair
2. Faulty healing rare	2. Faulty healing not uncommon
3. Rarely painful in puerperium	3. Pain in one third of cases for a few days
4. Dyspareunia rarely follows	4. Dyspareunia occasionally follows
5. Anatomical end-results almost always excellent	5. Anatomical end-results more or less faulty in some 10 per cent of cases (depending on operator)
6. *Third degree extension in two to five per cent of cases (depending on operator)*	6. *Third degree extension in less than one per cent of cases*

With proper selection of cases it is possible to secure the advantages of median episiotomy and at the same time reduce to a minimum its one disadvantage, namely, the greater likelihood of third degree extension. Thus, the likelihood of extension of a median episiotomy into the rectal sphincter is much greater when the baby is large, when the occiput is posterior, in midforceps deliveries and, in our experience, in breech deliveries. In addition, the size of the perineal body is related to the likelihood of third degree laceration, the accident being more probable naturally if it is short. It is our practice, in general, to use mediolateral episiotomy under the circumstances mentioned, but to employ the median incision otherwise. Even with this selection of cases, however, it must be avowed that the overall number of third degree lacerations sustained under this regime will be greater than would have been encountered with routine mediolateral episiotomy. In our opinion, nevertheless, the advantages gained more than offset the single objection of third degree extension. This brings up the question: Just how serious an accident is a third degree laceration?

Back in the days when most babies were born in the home it is understandable that a third degree laceration was a major catastrophe. With poor lighting, inadequate

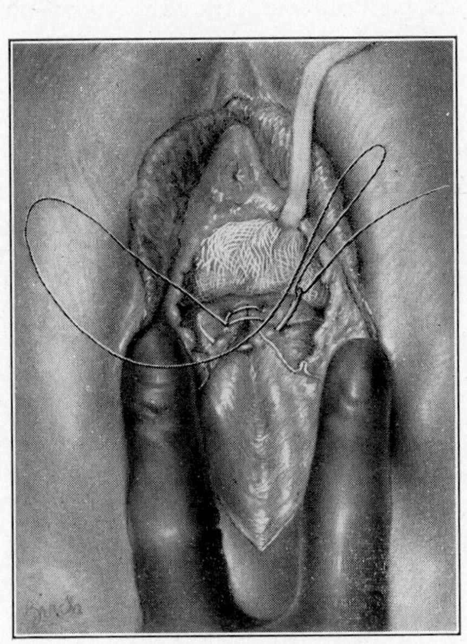

Fig. 296

Fig. 297

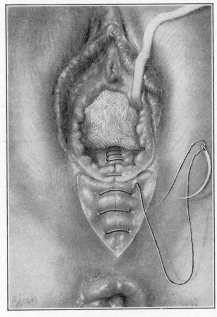

Fig. 296.—Repair of Median Episiotomy.

A half length of chromic catgut 00 or 000 is used as a continuous suture to close the vaginal mucosa.

Fig. 297.—Repair of Median Episiotomy.

Following closure of the vaginal mucosa and fourchet, the continuous suture is laid aside, and three or four interrupted sutures of 00 or 000 chromic catgut are placed in the fascia and underlying levator ani muscle.

exposure, a skimpy supply of instruments and no assistance, an inevitable sequel in most cases was incontinence of feces or a rectovaginal fistula; and it would require only three or four such tears to put the physician responsible for them pretty well out of business. It is no wonder that in those days a third degree laceration was a stigma and a disgrace. This stigma is still attached to the accident in the minds of most obstetricians. Under modern conditions of hospital delivery a third degree laceration, even though it extends up the rectum, is a much less serious accident than it was years ago. Thus, in a study of 710 third degree lacerations by Kaltreider and Dixon, all the patients having been managed under modern hospital conditions and in competent hands, repair of the laceration proved ultimately satisfactory in 99 per cent of the cases. The most serious complication, rectovaginal fistula, occurred in 16 patients or in 2.25 per cent. Of these, 10 healed spontaneously, 1 patient did not return and 5 underwent subsequent operations with ultimate cure of the fistula. To put it differently, a rectovaginal fistula needed repairing only once in 3,055 median episiotomies reported by these authors. Although it is still difficult for most of us to view a third degree laceration with equanimity, it is by no means a major catastrophe when properly repaired and, if all aspects of the question are considered,

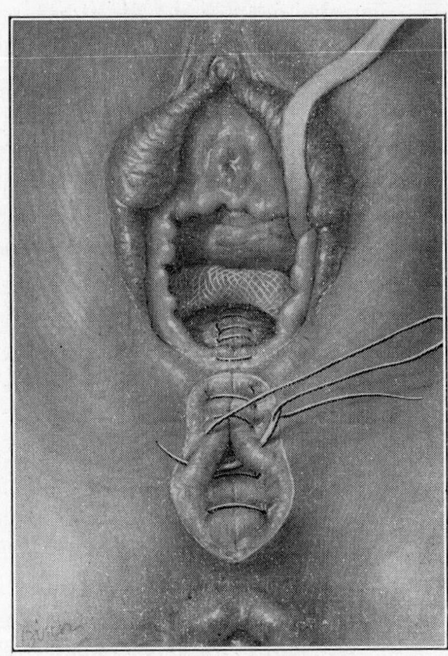

Fig. 298

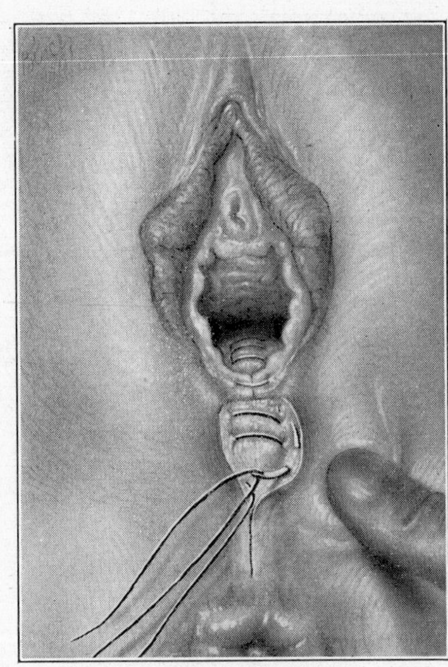

Fig. 299

Fig. 298.—Repair of Median Episiotomy.

The continuous suture is now picked up and carried downward to unite the subcutaneous fascia.

Fig. 299.—Repair of Median Episiotomy.

Finally, the continuous suture is carried upward as a subcuticular stitch. A large, straight cutting needle may be used to advantage instead of the curved needle shown.

median episiotomy despite its one drawback is a satisfactory procedure in 9 out of 10 deliveries. Let it be understood, however, that many authorities feel differently about this matter and employ mediolateral episiotomy routinely.

When Should Episiotomy Repair Be Done? The most general practice perhaps is to defer episiotomy repair until after the placenta has been delivered. This permits the obstetrician to give his undivided attention to the signs of placental separation and to expel the organ just as soon as it has separated. This early delivery of the placenta is believed to save blood loss since it militates against the possibility of a large retroplacental hematoma forming. Certainly, if ergonovine is administered with the anterior shoulder, it is obligatory to deliver the placenta at once. Moreover, Calkins, who has reported very low blood loss postpartum in his clinic, favors immediate delivery of the placenta in the belief that separation usually occurs within a minute or so after delivery of the infant. A further advantage of this program is that the episiotomy repair is not interrupted by the obvious necessity of delivering the placenta.

If, following delivery of the baby and a minute or two wait before clamping the cord, it is obvious that the placenta is separated and can be made visible in the vagina by gentle fundal pressure, it should be delivered immediately, of course. On the other hand, if it has not definitely separated during this minute or two, our practice has been to proceed with the repair, the fundus meanwhile being carefully watched by a competent attendant. In the course of the next few minutes, separation usually occurs and the placenta drops into the upper vagina where it is expressed when the repair has been completed. Occasionally, it becomes necessary to express the placenta in the midst of the repair but this is only a minor nuisance. We follow this course in the belief that it forestalls premature and injudicious efforts to hasten placental separation at this critical time. These efforts in our opinion constitute one of the most common causes of postpartum hemorrhage. This general policy has been followed in our last 25,000 cases with a reasonably low blood loss and without a single death from postpartum hemorrhage; hence we endorse it for general use. The fundus must be watched carefully by a competent person while the repair is being done.

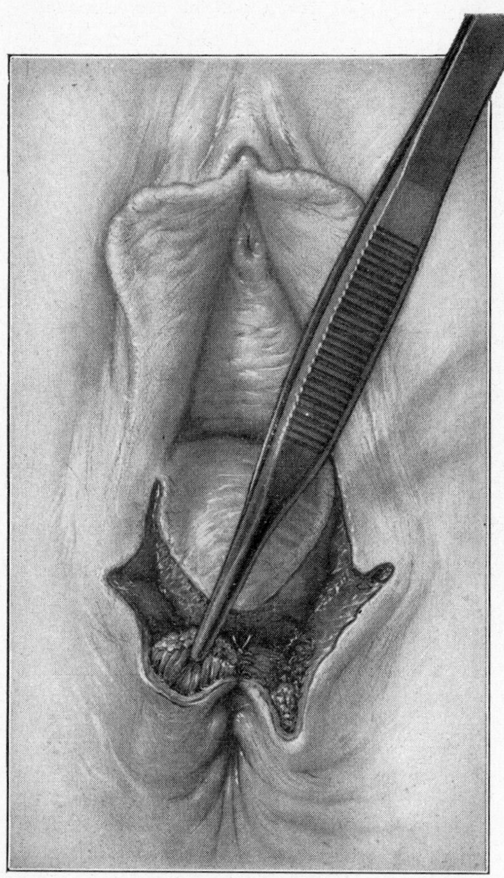

Fig. 300.—Third-Degree, or Complete, Perineal Tear.

The stump of the severed sphincter is identified.

Technic. The technic which we have employed for some years in episiotomy repair is shown in Figs. 296 to 299. This is but one of many methods which are equally satisfactory. The suture material ordinarily employed is catgut and it is important that it should be of the finest size which the operator can handle with facility. Either 00 or 000 chromic catgut is satisfactory, but some authorities even recommend 0000 catgut.

The technic of repairing a third degree laceration with extension into the wall of the rectum (Fig. 300) is shown in Fig. 301. Here again various technics have been recommended but all emphasize careful suturing of the rectal wall with sutures about one-half cm. apart, the covering of this layer of sutures with one of fascia and finally, careful isolation of the rectal sphincter with its suture by two or three ligatures. The remainder of the repair is the same as for ordinary episiotomy. Despite older ideas to the contrary, third degree lacerations require no especial attention in the puerperium except for the fact that enemas should be withheld. If enemas become absolutely necessary, the nozzle should be introduced most carefully by the obstetrician with its point directed posteriorly.

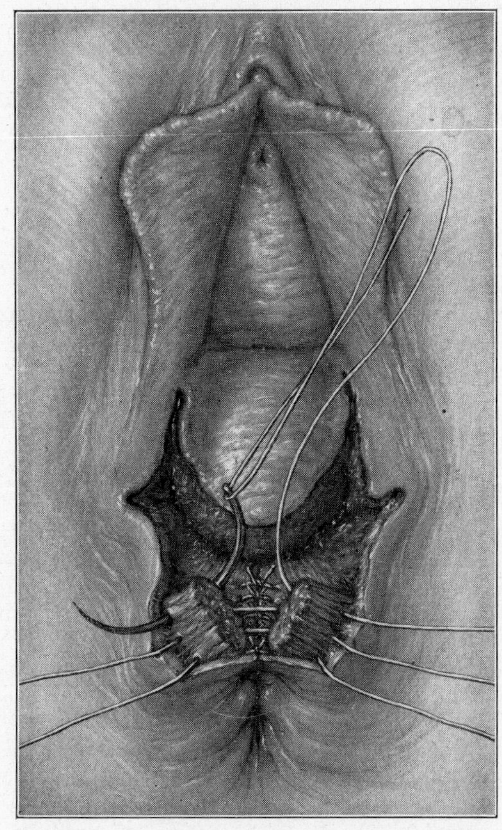

Fig. 301.—Repair of Complete Perineal Tear.
The rectal mucosa has been repaired with interrupted, fine chromic catgut sutures. The torn ends of the sphincter ani are then approximated with two or three interrupted chromic catgut sutures, after which the wound is repaired along the same lines as outlined in a second degree tear or an episiotomy.

HOME DELIVERY

As already indicated, once the physician has become well indoctrinated in the technic of aseptic delivery and has developed an "aseptic conscience," only a little ingenuity is necessary to apply the principles involved to home confinement. Circumstances in various communities and in different homes are so dissimilar, moreover, that the recommendation of any specific technic would carry little value. The following suggestions, including instructions to the nurse and lists of equipment necessary, are intended merely as reminders from which the physician can select items that are helpful and discard those which are not suitable to his own particular circumstances. If the patient is to be delivered at home, the room to be used for the confinement should be inspected in advance and suggestions made as to its arrangement. The obstetrician should also inquire as to the number of wash basins which are available; for with the increasing perfection of plumbing, the portable wash basin has become replaced by permanent washstands, so that in many modern homes it is difficult to find a sufficient number for disinfecting the hands and cleansing the patient.

For home delivery the patient is instructed to procure the following supplies which are needed for delivery:

1. A flat ironing board or table leaf or any board four feet long
2. Pail
3. Bedpan

4. Pitcher, one quart
5. Hand basins, two
6. Covered kettles, two (each holding about 6 qts.)
7. Soup ladle, one
8. Mason jar, one quart
9. Lysol, 4 oz.
10. Cotton, one lb.
11. Sanitary pads, two dozen
12. Bed pads (one large and eight small) (made of paper, covered with old linen)
13. Linen and clean blanket for bed
14. Towels (three Turkish and four cotton)
15. Gowns, two
16. Stockings (light color)
17. Washcloths, two
18. Electric bulb (100 wt.)
19. Some old newspapers

Below is given the card for the nurse containing directions for the preparation before and at the time of labor, as well as for the care of the mother and baby afterward:

DIRECTIONS FOR OBSTETRICAL NURSE

Preparations Before Labor

(a) If the patient is to be delivered at home, see that she has been instructed to provide herself with the following supplies: a bedpan, an enema bag, one pound absorbent cotton (Grade B), four dozen absorbent vulvar pads, two or three enamel basins, two kettles with covers, six newspaper pads (12 thicknesses) covered with unbleached muslin, rubber sheeting (1 x 2 yards) for protection of mattress (or newspapers may be used), Lysol (4 ounce bottle), albolene (1 pint).

(b) A week before the expected date of confinement prepare a sterile delivery pack to include one enamel basin, one cover (double unbleached muslin), three perineal pads, one binder, one cord dressing, two cord ties, five cotton balls, five gauze sponges (4 x 4 inches), two half sheets, two leggings, three towels, and one apron. The sterile bundle should be resterilized every ten days should it not be used within that period.

At Time of Labor

(a) If the patient is to be delivered in the hospital, take her there as soon as pains are definitely established, or the membranes rupture. If she is to be delivered at home notify the doctor and remain in constant attendance especially noting the character, duration and frequency of the pains.

(b) At the commencement of labor wash the hands and put on an apron, cap and mask. Prepare two large covered kettles of boiled water. Keep one hot and allow the other to cool.

(c) Make up the bed on the side best suited for delivery. Protect the entire mattress with rubber sheeting, oilcloth or newspapers. Protect the floor and other objects in the immediate vicinity with newspapers.

(d) When labor has definitely set in, give the patient a warm sponge bath and a soapsuds enema if it has been ordered by the doctor.

(e) To prepare the patient for delivery, shave the external genital and pubic regions. Then wash the genitalia thoroughly from above downwards (towards the anus), the abdomen to the umbilicus and the thighs to the knees with soap and warm water, taking care that the soapsuds and rinsings do not come in contact with the vaginal opening.

(f) Drape the patient with a clean sheet in order to minimize exposure, and when the birth of the child appears imminent, roll the patient's gown above the hips and put on the obstetrical leggings.

After Labor

(a) As soon as labor is over, cleanse the genitalia with cotton pledgets and sterile water, and then bathe with plain sterile water or Lysol solution (½ of 1 per cent), after which apply a sterile vulvar pad and place the patient upon a clean bed pad.

(b) Do not use an abdominal binder, unless especially ordered.

(c) Change vulvar pads as often as necessary, washing the genitalia each time with Lysol solution (½ of 1 per cent).

(d) Take temperature, pulse and respirations four times a day, unless otherwise directed, and record upon chart.

(e) On the day of delivery, secure the physician's orders regarding diet, medication, elimination, care of the mother's nipples, and the nursing schedule.

(f) Promptly report to the physician any abnormal condition of the mother and baby.

Care of Child

(a) Leave the baby alone until the mother is cared for, wrapping it in a receiving blanket and putting it in a safe place.

(b) The doctor will instill 1 per cent silver nitrate solution in the eyes.

(c) Cleanse the child thoroughly with albolene, but do not give it an initial bath. Afterwards, give a daily lap bath with castile soap and warm water, but do not give a full bath until the cord has come off.

(d) Dress the cord with a sterile gauze or alcohol dressing.

(e) Feeding: To conform to the physician's orders.

(f) Weigh the child twice a week and record the result.

Preparations on the Part of the Physician. When the physician has promised to attend an obstetrical patient he should hold himself in readiness to respond promptly at any hour and should instruct the patient as to the best method of communicating with him without delay. If he is obliged to leave town about that time, he should notify the patient and arrange for a competent substitute to take his place if necessary. He should also remember that the proper care of such cases requires a great deal of time, and frequently no small sacrifice of personal convenience, and if he is not willing to place himself at the disposal of his patients, as far as may be necessary, he should refuse to attend them. Undue haste is one of the most frequent causes of unsatisfactory results in this branch of medicine.

The physician in private practice should provide himself with an *obstetrical kit*, which should be neatly packed in an appropriate satchel and kept ready for immediate use. It should contain not only the instruments which he may need, but also the various drugs required for hand disinfection, anesthesia, and the usual emergencies, as well as a supply of sterile towels and dressings, in case the patient has failed to provide herself with such materials, and for emergency cases. A complete kit should contain the following:

Instruments	*Drapes and Accessories*	*Drugs*
Baumanometer	Ether mask	Green soap—50% solution
Flashlight	Rubber apron	Alcohol
Thermometer	Nail brush and stick	Acriflavine—1% solution
Syringes: 2 and 5 cc. size	Prep pads (3)	Esbachs solution
Needles:	Gowns (3 or more)	Lubricating jelly
one 1½″ 19 gauge	Leggings (2 pairs)	Ether
one 1½″ 22 gauge	Packing (6″ gauze) in tube	Aspirin, gr. v. tabs.
one ⅝″ 25 gauge	Towels (3 or more)	Aromatic spts. ammonia

Instruments	*Drapes and Accessories*	*Drugs*
Tracheal catheter	Gloves (3 pair or more)	Procaine 1% solution—50 cc. tube
Pelvimeter	Suture material chromic and plain	Morphine sulfate ¼ gr. tabs.
Razor and blades	Cord dressing	Codeine sulfate ½ gr. tabs.
Rubber catheter	Gauze wipes (4 pkgs. or more)	Ergonovine 1/325 gr. tabs.
Enema bag	Face masks	Pitocin 1 cc. amp.
Test tube	Applicators	Adrenalin 1 cc. amps.
Wassermann bottle	Brom-Thymol-Blue indicators	Caffeine Sodio-Benzoate, 7½ gr. amps.
Scale	Kelly pad	Atropine 1/100 gr. tabs.
Cord set: scissors, Kelly clamps (2), thumb forceps	Sterile cover for Kelly pad	Saline physiological sol. 5 cc. amps.
Perineal and cervical set: scissors, needle holder, artery clamps (4 or more), thumb forceps, long dressing forceps, tenaculum forceps, Sims reactor, assorted needles, medicine glass, sponge forceps (2)	Cotton (1 pkg.)	Lysol
	Tape measure	Silver nitrate 1% amp.
	Baby weighing blanket	Boric acid wipes or sterile water
	Glass slides	
	Vulva pads	

An ordinary Simpson forceps should be carried as well as one of the commercial units for the intravenous administration of glucose solution. This should be sterilized in advance and wrapped in a sterile towel so as to be ready for immediate use. Everything mentioned in the above list may be packed into a satchel measuring 20 x 10 inches at its base.

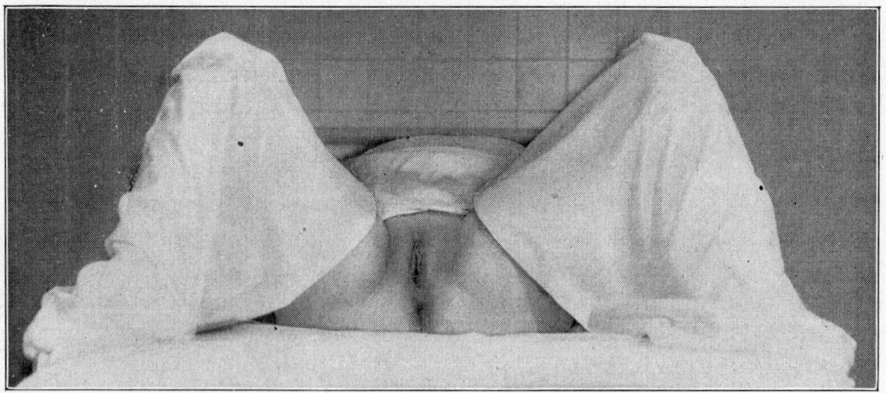

Fig. 302.—Patient Draped for Home Delivery.

Preparation of the Bed. If the patient is to be delivered at home, the bed should be prepared as soon as the pains become severe, since in the case of a multiparous woman the second stage of labor may be so short as to leave no time for such preparations. A high single iron bedstead is preferable, but one frequently has to be content with the ordinary double bed. In such circumstances one side of it should be prepared for the patient; whether the right or left depends upon which hand the physician expects to use for vaginal examination and the conduct of labor. A large piece of rubber sheeting, 1 x 2 yards, should be placed over the center of the mattress, covering its entire width, and over this a sheet is spread. A second piece of rubber sheeting, 1 x 1½ yards, is placed upon the side of the bed upon which the patient is to lie, in such a position that it will come directly under her buttocks. The entire bed is then covered by a draw-sheet; over this is placed a sterile bed pad, upon which the buttocks rest. With this arrangement, the upper sheet and the smaller piece of rubber cloth can be removed at the completion of labor, leaving the mattress protected

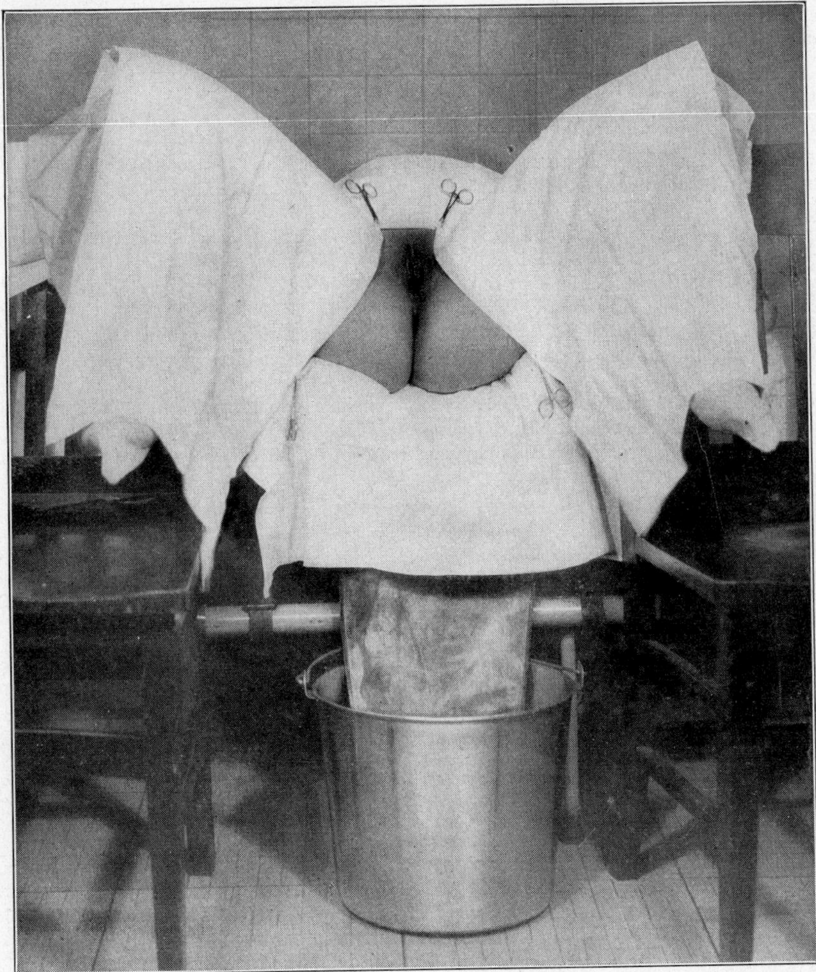

Fig. 303.—Alternate Position for Home Delivery.

by the large piece of rubber sheeting and the under sheet. An ironing board placed between the springs and the mattress aids greatly in preventing the patient's hips from sinking down into the bed.

The patient may be positioned either as shown in Fig. 302 or 303. The former position is recommended for vertex deliveries since it is less conducive to tears. The best analgesic agent for home delivery is probably rectal ether, supplemented by local infiltration anesthesia if outlet forceps have to be used.

BIBLIOGRAPHY

Abe, T. The Detection of the Rupture of Fetal Membranes with the Nitrazine Indicator. Am. J. Obst. & Gynec., 1940, 39:400.

Ballentine, G. N. Delayed Ligation of the Umbilical Cord. Pennsylvania M. J., 1947, 50:726.
Baptisti, A., Jr. Chemical Test for the Determination of Ruptured Membranes. Am. J. Obst. & Gynec., 1938, 35:688.
Bourgeois, G. A. The Identification of Fetal Squamas and the Diagnosis of Ruptured Membranes by Vaginal Smear. Am. J. Obst. & Gynec., 1942, 44:80.
Brandt, M. L. Mechanism and Management of the Third Stage of Labor. Am. J. Obst. & Gynec., 1933, 25:662.
Calkins, L. A. Management of the Third Stage of Labor. J.A.M.A., 1933, 101:1128.
Carroll, B. H., Meier, H. H., and Stone, O. H. Immediate Postpartum Hemorrhage due to Retained Secundines. Am. J. Obst. & Gynec., 1948, 55:620.
Davis, M. E., Adair, F. L., Rogers, G., Kharasch, M. S., and Legault, R. R. A New Active Principle in Ergot and Its Effects on Uterine Motility. Am. J. Obst. & Gynec., 1935, 29:155.
Davis, M. E., Adair, F. L., and Pearl, S. The Present Status of Oxytocics in Obstetrics. J.A.M.A., 1936, 107:261.
DeMarsh, Q. B., Alt, H. L., Windle, W. F., and Hillis, D. S. The Effect of Depriving the Infant of Its Placental Blood, on the Blood Picture during the First Week of Life. J.A.M.A., 1941, 116:2568.
DeMarsh, Q. B., Windle, W. F., and Alt, H. L. Blood Volume of Newborn Infant in Relation to Early and Late Clamping of Umbilical Cord. Am. J. Dis. Child., 1942, 63:1123.
Douglas, R. G., and Rhees, H. S. Experimental Evaluation of the Use of Some Vaginal Antiseptics during Labor. New York State J. Med., 1934, 34:996.
Grimes, W. H., Bartholomew, R. A., Colvin, E. D., and Fish, J. S. A Comparison of Intravenous Oxytocin and Ergonovine in the Control of Hemorrhage Attending Delivery. South. M. J., 1948, 41:980.
Haselhorst, G., and Allmeling, A. Die Gewichtszunahme von Neugeborenen infolge postnataler Transfusion. Ztschr. f. Geburtsh. u. Gynäk., 1930, 98:103.
Hofbauer, J. Die Verwertung der Hypophysenextrekte in der praktischen Geburtschilfe. München. med. Wchnschr., 1912, 59:1210.
Johnston, R. A., and Siddall, R. S. Is the Usual Method of Preparing Patients for Delivery Beneficial or Necessary? Am. J. Obst. & Gynec., 1922, 4:645.
Kaltreider, D. F., and Dixon, D. McC. A Study of 710 Complete Lacerations Following Central Episiotomy. South. M. J., 1948, 41:814.
Leff, M. The Comparative Action of Posterior Pituitary and Ergonovine in the Third and Fourth Stages of Labor; Observations Based on 5000 Deliveries. Am. J. Obst. & Gynec., 1945, 49:734.
Meleney, F. L., Zau, Zung-Dau, Zaytzeff, H., and Harvey, H. D. Epidemologic and Bacteriologic Investigation of the Sloane Hospital Epidemic of Hemolytic Streptococcus Puerperal Fever in 1927. Am. J. Obst. & Gynec., 1928, 16:180.
Moir, C. Clinical Comparison of Ergotoxine and Ergotamine. Brit. M. J., 1932, 1:1022.
——— and Dale, H. The Action of Ergot Preparations on the Puerperal Uterus. Brit. M. J., 1932, 1:1119.
Numers, C. Eine neue Methode, den Blasensprung zu diagnostizieren. Acta Obst. et Gynec. Scandinav., 1936, 16:249.
Odell, L. D., and Seski, A. Episiotomy Blood Loss. Am. J. Obst. & Gynec., 1947, 54:51.
Pastore, J. B. A New Method for Measuring the Blood Loss During the Third Stage of Labor. Am. J. Obst. & Gynec., 1935, 29:866.
——— A Study of the Blood Loss during the Third Stage of Labor and the Factors Involved. Am. J. Obst. & Gynec., 1936, 31:78.
——— The Use of Pituitrin Intravenously in the Third Stage of Labor. Am. J. Obst. & Gynec., 1936, 32:280.
——— A Satisfactory Cord Clamp. Am. J. Obst. & Gynec., 1940, 39:890.
——— and Stander, H. J. Hemorrhage in Obstetrical Patients. Texas State J. Med., 1939, 35:390.
Plass, E. D. Postpartum Care of the Perineum. Bull. Johns Hopkins Hosp., 1916, 27:107.
Read, G. D. Correlation of Physical and Emotional Phenomena of Natural Labor. J. Obst. & Gynaec. Brit. Emp., 1946, 53:55.
Smith, J. Causation and Source of Infection in Puerperal Infection. Department of Health for Scotland. Reports of the Scientific Advisory Committee on Medical Administration and Investigation. Published by His Majesty's Stationery Office, Edinburgh, 1931.
Thompson, M. R. The Pharmacology of Ergot. J. Am. Pharm. A., 1930, 19:705.
Thoms, H. Natural Childbirth. Connecticut M. J., 1949, 13:47.

17

ANALGESIA AND ANESTHESIA

The relief of pain in labor presents especial problems. These may best be appreciated by reviewing the several important respects in which it differs from surgical anesthesia.

1. In surgical procedures there is but one patient to consider, whereas in parturition there are two, the mother and the baby. The respiratory center of the latter is especially vulnerable to sedative and anesthetic drugs, and since these agents, if given systemically, regularly traverse the placenta, the possibility of their jeopardizing the initiation of respiration at birth is apparent. This is not a mere theoretical consideration, since some sluggishness of respiration is observed in the majority of infants whose mothers have received morphine or its derivatives, barbiturates, ether, or other such drugs in labor. Moreover, degrees of maternal anoxemia so slight as to be innocuous to the maternal organism are sometimes lethal to the fetus, whose blood, even under optimal conditions, has a low oxygen tension (Fig. 137). Fatal anoxia of the fetus may also result from rather minor degrees of maternal hypotension if at all prolonged. This especial sensitivity of the fetus to the effects, or occasional side effects, of almost all forms of maternal anesthesia poses one of the most difficult problems in obstetrics and one which, of course, does not exist in surgical anesthesia.

2. In major surgery, quite apart from humane considerations, anesthesia is essential to the safe and satisfactory execution of the technical procedures involved. In normal labor, on the other hand, anesthesia is not absolutely necessary because the baby will usually be born satisfactorily without any kind of medication, albeit the mother may suffer severe pain. Hence, to a peculiar degree, an anesthetic death in obstetrics is usually an unnecessary death. When any form of pain relief is administered in labor, therefore, *safety is the sine qua non.*

3. Surgical anesthesia is administered for the duration of the operation which lasts in most cases for no more than an hour or two. Pain relief in labor, to be efficient, must cover not only the procedure of delivery (called "obstetric anesthesia") but also a period prior to the actual delivery which may range from one to 12 or even 24 hours (called "obstetric analgesia").

4. Both in obstetric analgesia and obstetric anesthesia, it is important that the drugs used exert little effect on uterine contractions. If they do, labor may come to a standstill and progress stop. If uterine retraction is suppressed, postpartum hemorrhage will occur. These problems do not exist in surgical anesthesia.

5. In the majority of surgical operations there is ample time to prepare the patient for anesthesia, especially by the withholding of food and fluids for 12 hours or so. The great majority of labors begin without definite warning and, as a consequence, many obstetric anesthesias have to be administered within a few hours after a full

meal. Vomiting with aspiration of gastric contents is hence a frequent threat in obstetric anesthesia.

Because of the difficulties presented by the several circumstances enumerated, no completely safe and satisfactory method of pain relief in obstetrics has been developed. As a consequence, it is sometimes alleged that the hazards of pain relief in labor offset its advantages. This is untrue. Quite apart from humane objectives, a vast experience has shown that obstetric analgesia and anesthesia, when judiciously employed, may be beneficial rather than detrimental to both baby and mother, at least in the overall picture. The reason is this: pain relief forestalls the insistent importunities of the parturient and her family for premature operative interference; prior to the present era, premature and injudicious operative delivery, thus provoked, constituted the commonest cause of traumatic injury to both mother and infant. In the case of the mother, such injuries were occasionally fatal; in the case of the baby they were frequently so. The relief of pain itself, while commendable, would not justify the employment of methods which themselves are not without danger, were it not for the fact that they permit more meticulous, more gentle, and frequently easier deliveries, resulting in healthier mothers and more living babies.

General Principles. At the risk of belaboring a point already stressed (page 383), let it be remembered that the proper psychological management of the patient throughout prenatal care and labor is an indispensable basic sedative. A woman who is carefree, unafraid, and possessed of complete confidence in her obstetrician and nurses, usually enjoys a relatively comfortable first stage or requires a minimum of medication. This wholesome attitude toward parturition must be assiduously fostered at all times as an essential phase of pain relief.

The optimal time for starting medicinal analgesia demands astute judgment which can only be garnered from experience. A grave and common error is to initiate it too soon. On retrospect, many of our worst cases of prolonged labor may be charged to the premature use of sedative drugs or the premature employment of continuous caudal anesthesia. One rule should be absolute: such medication should never be started until positive proof exists that the cervix is showing progressive effacement and dilatation. In general, primigravidae should not be given analgesic medication until the pains are strong and the cervix is 3 cm. dilated, while in multiparae, it is prudent to do without it until the cervix is 4 cm. dilated. If an error is to be made, it will be a less costly mistake if the medication is started too late rather than too early. When pain relief is started appreciably later than the optimal time, the efficacy of the medication is diminished as a rule. This is especially true in rapid multiparous labors.

Patients under any form of analgesia require constant and meticulous attention. If left alone, a patient under barbiturate and scopolamine analgesia may throw herself out of bed or against a wall, or may vomit and aspirate the gastric contents. Numerous injuries and a few deaths are on record as a result of such negligence. Similarly, conduction anesthesia demands assiduous attention to the blood pressure and anesthetic levels if safety is to be achieved.

For an obstetrician to master many of the various technics which have been recommended for pain relief in labor is quite impossible and undesirable. Indeed, the more he can concentrate on one program, the better. Nevertheless, he will find it prudent to have at his disposal the following: (1) a method of systemic analgesia, such as a barbiturate and scopolamine, or rectal ether; (2) a method of systemic anesthesia such as gas-oxygen-ether, or pentothal sodium; and (3) a method of regional anesthesia such as saddle block, local infiltration, or continuous caudal.

PROGRAMS DESIGNED TO PROMOTE AMNESIA

The method of so-called analgesia most widely employed in this country is a combination of drugs designed to produce narcotic amnesia of everything which transpired in labor. The mainstay in such regimes is scopolamine. Almost always, however, this drug is used in combination with a sedative agent such as one of the barbiturates, rectal ether, paraldehyde, morphine, or Demerol, the last mentioned being a synthetic morphine substitute. Scopolamine does not raise the pain threshold nor does it enhance the analgesic action of other drugs such as morphine. The purpose of its use in labor is solely to produce amnesia. It is true that in patients without pain, scopolamine is primarily a depressant and that therapeutic doses usually promote drowsiness, fatigue and sleep. However, its action is variable and, especially in the presence of pain, it frequently produces excitement, restlessness, hallucinations, and delirium. Herein lies the rationale in obstetric analgesia of combining scopolamine with one of the sedative drugs, the purpose of the latter being largely to forestall, as much as possible, the restlessness which scopolamine often causes in the presence of labor pains. Conversely, scopolamine tends to counteract the respiratory depression which may follow the administration of a barbiturate or morphine.

Under any of the amnesic programs, when successful, the patient usually sleeps quietly between pains but may exhibit varying degrees of restlessness during contractions; not infrequently she may shriek, make grimaces, and show other evidence of pain, but upon awakening from the narcosis, will remember little or nothing about her labor and will vow that she experienced no discomfort whatsoever. However, the several disadvantages of these amnesic regimes must always be borne in mind when applying them to individual cases. (1) Narcosis of the infant with inhibition of respiration is common but is rarely serious provided the baby is at term. In premature infants, however, the deleterious respiratory effects may be a determining factor in the outcome and these drugs should not be employed in premature labor. (2) Uterine contractions, unless strong, are likely to be inhibited and care must be exercised, as already emphasized, not to initiate the program too early. (3) Restlessness is common and the patient must never be left alone for a second; restlessness is best forestalled, or minimized, by giving the sedative drug 20 to 30 minutes before the scopolamine is administered.

Scopolamine and Morphine, or "Twilight Sleep." This method of combating the pain of labor was introduced in 1902 by Steinbückel who reported that the hypodermic injection of scopolamine and morphine practically annulled the pains of labor. In 1907, Gauss reported its administration in 1,000 cases in Freiburg, and stated that by a proper regulation of dosage 80 per cent of the patients would pass into a semiconscious state, which he designated as "twilight sleep." In this condition, he pointed out, the patient appears to appreciate pain at the time, but has no recollection of it later. For this purpose he administered 0.3 mg. (1/200 grain) of scopolamine and 0.01 gm. (1/6 grain) of morphine hypodermically and repeated the scopolamine, but not the morphine, once or several times later if necessary. In this, as in other forms of amnesia, the indication for repetition of scopolamine is not afforded by the lapse of any specified length of time, but rather by the mental condition of the patient who should be kept in a state in which her speech is slurring and somewhat incoherent. It is this impairment of cerebration which must be taken as an index of the action of the drug, rather than the complaints of the patient; many of them complain bitterly with every pain yet afterwards have no recollection whatsoever of what occurred. Twilight sleep is of great historical importance because it was the forerunner of all modern amnesic regimes. It received wide acclaim in this country during the second decade of this century, but has been supplanted in large measure by the substitution of one or another of the barbiturates or Demerol for the morphine. Nevertheless, Krebs, Wulff, and Wassermann, as well as Bill, have reported favorable results in a large series of cases with scopolamine-morphine amnesia.

Scopolamine and Barbiturates. Fully 60 per cent of labors in which pain relief is used are conducted under some form of barbiturate or Demerol medication in association with scopolamine. Barbiturates with short or moderate duration of action are preferred, notably sodium amytal, sodium pentobarbital, and sodium seconal. These are hypnotics and produce relaxation from tension and absence of fear, but are not in themselves markedly analgesic. Thus, Wolff, Hardy, and Goodell have shown that 0.5 gm. of Evipal orally, an amount barely compatible with the waking state, raised the pain threshold only 21 per cent. It is quite probable that most of the barbiturates act in a similar manner. When combined with scopolamine, however, narcosis and amnesia result.

As soon as the patient has been examined and it is determined that she is in good labor with none of the contraindications mentioned above present, some thought can be given to the feasibility of this type of pain relief. If the patient complains of her pains and the cervix is effaced and 3 to 4 cm. dilated, 0.3 gm. (5 grains) of one of the above mentioned barbiturates is given by mouth. Twenty minutes later 0.3 or 0.4 mg. (1/200 to 1/150 grain) of scopolamine is given hypodermically. The patient is placed in a dimly lighted and quiet room. These drugs take effect rapidly, and within 20 to 30 minutes the patient should be asleep between pains. She will occasionally move around restlessly and sometimes cry out with contractions. Excitement will occur in about 10 per cent of cases. The attendant should keep the patient in bed, protect her from self-injury, but should not restrain her forcefully as this tends to increase the excitement stage. One hour after the initial dosage of the scopolamine it may be repeated to advantage in dosages of 0.1 or 0.2 mg. (1/600 to 1/300 grain), depending on the condition of the patient, as discussed under scopolamine-morphine amnesia. The injection of scopolamine can be repeated hourly in a dose of 0.1 mg. (1/600 grain) if necessary, but the maximum total dosage should not exceed 1.0 mg. (1/60 grain). The dosage of barbiturate may be repeated every four hours in 0.1 gm. amounts. This type of analgesia is usually not sufficient for delivery and some superimposed anesthesia must be employed.

Occasionally barbiturates are given intravenously. Lewis has had excellent results using rather large doses of intravenous sodium vinbarbital alone. It has been our experience, utilizing intravenous sodium pentobarbital and scopolamine, that the effect is more rapid and controllable and that the dose of the barbiturate is reduced by one-half as compared with oral methods. This technic is particularly effective in rapid multiparous labor. Usually 0.150 to 0.2 gm. (2½ to 3 grains) of the barbiturate is given slowly in the arm vein, the scopolamine being administered in the usual dosage hypodermically. Analgesia begins immediately and does not differ in any particular from that induced by oral methods. We have had no untoward results.

From our studies, those of Irving, Berman and Nelson, and those of Tollefson and many others, one can anticipate with the above regime good amnesia in from 70 to 85 per cent of patients. The respiratory activity of the baby at birth will depend in part on whether a general anesthetic has been superimposed for delivery. If it has, 60 to 70 per cent of the babies will breathe spontaneously; 15 to 20 per cent will show transient apnea and require the administration of oxygen, while from 5 to 10 per cent will show apnea for two minutes or more and require resuscitative efforts. However, statistical studies on very large series of cases indicate that the end results for these infants are satisfactory, provided judgment has been used in the dosages of the drugs administered. When the infant is delivered under saddle block anesthesia, low spinal, or local infiltration, its respiratory activity is decidedly better and apnea less frequent than when it has been narcotized by the combined action of a systemic analgesic program and a systemic anesthesia.

Scopolamine and Demerol. Demerol hydrochloride is a synthetic compound which resembles morphine in its analgesic properties and atropine in its antispasmodic effects. Hence, in labor it not only relieves pain but is believed to exert a relaxing effect on the cervix and so expedite dilatation. It is usually administered intramuscularly in dosages of 100 mg., and may be repeated once after four hours. A moderate sedative effect is produced, the patient usually sleeping between pains but awakening when addressed. Demerol, used alone, does not cause excitement or disorientation but rather a mental state of well-being or actual euphoria. Batterman and Himmelsbach point out that its effect on the pain threshold lies between that of morphine and codeine. A dose of 100 mg. of Demerol intramuscularly has been compared in its analgesic effect with that of 10 mg. of morphine, but the action of Demerol is of shorter duration since the drug is rapidly inactivated by the liver.

Demerol is usually employed in conjunction with 0.4 mg. (1/150 grain) of scopolamine and in that event the resultant effect is similar to that produced by the barbiturates and scopolamine. Schumann has administered 100 mg. of Demerol intramuscularly or intravenously, with scopolamine, in repeated doses throughout labor in 1,000 cases; satisfactory amnesia was obtained in 70 to 90 per cent of cases. It is his opinion that, while Demerol possesses other properties which make it more desirable for purposes of obstetric analgesia than the barbiturates, it falls slightly short of the barbiturates in producing satisfactory amnesia. In Schumann's opinion, Demerol exerts no depressant effect on either full-term or premature infants, whether administered by the intramuscular or intravenous route. Our experience with Demerol has not led to such a completely favorable conclusion about its effect on the infant, for it would be our reaction that the incidence of fetal apnea with Demerol is about the same as with the barbiturates.

Demerol may be used intravenously but certain precautions must be exercised. It must be given very slowly, taking at least two minutes by the clock to administer 50 mg. (the maximum single dose, in my opinion, which should be given by this route). If the Demerol-scopolamine mixture is given rapidly, the patient invariably vomits immediately, and over a transient 30 to 40 seconds the pulse becomes rapid, irregular and thready, with a gradual return to normal (Schumann). If the drug is given slowly about one quarter of the patients will experience transient nausea and may vomit. Whether administered intramuscularly or intravenously, the incidence of excitement (which is due primarily to the scopolamine) is about the same as with barbiturate-scopolamine combinations.

Paraldehyde. Paraldehyde, the action of which is fundamentally similar to alcohol, is a powerful hypnotic and has been used extensively for obstetric analgesia both alone and in combination with scopolamine, barbiturates and morphine. Although its main effect is to cause lethargy and sleep, dosages large enough to yield blood levels of 20 mg. per cent or more (30 cc. by mouth) produce also amnesia and a substantial raising of the pain threshold. The amnesic effects of paraldehyde appear to be greatly enhanced when it is employed in combination with morphine or one of the barbiturates. Thus, Kane and Roth obtained complete amnesia in 90 per cent of 611 cases after rectal administration of 12 cc. per 100 pounds body weight, followed 30 minutes later by morphine sulfate 16 mg. (¼ grain); the full initial dose of paraldehyde was repeated after one and one half hours. In the opinion of Colvin and Bartholomew, complete amnesia as to pain can be obtained in 98 per cent of cases by proper technic. As preliminary administration, they employed 0.2 gm. (3 grains) sodium pentobarbital or 0.4 gm. (6 grains) of sodium amytal, followed in 1 or 2 hours by 24 cc. of paraldehyde by mouth, taken a teaspoonful at a time in ice water.

The disadvantages of paraldehyde in obstetric analgesia are several. (1) It inhibits uterine contractions, and for this reason Colvin and Bartholomew stress especially the fact that it should not be administered until labor is well established and the cervix is thin and 4 to 5 cm. dilated. (2) It is sometimes vomited when given by mouth and expelled when administered per rectum. (3) It passes readily through the placenta, and fetal apnea is not uncommon. (4) Restlessness is occasionally observed and may be extreme. (5) Although paraldehyde possesses in general a wide margin of safety, some bizarre maternal deaths have occurred following minimal doses (Shorr; Kotz, Roth and Ryon). (6) It has a disagreeable, pungent taste and an unpleasant fusel-oil odor which may be noted on the mothers' and infants' breaths for as long as 24 hours. For these reasons paraldehyde has been superseded to a great extent by other types of analgesia but is still used with satisfaction in many clinics.

GAS ANESTHETICS

The narcotic gases—nitrous oxide, ethylene, and cyclopropane—are widely used in current obstetrical practice. They are of low toxicity and provide rapid relief of pain. Although these agents are, as a rule, safe in the hands of skilled anesthetists, they may, in the hands of the inexperienced, become suddenly dangerous to both mother and child.

Nitrous oxide is the only one of the three which should be used to provide intermittent pain relief during labor. Ethylene and cyclopropane are too explosive to permit frequent removal of the mask and, therefore, should be used only for delivery.

Nitrous Oxide. The concentration of nitrous oxide for the purpose of analgesia should never exceed 80 per cent. Eastman and others have shown that if the oxygen concentration is less than 15 to 20 per cent anoxemia of the fetus results. Furthermore, prolonged use of this gas in higher concentrations may result in fatal maternal accidents, as shown by Courville, Lowenberg, and others. Although nitrous oxide and oxygen are usually given through a closed machine where the degrees of concentration of the gas can be read directly from a gauge, even the most costly machine does not provide sufficient accuracy to guarantee the proper concentration of oxygen. While some authorities state that gas anesthesia may be continued safely for many hours during the first stage of labor, it is wiser to limit its use to the second stage. It has little effect on the uterine activity and may therefore be commenced as soon as the cervix becomes fully dilated. The method should be restricted to hospital use where trained assistants and adequate apparatus are available.

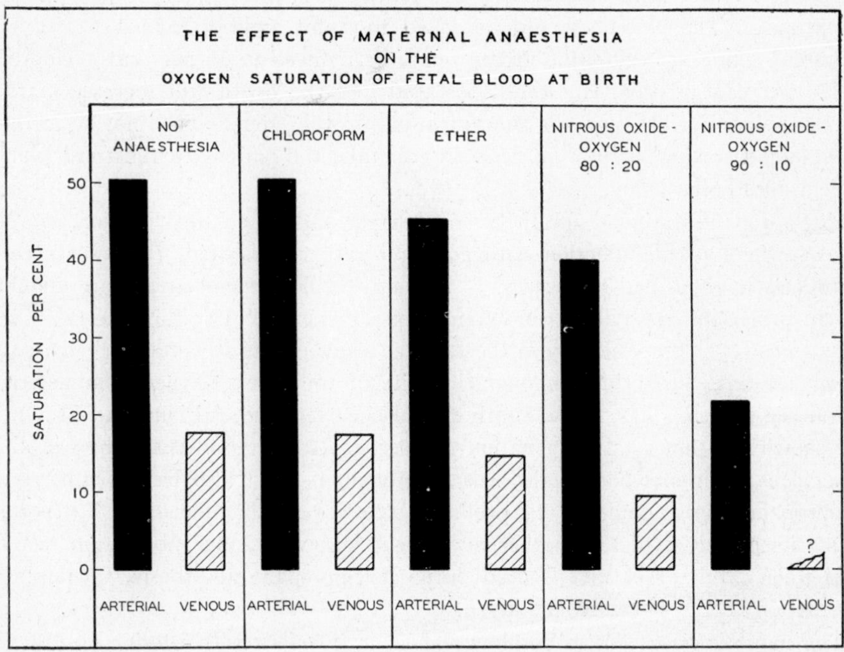

Fig. 304.—The Effects of Various Commonly Used Anesthetics, when Administered Continuously for Five Minutes or More, on the Oxygen Saturation of the Fetal Blood.

Note that, under these circumstances, very high concentrations of nitrous oxide-oxygen may produce fetal anoxemia.

When the patient indicates that a uterine contraction has begun, the mask is placed on her face and she is encouraged to take three deep breaths of an 80-20 mixture of nitrous oxide and oxygen. Frequently a concentration of more oxygen and less gas will suffice. The use of gas in this method may be continued until the head crowns, when the anesthetic is deepened by adding a little ether to aid controllability of the head and for the performance of an episiotomy if necessary.

Ethylene Anesthesia. Ethylene gas has been advocated enthusiastically for obstetrical use by Heaney, Plass, and others. The fact that analgesia can be obtained with slightly higher oxygen concentrations than with nitrous oxide should make it less prone to contribute to fetal anoxia. However, the fact that several explosions have occurred during its administration warrants caution. Henderson reported that the comparatively high dilution in which the gas is used for obstetrical anesthesia makes the risk of explosion much greater than with higher concentrations which are employed for surgical procedures.

Cyclopropane. Bourne as well as Morgan and his associates have reported extensively on the use of cyclopropane for delivery and cesarean section. It is usually given with a closed system. Three to 5 per cent concentration in oxygen will produce analgesia, while 6 to 8 per cent will produce unconsciousness. Twenty to 25 per cent concentration of the gas will maintain surgical anesthesia. Respiratory failure develops in concentrations between 30 and 42 per cent.

It is our practice to allow the patient to breathe for a short time from a bag containing 100 per cent oxygen. This concentration is then diluted 30 per cent with cyclopropane. The patient should be asked to count audibly from 1 to 20. When incoherent counting begins, the mixture may be reduced to 25 per cent cyclopropane and 75 per cent oxygen. Anesthesia is rapid and the depth will increase markedly between pains. For delivery, the concentration of cyclopropane need not be increased. For cesarean section, it may be necessary to take the patient to the third plane of surgical anesthesia.

Cyclopropane is a good anesthetic for delivery and for cesarean section, especially in cases where rapid induction with good relaxation is desired. It presents certain advantages in some bad risk cases. It is highly explosive and great care should be used in protecting the patient and the hospital personnel. For this reason it is our policy to use cyclopropane only in those instances where its advantages to the patient are outstanding. Surprisingly enough, in spite of the excess oxygen administered to the mother with this gas, C. A. Smith and also Rovenstine, Adriani, and Studdiford, have shown that low fetal oxygenation can occur. Resuscitation is required in almost 30 per cent of infants born under this anesthetic. It must also be remembered that cyclopropane has a tendency to produce excessive uterine bleeding. Furthermore, cardiac irregularities of the mother may occur and ventricular fibrillation has been noted when pituitary extract is used during cyclopropane anesthesia. Certainly this combination should never be employed.

The narcotic gases do not prolong labor or interfere with uterine contractions. Woodbury, Hamilton, and Torpin observed little effect of nitrous oxide or cyclopropane on uterine contraction patterns during the first and second stages of labor. While satisfactory analgesia can be produced with nitrous oxide, its routine use is impractical from the standpoint of personnel and it has largely been replaced by other types of analgesia in many institutions. Its greatest weakness is its lack of potency as an anesthetic agent in concentrations permitting adequate oxygenation of the child.

The narcotic gases should not be used unless the patient's stomach is empty, since deaths due to aspiration of stomach contents have been reported. The lack of adequate gas machines or trained personnel should also preclude the employment of narcotic gases. Inadequate precautions against explosion are definite contraindications to the use of ethylene and cyclopropane, while the requirement of deep relaxation should exclude nitrous oxide.

VOLATILE ANESTHETICS

Of the volatile anesthetics, ether, trichlorethylene, and chloroform merit consideration. These agents are powerful anesthetics. They cross the placenta readily and are capable of producing narcosis in the fetus. Ether and chloroform inhibit uterine contractions. With the exception of trichlorethylene, these compounds do not lend themselves to analgesia, being better suited to anesthesia for delivery or cesarean section.

Ether. The margin of safety is usually greater with ether than with any other anesthetic. This is especially true in the hands of the less experienced anesthetist. Administered by the open drop method with an adequate mixture of air to prevent any possibility of cyanosis, it is a relatively safe anesthetic even in the presence of severe cardiac or hypertensive disease. In the closed method of administration so frequently employed at the present time, it is possible to complement or indeed supplement nitrous oxide or ethylene anesthesia by ether when more relaxation or deeper anesthesia is required. As soon as the necessity for deeper anesthesia is removed the ether can be discontinued and the anesthesia maintained with the gas previously administered. Modern apparatus employed in the administration of anesthesia greatly facilitates such a procedure. Because of its relative safety, ether has been used extensively for cesarean section. However, Cole and Kimball showed a striking increase in fetal mortality due to asphyxia in elective cesarean sections done under ether, as compared with those under spinal. Hellman showed a similar higher fetal mortality in infants delivered by cesarean section under ether anesthesia, as compared with those under pentothal sodium. Ether is also conducive to uterine relaxation and bleeding.

Rectal Ether. Because of its irritating action on the upper respiratory passages, ether is not satisfactory for analgesic purposes when administered by inhalation. However, the pioneer observations of Gwathmey on the value of rectal ether for obstetric analgesia have been extended by McCormick with the development of a satisfactory and very safe method of pain relief. Especial emphasis should be placed on the fact that this is one of the few procedures which is feasible for home delivery. On the basis of a vast experience, McCormick reports most favorably on the method from the viewpoint of both safety and efficacy and has kindly permitted the reproduction here of the technic which he has recommended.

McCormick Technic of Rectal Ether

1. A cleansing enema of a 5 to 10 per cent solution of soda (1 to 2 grossly heaping tablespoonfuls of sodium bicarbonate to 1 quart of tepid water) is given at the beginning of labor, preferably not less than one hour before the instillation of rectal ether.

2. Early in labor the patient is addressed as follows: "Mrs. ———, we are desirous of making your labor as painless as possible, and are prepared to do so without danger to you or your baby. Our success in relieving you will depend somewhat upon your cooperation. Therefore, when your pains become uncomfortable let the nurse know and she will give you two, or perhaps three, capsules (pentobarbital sodium, each 0.1 gm.—1½ grains) to relieve you.

"When your pains again become uncomfortable notify her as before and she will give you another capsule or two (pentobarbital sodium), or maybe a hypodermic (morphine sulfate, 10 or 15 mg.—⅙ or ¼ grain).

"Later, when this medicine begins to lose its effect, let her know and she will inject a solution into your rectum (ether-oil or ether-paraldehyde-oil)."

Morphine is not used routinely; it is reserved for the occasional protracted case. It is not administered within four hours of the anticipated time of delivery and is avoided in cases of prematurity.

3. Formula No. I:

Ether	75 cc. (2½ ounces)
Olive or mineral oil	45 cc. (1½ ounces)

Formula No. II:

Ether	75 cc. (2½ ounces)
Paraldehyde	7.7 cc. (2 drams)
Olive or mineral oil	45 cc. (1½ ounces)

(Note the omission of quinine and alcohol.)

Formula No. II may be used to advantage in a restless or "stormy" labor, particularly during the second stage.

4. Rectal ether instillation is performed by using a special pressure instillator.

(A fair substitute for the instillator is a 4-ounce Asepto bulb syringe with a 22 French soft catheter attached or, better still, a 4-ounce hard-tipped Davol rectal syringe and catheter.)

Important Points in Technic. (1) The patient is placed on her left side with the thighs well flexed and the hips brought to the edge of the bed. (2) The physician puts a rubber glove on his right hand and lubricates the anal area and the catheter freely with lubricating jelly (seaweed or tragacanth—not petrolatum). (3) He guides the catheter past the presenting part with the gloved index finger, making certain the catheter does not curl. The finger is then removed. (4) The instillation is started immediately at the conclusion of a uterine contraction.

5. Rectal ether instillations are repeated as needed, in an hour if indicated. Analgesia is maximum in about 40 minutes and its usual duration is from two to six hours.

The average multipara requires but one or two instillations; the primigravida, two or three. (In one instance seven instillations were administered during a 48-hour labor without ill effect.)

6. If the patient is in extremely active labor when first seen, the pentobarbital sodium and the rectal ether are often administered simultaneously.

7. In order to maintain a desired amnesia 0.1 to 0.18 gm. (1½ to 3 grains) of pentobarbital sodium is sometimes given between the ether instillations as indicated; the total amount rarely exceeds 0.5 to 0.6 gm. (7½ to 9 grains) per case.

8. The labor room is not darkened, the patient's ears are not plugged and hushing conversation, closing the door, and the like are not necessary.

9. As a rule the analgesia is augmented during the perineal stage (especially in primigravidae) or the instrumentation period by inhalation ether, nitrous oxide or cyclopropane anesthesia. Only about one half of the usual amount of inhalation anesthetic is required. Chloroform is not used because of the narrow margin of safety.

10. As in dealing with any prolonged form of analgesia, three precautions are kept in mind: (a) the patient is guarded from falling out of bed (adjustable bedsides or vigilant nurse), (b) in protracted cases dehydration and exhaustion are prevented by free oral and intravenous administration of fluids and glucose, and (c) the bladder is observed regularly for overdistention and is emptied by catheter when necessary.

In regard to the value of rectal ether, McCormick says: "It may be stated that the advantages of simplicity of administration, high degree of efficiency, inexpensiveness, extreme safety for both mother and infant, equal adaptability to home and hospital use, and unusual freedom from contraindications, render rectal ether analgesia applicable to practically every woman in labor." Tew claimed 84 per cent pain relief with rectal ether. The method failed in his hands in only 3 per cent and excitement occurred in only 4 per cent. He stated that there was no increase in the duration of labor or in the percentage of operative deliveries. However, Bourne and Burn have shown that uterine contractions are impaired by ether as by other analgesic drugs. Tew found no deleterious effect on the infant.

Trichlorethylene. Although this gas (known as trilene) has had extensive use in the British Isles, it is little known in America. It is a sufficient anesthetic for delivery but will not provide any marked degree of relaxation. Its greatest advantage is that it can be self-administered with a very simple inhaler. The inhaled mixture is about 0.65 per cent trichlorethylene in air. This, as a rule, will produce only analgesia. If sleep is inadvertently induced, the patient's finger will slip from the air hole of the inhaler and only pure air can be inhaled. We have had little experience with this drug but because of the simplicity of its use and relative safety it seems to offer advantages.

Chloroform. Any prolonged administration of this drug is occasionally followed by pronounced central necrosis of the liver lobules, which may end fatally several days after delivery. In addition, there is an immediate danger during anesthesia because of its limited margin of safety as compared with other forms of anesthesia. Although chloroform is a superb anesthetic from the viewpoint of the fetus, because of the oxygenation which it permits, its dangers, as stated, have militated against its widespread use; nevertheless it is employed successfully in a number of clinics.

We have had no personal experience with either chloroform or trichlorethylene. Our results with ether as an anesthetic have been good, although in cesarean section there is some fetal narcosis. The margin of safety and the simplicity of administering ether anesthesia are impressive.

The inhalation of the volatile anesthetics is contraindicated when upper respiratory infection or pulmonary disease exists and after a full meal. In the presence of diabetes and, perhaps, heart disease, there are other methods of pain relief which should yield better results. This type of anesthesia is contraindicated in the presence of prematurity or when, for other reasons, one expects possible fetal asphyxia. There are few contraindications to rectal ether. However, if for any reason, fetal distress is suspected, other forms of analgesia may be preferable.

INTRAVENOUS ANESTHESIA

Sodium Pentothal. Intravenous sodium pentothal offers many advantages as an anesthetic agent in obstetrics. These include: ease and extreme rapidity of induction, ample oxygenation, ready controllability, minimal postpartum bleeding, and promptness of recovery without vomiting. The first and last mentioned of these advantages make it very popular with patients. As shown by Hellman, little pentothal traverses the placenta during the first eight minutes of administration and this allows ample time for low forceps delivery and even extraction of the infant at cesarean section, provided the anesthesia is not started until the patient is draped. As a supplement to local anesthesia in cesarean section, it may be begun a minute or two before the uterine incision is made, with the result that the infant receives a negligible quantity of the drug. Because of its short time duration, sodium pentothal finds several uses in obstetrics aside from delivery, notably for dilatation and curettage. It is not an ideal anesthetic for spontaneous delivery since the movements of the patient are likely to dislodge the needle.

The disadvantages of intravenous sodium pentothal in obstetrics are chiefly two in number: the possibility under certain circumstances of fetal narcosis; and maternal laryngospasm. In low forceps operations, where sodium pentothal finds its greatest usefulness for delivery, the infant rarely shows significant apnea provided that delivery is accomplished within eight minutes of the initiation of the anesthesia. When it is anticipated that as much as 8 or 10 minutes may intervene, it should not be used. Laryngospasm occurs occasionally and may present serious difficulties. This complication is apparently due to a respiratory parasympathetic action brought about by certain shorter-acting barbiturates. It can be prevented in most cases by premedication with atropine or scopolamine, which paralyze the parasympathetics. Sodium pentothal provides neither abdominal nor uterine relaxation and it is hence contraindicated in version and extraction. The relaxation is quite adequate, however, for cesarean section and, as a rule, for cesarean hysterectomy.

For frequent use of sodium pentothal on an active delivery floor, a routine method of preparation is desirable which will make the agent instantly available. The following program has proved satisfactory in our clinic. Each morning 20-cc. syringes are filled with a 2.5 per cent solution of sodium pentothal, a sufficient number being prepared to cover a 24-hour period. Two filled syringes are always present in each delivery room. They remain usable for approximately 48 hours. The anesthetic is administered in the routine manner, 1 to 3 cc. being given as a test dose. After a delay of 15 seconds the drug is given intermittently as required. The average amount required for vaginal delivery is 0.75 gm. (30 cc.). Either atropine or scopolamine is routinely used prior to the anesthetic and for all but the shortest procedures the patient should, in addition, receive oxygen. An emergency drug tray containing the usual analeptic drugs and cardiac stimulants should be part of the equipment in each delivery room. One of the standard adult resuscitators is essential on any modern delivery floor using a variety of anesthetic and analgesic technics.

In more than 5,000 deliveries conducted under sodium pentothal anesthesia in our clinic, about 85 per cent of which were low forceps, the results have been generally satisfactory. There were two maternal deaths, neither of which could be attributed to the anesthesia. The first 3,604 of these deliveries, analyzed by Hellman, showed that the total uncorrected mortality, including both stillbirths and neonatal deaths, was 3.7 per cent; for cases in which the fetal heart could be heard prior to anesthesia, it was 1.8 per cent, while the corresponding figure for full term infants was 0.9 per cent. Dippel and his associates have likewise found sodium pentothal a safe agent both for mother and child in a series of 350 vaginal deliveries. Two large series of cesarean sections under sodium pentothal anesthesia have been reported, namely that of Herrick and that of Gustafson and Gardiner. In the first series of 492 sections, there was no maternal death and it was found that 70 per cent of the infants cried spontaneously. Of the 15 infant deaths (3 per cent) it was felt that five may have been attributable to the anesthesia on the grounds that too long a period intervened in these five cases between the initiation of anesthesia and delivery. In Gustafson and Gardiner's 207 sections under pentothal, one maternal death occurred in association with eclampsia and the author is probably correct in concluding that it should not be used in severe toxemia of pregnancy. There was one stillbirth due to severe abruptio placentae and four neonatal deaths. Although, in 3 of the latter, 10 to 18 minutes intervened between the induction of anesthesia and delivery, the authors were unable to demonstrate any significant correlation, in their series as a whole, between duration of anesthesia and the condition of the infant at birth.

REGIONAL ANESTHESIA

The local anesthetic agents in common use are procaine, metycaine, nupercaine, and pontocaine, arranged in order of ascending duration of action. It can be said that with this group of drugs prolongation of action is roughly correlated with increased toxicity. They are, however, so similar in their effects that interest centers mainly about technics of administration, rather than their pharmacologic activity. Their short duration of anesthesia, the large area involved in obstetric pain, and the inaccessibility of the pathways of the pain, have somewhat limited their use in this field. However, the recent development of continuous technics, and the advancement of knowledge concerning the means of blocking the pathways of obstetric pain, have opened new horizons for the use of regional anesthesia.

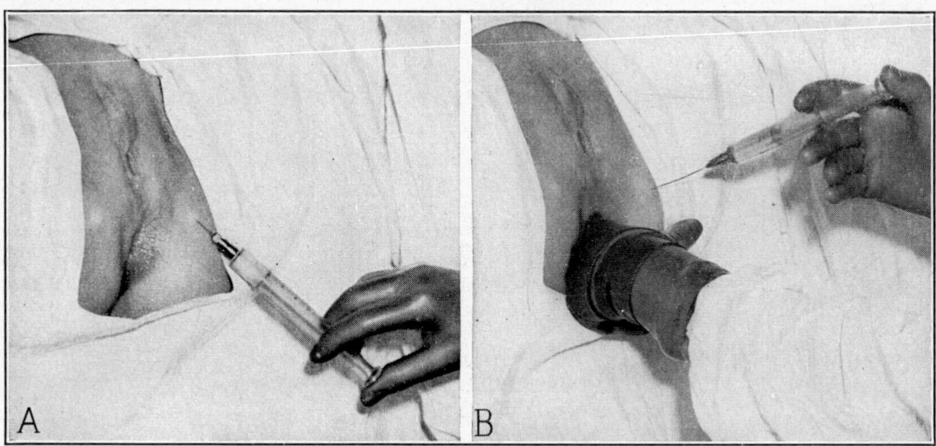

FIG. 305.—LOCAL INFILTRATION ANESTHESIA FOR EPISIOTOMY.

A. Intradermal wheals raised over ischial tuberosities.

B. Index finger in rectum for palpation of ischial spines and infiltration of internal pudic nerves. Infiltration of perineal fibers of the ilio-inguinal nerves and posterior cutaneous femoris nerves completes the procedure.

Local Infiltration. Procaine and metycaine are used for local infiltration. This technic is of no value for analgesia during labor, but may be employed for either vaginal or abdominal delivery. From the standpoint of safety, local infiltration anesthesia is pre-eminent. Its advantages were summarized by Greenhill in 1943 as follows:

1. There is practically no anesthetic mortality.
2. Fetal mortality or asphyxia from direct effect of the anesthetic agent is absent.
3. Simplicity of administration is obvious. It can be administered by the obstetrician and is suitable for home and hospital delivery.
4. Uterine contractions are not impaired.
5. There is no need to hurry through an operation.
6. The toxic effects are minimal.

Five-tenths to 1.0 per cent procaine hydrochloride or 1.0 to 1.5 per cent metycaine may be used. In spontaneous delivery the patient is placed in lithotomy position, a wheal is made as shown in Fig. 305 and the fourchet and the adjoining region injected with a 5 cm. long No. 20 needle. The injection is made on the right side of the patient, as shown in Fig. 305, using the needle in a fan-shaped manner and following the lower border of the vulva on each side. The anesthesia may be begun at the time delivery is imminent. If a more profound anesthesia is desired additional wheals may be made at the upper portion of each labium and a line of infiltration may be directed downward to join the previously infiltrated areas. As a rule, 30 cc. of solution should suffice. In using local anesthetic agents a more prolonged action may be obtained if epinephrine is added so that the final dilution of this substance is between 1:100,000 and 1:200,000.

In the event of operative delivery, more profound anesthesia may be obtained if the pudendal nerves are blocked. With the patient in lithotomy position, draped and prepared for delivery, bilateral wheals in the skin are made with a hypodermic needle midway between the anus and the tuberosity of the ischium. The index finger of the left hand is inserted into the rectum and the left ischial spine palpated. A No. 20 spinal needle 10 cm. long is passed horizontally through the wheal on the left side to a point just below and beyond the spine (Fig. 306, left side of patient). Injury of the rectum is prevented by the left index finger in the rectum. About 15 cc of solution is injected which anesthetizes the internal pudendal nerve. The needle is withdrawn to a point just beneath the skin, the direction is then changed laterally, and the needle inserted directly toward the tuberosity of the ischium until the bone is reached, where 5 cc. of solution is injected. The needle is again withdrawn to just beneath the skin and the labia on the left side infiltrated. With the right index finger in the rectum the procedure is repeated on the right side. Relaxation of the perineal muscles and anesthetization of the skin of the perineum follow in a few minutes. Uterine contractions are not interfered with so that the cooperation of the patient, in the way of voluntary expulsive efforts, may be utilized during the course of operation. In difficult forceps operations, it is sometimes advisable to block the ilio-inguinal nerve which supplies a few fibers to the anterior portion of the vulva and clitoris. This is easily done for the nerve runs directly beneath the fascia along Poupart's ligament.

Local infiltration of the abdominal wall for the performance of cesarean section is a most valuable procedure. It is especially advantageous in cases in which the infant is premature, in preeclampsia, and in conditions in which general or spinal anesthesia is contraindicated. To be successful with this technic, however, several general principles must be kept constantly in mind. In the first place, the utmost gentleness is essential in the handling of tissues and in all procedures executed; any manipulation which entails tugging on the uterine ligaments is particularly painful. In the second place, minute attention to detail in the injection of the anesthetic solution is necessary. Thirdly, it is most important to proceed slowly and to allow a sufficient period of time after injection to permit the solution to take effect before going ahead. Thus, after infiltration of the abdominal wall, a full 10 minutes should intervene before the incision is made. Similarly, a period of three to five minutes should transpire between injection of the fascia and invasion of the deeper structures. All this makes for a rather slow, drawn-out operation, but the great safety for mother and child more than compensates for the time and effort expended.

The solution most commonly employed is procaine in a 1 per cent dilution. The amount required will be about 200 cc. In order to prevent too rapid absorption, 1.0 cc. of a 1:1000 solution of epinephrine is added to 200 cc. of the procaine solution. The first step in the technic is the production of an intradermal wheal in the lower midline of the abdomen after all other preparations have been made for cesarean section. The skin is then infiltrated from the umbilicus through the suprapubic

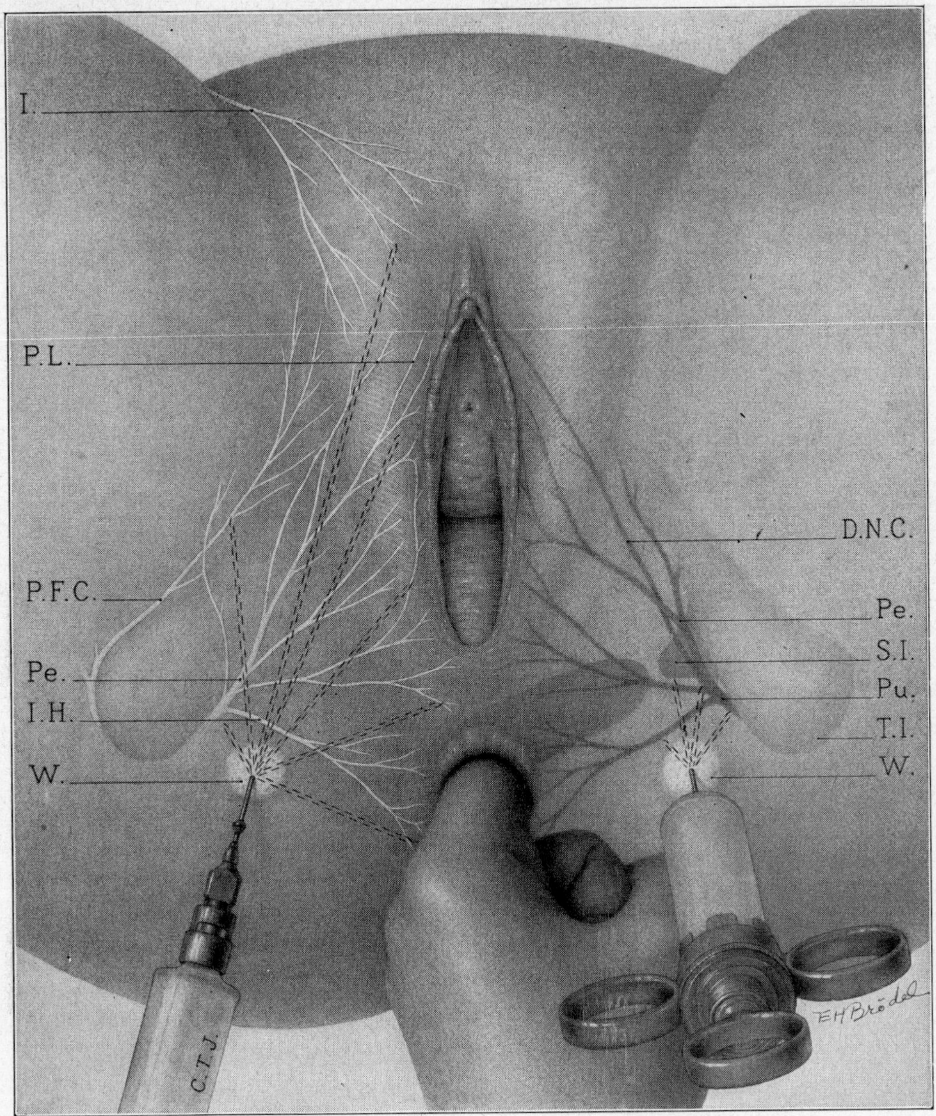

FIG. 306.—LOCAL INFILTRATION TECHNIC OF THE NERVES OF THE FEMALE PERINEUM.

Superficial and deep innervation is shown on the right and left sides of the patient, respectively. *I.,* Ilio-inguinal nerve; *P.L.,* posterior labial nerve; *P.F.C.,* posterior femoral cutaneous nerve, perineal branch; *Pe.,* perineal nerve; *I.H.,* inferior hemorrhoidal nerve; *D.N.C.,* dorsal nerve of clitoris; *Pu.,* pudendal nerve; *S.I.,* spine of ischium; *T.I.,* tuberosity of ischium; *W.,* wheal, intradermal. (From Griffin and Benson, *American Journal of Obstetrics and Gynecology.*)

region. Fan-wise injection of the upper angle and particularly of the lower angle above the symphysis is important. After waiting for 10 minutes, the fascia is exposed and is in turn infiltrated and subsequently incised. It is well, at this point, to infiltrate the fascia on either side for several centimeters lateral to the incision. The parietal peritoneum is carefully infiltrated and incised. An alternate and equally satisfactory procedure is fascial infiltration up and down the lateral border of the rectus muscles.

By blocking the nerves before they give off their terminal branches, these injections anesthetize the whole thickness of the abdominal wall from the skin to the peritoneum, inclusive. The incision should be adequate so that retraction of the incision margins is not necessary or can be reduced to a minimum. The peritoneum covering the uterus may also be injected before the latter is opened. This is especially useful under the peritoneal reflexion in low cervical section. Morphine (0.015 gm.) and scopolamine (0.4 mg.) given hypodermically 10 minutes before the baby is delivered add to the comfort of the patient. Less anesthetic solution is required and a more profound block of the abdominal wall may be obtained by the following technic. The tenth, eleventh, and twelfth intercostal nerves on each side are blocked with 3 to 5 cc. of anesthetic solution just posterior to the lateral cutaneous branches. Blockage of the ilio-inguinal nerve at a point medial to the anterior superior spine of the pelvis adds to the efficacy of the block. Occasionally, slight infiltration of the skin makes the anesthesia more effective. For details of this procedure the reader is referred to Pitkin's Conduction Anesthesia.

With gentleness and care, patients can be delivered by these methods with little pain. In general, they require larger amounts of anesthetic drugs than with the direct types of block, but toxic manifestations are uncommon. Nevertheless, a few rare cases of death have been reported in sensitive individuals. As far as is known, the infant is unaffected by the local anesthetic drugs.

The contraindications to the use of local anesthesia are few. They are: drug sensitivity, apprehension on the part of the patient, and the need for relaxation during the operative procedure.

Parasacral and Paravertebral Block. A number of attempts have been made to apply these technics in obstetrics. Several disadvantages, particularly the short duration of the anesthetic effect and the need for multiple injections, have rendered them unsatisfactory and they have been superseded by the continuous caudal and spinal methods. In addition, paravertebral block is not safe and deaths have been reported from perforation of the pleura and injection of the anesthetic agent directly into the pleural cavity.

Continuous Caudal Analgesia and Anesthesia. At the lower end of the sacrum and on its posterior surface there is a foramen resulting from the nonclosure of the laminae of the last sacral vertebra. It is screened by a thin layer of fibrous tissue. This foramen is called the sacral hiatus and leads to a space within the sacrum known as the caudal canal or caudal space. This space is actually the lowest extent of the bony spinal canal. Through it a rich network of sacral nerves passes downward after they have emerged from the dural sac a few inches above. The dural sac separates the caudal canal, below, from the spinal cord and its surrounding fluid, above.

By filling the caudal canal with a suitable anesthetic solution, pain sense in the sacral nerves is abolished and anesthesia of the pelvic region produced. This is called caudal anesthesia. In continuous caudal anesthesia a pliable needle with a rubber tube attached, or a fine catheter, is inserted, through the sacral hiatus and into the caudal space, and left there. The space is then kept filled with anesthetic solution. If the procedure is successful the patient experiences no pain in labor whatsoever and is conscious neither of uterine contractions nor of perineal distention. The continuous caudal technic provides both analgesia in the first and second stages and anesthesia for delivery.

Caudal anesthesia by the single dose method is not new in obstetrics, Stoeckel, Läwen, Baptisti, and many others having reported on the use of this method for delivery. However, the short duration of the anesthesia obtained, accidents due to inadvertent insertion of the needle into the spinal canal, and other technical difficulties seemed to be inherent and insuperable drawbacks and its use never achieved great popularity.

In 1945 Hingson reported satisfactory relief of pain in 92 per cent of 3,000 patients by the continuous caudal technic. This climaxed five years of work in an effort to improve and safeguard caudal anesthesia. The importance of Hingson's contribution lay not only in the development of the continuous caudal technic but also in the introduction of the principle of the test dose, which precludes the likelihood of introducing large and lethal amounts of anesthetic solution into the spinal canal.

When the patient is in good labor and the cervix at least 3 to 4 cm. dilated, she is placed on her side in a lateral Sims position. The sacral and coccygeal area is cleaned with ether and is prepared with one of the antiseptic tinctures. Considerable experience under supervision is necessary for accurate palpation of the sacral hiatus. Once the sacral hiatus has been identified, a small skin wheal is made over the area with an anesthetic solution. Using a slightly longer needle, the anesthesia is carried down and the fascia over the sacral hiatus injected. A 16 gauge Love-Barker needle, or for that matter any 16 gauge, 3 to 5 in. needle, is directed toward the sacral hiatus. It is then depressed and inserted into the canal for a distance of approximately 1 cm. Following this, a polyethylene or vinethyl catheter is passed through the needle and into the caudal canal for a distance of 3 to 5 cm. Once the catheter has passed the tip of the needle, care should be taken not to withdraw the catheter lest the end be severed. Following the placement of the catheter, the 16 gauge needle is withdrawn. The catheter is then attached to one of the closed systems currently in use for the administration of caudal anesthesia. All of the local anesthetics can be used. It has, however, been customary to employ metycaine in 1.5 per cent solution which is prepared in standard bottles. A small amount of sulfathiazole ointment is placed over the junction of the skin and the catheter and the catheter held in place with adhesive tape. Following this, the patient is permitted free movement. A test dose of 8 cc. of anesthetic solution is injected slowly. After a wait of five minutes the patient is tested for spinal anesthesia. If she possesses free movement of both legs and there is no sensory impairment, the caudal is then administered. We commonly use an initial dosage of 22 cc. This, plus the test dose, should give anesthesia to the umbilicus in about 20 minutes. The dosage of caudal is repeated as necessary. On the average, 20 cc. doses will have to be administered every 40 minutes. For a more detailed description of these technics, the reader is referred to the textbook on the subject by Lull and Hingson.

A summary of the results of 10,000 cases, based on the questionnaire by Hingson and Edwards, indicates that complete pain relief can be obtained in 81 per cent of women, partial relief in 12 per cent of women, and failure in 7 per cent. There is no question but that caudal analgesia impairs the frequency and intensity of uterine contractions. This was observed by Siever and Mousel and has since been studied in our clinic extensively. This alteration in uterine contractions is much more prevalent if the anesthesia is started very early in labor, or if the level is raised to the height of the seventh and eighth thoracic vertebrae. There is some prolongation of the second stage and the incidence of forceps delivery is increased. In most instances, however, the head will descend to such a level that the forceps delivery is simple and without danger to mother and child. In two studies carried on in different cities, Hingson compared caudal analgesia with other types of pain relief. In both studies there was a reduction in the stillbirths and neonatal mortality rate in the caudal group. This was true not only of full-term infants but prematures as well. Furthermore, in the Memphis study there was a diminution in the full-term and premature neonatal mortality rates in a caudal analgesia group, as compared with a control group to whom no pain relief was administered. Masters and Ross have compared a group of premature infants born under caudal anesthesia with those born under sedation analgesia plus general anesthesia; their caudal anesthesia group has also shown a very marked reduction in infant mortality rates. In all these studies, serious question can be raised about the validity of the control groups. However, there can be little doubt that this form of anesthesia exerts the least possible effect on the baby, *provided the maternal blood pressure does not fall below 100 mm. Hg,* a most important proviso. It is of particular advantage to the premature infant as it tends to retard rapid and forceful labor and enables the operator to perform a gentle and controlled delivery. For the healthy mature infant the choice of sedation, general anesthesia, or local infiltration makes little difference. For the infant whose life is endangered by any of a number of obstetrical hazards, caudal block presents many advantages.

One of the chief hazards of caudal anesthesia is the fall in maternal blood pressure. A fall of more than 20 mm. has been observed by Hingson in 20 per cent of patients. This can usually be controlled by alertness and prompt action on the part of the physician. The administration of epinephrine or of ephedrine will frequently meet the situation. Often the mere elevation of the patient's legs for a few minutes will restore the pressure to normal. The maintenance of the anesthetic level in the neighborhood of the umbilicus will preclude many of these drops in pressure.

Hingson has reported 43 maternal deaths in the course of 200,000 administrations of continuous caudal analgesia. Eleven of these were definitely related to the method. These deaths do not necessarily militate against the use of caudal analgesia but should call attention to the fact that caudal anesthesia is a tool for the experienced operator and is dangerous in the hands of the inexperienced.

Contraindications to this method of analgesia are several. Infection of the skin over the sacral area, especially the presence of an old pilonidal sinus, should preclude its use. Quite a few patients will express a desire to be asleep during the actual delivery and for these some other form of analgesia is preferable. In prolonged labors this type of pain relief is contraindicated because its use may become troublesome and inefficient after six to eight hours. Nor should it be employed in the presence of hemorrhage or shock, because of its vasodepressor tendencies. For the same reason it should be used cautiously in preeclampsia and eclampsia. Caudal analgesia is probably the method of choice when one is dealing with prematurity, cardiac disease, pulmonary disease, or diabetes.

Spinal Anesthesia. Spinal anesthesia, as used in obstetrics, falls into two major divisions. The first is a semi-terminal type of anesthesia which is employed for the latter part of labor and delivery and is provided by low dosage of a hyperbaric or isobaric solution. The second is a terminal type and is administered either by the single dosage method or the continuous technic; its largest field of employment is cesarean section. Although minute doses of spinal anesthesia can be given to provide pain relief throughout labor, this technic is difficult and, by and large, unsatisfactory. Too often labor is stopped by spinal anesthesia.

Low Dosage Hyperbaric Spinal (Saddle Block). This form of anesthesia is one of the most popular in the United States today. Nearly all the local anesthetic agents have been used in saddle block anesthesia, as shown in Table 12. By the addition of glucose to the solution of nupercaine or other anesthetic agent, localization and concentration of the drug in the conus of the dural sack are facilitated. Inasmuch as this anesthetic is of short duration, it is necessary to time its administration properly and delivery should be anticipated within an hour or so following the onset of anesthesia. With the patient in the sitting position, spinal puncture is made through the fourth lumbar interspace. A short-bevel 22 to 28 gauge needle is commonly used. When free flow of clear spinal fluid is obtained, a Leur-Lok syringe containing the properly prepared solution is attached to the needle, aspiration of 0.1 cc. of spinal fluid carried out, and solution rapidly injected. At the end of 10 seconds the needle is removed and at exactly the proper time indicated in Table 12, the patient is placed flat on her back with a pillow under her head to keep the neck sharply flexed. It is well to time the procedure so that it is carried out entirely between contractions of the uterus.

Drugs	Dose (mg.)	Method of Preparation	Time Sitting Up (Seconds)
1. (a) Nupercaine (buffered), 1:200 sol.	2.5	Draw up 2 cc. of 10% glucose, then 2 cc. of nupercaine. Mix. Discard all but 1 cc.	30
(b) Nupercaine (unbuffered), 2.5 mg./cc. in 5% glucose		Draw up 1 cc. of prepared solution. Use as such.	
2. Pontocaine, 1% sol.	5	Draw up 2 cc. 10% glucose, then 2 cc. of pontocaine. Mix. Discard all but 1 cc.	30
3. Novocain (Procaine), 20% sol.	50	Draw up 3 cc. 10% glucose, then 1 cc. of novocain. Mix. Discard all but 1 cc.	35
4. Metycaine, 10% sol.	33	Draw up 2 cc. 10% glucose, then 1 cc. of metycaine. Mix. Discard all but 1 cc.	35

TABLE 12. TECHNIC OF SADDLE BLOCK ANESTHESIA WITH VARIOUS DRUGS.

The dosages cited represent the maximum amounts which should be given. Current trends are toward using about two thirds or even half of these dosages. For instance, 35 mg. of procaine is usually adequate for low forceps, episiotomy and repair.

(From Andros and others, *American Journal of Obstetrics and Gynecology,* 1948, 55:806.)

This method was first described by Adriani and Roman-Vega and by Parmley and Adriani in 1946. In a series of 136 women in whom injection was usually made when the cervix was 5 to 6 cm. dilated, there was complete relief of pain during the remainder of labor and at delivery in 81 per cent. A momentary fall in blood pressure, sometimes to as low as 80 mm. Hg, occurred in one-half the patients; in the other half, lowering of the blood pressure averaged 10 mm. Hg. Little or no paralysis of the leg or thigh muscles or of the recti of the abdomen occurred; and, in general, the regions anesthetized corresponded to the parts of a horseback rider which are in contact with the saddle; hence the name.

Andros reports that 72.2 per cent of 719 cases received excellent pain relief, while in an additional 20 per cent the pain relief was adequate. The results were poor in 6.4 per cent. He reported an extremely low infant mortality rate of 0.85 per cent. Rarely, permanent nerve damage occurs with spinal anesthesia. Fall in blood pressure is a possible complication of any spinal anesthesia and should be watched for and vigorously combated. Andros reports a fall in systolic blood pressure of 20 mm. Hg or greater in 26 per cent of cases. A mean drop of 14.8 mm. occurred. One of the most troublesome complications of this type of anesthesia is the postpartum headache. Andros reports an incidence of headache in 14.5 per cent of all patients; 10.2 per cent had mild headache, 3.5 per cent moderate, and 0.8 per cent severe. These figures agree in general with those of our own clinic. It would seem, from the work of Franksson and Gordh, that spinal headache is due to continued leakage of spinal fluid through the puncture hole in the dura. The use of small 28 gauge needles makes continued leakage unlikely.

Low Dosage Isobaric Spinal. This differs from saddle block anesthesia in two respects. In the first place, the crystals of the anesthetic drug are dissolved in spinal fluid so that the resultant solution is approximately isobaric. In the second place, the patient is positioned on her side for the injection. This technic is preferred by many obstetricians because positioning the patient in the sitting posture (as in saddle block) at this critical time in labor is sometimes troublesome as well as distressing to the parturient. The dosage employed is the same as in saddle block anesthesia. The anesthetic agent is usually dissolved in about 2 cc. of spinal fluid and injected into the third or fourth interspace. The duration of anesthesia is about one hour, allowing ample time for a low forceps delivery and the repair of an episiotomy.

As is true of caudal analgesia, spinal anesthesia should never be given unless trained personnel is available to watch the patient and take proper steps to combat falls in blood pressure. It should never be given in cases of drug sensitivity or in the presence of central nervous system lesions. It is also contraindicated in any of the hemorrhagic complications of pregnancy, such as placenta previa, abruptio, etc.

Continuous, or Fractional, Spinal Anesthesia for Cesarean Section. While single injection technics of spinal anesthesia for cesarean section continue to be used, it is our opinion that the dosage necessary is so high that marked alterations in blood pressure are bound to occur at times and not a few maternal and fetal deaths will result. This is borne out by the numerous maternal fatalities which have been reported in the course of spinal anesthesia given for delivery. Dosages of anesthetic drugs which give reasonably safe results in surgical patients may lead, in obstetrical patients, to extremely high levels of spinal anesthesia and precipitous falls in blood pressure. Hence, we believe that, with the exception of the very small dosage of anesthetic drug employed in the methods just described, single injection technics of spinal anesthesia should be replaced with one of the continuous methods. At the present time we employ continuous spinal anesthesia in the majority of our cesarean sections.

As recommended by Lull, the blood pressure should be checked one-half hour before operation; if it is below 130 mm. Hg systolic, ¾ grain of ephedrine hydrochloride should be given, and if at any time during the operation the pressure reaches

90 mm. Hg or less, it should be repeated and intravenous glucose started. Cosgrove recommends that a continuous drip of glucose and sodium chloride solution be started routinely before any spinal anesthesia is given. It stabilizes the circulatory apparatus and establishes, moreover, a channel through which vasopressor drugs, oxytocics, supplemental anesthetics such as sodium pentothal, plasma, and blood may be readily used as indicated.

With the patient lying on her side, a Tuohy needle is inserted into the second or third lumbar interspace and passed into the spinal canal. Once the clear flow of fluid is obtained, a small plastic catheter is passed through the needle and for 2 to 3 cm. downward in the canal. The catheter is taped in place and 15 to 25 mg. of procaine or 10 to 25 mg. of metycaine are injected slowly. Five-minute blood pressure determinations should be made. If the pressure remains at 100 mm. Hg the operator may proceed with small additional doses as necessary. A careful check is maintained on the anesthetic level and when this has reached an area approximately at the costal margin the patient is ready for operation. Repeated small doses of the anesthetic agent will usually be necessary. A slow drip of 0.1 per cent sodium pentothal in glucose will maintain the patient in a slight degree of euphoria without producing any effect upon the fetus.

In 1,000 cesarean sections under continuous spinal anesthesia, reported by Lull, there was only one maternal death and that occurred as the result of leukemia 12 days after the operation. The uncorrected fetal mortality was 4.7 per cent. Among 986 infants born alive in this series, only one required actual resuscitation other than clearing out the upper respiratory passages. There were 27 failures, 10 being technical failures and 17 attributable to the fact that the anesthetic did not rise high enough to permit proceeding with the operation and supplemental anesthesia was necessary. It should be noted that Lull's average initial dose was 15 mg. of procaine. This large series of cesarean sections performed under continuous spinal anesthesia shows that with minimal dosage and judicious management this type of anesthesia possesses a high degree of safety both for mother and infant.

Spinal anesthesia is contraindicated in debilitated, severely anemic patients and in those with central nervous system lesions. In the presence of hemorrhage or shock, unless the blood loss can be made up with adequate transfusion, it is also hazardous. Drops in blood pressure are particularly prone to occur in hypertensive patients and, if used at all in such cases, the anesthesia level must be built up very slowly with the injection of only minute quantities of the agent at a time (for instance, no more than 15 mg. of procaine). If the blood pressure falls appreciably before an adequate anesthesia level is obtained, conduction anesthesia should be abandoned and some other technic used.

SUMMARY

From what has been said in the present chapter, it becomes evident that no single method is entirely satisfactory for the alleviation of pain during labor. At the same time it is recognized that there has been an increasing demand on the part of the laity, especially during the present century, for relief of suffering associated with childbirth. It is proper that these pains should be relieved, provided such relief can be administered with safety to both mother and child. But it must be emphasized everlastingly that safety is the prime desideratum. A satisfactory patient-physician relationship will often enable the obstetrician to carry his patient for some time during the early stages of labor without any need for pain-relieving agents. From this point on the advances in technic of the past decade have furnished the obstetrician with a multitude of methods for relieving pain, each with its own advantages and drawbacks. Vigorous and controlled research is now necessary so that the technics available can be properly evaluated from the standpoint of their effect on the physiology of the mother, on labor, and on the fetus. Only a beginning has been made in this direction.

BIBLIOGRAPHY

Adriani, J., and Roman-Vega, D. A. Saddle Block Anesthesia. Am. J. Surg., 1946, 71:12.

American Medical Association. Preliminary Report of the Council on Evipan Soluble. J.A.M.A., 1937, 108:1172.

Andros, G. J., Dieckmann, W. J., Ouda, P., Priddle, H. D., Smitter, R. C., and Bryan, W. M., Jr. Spinal (Saddle Block) Anesthesia in Obstetrics. Am. J. Obst. & Gynec., 1948, 55:806.

Baptisti, A., Jr. Caudal Anesthesia in Obstetrics. Am. J. Obst. & Gynec., 1939, 38:642.

——— Continuous Caudal Analgesia in Obstetrics. Am. J. Obst. & Gynec., 1944, 48:103.

Batterman, R. C., and Himmelsbach, C. K. Demerol—A New Synthetic Analgesic. J.A.M.A., 1943. 122:222.

Belinkoff, S. Cyclopropane-pituitrin Incompatibility. Am. J. Obst. & Gynec., 1944, 48:109.

Bernstine, J. B., and Prince, L. N. Vinbarbital Sodium for Obstetric Amnesia and Analgesia. Am. J. Obst. & Gynec., 1943, 45:851.

Bill, A. H. Analgesia and Anesthesia and Their Bearing upon the Problem of Shortened Labor. Am. J. Obst. & Gynec., 1937, 34:868.

Bourne, A. W., and Burn, J. H. Action on the Human Uterus of Anesthetics and Other Drugs Commonly Used in Labor. Brit. M. J., 1930, 2:87.

Bourne, W. Analgesia and Anesthesia in Obstetrics. New York State J. Med., 1937, 37:1905.

——— Cyclopropane Anesthesia in Obstetrics. Lancet, 1934, 2:20.

Channing. A Treatise on Etherization in Childbirth. Boston, 1848.

Cleland, J. G. P. Paravertebral Anesthesia in Obstetrics. Surg., Gynec. & Obst., 1933, 57:51.

Cole, W. C. C., and Kimball, D. M. Relationship of Maternal Ether Anesthesia to Inauguration of Fetal Respiration. Nebraska M. J., 1943, 28:200.

Colvin, E. D., and Bartholomew, R. A. Improvements in the Paraldehyde Method of Relief of Pain in Labor. Am. J. Obst. & Gynec., 1938, 35:589.

Cosgrove, S. A., Hall, P. O., and Gleeson, W. J. Spinal Anesthesia with Particular Reference to Its Use in Obstetrics. Anesth. & Analg., 1937, 16:234.

Courville, C. B. Asphyxia as a Consequence of Nitrous Oxide Anesthesia. Medicine, 1936, 15:1.

Crawford, M. D. Clinical and Biochemical Findings in Delayed Chloroform Poisoning. J. Obst. & Gynaec. Brit. Emp., 1942, 49:549.

Daichman, I., Kornfeld, G., and Shir, M. M. A. Comparative Study of Sodium Amytal, Sodium Amytal and Scopolamine, Gwathmey (Ether in Oil) and Avertin. Am. J. Obst. & Gynec., 1934, 28:101.

Dippel, A. L., Helman, R. J., Wolters, C. E., Wall, H. A., and Hairston, F. H. Sodium Pentothal Anesthesia for Selected Vaginal Obstetrics. Surg., Gynec. & Obst., 1947, 85:572.

Drabkin, D. L., Ravdin, I. S., Hirst, J. C., and Latham, M. E. The Effect of Amytal Anesthesia upon the Uterus and Its Use in Obstetrics. Am. J. M. Sc., 1929, 178:379.

Eastman, N. J. The Role of Anesthesia in the Production of Asphyxia Neonatorum. Am. J. Obst. & Gynec., 1936, 31:563.

Edwards, W. B., and Hingson, R. A. Continuous Caudal Anesthesia in Obstetrics. Am. J. Surg., 1942, 57:459.

Evans, J. R. Intravenous Administration of Vinbarbital Sodium for Induction of Obstetric Amnesia. Am. J. Obst. & Gynec., 1944, 47:821.

Franksson, C., and Gordh, T. Headache after Spinal Anesthesia and Technique for Lessening Its Frequency. Acta chir. Scandinav., 1946, 94:443.

Galloway, C. E., and Smith, P. H. A Study of Nembutal and Scopolamine for the Relief of Pain in Five Hundred Deliveries. Am. J. Obst. & Gynec., 1935, 29:207.

Gauss, C. J. Geburten im künstlichen Dämmerschlaf. Arch. f. Gynäk., 1906, 78:579.

Gilbert, G., and Dixon, A. B. Observations on Demerol as an Obstetric Analgesic. Am. J. Obst. & Gynec., 1943, 45:320.

GREENHILL, J. P. The Use of Local Infiltration Anesthesia in Obstetrics and Gynecology. S. Clin. North America, 1943, 23:143.

——— Anesthesia in Obstetrics. Am. J. Obst. & Gynec., 1947, 54:74.

GRIFFITH, H. R. Cyclopropane Anesthesia; Clinical Record of 350 Administrations. Canad. M. A. J., 1934, 31:157.

——— The Management of Complications Arising during Cyclopropane Anesthesia. New York State J. Med., 1940, 40:209.

——— and GOODALL, J. R. Analgesia and Anaesthesia in Obstetrics. J. Obst. & Gynaec. Brit. Emp., 1941, 48:323.

GUSTAFSON, G. W., and GARDINER, S. H. The Use of Pentothal Sodium Anesthesia for Cesarean Section. Am. J. Obst. & Gynec., 1949, 58:246.

GWATHMEY, J. T., and others. Painless Childbirth by Synergistic Methods. Bull. Lying-In Hosp., N. Y., 1924, 13:83.

HEANY, N. S. Ethylene and Oxygen Anesthesia for Gynecological and Obstetrical Work. Am. J. Obst. & Gynec., 1924, 8:416.

——— The Relief of Labor Pains by the Use of Paraldehyde and Benzyl Alcohol. J.A.M.A., 1936, 107:1710.

HELLMAN, L. M., SHETTLES, L. B., MANAHAN, C. P., and EASTMAN, N. J. Sodium Pentothal Anesthesia in Obstetrics. Am. J. Obst. & Gynec., 1944, 48:851.

HELLMAN, L. M., SHETTLES, L. B., and STRAN, H. A Quantitative Method for the Determination of Sodium Pentothal in Blood. J. Biol. Chem., 1943, 148:293.

HENDERSON, Y. The Hazard of Explosion of Anesthetics. Report of the Committee on Anesthesia Accidents. J.A.M.A., 1930, 94:1491.

——— and LUCAS, G. H. W. Cyclopropane; New Anesthetic. Anesth. & Analg., 1930, 9:1.

HERRICK, F. L. Pentothal Sodium Anesthesia for Cesarean Section. Am. J. Obst. & Gynec., 1948, 55:883.

HERSHENSON, B. B. Premedication and Anesthesia in Obstetrics; Current Practices at the Boston Lying-In Hospital. New England J. Med., 1948, 239-429.

HINGSON, R. A. Contraindications and Cautions in the Use of Continuous Caudal Analgesia. Am. J. Obst. & Gynec., 1944, 47:718.

IRVING, F. C., BERMAN, S., and NELSON, H. B. The Barbiturates and other Hypnotics in Labor. Surg., Gynec. & Obst., 1934, 58:1.

JORGENSEN, C. L., GRAVES, J. H., and SAVAGE, J. E. Saddle Block Anesthesia for Delivery. Report of 1000 Cases. South. M. J., 1948, 41:830.

KANE, H. F., and ROTH, G. B. The Use of Paraldehyde in Obtaining Obstetric Analgesia and Amnesia. Am. J. Obst. & Gynec., 1935, 29:366.

KELLOGG, K., and PARRETT, V. The Residual Effect of Prolonged Caudal Anesthesia upon the Neuromuscular System in Dogs. Am. J. Obst. & Gynec., 1944, 47:327.

KIRSCHBAUM, H. M. Scopolamine in Obstetrics. Am. J. Obst. & Gynec., 1942, 44:664.

KNIGHT, R. T. Cyclopropane Anesthesia in Obstetrics. Anesth. & Analg., 1936, 15:63.

KOTZ, J., ROTH, G. B., and RYON, W. A. Idiosyncrasy to Paraldehyde. J.A.M.A., 1938, 110:2145.

KREBS, O. S., WULFF, G. L., JR., and WASSERMANN, H. C. Scopolamine-Morphine Seminarcosis with Modification. J.A.M.A., 1936, 107:1704.

KRETZSCHMAR, N. R., TOWSLEY, H. A., STODDARD, F. J., and ENGELFRIED, J. A Study of Intrauterine Oxygen Exchange. Am. J. Obst. & Gynec., 1941, 42:677.

LABAT, L. G. Regional Anesthesia, 2nd ed. Philadelphia, 1928.

LANIER, V. S., MCKNIGHT, H. E., and TROTTER, M. Caudal Analgesia: An Experimental and Anatomical Study. Am. J. Obst. & Gynec., 1944, 47:633.

LEVINE, W., HERZLICH, J., HALPERIN, J., and TALLER, H. Continuous Caudal Anesthesia in Obstetrics. Am. J. Surg., 1944, 64:31.

LEWIS, M. S. Vinbarbital Sodium for Obstetric Amnesia, Analgesia and Anesthesia. Am. J. Obst. & Gynec., 1946, 51:395.

LÖWENBERG, K., WAGGONER, R. W., and ZBINBEN, T. Destruction of the Cerebral Cortex following Nitrous Oxide Anesthesia. Ann. Surg., 1936, 104:801.

LULL, C. B., and HINGSON, R. A. Control of Pain in Childbirth, 3rd ed. J. B. Lippincott Co., Philadelphia, 1948.

LULL, C. B., and ULLERY, J. C. Cesarean Section under Continuous Caudal Analgesia. A Supplementary Report. Am. J. Obst. & Gynec., 1944, 48:235.

MAYER, E. The Toxic Effects following the Use of Local Anesthetics. J.A.M.A., 1924, 82:876.

MCCORMICK, C. O. A New Rectal Ether Analgesia Apparatus. Am. J. Obst. & Gynec., 1930, 20:411.

——— HUBER, C. P., SPAHR, J. F., and GILLESPIE, C. F. An Experience with One Hundred Cases of Continuous Caudal Analgesia. Am. J. Obst. & Gynec., 1944, 47:297.

MENGERT, W. F. Morphine Sulfate as an Obstetric Analgesic. A Clinical Analysis. Am. J. Obst. & Gynec., 1942, 44:888.

——— Continuous Caudal Anesthesia with Procaine Hydrochloride in 240 Obstetric Patients. Am. J. Obst. & Gynec., 1944, 48:100.

MILLER, L. L., and WHIPPLE, G. H. Chloroform Liver Injury Increases as Protein Stores Decrease. Studies in Nitrogen Metabolism in Dogs. Am. J. Med. Sc., 1940, 199:204.

MONTGOMERY, T. L. Obstetric Amnesia, Analgesia and Anesthesia. Their Relationship to Sudden Death in Labor. J.A.M.A., 1937, 108:1679.

MORGAN, G. S., EAMAN, S. G., and GRIFFITH, H. R. Cyclopropane Anesthesia for Cesarean Section. Anesth. & Analg., 1937, 16:113.

NORTON, J. F. A Mortality Study of 187 Deaths in 66,376 Live Births. Am. J. Obst. & Gynec., 1945, 49:554.

PARMLEY, R. T., and ADRIANI, J. Saddle Block Anesthesia with Nupercaine in Obstetrics. Am. J. Obst. & Gynec., 1946, 52:636.

PITKIN, G. P. Conduction Anesthesia. J. B. Lippincott Co., Philadelphia, 1946.

PLASS, E. D., and SWENSON, C. N. Ethylene in Obstetrics. J.A.M.A., 1926, 87:1716.

ROSENFELD, H. H., and DAVIDOFF, R. B. Paraldehyde as a Factor in Painless Labor. Surg., Gynec. & Obst., 1935, 60:235.

ROVENSTINE, E. A., ADRIANI, J., and STUDDIFORD, W. E. Gas Changes in Maternal and Fetal Blood during Cyclopropane Obstetric Anesthesia. California and West. Med., 1940, 53:59.

SCHMIDT, E. R., and WATERS, R. M. Cyclopropane Anesthesia. Postoperative Morbidity in 2,200 Cases. Anesth. & Analg., 1935, 14:1.

SCHUMANN, W. R. Demerol (S-140) and Scopolamine in Labor. A Study of 1,000 Cases. Am. J. Obst. & Gynec., 1944, 47:93.

SHOOR, M. Paraldehyde Poisoning. J.A.M.A., 1941, 117:1534.

SIEVER, J. M., and MOUSEL, L. H. Continuous Caudal Anesthesia in Three Hundred Unselected Obstetric Cases. J.A.M.A., 1943, 122:424.

SIMPSON, J. Y. On the Employment of the Inhalation of Sulphuric Ether in the Practice of Midwifery. Month. J. Med. Sc., 1846, 7:721.

SMITH, C. A. The Effect of Obstetrical Anesthesia upon the Oxygenation of Maternal and Fetal Blood with Particular Reference to Cyclopropane. Surg., Gynec. & Obst., 1939, 69:584.

——— and BARKER, R. H. Ether in the Blood of the Newborn Infant. A Quantitative Study. Am. J. Obst. & Gynec., 1942, 43:763.

SNYDER, F. F. Obstetric Analgesia and Anesthesia. Their Effects on Labor and the Child. W. B. Saunders Co., Philadelphia, 1949.

——— and GEILING, E. M. K. Action of Morphine in Obstetric Analgesia. Am. J. Obst. & Gynec., 1943, 45:604.

TEW, C. R. Rectal Analgesia in Obstetrics. Am. J. Surg., 1935, 27:289.

TOLLEFSON, D. G. Analgesia and Anesthesia in Labor. West. J. Surg., 1941, 49:44.

URNES, M. P., and TIMERMAN, H. J. Breech Delivery. A Comparative Study of Local and General Anesthesia. J.A.M.A., 1937, 109:1616.

WEINTRAUB, F., and MERRIAM, M. S. Spinal Anesthesia for Cesarean Section. Am. J. Obst. & Gynec., 1943, 46:836.

WOLFF, H. G., HARDY, J. D., and GOODELL, H. Measurement of Effect on Pain Threshold of Acetylsalicylic Acid, etc. J. Clin. Investigation, 1941, 20:63.

WOODBRIDGE, P. D. Incidence of Anesthetic Explosions. J.A.M.A., 1939, 113:2308.

WOODBURY, R. A., HAMILTON, W. F., and TORPIN, R. The Effect of Cyclopropane on the Uterine Contractions. Am. J. Physiol., 1938, 121:640.

Section Five: THE PUERPERIUM AND THE NEWBORN

18

THE PUERPERIUM

The term puerperium or puerperal state (from *puer,* a child; and *parere,* to bring forth) comprises the period elapsing between the termination of labor and the return of the generative tract to its normal condition and refers to the six weeks following the completion of labor. Although the changes occurring during this period are considered as physiologic, they border very closely upon the pathologic, inasmuch as under no other circumstances does such marked and rapid tissue catabolism occur without a departure from a condition of health.

ANATOMICAL CHANGES IN THE PUERPERIUM

Involution of the Uterus. Immediately following the expulsion of the placenta, the contracted and retracted body of the uterus forms a hard muscular tumor, the apex of which lies about midway between the umbilicus and symphysis, usually 12 cm. (4¾ inches) above the latter. At autopsy, shortly after labor, it consists of an almost solid mass of tissue containing in its center a flattened cavity, whose anterior and posterior walls are in close apposition, each of which measures 4 to 5 cm. in thickness. Owing to the compression of its vessels by the retracted muscle fibers, the puerperal uterus on section presents an anemic appearance, as contrasted with the purplish pregnant organ. During the next two days the uterus remains apparently stationary in size, after which it atrophies so rapidly that by the tenth day it has descended into the cavity of the true pelvis, and can no longer be felt above the symphysis. It regains its normal size by the end of five or six weeks. Some idea of the rapidity with which the process goes on may be gained by recalling the fact that the freshly delivered uterus weighs about 1,000 gm., one week later 500 gm., at the end of the second week 375 gm., and at the end of the puerperium only 40 to 60 gm.

This rapid decrease in size is due to what is designated as *involution,* and is the most striking example of atrophy with which we are acquainted; in that the organ becomes reduced to one twentieth or one twenty-fifth of its original size within a few weeks.

It was formerly believed that the muscle cells underwent fatty degeneration during involution, and that large numbers of them completely disappeared. Sänger, however, was the first to show that only the excess of protoplasm is removed, and that the actual number of individual cells is not greatly diminished. Stieve, however, contends that many of the cells completely disappear. Sänger estimated that during the process the individual cells decrease from 208.7 to 24.4 microns in length.

It is now held that involution is effected by autolytic processes by which the protein material of the uterine wall is in great part broken down into simpler components, which are then absorbed and eventually cast off through the urine. The evidence in favor of such a view is afforded by the study of the nitrogen content of the urine. For the 24 hours immediately following labor 7 to 9 gm. of nitrogen are excreted, but some time during the second or third day an increase of 30 to 50 per cent is noted. This excess output continues for a number of days, but gradually returns to normal at about the time the uterus has disappeared into the pelvic cavity.

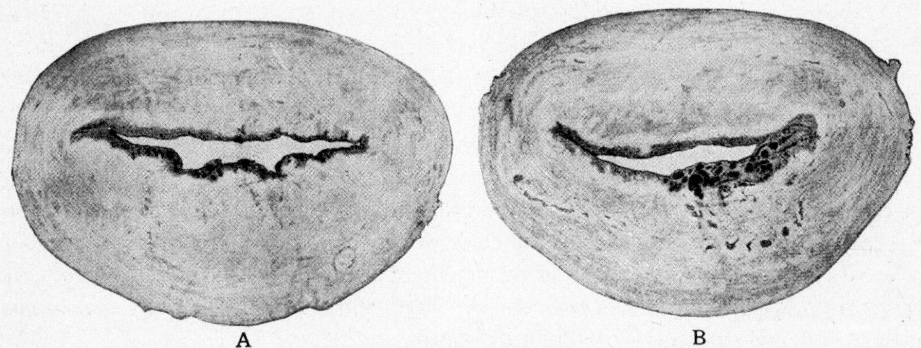

FIG. 307.—THE PLACENTAL SITE.

A, at delivery; B, 8 hours postpartum.

(From Williams, *American Journal of Obstetrics and Gynecology.*)

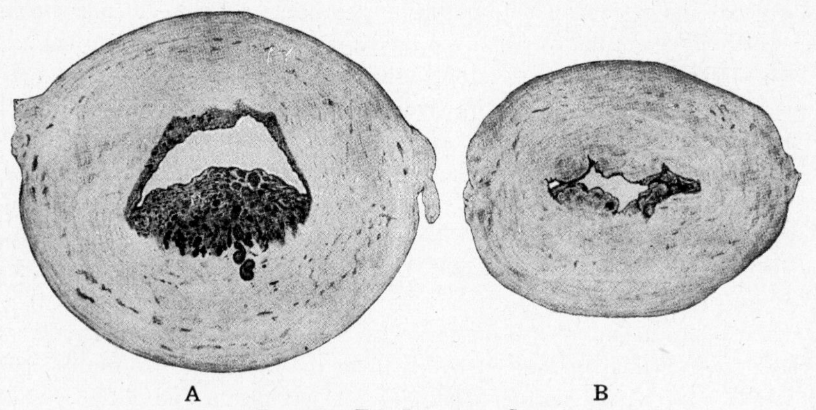

FIG. 308.—THE PLACENTAL SITE.

A, 8 days postpartum; B, 14 days postpartum.

(From Williams, *American Journal of Obstetrics and Gynecology.*)

That this phenomenon is not entirely attributable to the removal of other products of pregnancy was clearly shown by Slemons, who, in a patient, from whom the uterus had been removed at cesarean section, found that the characteristic increase in the nitrogen output was lacking, and that the difference practically corresponded to the quantity of nitrogen contained in the uterus. Harding and Montgomery, on the other hand, contend that the negative nitrogen balance is in great part connected with lactation, and in certain patients, at least, can be overcome by greatly increasing the nitrogenous constituents of the diet.

As has been said before, the separation of the placenta and its membranes occurs in the outer portion of the spongy layer of the decidua, and accordingly a remnant of the latter remains in the uterus after their expulsion. It presents striking variations in thickness, an irregular, jagged appearance, and is markedly infiltrated with blood, especially at the placental site. As the result of hyaline and fatty degeneration, the greater portion of this tissue is cast off in the lochia, leaving behind only the fundi of the glands and a minimal amount of connective tissue, from which the new endometrium is regenerated.

Within two or three days after labor, the portion of decidua remaining in the uterus becomes differentiated into two layers, the one adjoining the uterine cavity being necrotic, and the other adjoining the muscularis being well preserved. The former is cast off in the lochia, while the latter, which contains the fundi of the glands, remains in situ and constitutes a matrix from which the new endometrium is regener-

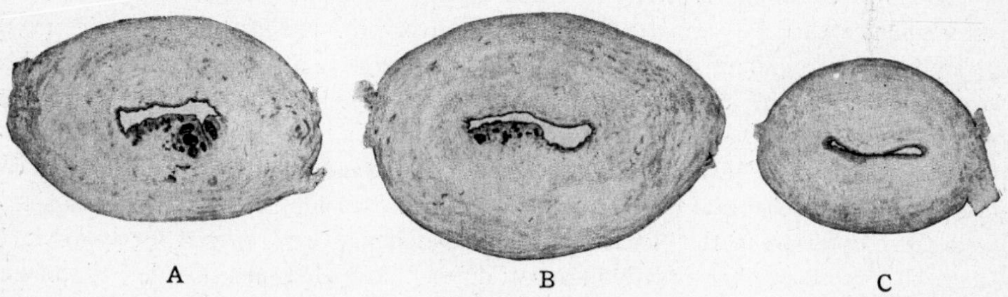

Fig. 309.—The Placental Site.
A, 17 days postpartum; B, 24 days postpartum; C, 120 days postpartum.
(From Williams, *American Journal of Obstetrics and Gynecology.*)

ated, its epithelium resulting from the proliferation of the gland cells, and its stroma from the connective tissue between them. The process of regeneration is rapid except at the placental site. Elsewhere, the free surface becomes covered by epithelium within a week or ten days, and the entire endometrium is restored by the end of the third week. On the other hand, six to seven weeks are required for the disappearance of the placental site in the normal puerperal woman, and according to Williams "it is not effected by absorption in situ, but rather by a process of exfoliation which is in great part brought about by the undermining of the placental site by the growth of endometrial tissue. This is effected partly by extension and down growth of endometrium from the margins of the placental site and partly by the development of endometrial tissue from the glands and stroma left in the depths of the decidua basalis after the separation of the placenta." Williams concluded that "such a process of exfoliation should be regarded as very conservative, and as a wise provision on the part of nature; otherwise great difficulty might be experienced in getting rid of the obliterated arteries and organized thrombi, which if they remained in situ would soon convert a considerable part of the mucosa into a mass of scar tissue, with the result that after a few pregnancies it would no longer be possible for it to go through its usual cycle of changes, and the reproductive career would come to an untimely end."

Changes in the Uterine Vessels. Immediately after the completion of the third stage of labor, the placental site is represented by an irregular, nodular, elevated area of about the size of the palm of the hand, the elevations being due to the presence of thrombosed vessels. This area decreases rapidly in size, so that it measures 3 to 4 cm. in diameter at the end of the second week, and only 1 to 2 cm. at the completion of the puerperium, although it still remains elevated above the general surface of the interior of the uterus and is tinged with blood pigment. Its original position remains recognizable for quite a long period, and even six months after childbirth appears as a slightly elevated pigmented area.

According to Hinselmann, the sinuses at the placental site do not undergo thrombosis during pregnancy, but the process becomes inaugurated during the latter portion of the second stage, during the third stage and particularly after completion of the third stage of labor, although many sinuses never become thrombosed, but are simply compressed by the contracting uterine muscle. The thrombi become organized by the proliferation of the intima of the vessels, and eventually are converted into typical connective tissue.

As the pregnant uterus requires a much more abundant blood supply than the nonpregnant organ, it is apparent that after delivery the lumens of its arteries must undergo a corresponding diminution in caliber. Formerly it was thought that this was brought about by a *compensatory endarteritis,* which disappeared in subsequent pregnancies. Now, however, the prevailing belief is that the larger vessels are completely obliterated by hyaline changes, and that new and smaller vessels develop in their stead. The absorption of the hyaline material is accomplished by processes similar to those observed in the ovaries, although the changes may persist for years, and under the microscope offer a ready means of differentiating between the uteri of women who have, and those who have not, borne children.

Changes in the Cervix, Vagina, and Vaginal Outlet. Immediately after the completion of the third stage, the cervix and lower uterine segment are represented by a soft, collapsed, flabby structure, whose boundaries can be made out only with difficulty. The margins of the external os are usually marked by depressions indicating the seat of lacerations. Its opening contracts slowly. For the few days immediately following labor it readily admits two fingers, but by the end of the first week it has become so narrow as to render difficult the introduction of one finger. What remains of the retraction ring comes in contact with the upper portion of the cervical canal, so that in digital examination the lower margin of the former may be mistaken for the internal os.

Stieve has pointed out that the body of the uterus and the cervix behave diametrically differently during the puerperium, in that the former undergoes involution, whereas in the latter a very considerable new formation of muscle cells occurs. Concomitant with this muscle hyperplasia and retraction of the cervix, healing of the lacerations occurs. Following the completion of involution, the external os does not assume its pregravid appearance in entirety, and varying degrees of an increase in the external opening and depressions at the site of the lacerations represent permanent changes, which are characteristic of women who have given birth through normal passages.

The vagina requires some time to recover from the distention to which it has been subjected. In the first part of the puerperium it is represented by a capacious smooth-walled passage, which gradually diminishes in size, though it rarely returns to its virginal condition. The rugae begin to reappear about the third week. The vaginal outlet is also markedly distended, and in primiparae usually bears the signs of more or less extensive laceration. The hymen, as such, has disappeared, and its place is taken by a number of small tags of tissue, which, as the process of cicatrization goes on, become converted into the *carunculae myrtiformes,* which are characteristic of the vaginal opening of parous women. The labia majora and minora become flabby and atrophic, as compared with their condition before childbirth.

Changes in the Peritoneum and Abdominal Wall. While these changes are taking place in the uterus and vagina, the pelvic peritoneum and the structures of the broad ligaments are accommodating themselves to the changed conditions of affairs. For the first few days after labor the peritoneum covering the lower part of the uterus is arranged in folds, which soon disappear. The broad and round ligaments are much more lax than in the nonpregnant condition, and require considerable time to recover from the stretching and loosening to which they have been subjected.

As a result of the changes in the abdominal wall including hyperplasia and hypertrophy of the muscle fibers, the rupture of the elastic fibers of the cutis and the prolonged distention due to the presence of the enlarged pregnant uterus, the abdominal walls remain soft and flabby for some time. The process of involution of these structures requires at least six weeks. Except for the presence of silvery striae, they gradually return to their original condition provided the abdominal muscles have retained their tonicity; but when this is much impaired they always remain lax and flabby. In not a few instances, particularly in small women of the hypoplastic type, there may be a marked separation or *diastasis of the recti muscles,* so that a considerable portion of the abdominal contents is covered simply by peritoneum, thinned-out fascia, and skin.

Changes in the Urinary Tract. Cystoscopic examination soon after delivery shows not only edema and hyperemia but frequently submucous extravasation of blood. At times the edema of the trigone is so marked as to be the cause of obstruction of the urethra and acute retention. In addition to these factors the puerperal bladder has an increased capacity and is not as sensitive to intravesical fluid tension as in the nonpregnant state, so that overdistention and incomplete emptying with the establishment of residual urine are common. The paralyzing effect of anesthesia and the temporarily disturbed function of the nerve supply to the bladder are undoubtedly contributory factors. Residual urine with the presence of bacteriuria in a traumatized bladder present the optimum conditions for the development of bladder infection. Taussig found the incidence of cystitis to be 3.8 per cent, while Prather reports 1.1 per cent. Following delivery the dilatation of the ureter and kidney pelvis undergoes involution rapidly in normal women and is complete within four to six weeks. The stretching and dilatation do not continue long enough to impair permanently the elasticity of the ureter unless infection has supervened.

Anatomy of the Breasts and Lactation. Each breast is made up of from 15 to 24 lobes, which are arranged more or less radially, and separated from one another by a varying amount of fat, to which the size and shape of the organ are in great part due. Each lobe consists of several lobules, which in turn are made up of large numbers of acini. These last are composed of a single layer of epithelium, beneath which is a small amount of connective tissue richly supplied with capillaries. Every lobule is provided with a small duct, which, meeting others, unites to form a single larger canal for each lobe. These so-called *lactiferous ducts* make their way to the nipple and open separately upon its surface, where they may be distinguished as minute isolated orifices. The acini represent the functioning portion of the breasts, and it is from their epithelium that the various constituents of the milk are formed.

We have already referred to the changes occurring in the breasts during pregnancy, and their condition remains much the same for the first two days after labor. At this time they do not contain milk, but a small amount of colostrum can be expressed from the nipples. This is a thin, yellowish fluid, which has a specific gravity of 1.030 to

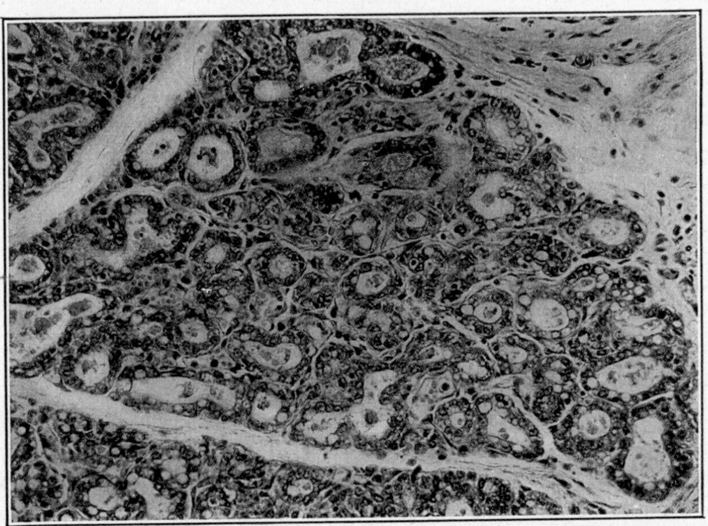

FIG. 310.—SECTION OF BREAST IN LATE PREGNANCY.

The lobules are large and the acinar cells contain fat droplets. (From Bell, *Textbook of Pathology,* Lea & Febiger, Philadelphia.)

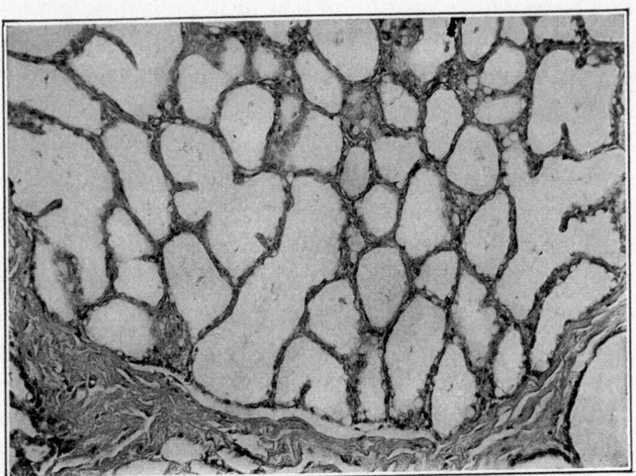

FIG. 311.—SECTION OF BREAST DURING LACTATION.

The acini are distended and the cells are filled with fat. (From Bell, *Textbook of Pathology,* Lea & Febiger, Philadelphia.)

1.035 and is alkaline in reaction. When examined under the microscope, colostrum is seen to consist of a fluid in which are suspended numerous round bodies, 0.001 to 0.025 mm. in diameter (the so-called *colostrum corpuscles*), which represent castoff epithelial cells which have undergone fatty degeneration. The fluid portion is a transudate which consists in great part of serum albumin, and coagulates on heating. Colostrum contains more protein material and salts, but less fat, than normal milk; while its sugar content is about the same.

Colostrum possesses only slight nutritive properties but acts as a mild cathartic. It has been suggested that its chief value consists in its euglobulin content, which can pass directly into the blood and apparently carries with it certain protective antibodies in which the child is deficient. According to this view, it is desirable for the newborn to receive its full ration of colostrum, whereby its immunity to various infections is increased. Doubtless, this may be correct in ruminants in which the structure of the cotyledonary placenta makes unlikely the transmission of such substances from mother to child, but it would appear improbable in man where the conditions for intra-uterine transmission are much more favorable.

The physiology of the phenomenon of lactation has in the past remained obscure. Extensive research in recent years has thrown considerable new light on the subject. The present conception of the process is that the development of the breast tissue during pregnancy is a necessary prerequisite. The alveolar cells, after completion of growth, begin to show secretory activity at about the middle of pregnancy. The growth of the duct system is evidently dependent upon the estrogenic hormone which probably stimulates the pituitary gland to produce increasing amounts of the duct-growth principle (Mammogen I), while the growth of the lobule-alveolar system is brought about by a second mammogenic hormone (Mammogen II), the production of which is dependent upon stimulation of the hypophysis by either progesterone alone or progesterone and estrone acting together. The experimental data, upon which this theory is based, are still incomplete. Nevertheless, we can state definitely that the growth of the mammary gland during pregnancy is dependent upon the interaction of the ovarian and mammogenic hormones.

After full proliferation of the gland is attained, as a result of these hormonal influences, lactation is induced and maintained by the lactogenic hormone of the anterior pituitary, although initiation of lactation may require the additional stimulus of the adrenal cortical hormone.

It appears then that the pituitary, through the ovarian hormones, regulates the necessary growth of the mammary gland system and provides the stimulus for actual milk secretion. Turner aptly writes: "No less important in the secretion of milk, however, is the indirect influence of the pituitary in regulating general metabolism (thyroid), and the metabolism of carbohydrate, fat, protein, and mineral matter. The abundance and availability of the precursors of milk in the blood make possible maximum milk production. While only the outline of this control mechanism is known, the studies with hypophysectomized animals are beginning to light a far reaching control system in which the pituitary and the other glands and organs act and react as the needs of the organism vary during the cycles of sexual activity, reproduction, and lactation."

Milk. On the third or fourth day after labor and occasionally on the second, the breasts suddenly become larger, firmer, and more painful. This indicates the establishment of the lacteal secretion, and on pressure a small amount of bluish-white fluid (the *milk*) will exude from the nipples. Coincident with these changes the patient experiences more or less lassitude, and may suffer from headache. At the same time she has throbbing pains in the breasts, which may extend into the axillae, and the pulse becomes slightly accelerated. There is rarely any elevation of temperature. It was formerly believed that the establishment of the milk flow was associated with marked constitutional disturbances, which were regarded as manifestations of the so-called *milk fever*. As has already been said, this is very exceptional, and usually a rise of temperature at this time is indicative of infection.

Mother's milk is usually bluish-white in color, though it sometimes has a yellowish tinge. It is slightly alkaline in reaction, and has a specific gravity of from 1.026 to 1.036, the average being 1.031. Under the microscope it appears as a clear fluid in which are suspended large numbers of small round bodies, 0.008 mm. in diameter (the so-called *milk corpuscles*). These consist of minute drops of fat surrounded by a membrane. Chemical examination shows that they are made up of the triglycerides of olein, palmitin, and stearin. The fluid portion of the milk is a transudate, and consists of protein material, milk sugar, salts, and water. Milk, therefore, represents an emulsion of fine fat droplets in a fluid medium.

The protein material in milk serum consists of one third casein and two thirds lactalbumin, which are direct metabolic products of the mammary epithelium, and differ from serum albumin in that they do not coagulate on heating. The fat and lactose, or milk sugar, are also products of the epithelial cells. The milk serum contains a considerable amount of mineral matter, one half of which, according to the investigations of Holt, consists of calcium phosphate and potassium carbonate, while the remainder is made up of sodium chloride, potassium chloride, potassium sulfate, magnesium carbonate, and minute quantities of several other salts, including iron.

The average composition of milk is as follows: proteins, 1 to 2 per cent; fats, 3 to 5 per cent; sugar, 6.5 to 8 per cent; salts, 0.1 to 0.2 per cent; the rest being water. According to Holt, the average composition of 17 twenty-four hour specimens of mature milk was as follows: proteins, 1.15; fat, 3.26; sugar, 7.5; and ash, 0.206 per cent, respectively; while in the so-called transitional period (from the end of the first to the fourth week) the protein and fat content is considerably greater, 1.56 and 4.37 per cent, respectively. Milk also contains a not inconsiderable number of bacteria, which, according to the researches of Köstlin, are derived from the terminal ends of the lactiferous ducts and the surface of the nipples; it is questionable whether they are present in the deeper portions of the breast.

Nutritious mother's milk varies markedly in its composition, not only in different individuals, but also in the same individual at various times. The variation in the composition of the milk of the same woman at different times is dependent upon various factors, principally the diet, the amount of exercise, and the mental condition. The quantity of milk varies to a large extent with the amount of fluid ingested by the patient, and a general diet rich in cow's milk conduces to increased mammary activity. The total diet should have an additional 1,000 calories to cover energy requirements in the secretion of milk and the caloric value of the milk itself.

There are large numbers of preparations on the market which are known as *galactagogues,* and are vaunted as increasing the amount of milk; but whatever virtue they may possess is due in great part to the quantity of fluid taken with them. Exercise in the open air also increases the milk flow, and it is frequently observed that a woman who has but a small quantity, so long as she is confined to her room, will secrete an abundant supply as soon as she begins to take outdoor exercise.

The quantity of the milk is likewise dependent in great part upon the food taken by the mother. It is a matter of experience that a diet rich in proteins increases the ratio of the fats, while excessive exercise diminishes the amount of protein material. Marked alterations in the quality and quantity of protein frequently result from nervous and mental influences, and it is not unusual for some profound emotion to lead to almost complete suppression of the lacteal secretion, or to so change its quality as to render it temporarily unfit for the use of the infant. Certain drugs also exert a marked influence upon the milk flow, and it is well known that the use of belladonna or atropine markedly diminishes it. Many substances ingested by the mother may be transmitted through the milk, and thus exert their physiologic influence upon the child. This is particularly true of opium and its derivatives, atropine, salicylates, iodides, bromides, quinine, lead and mercury. Alcohol, especially when consumed in large quantities, is secreted in the milk. Some allergens and immune bodies such as diphtheria antitoxin and typhoid agglutinins are known to be present at times in mother's milk.

It is generally believed that the occurrence of menstruation, or the onset of another pregnancy during lactation, exerts a very deleterious effect upon the quality of the milk, in some cases rendering it necessary to wean the child. When it is remembered how large a proportion of women menstruate while suckling, and how often the first indication of the occurrence of pregnancy in a nursing mother consists in the perception of fetal movements, it is apparent that the deleterious effect of such occurrences is overestimated. However, when the diagnosis of pregnancy is made it is usually advisable to wean the nursing infant for maternal reasons.

Nursing. The ideal food for the newborn child is the milk of its mother, and, unless lactation be contraindicated by some physical defect, it is the physician's duty to urge that every woman should at least attempt to suckle her child. In many instances where the supply of milk at first appears insufficient, it becomes increased in amount if sucking is persisted in. The act itself also exerts a beneficial influence upon the involution of the uterus, as it is well known that the repeated irritation of the nipples results in reflex stimulation of the uterus, and Temesváry has further proved by actual measurement that involution occurs more rapidly in nursing women.

CLINICAL ASPECTS OF THE PUERPERIUM

Postpartum Chill. Quite frequently the patient may have a more or less violent rigor, coming on shortly after the completion of the third stage of labor. This may be a nervous or vasomotor phenomenon, without prognostic significance. In this respect it stands in marked contrast to a chill occurring later in the puerperium, which usually indicates the onset of an acute infectious process. However, in a not inconsiderable percentage of patients exhibiting a postpartum chill blood cultures have proven the presence of bacteria in the circulating blood. Whether this phenomenon is purely nervous, vasomotor or due to a temporary bacteremia or some other cause such as the introduction into the circulation of foreign protein through the uterine veins, or the absorption of the metabolic products of the overworked uterine muscle cells, cannot be stated at the present time.

Temperature. The temperature should remain within normal limits during the puerperium; hence any rise should be regarded as abnormal, and considered as a sign of puerperal infection until convincing evidence to the contrary can be adduced. Occasionally the temperature may become slightly elevated toward the end or just after the completion of a difficult labor, but rarely goes above 100.4° F. (38° C.); it usually falls to normal within 24 hours, and does not rise again. A higher temperature occurring during labor usually indicates intrapartum infection, associated with bacterial invasion of the placenta, fetal membranes, liquor amnii or maternal tissues.

Owing to the fact that slight rises of temperature occur frequently during the puerperium without apparent cause, it is customary to designate as normal all puerperia in which the temperature remains below 100.4° F. (38° C.). Febrile puerperia, on the other hand, should include all patients in whom the temperature exceeds that limit in *any* two 24-hour periods of the puerperium, the first 24 hours postpartum only being excluded. Such a definition of puerperal morbidity is of value only when the temperature is accurately recorded *every four hours* and should include at least five readings per day; the sixth reading may be omitted at night if the patient can enjoy an otherwise uninterrupted sleep. This practice should be continued throughout the *entire* period of hospitalization. The practice of taking temperatures twice daily or at other irregular or infrequent intervals does not give by any means a true picture of the incidence of puerperal morbidity or afebrile puerperia. A review of the records of patients recently delivered in the New York Lying-In Hospital demonstrated that the incidence of puerperal morbidity would be only *one third* as high if the temperature had been recorded twice daily instead of every four hours. Stout found that in home deliveries where the temperature was recorded only once daily the morbidity was approximately *one tenth* that of the figure obtained when the four-hour system of recording temperatures was employed. This arbitrary differentiation between normal and febrile patients does not by any means preclude the existence of puerperal infection in the so-called normal patients. Indeed, we have encountered instances of serious thrombophlebitic types of infection where the temperature never exceeded 99.7° or 100° F. (37.6° or 37.8° C.). Such elevations in the temperature usually occurred daily. In still other cases a low-grade infection may be indicated by a repeatedly fluctuating temperature although it may never exceed the upper limits of normal; the daily variation is often one to two degrees centigrade.

It was formerly believed that the establishment of the lacteal secretion on the third or fourth day of the puerperium was naturally attended by a slight rise in temperature. Indeed, so prevalent was this idea that in preantiseptic times the so-called *milk fever* was regarded as a normal phenomenon. At present it is realized that no such entity exists, but on rare occasions extreme vascular and lymphatic engorgement may cause a sharp peak of fever for a few hours; this never lasts longer, however, than 12 hours at the most and, in general, any rise of temperature in the puerperium should excite the suspicion of endometritis.

Pulse. During the puerperium the pulse may be somewhat slower than at other times, averaging between 60 and 70. In nervous women, however, and in those who have had difficult labors or have suffered any considerable loss of blood, a more rapid rate than normal is not infrequent. In a certain number of cases, on the other hand, a day or two after the birth of the child, the pulse becomes unusually slow, and sometimes falls to 50, 40, or even fewer beats to the minute. Fehling has reported a case in which the rate was only 36. Ordinarily this phenomenon is quite transient and the pulse attains its normal rate by the end of the first week or 10 days. The slow pulse is usually regarded as a favorable prognostic sign, whereas a rapid heart action, unless it can be accounted for by hemorrhage or cardiac disease, should be looked upon with suspicion. This puerperal bradycardia is usually regarded as a characteristic phenomenon. In a series of cases reported by Lynch, a slowing of 10 or more beats per minute, as compared with pregnancy, was noted in 20.5 per cent, and occurred more than twice as frequently in multiparous as in primiparous women.

Numerous theories have been advanced from time to time in the attempt to explain its mode of production, but none of them is wholly satisfactory. It is conceivable that the change in the posture of the heart which occupies a position more medial and inferior to its prelabor position may play a role in the phenomenon. It is not impossible that the solution is quite simple, and may depend upon two factors: the absolute rest in bed, together with the great diminution in work which the heart is called upon to perform after the elimination of the uteroplacental circulation.

After-pains. In primiparous women the puerperal uterus tends to remain in a state of tonic contraction and retraction, unless it has been subjected to unusual distention, or blood clots or other foreign bodies have been retained in its cavity, as a consequence of which active contractions occur in the effort to expel them. In multiparous women, on the other hand, the uterus has lost part of its initial tonicity, so that persistent contraction and retraction cannot be maintained, and consequently it contracts and relaxes at intervals, the contractions giving rise to painful sensations, which are known as after-pains, and which occasionally are so severe as to require the administration of a sedative. In many patients these are particularly noticeable when the child is put to the breast, and may last for days, but ordinarily they lose their intensity and become quite bearable after the 48 hours immediately following delivery.

Lochia. During the first part of the puerperium there occurs normally a variable amount of vaginal discharge—the lochia. For the first few days after delivery it consists of blood-stained fluid—*lochia rubra;* after three or four days it becomes paler—*lochia serosa;* and after the tenth day, owing to a marked admixture with leukocytes, it assumes a whitish or yellowish-white color—*lochia alba.* It has a peculiar fleshy odor, suggesting fresh blood. In normal cases the total quantity of lochia varies between 500 and 1,000 gm., being less profuse in women who suckle their children. Foul-smelling lochia indicates infection with putrefactive bacteria. In many instances the reddish color is preserved for a longer period, but when it persists for more than two weeks it indicates the retention of small portions of the after-birth, or imperfect involution, which is frequently associated with retroflexion of the uterus. When examined under the microscope during the first few days, the lochia consists of red blood corpuscles, leukocytes, fatty epithelial cells, shreds of degenerated decidual tissue and bacteria. Micro-organisms can always be demonstrated in the vaginal lochia and are present in the majority of cases when the discharge has been obtained from the uterine cavity. Thus, in uterine cultures carried out on 37 normal, afebrile puerperas three days postpartum, Douglas and Rhees obtained sterile results in only 21.6 per cent of the cases. The organism most frequently found was the anaerobic streptococcus which was demonstrable in 56.7 per cent of the cultures. Similar results have been obtained by Guilbeau, Schaub and Andrews at the Johns Hopkins Hospital. Using a special technic (page 956) designed to eliminate vaginal contamination, these investigators carried out uterine cultures on 32 normal afebrile puerperas from 36 to 72 hours postpartum and obtained sterile cultures in only 6.2 per cent of the cases, the anaerobic streptococcus being present in 81.3 per cent. The colon bacillus, various anaerobic gram negative bacilli, staphylococci and gas bacilli are also encountered occasionally. It should be noted, however, that the aerobic beta-hemolytic streptococcus is never encountered in normal puerperas. Noguchi and Kalaki have shown that darkfield examination of normal vaginal lochia frequently reveals the presence of spirochetes, similar to those found in the mouth. They are usually of no pathogenic significance but may lead to serious diagnostic error unless this fact is realized.

Kessler, who has studied the hydrogen-ion concentration of the vaginal secretion, found that its pH changes from 4 to 5 during pregnancy to 6 to 7 during the puerperium, and that the normal acidity is not regained until five or six weeks after delivery.

Urine. One of the most striking phenomena of the puerperium is the diuresis which regularly takes place between the second and sixth days. As already noted, pregnancy is associated with an increased tendency of the body to retain water and this diuresis of the puerperium represents simply a reversal of this process and a return to normal of the water metabolism. It may amount to over 3,000 cc. a day.

In the majority of cases the examination of urine, removed by catheterization immediately after the completion of labor, shows a slight amount of albumin and numerous hyaline casts, even though both may have been absent throughout pregnancy. In a series of patients studied by Little, traces of albumin were noted in 89 per cent, and casts in 41 per cent. This is a transient phenomenon resulting from the systemic strain caused by labor and usually disappears within 24 hours, though in a certain number of cases traces of albumin persisted for some days, but always disappeared by the end of the second week, unless the patients were suffering from toxemia or chronic nephritis. It should be remembered that such statements apply only to urine obtained by catheterization, as voided specimens very frequently contain albumin so long as the lochia persists.

Dodds in a study of 281 normal patients has shown that the cultures of carefully obtained catheterized specimens of urine, secured on the third and ninth days, were sterile in 85.4 per cent. A colon bacilluria was present in 4.9 per cent, and bacteriuria due to other organisms was present in 9.6 per cent of her cases. No clinical evidence of infection in the urinary tract was present in any of these patients.

Occasionally substantial amounts of sugar may be found in the urine during the first weeks of puerperium. Careful investigation has shown that the reaction is due to the presence of lactose, or milk sugar, which is supposed to be absorbed from the mammary glands, so that the condition has no connection with diabetes. Ney observed it in 77 per cent of his cases, while McCann and Turner detected it in small quantities in every case which they examined. The question will be considered more fully in the section on glycosuria and diabetes in pregnant women.

A marked increase occurs in the amount of acetone in the urine immediately after labor, which disappears within the next three days. It may be found in 94 per cent of cases, and is most abundant after difficult and prolonged labors. Its production is due to the excessive breaking-up of carbohydrates resulting from the increased muscular activity incident to parturition and starvation.

Eastman and Lee have studied the creatine excretion during the puerperium. They found that the excretion of creatine in lactating women during the first two weeks of the puerperium started at a low level on the second day and increased rapidly until a very high level of excretion was reached by the end of the first week. In nonlactating women, on the other hand, the excretion rate is very high on the second day postpartum, and at the end of the first week only traces were excreted. These authors also differentiated puerperal creatinuria from the creatinuria found in patients with starvation and inanition, and exophthalmic goiter. Furthermore, they call attention to the parallelism between this condition and the establishment of lactation.

Blood. Most of the blood and metabolic alterations characteristic of pregnancy disappear within the first two weeks of the puerperium. An exception is found in blood fibrinogen which increases during the first week postpartum. Paralleling this trend, the blood sedimentation rate increases in rapidity; and in a series of cases studied at the New York Hospital, only two thirds had values within normal limits at the six weeks examination. Subinvolution and bleeding, however, were nearly always associated with an increased rate at that time.

A decided leukocytosis occurs during and just after labor, as shown by Hofbauer. He demonstrated that the leukocytes gradually increase in number from the onset of labor and reach a maximum 10 or 12 hours after its conclusion, at which time they are nearly twice as abundant as during pregnancy. Following long labors the count not infrequently reaches as high as 30,000. The lymphocytes show a marked relative and usually an absolute decrease in number. The eosinophiles are decreased or absent. The picture gradually returns to normal, as a rule, by the end of the first week postpartum, but even then, counts of 15,000 are occasionally met in entirely normal puerperas. During labor there is a tendency for the icterus index to increase. This is particularly true in prolonged labor when the icterus index may reach a value of 8 or even 10 units without any other evidence of pathologic change.

Loss of Weight. In addition to the loss of 6 to 6½ kg., which results from the evacuation of the contents of the uterus, there is generally a still further loss of body weight during the puerperium, which, according to Gassner, amounts to 4,500 gm. in the first week. Heil estimated it at 2,000, and Klemmer at only 900, gm. This apparent contradiction is due to the fact that at the time of Gassner's studies, the diet postpartum was greatly restricted. At present, when it is more liberal, the loss of weight is much less, and in many instances does not occur at all if sufficient food is taken. In normal women the loss is sometimes regained by the end of the puerperium. In an investigation of 2,502 normal pregnancies carried out by Stander and Pastore in the New York Lying-In Hospital, the average loss coincident with delivery was 5.35 kg. or 7.74 per cent of the body weight. An additional loss of 2.30 kg. or 3.77 per cent was noted during the first ten days of the puerperium. A further loss of 680 gm. or 1.11 per cent was sustained during the last five weeks of the puerperium. In other words, the total loss of weight from onset of labor to the sixth week postpartum averaged 8.33 kg. The primipara did not as a rule return to her original nonpregnant weight. Peckham has shown that approximately one half of the patients in his study gained weight during the year following discharge from the hospital.

General Functions. The function of the skin is markedly accentuated, as is demonstrated by the profuse sweating which frequently characterizes this period. It is most marked at night, and it is not unusual for the patient to awake from a sound sleep to find her nightgown drenched with perspiration. It passes off spontaneously and does not require treatment. The appetite is usually diminished during the first few days after labor, and the patient experiences little desire for food. At the same time, owing to the marked diaphoresis and the quantity of fluid lost through the lochial discharge, thirst is considerably increased. The bowels are nearly always constipated during the first days of the puerperium. This is due partly to inactivity, but principally to the relaxation of the abdominal walls and their consequent inability to aid in evacuating the intestinal contents.

CARE OF THE PATIENT DURING THE PUERPERIUM

Attention Immediately after Labor. After carefully examining the placenta just after its expulsion, to make sure that it is intact, the physician should devote his undivided attention to the patient in general and the condition of the uterus in particular. If all is well, any necessary perineal repair may be proceeded with. At this time the uterus should form a hard, round, resistant tumor, whose upper margin lies below the umbilicus. As long as it remains in this condition, there is no danger of postpartum hemorrhage from uterine atony, which becomes imminent if the uterus should grow soft and flabby. To guard against such an occurrence, the uterus should be gently palpated through the abdominal wall immediately after the conclusion of the third stage, and the maneuver repeated at frequent intervals. If the size and consistency remain unaltered it should be left absolutely alone; but if any tendency toward relaxation is detected, the organ should be grasped through the abdominal walls and gently massaged until it remains persistently contracted; at the same time pituitary extract or ergot should be administered hypodermically.

Intelligent interpretation of the condition of the uterus is essential to the successful management of this most critical time. The firm, hard, round uterus is due primarily to retraction of the muscle of this organ. Following this phenomenon the uterus contracts at more or less regular intervals. Unnecessary stimulation, in the absence of bleeding or increase in the size of the fundus, may stimulate premature contractions and cause undue fatigue which may later result in relaxation and hemorrhage.

Even in normal cases, the physician should not leave the patient immediately after the completion of labor, but should remain in constant attendance for at least one hour, so as to be available should any complication arise. If at the end of that period the uterus remains satisfactorily contracted, the patient can be safely left, but, if it is not, contractions should be stimulated by appropriate measures, and the behavior of the organ carefully watched until the physician feels assured that all danger of hemorrhage has passed. Occasionally, this may necessitate a wait of several hours. This type of bleeding may be concealed, the blood accumulating within the uterus, without external evidence of bleeding. This condition may be guarded against by the frequent palpation of the fundus at regular intervals during the first few days postpartum.

Toilet of the Vulva. Shortly after completion of the third stage of labor and any necessary repair of the perineum, the drapings and soiled linen beneath the patient are removed, providing there is no excessive bleeding or other reason to keep the patient in the lithotomy position. The external genitalia and buttocks are then bathed with an antiseptic solution. A sterile vulva pad, made of cotton wrapped in gauze, is then applied over the genitalia and held in place by a "T" bandage, being replaced by a clean one whenever necessary. The number of pads required in 24 hours varies according to the amount of lochial discharge, and affords a fairly accurate means of estimating its quantity. Twice daily, after each movement of the bowels, prior to catheterization and before any local treatment or examination, the external genitalia should be cleansed with sterile cotton pledgets, using liquid soap, followed by an antiseptic solution or sterile water, care being taken that the parts are washed from above downwards, the pledgets being discarded after a single application so as to avoid contamination from the rectum.

The vulvar pad not only absorbs the lochia and prevents contamination of the vulva from without, but also makes it difficult for the patient to touch her genitalia, a practice very common among the uneducated classes, and one that occasionally gives rise to infection.

Binder. An abdominal binder is unnecessary although it used to be thought that it aided involution and helped restore the patient's figure. It is now the consensus that it has no effect on the former process and may actually retard the latter by inhibiting the movements of the abdominal wall. If, however, the abdomen is unusually flabby or pendulous, or if the patient believes she would feel more comfortable with a binder, one may be applied for the first week of the puerperium.

After-pains. Since after-pains occur less frequently in primiparae it is not usually necessary to provide for their relief after the birth of a first child. On the other hand, after the delivery of a multiparous patient, it is often necessary to prescribe codeine and aspirin or other analgesic at intervals during the first few days of the puerperium, if the pains are severe. Not infrequently the uterine contractions are accentuated during nursing, giving rise to an increase of the symptoms at this time.

Early Ambulation. During the past decade important changes have taken place in the management of the puerperium in the direction of early ambulation. It is now the general (although not the universal) custom to allow normal patients out of bed 24 to 72 hours postpartum. The first day up, the puerpera usually sits in a chair in the morning and afternoon for a few minutes to half an hour; the next day, she walks a little about her room, followed by further walking on the next day. The advantages of early ambulation are many and appear to be confirmed by numerous well-controlled studies. Under this regime patients get their strength back much sooner; thus, multiparae, whose previous deliveries have been followed by 7 to 14 days entirely in bed, state that they feel better and stronger with early ambulation. Another advantage relates to bladder and bowel function. Thus, bladder complications leading to catheterization are greatly reduced, while constipation and distention are also less frequent.

The objections which have been raised against early ambulation have been shown to be more theoretical than actual. For instance, Rosenblum, Melinkoff and Fist find less abnormal bleeding in early risers, report uterine involution as being uniformly good, find no effects on episiotomies or abdominal wounds and have encountered no increase in uterine prolapse or retroversion at later examination. In a similar investigation Guerriero reports comparable findings and concludes that early ambulation offers advantages to the obstetric patient without imposing any disadvantages. The experience of others, including ourselves, has been similar.

With this regime it is possible to send patients home much earlier than was formerly the custom and, when the pressure for beds is great, it is not unusual for women to be released from the hospital as early as the fourth or fifth day; and discharge on the sixth or seventh day is common. In this connection it should be recalled that early ambulation and the duration of hospital stay are two different matters and that the former does not necessarily entail early release from the hospital. The manifold duties and responsibilities which most mothers assume when they go home, are sufficiently onerous as to make extremely early discharge detrimental in some cases and it is my opinion that the optimal hospital stay is 10 days even with early ambulation. Certain advantages accrue also to the baby from more prolonged hospitalization.

Diet. Formerly it was the custom to restrict to a minimum the diet of the puerperal woman, and, as has already been said, this limitation goes far to explain the loss of weight which was frequently observed during the first few days. At present, however, a more liberal allowance is customary, and the patient is encouraged to take plenty of plain nourishing food.

If not nauseated, she should be given a glass of milk or a cup of tea soon after labor. For the first few days the appetite is not vigorous, but small quantities of easily digested food may be taken at frequent intervals. A liquid diet is usually employed on the day of delivery followed by a soft diet of approximately 2,500 calories on the first day postpartum, and during the remainder of the puerperium a general diet containing about 3,000 calories which includes at least one and one-half quarts of milk. Intermediate fluid nourishment with a milk or fruit juice base is given three times daily. The total daily fluid intake should reach at least 3,000 cc.

The diet of the lactating mother should be like that taken during her antepartum period, with the addition of a pint of milk, bringing her total milk intake up to a quart and a half a day. Again it should be stressed that this need not all be taken as fluid milk, but that some may be incorporated in cooking. Such a diet will supply the nutritional requirements for lactation recommended by the Committee on Food and Nutrition of the National Research Council.

Temperature. The temperature should be carefully watched during the first two weeks of the puerperium, as fever is usually the first symptom of the onset of an infectious process. If the patient is in a hospital or in the charge of a trained nurse the temperature should be taken five times daily—at 6 A.M., 10 A.M., 2 P.M., 6 P.M., and 10 P.M., and recorded upon a suitable chart. The physician should be immediately notified if it rises above 100° F. But when the patient is cared for at home and a nurse is not available, the temperature should be taken by the physician himself, morning and evening, for the first five days. This, of course, means that during that time he must visit the patient twice a day, once a day for the following two or three days, and afterward at less frequent intervals. But if a competent nurse is in attendance, a single daily visit will suffice, unless untoward symptoms develop. It is well, whenever possible, that the patient be seen within the first 12 hours following delivery.

Urination. Every effort should be made to induce patients to void within six hours after delivery. A voiding must measure 100 cc. to be considered satisfactory. If, within the first eight hours after delivery, the patient does not void 100 cc. at any one time, she should be catheterized and earlier than eight hours if there is any suspicion that the bladder is distended. Routine catheterization should be continued every eight hours unless the patient is able to void 100 cc. or more at a time, and only then may it be discontinued. Moreover, if at any time there is evidence of bladder distention, one should not await the end of the eight-hour period mentioned, but catheterize at once. It should be emphasized that patients who are having or who recently have had intravenous fluids, are very likely to develop a full bladder.

They should be watched especially in this regard and treated accordingly. Moreover, patients who have had analgesia in labor may not be aware that the bladder is full and should be observed for this condition with particular care.

Bowels. In view of the sluggishness of the bowels in the puerperium, a mild cathartic should be administered on the evening of the second day, unless they have previously moved spontaneously. If evacuation has not occurred by the morning of the third day, a soapsuds enema should be employed. With early ambulation, constipation in the puerperium is less a problem than formerly, but it is frequently necessary to repeat the laxative or the enema from day to day.

Care of the Nipples. Contrary to previous attitudes, the nipples require little attention in the puerperium other than simple cleanliness and attention to fissures. Since crustations from dried milk are likely to accumulate and irritate the nipples, cleansing of the areolae with sterile water and soap before each nursing is desirable. Sore nipples are a frequent complaint. They are best treated with tincture of benzoin, lanolin, penicillin ointment, or one of the commercial preparations compounded for the purpose. Occasionally it is necessary to resort to a nipple shield for 24 hours.

Posture and Exercises. All normal patients should have one hour's rest in the midday. During this rest hour they are instructed to lie on their abdomens. This posture should be assumed by all puerperal women because of the high incidence of retroversion of the uterus in the puerperium.

Because of the extensive changes in the abdominal wall already referred to, physical exercises directed toward strengthening the abdominal wall muscles may be desirable. The most important of these, such as deep breathing, head and shoulder raising exercises, may be commenced between the fifth and seventh day. If these exercises are practiced, they should be carried out twice daily and continued until the end of the fifth or sixth week.

Reappearance of Menstruation. If for any reason the woman does not suckle her child, the menstrual flow will probably return within eight weeks after labor. On the other hand, it is generally believed that the flow ordinarily does not appear so long as the child is suckled, or at least not until it is nearly a year old. In our experience, the greatest possible variations are observed in this respect, as in lactating women the first period may occur as early as the second or as late as the eighteenth month following delivery, with the most usual time during the fourth month. It is, likewise, generally believed that ovulation does not occur during lactation, and many women suckle their children for long periods in the hope of avoiding conception. That the belief is not justified is shown by the fact that not a few women conceive in such circumstances. Pinard stated that from 40 to 73 per cent of his patients menstruated within six months after the birth of the child, and that the function becomes re-established later in multiparous than in primiparous women. Ehrenfest, in 1915, stated that 51.3 per cent of his patients menstruated within three months and 71 per cent within six months after delivery; while in 80 per cent menstruation occurred before the cessation of lactation. Peckham in a study of 2,885 patients, who were examined one year postpartum, found that menstruation returned prior to the cessation of lactation in 71.45 per cent of his cases. Furthermore, in 35.09 per cent of instances menstruation occurred seven or more months prior to the end of lactation. He also found that the average duration of lactation was almost three months more than the mean time interval between delivery and menstruation. Following the cessation of lactation, if menstruation has not already returned, it is usual for it to do so within two months.

Follow-up Examination. The patient should return for examination about six weeks postpartum. At this time the general physical condition of the patient should be investigated, the blood pressure taken, the urine examined for albumin, the condition of the abdominal walls noted, the breasts inspected and a thorough pelvic examination carried out. Any abnormalities found, such as cervicitis, can be treated at this time and arrangements made for further treatment or examinations if indicated.

BIBLIOGRAPHY

DODDS, G. H. Bacteriuria in Pregnancy, Labor and the Puerperium. J. Obst. & Gynaec. Brit. Emp., 1931, 38:773.

DOUGLAS, R. G., and RHEES, H. S. Bacteriological Findings in the Uterus during Labor and the Early Puerperium. Am. J. Obst. & Gynec., 1934, 27:203.

EASTMAN, N. J., and LEE, S. W. Puerperal Creatinuria. Chinese M. J., 1932, 46:143.

EHRENFEST, H. The Reappearance of Menstruation after Childbirth. Am. J. Obst., 1915, 72:577.

FAHRAEUS, R. The Suspension Stability of the Blood. Acta. med. Scandinav., 1921, 55:1.

GASSNER. Ueber die Veränderungen des Körpergewichtes bei Schwangeren, Gebärenden u. Wöchnerinnen. Monatschr. f. Geburtsh., 1862, 15:1.

GOODALL, J. R. The Involution of the Puerperal Uterus. Am. J. Obst., 1909, 60:921.

GUERRIERO, W. F. Early Controlled Ambulation in the Puerperium. Am. J. Obst. & Gynec., 1946, 51:210.

GUILBEAU, J. A., SCHAUB, I., and ANDREWS, M. C. Penicillin Treatment in the Obstetrical Patient. A Study of Its Effect on the Bacterial Flora of the Postpartum Uterus. Am. J. Obst. & Gynec., 1949, 58:101.

HARDING, V. J., and MONTGOMERY, R. C. Nitrogen Metabolism in the Puerperium. J. Biol. Chem., 1927, 73:27.

HEIL, K. Untersuchungen über die Körpergewichtsverhältnisse normaler Wöchnerinnen. Arch. f. Gynäk., 1896, 51:18.

HINSELMANN, H. Die angebliche, physiologische Schwangerschaftsthrombose, etc. Ztschr. f. Geburtsh. u. Gynäk., 1913, 73:146.

HOFBAUER, J. Zur Physiologie des Puerperiums. Monatschr. f. Geburtsh. u. Gynäk., 1897, V. Ergänzungsheft, ff. 52.

HUBBARD, R. S., and BROCK, H. J. Lactose in the Plasma of Pregnant and Lactating Women. J. Biol. Chem., 1935, 110:411.

LYNCH, F. W. The Bradycardia of the Puerperium. Surg., Gynec. & Obst., 1911, 12:441.

——— Retroversions of the Uterus following Delivery. Am. J. Obst. & Gynec., 1922, 4:362.

MCCANN, F. S., and TURNER, W. A. On the Occurrence of Sugar in the Urine during the Puerperal State. Tr. Obst. Soc., 1892, 34:473.

NEUMANN, H. O. Die Senkungsgeschwinddikeit der roten Blutkoerperchen unter der Geburt und im Wochenbett. Zentralbl. f. Gynäk., 1925, 49:586.

NOGUCHI, H., and KALAKI. The Spirochetal Flora of the Normal Female Genitalia. Stud. Rockefeller Inst. M. Research, 1920, 32:141.

NOVAK, J., and JETTER, L. Beitrag zur Kenntniss der puerperalen Bradycardia. Monatschr. f. Geburtsh. u. Gynäk., 1910, 32:531.

PECKHAM, C. H. An Investigation of Some Effects of Pregnancy Noted Six Weeks and One Year After Delivery. Bull. Johns Hopkins Hospital, 1934, 54:186.

PIZZOLATO, P., and BEARD, H. H. Creatine-creatinine Metabolism and the Hormones. Endocrinology, 1939, 24:358.

PRATHER, G. C. Postpartum Bladder Complications. Am. J. Obst. & Gynec., 1929, 17:215.

ROSENBLUM, G., MELINKOFF, E., and FIST, H. S. Early Rising in the Puerperium. J.A.M.A., 1945, 129:849.

SLEMONS, J. M. Involution of the Uterus and Its Effect upon the Nitrogen Output of the Urine. Bull. Johns Hopkins Hosp., 1914, 21:195.

TEACHER, J. H. On the Involution of the Uterus Post Partum. J. Obst. & Gynaec. Brit. Emp., 1927, 34:1.

WILLIAMS, J. W. Regeneration of the Uterine Mucosa after Delivery with Especial Reference to the Placental Site. Am. J. Obst. & Gynec., 1931, 22:664.

19

THE NEWBORN

The Cause of the Onset of Respiration at Birth. Normally, the newborn infant begins to cry almost immediately after its exit from the vulva. This act indicates the establishment of active respiration, which is accompanied by important modifications in the circulatory system. The mode of production of the first breath has given rise to much speculation but has remained, at least until recent years, something of an enigma. Of the various explanations which have been advanced, the most noteworthy are as follows:

Physical Stimulation. This is the nineteenth century theory of Preyer which postulates that the handling of the infant incident to delivery, its contact with air and with various surfaces which are rough in comparison to the amnion, provokes respiration through stimuli reaching the respiratory center from the skin. *Objection:* Rough abdominal palpation, the application of forceps to the infant's head and attempts at version and extraction do not initiate breathing as long as the fetus is in utero with the placental circulation intact. The view that skin irritation as the result of exposure to air and change of temperature causes the infant to breathe was refuted by Ahlfeld, who delivered several women in warm saline baths and found that respiration began as usual.

Compression of Fetal Thorax Incident to Delivery. In the x-ray studies of Warnekros, he noted an almost conical compression of the thorax during the second stage, and suggested that the expansion which must inevitably follow the delivery of the shoulders would afford a possible explanation for the first inspiratory movement. *Objection:* Babies born at cesarean section usually cry satisfactorily and sometimes just as quickly as babies born vaginally. Nevertheless, it is well known that cesarean section babies do not regularly breathe as promptly or as satisfactorily as infants born per vaginam and it may well be that the compression of the thorax incident to vaginal delivery constitutes an auxiliary factor in the initiation of respiration.

Carbon Dioxide Accumulation. Since theories based on physical processes such as the above, fail to furnish a rational explanation of the onset of respiration, attention for many years centered on biochemical interpretations of this phenomenon. This trend would seem only logical in view of the known chemical factors which influence respiration in the adult. One of these has to do with the effects of increased tension of carbon dioxide in the blood. During the interval between the interruption of the placental respiratory exchange and the establishment of pulmonary respiration, it is obvious that this gas would tend to rise in the infant's blood and, since it is a recognized respiratory stimulant, it would seem a logical presumption that its increased tension brings about the first breath. In studies which I carried out a number of years ago on this question, and in which the carbon dioxide tension of the blood in infants at birth was studied, it was discovered that respiration began just the same whether the tension of this gas was high or low and seemed indeed to bear no relationship to the carbon dioxide tension whatsoever. Accordingly, as a sole explanation of the onset of respiration at birth, this hypothesis seems to me unlikely, but along with other factors it may well play a role.

Oxygen Deprivation. It is Barcroft's opinion, as the result of experimental work done on the goat, that lack of oxygen is the cause of the onset of respiration at birth and, as he phrases it, "We are faced with the remarkable paradox that the dying (that is, anoxemic) gasp of the fetus is the earnest of life to the individual." *Objection:* A vast amount of experimental work, as well as many observations on aviators at high altitudes, has made it clear that profound lack of oxygen regularly produces apnea. If minor degrees of anoxemia produce the first respiration of the fetus at birth, some certain facts become difficult to explain. In the first place, when nitrous oxide oxygen anesthesia is administered to pregnant women, the fetus, as we have emphasized in a previous chapter, always suffers considerable anoxemia, and if minor levels of oxygen want constitute the sole cause of respiration at birth we would expect such fetuses to make violent respiratory efforts in utero. There is no evidence that they do. Actual studies of the oxygen content of the blood at birth show no relationship between the concentration of this gas and respiration except possibly the circumstance that infants with high oxygen levels breathe more readily and those with extremely low oxygen, as has been stated, are apneic. Moreover, all chemical theories of the onset of respiration at birth break down in the face of the following evidence: at low cervical cesarean section performed under local or spinal anesthesia, it is possible through a small incision in the lower uterine segment to expose the baby's face and observe it crying vigorously in utero.

Intra-uterine Respiration. The above observation that at low cervical cesarean section, the baby may be observed to cry in utero, is in keeping with only one explanation of the onset of respiration at birth, namely, that it is simply the continuation of intra-uterine respiratory movements which have been occurring throughout the greater part of pregnancy. This topic has already been discussed on page 181. Although shallower, these respiratory movements resemble qualitatively the respiratory movements observed after birth. There is great variation in respiratory activity among rabbit fetuses in the same uterine horn, some being quiescent, others respiring at independent rates up to 60 per minute. The rate usually increases during the first half hour of an experiment and thereafter remains fairly constant. In general, respiratory activity increases near term with the age of the fetus. It is important to note that a number of anesthetic agents—ether, paraldehyde, sodium phenobarbital, and sodium pentobarbital—given to the mother in amounts that do not impair her respiration but merely induce light anesthesia are nevertheless found to depress seriously or even to inhibit completely the intra-uterine respiration in the fetus. That these same drugs when given to the human parturient tend to retard the onset of respiration in the infant at birth, is in keeping with the viewpoint that the onset of breathing immediately after delivery is dependent, at least to a certain extent, on the unimpaired activity of these intra-uterine respiratory movements. Snyder and Rosenfeld have obtained no evidence of stimulation or initiation of intra-uterine respiration by oxygen want. Thus, anoxemia induced in the mother by administration of a gas mixture containing 4 per cent oxygen and 5 per cent carbon dioxide in nitrogen produced immediate slowing or cessation of fetal respiratory movements though the maternal respiration was greatly stimulated. Upon replacement of the low oxygen mixture by air, fetal respiration usually returned to normal, but prolonged or excessive anoxemia caused permanent impairment. Moreover, carbon dioxide in 5 and 7.5 per cent concentrations in air and in oxygen, administered to the mother for periods up to 15 minutes, failed to influence fetal respiration to a significant degree though an occasional increase in rate was noted.

On the basis of these studies, Snyder and Rosenfeld regard the onset of postnatal respiratory activity not as an event initiated abruptly at birth but rather as a transition from the type of respiratory movement discernible during intra-uterine life.

As already indicated, the whole phenomenon of intra-uterine respiration and its bearing on the onset of respiration at birth, is not universally accepted. Indeed, one of the most competent and assiduous students in this field, Windle, questions it seriously. Experiments carried out by Windle and his associates, contrary to the findings of Snyder and Rosenfeld, indicate that experimental anoxemia induces aspiration on the part of some, but not of all the intra-uterine fetuses. They also point out the well-known clinical fact that difficult labor with consequent fetal asphyxia often produces aspiration of amniotic fluid and that such aspiration of amniotic fluid has long been regarded both by obstetricians and pathologists as a not uncommon cause of intra-uterine and early neonatal death. This question is therefore a moot one, but after extensive contact with the problem, it is my opinion that Snyder and Rosenfeld are essentially correct and that intra-uterine respiration of the fetus probably constitutes the most important, although possibly not the only, factor in the initiation of respiration at birth.

Circulatory Changes. As soon as the lungs begin to function, the blood which is brought by the inferior vena cava to the right auricle no longer passes through the foramen ovale, but makes its way directly through the right ventricle, whence it is carried to the lungs by means of the pulmonary arteries. Coincident with the establishment of the pulmonary circulation, there ensues a marked increase in the pressure in the left auricle. This in turn brings about the closure of the valve of the foramen ovale, which after a few months fuses with the periphery of the opening. At the same time the blood ceases to flow through the ductus Botalli into the aorta, and the canal itself gradually becomes obliterated. According to Strassmann, the primary cause for this change is to be found in the fact that the ductus traverses the wall of the aorta in an oblique direction, so that, as soon as the pressure in the aortic arch is increased, its wall acts as a valve and in this way occludes the distal end.

The circulation through the umbilical arteries normally ceases in from 5 to 15 minutes after birth, pulsation disappearing first at the maternal end of the cord. This is brought about by the contraction of the thick muscular walls, which practically obliterate the lumens of the arteries. Occasionally, however, when the cord has not been ligated sufficiently tightly, secondary hemorrhage may occur from its fetal end after the child has been placed in a warm bed. To guard against such an occurrence the cord should be reinspected before the physician leaves the patient.

The child passes urine almost immediately after birth, and frequently while in the act of being born. In a considerable number of cases a certain amount of meconium is also discharged. As a result of the cooling of the surface of the child on coming into the world, its temperature becomes reduced by a few degrees, which, however, are promptly regained after it has been bathed and placed in a warm bed. For the first few days of life the temperature is in very unstable equilibrium, and a very slight cause may give rise to considerable fluctuations above or below the normal level.

The Umbilical Cord. Immediately following delivery the child is grasped securely by the ankles and suspended while any mucus is sponged out of the mouth with the other hand. The cord is then doubly clamped about 5 to 6 cm. from the

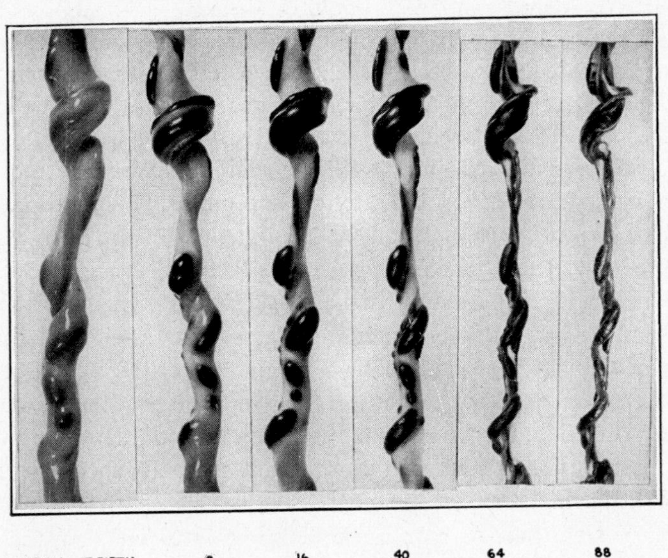

FIG. 312.—DESICCATION OF A SEGMENT OF UMBILICAL CORD WHEN LAID ON A NONABSORBENT SURFACE AND EXPOSED TO AIR.

abdomen and cut between the clamps. A ligature of sterilized bobbin or tape should be placed about it and tied tightly in two places, about 2 and 4 cm., respectively, from the surface of the abdomen, the cord being bent upon itself. It is then covered with a dry, sterile dressing.

Owing to the absence of circulation, what is left of the cord undergoes a process of mummification. Within 24 hours it loses its characteristic bluish-white moist appearance, and soon becomes dry and almost black (Fig. 312). Gradually a line of demarcation appears just beyond the skin surface of the abdomen, until in a few days the stump sloughs off, leaving behind a small granulating wound, which, after healing, forms the umbilicus.

This separation usually takes place within the first two weeks after birth, separation taking place most frequently on the tenth day, but it is not unusual for it to require a longer time, and occasionally several weeks may elapse before it occurs. In the very rare instances in which the stump is still adherent at the end of the puerperium, it may become necessary to clip it off with a pair of scissors.

Formerly the care of the cord was considered a very trivial matter, and the midwife, as a rule, would wrap it in a piece of greased or singed linen, after which little or no attention was paid to it. This practice, however, and the total neglect of aseptic precautions frequently resulted in an infection which was transmitted through the umbilical vessels, so that in times past large numbers of children perished from so-called "puerperal fever," as well as from tetanus neonatorum. Even now, when the necessity for proper treatment is generally recognized, umbilical infections are not unknown. In a study of all neonatal deaths occurring among 32,290 babies born in the New York Lying-In Hospital during the 11 years immediately prior to September first, 1943, one death was ascribed to this cause but in this instance the umbilicus was not positively proven the source of the peritoneal infection.

Usually these umbilical infections indicate gross lack of care, but occasionally they occur in spite of every precaution. As the umbilical stump in such cases frequently presents no outward sign of infection, the condition cannot be diagnosed definitely without a thorough autopsy. Accordingly, it may be stated as a safe general rule that, whenever children die without any appreciable cause within three weeks after birth, such an infection should be suspected, and, if an autopsy is performed, examination of the intra-abdominal portion of the umbilical vessels will frequently show that they are filled with purulent thrombi, in which pyogenic micro-organisms can be demonstrated. In view, therefore, of the not inconsiderable danger of infection from this source, strict aseptic precautions should be observed in caring for the cord. The reader is referred to Ploss' work for interesting details concerning its treatment in various countries and by aboriginal peoples.

Following ligature of the cord it is covered with a sterile dressing saturated with 70 per cent alcohol. The cord is inspected daily and a dry sterile dressing applied until the cord is separated and the umbilicus dry. At the time of dressing it is important to direct the stump of the cord upward which diminishes the frequency of soiling of the dressings with urine especially in male infants.

From time to time various methods have been recommended in place of the time-honored ligature as, for instance, cutting the cord with red hot scissors, compressing it by powerful forceps, as in angiotripsy, the use of specially devised metallic clamps such as those of Kahn, Hesseltine and White, of rubber bands (Carrington and Kanner) or of Ziegler's ingenious rubber device. A recent comparative study conducted in the New York Hospital showed that the new all-metal Ziegler clamp and one devised by Pastore gave better results than ligatures. The cord clamps prevented subsequent hemorrhage, reduced the amount of care of the cord, gave uniformly better results and resulted in a marked increase in the percentage of babies with cords separated at the time of discharge from the hospital. On the other hand, after trying out various clamps, we have reverted to the use of ligatures at the Johns Hopkins Hospital on the grounds that in our hands, at least, they are simpler, safer and as satisfactory in general as the clamp.

Care of the Eyes. In view of the frequency with which the eyes of the newborn child become infected when passing through the birth canal of women suffering from gonorrhea, Credé in 1884 introduced the practice of instilling into each eye immediately after birth one drop of a 1 per cent solution of silver nitrate, which was afterward washed out with salt solution. This procedure has led to a marked decrease in the frequency of gonorrheal ophthalmia and the cases of blindness resulting from it, and should be followed as a matter of routine as soon as the cord is cared for. The following technic is recommended:

As a preliminary precaution the region about each eye should be irrigated with sterile water. This should be applied to the side of the eye nearest the nose and allowed to run off from the opposite side. Then, the lower lid should be drawn down and the silver solution dropped into the lower cul-de-sac, whence in the course of two minutes it diffuses itself over the entire conjunctiva. At the expiration of that time the lids should be held apart and the conjunctival sac freely flushed with warm normal salt solution by means of a rubber eye syringe. This serves the double purpose of washing out the excess of silver nitrate, and of forming an insoluble compound with any fraction of it which by chance should be retained.

Cohn estimated, in 1876, that 30 per cent of the patients in the blind asylums of Germany, Austria, Holland, and Switzerland owed their trouble to ophthalmia neonatorum. Twenty years later these figures had become reduced to 19 per cent; while Credé-Hörder, in 1912, reported a further diminution to 12.39 per cent. J. J. Carroll stated that 30 per cent of the inmates of the Maryland School for the Blind, in 1909, owed their blindness to the same cause, and that its incidence had increased rather than decreased during the previous twenty years. The more general adoption of prophylactic measures, following state laws and health department regulations which are now existent in nearly all states and provinces of the United States and Canada, has caused a great decrease in the incidence of blindness due to ophthalmia neonatorum. The percentage of new pupils in United States schools for the blind whose blindness was due to this disease has fallen from 28.2 per cent in 1906 to 5.6 per cent in 1942.

In the New York Lying-In Hospital between 1935 and 1945, gonorrheal ophthalmia developed in 6 among 32,290 newborn, an incidence of 0.02 per cent, or once in 5,380 cases, despite the prophylactic treatment described above. In 35,000 newborn observed at the Johns Hopkins Hospital between 1925 and 1946, who were treated by the same technic, there were 14 cases, an incidence of 0.04 per cent, or once in 2,500 cases. In pre-penicillin days, the frequency of the disease throughout the country was probably similar to these percentages. With the advent of penicillin, however, it would be difficult to ascertain even the approximate frequency of the condition since today any infant with substantial conjunctival discharge usually receives this antibiotic at once, often without bacteriologic examination, and since immediate cure is the rule, few cases last long enough to become established. The frequency with which gonorrheal ophthalmia develops despite silver nitrate prophylaxis will depend in large measure on whether or not the solution actually gets into the conjunctival sac. It seems probable, indeed, that the occasional failures of this preventive measure are not to be charged against silver nitrate per se, but against faulty technic in its instillation.

Zweifel, in 1900, advocated substituting a 1 per cent solution of silver acetate for the nitrate, and reports that, in a series of 5,222 children so treated, ophthalmia was observed in only 0.23 of 1 per cent. The employment of protargol, argyrol, sophol, and various other preparations of silver has been suggested, but experience has shown that they give no better results than silver nitrate. Care should be taken that only fresh solutions are employed, as they rapidly deteriorate on keeping, especially when exposed to the light. The technic can be simplified and made safer by the use of wax ampules which are extensively used at the present time. Because of the possibility of error in the strength of solution instilled, the wax ampule is preferable to bottled solutions. Hartman has suggested the use of silver acetate instead of the nitrate solution, in order to prevent the chemical conjunctivitis sometimes caused by the latter salt.

The silver nitrate procedure produces a discernible chemical conjunctivitis in over half the cases. Thus, in 716 infants in our clinic, who were treated with silver nitrate and who were inspected daily in regard to ocular status, 55.6 per cent showed one or more signs of irritation, such as redness, edema or discharge. Redness was demonstrable in 49.7 per cent, edema in 48.3 per cent and discharge in 32.1 per cent. These signs of irritation, however, were transient and in no case caused any permanent damage. Indeed, in the whole history of our clinic, covering over 70,000 deliveries, no single instance has occurred in which the prophylactic use of silver nitrate *in the correct concentration,* produced any permanent injury to the infant's eyes.

With the demonstration that penicillin was highly gonococcocidal, the question naturally arose as to whether it might not be preferable to silver nitrate as a prophylactic agent against ophthalmia neonatorum. Over the past three years this problem has been studied in Baltimore at the Johns Hopkins Hospital and at Sinai Hospital. On the basis of over 10,000 cases in which penicillin, either intramuscularly or as an ointment, has been employed instead of silver nitrate, our impressions are as follows:

1. Since no case of gonorrheal ophthalmia has developed in these 10,000 cases, the efficacy of penicillin for this purpose, whether given intramuscularly or instilled locally as an ointment, cannot be questioned. It is probably, indeed, a more effective prophylactic agent than silver nitrate. Support is lent to this statement by the fact that whenever a case of gonorrheal ophthalmia does develop today, penicillin cures it within a few hours, whereas silver nitrate (whose record as a therapeutic agent in the old days was poor) has long since been abandoned for this purpose.
2. The incidence of chemical irritation with penicillin ointment or with penicillin intramuscularly is much less than with silver nitrate. Among 706 infants treated with penicillin ointment in our clinic, one or more signs of irritation were present in 16.6 per cent and among 705 managed with intramuscular penicillin, in 20.0 per cent, as compared with 55.6 per cent in the silver nitrate series. In those cases in which irritation did occur, it was milder.
3. On the other hand, penicillin has the disadvantage that it is not suitable for home obstetrics since, at the present writing, solutions of it must be kept in a refrigerator.
4. Care must be exercised that penicillin is not used beyond the expiration date.
5. Penicillin sensitivity may be produced but in our experience this is rare.
6. When given intramuscularly to syphilitic babies pencillin may give rise to Herxheimer reactions.

In sum, there are certain advantages and disadvantages to each technic. The most grave objection to silver nitrate, unless wax ampules are used, is the possibility of error in its preparation, a 10 per cent solution being compounded instead of a 1 per cent. Many such mistakes have been made throughout the country and a number of babies blinded thereby. At the present time, the use of a silver preparation is mandatory by statute in most states and whether these regulations will be changed to sanction the hospital use of penicillin for this purpose, whenever the physician prefers it to silver nitrate, remains to be seen.

Care of the Skin. The necessity for strict aseptic precautions at all times is of the greatest importance especially in hospital practice. Laundering of infant clothing demands meticulous care, following which sterilization should be effected. The hands of every attendant coming in contact with the infant should be carefully washed beforehand.

Keiffer considers that the vernix caseosa represents a secretion from the amniotic epithelium, and is absorbed by the skin of the child. For this reason he recommends that it not be removed, as he believes that it has a nutritional function and tends to diminish the initial loss of weight. Although Keiffer's recommendation was made many years ago, it has not been widely accepted until the past decade when removal of the vernix has been rather generally abandoned. The blood, any meconium and excess vernix are removed with cotton pledgets shortly after birth. Handling of the baby is reduced to a minimum; the skin folds are inspected each day, and following change of diapers a bland, lanolin-petrolatum base lotion is applied to the groin and is also used to cleanse the baby after a bowel movement. To the cord a dry dressing is applied in the delivery room, to be followed by an alcohol dressing when the initial care is given in the nursery. The daily care of the cord consists of inspection and if found dry no further alcohol is applied, while if moist the area is cleansed with 75 per cent alcohol and a dry dressing applied.

Stools and Urine. For the first few days after birth the intestinal contents are represented by a brownish or brownish-green, soft material—the meconium. It is made up of cast-off epithelial cells from various portions of the intestinal tract, a few epidermal cells and lanugo hairs which have been swallowed with the amniotic fluid. Its peculiar color is due to the presence of bile pigments. During pregnancy and for a few hours after birth the intestinal contents are sterile, but bacteria soon gain access to them and are afterward present throughout life. The passage of meconium and urine in the minutes immediately following birth or the next few hours usually indicates patency of the respective tracts. On the other hand failure to eliminate meconium or urine should facilitate early recognition and treatment of congenital defects.

After the third or fourth day, with the establishment of the mammary secretion, the meconium disappears, and its place is taken by feces, which are light yellow in color, homogeneous in consistence, and possess a characteristic odor. For the first few days the stools are not formed, but after a short time they take on the characteristic cylindrical shape. The bowels, as a rule, move twice daily, but a single large dejection is sufficient.

If the child is not gaining weight satisfactorily, the physician should make it a rule to inspect the stools at each visit, and instruct the nurse to save a napkin in anticipation of his arrival, as in this way important information may be gained concerning disturbances of the digestive process.

Icterus. Not infrequently in the first days of life, the skin and conjunctivae of the child take on a yellowish hue, which may vary from a scarcely visible discoloration to an intense jaundice. It is regarded as physiologic, and has been called icterus neonatorum, and occurs in 15 to 80 per cent of the newborn infants according to various authors. Race, light conditions, and individual interpretation make accurate recording of the jaundice difficult. At the New York Lying-In Hospital, 10.5 per cent of 5,748 infants showed definite icterus on two or more successive days.

Hyperbilirubinemia occurs in the newborn infants, and may or may not be associated with clinical jaundice. Waugh and co-workers using the Evelyn photoelectric colorimeter technic, found that the total bilirubin (indirect) content of cord blood plasma of normal infants averaged 1.35 mg. per cent, with a gradual increase to an average of 6.32 mg. per cent on the fourth day, followed by a gradual decrease thereafter. Clinical jaundice was usually reported when the bilirubin level was greater than 5 mg. per cent, although some infants had clinical jaundice with lower values.

The direct bilirubin content of cord blood plasma was 0.51 mg. per cent according to Waugh, and remained constant in the first days of life.

The icterus index as originally described by Meulengracht, with subsequent modification of technic rather than principle, is a less accurate method for the determination of bilirubin, but is simpler and therefore more practical. The index at birth varied from 7 to 28 in cases studied by Goldbloom and Gottlieb. In our clinic an average value of 18 was obtained in a large number of cord blood serum analyses. The frequency of hemolysis of cord blood is a drawback to the test. Gordon and Kemelhor report average readings of 21 units for the second day, with a gradual increase to 28 on the sixth day, and a gradual decline thereafter.

According to Virchow, Hofmeier, Gordon and Kemelhor, and others, the condition is of hematogenous origin, and is due to the breaking down of large numbers of red cells whose hemoglobin is no longer necessary for extra-uterine life. Goldbloom and Gottlieb state that the lower oxygen tension in utero is responsible for the fetal polycythemia, and that after birth, the higher oxygen tension produces red cell destruction with a rise in the blood bilirubin. Following the work of Aschoff, McNee, and Lepehne, it is likely that the breakdown occurs in the reticuloendothelial system of the spleen. Many authors hold that the icterus is of hepatogenous origin, and that physiologic insufficiency and functional immaturity of the liver in the newborn make impossible the utilization of increased amounts of bilirubin. Yllpo and Hirsch have regarded this as the cause of the jaundice, since the urine and stools of icteric and nonicteric infants contained similar amounts of bile pigment. This view is illustrated clinically by the higher incidence of jaundice in premature infants. It seems more than probable that hyperbilirubinemia is both hematogenous and hepatogenous in origin; is present with or without visible signs of icterus; is evidence of the adjustment to postnatal life; and is without clinical significance.

When the jaundice becomes intense or prolonged, an attempt should be made to differentiate physiologic from pathologic causes, such as: erythroblastosis fetalis (icterus gravis), congenital malformations of the bile ducts, congenital syphilis, and sepsis of the newborn. Repeated red cell counts and hemoglobin determinations may become necessary, even in the infants with physiologic icterus, in order to forestall dangerously low levels by giving transfusions of compatible blood. Hemorrhagic disease of the newborn and related conditions, such as hypoprothrombinemia, birth trauma and asphyxia, are discussed in a later section.

Initial Loss of Weight. Owing to the fact that the child receives little or no nutriment for the first three or four days of life, and at the same time casts off considerable quantities of urine, feces, and sweat, it progressively loses weight until the milk flow becomes established; the total loss is usually said to be approximately 7 per cent of the birth weight. In our experience the initial weight loss can be reduced to a minimum by offering the infant 30 cc. of a 5 per cent lactose solution in recently boiled water every four hours until the establishment of lactation. A recent survey of initial weight loss in the newborn carried out in the New York Lying-In Hospital reveals the weight loss to be about 6 per cent.

If the child is nourished properly, this is usually regained by the end of the tenth day, after which the weight should increase steadily at the rate of about 25 gm. (6 drams) a day for the first few months, so that it becomes doubled by the time the child is five months of age.

Frequency of Feeding. In spite of the small quantity of colostrum available and the somewhat limited nutritive properties, it is advisable, because of the stimulating effect of nursing on mother and child, to commence regular nursing about 12 hours postpartum. Most infants thrive best when fed at intervals of four hours, and upon a definite schedule. This is best arranged with reference to the daily bath, so that if it is given a little before 10 A.M., the first feeding would come at 6 A.M., with the evening feeding at the parent's bedtime, and a single one during the night. By this arrangement six feedings will be given each day, which can frequently be reduced to five, as many children can be trained to sleep the entire night without awakening. This, however, can only be accomplished by feeding it at regular intervals during the day, so as to insure that it receives the proper amount of nutriment in the 24 hours. Premature or frail infants not infrequently require nursing at a shorter interval and in most instances a three-hour interval is satisfactory. As soon as conditions warrant a change, the four-hour interval should be commenced.

Just before each feeding the napkin should be changed and the child made comfortable, but as soon as it is taken from the breast it should be placed in bed and not disturbed. It should not be allowed to sleep at its mother's breast, nor should it be rocked or fondled after feeding. The infant should be supported in the upright position by the nurse while the back is gently stroked to encourage the eructation of swallowed air. This is always advisable at the conclusion of nursing and sometimes it is necessary to interrupt the feeding for this purpose. If these regulations are persisted in, the child will usually go to sleep within a few minutes after being put to bed, and if it wakes before the next feeding is due it will generally remain quiet. The importance of following these directions cannot be overestimated, for it is only by rigid adherence to such details that the child can be given regular habits, and its care prevented from becoming a strain upon all concerned.

Duration of Feeding. Definite rules cannot be given concerning the proper length of each feeding, as this point is dependent upon several factors such as the quantity of milk, the readiness with which it can be obtained from the breast, and the avidity with which the child nurses. Generally speaking, it is advisable to allow the child to remain at the breast for 10 minutes at first, and to lengthen or decrease the time according to circumstances, four or five minutes being sufficient for some children, while 15 or 20 minutes will be required by others. Our practice is to have the baby nurse for five minutes at each breast for the first four days, or until the mother has a supply of milk. After the fourth day the baby nurses up to 10 minutes on each breast. A child which is receiving the proper amount of nourishment should not spit up its food, should increase steadily in weight, and should have normal yellow homogeneous stools.

In the hospital, the child should be weighed daily, but only once a week at home; as minor variations in the weight curve may be the cause of great unhappiness to the untrained mother. As has already been said, the child should regain its birth weight by the end of the tenth day, and from then on it should gain approximately 25 gm. a day, or, roughly speaking, 5 ounces a week. After the first few months the increase is more gradual, the average child doubling its weight at the fifth and trebling it at the twelfth month.

Artificial Feeding. The frequency with which artificial feeding as a complement to the breast supply or as a supplement for it becomes necessary has a direct relationship to the social and economic status of the patient. Approximately 90 per cent of the women living in tenements, often in unsanitary surroundings and with inadequate and poorly balanced diets, are able to nurse their infants. In the New York Lying-In Hospital, on the ward service about two thirds, and on the private service less than one third, of the women respectively are able to supply all the food requirements of their infants by means of nursing. When the supply of mother's milk is defective, or when abnormalities of the nipples or constitutional disease renders nursing inadvisable, artificial feeding must be resorted to. Numerous so-called infant foods are advertised for this purpose, but most of them are very defective, so that for practical purposes *cow's milk* in some form is the only advisable substitute for the mother's milk. Unfortunately, however, it differs markedly from the latter in composition, and thus must be modified when used as a substitute for mother's milk. It is usually slightly acid in reaction, and has a specific gravity of 1.029 to 1.033. Its average composition is: proteins, 3.5 per cent; fats, 3.5 per cent; sugar, 4.75 per cent, and salts, 0.7 per cent. It is apparent, therefore, that it contains less fat and sugar, and more protein material and salts, than mother's milk, and consequently cannot be used in its natural form, but must first be modified in some way.

If the child is healthy, satisfactory results are frequently obtained by diluting cow's milk with various proportions of water and adding sugar. Such preparations contain approximately the normal amount of proteid materials and sugar, but are lacking in fat. Such a formula, which is simple and useful in a large majority of infants, is one containing three parts whole milk, one part water and sufficient cane sugar to give a five per cent solution. *Only* pasteurized milk should be used for this purpose. The formula can conveniently be made daily and divided into the number of bottles required. It is necessary that the mixture be boiled for five to 10 minutes and that the bottles, nipples and utensils be boiled for the same length of time.

Rooming-in. By "rooming-in" is meant a program in which the infant is kept in a crib at the mother's bedside rather than in the nursery. It is an outgrowth in part of early ambulation, which permits the mother to be up and take care of the baby herself. It stems in part also from the modern trend to make all phases of childbearing as "natural" as possible and to foster proper mother-child relationships at an early date. By the end of 24 hours the mother is generally out of bed and thereafter, under this regime, conducts practically all the routine care of herself and the infant. An outstanding advantage of this program is that the mother, when she goes home, is much better able to assume care of the baby than she would otherwise be. Rooming-in has been endorsed especially by Montgomery and his associates and is now under trial in many hospitals, but at the present writing is not a generally accepted practice.

BIBLIOGRAPHY

Aschoff, L. Fortbildungsvortrage und Uebersichstreferate das reticulo-endotheliale System und seine Beziehungen zur Gallenfarbstoffbilding. Munchen. Med. Wchnschr., 1922, 69:1352.

Barcroft, J., and Barron, D. H. The Genesis of Respiratory Movements in the Fetus of the Sheep. J. Physiol., 1936, 88:56.

Barcroft, J., Elliott, R. H. E., Flexner, L. B., Hall, F. G., Herkel, W., McCarthy, E. F., McClurkin, T., and Talaat, M. Conditions of Fetal Respiration in the Goat. J. Physiol., 1934, 83:192..

Barcroft, J., Kramer, K., and Millikan, G. A. The Oxygen in the Carotid Blood at Birth. J. Physiol., 1939, 94:571.

BERENS, C. Ophthalmia Neonatorum. With Special Reference to the Sulfonamides in Treatment and the Continued Importance of Silver Preparations in Prevention. Am. J. Obst. & Gynec., 1944, 47:855.

BLUMBERG, M. L., and GLEICH, M. The Simplified Treatment of Gonococcic Ophthalmia Neonatorum with Chemotherapy. J.A.M.A., 1943, 123:132.

CARRINGTON, G. L. Use of Rubber Band for Tying Umbilical Cord. Am. J. Obst. & Gynec., 1937, 33:698.

CARROLL, J. J. Why Does Ophthalmia Neonatorum Continue to Cause So Much Blindness? Maryland M. J., 1909, 52:489.

COMMITTEE ON CONSERVATION OF VISION. Prevention of Blindness in Newborn Babies. Proceedings Of the Forty-Fifth Annual Meeting of the Conference of State and Provincial Health Authorities of North America, 1930. (Revised to 1934.)

CREDÉ, C. S. F. Die Verhütung der Augenentzündung der Neugeborenen. Berlin, 1884.

CREDÉ-HÖRDER, C. Hat die Blennorrhœa neonatorum Abgenommen? Zentralbl. f. Gynäk., 1912, 1503.

EASTMAN, N. J. Fetal Blood Studies. I. The Oxygen Relationships of Umbilical Cord Blood at Birth. Bull. Johns Hopkins Hosp., 1930, 47:221.

EVELYN, K. A. A Stabilized Photoelectric Colorimeter with Light Filters. J. Biol. Chem., 1936, 115:63.

GOLDBLOOM, A., and GOTTLIEB, R. Icterus Neonatorum. Am. J. Dis. Child., 1929, 38:57.

——— Studies on Icterus Neonatorum. J. Clin. Invest., 1930, 8:375.

GORDON, M. B., and KEMELHOR, M. Icterus Neonatorum. J. Ped., 1933, 2:685.

HANNES. Icterus neonatorum. Ber. ü. r. ges. Gyn. u. Geburtsh., 1924, 5:193.

HARTMAN, W. F. The Prophylaxis of Ophthalmia Neonatorum with Silver Acetate. Penn. M. J., 1940, 43:639.

HESSELTINE, H. C. Simple, Safe and Economical Cord Clamp. Am. J. Obst. & Gynec., 1937, 33:884.

HIRSCH, A. Icterus Neonatorum. Ztschr. f. Kinderh., 1913, 9:196.

HOLT, L. E., COURTNEY, A. M., and FALES, H. L. A Chemical Study of Woman's Milk. Am. J. Dis. Child., 1915, 10:229.

HOLT, L. E., and MCINTOSH, R. Holt's Disease of Infancy and Childhood. Eleventh Edition. D. Appleton-Century Co., Inc., New York, 1940.

JASCHKE and LINDIG. Zur Biologie des Colostrums. Ztschr. f. Geburtsh. u. Gynäk., 1916, 78:188.

KAHN, M. E. Improved Umbilical Cord Clamp; Preliminary Report. Am. J. Obst. & Gynec., 1936, 32:513.

KANNER, H. M. Simple, Safe and Economical Cord Tie. Am. J. Obst. & Gynec., 1939, 37:509.

KEIFFER, H. Recherches sur la Physiologie de l'Amnios Humain. Gynéc. et. obst., 1926, 14:1.

KELLER, C. Die Nabelinfektion, etc. Ztschr. f. Geburtsh. u. Gynäk., 1906, 58:454.

KURZROK, R., BATES, R. W., RIDDLE, O., and MILLER, E. G. The Clinical Use of Prolactin. Endocrinology, 1934, 18:18.

LEPEHNE, G. Untersuchungen über Gallenfarbstoff im Blutserum des Menschen. Deutsches Arch. f. Klin. Med., 1920, 132:96.

LEWIS, J. H., and WELLS, H. G. The Function of the Colostrum. J.A.M.A., 1922, 78:863.

LINZENMEIER, G., and LILIENTHAL, F. Zur Frage des Icterus neonatorum. Zentralbl. f. Gynäk., 1922, 46:1873.

MCNEE, J. W. The Use of the van den Bergh Test in the Differentiation of Obstructive from Other Types of Jaundice. Brit. Med. J., 1922, 1:716.

——— and KEEFER, C. S., The Clinical Value of the van den Bergh Reaction for Bilirubin in Blood: with Notes on Improvements in Its Technique. Brit. Med. J., 1925, 2:52.

MEULENGRACHT, E. Die klinische Bedeutung der Untersuchung auf Gallensfarbstoff im Blutserum. Deutsches Arch. f. Klin. Med., 1920, 132:285.

MONTGOMERY, T. L., STEWARD, R. E., and SHENK, E. P. Observations on the Rooming-In Program of Baby with Mother in Ward and Private Practice. Am. J. Obst. & Gynec., 1949, 57:176.

PLOSS, H. H., BARTELS, M., and BARTELS, P. Woman. C. V. Mosby Co., St. Louis, 1936.

POTTER, E. L., and BOHLENDER, G. P. Intrauterine Respiration in Relation to Development of the Fetal Lung. Am. J. Obst. & Gynec., 1941, 42:14.

SIEVERS, J. J., KNOTT, L. W., and SOLOWAY, H. M. Penicillin in the Treatment of Ophthalmia Neonatorum. J.A.M.A., 1944, 125:690.

SMITH, C. A. Physiology of the Newborn Infant. Charles C. Thomas, Springfield, Ill. 1946.

SNYDER, F. F., and ROSENFELD, M. Intrauterine Respiratory Movements of the Human Fetus. J.A.M.A., 1937, 108:1946.

SNYDER, F. F., and ROSENFELD, M. Direct Observation of Intrauterine Respiratory Movements of the Fetus and the Role of Carbon Dioxide and Oxygen in their Regulation. Am. J. Physiol., 1937, 119:153.

STEELE, A. G., and WINDLE, W. F. Some Correlations Between Respiratory Movements and Blood Gases in Cat Fetuses. J. Physiol., 1939, 94:531.

TURNER, C. W., and ALLEN, E. The Normal and Experimental Development of the Mammary Gland of the Monkey (Macacus rhesus). Anat. Rec., 1933, 55:80.

TURNER, C. W., FRANK, A. H., GARDNER, W. U., SCHULTZE, A. B., and GOMEZ, E. T. The Effect of Theelin and Theelol on the Growth of the Mammary Gland. Anat. Rec., 1932, 53:227.

TURNER, C. W., and GOMEZ, E. T. The Experimental Development of the Mammary Gland. I. The Male and the Female Albino Mouse. II. The Male and Female Guinea Pig. Mo. Agr. Exp. Sta. Res. Bull., 1934, 206.

——— The Effect of Ovariectomy upon Lactation in the Albino Rat. Mo. Agr. Exp. Sta. Res. Bull., 1936, 370.

——— The Development of the Mammary Gland of the Goat. Mo. Agr. Exp. Sta. Res. Bull., 1936, 240.

WARNEKROS, K. Schwangerschaft und Geburt in Roentgenbilde. München, 1921.

WAUGH, T. R., MERCHANT, F. T., and MAUGHAN, G. B. Blood Studies on the Newborn: II. Direct and Total Blood Bilirubin: Determinations Over a Nine-day Period, with Special Reference to Icterus Neonatorum. Am. J. M. Sc., 1940, 199:9.

WHITE, M. R. Umbilical Cord Clamp. Am. J. Obst. & Gynec., 1939, 37:345.

WINDLE, W. F. Physiology and Anatomy of the Respiratory System in the Fetus and Newborn Infant. J. Pediat., 1941, 19:437.

——— MONNIER, M., and STEELE, A. G. Fetal Respiratory Movements in the Cat. Physiol. Zool., 1938, 11:425.

YLLPO, A. Icterus Neonatorum. Ztschr. f. Kinderh., 1913, 9:208.

ZIEGLER, C. E. New All Metal Umbilical Cord Clamp. Am. J. Obst. & Gynec., 1936, 32:884.

Section Six: ABNORMALITIES OF PREGNANCY

20

ABORTION AND PREMATURE LABOR

DEFINITIONS

Abortion is the termination of a pregnancy at any time before the fetus has attained a stage of viability. Interpretations of the phrase "stage of viability" have varied between fetal weights of 400 gm. (about 20 weeks of gestation) and 1,000 gm. (about 28 weeks of gestation). In support of the former figure, it may be stated that an infant reported by Monro, weighing only 397 gm., actually did survive, and therefore, speaking very strictly and on the basis of this single precedent, an infant weighing 400 gm. or above may be regarded as capable of living. However, the survival of an infant weighing even 700 or 800 gm. is so rare as to be miraculous and as a consequence, the 1,000 gm. figure is widely used as demarcating the stage of viability. The rationale of this figure is that infants below this weight possess very little chance of survival, while those weighing above 1,000 gm. have a substantial chance of living which increases sharply with each 100 gm. increment. This is a variable matter, however, and the refinements of pediatric care have made it possible for smaller and smaller infants to survive. In our clinic, an abortion is defined as the termination of pregnancy at any time when the fetus weighs less than 400 gm. Infants weighing between 400 and 999 gm. are called "immature" but, as indicated, in many clinics this group is included under the definition of abortion.

Premature infants are those born after the stage of viability has been reached but before they have the same chances of survival as a full term infant. The consensus has put the upper limit for this group at 2,500 gm. or 5.5 pounds. The lower limit will depend on the definition employed for abortion but, as stated, the 1,000 gm. figure is the one most frequently used.

Since the term abortion suggests to the layman a criminal interruption of pregnancy, he uses the word "miscarriage" to refer to this accident. It is prudent, therefore, to employ the latter term in speaking to patients or their families, but it is rarely used in medical parlance.

Abortion may be subdivided into its two main forms: spontaneous and induced. *Spontaneous abortion* is the termination of a previable conception through natural causes and without the aid of mechanical or medicinal agents. *Induced abortion* has two forms: therapeutic and criminal. *Therapeutic abortion* is the instrumental termination of pregnancy because of some grave maternal disease which would make continuation of gestation extremely hazardous to the mother. *Criminal abortion* is the termination of pregnancy without medical and legal justification. As a consequence of certain aberrations in the clinical course of abortion, the following conditions also are distinguished: a *complete abortion* is one in which the entire products of conception have been expelled. An *incomplete abortion* is one in which part of the products of conception have been passed but part (usually the placenta) remains in the uterus. A *missed abortion* is one in which the fetus dies in utero but the products of conception, instead of being expelled, are retained in utero for two months or longer. *Habitual abortion* is a condition in which abortion occurs in a number of successive pregnancies, usually specified as three.

SPONTANEOUS ABORTION

Incidence. The incidence of spontaneous abortion in general has been established as very close to 10 per cent of all pregnancies. This figure is based in part on the findings in several large series of private patients. Such women present peculiar advantages for any such study, since they usually report for prenatal care very early and, having done so, are not likely to undergo criminal abortion without the knowledge of their obstetricians. This tends to eliminate two important sources of error: (1) early unreported abortions occurring at home, and (2) criminal abortions camouflaged as spontaneous. Danforth's and Galloway's abortion rate for their private practices was 11 per cent. Hertig has examined all the abortion specimens from a large obstetric practice in Boston over a period of six years and found the incidence of spontaneous abortion to be 10.6 per cent in the 1,150 cases of full term pregnancy and spontaneous abortion combined. Hertig also summarized the observations of five American authors and concluded that this combined experience showed an average incidence of 9.8 per cent for spontaneous abortion. In a series of 1,100 private obstetrical cases reviewed by Guttmacher, the rate was also 9.8 per cent. Publications on the incidence of spontaneous abortion among clinic patients show surprisingly similar figures: Stix, 10.9 per cent; Pearl, 11.8 per cent; and Wiehl and Berry, 9.7 per cent. Neither race, social status, nor parity seems to affect this incidence.

Month	Spontaneous	Self-induced	Criminal	Per cent Total
1	64	25	3	9.2
2	249	158	18	42.8
3	203	119	17	34.0
4	33	34	8	7.5
5	35	18	2	5.4
6	7	2	0	0.9

Table 13. Incidence of Abortion According to the Duration of Pregnancy. (Simons.) Therapeutic abortions are excluded.

In a statistical analysis of 1,000 abortions, Simons has demonstrated that about 75 per cent of all such abortions occur during the second and third months of pregnancy, that is, before the twelfth week. Simons' data in full are reproduced in Table 13. Although it is sometimes stated that spontaneous abortion is most likely to occur at the precise time of either the second or third missed periods, there is actually very little evidence to support this viewpoint.

Etiology. In the early months of pregnancy spontaneous expulsion of the ovum is nearly always preceded by the death of the fetus. For this reason the consideration of the etiology of early abortion practically resolves itself into determining the cause of fetal death. In the later months, on the other hand, the fetus is frequently born alive and other factors must be invoked to explain its expulsion. Fetal death may be due to abnormalities occurring in the ovum itself, to abnormalities of the generative tract, or to systemic disease on the part of the mother and occasionally of the father.

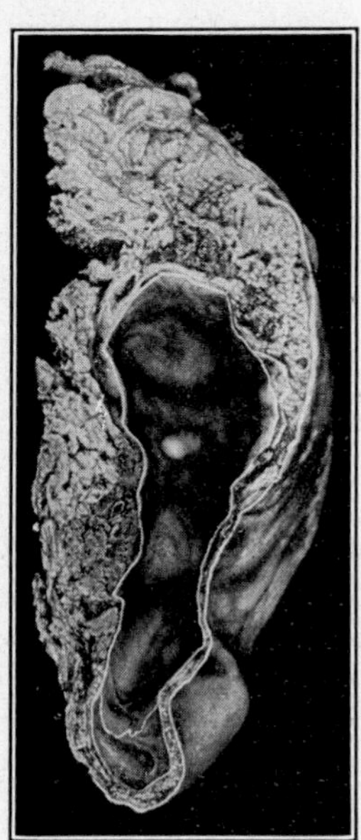

Fig. 313.—Abortion Due to Defective Germ Plasm. × 1.

Note degenerated embryo in center.

Abnormal Development. The most usual cause for the death of the fetus is to be found in abnormalities of development which are inconsistent with life. The investigations of Mall, Streeter and Hertig indicate that such conditions are present in a large percentage of all early abortions. In an analysis of 1,000 spontaneous abortions Hertig noted pathological ova ("blighted ovum") in 48.9 per cent, embryos with localized anomalies in 3.2 per cent and placental abnormalities in 9.6 per cent of his cases. It is also of significance that he observed hydatidiform degeneration in 63 per cent of abnormal ova. The incidence of abnormal ova among spontaneous abortions is known to decrease markedly from the first to the fourth month of gestation. We are as yet completely ignorant concerning the causation of such abnormalities in human beings, but reasoning from the results obtained in experimental teratology, it would seem probable that two main sets of factors are concerned: abnormalities in the earliest stages of segmentation of the ovum, and changes in its environment. In the case of a pathological fetus, Hertig found the average date of expulsion of the abortus to be 10.2 weeks menstrual age. Invariably the embryo had been dead for a period of weeks—average, six weeks—before the abortion is completed.

Pending more precise knowledge, abnormalities in the early stages of segmentation are attributed to defective germ plasm, which of course implies that the defect may originate in the germ cells of mother or father, or of both. In many such cases the embryo is lacking or is represented by a formless mass of tissue, while the fetal membranes appear normal. In such circumstances it would seem that the defect had implicated the cells making up the internal cell mass, but had not affected the main body of trophoblast from which the membranes are formed. On the other hand the entire trophoblast may be implicated, and Grosser considers whenever the entire periphery of chorionic vesicles, under 5 cm. in diameter, is not thickly covered with villi that we have to deal with a primary trophoblastic defect, and consequently that normal development will not occur. In an attempt to differentiate between the cases with and without blighted ova, Rutherford studied, by means of decidual biopsy, 100 cases of bleeding during the first four months of pregnancy and found that a diagnosis could be made on such criteria as difference in staining reaction, vascular thrombosis and infiltration of erythrocytes and leukocytes into the stroma.

The most conclusive evidence in favor of defective germ plasm is afforded by the occurrence of double-ovum twins, in which one vesicle contains a normal and the other a rudimentary embryo. In such cases the abnormality cannot be attributed to a defect in implantation, as both ova were implanted upon the same decidua. In most cases, however, the evidence is more inferential and is based upon the condition of the

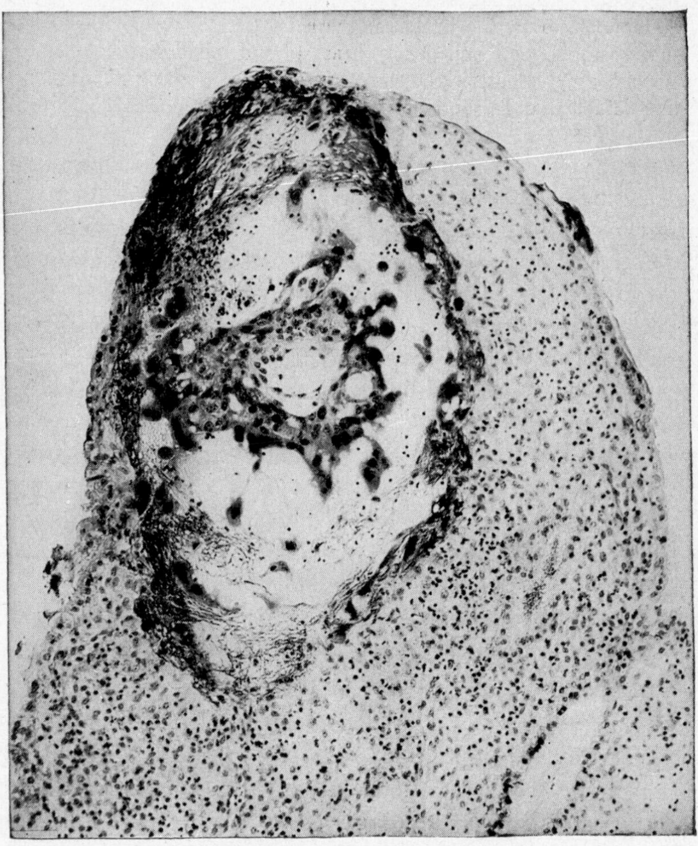

FIG. 314.—ABNORMAL OVUM.

A cross section of a defective ovum showing an empty chorionic sac embedded within a polypoid mass of endometrium. (From Hertig and Rock, *American Journal of Obstetrics and Gynecology.*)

embryo as contrasted with the rest of the product of conception. In this way Streeter concluded that defective germ plasm was the essential cause for 81 out of the 104 abortions reported by Huntington. Even when the abortion is produced by the action of chemical agents, a similar explanation may be invoked, as Datnow found that when abortions are provoked in rabbits by colloidal lead, changes in the trophoblast constitute the striking feature.

The failure of ova to be fertilized, and the failure of fertilized ova to develop normally are found in all mammals. In animals producing multiple young, the extent of these anomalies may be determined by counting the number of embryos or the number of young in a litter and comparing this number to the total corpora lutea in both ovaries of the mother. The discrepancy is termed ova loss. A second method of study is the recovery of batches of ova from the fallopian tubes and by microscopic examination to determine the number of normal segmenting eggs, unfertilized eggs and abnormal fertilized eggs. By the first method Corner found a 24 per cent ova loss in the sow, and by the second method Hartman found a 35 per cent loss in the opossum. In mammals bearing multiple young, the failure of some ova to be fertilized and of others to develop, is in large part a germ plasm defect.

These failures in fertilization and development are not confined to animals alone, but occur in the vegetable kingdom as well. All the proof one needs can be furnished by opening a few pods of table peas. In the majority there is one undeveloped ovum—a runty pea. Fruit trees, such as apple, pear and peach, bear stunted, abnormal fruit on the same limb with perfect specimens. Just as in the case of the human, these abnormal specimens are likely to become detached and drop early, months before the normal, mature fruit.

The recognition of the effect of abnormal germ plasm is simpler than explaining its exact mechanism. The causes can be divided into two main groups, those arising from defective chromosomes and genes, and those arising from faults in intra-uterine environment. Both of these factors are based on theory and analogy and they can not be demonstrated in the human by the microscope or the test tube.

We know from experimental biology, especially from the work on the fruit fly *Drosophila* that when defective genes of the sperm are properly aligned so as to be coupled with similar defective genes of the egg, distinct abnormalities will appear in the offspring. Defective genes, if of sufficient magnitude, may cause a totally abnormal embryo or even an embryo which succumbs. When the defect in the genes is more circumscribed, only certain organ-systems or specific organs may be involved. When one realizes that the placenta is a fetal organ, then it is clear how the placenta alone, or in combination with the embryo, may be affected by defective chromosomes and genes.

The question of primary importance is: What causes abnormal chromosomes and genes? Unfortunately, a categorical answer cannot be given. Probably everyone carries a certain number of abnormal genes in each of his gametes, defects transmitted through heredity, passed directly from remote ancestors through immediate progenitors. And when, by ill chance, in the process of fertilization the defective genes of a sperm are matched by identical defective genes in an ovum, the genetic character presided over by these genes is made defective. If at fertilization the defective genes of one gamete are matched by normal genes in the gamete of the opposite sex, then the character involved usually appears normal. A second question is: What affects genes and chromosomes other than heredity? Nothing, as far as we know. The idea that chronic poisoning of the male from excessive alcohol and tobacco, or exposure to the fumes of heavy metals, adversely affects spermatozoa and causes defective germ plasm abortions, or congenitally malformed children, lacks clear proof. One would have to premise that these agents cause actual chromosomal mutations, as Muller has produced by x-ray in *Drosophila*.

If we pause to consider the complexities of implantation and early fetal nutrition, it is no surprise that faulty intra-uterine environment may in turn cause defects in the conceptus. The delicate hormonal control of tubal and uterine peristalsis, the multiple endocrine factors associated with progestational changes in the endometrium and the ill-understood process of the dissolving action of the ovum itself in sinking beneath the uterine epithelium, all inspire us with wonder that in so high a percentage of cases these multiple factors integrate sufficiently to produce implantation.

Furthermore, after properly implanting, the ovum immediately faces the vicissitudes connected with attaining nutriment, the utilization of glycogen, tapping of maternal capillaries to surround itself with lakes of blood and the development of functioning villi. If any of these several mechanisms goes awry, the growth and continued existence of the embryo and trophoblast are seriously affected. Then fetal death and spontaneous abortion occur.

The factors which affect intra-uterine environment are only partially understood. Dareste and Fischer in the nineteenth century, and Stockard in the present century, have shown that fertilized eggs of *Fundulus* and other marine animals are very susceptible to changes in both the oxygen content and temperature of their fluid environment. The magnitude of the alteration and the time of its occurrence determine whether the ova die, whether the embryos are retarded, whether they undergo duplication in part or total, or are otherwise malformed. Steffko showed that alterations in the hydrogen-ions of the human uterine contents following the introduction of fragments of silkworm gut lead to degenerative changes in the embryo and its surrounding membranes. Evans and his associates showed that vitamin E deficiency in the pregnant rat leads to death of the embryos and their resorption. There is suggestive clinical evidence that such avitaminosis may play a role in cases of human habitual abortion. These, then, are just a few of the environmental factors affecting the early egg; there must be many more.

Abnormalities of the Placenta. Later in pregnancy, probably from the twentieth week on, certain diseases and abnormalities of the placenta may lead to abortion, but more usually they lead to premature labor. Endarteritic changes, independent of syphilis, may develop in the blood vessels of the villi, and interfere sufficiently with placental transmission to cause fetal death. Very large infarcts may put enough placental tissue out of commission so that the organ will no longer be adequate to meet fetal needs. Occasionally such abnormalities as placenta previa, premature separation and velamentous cord may so interfere with the fetal circulation that death of the embryo occurs.

Maternal Disease. Severe Acute Infections—notably pneumonia, typhoid, and pyelitis—occasionally lead to abortion, though they are more likely to bring about premature labor. Either toxins from the mother or specific bacterial invasion may make the fetus ill, cause its death and later its expulsion. Moreover, a severe toxic condition of the mother may initiate labor, even when the fetus appears unaffected. This is especially true in severe pneumonia. Poisoning with heavy metals or illuminating gas also occasionally produces abortion.

Chronic Wasting Diseases in early pregnancy, such as tuberculosis or carcinomatosis, rarely cause abortion, the patient often dying undelivered. In later pregnancy premature labor is not uncommon with these conditions. The toxemias of pregnancy are almost never associated with abortion, but they are an occasional cause of premature labor.

Syphilis. This disease was formerly imputed to be a common cause of abortion. However, studies have shown that the spirochete does not cross the placental barrier to invade the fetus until after the twentieth week. And, since it requires several weeks of syphilitic fetal infection to bring about the death of the embryo or its expulsion, we have come to realize that syphilis rarely, if ever, causes abortion. However, it is still a common cause of premature stillbirth.

Endocrine Dyscrasias or Imbalances, which are occasionally convenient terms to cloak ignorance of exact factors, may also cause abortion. The various endocrine glands behave as though connected in series, like Christmas tree lights, and when one functions abnormally it in turn maladjusts the others. In many cases it is assumed that the secretion of progesterone by the corpus luteum, or the secretion of a progesterone-like substance by the trophoblast, is deficient in amount or quality. Since progesterone maintains decidual development, its relative paucity would theoretically interfere with the nutrition of the conceptus and so conduce to its death. Other endocrine glands, especially the thyroid, may also be involved in some cases of abortion. This theoretical endocrine basis for habitual abortion is taken into account in the therapy of the condition (see section on therapy of habitual abortion).

Laparotomy. The trauma of laparotomy may occasionally provoke abortion. The nearer the site of surgery is to the pelvic organs, the more likely the abortion. However, ovarian cysts and pedunculated fibroids may be removed during pregnancy without interfering with the gestation as a rule. Postoperative sedation and the daily administration of progesterone for the first week or 10 days diminish the probability of postoperative abortion.

Abnormalities of the Reproductive Organs. Local abnormalities and diseases of the generative tract are only infrequently responsible for abortion. An infantile uterus, adnexal inflammation, tumors of the uterus and endocervicitis are important causes of sterility, but it is rare for them to cause abortion.

Displacements of the uterus, such as a retrodisplacement, rarely cause abortion. However, in instances of incarceration, abortion is the rule, unless the uterus is freed from the pelvis.

Fibromyoma of the uterus usually does not cause abortion. The position which the fibroid occupies is more likely to affect this issue than the size of the tumor. Submucosal tumors and those situated in the lower segment are the most likely to cause abortion. It is amazing how sometimes the most gnarled and nodular uterus carries a pregnancy to term. The only way one can determine how a uterus with fibroids will behave in pregnancy is to give it the clinical test. Without such a test, prognostication is difficult and often fallacious.

An important lesion of the generative tract, in the etiology of abortion, is a congenitally short cervix, or one which is shortened by surgical amputation. One can not deplore too strongly the tendency of some operators to amputate the cervix during the childbearing years. Long cervical tears, which are not properly approximated at the time of delivery, or which heal badly, may also cause a late abortion.

Psychic and Physical Trauma. Everyone, doctor and layman alike, seeks a tangible, simply understood cause for the more commonplace medical phenomena. A woman aborts. Why? It must have been related to some immediate joy, sorrow or fright, or perhaps to a recent fall, bump or blow. The woman, the husband and the doctor all forget the multiple traumata which have not interrupted the pregnancy previously. They only remember the particular one which appeared to have a time relationship to the abortion. An important argument against the role of trauma in causing spontaneous abortion is the fact that most spontaneous abortions occur six weeks or so after fetal death, and if trauma were the cause it would not be a recent incident, but one which happened some six weeks before the abortion occurred, as a rule. That the traumatic factor may be overemphasized is borne out by Hertig and

Sheldon's analysis of 1,000 cases of abortion, in only one of which he was definitely able to ascribe the cause to external trauma and psychic shock.

Contagious Abortion. It has been suggested by some authorities that the *Bacillus abortus* of Bang, the causative agent of contagious abortion in cattle, produces repeated abortion in humans as well. This view gained impetus when it was shown that the cattle micro-organism is responsible for many cases of human undulant fever and Malta fever. There is no question that some women affected with habitual abortion show positive agglutination for the Bang organism, but it is not proved that the Bang infection causes them to abort. Since undulant fever is so common, it is just as likely that the two conditions are coincidental. In cattle the bacilli congregate beneath the placenta and in some unknown way cause the death of the fetus. The fetus itself develops no specific lesions. The whole topic of human abortion and infection with the Bang group of micro-organisms is far from clear, and we must maintain an open mind about it.

Pathology. The most frequent lesion in spontaneous abortion is hemorrhage into the decidua basalis, followed by necrotic changes in the tissues adjacent to the bleeding. This in turn sets up an inflammatory reaction. Owing to the hemorrhage and necrosis, the ovum becomes detached in part or whole and acts as a foreign body in the uterus, eventually initiating contractions which result in its expulsion. Until recently it was generally accepted that the decidual hemorrhage was the primary lesion and the death of the embryo secondary. However modern studies have demonstrated that the reverse is usually true. The death of the embryo is primary and the decidual hemorrhage secondary. A typical early specimen consists of thickened, opaque, slightly blood-infiltrated membranes, with a thicker area at one point, representing the placenta. The expelled intact ovum is fluid-filled, and its walls seem rather lax and under little internal pressure. Upon opening the membranes, clear fluid is found, with a small macerated fetus sunk back against a many-pleated, grayish amnion.

If the villi are studied under a dissecting microscope, they will often appear thick and distended with fluid, the ends of the villous branches resembling little sausage-shaped sacs. In some the sac-like termination seems about to drop off, since the base where it arises from the villous stem is often constricted. Such fluid-filled villi are undergoing hydatid degeneration. This degeneration probably follows the death of the fetus and is caused by the imbibition of tissue fluid.

Before the tenth week, the ovum is likely to be expelled as an intact sac, often with the decidual cast of the uterus adherent to it. This is attributable to the fact that prior to that time the anchoring villi of the chorion have not yet attached themselves securely to the decidua and separation in toto of the loosely attached ovum is easy. Between the eighth and twelfth weeks, however, the chorion develops markedly and its anchoring villi establish firm connection with the decidua, making for retention of chorionic elements in many of these later abortions.

In addition to the more typical abortion specimen mentioned in the first paragraph of this section, there are several atypical forms, which we shall describe briefly.

Blighted or dropsical ovum is the name applied to a small, relatively hydramniotic sac, in which the fetus is completely absent or represented by a small amorphous mass.

Blood or carneous mole is an ovum which is surrounded by a capsule of clotted blood of varying thickness, with degenerated chorionic villi scattered through it. The small, fluid-containing cavity within it appears compressed and distorted by the thick walls of old blood. This specimen is associated with an abortion that occurs rather leisurely, giving the blood collecting between the decidua and chorion the opportunity to coagulate and form in layers.

Tuberous mole, ovum tuberculosum and tuberous subchorial hematoma of the decidua are different names applied to the same type of specimen. The characteristic feature is a highly nodular, almost boulder-like appearance of the amnion, which is due to the lifting up of the amnion by localized hematomas of varying size, beneath the amnion and the chorionic membrane.

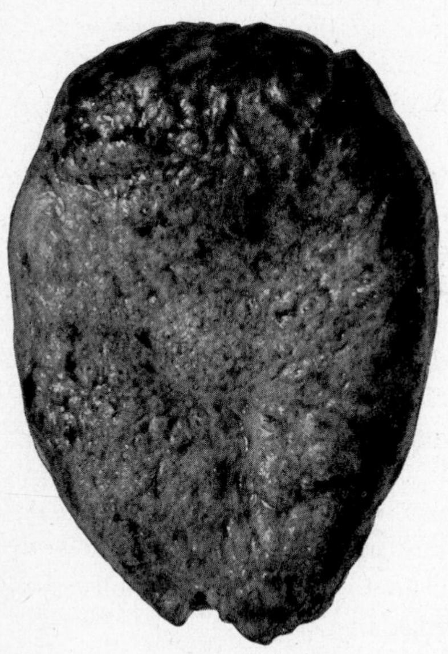

Fig. 315.—Blood Mole of a Complete Abortion.

Dissolution of the dead fetus is possible only in the early weeks of pregnancy. In abortions occurring after the fetus has attained any considerable size, several outcomes are possible. In the first place, the amniotic fluid may be absorbed, when the fetus becomes compressed upon itself and assumes a desiccated appearance—*fetus compressus.* At the same time the placental circulation becomes abolished, degeneration results, and the whole structure takes on a dry, whitish appearance. Occasionally, the fetus becomes so dry and compressed as to resemble parchment, when the process is designated as *mummification.* Although this is rarely observed in ordinary abortion, it occurs relatively frequently in twin pregnancy, particularly when one fetus has died at an early period, while the other has gone on to full development—*fetus papyraceus.*

In other cases the retained fetus may undergo *maceration.* In such circumstances, the bones of the skull collapse, the abdomen becomes distended with a blood-stained fluid, and the entire fetus takes on a dull reddish color due to staining with blood pigment. At the same time the skin softens and peels off at the slightest touch, leaving behind the bright-red corium. The internal organs degenerate and become soft and friable, losing their capacity for taking up the usual histologic stains.

Very exceptionally, and particularly when the membranes have long since ruptured and a mild but chronic infectious process has become established, the soft parts of the embryo may undergo dissolution and digestion, so that when the process is terminated all that remains is the skeleton, which sometimes resembles a shrimp more nearly than a fetus. Once in many thousand cases, although we have never observed it, the fetus may be retained in utero for a long period, until the deposition of lime salts converts it into what is known as a *lithopedion.* This phenomenon is relatively common in certain lower animals, and is a recognized, but rare, termination of extra-uterine pregnancy.

Clinical Aspects. The clinical aspects of spontaneous abortion are most conveniently discussed under five subgroups: threatened, imminent, inevitable, incomplete and missed.

An abortion is presumed *threatened* when any bloody vaginal discharge or frank vaginal bleeding occurs during the first 20 weeks of pregnancy. A threatened abortion may or may not be accompanied by mild, menstrual-like cramps or backache. This interpretation of threatened abortion makes it an extremely commonplace phenomenon, since 2 out of 10 pregnant women have vaginal spotting or actual bleeding

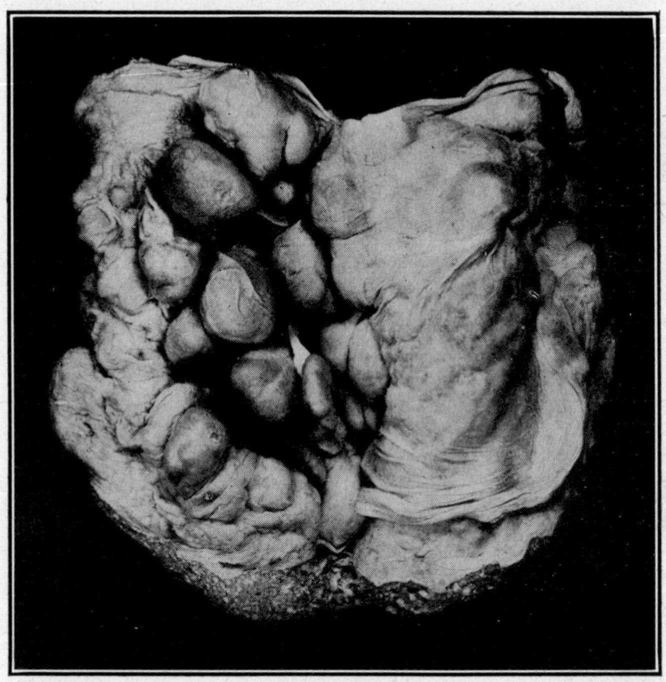

Fig. 316.—Tuberous Subchorial Hematoma. (After H. Dumler.)

during the early months of gestation. Yet of these two who bleed, only one actually aborts. There is reason to believe, indeed, that many cases termed threatened abortion are not threatening to abort at all. Many are probably instances of physiologic bleeding, bleeding which is analogous to the placental sign described by Hartman in the macacus rhesus monkey. In these animals there is always at least a microscopic amount of bleeding. The blood seems to make its way from ruptured paraplacentally situated blood vessels and eroded uterine epithelium into the uterine cavity. It begins most commonly 17 days after conception, or about 29 days after the pregnant monkey's last menses. In many of Hartman's animals the bleeding was sufficient to be observed grossly for several days. Microscopic evidence lasted on the average for 23 days. Then, too, in the human, inflammatory lesions of the external os are prone to bleed in early pregnancy, especially postcoitum. Polypi presenting at the external os also tend to bleed in early gestation. It is almost impossible to differentiate clinically these benign types of pregnancy bleeding—abbreviated menses, placental-sign, erosions, polypi, etc.—from actual instances of threatening abortion.

It is this confusion which makes most physicians term all bleeding in early pregnancy threatened abortion, and it is this circumstance which gives the treatment of so-called threatened abortion so great a likelihood of success. Most women who actually threaten to abort, probably progress into the next stage of the process—imminent abortion—no matter what is done. On the other hand, if the bleeding is due to some of the benign causes mentioned, it is likely to disappear, no matter what is done or not done.

The bleeding of threatened abortion is frequently slight in amount and may persist for many days, or even weeks. At times it is fresh, and therefore red in color, the color intensity varying with the amount of mucus admixed. At other times, when the discharge is made up of old blood seeping out, the color is a dark, dirty brown. A truly threatened abortion is frequently accompanied by either lower abdominal cramps or persistent backache, or both. These symptoms are lacking in the benign bleeding group.

Imminent abortion is marked by rather copious vaginal bleeding, often with the passage of clots. At the same time there are severe cramplike abdominal pains, caused by uterine contractions. The cervix now begins to dilate and after this has occurred it is extremely rare for the process to subside and pregnancy to continue. Usually, after an hour or two, an imminent abortion is terminated by the expulsion of the conceptus.

Inevitable abortion is signalized by the rupture of the membranes in the presence of cervical dilatation. Under these conditions abortion is certain to occur. Very rarely a gush of fluid occurs during the first half of pregnancy and nothing dire follows. Such cases may be explained in several ways: the membranes may seal over the defect; fluid may collect between the amnion and chorion, with subsequent rupture of the chorion, the amnion remaining intact; finally, incontinence of urine may be confused with the rupture of the membranes, in late or early pregnancy.

Incomplete Abortion. As stated previously, the fetus and placenta are likely to be passed together before the tenth week and separately thereafter. Even if the fetus and placenta appear to be expelled as one intact ovum, some of the placenta may tear loose and remain behind, adhering to the uterus. When the placenta, in whole or in part, is not expelled, bleeding ensues sooner or later and constitutes the main, and usually the only, symptom of incomplete abortion. Bleeding is invariable in this condition, is often profuse and may occasionally be massive to the point of profound shock. Such hemorrhage is understandable when it is recalled that bleeding into the spongy layer of the decidua basalis occurs as one of the earliest alterations in every abortion. As a result, more or less separation of the ovum from the decidua occurs with opening of the underlying venous sinuses. As the process of abortion continues, the uterine contractions, together with the expulsion of the fetus and amniotic fluid, produce still further separation. If the placenta separates completely, the muscle fibers clamp down on the blood vessels lying in their interstices and stop blood loss. If, however, placental tissue is partly attached and partly separated, the splintlike action of the attached portion of placenta interferes with myometrial retraction in the immediate vicinity and the vessels in the denuded segment of the placental site, thus without benefit of constriction by muscle fibrils, bleed profusely.

This general principle that a partially separated placenta causes bleeding—often profuse hemorrhage—is one of the most important in all obstetrics. With a completely attached placenta, bleeding from the placental site is obviously impossible. With a completely detached placenta, hemorrhage from the placental site is usually controlled effectively by myometrial retraction. But a partially separated placenta always provokes bleeding and is a common cause of obstetric hemorrhage. Indeed, it constitutes the mechanism responsible for blood loss in four of the most important hemorrhagic complications of childbearing: third stage hemorrhage, abruptio placentae, placenta previa, and incomplete abortion.

A *missed* abortion is the retention, two months or more after its death, of an early intra-uterine pregnancy. In the typical instance, the first few months of pregnancy are completely normal: amenorrhea, nausea and vomiting, breast changes and growth of uterus. All goes well until the ovum dies, when there may, or may not, be vaginal bleeding or even symptoms denoting a threatened abortion, which subside. It is then noted that the uterus seems to remain stationary in size and the breasts regress. The patient is likely to lose a few pounds in weight. Careful palpation and measurement of the uterus reveal the fact that it has not only ceased to enlarge, but is growing smaller, from the absorption of amniotic fluid and maceration of the fetus. Most patients are symptomless during this period, except for the persistence of amenorrhea. Some, however, complain of lassitude and depression. If the missed abortion terminates spontaneously, as most do, the process of expulsion is quite the same as in any ordinary abortion. The product, if retained several weeks after fetal death, is a shrivelled sac containing a highly macerated embryo, and if retained for months or years it appears to be a mass of old tissue and blood, with areas of dense calcification. The cause of missed abortion is not known.

The most accurate observations on this condition are those of Streeter who reported upon a series of 437 cases of retention of the dead fetus. By comparing the size of the fetus and thus its actual period of growth, with the menstrual age, he was able to point out the probable time-discrepancy between the death of the fetus and its birth. This he found to be about six weeks, as an average, although it was usually somewhat shorter in the early stages of pregnancy and apt to be longer in advanced gestation. In a small number the retention in utero was markedly prolonged to a varying number of months. From this study and those of Seitz, Litzenberg and others, it would seem that in abortion the product of conception is usually tolerated in utero for varying periods of time up to about eight weeks as a maximum, while in the occasional instance this period may be considerably exceeded, in which case we may properly use the term *missed abortion.*

Treatment. *Threatened Abortion.* For the sake of clarity threatened abortions will be divided into two categories, those with vaginal bleeding and no pain, and those with vaginal bleeding plus pain.

VAGINAL BLEEDING WITHOUT PAIN, IN EARLY PREGNANCY. A patient should be instructed to notify her physician immediately whenever vaginal bleeding occurs during pregnancy. In early pregnancy it requires the utmost medical acumen to determine whether the bleeding is benign in type, or whether it presages abortion. In either event, the patient should be put to bed, prescribed a light diet, cautioned against straining at stool, and advised to save for the doctor's inspection the perineal pads and all clots and tissue that she may pass. If the patient is apprehensive, 0.5 grain of phenobarbital every four hours should be prescribed and a stronger sedative, such as 1.5 grains of seconal or nembutal, before she attempts to sleep for the night,

If the bleeding diminishes or disappears within 48 hours, she is allowed out of bed, but must not go up and down stairs for 24 hours more. She is then cautioned to limit her activities for another two or three days. Coitus is interdicted for two weeks following the last bleeding. If the bleeding continues unchanged after 48 hours of bed rest, it is wise to explain to the patient that she may abort, and if about to abort little can be done to prevent it, continued bed rest simply postponing the inevitable a few days longer. On the other hand, if the bleeding is of a benign variety, its continuance is of no grave moment. In either instance, getting out of bed is indicated, for if abortion is threatened, getting up may precipitate the issue and save wasted days of inactivity. This apparently radical procedure is dictated by the fact that most abortions are germ plasmic in origin, and it is a conservative act to get them over promptly. If the bleeding is benign, getting up will not cause abortion. Exposure of the cervix with a sterile bivalve speculum may reveal a cervical polyp or erosion as the source of blood. Either may safely be treated in early pregnancy. The polyp may be twisted off and its base cauterized, and the erosion gently cauterized with silver nitrate or the actual cautery.

Vaginal Bleeding with Pain, in Early Pregnancy. Usually the vaginal bleeding begins first and the pain begins later; it may be a few hours later or several days later. The pain may be anterior and clearly rhythmic in type, simulating diminutive labor pains; it may be a persistent low backache, associated with a feeling of pelvic pressure, or it may be a dull, midline, suprasymphyseal discomfort, accompanied often by urinary frequency and tenderness over the uterus. No matter which of the three forms the pain takes, the prognosis is poor for continuation of the pregnancy. Usually, when abortion threatens to this extent, it progresses to the stage of imminent abortion and finally to abortion itself. However, some threatened abortions with pain clear up and go through a normal pregnancy; accordingly, it may be worth while to try to save the pregnancy, since no harm can be done except prolonging the unpleasant process by several hours or days. The patient is ordered to bed and a teaspoon of paregoric given pending the doctor's arrival. An ice cap is placed on the lower abdomen. When the doctor arrives and he finds the bleeding slight and the cervix undilated, he injects $\frac{1}{4}$ grain or $\frac{1}{6}$ grain of morphine. The paregoric is repeated every 6 hours during the first 24 hours; by the end of this time the process either will have progressed to the stage of imminent abortion or the pains will have disappeared. In the latter instance, the patient is then treated like a case of vaginal bleeding without pain. Progesterone and vitamin E therapy might be added to the above regimen. Ten milligrams of progesterone are injected intramuscularly, twice during the first day, then 10 mg. daily until bleeding ceases, followed by 10 mg. every other day for one week. Pregnanenolone, 50 mg. by mouth, may be used instead of injections if desired, and is more convenient. If vitamin E concentrate in the form of the mixed tocopherols is available, 40 mg. may be given by mouth daily, until fetal movements appear. The efficacy of these two therapeutic agents in preventing a truly threatened abortion from progressing to actual abortion is still unsettled.

In occasional instances, notwithstanding appropriate treatment and rest in bed, slight hemorrhage may persist for weeks; and it then becomes essential to determine whether there is any possibility of the pregnancy continuing. If two consecutive chorionic gonadotrophin determinations on blood or urine are negative, it can be assumed that the outlook is hopeless. Positive findings, however, indicate simply that there is living trophoblast still present and mean little or nothing in respect to whether the fetus is alive or dead. In the latter event the problem cannot be settled at once, but necessitates a delay of several weeks and repeated bimanual examinations. If at the end of this period one is convinced that the uterus has not increased in size, or even has become smaller, one is usually justified in concluding that the fetus is dead while, on the other hand, an increase in size probably indicates that it is still alive. As soon as one is convinced that the fetus is dead, the uterus should be emptied.

Imminent Abortion. Since an imminent abortion is almost certain to terminate in actual abortion, it is wise to hospitalize the patient at once. She should be grouped and matched for possible transfusion as soon as she arrives. If the bleeding is not profuse and the pain not severe, temporization may be carried out by administering ⅙ grain of morphine and awaiting developments. If bleeding and pain persist unabated for six hours, it is probably best to face the reality of abortion and encourage its occurrence by injecting 0.5 cc. of pituitrin every half-hour, for six doses. Since this is likely to increase the pain, it is well to precede the injections with 3 to 4.5 grains of nembutal, seconal or amytal. All tissue passed should be kept and carefully studied; first, to see whether the abortion is complete, and second, to determine whether the abortion is caused by germ plasm defects or some other factor which has caused the uterus to empty itself of a normal ovum. If the patient is afebrile and the pituitrin does not succeed in making the pregnancy abort, the patient should be taken to the operating room and a curettage done, under anesthesia. Intravenous pentothal sodium anesthesia is quite ideal, in our hands, for such a short procedure, in which anesthesia is the prime requisite and not complete muscular relaxation. If the patient is febrile, further temporization is obligatory, unless the bleeding is too severe to permit it. Whenever possible, the expectant treatment should be pursued in febrile cases until the patient has been afebrile for 72 hours. Administration of penicillin is a great boon in the infected case, and should be continued for several days after the curettage.

Inevitable Abortion. If in early pregnancy the sudden discharge of fluid, suggesting rupture of the membranes, occurs before any pain or bleeding, the patient is put to bed and observed. If, after 48 hours, there is no further fluid and no bleeding or pain, the patient may get up and, after 48 hours more, continue her usual activities.

On the other hand, if the gush of fluid is followed by bleeding and pain, or if it occurs after pain and bleeding have already begun, abortion is inevitable. The patient should be hospitalized, matched for transfusion, and the pituitrin injections, described above, carried out. If pituitrin is ineffective, curettage should be done, as detailed above.

Incomplete Abortion. A patient with an incomplete abortion should be hospitalized, matched for transfusion and, if afebrile, the retained tissue removed promptly. Since pituitrin is seldom effective in these cases, surgical completion of the abortion should be resorted to at once. In many cases the unpassed placental tissue simply lies loose in the cervical canal and can be lifted from an exposed external os with ovum forceps. If not, ordinary curettage is performed. In an incomplete abortion, it is often unnecessary to dilate the cervix preliminary to curettage. The technic of completion of an incomplete abortion is described on page 1045.

Hemorrhage from incomplete abortion is occasionally severe, acute and shocking, but rarely, if ever, fatal. Apparently when the blood pressure drops low enough the bleeding from the uterus stops temporarily. Such patients will do best if transfused while being curetted.

Missed Abortion. The safest treatment of missed abortion is simply to wait for nature to take its course, which finally eventuates in a normal, spontaneous abortion. Although the importunities of the patient and her relatives for interference may make this course difficult, the wise physician will stand firm in the matter because dilatation of the cervix and curettage are more difficult in these cases and fraught with a greater likelihood of uterine perforation. The old notion that these patients absorb toxic products from the products of conception is without foundation, and any symptoms which suggest this genesis are probably the result of the psychological reaction of the patient.

HABITUAL ABORTION

The general connotation of the term "habitual abortion" is sufficiently clear, namely, sequential abortion in such number as to leave little doubt that some recurrent etiological factor is responsible. In order to convert this generalization into a usable definition it obviously becomes necessary to know how many consecutive abortions a woman must have had before there is little doubt that some recurrent etiological factor is responsible. With data now available it is possible to do this in a logical and fairly accurate manner.

The incidence of spontaneous abortion in general, as already discussed, is very close to 10 per cent of all pregnancies. As pointed out by Malpas, all cases of spontaneous abortion may be regarded as falling into two main categories. On the one hand, there is a group in which abortion is the result of random or fortuitous factors which are not likely to repeat themselves in a succeeding pregnancy except, again, by chance On the other hand, there is a group in which some condition inimical to the growth of the ovum recurs in each pregnancy. In Hertig's opinion the proportion of habitual abortions in all spontaneous abortions probably lies somewhere between 3.6 and 9.8 per cent. If Bishop's figure of 0.41 per cent as representing the absolute incidence of habitual abortion in pregnancy is used and it is recalled that 10 per cent of all pregnancies abort spontaneously, the percentage of spontaneous abortions that are due to recurrent factors is 4.1. Other figures reported are of the same order.

On the basis of the above estimates it would appear, then, that about 9.6 per cent of all pregnancies terminate in abortion as the result of random factors and that 0.4 per cent, approximately, end in abortion as the result of recurrent causes. With these figures in mind let us follow 100,000 women through successive pregnancies and calculate the incidence with which repeated abortion might be expected to occur. As shown in Table 14, 9,600 of these women would abort in their first pregnancies as the result of random factors and 400 because of recurrent causes, a total of 10,000 abortions, or 10 per cent. Now, if these 10,000 women, each with a history of one abortion, are followed in similar manner through their second pregnancies, 922 (9.6 per cent of 9,600) will abort from chance causes, while the same 400 who aborted in the previous pregnancies from recurrent factors will do so again. In other words, only 13.2 per cent of these patients with one previous abortion repeat in the next pregnancy. Since 86.8 per cent do not abort, the spontaneous cure rate is 86.8 per cent.

Number of Cases	Previous Abortion	Will Abort from Accidental Causes	Will Abort from Recurrent Causes	Total Abortions	Per cent Will Abort	Spontaneous Cure Rate
100,000	0	9,600	400	10,000	10.0	—
10,000	1	922 (9.6% of above figure)	400 (Same 400)	1,322	13.2	86.8
1,322	2	88 (9.6% of above figure)	400 (Same 400)	488	36.9	63.1
488	3	8 (9.6% of above figure)	400 (Same 400)	408	83.6	16.4

TABLE 14. SHOWING HOW 100,000 WOMEN WILL BEHAVE IN SUCCESSIVE PREGNANCIES IN RESPECT TO REPEATED ABORTION.

The calculations are based on the assumption that 10 per cent of all pregnancies terminate in spontaneous abortion, 9.6 per cent from accidental causes and 0.4 per cent from recurrent factors. Even though the figures, 9.6 and 0.4, are changed considerably, the result is about the same. Thus, Malpas, who first suggested this approach, employed 17 and 1 and calculated spontaneous cure rates of 78.4 62.0, and 27.0 per cent respectively, instead of those given in the right-hand column.

Table 14 follows these same women through four pregnancies and shows that after two consecutive spontaneous abortions, a patient in any third gestation has almost two chances out of three (63.1 per cent) of a successful term pregnancy without any therapy whatsoever. This fact is important for several reasons: (1) In dealing with patients who have had two previous abortions a physician is justified in offering a fairly optimistic outlook for any third gestation. (2) In the evaluation of any therapy given to such women in their third pregnancies, the physician must be wary because two out of three will go to term satisfactorily without treatment. (3) Any definition of habitual abortion based on two consecutive spontaneous abortions is inept and misleading. On the one hand it gives rise to undue pessimism in regard to the natural outcome of subsequent pregnancies in such cases; and, on the other, it may result in unjustified optimism in the evaluation of therapy.

Between a woman who has had two consecutive abortions and one who has had three, there is a great difference in prognosis, the spontaneous cure rate falling from 63.1 to 16.4 per cent. Certainly, when the outlook for a subsequent pregnancy is as poor as it is in this latter group, with only one chance in six of success in any subsequent gestation, we are fully justified in postulating a recurring factor. There is good reason for believing, accordingly, that habitual abortion should be defined as *a condition in which a woman has had three or more consecutive, spontaneous abortions*. As indicated in the preceding paragraph, the definition of this condition is not merely of academic interest but has far-reaching clinical implications, particularly in regard to the evaluation of therapy.

Etiology. Few subjects rest upon such an uncertain and unsatisfactory basis as does the etiology of habitual abortion. Obviously, there can be only two main causes, defective germ cells and faulty maternal environment. As will be seen, the latter may be due to a multitude of factors.

Defective Germ Cells. Either the spermatozoa or the ova are regularly so defective that a pathologic conceptus results from every fertilization and is aborted. The fact that periods of sterility are often interspersed with abortions tends to support this idea of ineffectual germ cells.

Faulty Maternal Environment. It is well known that 50 to 80 per cent of all abortuses are pathologic, often lacking an embryo altogether. Whether this is usually due to a primary defect in the germ cells, as suggested above, or to faulty maternal environment, is an old and moot question, but in habitual abortion at least there is considerable evidence to suggest that maternal causes are responsible for many cases. These causes may be of various kinds, as follows:

Thyroid Deficiency. In a careful study of 43 cases of habitual abortion studied in our clinic by Delfs and Jones, it was found that low thyroid function was by far the most common deficiency encountered since it occurred in 31 (72 per cent) of the 43 cases and was the sole factor in 19 (44 per cent). Litzenberg pointed out the importance of thyroid in reproduction many years ago but recently it has been overshadowed by the newer and more popular steroid hormones.

Progesterone and Estrogen Deficiency. Since these two hormones are responsible for the maintenance of the decidual bed which in turn maintains the conceptus, it is understandable that a shortage in either might conceivably cause the death of the embryo. The data of Delfs and Jones mentioned above suggest that the deficiency of progesterone alone is rare and, even when associated with other deficiencies, was demonstrable in but 17 per cent of their cases. Nevertheless, a large number of reports have purported to show that progesterone therapy in habitual abortion is efficacious in many cases.

Vitamin E Deficiency. Female rats on a vitamin E deficient diet conceive satisfactorily but absorb or abort the fetuses about the twelfth day of pregnancy. Although this phenomenon does not ensue in certain other species, although human diets are rarely deficient in vitamin E and although serum vitamin E values are not ordinarily reduced in habitual abortion, this theory is widely held, and some form of vitamin E is usually employed in therapy. It may be concerned in progesterone manufacture and action.

Uterine Abnormalities. Both hypoplasia of the uterus and partial septa which bulge down into the cavity are known causes of habitual abortion.

Fibromyomata. These may be causes of habitual abortion if situated near the endometrium.

Cervical Lacerations and Previous Operations on Cervix. Cervical injury, whether from childbirth or operation, is an occasional cause of late abortion.

Retroflexion of Uterus. If present in extreme degree, retroflexion of the uterus may cause abortion as a result of the associated passive congestion of the endometrium.

Syphilis. Although never a cause of abortion before the fourth month, syphilis was formerly a common cause of late abortion and still possesses this potentiality if untreated.

Hypertensive Vascular Disease. Late abortions, fetal death in utero, and premature delivery, often as the result of abruptio placentae, are rather common accompaniments of this condition, particularly if there is an associated nephritis.

Finally, as far as we are able to ascertain at the present time, Rh incompatibility does *not* cause abortion.

Treatment. *Preliminary Investigation.* Patients with a history of repeated abortion should have a thorough study before another pregnancy is undertaken. General and pelvic examinations should be carried out with correction of any contributory factors such as infection or anemia. Weight and nutritional status should also be evaluated. Many of these women show slight to moderate obesity and an occasional one is underweight. Dietary measures should be directed toward an ideal weight. All patients with reproductive difficulties should have a high protein, high vitamin diet, with adjustment of total calories to favor loss or gain as the situation indicates. Inquiry should be made into the habits of the patient. Excessive fatigue, insufficient sleep, nervous tension due to overwork or social activities, should be corrected. Immoderate drinking and smoking should be eliminated, particularly as the latter often interferes with good nutrition. If the husband's semen examination, which should always be carried out, shows abnormalities, a similar dietary and hygienic regime should be instituted for him. Vigorous sports, strenuous activity and hard work are prohibited throughout pregnancy. Bed rest is generally unnecessary for long periods but it should be advised for episodes of uterine irritability, cramping or bleeding. Coitus should be omitted for the first four months of pregnancy and should be discontinued entirely if followed by discomfort or cramps

These measures directed at the general health of the patient are of more value in many cases than the supposedly specific types of therapy listed below; and certainly they should comprise part of the instructions given to all these patients.

Thyroid Extract. Basal metabolism and blood cholesterol determinations should be carried out before pregnancy is begun. Treatment may be considered indicated if the cholesterol is over 225 mg. per cent, or if the basal metabolic rate is below zero. It is recognized that the latter criterion varies from the usual allowance of minus 10 for the lower limit of normal and therefore includes a few patients who may be low normals. This is justifiable therapy in individuals who give a history of abortions, as there is some evidence that reproductive difficulty may be the most sensitive indicator of thyroid deficiency and may be manifest long before other clinical signs. Most of these patients never develop symptoms and signs of definite myxedema. Dosage of thyroid should be adjusted to the need but large amounts are rarely required. Most patients respond well in the range of one-half grain to 2 grains daily. Thyroid treatment should be maintained three to four months before pregnancy is attempted. This point of treatment with thyroid some months before pregnancy has been overlooked frequently and may account for some disappointments in its use. It should be continued throughout pregnancy though reduction in dosage may be necessary occasionally in the last trimester.

Progesterone. The most logical use of progesterone in habitual abortion would seem to be prophylactic treatment in the premenstrual period and through the early weeks of pregnancy as suggested by Rutherford. This aids in building up and maintaining a succulent progestational endometrium during the critical stage of implantation and rapid early fetal development. Satisfactory dosage is 30 mg. daily of one of the oral preparations, divided into three doses beginning 7 to 10 days before the expected menstrual period. If the menstrual period occurs, indicating that pregnancy is not present, medication is discontinued until the latter part of the next cycle. If pregnancy occurs, the therapy is continued in the same dosage until the fourth or fifth month of pregnancy when it may be tapered off, although there is no objection, aside from its expense, to carrying it on to the last month.

Estrogen and Combined Estrogen Progesterone. As the results of the observations of Karnaky, Vaux and Rakoff and of Smith and Smith, estrogen alone or in combination with progesterone is being used widely in the treatment of habitual abortion. The rationale of the combined employment of estrogen and progesterone as stated by Vaux and Rakoff is as follows: (1) Progesterone and estrogen are believed to come from the same sources throughout gestation, and their concentrations throughout gestation roughly parallel each other. (2) It is logical to assume that a deficiency in progesterone would be accompanied by a deficiency in estrogen. (3) In the experience of Vaux and Rakoff such double deficiencies of estrogen and progesterone frequently occur in abortion patients, often appearing early in the gestation and persisting in many cases throughout the period of pregnancy. (4) There are good reasons to believe that estrogen and progesterone influence the normal reactions of each other upon the uterus and are involved in the normal metabolism of each other. Smith and Smith recommend estrogen alone in the belief that it stimulates the secretion both of estrogen and progesterone. The latter authors employ estrogen in the form of diethylstilbestrol and recommend the following dosage schedule: 5 mg. by mouth is started during the sixth or seventh week counting from the beginning of the last menstrual period; the daily dosage is increased by 5 mg. at two weekly intervals to the fifteenth week when 25 mg. daily are given; thereafter the daily dosage is increased by 5 mg. at weekly intervals; administration is discontinued at the end of the thirty-fifth week. Smith and Smith emphasize the fact that these dosages are not large enough per se to raise the estrogen level above the physiologic norm of pregnancy.

Vitamin E. In the study by Delfs and Jones mentioned above, only 16 per cent of the patients showed vitamin E levels below the normal range and it is very questionable whether vitamin E deficiency plays any appreciable role in the causation of habitual abortion. Nevertheless it is harmless and relatively inexpensive and may be used prophylactically before and during pregnancy despite the fact that it is probably unnecessary. Alpha-tocopherol in 25 mg. dosage daily is satisfactory and will raise low vitamin E levels to normal.

Prognosis. As Table 14 and many reports attest, the outlook for a successful pregnancy after two consecutive abortions is relatively good, being of the order of 65 per cent, even without treatment. With proper management, three fourths of these patients or more should be able to go through pregnancy satisfactorily. Following three consecutive abortions, the prognosis is less hopeful but even in this group, Delfs and Jones have reported 67 per cent success in 43 pregnancies in which the therapy consisted chiefly in hygienic measures, thyroid, and in some cases, progesterone. Many similar series are on record with equally good or better results. After four consecutive abortions, the outlook is decidedly worse but it should be emphasized that in the absence of clear-cut anatomical derangements (such as an amputated cervix), the prognosis is rarely altogether hopeless. Thus, it is not unusual to see patients who have had six or seven consecutive abortions and who, without treatment or other adequate explanation, go through a full term pregnancy without mishap.

INDUCED ABORTION

Therapeutic abortion is discussed in Chapter 39.

Criminal Abortion. The incidence of criminal abortion, for obvious reasons, cannot be estimated with accuracy, but most observers believe that it is appallingly frequent. In 1936 Taussig concluded that there was 1 abortion to every 2.5 viable births in the urban communities of this country, and 1 abortion to every 5 births in the rural areas, yielding a total of 681,000 abortions annually, an abortion rate of 22 per 100 pregnancies. Since the spontaneous abortion rate is approximately 10 per 100 pregnancies, and since the incidence of therapeutic abortion is well under 1 per 100 pregnancies, the conclusion seems justifiable, according to Taussig, that some 11 or 12 per cent of the total pregnancies in the United States are terminated by criminal interference. Tietze has recently reviewed 10,397 of our obstetric case records which provide histories of 30,133 previous pregnancies. Of these, 5,124, or 17.0 per cent, ended in abortions. By employing the same kind of reasoning as is used above, it may be concluded that some 7 per cent of these abortions were criminal. Similar studies on case histories at certain New York birth control clinics, show a much higher frequency of criminal abortion, namely, about 20 per cent (Stix, Kopp). On the other hand, Wiehl and Berry, in a study of a population sample from the five Boroughs of New York City, report a rate of only 4 per cent.

Wiehl and Berry cite a very high incidence of criminal abortion for third and fourth pregnancies in women of the low income group. Moreover, Taussig writes: "The vast majority of all (criminal) abortions, equalling 90 per cent, occur among married women, especially those between 25 and 35 years of age who have had several children." According to the study of Stix, 75 per cent of illegal abortions are induced by persons designated by the patients as doctors, 19 per cent by midwives and 6 per cent are self-induced. Taussig states that over 50 per cent are performed by doctors, 20 per cent by midwives and less than 30 per cent by the patient herself.

Criminal abortion is one of the most important causes of maternal death. In 1936 Taussig estimated that at least 8,000 fatalities in the United States stemmed annually from this source; and although chemotherapy has reduced the figure, the toll is still high. Moreover, for every woman who dies as the result of criminal abortion, several are disabled or rendered sterile. The high death rate associated with criminal abortion is attributable to three main causes: (1) postabortal infection; (2) hemorrhage; and (3) perforation of the uterus. (See below.)

THE DANGERS OF LEGITIMATE AND CRIMINAL ABORTION

Postabortal Infection. Puerperal infection following abortion is the chief cause of abortion mortality, being responsible for about three quarters of all such deaths. Postabortal infection is largely a problem of induced abortion, especially criminal abortion, for it rarely complicates true spontaneous abortion. The clinical as well as the pathological picture of postabortal infection resembles puerperal infection as discussed in Chapter 35. Moreover, except for the problem of emptying the uterus, the treatment is the same.

There is a great difference of opinion in regard to the advisability of immediate evacuation of the uterus in cases in which the infected abortion is incomplete. It is rather generally agreed that if the infection has extended beyond the uterus, it is best to abstain from interference unless one's hand is forced by life-threatening hemorrhage. On the other hand, if careful pelvic examination shows the septic process well localized within the uterus, one school favors immediate evacuation of the uterus while the other practices continued temporization with perhaps the administration of oxytocic drugs. The danger of instrumental emptying of the uterus under these circumstances lies, of course, in the likelihood of disseminating infection to distant foci. The advent of chemotherapy, especially the antibiotics, has greatly reduced but by no means eliminated this hazard. Our present management of cases of infected incomplete abortion is as follows. Immediately upon admission to the hospital, the patient is given massive doses of penicillin or aureomycin together with therapeutic doses of sulfadiazine. If bleeding is substantial, evacuation of the uterus is performed, preferably by means of a sponge forceps; in some cases, however, it is necessary to employ a curet, despite the infection. If the amount of bleeding is inconsequential, the chemotherapy is continued and, as a rule the temperature returns to normal within 24 or 48 hours. After the temperature has remained normal for 48 hours, the uterus is emptied by means of a sponge forceps and curet.

Hemorrhage. In hospital practice fatal hemorrhage from abortion is extremely rare. Thus, we have treated over 2,500 cases of abortion at the Johns Hopkins Hospital without a single death which was directly attributable to bleeding; many of these patients were admitted in an alarming state of exsanguination, but the bleeding invariably stopped before the blood loss assumed lethal proportions. Other clinics can cite similar records, and in general it would appear that in hospital practice not one abortion death in a hundred is the direct result of hemorrhage. In sharp variance with this statement is the fact that maternal mortality surveys for the country at large invariably attribute a substantial proportion of abortion deaths to hemorrhage. This curious discrepancy needs explanation. Although it would be difficult to prove, it seems probable that some of the deaths charged to abortion hemorrhage in the mortality surveys were actually cases of uterine perforation and shock consequent to criminal abortion.

From a practical viewpoint the importance of abortion hemorrhage is twofold: (1) it necessitates evacuation of the uterus, even in a febrile patient when this would not otherwise be done; (2) it makes the patient an easy prey to infection. In assessing the need for evacuating the uterus, individual attention must be given each patient, the chief points to be considered being the amount of blood being lost, the degree of anemia already present, the presence of infection, the probability of rapid spontaneous expulsion of the products of conception, and the extent of the manipulations which will be necessary in order to procure evacuation. In the presence of infection, the simplest method which will control the bleeding is the best, intra-uterine manipulation being avoided if at all possible. The common procedures employed to meet this situation are: (1) The administration of pituitary extract or pitocin in an effort to promote spontaneous expulsion of the uterine contents. (2) Inspection of the cervix, which will often be found dilated, with the product of conception in its rim, whence it can be easily removed without uterine invasion. (3) If the above measures fail, uterine tamponade may occasionally prove helpful, the gauze being removed after 12 hours; following this period the product of conception is usually completely separated and is either in the vagina or can be removed from the uterus without extensive manipulation. (4) As stated above, the advent of chemotherapy has lessened the danger of instrumental evacuation of the uterus in the presence of infection and with the protection afforded by these agents, any substantial degree of hemorrhage is best met by the removal of the ovum by means of sponge forceps and/or the curet.

Uterine Perforation. Perforation of the uterus in the induction or completion of an abortion is ordinarily due to mistakes in judgment or technic on the part of the operator. In the hands of well-trained operators, in good clinics, the frequency has been variously estimated from 1 to 150 to 1 in 1,000 evacuations of the uterus. In the hands of less-skilled persons, under clandestine circumstances, it must be far more frequent. It is estimated that every second or third perforation ends fatally. Most perforations are committed by physicians; for curets, metal dilators, ovum forceps and sounds are the main offenders in the order named, and these tools are rarely used by lay abortionists. They rely on rupture of the membranes, the injection of fluids and pastes, and the introduction of laminaria and bougies. It is well to remember that one is unlikely to perforate a well-contracted uterus, and therefore 1 cc. of intramuscular pituitrin, given just before the operation, will help safeguard against this accident.

Simple perforation through the fundus may cause no difficulty, unless bacteria from within the uterus contaminate the peritoneum. If simple perforation occurs in a clean case, in good hospital surroundings, it is wise simply to observe the patient and refrain from laparotomy unless evidence of hemorrhage appears. If the case is sent in from the outside, and if the perforation is less than 24 hours old, a laparotomy should be done. The type of operation performed will depend on the condition met—a hysterectomy may be necessary, sometimes even intestinal resection.

Frequently, the perforation damages the parametrium and initiates severe hemorrhage. One of the commoner serious accidents is for the operator to pull down with an ovum forceps loops of intestine, or parts of the omentum, through the uterine rent, and to tear off or cut off pieces before he realizes what has happened. Obviously, laparotomy holds out the only hope in such cases.

PREMATURE LABOR

As pointed out in Chapter 1, premature birth is by far the most common cause of neonatal mortality, being responsible for one half of all such deaths. The incidence of premature labor in 3,331 cases observed at the Johns Hopkins Hospital was 11.7 per cent, but this is probably higher than obtains in the population at large. Dana's figure for the New York Lying-In experience was 2.95 per cent and our own in unselected private patients was 5.3 per cent. Only in some 40 per cent of these cases can the cause of the premature delivery be demonstrated definitely. On the basis of the Johns Hopkins Hospital series cited previously, the maternal diseases which most frequently initiate the onset of premature labor are chronic hypertensive vascular disease, abruptio placentae, placenta previa and untreated syphilis. In other cases certain diseases, especially preeclampsia, demand termination of pregnancy prior to viability of the fetus in order to safeguard the mother's life. If cases of multiple pregnancy and congenital abnormalities be added to these two groups, the total number of cases of premature labor in which the causative factor can be definitely demonstrated is less than 40 per cent. While this percentage must be regarded as an approximation only, there is general agreement that a large proportion of premature labors, in the neighborhood of one-half, are without explanation.

In view of the high mortality rate of premature infants and the consequent wastage of infant life associated with premature labor, the factors responsible for these many unexplained premature births constitute an important problem. There is suggestive evidence that in many of the cases nutritional deficiencies play a role, but this evidence is not altogether conclusive and, at best, difficult to prove.

Premature labor is often signalized by rupture of the membranes at or before its onset, this accident being noted in one third of Dana's cases at the New York Lying-In Hospital. In 20.2 per cent of her entire series premature rupture of the membranes occurred in the absence of any other complication and she feels that this sudden escape of fluid may in itself constitute an actual causative factor in precipitating premature labor. Whether in such cases the forces concerned in labor, such as increased uterine contractility and cervical effacement, have already been mobilized so that rupture of the membranes occurs simply as the result of these processes, or whether the rupture of the waters itself is the primary etiological factor, as Dana believes, cannot be stated definitely. If she is correct in her viewpoint, one sixth to one fifth of premature labors could be charged against this sheer accident.

Management of Premature Labor. Because of the tenuous hold which premature infants have on life it is of the utmost importance that nothing be done in labor to narcotize or traumatize them. One of the most common errors made in the management of premature labor is an effort to stop it by the administration of morphine or some other sedative drug. This is not only futile, as a rule, but is often followed in a few hours by the delivery of a heavily drugged infant. Patients who rupture their membranes prematurely should be left alone, preferably in the hospital, and no attempt made to bring on labor. They will often go for weeks with ruptured membranes and finally go into labor near term without event. The chief potential danger is intra-uterine infection, especially if coitus should take place. If all possibility of the latter can be eliminated, the patient can stay at home. We have handled several hundred cases of premature rupture of the membranes in this manner without complication, but now and then penicillin may be necessary because of infection. No greater error can be made than to try to induce labor in these cases because no end of maternal difficulties may result and in addition many infants lost from prematurity. It is now widely recognized that interference is rarely necessary in these cases.

Patients in premature labor should be permitted no form of analgesia except continuous caudal or spinal anesthesia. Likewise, the delivery should be effected by caudal, spinal or local infiltration anesthesia. Delivery should be preceded by a liberal median episiotomy.

In regard to the best way to effect the actual delivery of a premature infant, especially a small one, the ideal procedure, in my opinion, is as follows: with the head on the perineum and the vulvar ring just beginning to distend, a median episiotomy is made and this is followed by gentle fundal pressure. This usually suffices for most cases but with some of the larger prematures, gentle forceps extraction may be advisable. When possible we prefer spontaneous delivery, assisted by fundal pressure, to forceps. The cord should not be clamped until pulsations cease since these infants, due to their tendency to develop anemia, need all the blood they can get. The infant now becomes a pediatric problem, but it should be remembered by obstetricians as well as pediatricians that the main immediate desiderata are: a clear airway, oxygen, warmth and as little handling as possible.

BIBLIOGRAPHY

American Medical Association, Council on Pharmacy and Chemistry. The Treatment of Habitual Abortion with Vitamin E. J.A.M.A., 1940, 114:2214.

Bishop, P. M. F. Studies in Clinical Endocrinology: "Habitual Abortion"; Its Incidence and Treatment with Progesterone and Vitamin E. Guy's Hosp. Rep., 1937, 87:362.

Breus, C. Das tuberöse subchoriale Haematom der Decidua. Leipzig u. Wien, 1892.

Corner, G. W. Embryonic Pathology in Mammals, with Observations upon Intra-uterine Mortality in the Pig. Am. J. Anat., 1923, 31:523.

Dana, E. S. Premature Delivery, Causes and Results. Am. J. Obst. & Gynec., 1946, 51:329.

Datnow, M. M. An Experimental Investigation Concerning Toxic Abortion Produced by Chemical Agents. J. Obst. & Gynaec. Brit. Emp., 1928, 35:693.

Delfs, E., and Jones, G. E. S. Some Aspects of Habitual Abortion. South. M. J., 1948, 41:809.

——— Endocrine Patterns in Abortion. Obst. & Gynec. Survey, 1948, 3:680.

Eastman, N. J. Habitual Abortion. Chapter 4 in Progress in Gynecology, Grune and Stratton, New York, 1946.

——— Prematurity from the Viewpoint of the Obstetrician. Am. Practitioner, 1947, 1:343.

Evans, H. M., Burr, G. O., and Althausen, T. L. The Antisterility Vitamine Fat Soluble E. Memoirs of the University of California, 1927, Vol. 8.

Galloway, C. E. Discussion of Simons' Paper. Am. J. Obst. & Gynec., 1939, 37:848.

Grosser, O. Trophoblastswäche und zottenarme Menscliche Eier. Ztschr. f. mikr.-anat. Forsch., 1926, 5:197.

Guttmacher, A. F. An Analysis of 521 Cases of Twin Pregnancy. II. The Hazards of Pregnancy Itself. Am. J. Obst. & Gynec., 1939, 38:77.

Hartman, C. G. The Interruption of Pregnancy by Ovariectomy in the Aplacental Opossum. Am. J. Physiol., 1925, 71:346.

——— Studies in the Reproduction of the Monkey. Carnegie Inst. of Wash., 1932, Contrib. to Embryology, No. 134.

Hertig, A. T., and Edmonds, H. W. Genesis of Hydatidiform Mole. Arch. Path., 1940, 30:260.

Hertig, A. T., and Livingstone, R. G. Spontaneous, Threatened and Habitual Abortion. Its Pathogenesis and Treatment. New England J. Med., 1944, 230:797.

Hertig, A. T., and Sheldon, W. H. Minimal Criteria Required to Prove Prima Facie Case of Traumatic Abortion or Miscarriage. Ann. Surg., 1943, 117:596.

Huntington, J. L. A Review of the Pathology of 104 Consecutive Miscarriages in Private Obstetric Practice. Am. J. Obst. & Gynec., 1929, 17:32.

Karnaky, K. J. The Use of Stilbestrol for Treatment of Threatened and Habitual Abortion and Premature Labor. South. M. J., 1942, 35:838.

Kopp, M. E. Birth Control in Practice. Robert M. McBride and Co., New York, 1934.

Liepmann, W. Die Abtreibung. Berlin u. Wien, 1927.

Litzenberg, J. C. Missed Abortion. Am. J. Obst. & Gynec., 1921, 1:475.

Mall, F. P., and Meyer, A. W. Studies on Abortuses: A Survey of Pathologic Ova in the Carnegie Embryological Collection. Carnegie Inst. of Wash., 1921, Publ. No. 275, Vol. 12.

Malpas, P. A Study of Abortion Sequences. J. Obst. & Gynaec. Brit. Emp., 1938, 45:932.

Monro, J. S. Premature Infant Weighing Less than One Pound at Birth Who Survived and Developed Normally. Canad. M. A. J., 1939, 40:69.

Muller, H. J. Quoted by Castle, W. E. Genetics and Eugenics. Harvard University Press. Cambridge, 1931, p. 246.

Rock, J., and Hertig, A. T. Some Aspects of Early Human Development. Am. J. Obst. & Gynec., 1942, 44:973.

Rutherford, R. N. The Significance of Bleeding in Early Pregnancy as Evidenced by Decidual Biopsy. Surg., Gynec. & Obst., 1942, 74:1139.

Simons, J. H. Statistical Analysis of One Thousand Abortions. Am. J. Obst. & Gynec., 1939, 37:840.

Smith. O. W. Diethylstilbestrol in the Prevention and Treatment of Complications of Pregnancy. Am. J. Obst. & Gynec., 1948, 56:82.

Stix, R. K. A Study of Pregnancy Wastage. Milbank Memorial Fund Quart., 1935, 13:347.

Stockard, C. R. Developmental Rate and Structural Expression; an Experimental Study of Twins, etc. Am. J. Anat., 1921, 28:115.

Streeter, G. L. Focal Deficiencies in Fetal Tissues and Their Relation to Intra-Uterine Amputation. Carnegie Inst. of Wash., 1930, Publ. No. 414. (Data on fetal retention tabulated on page 5.)

Taussig, F. J. Abortion. Spontaneous and Induced. Medical and Social Aspects. C. V. Mosby Co., St. Louis, 1936.

Tietze, C. An Investigation into the Incidence of Abortion in Baltimore. Am. J. Obst. & Gynec., 1948, 56:1160.

Vaux, N. W., and Rakoff, A. E. Estrogen-Progesterone Therapy: A New Approach in the Treatment of Habitual Abortion. Am. J. Obst. & Gynec., 1945, 50:353.

Wall, R. L., and Hertig, A. T. Habitual Abortion, Am. J. Obst. & Gynec., 1948, 56:1127.

Wiehl, D. G., and Berry, K. Pregnancy Wastage in New York City. Milbank Memorial Fund Quart., 1937, 15:229.

21

ECTOPIC PREGNANCY

By *ectopic pregnancy* is meant any gestation located outside the uterine cavity. It is a broader term than *extra-uterine pregnancy* since it includes gestations in the interstitial portion of the tube, those situated in a rudimentary horn of a uterus (cornual pregnancy) and cervical pregnancies as well as tubal, abdominal and ovarian gestations. The vast majority of ectopic pregnancies, over 95 per cent, are tubal gestations; as a consequence, the term "ectopic" is often used colloquially to mean tubal pregnancy but actually, as indicated, the two terms are not synonymous, tubal pregnancy being a type of ectopic gestation.

TUBAL PREGNANCY

Incidence. The frequency of tubal gestation is approximately once in every 250 pregnancies. Schumann calculated that the condition occurred once in every 303 pregnancies in Philadelphia during the year 1918. In 34,356 obstetric cases observed at the New York Lying-In Hospital, there were 128 instances of extra-uterine pregnancy, a frequency of one in 268 pregnancies. The condition is somewhat more common among Negresses than in white women. Thus, Anderson studied all the tubal pregnancies occurring in Baltimore over a five-year period in relation to all viable deliveries and found that the ratio of tubal pregnancies to viable deliveries in white women was 1:177, whereas in Negresses it was 1:121. This differential is believed to be due to a higher incidence of pelvic inflammatory diseases in Negresses.

Etiology. The causes of ectopic pregnancy may be classified as follows:

I. *Conditions which prevent or retard the passage of the fertilized ovum into the uterine cavity.*

(a) Chronic salpingitis, through causing agglutination of the arborescent folds of the tubal mucosa with narrowing of the lumen or the formation of blind pockets.

(b) Congenital and postembryonic developmental abnormalities of the tube, especially diverticula, accessory ostia and hypoplasia.

(c) Peritubal adhesions subsequent to postabortal or puerperal infection causing kinking of the tube with narrowing of the lumen.

(d) Tumors pressing from outside against the tube.

(e) Previous plastic operations on the tube.

(f) External migration of the ovum. By retarding the entry of the fertilized ovum into the tube, external migration allows time for the growth of the trophoblast (the burrowing apparatus) while the ovum is still in the tube. Normally the trophoblast does not develop until the ovum is in the uterine cavity.

II. *Conditions which increase the receptivity of the tubal mucosa to the fertilized ovum.*

(a) Ectopic endometrial elements in the tubal mucosa.

Although salpingitis is generally recognized as an important cause of tubal gestation, there is a divergency of opinion as to what proportion of cases can be attributed to it. Mahfouz has reported that in more than half of his series of 120 cases of tubal pregnancy there was a history of previous salpingitis and sterility. Tyrone, Romano, and Collins found salpingitis in 35 per cent of 309 cases. In 129 tubal pregnancies recently studied by Jarcho, salpingitis was demonstrable in 52.8 per cent. In a study of 141 cases of ectopic gestation observed at the New York Lying-In Hospital, Marchetti, Kuder and Kuder report a definite history of previous pelvic infection in 26.9 per cent of their cases. Langman and Goldblatt, in a study of 310 cases of ectopic pregnancy operated on in a large metropolitan hospital, report that less than 20 per cent had a history of pelvic infection but microscopic examination raised the incidence to more than 50 per cent. Other authors find that salpingitis plays a less important role in the etiology of ectopic pregnancy and point out moreover that the effusion of blood in this condition may cause irritative changes which simulate histologically the picture of salpingitis. In a study of salpingitis as an etiologic factor in ectopic pregnancy Van Etten found that only 10.4 per cent of the cases studied by him showed signs of previous or concurrent tubal inflammation. In MacFarlane and Sparling's series of 110 cases, only 17.2 per cent gave a history of pelvic infection, while less than 10 per cent of the specimens examined by Litzenberg showed salpingitis when subjected to pathological examination. Edward Allen, moreover, has adduced various evidence to support the viewpoint that salpingitis is an infrequent cause of tubal pregnancy. Thus he emphasizes such circumstances as the mobility of the affected tube in early ectopic pregnancy, the absence of external evidence of firm adhesions to the serosal coat of the tube and the normalcy of the tubal mucous membrane at some distance from the site of implantation. To summarize all this evidence, including Anderson's study mentioned above, it seems probable that salpingitis, although an important cause of tubal pregnancy, is responsible for only a minority of the cases, perhaps one-quarter.

Osiakina-Rojdestvenskaia has studied the tubes from 100 cases of tubal gestation by a meticulous histologic technic which made it possible for him to examine all the obstacles which might have interfered with the progress of the ovum and all the changes in the various layers along the entire length of the tube. He lists the etiologic factors in this series as follows: defective tubal development of postembryonic origin, 21 cases; adhesions between tubal folds due to insufficient differentiation of the tubal mucous membrane, 21 cases; adenomyosis, 19 cases; inflammation, 14 cases; and tumors, 3 cases. Seventy-six of the 100 cases, accordingly, were the result of mechanical obstacles in the tube. Ten additional cases are explained on the grounds that external migration of the ovum had occurred with the result that the ovum had time to develop its capacity to implant before reaching the uterus. Of the 14 cases attributed to inflammatory changes in the tube, six were due to perisalpingitis. In such cases the author found, in addition to adhesions which caused curvature of the tube, numerous scars in the muscular tissue which doubtless interfered with motor activity. Partial obliteration of the tubal lumen secondary to inflammatory processes, he encountered in only three cases. The author concludes that the most important factor in the causation of ectopic pregnancy is defective, postembryonic development of the tube.

Various observers have demonstrated healthy endometrial tissue in tubal lumina. Sampson and Jacobsen, and others, have proved beyond doubt that such endometrial tissue, escaping through the tubes during menstruation, becomes implanted elsewhere and continues to grow. Frankel and Schenck are of the opinion that all ectopic preg-

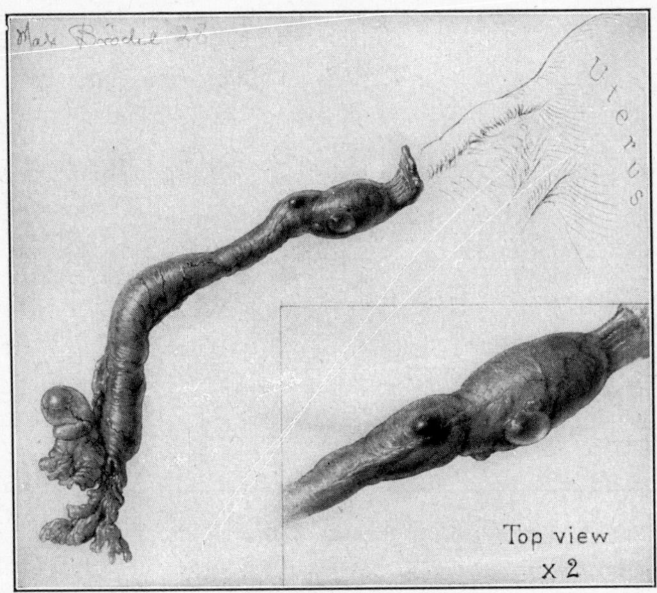

Fig. 317.—A Very Early Tubal Pregnancy.
(From Cullen, *Journal Missouri State Medical Association.*)

nancies, tubal or otherwise, occur because of nidation of the fertilized ovum in a locus of ectopic endometrial tissue to which the ovum is chemotactically attracted. In the 16 pregnant tubes examined by these authors, well-defined decidual tissue was present at the implantation site in 14 cases, and there only, while two tubes were so distended with old clotted blood that accurate identification of tissues was impossible. In one case they succeeded in finding endometrial glands in this decidual tissue, proving that they were dealing with actual endometrial elements and not with changes which the tubal mucosa had undergone. In the examination of a series of nonpregnant tubes they found ectopic endometrial tissue in one of 204 cases, an incidence of 0.5 per cent. The ratio of ectopic pregnancy to intra-uterine pregnancy was one in 303 in Schumann's series, 4 in 309 in Farrar's series, a suggestive correspondence of statistics. Villard, Regad, and Contamin also believe that the endometrial theory is the most adequate and only physiologic explanation of the condition.

Anatomic Considerations. The ovum may develop in any one of the several portions of the tube, giving rise to ampullar, isthmic and interstitial pregnancies, respectively. In rare instances it may be implanted on the fimbriated extremity, and occasionally even on the fimbria ovarica. From these primary types certain secondary forms occasionally develop: tubo-abdominal, tubo-ovarian and broad ligament. The ampulla is the most frequent site of implantation and the isthmus the next most common. Interstitial pregnancy is uncommon, being observed in only 3 to 4 per cent of all tubal gestations. Jarcho has analyzed 1,225 cases of ectopic pregnancy of all types, as reported by nine authors, and found that the location of the ectopic ovum was as follows: ampulla, 578; isthmus, 265; fimbriated extremity, 71; interstitial portion, 45; infundibula, 31; entire tube (including hematosalpinx containing products of conception), 17; abdomen, 17; distal half of tube, 10; distal two thirds of tube, 6; broad ligament, 5; entire tube and ovary, 5; cornu, 5; tubo-ovarian, 2; and rudimentary horn, 1. In 164 cases the site was not stated or, if stated, not proven.

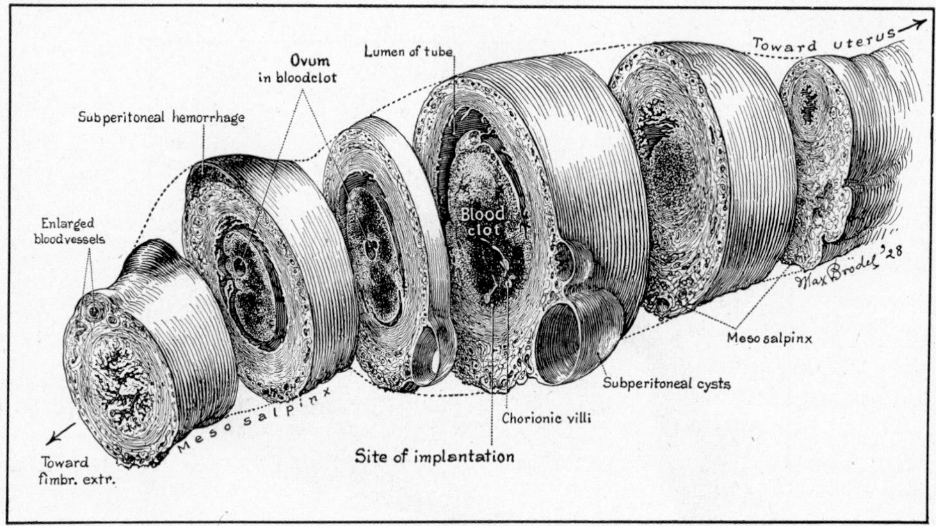

FIG. 318.—CROSS SECTION OF TUBE IN FIG. 317.

(Courtesy of Dr. Thomas S. Cullen.)

Mode of Implantation of the Ovum. The ovum may become implanted in one of two ways, columnar or intercolumnar. In the first, which is very rare, the ovum becomes attached to the tip or side of one of the folds of the mucosa; while in the second, implantation occurs at the peripheral portion of the lumen in a depression between two folds. In either event the ovum does not remain upon the surface but at once burrows through the epithelium and comes to lie in the tissue just beneath it. At that time its periphery is made up of a capsule of rapidly proliferating trophoblast the cells of which invade the surrounding tissues. The invasive and corrosive properties of these ectodermal cells bring about degeneration of the muscle and connective-tissue cells which eventually become converted into fibrin. At the same time maternal blood vessels are opened up and the blood is poured out into spaces of varying size lying entirely within the trophoblast or between it and the adjacent tissue. Young considers that edema and necrosis occur before the maternal tissue is reached by the fetal cells, and are probably due to the action of chemical substances secreted by the latter.

In the usual intercolumnar mode of implantation owing to the absence of a submucosa and the absence of a decidual membrane in the tube, as soon as the ovum penetrates the epithelium it comes to lie in the muscular wall and is separated from the lumen by a layer of tissue of varying thickness—the capsular membrane, or pseudocapsularis. On the other hand, in the rare columnar mode of implantation the ovum lies in the interior of a fold of mucosa and, except at its base, is surrounded on all sides by tubal epithelium so that it has but slight space for expansion.

The further development of the pregnancy depends in great part upon the portion of the tube in which implantation has occurred. When in the ampulla, the growing ovum pushes the capsular membrane forward into the tubal lumen so that the latter may eventually become so compressed as to appear as a mere crescentic slit. Later, if the course of the pregnancy is not interrupted, the capsular membrane may fuse with the neighboring mucosa, so that the lumen of the tube becomes obliterated in the immediate vicinity of the ovum.

However, when implantation occurs in the isthmus, and particularly in the portion immediately adjoining the uterus, the small size of the lumen precludes the possibility of such expansion. As a consequence the ovum distends the tube wall eccentrically, so that the lumen may eventually become completely separated from the underlying muscularis and be surrounded by fetal tissue and villi, with the result that intraperitoneal rupture frequently occurs before the patient is aware that she is pregnant. Connors, Cresci and Glass have recently reported the occurrence of tubal pregnancy in a woman who, four years previously, had been subjected to a supracervical hysterectomy.

Decidua. The tube does not undergo extensive decidual reaction but it is possible by careful study to distinguish decidual cells and to differentiate clearly between them and fetal cells. The former are usually found in discrete patches in the tips of some of the folds of the mucosa in the neighborhood of the ovum. Furthermore, one can occasionally find decidual cells scattered among the fetal tissues at the placental site, but a continuous decidual membrane analogous to the decidua in uterine pregnancy is never seen.

The absence, or comparative scantiness, of the decidual reaction is of interest not only from a scientific point of view, but also has a distinctly practical bearing, as it would seem to offer a satisfactory explanation for the invasion and destruction of the tubal wall by the fetal elements. In uterine pregnancy such an invasion is noted only in the rare instances of placenta accreta which is believed to result from defective development of the decidua. Consequently, it would appear that one of the main purposes of decidua formation is to protect the maternal tissues against the invasive and corrosive action of the fetal cells.

Decidua Capsularis. In view of the general scantiness of the decidual reaction, it is evident that one could not reasonably expect the formation of a structure identical with the decidua capsularis of uterine pregnancy. On the other hand, in all intact early tubal pregnancies, the ovum is separated from the lumen of the tube by a layer of connective and muscular tissue, which may contain a few isolated decidual cells. As the pregnancy advances this membrane becomes invaded by fetal cells, undergoes fibrinoid degeneration, and, if rupture does not occur, eventually fuses with the mucosa of the opposite side of the tube. As this structure is only superficially analogous to the decidua capsularis, it is better designated as the pseudocapsularis or capsular membrane.

Placenta. As the early stages of the development of the placenta are identical in both tubal and uterine pregnancy, the different outcome in the former is dependent upon the absence or scanty development of a decidual reaction. As a consequence the tissues of the tubal wall in contact with the ovum offer but slight resistance to the invasive properties of the fetal elements and soon undergo degenerative change. The chorionic villi and fetal cells invade this tissue, almost like a malignant growth, and at the same time open up maternal blood vessels. In many cases they penetrate directly through the peritoneal surface or through the capsular membrane, and give rise to intraperitoneal rupture or tubal abortion, as the case may be. In other instances, however, early rupture is due to the sudden opening up of a large vessel, when the weakened tubal walls yield to the increased pressure. Werth has aptly expressed the process by stating that the ovum, in making its bed, digs its own grave.

The microscopic structure of the fetal portion of the placenta is identical with that observed in uterine pregnancy. Even more frequently than in that condition, masses of Langhans' cells, syncytium, or even fragments of villi become broken off, and are carried by the veins to the general circulation. This process of deportation can be shown in almost every specimen by cutting serial sections. Moreover, Veit described as deportation the growth into venous channels of chorionic villi which retain their connection with the placenta, and believed that it plays an important part in the production of rupture, as such a clogging of the venous channels may so raise the pressure in the intervillous space that the weakened tubal walls necessarily give way.

Structure of the Fetal Sac. In tubal pregnancy there is a marked increase in the vascularity of the affected tube, the larger arteries and veins being much hypertrophied, while the smaller vessels, especially in the neighborhood of the placental site, are engorged.

Microscopic sections through the sac in the early months show a definite hypertrophy of the muscle cells, but no apparent increase in their number. Except at the placental site, the tube wall is considerably thickened and its cells are spread apart by edema. At a still more advanced period, the muscular constituents of the gestation sac appear to diminish in number, so that at full term almost its entire thickness is made up of a connective tissue poor in cells, with only here and there a muscle fiber. This indicates that the muscularis of the tube has not the same tendency to hypertrophy as that of the uterus, though occasionally it is quite marked.

In many advanced cases the exterior of the tube gives evidence of peritonitic involvement and often a considerable portion of the thickness of the fetal sac is due to peritoneal adhesions. Now and then, discrete patches of decidual formation result from the hypertrophy of the connective-tissue cells of such adhesions.

Uterine Changes. In the first three months the uterus undergoes considerable hypertrophy and its endometrium becomes converted into a decidua vera just as in uterine pregnancy, and differing from it only in a less marked development of the spongy layer and a greater abundance of blood spaces just beneath its free surface. Careful study of its histologic structure was reported by Sampson, in 1915. Soon after the death of the fetus, the decidua degenerates and usually comes away in small pieces, but occasionally it is cast off intact, representing a *decidual cast* of the uterine cavity

(Fig. 319). Its discharge is considered of marked diagnostic significance, so much so that in the past, various writers recommended curetting the uterus in doubtful cases, and basing their diagnosis upon the presence or absence of decidual tissue. This, however, is a useless practice, as within a few weeks after the death of the product of conception the decidua will be displaced by normal endometrium.

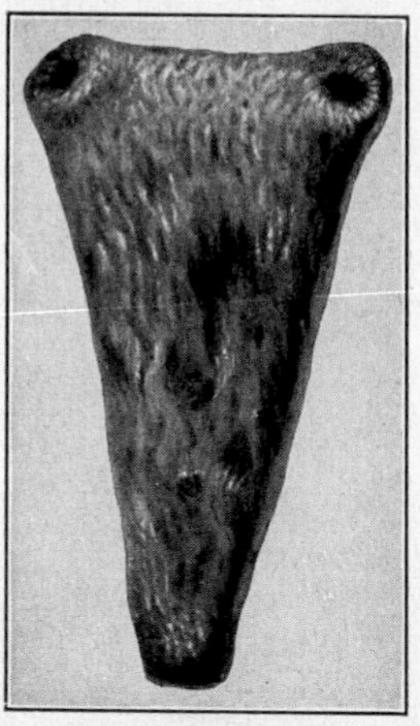

Fig. 319.—Decidual Cast of Uterus in Extra-uterine Pregnancy. (Zweifel.)

The external bleeding present in many cases of tubal pregnancy is uterine in origin and associated with involution of the uterine decidua, according to Jones and Brewer. These authors state that involution results from constriction in the spiral arteries and may reduce the thickness of the decidua by 50 per cent before sloughing occurs.

Termination of Tubal Pregnancy. *Tubal Abortion.* The most common termination of tubal pregnancy is rupture into the tubal lumen with subsequent extrusion into the peritoneal cavity through the fimbriated extremity. This occurs, as a rule, between the sixth and twelfth weeks. The frequency of tubal abortion depends in great part upon the site of implantation of the ovum. In ampullar pregnancy it is the general rule whereas intraperitoneal rupture is the usual outcome in isthmic pregnancy. This difference is due to the fact that in the former location the tubal lumen is sufficiently capacious to permit of a considerable degree of expansion of the fetal sac, whereas in the latter the lumen is so small that this is impossible; and as expansion can occur only toward the periphery, early rupture is the usual termination.

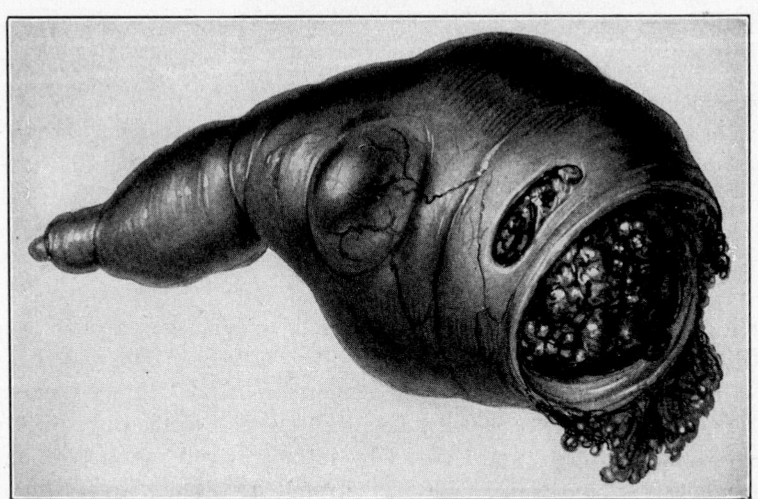

Fig. 320.—Tubal Abortion, Ovum Being Extruded through Fimbriated Extremity. × 1 (Kelly).

Tubal abortion results from the perforation or rupture of the capsular membrane or pseudoreflexa by the growing chorionic villi and therefore does not differ essentially from intraperitoneal rupture, except in the fact that in one case the accompanying hemorrhage occurs into the lumen of the tube, whereas in the other it takes place into the peritoneal cavity. Accordingly, the term "tubal abortion" could be well replaced by that of intratubal rupture, as suggested by Berkeley and Bonney.

The immediate consequence of the hemorrhage is the loosening of the connection between the ovum and the tube wall, the ovum becoming completely or partially separated from its site of implantation. If separation is complete, the entire ovum is extruded into the lumen of the tube and is gradually forced by the effused blood toward the fimbriated end through which it may be extruded into the peritoneal cavity, whereupon the hemorrhage usually ceases. In partial separation, on the other hand, the ovum remains in situ, and the hemorrhage continues. Accordingly, we distinguish between *complete* and *incomplete tubal abortions,* the latter occurring ten times more frequently than the former, according to Wormser.

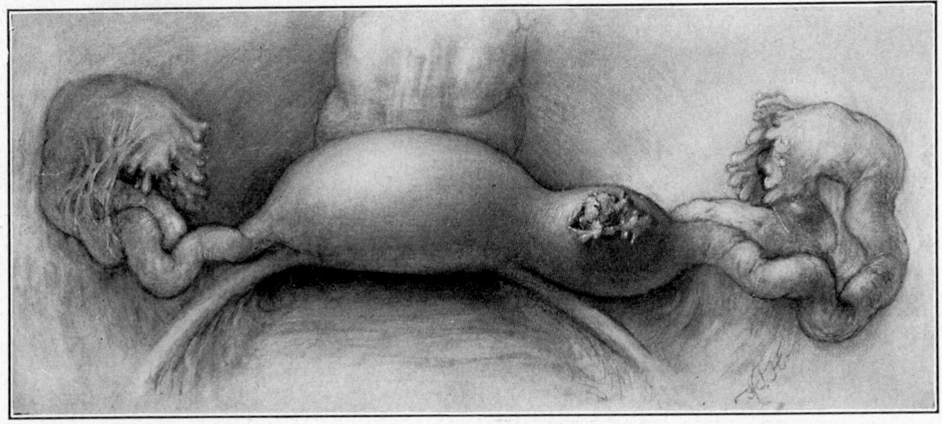

Fig. 321.—Tubal Pregnancy, Isthmic Portion, with Rupture.

In incomplete tubal abortion, when the hemorrhage is moderate in amount, the ovum may become infiltrated with blood and becomes converted into a structure analogous to the blood or fleshy mole observed in uterine abortions. Slight bleeding usually persists as long as the mole remains in the tube, and the blood slowly trickles from the fimbriated extremity into Douglas' cul-de-sac, where it becomes encapsulated, giving rise to a *hematocele.* If the fimbriated extremity is occluded, the tube may gradually become distended by blood—*hematosalpinx.*

After incomplete abortion, small particles of the chorion may remain attached to the tube wall and, becoming surrounded by fibrin, give rise to a placental polyp just as is often noted after an incomplete uterine abortion.

Rupture into the Peritoneal Cavity. Less than one half of the cases of tubal pregnancy end within the first twelve weeks by intraperitoneal rupture, which usually occurs spontaneously, but occasionally is the result of violence. Generally speaking, when rupture occurs in the first few weeks, the pregnancy is situated in the isthmic portion of the tube a short distance from the cornu of the uterus (Fig. 321). On the other hand, when the ovum is implanted in the interstitial portion of the tube, rupture usually does not occur until later and sometimes not until the fourth month. This difference is due to the fact that the interstitial portion of the tube is surrounded by a thick layer of uterine musculature, which reacts promptly to the stimulation of pregnancy, and by its hypertrophy allows the ovum to attain a considerable size before rupture occurs.

The prime factor in the causation of rupture is the intramural embedding of the ovum, and the consequent invasion of the tube wall by chorionic ectodermal elements, with consequent fibrinoid degeneration of the muscular layer. Its direct cause may be violence, such as vaginal examination, defecation, coitus, a fall, or even mere over-exertion, though in the great majority of cases it occurs spontaneously. In the latter

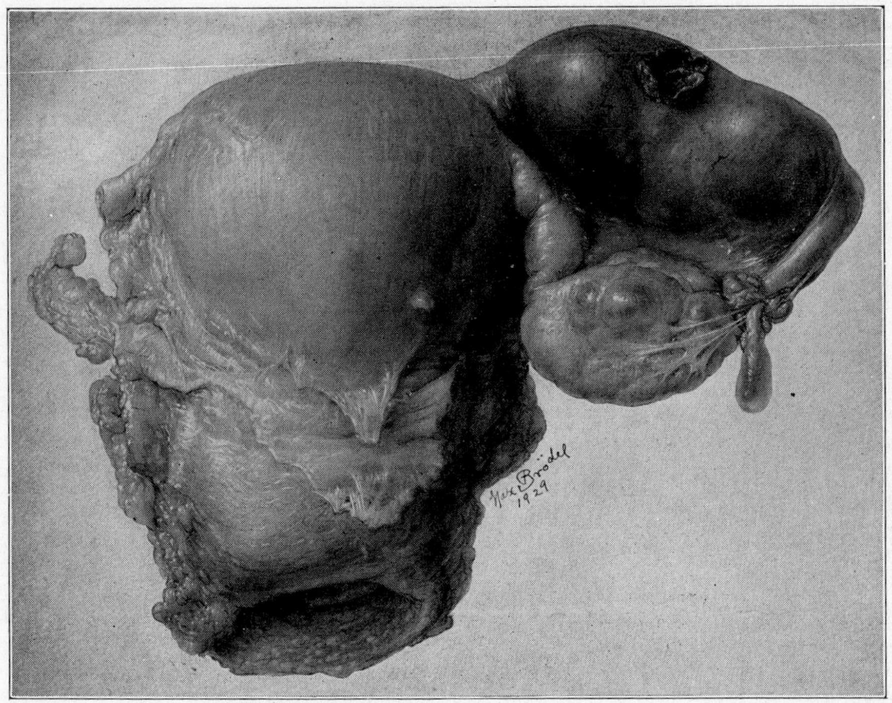

FIG. 322.—RUPTURED TUBAL PREGNANCY. × 4/5.

Death from hemorrhage immediately after admission to hospital. Left appendages had been removed on account of tubal pregnancy several years previously.

event, rupture is brought about either by direct perforation by the growing villi, or by the weakened tube wall yielding to a sudden increase of pressure in the intervillous spaces, following the sudden opening up of a large vessel or the clogging of venous channels by the chorionic villi. The evidence available seems to indicate that the latter is the more usual factor.

If rupture occurs in this way in a tube with an approximately normal lumen, it is apparent that it will be likely to occur at a much earlier period if the ovum is arrested in a diverticulum from the tubal lumen, as in that event the ovum will have only a portion of the tube wall to penetrate, instead of its entire thickness.

Occasionally, when the fimbriated end of the tube is occluded, secondary rupture may occur after a primary abortion. In such circumstances the weakened tubal wall yields to the pressure of the blood which has been poured into its lumen and can find no other means of escape.

Rupture usually occurs in the neighborhood of the placental site, and either into the peritoneal cavity or between the folds of the broad ligament, depending upon the original site of the ovum. The terminations of the two conditions differ so markedly that it will be necessary to consider them separately.

In intraperitoneal rupture the entire ovum may be extruded from the tube but, if the rent is small, profuse hemorrhage may occur without its escape. In either event the patient immediately shows signs of collapse. If death from hemorrhage does not

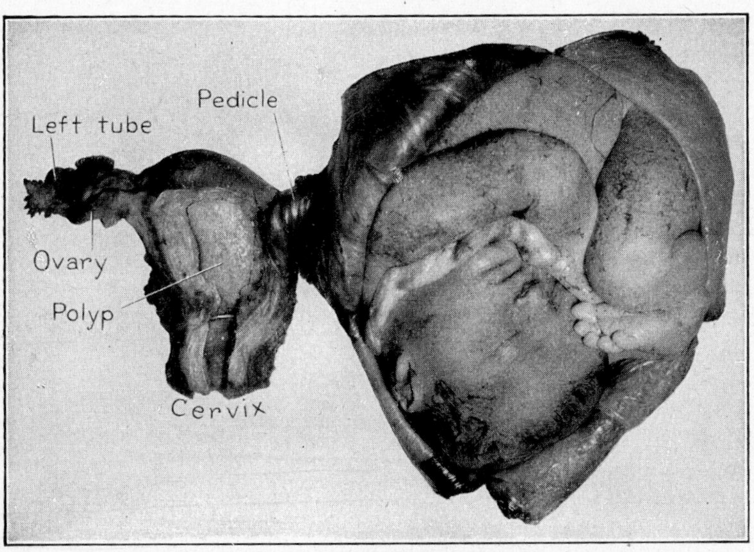

FIG. 323.—BROAD LIGAMENT PREGNANCY AT TERM.

The sac has been opened to expose the fetus, thus hiding most of proximal and all of distal ends of elongated right tube which almost encircles the sac. In the region of the isthmus the tube cannot be traced for some distance as it merges with the wall of the sac, and it is probably at this site that early rupture occurred. The torn distal end of the tube has been carried laterally by the growing fetus. In the photograph the right ovary and ruptured vessels are hidden on the under surface of the sac near the cervix. (Courtesy of Dr. Thomas J. Sims, University of Kansas School of Medicine.)

follow, the effect of rupture varies according to the amount of damage sustained by the ovum. If expelled intact into the peritoneal cavity, the death of the fetus is inevitable; and unless the pregnancy has advanced beyond the third month, the product of conception will be rapidly absorbed.

It is still thought by many that in such circumstances the ovum may become re-attached to any portion of the peritoneal cavity, and there establish vascular connections which will render further development possible. It is unlikely that this could occur, because the ovum would probably become irreparably damaged before such connections could be made.

On the other hand, if only the fetus escapes at the time of rupture, the effect upon the pregnancy will vary according to the extent of injury sustained by the placenta. If much damaged, death of the fetus and termination of the pregnancy are inevitable; but if the greater portion of the placenta still retains its attachment to the tube further development is possible, and the fetus may go on to full term giving rise to a secondary abdominal pregnancy. In such cases the tube may close down upon the placenta and form a sac in which it remains during the rest of the pregnancy. Or, while a portion of the placenta remains attached to the tube wall, its growing periphery extends beyond it and establishes connections with the surrounding pelvic organs. In such circumstances the placenta may be attached partly to the uterus, pelvic floor, rectum, or even the intestines.

When the fetus escapes from the tube, following rupture, it is nearly always surrounded by its membranes, and most authorities believe that further growth is impossible unless it is enclosed within the amnion, although several cases have been reported in which a full-term fetus lay perfectly free in the peritoneal cavity, and all that was left of its membranes was found in the tubal sac.

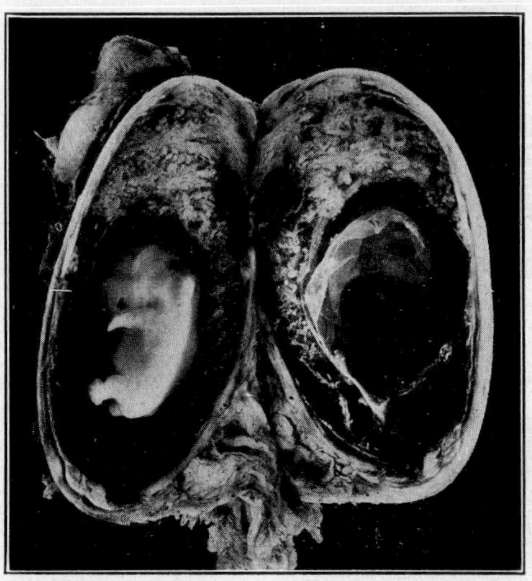

Fig. 324.—Tubal Pregnancy. × 1.

Estimated age six weeks. Note amnion, chorion and villous formation. (Carnegie Col. 6768.)

Rupture into the Broad Ligament. In a small number of cases, especially when the original insertion of the ovum was basiotropic, as Lichtenstein designates it, rupture may occur at the portion of the tube uncovered by peritoneum, so that the contents of the gestation sac are extruded into a space formed by the separation of the folds of the broad ligament. Generally speaking this is the most favorable variety of rupture, and may terminate either by the death of the ovum and the formation of a *broad-ligament hematoma,* or by the further development of the pregnancy.

The outcome depends largely upon the degree of completeness with which the placenta has been separated. If it still remains attached to the interior of the tube, it generally becomes displaced upward as pregnancy advances, and comes to lie above the fetus. But when it is situated near the point of rupture it gradually extends down between the folds of the broad ligament, being implanted partly upon the interior of the tube and partly upon the pelvic connective tissue. In either event, the fetal sac lies entirely outside the peritoneal cavity, and as it increases in size the peritoneum is gradually dissected up from the pelvic and abdominal walls. This condition is designated as *extraperitoneal* or *broad-ligament pregnancy.* Occasionally, the broad-ligament sac may rupture at a later period and the child is extruded into the peritoneal cavity, while the placenta retains its original position—*secondary abdominal pregnancy.*

The so-called *tubo-uterine pregnancy* results from the gradual extension into the uterine cavity of an ovum which was originally implanted in the interstitial portion of the tube. *Tubo-abdominal pregnancy,* on the other hand, is derived from a tubal pregnancy in which the ovum has been inserted in the neighborhood of the fimbriated extremity and gradually extends into the peritoneal cavity. In such circumstances, the portion of the fetal sac projecting into the peritoneal cavity forms adhesions with the surrounding organs, which often seriously complicate its removal at operation.

Neither of these conditions is common, nor do they deserve to be classified separately; in reality they are merely pregnancies developing at unusual portions of the tubes.

The term *tubo-ovarian* pregnancy is employed when the fetal sac is composed partly of tubal and partly of ovarian tissue. Such cases owe their origin to the development of an ovum in a tubo-ovarian cyst, or in a tube whose fimbriated extremity was adherent to the ovary at the time of fertilization. They are therefore primarily either tubal or ovarian in origin.

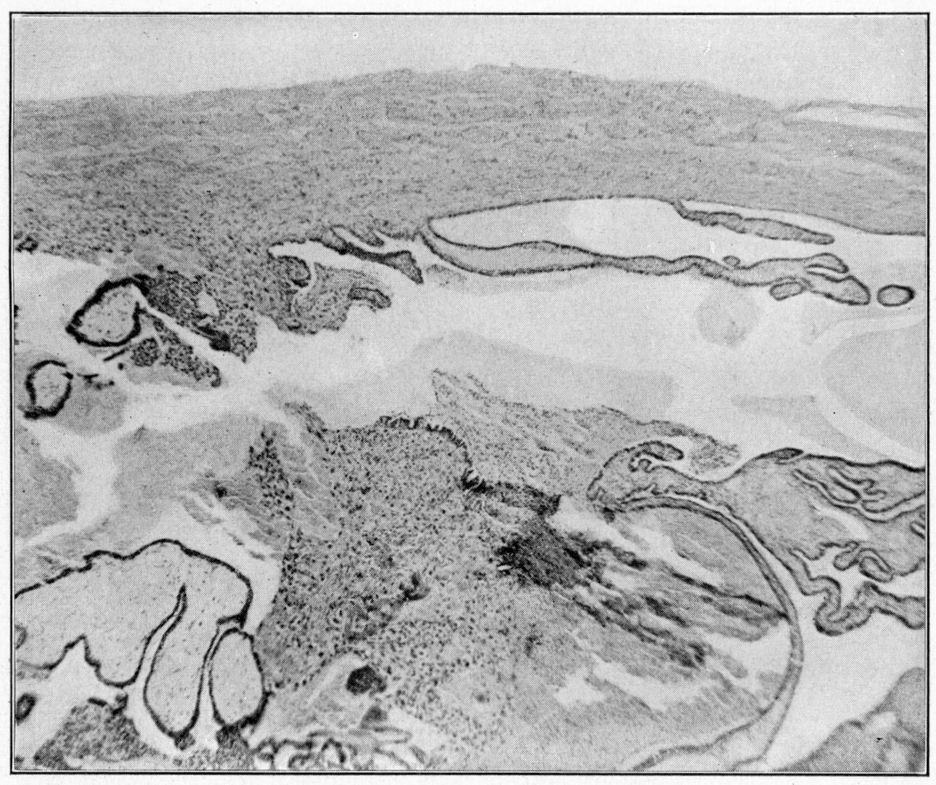

FIG. 325.—TUBAL PREGNANCY.
Section showing attachment of chorion to tube wall above.

Signs and Symptoms. The manifestations of an unruptured tubal pregnancy are not characteristic, and the patient and her physician are frequently unaware of the existence of any abnormality until death of the fetus, rupture, or tubal abortion occurs. Ordinarily the patient considers herself pregnant, presents the usual subjective symptoms and possibly suffers from slight pains in one or the other ovarian regions, which she regards as the usual concomitants of her condition. Occasionally, however, an astute examiner will make the correct diagnosis and in some clinics unruptured ectopic pregnancies constitute a substantial part of all their cases of this complication.

Almost all the symptoms and signs produced by tubal pregnancy are caused by ultimate rupture of the tubal wall and resultant hemorrhage into the peritoneal cavity. Hence, when one speaks of the symptoms and signs of tubal pregnancy, reference is usually made to the clinical picture encountered in a tubal gestation which has ruptured.

In the so-called "typical" or "textbook" case of ruptured tubal pregnancy, the woman misses a period or two, has slight vaginal bleeding occasionally (usually referred to as "spotting") and then suddenly is stricken with severe unilateral abdominal pain, frequently described as sharp, stabbing or tearing in character, but it may be cramplike. Vertigo ensues and sometimes actual fainting. Examination shows a pallid woman, obviously in shock. Abdominal palpation reveals tenderness and vaginal examination, especially motion of the cervix, causes exquisite, intolerable pain. To one or another side of the uterus is a tender, boggy mass.

A certain proportion of cases of tubal pregnancy present just such a picture and in that event there can be no question whatsoever about the diagnosis. Unfortunately, however, these classical cases are in the minority and, as pointed out by Tyrone, Romano and Collins, the most frequently seen case is the "atypical" one. This paradox finds ready explanation in statistical studies of the condition, which show that no single sign or symptom, with the exception of pain, is present in any great preponderance of cases. This makes it advisable to review the various symptoms and signs of ruptured tubal pregnancy and to state the approximate frequency with which they are met.

Pain. Pain is present in almost all cases, being noted in 100 per cent of Lavell's series of 410 cases, in 98.5 per cent of Marchetti's series and in excess of 90 per cent in most reports. It may be unilateral but is about as likely to be generalized over the abdomen. It may be lancinating or cramplike. Extension of the pain to the region of the shoulders is a common complaint. It is often precipitated by lifting a heavy object, by defecation or any other activity which increases abdominal pressure, but may start while the patient is at rest. It bears no constant time relationship to vaginal bleeding. Thus, in those cases in which the latter occurs, in about one third the pain precedes the spotting, in a third it occurs simultaneously with the first spotting, while in another third it follows the initial vaginal bleeding. Moreover, in at least a quarter of the cases, no vaginal bleeding whatsoever occurs.

Amenorrhea. Hospital records indicate that a history of amenorrhea is not obtained in a quarter of the cases or more. One reason for this is that the patient mistakes the pathologic bleeding which so frequently occurs in tubal pregnancy for a true menstrual period and so gives an erroneous date for the last period. This important source of diagnostic error can be eliminated in many cases by more careful history taking. It is extremely important that the character of the last period be investigated in detail in respect to duration, amount and as to whether it impressed the patient as being abnormal in any way. As suggested by Brady, it may be that true amenorrhea is less frequent in tubal pregnancy because the insecure implantation of the ovum does not bring about the necessary endocrine action to prevent menstruation. Although the reason for this phenomenon may be obscure, the important fact to remember is that no history of amenorrhea has been obtained in a quarter to a half of the recorded cases and that the absence of a missed period by no means rules out tubal pregnancy.

Vaginal Spotting or Bleeding. The incidence of vaginal bleeding is about the same as that of amenorrhea, namely, in the neighborhood of 75 per cent. As long as the ovum remains intact, uterine bleeding is usually absent, but with the disturbance or death of the ovum, the chain of endocrine relationships which maintain the uterine decidua is broken and the collapsed uterine mucosa bleeds. The bleeding is usually scanty in amount, dark brown in color and may be either intermittent or continuous. Although profuse vaginal bleeding suggests an incomplete intra-uterine abortion rather than an ectopic gestation, severe vaginal hemorrhage occurs in about 5 per cent of tubal gestations.

Syncope and Shock. The pallid, shocked patient, so inseparably associated in most physicians' minds with the picture of ruptured tubal pregnancy, is seen in the minority of cases only. Although faintness and weakness occurred in 47 per cent of Jarcho's series, it is usually recorded less frequently. Thus, Marchetti, Kuder and Kuder noted such symptoms in 29.1 per cent; while in Langman and Goldblatt's series of 310 cases, 133 patients complained of weakness and 91 fainted. Actual shock occurs in but 10 to 20 per cent of cases.

Nausea and Vomiting. As the result of peritoneal irritation, nausea and vomiting are common symptoms, being observed in about a third of the patients. Langman and Goldblatt regard nausea as the most frequent general symptom and in 310 cases encountered nausea in 162 patients and vomiting in 142.

Urinary Disturbances. Because of the peritoneal irritation induced by pelvic hemorrhage, frequency of urination is an occasional complaint. Although this symptom was reported in but 6.35 per cent of Jarcho's series, Meagher observed it in 76 of 247 cases, or almost one third.

Vaginal Tenderness. By far the most common physical finding in ruptured tubal pregnancy is exquisite tenderness on vaginal examination, especially on motion of the cervix. This is demonstrable in over three quarters of the cases, but occasionally may be absent. Abdominal tenderness and rigidity are present in about the same proportion of cases.

Pelvic Mass. A number of studies indicate that a pelvic mass is palpable in about one half of the cases only. Several authors report this finding more frequently, Marchetti and his associates finding a mass in 70.2 per cent of those cases in which vaginal examination was done. The mass varies in size, consistency and position. It ranges as a rule between 5 and 15 cm. in diameter and may be soft and elastic. With extensive infiltration of the tubal wall with blood, however, it may be firm. It is rarely anterior to the uterus but almost always either posterior or lateral.

Uterine Changes. Because of the action of estrogen produced by the placenta, the empty uterus grows during the first three months of a tubal gestation to about the same size as it does with an intra-uterine pregnancy and its consistency also is similar as long as the fetus is alive. These uterine changes will depend on the duration of the pregnancy but may be altogether absent if the fetus is dead. The position of the uterus may be pushed to one or the other side by the fetal mass. In broad ligament pregnancies or if the broad ligament is filled with blood, the uterus may be greatly displaced with the cervix high up behind the symphysis pubis. This position of the cervix is in general a rather dependable sign of a broad ligament mass of some kind. As already noted, uterine casts are passed by a small minority of patients, possibly by 5 or 10 per cent.

Blood Pressure and Pulse. As might be expected, the blood pressure falls in proportion to the amount and the suddenness of the intra-abdominal hemorrhage. In a sense this drop in blood pressure is a protective mechanism since it favors hemostasis; as a consequence a rise in pressure often follows the fall, but as the pressure returns again toward normal, it produces a renewal of the bleeding with another drop. This is a frequent sequence in ruptured tubal gestation. In the cases which rupture suddenly, the systolic pressure is usually below 100, and in 22 of Jarcho's total 147 cases, or in 15 per cent, it fell below 70 mm. Hg; in 71, or in 48.3 per cent, it ranged between 70 and 90 mm. Hg. The latter figures represent the usual picture in acute rupture. A rapid pulse is one of the most characteristic signs of rupture of tubal pregnancy as emphasized especially by Ware and Winn. These authors rightly regard the rate and volume of the pulse as a more reliable index of the condition of the patient who has recovered from the initial shock than blood pressure readings.

Hemoglobin. Following a severe hemorrhage the depleted blood volume is made up to normal by the passage of water from the tissues to the blood stream, but this is a gradual process extending over a day or two. Even after a substantial hemorrhage, therefore, the hemoglobin concentration may show only a slight reduction within the next few hours. This behavior of the hemoglobin is strikingly shown by cases in which it may be decidedly lower three days after operation than at the time of operation despite several blood transfusions in the interim. For the first few hours after an acute hemorrhage, therefore, the hemoglobin reading is not a reliable index of the degree of blood loss. But because of this factor of progressive blood dilution, a rapid decrease in hemoglobin concentration while the patient is under observation is a more valuable sign of blood loss than the initial reading, a most important practical point. Of course, in cases in which a pelvic hematocele has been gradually forming over a period of a week or more, extremely low hemoglobin levels may be met.

Temperature. Following acute hemorrhage the temperature may be low but with recovery from shock it sometimes shows a tendency to rise slightly as the result of absorption of blood. As a consequence, temperatures between 100 and 101 F. are seen in about one patient in three, but it is rare for this temperature level to be exceeded in the absence of infection. This is an important distinguishing sign between ruptured tubal pregnancy and acute salpingitis (frequently confused with tubal pregnancy) in which the temperature is usually above 101 F.

Leukocyte Count. The leukocyte count shows extreme variations in ruptured ectopic pregnancy. In about half the cases it is normal, but in the remainder all degrees of leukocytosis may be encountered up to 30,000. While the leukocyte count is therefore of little diagnostic import, it may be helpful in pointing to the type of bleeding which has occurred. As a general rule, in cases of old rupture or slow leakage, the count is likely to be normal whereas after sudden massive hemorrhage it usually exceeds 15,000.

Cullen's Sign. This is a blue discoloration of the skin in the region of the umbilicus as the result of intraperitoneal hemorrhage. This is a rare sign but is occasionally discernible in thin women or in patients with an umbilical hernia. Only twice has it been seen in my personal experience and in both instances it was too faint to be recorded photographically.

Picture in the So-called "Chronic" Case. In many cases of ruptured tubal pregnancy, a gradual disintegration of the tubal wall occurs followed by a very slow leakage of blood into the tubal lumen and/or the peritoneal cavity. Acute symptoms are hence mild. Even these may subside; but gradually the trickling blood collects in the pelvis, becomes more or less walled off by adhesions and a pelvic *hematocele* results. In some cases the hematocele is eventually absorbed and the patient recovers without operation. In others it may rupture into the peritoneal cavity followed by an acute picture of shock. In others it may become infected with abscess formation. In still others, and most commonly, the hematocele causes continual pain and finally the physician is consulted weeks or even months after the original rupture. These cases present the most atypical manifestations and since all gradations exist between this type and the type with acute rupture, it is understandable that tubal pregnancy may exhibit a wide and often confusing variety of clinical syndromes.

Diagnosis. Diagnosis in ruptured tubal pregnancy is all important. Indeed, it is failure to make the correct diagnosis promptly that accounts for almost all deaths in this condition. Unfortunately, however, there is no disorder in all obstetrics and gynecology which may present so many diagnostic pitfalls and blind alleys. Documentation of this statement is found in the following facts: If the many reports on ectopic pregnancy are surveyed, it will be found that the pre-operative diagnosis of ruptured tubal pregnancy is shown at operation to be wrong in about 20 per cent of cases; moreover, among all ectopic pregnancies found at the operating table, the pre-operative diagnosis is something else in about 20 per cent of cases.

The conditions most frequently confused with tubal pregnancy are: pelvic inflammatory disease, threatened or incomplete abortion, torsion of an ovarian cyst, appendicitis and spontaneous rupture of a follicle cyst or corpus luteum with intra-abdominal hemorrhage.

The disease most commonly mistaken for ruptured tubal pregnancy is pelvic inflammatory disease. In salpingitis there is often a past history of similar attacks. There is usually no missed period. In salpingitis there may be a history of metrorrhagia but this is not nearly so common as the spotting characteristic of tubal gestation. Pain and tenderness are more likely to be bilateral in pelvic inflammatory disease. A pelvic mass in tubal pregnancy, if palpable, is unilateral, whereas in salpingitis both fornices are prone to be equally resistant and tender. The fever in acute salpingitis usually exceeds 101° F., whereas in tubal pregnancy it is either absent or ordinarily below 101° F. A positive hormonal test for pregnancy is rare in salpingitis but not uncommon in recently ruptured tubal pregnancies; however, a negative test may be obtained in either condition and hence is meaningless.

In threatened or incomplete abortion, the vaginal bleeding is usually more profuse and the blood more likely to be red. If shock is present it is in proportion to the amount of vaginal hemorrhage, but in tubal pregnancy shock is almost always far in excess of what might be expected from vaginal blood loss. The pain in abortion is milder and located in the lower midline of the abdomen, whereas in tubal pregnancy it is unilateral or generalized. Abdominal as well as vaginal tenderness is usually lacking in abortion and a unilateral mass is not felt. The uterus is larger and softer than in tubal pregnancy, while in incomplete abortion the cervix is more or less open.

In torsion of an ovarian cyst and appendicitis, the signs and symptoms of pregnancy, including amenorrhea, are usually lacking. There is rarely a history of vaginal bleeding. The mass formed by a twisted ovarian cyst is discrete and ovoid while that of a tubal pregnancy is less well defined. In appendicitis there is no mass on vaginal examination and tenderness is either lacking or decidedly less than in ruptured tubal pregnancy, being localized higher over McBurney's point. If either of these conditions is mistaken for a tubal pregnancy, the error is not a costly one since both also call for prompt operation.

Rupture of a follicle cyst or corpus luteum with bleeding into the peritoneal cavity is almost indistinguishable from a ruptured tubal gestation. Fortunately, the condition is uncommon but several hundred cases have been reported.

Because of the difficulties of establishing the diagnosis of ruptured tubal pregnancy in certain cases, especially in the less acute ones, various diagnostic aids have been utilized. Hormonal tests for pregnancy are without value if negative, but point to the existence of active chorionic tissue somewhere in the body if positive. The more rapid *Rana pipiens* test, if positive, may sometimes be a helpful adjunct in differentiating tubal gestation from conditions unassociated with pregnancy. Various methods of puncturing the posterior fornix for the purpose of demonstrating blood have been employed, namely, needle puncture, posterior colpotomy and the culdescope. Since the condition most frequently mistaken for a ruptured ectopic pregnancy is pelvic inflammatory disease, which may occasionally bind intestines and other structures in the cul-de-sac, the blind introduction of a sharp instrument into the posterior fornix is not without danger. Moreover, the needle sometimes punctures a vein, with misleading results. While these methods have many advocates, it is my feeling that in doubtful cases abdominal exploration is safer and much more certain. The only disadvantages are a scar in the abdomen and a period of hospitalization which (with early ambulation) is only a few days longer than after cul-de-sac puncture.

Finally, let it be emphasized that the two main secrets of success in the diagnosis of ruptured tubal pregnancy are: (1) everlasting remembrance that lower quadrant pain in any woman between 15 and 50 may mean tubal pregnancy; (2) everlasting vigilance in securing a detailed and accurate history. The history is more important than the findings on pelvic examination and if one contradicts the other, it is better in general to rely on the history.

Prognosis. Ectopic pregnancy is an important cause of maternal death. Every eighteenth such death in Philadelphia, every sixteenth in New York City and every twelfth in Chicago was due to this condition during the decade of 1931 to 1940, as reported by Williams and Corbit. The mortality in the country at large is probably between 2 and 3 per cent. In a series of 3,343 American cases collected from the literature between 1925 and 1935, Gordon found an average mortality rate of 4.6 per cent. In 20 series analyzed by Jarcho including tubal, ovarian and abdominal gestations, reported between 1938 and 1947, there was a total of 2,634 cases, with 63 deaths, a mortality rate of 2.4 per cent. This average rate agrees with that of 2.4 per cent reported by Litzenberg in 1947 on the basis of an analysis of 1,421 cases from six teaching clinics. Newberger reports the occurrence of 398 cases of ectopic gestation with 17 deaths in Illinois during 1944. This represents a mortality rate of 4.27 per cent. Most of these reports point out that the common factors responsible for mortality in ruptured ectopic pregnancy are: failure of the family physician to recognize the acute emergency nature of the condition, delay in hospitalization, tardiness of operation in the hospital and too late and too little blood transfusion.

The most recent statistics on the mortality of ectopic pregnancy are those of

Anderson who has analyzed all the cases occurring in Baltimore over a five-year period ending in 1948. In 862 ectopic gestations, managed in 16 hospitals, there were 14 deaths, a gross mortality rate of 1.6 per cent. The death rate was much higher in Negresses, however, being 2.6 per cent in 258 cases, in contrast to 0.7 per cent in 604 cases in white women. The much lower mortality figure in white women probably reflects earlier reporting of symptoms and hence earlier diagnosis and earlier operation.

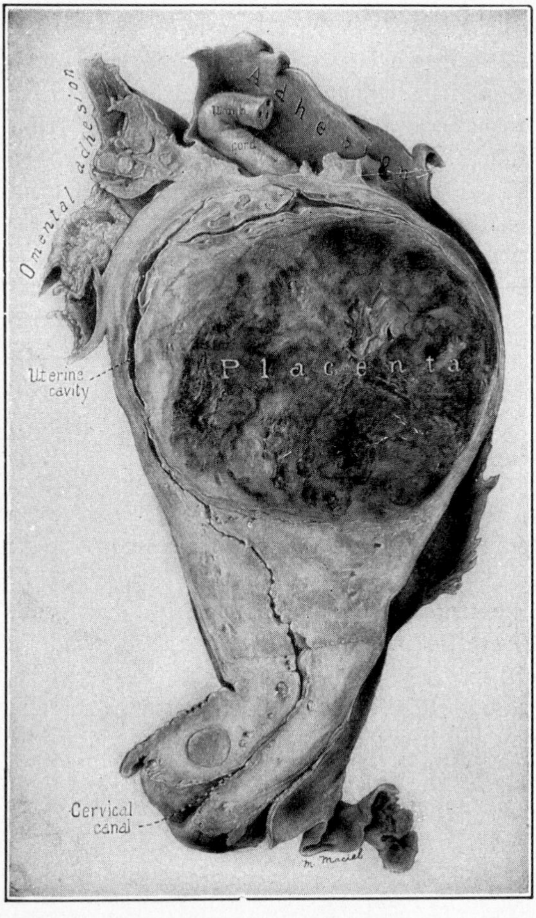

Subsequent Pregnancies. Since the tubal abnormalities which predispose to ectopic pregnancy are usually bilateral, notably pelvic inflammatory disease and developmental abnormalities, it is understandable that a substantial number of women are either sterile after this condition or develop another extra-uterine pregnancy in the remaining tube. The extensive literature on this topic may be summarized as follows: Of women who are operated upon for ectopic pregnancy and are left in a condition in which future pregnancies are a theoretical possibility, only about one third subsequently become pregnant. Of these subsequent pregnancies 1 in 10, approximately, terminates in another ectopic pregnancy. It will be noted that this is 30 times the usual incidence of this complication.

FIG. 326.—INTERSTITIAL PREGNANCY. × ½.

Note placenta in posterior wall of uterus, and umbilical cord protruding through fundus. Rupture had occurred at the fourth month, and fetus remained alive in the abdominal cavity until shortly before the death of the patient at the eighth month.

Treatment. The treatment of tubal pregnancy is immediate salpingectomy coupled, as a rule, with simultaneous blood transfusion. Before the transfusion era, it was customary to allow a patient in shock to "rally" before operation so that it could be performed on a rising blood pressure. Blood transfusion has removed the necessity for these delays but the general principle involved should be borne in mind because it is unwise to start operating on a shocked woman until blood is actually running into her veins. The response of most patients to the operation is dramatic, the blood pressure starting to rise just as soon as the major vessels are clamped.

A certain minority of the operations undertaken for ectopic pregnancy will prove at the operating table to be unnecessary because of an erroneous diagnosis. This must be accepted with equanimity because, as Dannreuther has stressed, it is better to operate on 10 patients and discover that the diagnosis was wrong than to make a single error of omission.

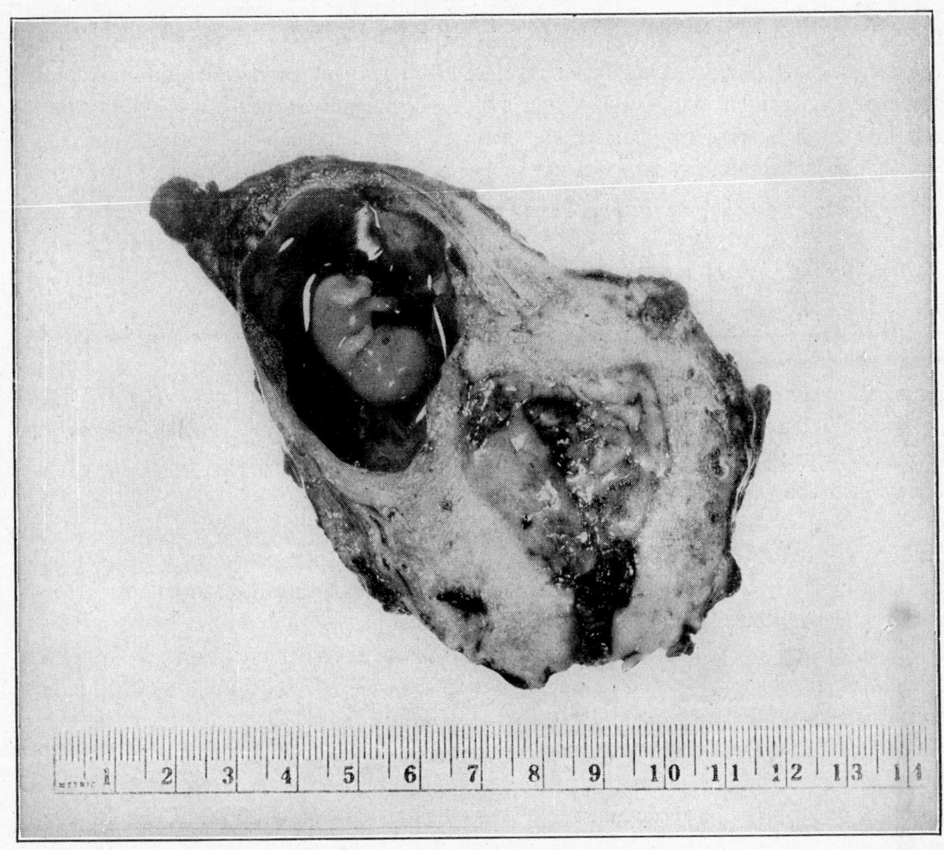

FIG. 327.—INTERSTITIAL PREGNANCY WITH FETUS IN SITU.
Note thick decidua in empty uterus.

Interstitial Pregnancy. When the fertilized ovum becomes implanted in that segment of the tube which penetrates the uterine wall an especially grave form of tubal gestation results, *interstitial pregnancy*. As stated, this occurs in 3 to 4 per cent of all tubal gestations. Because of the location of the implantation, no palpable tubal mass is found but simply an asymmetrical uterus which is difficult to differentiate from the findings in intra-uterine pregnancy. Hence, the early diagnosis is even more frequently overlooked than in other types of tubal implantation. Because of the greater elasticity of the myometrium in comparison to the tubal wall, rupture is prone to occur somewhat later, that is, between the end of the second and the end of the fourth months. Owing to the great vascularity of the surrounding muscle, the hemorrhage which attends the rupture may be fatal within an hour; and most tubal pregnancies in which death occurs before the patient can be brought to the hospital fall into this group.

Combined and Multiple Pregnancies. In rare instances tubal pregnancy may be complicated by a coexisting intra-uterine gestation, a condition designated as *combined pregnancy*. In 1926 Novak was able to collect 276 such cases from the literature.

Twin tubal pregnancy has been observed, both embryos being sometimes found in the same tube, while in other cases there is a fetus in each tube, both showing the same development. Arey has considered the subject in detail, and makes the surprising statement that single ovum twins occur many times more commonly in tubal than in uterine pregnancy. He explains the phenomenon by supposing that, in view of the difficulties experienced in becoming implanted, the rate of growth of the ovum is so retarded that two embryonic areas develop instead of one.

ABDOMINAL PREGNANCY

Although abdominal pregnancy is a rare condition its gravity, as well as certain other circumstances, gives it special interest. It occurs once in every 15,000 pregnancies approximately. Thus, Douglass and Kohn found in Baltimore that the ratio of abdominal pregnancies to live births was 1 to 16,370. Other reports cite figures of a similar order. Almost all cases are secondary to an early rupture of a tubal pregnancy into the peritoneal cavity. In most such cases the trophoblast, after rupture of the tubal wall, manages to maintain its previous tubal attachment and then gradually extends its implantation over the surrounding peritoneum. Meanwhile the fetus, usually within the amnion and chorion but sometimes not, undergoes growth within the peritoneal cavity. Under such circumstances the placenta is found over the general region of the tube (not now identifiable grossly) and over the posterior aspects of the broad ligament and uterus. In other cases the implanted ovum apparently escapes entirely from the tube after rupture and implants itself de novo on one or another site in the peritoneal cavity. Primary implantation of the fertilized ovum in the peritoneal cavity is extremely rare but has been reported by some authors, one of the best documented cases being that of Studdiford. E. L. King has directed attention to a very rare cause of abdominal pregnancy, postoperative separation of the uterine wound of a previous cesarean section. In three of his four cases reported, the ovum had become implanted upon the omentum filling the uterine defect, while the fourth had attached itself to the abdominal wall. He is of the opinion that in each case the fertilized ovum, escaping through the uterine wall defect, became implanted as a primary abdominal pregnancy.

Since early rupture of a tubal pregnancy is the usual genesis of abdominal pregnancy, a past history suggestive of the accident can be obtained in many cases. Thus, a history of early spotting or irregular bleeding is found in the great majority of cases. The course of gestation is prone to be uncomfortable as the result of peritoneal irritation; and nausea, vomiting, flatulence, constipation and diarrhea, as well as varying degrees of abdominal pain, are common. Multiparae state that the pregnancy does not "feel right." Late in pregnancy fetal movements may be very painful. When term is reached the empty uterus frequently goes into spurious labor. Many observations attest this fact which is a strong argument in favor of an endocrine cause for the onset of labor.

The fate of the fetus in abdominal pregnancy is exceedingly precarious since the great majority of the infants succumb. Thus, in 130 cases reviewed by Beacham and Beacham, the fetal mortality was 85 per cent. In an analysis of 249 cases reported in the literature since 1935, Ware found a total fetal mortality of 75.6 per cent. Of the 251 infants in his series, 140 died while still in the abdomen and 50

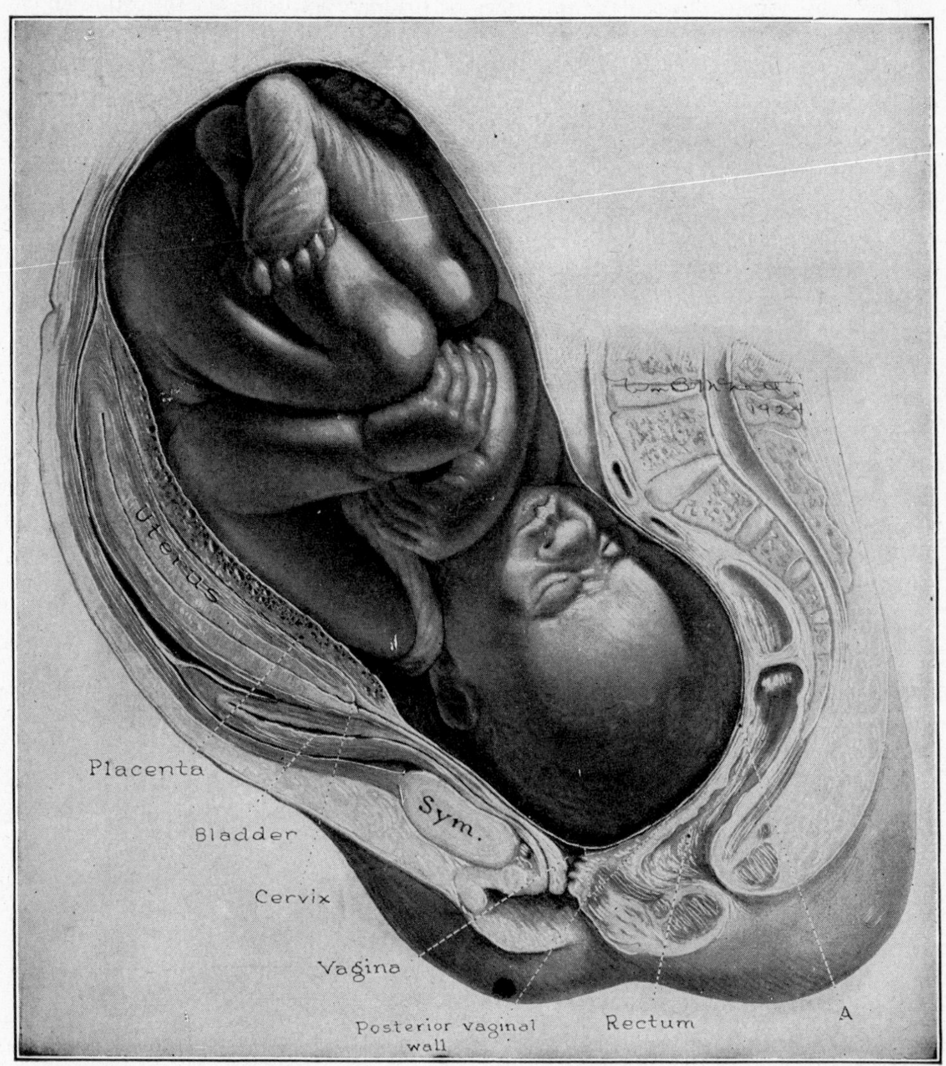

Fig. 328.—Extra-uterine Pregnancy at Term.

Uterus and bladder have been displaced upward out of pelvis by development of fetal head. Its growth has stretched out the septum between vagina and Douglas' pouch to resemble the fetal membrane. (From Rowland. By permission of *Surgery, Gynecology, and Obstetrics.*)

within a few hours or days after birth. Moreover, a large percentage of the infants show congenital malformations. Although this is questioned by some authors, others put the incidence as high as 50 per cent. When the fetus has attained a certain size before death, it cannot be absorbed and must eventually partake in one of the following outcomes: suppuration, mummification, calcification or adipocere transformation. Pyogenic bacteria often gain access to a gestation sac, particularly when it is adherent to the intestines, and give rise to suppuration of its contents. Eventually the abscess perforates at the point of least resistance and, if the patient does not die from septicemia, portions of the fetus may be extruded through the abdominal wall or more commonly into the intestines or bladder, according to the situation of the perforation. This outcome is particularly frequent in broad ligament pregnancies, on account of their proximity to the rectum. Mummification and lithopedion formation (calcification) occasionally ensue and in many instances the calcified product of conception has been carried for years as a benign foreign body and may do no harm unless it gives rise to dystocia in a subsequent pregnancy or produces mechanical pressure symptoms. The literature contains numerous instances in which a period of 20 to 30 years elapsed before its removal at operation or autopsy. Much more rarely the fetus may become converted into a yellowish, greasy mass to which the term "adipocere" is applied. The fatty material is supposed to be an ammoniacal soap, but a satisfactory explanation of its formation has not yet been advanced.

Examination late in pregnancy often reveals a fetus high in the abdomen which is frequently in transverse presentation, but abdominal tenderness sometimes precludes satisfactory palpation. The fetal parts can be felt with unusual ease and the whole fetus can be moved about in the abdomen freely; the fetal heart tones in cases in which the infant is alive tend to be loud. Braxton Hicks contractions are naturally absent, a most important diagnostic sign; nor are the round ligaments palpable. The cervix is usually displaced but this will depend in part on the position of the fetus. The cervix may undergo as much as 2 cm. dilatation in spurious labor but effacement does not occur. If the examiner is fortunate he may be able to map out the uterus, but this can be done with certainty in only a minority of the cases. Palpation of the fornices may reveal small parts or the fetal head clearly outside the uterus.

In patients near term the diagnosis of abdominal pregnancy can often be ruled out in a simple manner by introducing the tip of the finger into the cervix and palpating the presenting part of an intra-uterine fetus. If the cervix will not permit the introduction of a fingertip the cautious insertion of a sound until resistance is met, will usually demonstrate whether or not the uterus is empty. An x-ray taken with the sound in the uterus affords further information. More clear-cut verification of an empty uterus and an extra-uterine fetal skeleton may be had by the instillation of radio-opaque substances into the uterus for the purpose of obtaining uterograms or hysterosalpingograms. Although this procedure should not be used indiscriminately, it appears to be a relatively safe one and is recommended by most authors.

The operation for abdominal pregnancy frequently precipitates the most violent and colossal hemorrhage known to surgery. Thus, in a case at Sinai Hospital in Baltimore, the measured blood lost exceeded 4,000 cc. and in addition there was an estimated blood loss of several thousand centimeters; 8,000 cc. of blood was administered during the course of 6 hours and the patient recovered. The amount of hemorrhage may be surmised by the fact that, despite this stupendous amount of blood transfused, the patient's hemoglobin was lower three days after the operation than before. Without massive blood transfusion the outlook for many such patients is hopeless. Hence, it is mandatory that preparations for operation should include: first, the presence in the operating room of 2,000 cc. of blood ready for use; and second, facilities for rapid transfusion, the most satisfactory of which is probably a 3-way stopcock inserted in the transfusion tubing so that blood can be pumped in by means of a 50 cc. syringe connected with the stopcock.

The massive hemorrhage which often occurs in the course of operations for abdominal pregnancy is understood when it is recalled that there is no mechanism

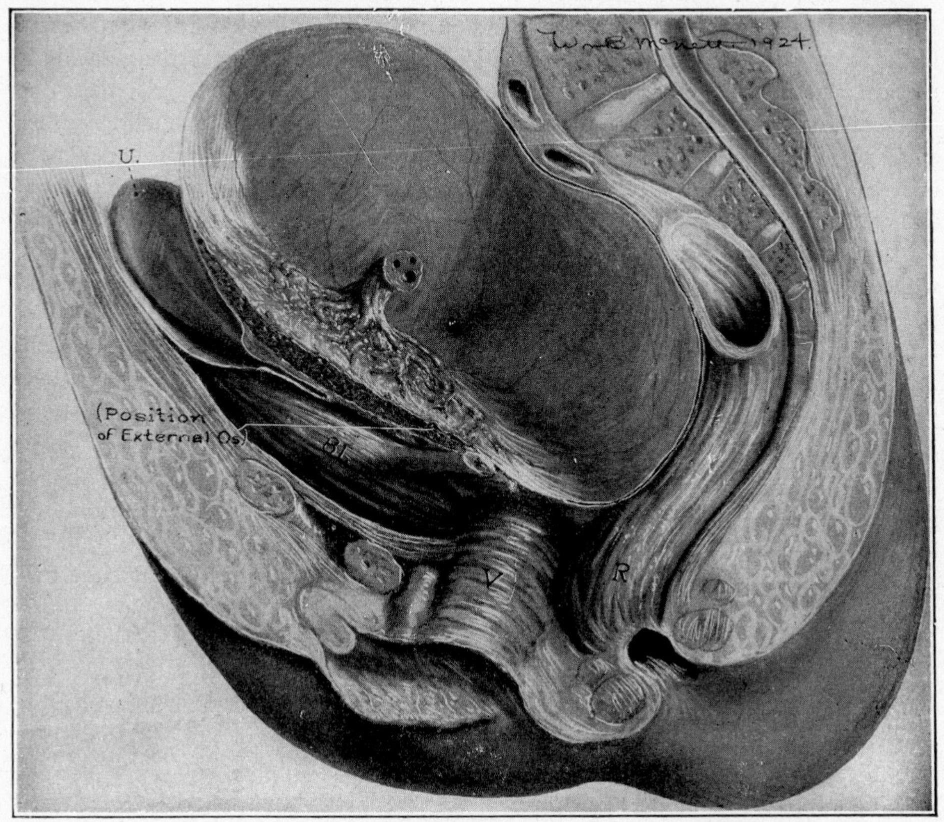

Fig. 329.—Relationships Immediately after Delivery of Live Child by Laparotomy.

Drawing shows how development of the head prevented downgrowth of the placenta which was attached chiefly to the posterior surface of the broad ligaments and uterus. The latter was removed with the placental mass. (From Rowland. By permission of *Surgery, Gynecology, and Obstetrics.*)

present to occlude the hypertrophied and open vessels of the placental site after placental separation. Because of this fact, it has been recommended that operation be deferred until the fetus is dead in the anticipation of placental death with diminished vascularity of the site of implantation. It is my feeling and that of Ware and others that, regardless of the infant, there is more to be lost than gained by this waiting policy. Thus, partial separation of the placenta with hemorrhage occasionally occurs spontaneously in the interval of waiting. Moreover, even though the fetus be dead several weeks, bleeding may still be torrential. Hence, in my opinion, immediate operation should be done just as soon as the diagnosis is established.

Aside from the urgency of blood transfusion already stressed, the most important injunction in the operative management of these cases is this: the placenta should be left in situ and the abdomen closed without drainage whenever removal of the placenta may cause hemorrhage or damage to a vital organ. Since removal of the placenta in abdominal pregnancy always carries risk of hemorrhage, this is tantamount to saying that it should be left in place unless the placental blood supply can be easily tied off or unless bleeding from partial separation necessitates its removal. As stated, in rare instances partial separation may occur spontaneously; it is more likely to occur as the result of manipulations incidental to the operation; and it is especially prone to develop as the result of exploration to ascertain just where the placenta is attached. Hence, by and large, the best results will be obtained by avoiding unnecessary exploration of the surrounding organs; the infant is simply delivered, the cord tied with catgut close to the placenta and the abdomen closed without drainage.

In the majority of cases the placenta is absorbed from its peritoneal attachment without causing elevation of temperature or adhesions. However, this is not always the case and complications sometimes ensue. Infection may develop with abscess formation and prolonged drainage through the abdominal incision; occasionally such abscesses point above the inguinal ligament or in the cul-de-sac and have to be opened. In other cases, such as one of ours, the placenta caused pain and tenderness and had to be removed two months later. While these complications may prove troublesome they are much less grave than the hemorrhage which often attends placental removal. Ware reports that when the placenta is allowed to remain in situ, the Friedman test may remain positive for as long as 35 days.

In Ware's series of 249 cases collected from the literature since 1935, the maternal mortality was 14.85 per cent. With the greater use of massive blood transfusion and a more cautious policy in regard to placental removal, this figure can doubtless be reduced substantially, but abdominal pregnancy will always remain one of the most grave complications in obstetrics both to mother and infant.

OVARIAN PREGNANCY

Up to 1878, there had existed no definite criteria by which specimens of supposed ovarian pregnancy could be judged, and many were described as examples of ovarian pregnancy which had no claim whatsoever to such a title. In that year, however, Spiegelberg formulated certain criteria which he held must be fulfilled in order to justify such a diagnosis. He demanded (1) that the tube on the affected side be intact; (2) that the fetal sac occupy the position of the ovary; (3) that it be connected with the uterus by the ovarian ligament; and (4) that definite ovarian tissue be found in its wall. When judged by these criteria, the majority of cases which had been described up to his time were found wanting, and subsequent investigation has shown that a number of cases which he considered conclusive are likewise open to very considerable doubt.

Meyer and Wynne, in 1919, were able to collect 42 cases of ovarian pregnancy from the literature, and since then several additional authentic specimens have been described each year. Consequently the possibility of ovarian pregnancy is now universally admitted but at the same time it is recognized that it occurs comparatively rarely.

In a considerable number of the cases recorded the pregnancy had gone to full term, and in several instances had eventuated in the formation of lithopedia which had been carried for years before being removed. This would appear to indicate that the ovary can accommodate itself more readily than the tube to the growing pregnancy. Full literature upon this aspect of the subject will be found in the article of Säntii (1928). However, rupture at an early period is the usual termination. The product of conception may undergo degenerative changes at an early period without rupture, and give rise to a tumor of varying size, consisting of a capsule of ovarian

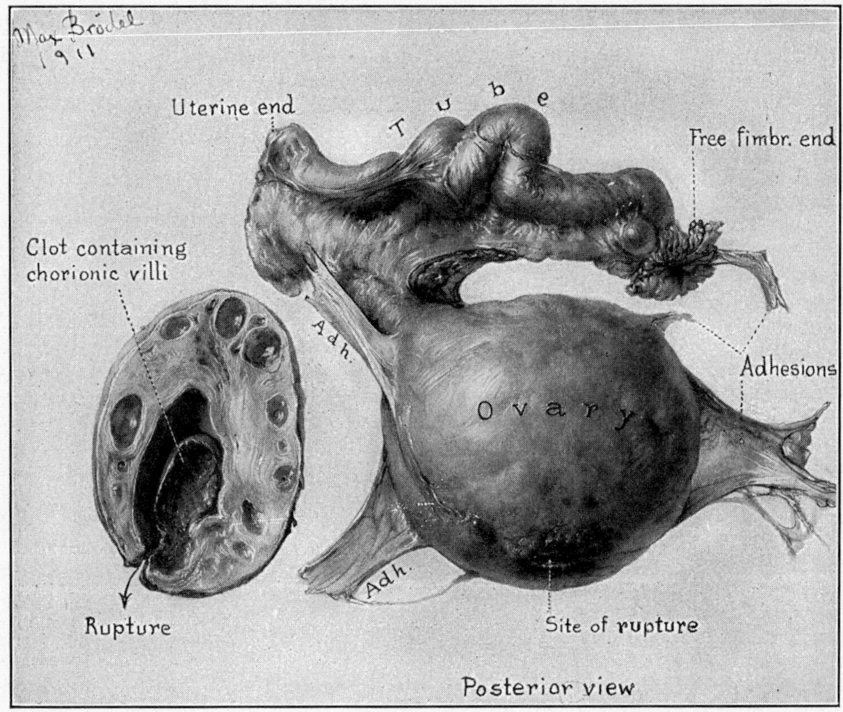

FIG. 330.—E. K. CULLEN'S SPECIMEN OF OVARIAN PREGNANCY. × 1.

tissue inclosing a mass made up of blood and chorionic villi, which may or may not contain an amniotic cavity. Such observations render it probable that a certain proportion of ovarian hematomata may actually represent the remains of an early pregnancy, but such a diagnosis should not be considered unless microscopic examination definitely reveals the presence of chorionic villi. In ovarian pregnancy the ovum itself and its mode of implantation do not differ essentially from that observed in the uterus, except that a definite decidual membrane is lacking so that the trophoblast invades the ovarian stroma directly.

CERVICAL PREGNANCY

Cervical pregnancy is a complication which is rarely encountered in obstetrics. In a recent review of the literature Studdiford found less than 50 cases reported. The site of the nidation of the ovum is in the cervical mucosa. Inasmuch as this mucosa reacts poorly to the proliferative activity of the trophoblastic epithelium associated with implantation, it is readily destroyed. Hence, as the placenta develops, it becomes anchored to the muscularis.

Usually, painless bleeding, which appears shortly after nidation, is the first sign of this abnormal pregnancy. As the pregnancy progresses, one finds a distended, thin-walled cervix with the external os partially dilated. Situated above the cervical mass, one may palpate a slightly enlarged uterine fundus.

Cervical pregnancy rarely goes beyond the twentieth week of gestation and usually is terminated surgically because of bleeding. Since the removal of the placenta is difficult and is associated with seriously profuse hemorrhage, packing of the cervix, large transfusions and even total hysterectomy is the treatment that is required.

BIBLIOGRAPHY

ALLEN, E. Ectopic Pregnancy. Clinics, J. B. Lippincott Co., Philadelphia, 1945, 4:648.

ANDERSON, G. W. The Racial Incidence and Mortality of Ectopic Pregnancy. (In press.)

AREY, L. B. The Cause of Tubal Pregnancy and Tubal Twinning. Am. J. Obst. & Gynec., 1923, 5:163.

BEACHAM, W. D., and BEACHAM, D. W. Abdominal Pregnancy. Obst. & Gynec. Surv., 1946, 1:777.

BERKELEY, C., and BONNEY, V. Tubal Gestation: A Pathological Study. J. Obst. & Gynec. Brit. Emp., 1905, 7:77.

BRADY, L. A Clinical Study of Ectopic Pregnancy. Bull. Johns Hopkins Hosp., 1923, 34:152.

BUFE, W. A Case of Unruptured Interstitial Pregnancy with Termination in the Formation of a Carneous Mole. Zentralbl. f. Gynäk., 1935, 59:1443.

CONNORS, D. A., CRESCI, J. V., and GLASS, M. Vaginal Delivery of a Six Months' Living Child Four Years after Supravaginal Hysterectomy. Am. J. Obst. & Gynec., 1943, 45:309.

CORNELL, E. L., and LASH, A. F. Abdominal Pregnancy. Internat. Abst. Surg. (Supplement to Surg., Gynec. & Obst.), 1933, 57:98.

CULLEN, T. S. Bluish Discoloration of the Umbilicus as a Diagnostic Sign when Ruptured Extrauterine Pregnancy Exists. Contributions to Medical and Biological Research (Osler volume). 1919, Vol. I, p. 420.

DANNREUTHER, W. T. The Enigma of Ectopic Pregnancy. J.A.M.A., 1927, 88:1302.

DOUGLASS, L. H., and KOHN, S. G. Abdominal Pregnancy. West Virg. Med. J., 1947, 43:307.

FARRAR, L. K. P. The Value of the Leucocyte Count as an Aid to Diagnosis in Ectopic Gestation. Surg., Gynec. & Obst., 1925, 41:655.

FRANKEL, J. M., and SCHENCK, S. B. The Endometrial Therapy of Ectopic Pregnancy. Am. J. Obst. & Gynec., 1937, 33:393.

GORDON, C. A. The Reduction of Mortality in Ectopic Gestation. Am. J. Obst. & Gynec., 1936, 31:280.

HELLMAN, A. M., and SIMON, H. J. Full Term Intra-abdominal Pregnancy. Am. J. Surg., 1935, 29:403.

HOLTZ, F. Einiges über Ätiologie, Symptomatologie und Behandlung der Tubergravidität. Acta obst. et gynec. Scandinav., 1936, 16:509.

JARCHO, J. Ectopic Pregnancy with Special Reference to Abdominal Pregnancy. Am. J. Surg., 1949, 77:273 and 423.

JONES, H. O., and BREWER, J. I. The Arterial Phenomena Associated with Uterine Bleeding in Tubal Pregnancy. Am. J. Obst. & Gynec., 1939, 38:839.

KING, E. L. Postoperative Separation of the Cesarean Section Wound, with Subsequent Abdominal Pregnancy. Am. J. Obst. & Gynec., 1932, 24:421.

LANGMAN, L., and GOLDBLATT, M. Ectopic Pregnancy; a Review of 310 Operative Cases. Surg., Gynec., & Obst., 1939, 69:65.

LAVELL, T. E. Diagnosis of Ectopic Gestation from Clinical Analysis of 410 Cases at Bellevue Hospital. Am. J. Obst. & Gynec., 1929, 18:379.

LAZARD, E. M. Hysterography as an Aid to Diagnosis of Abdominal Pregnancy. Case Report and Review of Literature. West. J. Surg., 1937, 45:653.

LICHTENSTEIN, F. Basiotrope Placentation, etc. Zentralbl. f. Gynäk., 1920, 44:657.

LITZENBERG, J. C. Microscopical Studies of Tubal Pregnancy. Am. J. Obst. & Gynec., 1920, 1:223.

——— Some Fallacies in Regard to Ectopic Pregnancy. South. Surg., 1937, 6:1.

——— Synopsis of Obstetrics, 3rd Edit. C. V. Mosby Co., St. Louis, 1947.

MacFarlane, K. T., and Sparling, D. W. Ectopic Pregnancy; Selected Data from 110 Cases Including a Report of Two Unusual Cases. Am. J. Obst. & Gynec., 1946, 51:343.

McNally, F. P. The Association of Congenital Diverticula of the Fallopian Tube with Tubal Pregnancy. Am. J. Obst. & Gynec., 1926, 12:303.

Mahfouz, N. P. Ectopic Pregnancy. J. Obst. & Gynaec. Brit. Emp., 1938, 45:209.

Mall, F. P. The Cause of Tubal Pregnancy and the Fate of the Enclosed Ovum. Surg., Gynec. & Obst., 1915, 21:289.

——— On the Fate of the Human Embryo in Tubal Pregnancy. Carnegie Inst. of Wash., 1915, Publ. No. 221, p. 104.

——— and Cullen. An Ovarian Pregnancy Located in the Graafian Follicle. Surg., Gynec. & Obst., 1913, 17:698.

Marchetti, A. A., Kuder, K., and Kuder, A. A Clinical Evaluation of Ectopic Pregnancy. Am. J. Obst. & Gynec., 1946, 52:544.

Meagher, W. C. When to Operate in Ruptured Ectopic Gestation: An Analysis of 247 Cases. Am. J. Obst. & Gynec., 1935, 29:541.

Meyer, A. W. Hydatidiform Degeneration in Tubal Pregnancy. Surg., Gynec. & Obst., 1919, 28:293.

——— and Wynne, H. M. N. Some Aspects of Ovarian Pregnancy. Bull. Johns Hopkins Hosp., 1919, 30:92.

Moritz, A. R., and Douglass, M. A Study of Uterine and Tubal Decidual Reaction in Tubal Pregnancy. Surg., Gynec. & Obst., 1928, 47:785.

Newberger, C. An Analysis of Obstetric Activities in the Hospitals of Cook County during 1944. Am. J. Obst. & Gynec., 1946, 51:372.

Novak, E. Combined Intrauterine and Extrauterine Pregnancy, with a Report of 276 Cases. Surg., Gynec. & Obst., 1926, 43:26.

Osiakina-Rojdestvenskaia, A. J. The Etiology of Extra-uterine Pregnancy. Surg., Gynec. & Obst., 1938, 67:308.

Sampson, J. The Influence of Ectopic Pregnancy on the Uterus. Tr. Am. Gynec. Soc., 1913, 38-121.

Säntii. Ein Fall von ausgetragener Eierstockschwangerschaft, etc. Acta gyn. Scandinav., 1928, 7:207.

Schumann, E. A. Extra-uterine Pregnancy. D. Appleton and Co., New York, 1921.

Siddall, R. S. The Occurrence and Significance of Decidual Changes of the Endometrium in Extrauterine Pregnancy. Am. J. Obst. & Gynec., 1936, 31:420.

Spiegelberg, O. Zur Casuistik der Ovarialschwangerschaft. Arch. f. Gynäk., 1878, 13:73.

Studdiford, W. E. Primary Peritoneal Pregnancy. Am. J. Obst. & Gynec., 1942, 44:487.

——— Cervical Pregnancy. Am. J. Obst. & Gynec., 1945, 49:169.

Tyrone, C. H., Romano, S. A., and Collins, C. G. Tubal Gestation. A Statistical Study Based on 309 Cases. Am. J. Obst. & Gynec., 1935, 30:112.

Van Etten, R. C. Is Salpingitis a Factor in the Incidence of Tubal Pregnancy? Am. J. Obst. & Gynec., 1931, 22:645.

Villard, E., Regad, J., and Contamin, R. Du Rôle des États Endometroides dans la Pathogenie de la Grossesse Tubaire. Gynéc. et obst., 1936, 33:305.

Ware, H. H. Observations on Thirteen Cases of Late Extrauterine Pregnancy. Am. J. Obst. & Gynec., 1948, 55:561.

——— and Winn, W. C. A Study of 150 Consecutive Cases of Ectopic Pregnancy. Am. J. Obst. & Gynec., 1941, 42:33.

Williams, J. W. Contribution to the Normal and Pathological Histology of the Fallopian Tubes. Am. J. M. Sc., 1891, Oct.

Williams, P. F., and Corbit, J. D. An Analysis of 101 Fatalities from Ectopic Pregnancy. Am. J. Obst. & Gynec., 1944, 48:841.

Young. The Anatomy of the Pregnant Tube. Edinburgh M. J., 1909, 3:118.

22

DISEASES AND ABNORMALITIES OF THE FETAL MEMBRANES AND PLACENTA

HYDATIDIFORM MOLE AND CHORIONEPITHELIOMA

Hydatidiform mole and chorionepithelioma are, respectively, benign and malignant neoplasms of the chorion. The former is uncommon and the latter very rare, but the nature of these conditions has stimulated interest in them greater than their incidence alone would dictate. The frequently bizarre clinical behavior of the growths, the pathological variations between benign moles and extremely malignant chorionepitheliomas, the relationship of both to normal trophoblast with its invasive tendencies, and the similar biological activity in all, raise many interesting problems.

HYDATIDIFORM MOLE

Pathology. In this condition part or all of the chorionic villi are converted into a mass of clear vesicles. Usually no embryo is present, though in occasional cases mole occurs in part of the placenta in association with a normal fetus. The vesicles vary in size from less than a millimeter to more than a centimeter in diameter and hang in grapelike clusters from thin pedicles (Fig. 331). The mass may attain great size, at times filling a uterus to the size of a six or seven months pregnancy.

The microscopic structure is characterized by alterations in the trophoblast, the stroma and the blood vessels (Figs. 332 and 333). The first is the definitive change though sometimes not the most obvious one. Both layers of the trophoblast undergo proliferation, the Langerhans' cells being recognized as well defined polyhedral cells with heavily stained nuclei and the syncytium being made up of masses of cytoplasm with clusters of nuclei frequently forming buds or syncytial giant cells. The areas of proliferation are most marked in the deep layers near the uterine wall and are often absent in the vesicular mass in the cavity far removed from blood supply. The amount of proliferation varies considerably in different moles. The stroma of the villi becomes hydropic and degenerates with very few stromal cells and rare blood vessels to be seen. Most of the vesicles are made up of such stroma surrounded by a very thin layer of trophoblast.

That hydatidiform mole was formerly thought to be a degenerative rather than neoplastic lesion is mirrored in such terms as myxoma chorii and cystic degeneration of the chorion. In his classical study in 1895, Marchand demonstrated that trophoblastic proliferation is the essential feature and this viewpoint is held by most investigators at present. The mole may be considered a pathological pregnancy with the primary defect in the ovum.

Some difference of opinion remains as to whether all hydatid change in the villi is true hydatidiform mole or whether there may be a type of degenerative reaction that merely resembles mole in its early stage. Hertig and Edmonds, in a study of pathological ova, found two thirds to show early hydatid degeneration.

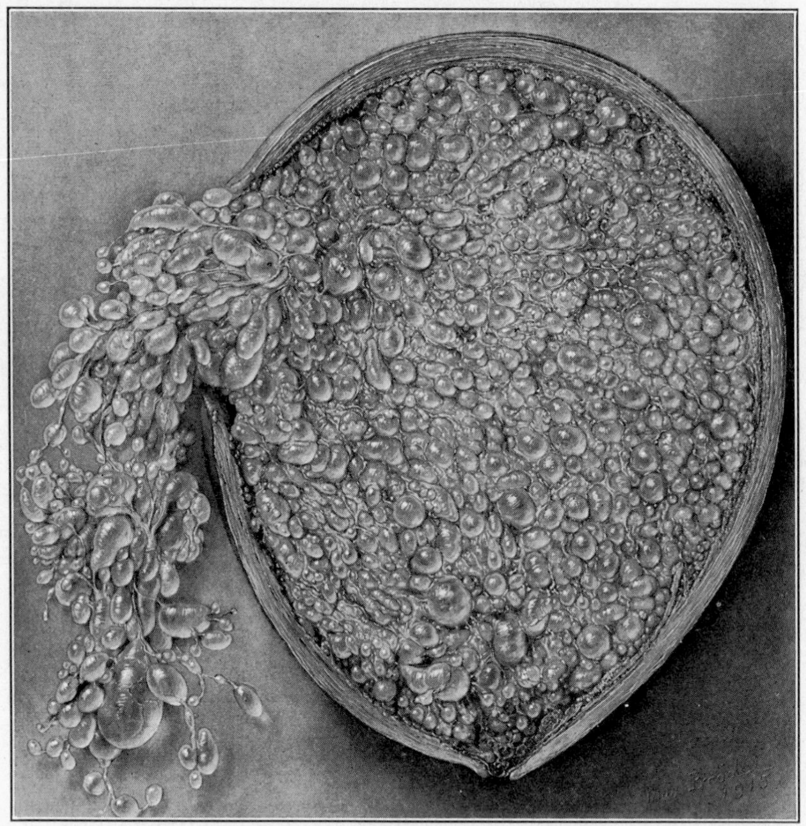

Fig. 331.—Uterus Containing a Hydatidiform Mole.

Transition from so-called hydatid degeneration to typical hydatidiform mole is equivocal.

Attempts have been made to relate the histological structure of hydatidiform moles to their potential malignant tendencies. Many pathologists feel that no reliable criteria exist for such differentiation. In general, hydatidiform moles which show a well-developed villous pattern, edematous stroma and scanty trophoblastic proliferation are usually benign; those which show hyperplastic growth of trophoblast in formless sheets with tendency to penetrate the stroma or invade the uterine wall or tendency to anaplastic cell changes are more likely to become malignant. Hertig studied 200 moles using such criteria and was able to show marked, though not absolute, correlation between the pathological and clinical malignancy.

In many cases of hydatidiform mole the ovaries show multiple lutein cysts (Fig.

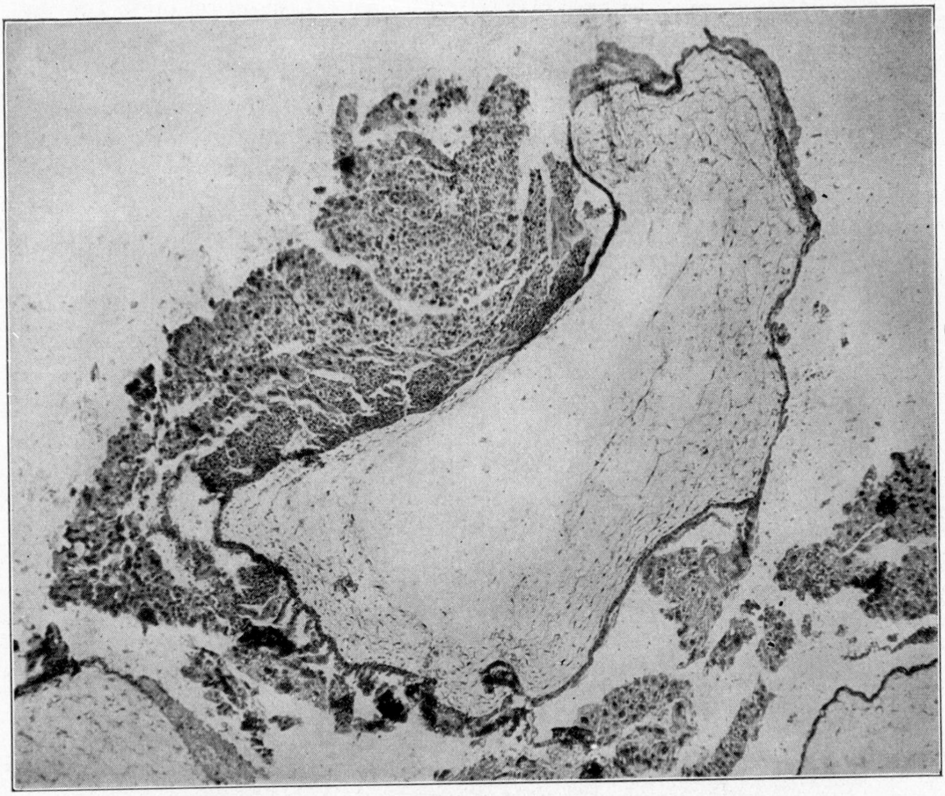

Fig. 332.—Section of Hydatidiform Mole Showing Proliferation of Trophoblastic Epithelium. × 65.

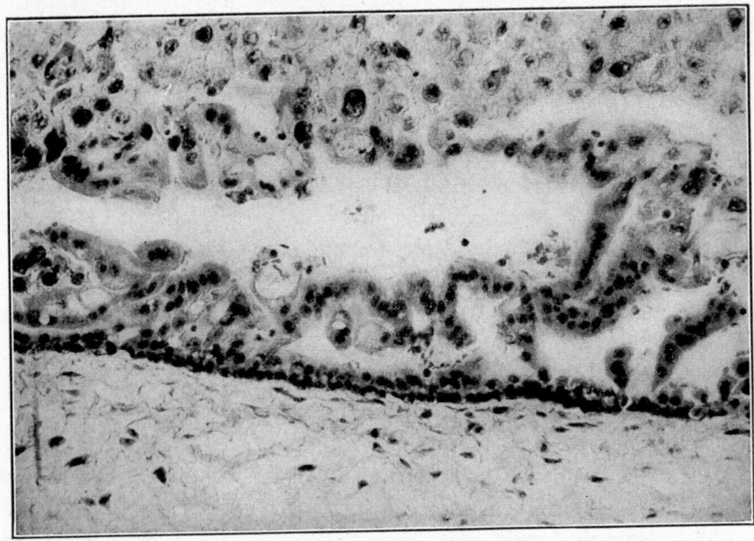

Fig. 333.—Hydatidiform Mole, Benign (× 245), Showing Trophoblastic Proliferation of Syncytium and Langhans' Cells and Edema of Stroma.

334). These may vary from microscopic size to 10 cm. or more in diameter. The surfaces of the cysts are smooth and often yellowish in color, being lined with lutein cells. The incidence of such cysts in association with mole has been stated to be from 25 per cent to as high as 60 per cent. The variation in figures depends on the criteria used; Novak has emphasized that most of the ovaries lacking gross cysts show microscopic cystic change and luteal hyper-reaction which often involves both thecal elements and granulosa.

It is believed that the lutein cysts of the ovaries are the result of overstimulation of lutein elements by large amounts of chorionic gonadotrophin secreted by the proliferating trophoblast. That such extensive ovarian changes are not seen in normal

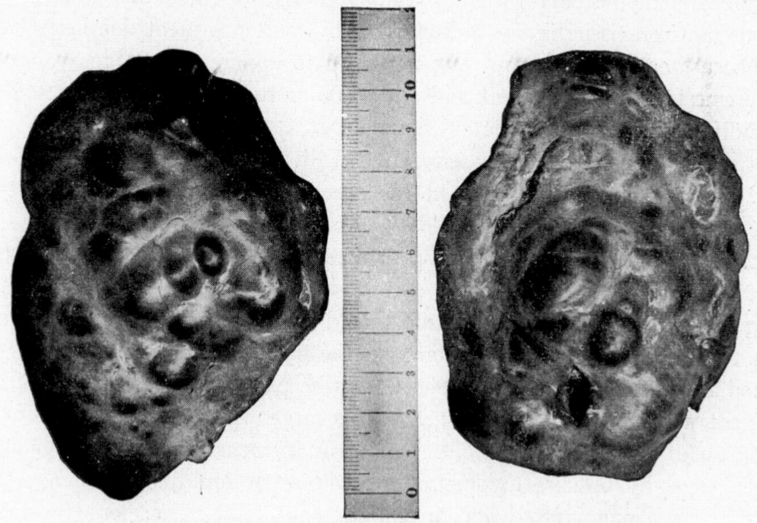

FIG. 334.—LUTEIN CYSTOMATA, BILATERAL, ASSOCIATED WITH HYDATIDIFORM MOLE. (Removal at operation no longer practiced.)

pregnancy may be explained on the basis that very high levels of gonadotrophin are not maintained for such long periods of time. In general, extensive cyst formation is usually associated with the larger hydatidiform moles and a long period of stimulation. The cysts regress after delivery of the mole and eventually disappear.

Clinical History. Hydatidiform mole occurs about once in 2,000 pregnancies. The age incidence is that of the reproductive period though some studies seem to show increased frequency after 40 years.

In the early stages of development of mole there are no characteristics distinguishing it from normal pregnancy. If early abortion does not occur, the growing uterus often enlarges more rapidly than usual so that its size exceeds that expected from the supposed duration of gestation. This is true of about one half of cases, the remainder being of average or smaller size. Uterine bleeding is the outstanding symptom and may vary from spotty to profuse hemorrhage. It may appear just before abortion but more often occurs intermittently for weeks or even months. Occasionally hydatid vesicles may be passed. Sooner or later the mole is aborted or removed by operation. Spontaneous expulsion is most apt to occur at about the third month and rarely is delayed beyond the sixth month.

In an occasional case, the great predilection of the trophoblast for venous channels may carry the mole deep into the uterine muscle. The so-called destructive mole may grow through to perforate the peritoneum, giving rise to hemorrhage and infection with acute abdominal signs. In rare instances, either before or after expulsion of a mole, small purplish tumors may be found in the vagina or vulva. These consist mostly of blood interspersed with characteristic hydatidiform villi. Since permanent recovery may follow local excision of these growths, it has been suggested that they may be due to simple transportation of benign villi rather than true metastases of malignant type.

Uterine infection is common with mole, which is understandable when a period of threatening abortion occurs with a patulous cervix, bleeding and a large mass of poorly vascularized tissue in the uterus. Anemia is often present due largely to blood loss but occasionally may be out of proportion to apparent bleeding.

Hyperemesis is more frequent and apt to be more severe and protracted in cases of hydatidiform mole than in normal pregnancy.

Severe preeclampsia is often associated with mole, especially with the larger growths. Toxemia may arise early in the second trimester when such a condition would not be expected ordinarily.

Jaundice may be present and disappear after passage of the mole, suggesting that it is not due to metastatic lesion.

Diagnosis. Often hydatidiform mole is diagnosed only when the specimen is expelled. As bleeding is the usual symptom, the initial diagnosis is commonly simple threatened abortion. Occasionally vesicles may be passed making the diagnosis clear. In a patient with persistent bleeding, a uterus larger than the expected size arouses the suspicion of mole. The possibilities of error in menstrual data, pregnant uterus unduly enlarged by obscure myomata, hydramnios or multiple pregnancy, must be considered. If pregnancy is advanced, palpation for fetal parts, perception of movements or heart tones and visualization of fetal skeleton by x-ray may be useful. Positive evidence is reliable; negative is less reliable, since routine x-ray occasionally fails to demonstrate a fetus at five months.

Hydatidiform moles produce large amounts of chorionic gonadotrophin. This originates from the extensive growth of trophoblast as evidence points to the Langerhans' cell as the site of production of this substance. Therefore, a biological test for chorionic gonadotrophin may be the decisive factor in the diagnosis of mole. There has been much discussion about the value of the test but it can be very useful if certain criteria are met: (1) a reliable quantitative method of assay must be used; (2) there must be a correlation with clinical data taking cognizance of the curve of gonadotrophin secretion in normal pregnancy.

Assays should be made on serum as it is subject to fewer variables than is the gonadotrophin in the urine. In our clinic we have found the immature rat uterine weight method of assay the most reliable. The assay result should be compared to the serum gonadotrophin curve for normal pregnancy at the supposed duration (Fig. 127). If it is far above the normal range for that stage of pregnancy, mole may be diagnosed. (It should be kept in mind that the decline of the curve from the peak is a little retarded in multiple pregnancies but the character of the curve is the same as for single pregnancy.) It is clear from the gonadotrophin curve for normal pregnancy that no *single* value can be set up as the borderline between normal and abnormal pregnancy. Very high values in the first two or three months mean nothing as they are encountered frequently in normal pregnancy. Thus the biological test is not of use in diagnosing mole in the early case. However, beyond 100 days after the last menstrual period, normal pregnancy shows a rapid decline in gonadotrophin, so that persistently high or rising levels at that time are strong evidence of abnormal growth of trophoblast. If the slightest doubt exists one or more repeat assays at intervals of a week will clarify the trend.

Formerly it was suggested that chorionic gonadotrophin in the spinal fluid was indicative of hydatidiform mole or chorionepithelioma. It is likely, however, that the presence of this substance in the spinal fluid is merely associated with a high blood level. The chorionic gonadotrophin reaction of the spinal fluid is sometimes negative in hydatidiform mole (as well as in chorionepithelioma) and occasionally positive in normal pregnancy. Thus, Hashimoto has reported positive Aschheim-Zondek reactions in five cases of normal pregnancy, using 18 to 20 cc. of spinal fluid, while Palmer found six positive tests in the spinal fluid among 42 normal pregnant women and one negative spinal fluid reaction in a patient with chorionepithelioma.

Prognosis. The immediate mortality from hydatidiform mole was formerly as high as 10 per cent due chiefly to hemorrhage, infection and uterine perforation. In a collective review of 576 cases in the late 1930's, Mathieu found an immediate mortality of only 1.4 per cent. This mortality should be practically eliminated with ample use of blood transfusion and chemotherapy.

The incidence of malignant transformation of mole to chorionepithelioma has been variously reported from 1 or 2 per cent to more than 10 per cent. Differences in pathological interpretation may account for some of the variation, but the smaller figure is probably more nearly correct for true chorionepithelioma.

Treatment. The treatment of hydatidiform mole has two phases, the immediate abortion or evacuation of the mole, and the later follow-up for detection of chorionepithelioma, if it should ensue. In the majority of cases of mole, abortion is imminent or in process when diagnosis is made and treatment is directed at completion of the abortion. Pituitrin stimulation may be useful. If bleeding is profuse evacuation of the uterus by ovum forceps and completion by curettage may be necessary but must be done with great caution as the uterus may be very soft and hence easily perforated. Hemorrhage may be severe and ample blood for transfusion should be available. If hemorrhage does not force intervention, spontaneous completion should be encouraged with curettage deferred until several days later when beginning involution has rendered the uterus firmer. Presence of infection also dictates deferring curettage until the infection has been controlled by chemotherapy. However, at some time in the early puerperium, before the patient is discharged from the hospital, a careful curettage should be done. This may save confusion both in the clinical and bio-assay follow-up as retained fragments of trophoblast may give rise to bleeding and positive tests for chorionic gonadotrophin which may be wrongly interpreted as new growth.

Use of hysterotomy or hysterectomy for mole has been recommended by some but is warranted only in special cases. In an occasional case where diagnosis of mole is unequivocal with no sign of impending spontaneous abortion and the uterus rises to the umbilicus or above, hysterotomy may be the best treatment. The operative evacuation of such a large mass through a slightly dilated cervix carries considerable risk of hemorrhage and trauma. If the abdominal approach is necessary in a patient of considerable parity, hysterectomy may be preferable as it meets the immediate problem and minimizes future risk of chorionepithelioma.

During the period of follow-up after hydatidiform mole, patients should be given reliable contraceptive advice, as the occurrence of a new pregnancy may confuse the picture and lead to an erroneous suspicion of chorionepithelioma. Several such cases of normal pregnancy treated mistakenly by hysterectomy have been reported.

Quantitative assays for chorionic gonadotrophin should be carried out after passage of any hydatidiform mole. Ideally these assays should be done weekly or biweekly until the result is negative, and then monthly up to one year. In about two thirds of cases of mole, chorionic gonadotrophin will be absent by 60 days, the majority being negative as early as 30 days after evacuation. Some of the remaining cases will show slow but steady decrease in gonadotrophin requiring several months to become negative but demonstrating no further abnormality. A smaller group of cases, in the neighborhood of 10 per cent, have a persistent elevation of gonadotrophin level or a rising titer. Such biological behavior indicates an undue persistence of living trophoblast or, in the presence of a rising titer, active proliferative growth. Clinical symptoms, especially irregular bleeding, are often but not invariably present. In this small group of cases exploratory laparotomy and hysterectomy should be carried out. Repeated curettages are apt to be misleading as the dangerous trophoblast may lie deep in the myometrium beyond the reach of the curette. A few of these cases will prove to be true chorionepithelioma, while others will be so-called destructive or invasive moles or intermediate pathological types, but are sufficiently uncertain in prognosis to warrant removal.

CHORIONEPITHELIOMA

Pathology. This extremely malignant tumor arises from the chorion and is thus of embryonic rather than uterine origin. It may be considered to be a carcinoma of the chorionic epithelium although some of its growth and metastatic behavior resembles sarcoma. The factors involved in such malignant transformation of the chorion are unknown. In chorionepithelioma the tendencies of normal trophoblast toward invasive growth and blood vessel erosion are greatly exaggerated. The characteristic gross picture is that of a rapidly growing mass invading both uterine muscle and blood vessels with areas of hemorrhage and coagulation necrosis. The tumor is dark red or purple with a ragged, friable structure. If it is present on the endometrium, bleeding, sloughing and infection of the surface usually occur early. Masses of tissue buried in the myometrium may extend outward, appearing on the uterus as dark, irregular nodules which eventually perforate the peritoneum.

Microscopically, columns and sheets of trophoblast are seen penetrating the muscle and blood vessels in a lawless manner interspersed with areas of clotted blood. An attempt at villous formation may be present in some areas but this is variable and often absent entirely. Both Langerhans' and syncytial cells are involved although one or the other may predominate and the former is believed to be the more malignant. Anaplastic cell changes are usually present in some degree and may be marked. However, such cell changes are often not as definitive in differentiating benign and malignant growth of the trophoblast as in other tumors. This difficulty of evaluating the cytology is one of the factors which makes for error in diagnosis of chorionepithelioma from uterine curettings where the general growth pattern may not be apparent. Cells of normal trophoblast burrowing into the placental site have been erroneously diagnosed as chorionepithelioma.

Metastasis is often very early and is generally blood-borne due to the affinity of trophoblast for blood vessels. The most common site is the lungs (over 75 per cent) and the second most common the vagina (about 50 per cent). The vulva, kidneys, liver, ovaries and brain also show metastases in many cases. Lutein cystomata are present in over one third of the cases.

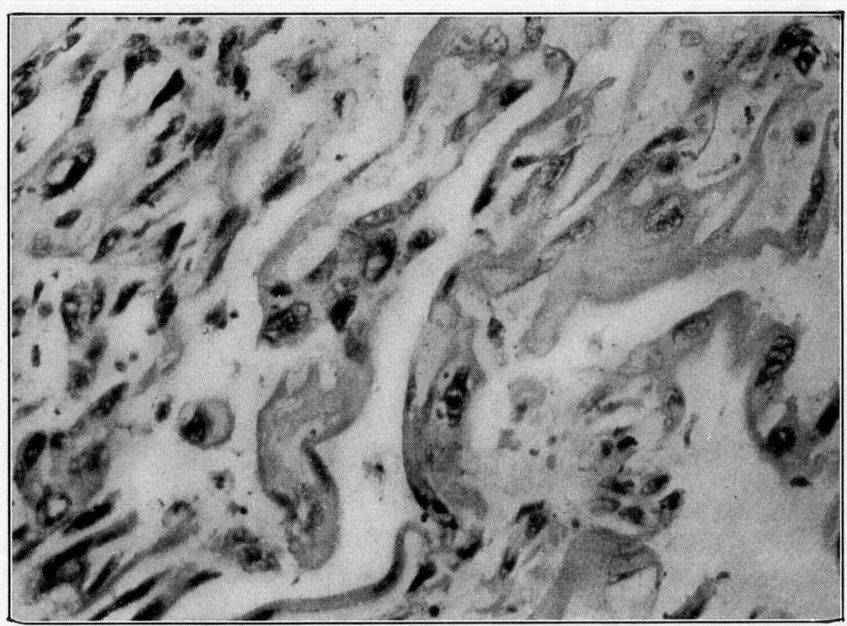

Fig. 335.—Chorionepithelioma, Malignant (× 245), Showing Invasive Proliferation of the Trophoblast, Langhans' and Syncytial Cells.

Clinical History. Chorionepithelioma occurs only once in many thousands of pregnancies, so that incidence figures mean little. The age incidence is that of the reproductive period since, except for rare cases arising in teratomata, it always follows pregnancy. Approximately 50 per cent of cases occur after hydatidiform mole, 25 per cent after abortions and 25 per cent after term pregnancies. It may result from ectopic as well as intra-uterine pregnancy. Chorionepithelioma may rarely coexist with the pregnancy but in most cases develops immediately afterwards. Occasionally it seems to lie dormant for long periods before undergoing active growth. One may question many such reported cases, however, as often a subsequent pregnancy with early unrecognized abortion may have occurred in the interim.

Frequently there is no evidence of the malignancy immediately after the pregnancy. The most common though not constant symptom is irregular bleeding after the immediate puerperium. It may be continuous or intermittent with sudden and even massive hemorrhages. Perforation of the growth through the uterus may cause intraperitoneal hemorrhage. Extension into the parametrial tissues may cause pain and fixation suggestive of inflammatory disease. Secondary infection is a common accompaniment.

In many cases the first indication of the condition may come from the metastatic lesions. Vaginal or vulvar tumors may be found. The patient may complain of pulmonary symptoms such as a cough and bloody sputum arising from pulmonary metastases. In a few cases it has been impossible to find chorionepithelioma in the uterus or pelvis, the original lesion having disappeared, leaving only distant metastases growing actively.

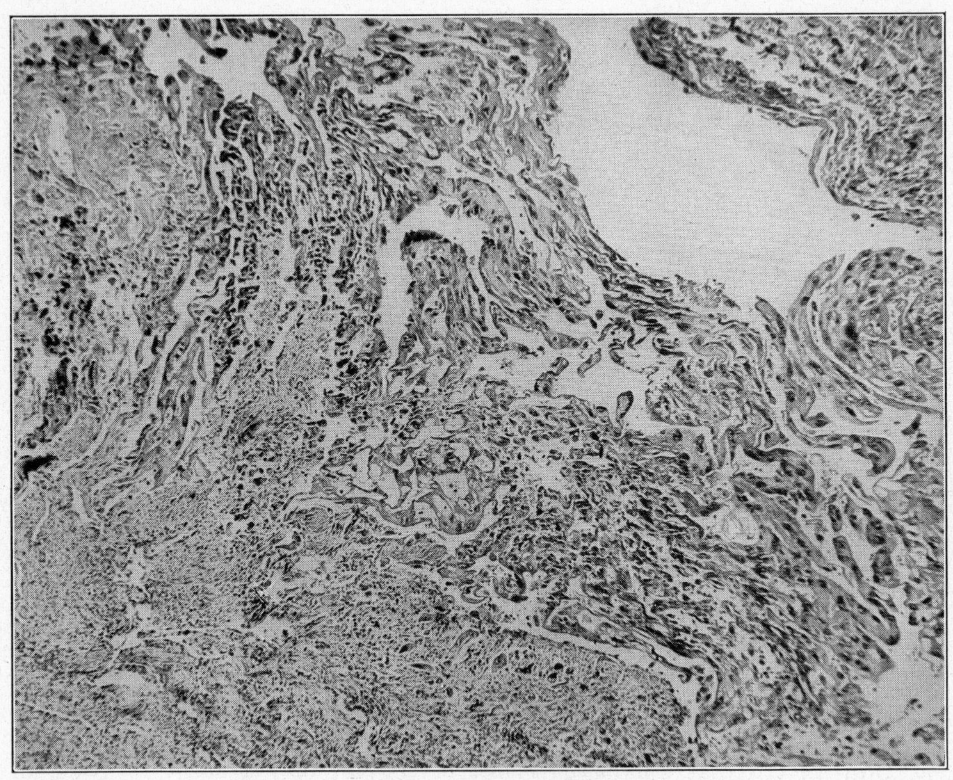

FIG. 336.—CHORIONEPITHELIOMA.

Note invasion and destruction of uterine musculature by trophoblastic cells. × 55.

Perforation of the uterine wall by chorionepithelioma with free and sometimes massive bleeding into the peritoneal cavity is probably a more common complication of this invasive neoplasm than is generally realized. Thus, Acosta-Sison and Espaniola encountered 8 examples of this accident in 32 cases of chorionepithelioma, or in 25 per cent. In Karl Wilson's series of 5 cases there was one such perforation. In 1942, Rosenbloom reported a dramatic case of fatal intra-abdominal hemorrhage following penetration of the uterine wall by chorionepithelioma in which the hole made by the growing neoplastic mass was 4 by 2 cm. Perforating chorionepithelioma has been discussed in some detail by Anspach and Hoffman in a paper which analyzed seven cases from the literature and one of their own. They point out that the clinical course of most of these cases so closely resembled a ruptured ectopic pregnancy that this diagnosis was made five times in the 8 cases reported. In 3 cases uterine hemorrhage previous to the rupture was noted; in 3 there had been a period of amenorrhea; and in two there was spotting. It is significant and worthy of note that in 3 cases the acute symptoms developed almost immediately after a pelvic examination and the authors advise therefore that great care should be taken in making pelvic examinations in suspected cases.

If unmodified by treatment, the course of chorionepithelioma is rapidly progressive and death occurs within a few months to one year in the majority of cases.

Diagnosis. Recognition of the possibility of the lesion is the most important factor in diagnosis. All cases of hydatidiform mole are under suspicion and should be followed as indicated under that subject. In any case of unusual bleeding after term pregnancy or abortion, the possibility should be kept in mind and investigated by curettage and bio-assay.

It is stressed that absolute reliance cannot be put in curettings. There must be great experience and much caution in making a positive diagnosis of chorionepithelioma from curettings unless the pattern is one of obvious malignancy for, as pointed out above, normal trophoblast may often penetrate deeply into the uterine wall at the implantation site simulating tumor growth. Conversely, malignant growth may lie below the surface of the uterus and be missed by the curet.

Chorionic gonadotrophin normally disappears from the serum and urine a few days after term delivery or simple abortion, provided that the latter is complete. Therefore, if assay shows persistent or rising titer of gonadotrophin after this period, it is diagnostic of new growth. Correlation must be made with clinical data and the possibility of a new pregnancy ruled out. Repeat assay should be made to eliminate the possibility of laboratory error before radical treatment is undertaken. In cases where distant inaccessible metastases, such as those in the lung, raise the question of chorionepithelioma, the positive gonadotrophin assay verifies the diagnosis.

Treatment. When the diagnosis of chorionepithelioma is made, hysterectomy should be done. Any localized metastases in the pelvis, vagina and vulva which can be excised should be removed. Contrary to usual practice with other malignancies, it is justifiable to use surgery in cases of chorionepithelioma already involved with distant metastases as there are a few reported cases in which metastases have regressed after removal of the primary tumor. Metastases which cannot be removed should be radiated; some good results have been reported with radiation of metastases but many cases do not respond at all.

HYDRAMNIOS

By hydramnios is understood the presence of an excessive quantity of liquor amnii. According to Lehn the normal amount of amniotic fluid is 1,000 cc. in primigravidae and 1,200 cc. in multiparae so that, generally speaking, a quantity greater than 2 liters may be considered excessive. In rare cases the uterus may contain an almost incredible amount of liquor amnii, Küstner having observed 15 liters and Schneider 30 liters at the fifth and sixth months of pregnancy respectively. In most cases the increase in the amount of amniotic fluid is gradual, in which instance this condition is commonly called *chronic hydramnios*. When it takes place very suddenly, so that the uterus may become immensely distended within a few days the condition is called *acute hydramnios*. The fluid in hydramnios is usually identical in appearance and composition with that normally present in the amniotic cavity.

Incidence. Minor degrees of hydramnios, 2 to 3 liters, are common, but the more marked grades are not frequent. Because of the difficulty of collecting amniotic fluid with any degree of completeness, the diagnosis is usually made on clinical impression only and in borderline cases the justification of the diagnosis will vary with the individual observer. For this reason the published statistics on the incidence of hydramnios are in poor agreement and range from 1 case in 200 pregnancies to 1 in 750. In 63,636 deliveries at the Johns Hopkins Hospital, 178 cases were classified as hydramnios, an incidence of 1 case in 358 deliveries. At the New York Lying-In Hospital, Mueller has reported 66 cases (acute and chronic) in 49,793 deliveries, a frequency of 1 in 754. Cases of hydramnios of sufficient degree to be of clinical significance, that is cases with 3,000 cc. or more, are less frequent than the above data would indicate and occur perhaps 1 in every 1,200 pregnancies or so. In the Johns Hopkins series mentioned above there were 57 such cases, a frequency of 1 in 1,164 cases. The acute variety is quite rare, Mueller having encountered only 4 cases in his series, or 1 in 12,500 deliveries.

The incidence of hydramnios in cases of fetal malformations, especially central nervous system defects, is very high and anencephalus is accompanied by it in over half the cases. In the 178 cases of hydramnios seen in our clinic, 31 or 17.4 per cent occurred in association with fetal deformities. In severe hydramnios this percentage is much higher. In our 57 cases in which the amount of fluid exceeded 3,000 cc., 15, or more than one-quarter, were accompanied by fetal malformations. The incidence of congenital anomalies in Mueller's cases of hydramnios was 29 per cent. Excessive amniotic fluid is also very common in twin pregnancies. Multiple gestation existed in 22 of our 178 cases of hydramnios, or in 12.5 per cent. In Guttmacher's study of 573 twin pregnancies observed in our clinic, he found that hydramnios was diagnosed in 40, an incidence of 7 per cent. Most investigators have observed that hydramnios is more frequent in single ovum twinning than in the dizygotic variety. However, of the 31 cases of hydramnios studied by Guttmacher in which the relations of the membranes were definitely determined, 7, or 22.6 per cent, were single ovum and 24, 78.4 per cent, were double ovum; this is approximately the proportion of single to double ovum pregnancies in the whole series. The incidence of hydramnios is also especially high in the hydrops variety of erythroblastosis and in pregnancies complicated by diabetes. It appears to be somewhat increased also in preeclampsia and eclampsia.

Etiology. Very little is known about the underlying mechanism of hydramnios. While the source of the amniotic fluid is to be interpreted with reasonable certainty as the amniotic epithelium, no histologic changes in the amnion or chemical changes in the amniotic fluid in cases of hydramnios have been found to explain its occurrence. In cases of anencephalus and spina bifida it is widely believed that an increased transudation of fluid from the exposed meninges into the amniotic cavity is responsible for the condition. Since, as Taussig has pointed out, there is ample evidence to indicate that anencephalic fetuses do not swallow amniotic fluid, the theory has been advanced that this may account for the excessive accumulation of liquor amnii. The absence of swallowing of amniotic fluid as a factor in hydramnios is further emphasized by the cases of this condition which have been reported in association with stricture of the esophagus, stroma blocking the esophagus and various other disorders in which the lumen of the esophagus is impinged upon.

As another explanation of the frequency of hydramnios in anencephalus, the theory has been advanced that the superabundant fluid results from excessive urinary secretion, which is brought about by the stimulation of cerebral or spinal centers which have been deprived of their usual coverings, just as happens in the piqûre experiments of the physiologists. This general idea that disturbances of swallowing or urination may have something to do with hydramnios receives some slight plausibility perhaps from the fact that anencephalus and other defects which interfere with swallowing are frequently associated with hydramnios, whereas defects of the urinary organs which cause anuria are almost equally frequent in cases of oligohydramnios. In hydramnios associated with monozygotic twin pregnancy the hypothesis has been advanced that one fetus usurps the greater part of the circulation common to both twins, develops cardiac hypertrophy, which in turn is followed by renal hypertrophy with increased secretion. As has been indicated, however, our own statistics indicate that hydramnios is no more frequent with monozygotic twins than it is with double ovum twinning and, as far as I am aware, no explanation whatsoever has been advanced as to the cause of excessive amniotic fluid so frequently seen in the latter type of multiple pregnancy.

The weight of the placenta tends to be high in hydramnios, a fact which has been emphasized especially by Taussig. Our own experience confirms this observation since the placenta weighed more than 800 gm. in 40 per cent of our cases and more than 900 gm. in 22 per cent. Because of this fact the suggestion has been advanced that the increased area of chorionic villi available for transudation of fluid may in some way be responsible for certain cases of hydramnios.

Symptoms. The symptoms accompanying hydramnios arise from purely mechanical causes and are due chiefly to the pressure exerted by the overdistended uterus upon adjacent organs. The effects are particularly marked in the respiratory functions, and, when the distention is excessive, the patient may suffer from severe dyspnea and cyanosis, and in extreme cases be able to breathe only in an upright position. Edema often occurs especially in the lower extremities, about the vulva and in the abdominal wall. As the result of overstretching of the muscular fiber, presumably, generalized pain in the uterus itself is not uncommon and in my own experience has been a more frequent and distressing symptom than respiratory distress. It is surprising what great degrees of abdominal distention can sometimes be borne by the patient with comparatively little discomfort, although this is the case only when the accumulation of fluid has taken place gradually. On the other hand, in acute hydramnios, the distention may lead to disturbances sufficiently serious to threaten the life of the patient. Acute hydramnios tends to occur earlier in pregnancy than the chronic form, often makes its appearance as early as the fourth or fifth month and rapidly expands the uterus to enormous size. Pain may be intense and the dyspnea so severe that the patient is unable to lie flat; edema of the abdomen, vulva and thighs, together with nausea and vomiting may also be observed and, all in all, the picture may be a most alarming one. As a rule acute hydramnios terminates in labor before the twenty-eighth week, or the symptoms become so dire that intervention becomes mandatory.

Wieloch has demonstrated that the pressure symptoms are due entirely to the size of the uterus and not to any increase of pressure within it. Upon puncturing the uterus through the abdominal wall, and measuring the pressure by means of a lumbar puncture apparatus, he found that in hydramnios it was in no way increased over that obtaining a normal pregnancy, which is surprisingly low. For this reason, it seems improbable that the frequent occurrence of premature labor, which so often complicates the condition, can be ascribed to greatly increased intra-uterine pressure, and consequently it must be due to mere passive overdistention of the uterine wall by the abnormal size of the amniotic mass.

Diagnosis. Unusual uterine enlargement in association with difficulty in palpating fetal small parts and in hearing fetal heart tones, and easy ballottement of the fetus are the main diagnostic signs of hydramnios. In severe cases the uterine wall may be so tense and tender that it is quite impossible to palpate any part of the fetus. Such findings call for an immediate x-ray of the abdomen to rule out or establish the presence of a fetal abnormality or a multiple pregnancy. The differentiation between hydramnios, ascites, and giant ovarian cyst can usually be made without difficulty as soon as the roentgenogram is studied, since the issue here hangs chiefly on the existence or nonexistence of pregnancy.

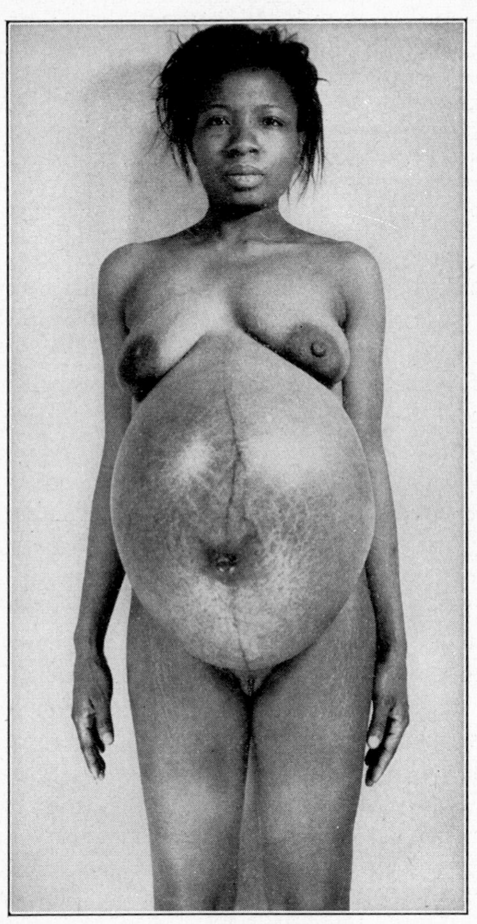

FIG. 337.—ADVANCED DEGREE OF HYDRAMNIOS, 5,500 CC. OF AMNIOTIC FLUID BEING MEASURED AT DELIVERY.

Prognosis. The outlook for the infant in substantial degrees of hydramnios is notoriously poor and, even though the x-ray shows a normal appearing fetus, the prognosis must be guarded. As already indicated, the incidence of fetal malformations incompatible with life is at least 20 per cent. Superimposed on this there may be anticipated an increased death rate from prematurity since the frequency of premature births in this complication is more than doubled. Prolapse of the umbilical cord, erythroblastosis and the well-known difficulties which encounter the baby of the diabetic mother, add still further to the death rate. As the result of these several factors, the total fetal loss in hydramnios exceeds 50 per cent. Vogt found that the fetal mortality exceeded 50 per cent in 237 cases which he analyzed and that 97 of the babies were premature and 25 presented some malformation. Mueller's fetal death rate at the New York Lying-In Hospital was 51 per cent, while that in the entire Johns Hopkins series mentioned above was almost identical, namely, 48.3 per cent. In our cases in which the amount of fluid exceeded 3,000 cc., however, the mortality rate rose to 68.1 per cent and, in general, the more severe the hydramnios, the more grave is the fetal outlook.

The hazards imposed by hydramnios on the mother are several and substantial but they can usually be combatted without serious threat to her life. The most frequent maternal complications are abruptio placentae, uterine inertia, postpartum hemorrhage and adherence of the placenta. The first of these sometimes follows massive escape of the liquor amnii and is understandable on the grounds that the pressure against the placenta is suddenly released. The last three complications are the result of uterine atony consequent upon overdistention. Abnormal presentations are more common as the result of the excessive amount of amniotic fluid so that operative interference will become imperative more frequently than under normal conditions.

Treatment. Minor degrees of hydramnios rarely require active treatment. Even moderate degrees of the complication, including cases in which some modicum of discomfort is present, can usually be carried along without intervention until labor starts or until the membranes rupture spontaneously. If there is any degree of dyspnea, abdominal pain or edema of the abdominal wall, or if ambulation is difficult, hospitalization becomes essential. Such patients should have complete bed rest, a salt-poor diet (less than 3.0 gm. per diem) and mild sedation at night if sleep is interfered with. Large doses of ammonium chloride (75 to 90 grains a day in enteric-coated tablets) as recommended by Abrams and Abrams are worthy of trial.

If the above measures fail and acute discomfort develops as the result of the growing uterine mass, puncture of the sac through the cervix (usually well dilated in such cases) becomes necessary. If at all possible the sac should be ruptured several inches above the edge of the os and the fluid allowed to drain away slowly. This may sometimes be effected by introducing a small trocar, such as is used for ovarian cysts, upward between the uterus and membranes, followed by puncture and release of fluid slowly through the trocar. Not infrequently, however, the membranes tear with sudden release of fluid and in that event the presenting part should be held as snugly as possible against the cervix to reduce the rate of flow. Blood should be available because of the frequence of postpartum hemorrhage and preparations made for dealing with the maternal complications already described.

In cases in which the child is not yet viable and no abnormality appears to be present on x-ray examination, abdominal puncture of the amniotic sac has been recommended by various British and European obstetricians. The literature on abdominal aspiration of amniotic fluid has been reviewed by Mueller who reaches the conclusion that there is nothing to be gained in fetal salvage by this technic; and the procedure is not, of course, without some danger. In five cases in which we have employed it, our results have scarcely been gratifying since labor ensued promptly in four of them. It cannot be recommended, accordingly, on the basis of the data now available.

OLIGOHYDRAMNIOS

In rare instances the amount of amniotic fluid may fall far below the normal limits, and occasionally it may be represented by only a few cubic centimeters of thick, viscid fluid.

The etiology of this condition is even less well understood than that of hydramnios. Jaggard, in 1894, reported a case in which the fetus presented an imperforate urethra with absence of one kidney and cystic degeneration of the other, and he therefore concluded that the lack of amniotic fluid was the result of nonsecretion of urine. Since then numerous similar cases have been reported. On the other hand, abnormalities of the urinary tract cannot be regarded as the sole cause of the condition, as Hüssy and others have found that hydramnios may accompany such conditions.

Forssell is inclined to attribute oligohydramnios to necrosis of the amniotic epithelium, which he believes favors undue absorption of the amniotic fluid. It is evident that substantial evidence is lacking with regard to this theory.

When oligohydramnios occurs early in pregnancy it is attended by serious consequences to the fetus, as adhesions may be formed between its external surface and the amnion and give rise to serious deformities. When occurring later, its effect upon the fetus, though less marked, is quite characteristic. Under such circumstances the fetus is subjected to pressure from all sides and takes on a peculiar appearance, and many minor deformities, such as clubfoot, are frequently observed.

In some cases of oligohydramnios the skin of the fetus is markedly thickened and presents a dry, leathery appearance. Most authorities attribute this to the lack of amniotic fluid, but Ahlfeld is inclined to believe that it is the cause and not the result of the condition, since the skin lesion may be so marked as to interfere with the normal cutaneous functions and thus do away with one of the sources of the liquor amnii.

INTRA-UTERINE AMPUTATION

Since Chaussier in 1812 first directed attention to such local deficiencies of the fetus as amputation of fingers, toes, arms and legs, encephalocele, hemicephalus, fissures of face, jaw or lips, ectopia cordis, extrophy of the bladder and umbilical hernia with eventration, these anomalies have usually been ascribed to adhesions between the amnion and various portions of the germinal disc. However, as a result of the investigations of Streeter it now seems that the majority of these anomalies have quite a different origin.

Streeter postulates that there is a normal disparity in the vitality of the different tissues of the body which is hereditary and transmitted by the germ plasm. For this reason, occasionally, extreme disparities between excessive growth potency and defective growth capacity must occur and as a result overgrowth is seen in some anomalies as well as lack of growth or complete absence in others. In between these two groups is a third in which, though a part is normal in size, it is aberrant in form. Examples are the various forms of doubling of digits such as extra fingers, webbed fingers, short fingers and anomalous joints. Whether an extremity is to grow too large or have abnormal form or is to be too small, is dependent on the growth characteristics of the specific limb-bud tissue from which it originates. It can be surmised, because of this, that these anomalies bear a definite relation to one another and are frequently blended or may be associated with abnormalities in other parts of the body.

Related to the above types of deficient or abnormal development is another condition which results in so-called intra-uterine amputation. Here sharply circumscribed areas of limb-bud tissues are of such inferior quality that only partial histogenesis occurs and the process ceases in the earlier weeks of pregnancy. As early as the fourteenth week, they may be seen as macerated masses of tissue sloughing away from normal adjacent tissue. Later on they are recognizable in the healing stage with ectoderm closing over the raw stump or surfaces. At birth all that remain are traces of the process in the form of depressions, healed stumps or grooves. The occasional residual strands of the degenerated hyalinized tissue still adherent to the affected regions account completely for the older concept that the deformity was due to amniotic bands or adhesions.

The defects are most common in the subcutaneous connective tissue although they are seen frequently in all those of mesenchymal origin. When the defects are extensive, skin, muscle and bone are also involved. The character of the damage depends upon the extent as well as the location of the area involved. Accordingly, if all of the soft tissues of a finger or foot are concerned, that portion sloughs off, subsequently heals and the process is characterized as "amputation." On the other hand, if an annular zone of subcutaneous connective tissue is involved to such an extent that

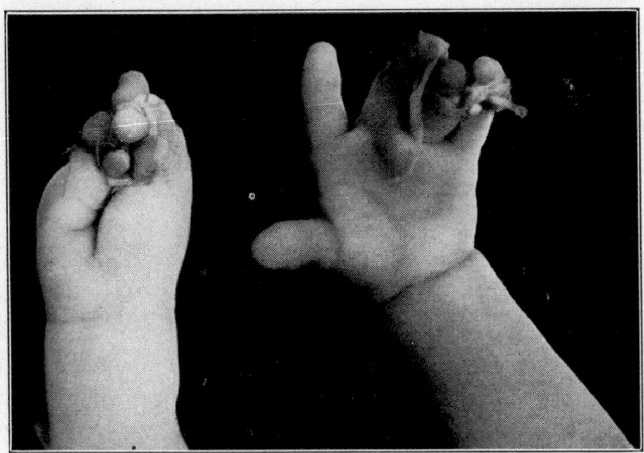

Fig. 338.—Hands of Sixteen Weeks' Fetus Showing Digits Entangled in Masses of Degenerate Fibrous Material. (So-called Amniotic Adhesions.)

Some of the digits are distorted and defective showing annular areas of necrosis which undoubtedly would have produced amputation had the fetus lived to term. (From Streeter, *Contributions to Embryology,* Carnegie Institution.)

the distal portions are deprived of nourishment, then that portion succumbs and is actually amputated. Frequently the annular areas are not of sufficient depth to bring about the foregoing result or even to disturb the circulation to any serious extent. Then the distal foot, hand or finger survives and evidence of the damage remains as a crease. When extensive, the crease may completely encircle the extremity while, if small, no mark may remain.

OTHER DISEASES OF THE AMNION

Inflammation of the Amnion. Occasionally inflammatory processes implicate the amnion. These are usually associated with similar changes in the chorion and decidua, and result from preexisting gonorrhea, from attempts at criminal abortion or from the extension of an intrapartum infection.

Cysts of the Amnion. Now and again small cystic structures, lined by typical epithelium, may be formed in the amnion. They generally result from the fusion of amniotic folds with subsequent retention of fluid.

Amniotic Caruncles. Under this name have been described certain nodules which occur upon the fetal surface of the placenta as well as upon the free amnion. Usually they appear in the neighborhood of the insertion of the cord as multiple, rounded or oval, opaque elevations, which vary from less than 1 to 5 or 6 mm. in diameter. Under the microscope they are seen to be made up of typical stratified epithelium. The lowest layer is cuboidal in shape and is continuous with the amniotic epithelium, while the upper layers become more and more flattened and stain less and less well as the surface is approached. Such structures were found by Solon B. Dodds in 60 per cent of a large series of placentas. As yet we are ignorant of their significance although in the ruminants, in which they are very abundant and attain considerable proportions, they contain large quantities of glycogen.

ABNORMALITIES OF THE PLACENTA

Abnormalities in Size, Shape, and Weight. The normal placenta is a flattened, roundish, or discoid organ, which averages from 15 to 20 cm. in diameter, and from 1.5 to 3 cm. in thickness. As compared with the fetus it is relatively larger in the earlier months of pregnancy rather than the later months, and varies considerably in size at term though, generally speaking, the thickness is in inverse proportion to its area. Now and again, when inserted in the neighborhood of the internal os, the placenta takes on a horseshoe-like appearance, its two branches running partially around the orifice.

The normal full term placenta on an average weighs about one-sixth as much as the child, that is, about 500 gm. In diseased conditions, on the other hand, this proportion no longer holds good, and in syphilis the placenta may weigh one-fourth, one-third, or even one-half as much as the fetus. The largest placentas usually encountered are observed in cases of erythroblastosis of the fetus and placenta. In one of Stander's cases of this character the fetus and placenta weighed 1,140 and 1,200 gm. respectively, and in another the placenta weighed over 2,000 gm. (See Fig. 527.)

Multiple Placentas in Single Pregnancies. Occasionally in a single pregnancy the placenta is divided into several parts which are absolutely distinct or closely united.

In rare instances the placenta is oblong with an aperture of varying size somewhere in the neighborhood of its center. To this abnormality Hyrtl applied the term *placenta fenestrata*. More frequently the organ is divided more or less into two lobes. When the division is incomplete and the vessels extend from one lobe to the other before uniting to form the umbilical cord, we speak of a *placenta dimidiata* or *bipartita*. Again, the two lobes may be quite separate, the vessels being perfectly distinct and not uniting until just before entering the cord. This is termed the *placenta duplex*. Occasionally the organ may be made up of three distinct lobes, otherwise called the *placenta triplex;* while in very rare instances it may consist of a number of small lobes, *placenta septuplex*. (Hyrtl has described as many as seven.)

All of these conditions result from abnormalities in the blood supply of the decidua. Generally speaking, the portion of the ovum which is to become converted into the chorion frondosum, and later into the fetal portion of the placenta, is that which is in contact with the most highly vascularized portion of the decidua. If the vascularization, instead of being practically limited to a single area, develops in several separate portions of the decidua, some such anomaly is bound to occur. Küstner believes that certain cases of placenta bipartita or duplex owe their origin to extensive infarct formation by which the intervening tissue is destroyed; but such an explanation cannot be accepted when the several lobules are separated from one another by apparently normal membranes.

Placenta Succenturiata. An important and not infrequent anomaly is the so-called *placenta succenturiata,* in which one or more small accessory lobules are developed in the membrane at some distance from the periphery of the main placenta. Ordinarily they are united to the latter by vascular connections; occasionally, however, these are lacking and as a result we have what are known as *placentae spuriae.*

The placenta succenturiata is of considerable clinical importance because the accessory lobules are sometimes retained in the uterus after the expulsion of the main

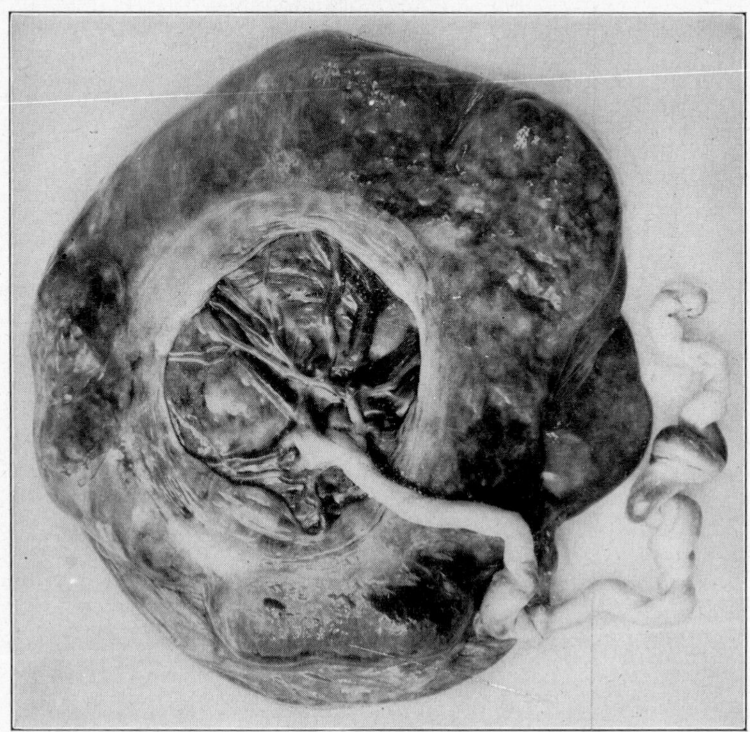

Fig. 339.—Placenta Circumvallata. × ½.

placenta and may give rise to serious hemorrhage. For this reason, one should always bear in mind the possibility of their existence and, in examining the after-birth, the membranes should be inspected as well as the placenta. Should small, roundish defects be present a short distance from the placental margin, the retention of a succenturiate lobe should be suspected. In fact this becomes a certainty if vessels extend from the placenta to the margins of the tear. In such cases, even if no hemorrhage occurs, the hand should be introduced into the uterus for the purpose of locating and removing the offending structure.

Placenta Membranacea. In rare instances the decidua capsularis is so abundantly supplied with blood that the chorion laeve in contact with it fails to undergo atrophy. In such circumstances, the entire periphery of the ovum is covered by functioning villi so that the placenta, instead of being a discoidal organ limited to the decidua basalis, is a thin membranous structure occupying the entire periphery of the chorion —*placenta membranacea.* This abnormality does not interfere with the nutrition of the ovum, but occasionally gives rise to serious complications during the third stage of labor, involving profuse hemorrhaging since the thinned-out placenta does not readily separate from its area of attachment. This necessitates manual removal which is sometimes very difficult.

Placenta Circumvallata. In exceptional instances the fetal surface of the placenta presents a central depression surrounded by a thickened, whitish ring, which is situated at a varying distance from the margin of the organ. According as the ring is

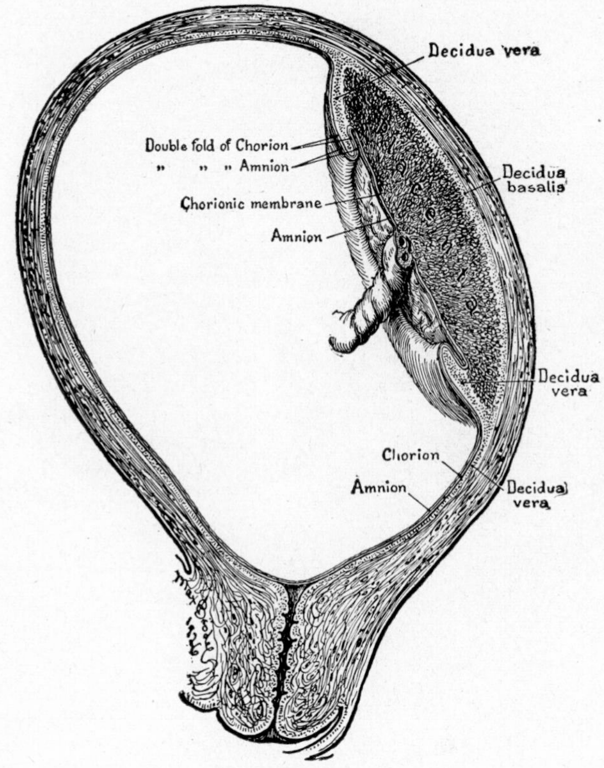

Fig. 340.—Diagram Showing Circumvallate Placenta in Situ.
Note relations of chorionic membrane, extrachorionic decidua and duplication of membranes.

complete or incomplete, we have to do with a complete or incomplete circumvallate placenta. When the ring coincides with the placental margin, the condition is sometimes described as a placenta marginata. Within the ring, the fetal surface presents the usual appearance, gives attachment to the umbilical cord, and shows the usual large vessels. These, however, instead of coursing over the entire fetal surface, terminate abruptly at the margin of the ring. The ring itself is composed of a double layer of amnion and chorionic membrane, which has undergone infarction; while the surface of the placenta outside of it is covered by a layer of decidua, which in turn is covered by the deflected membranes on their way to line the interior of the uterine cavity. Figure 340 gives a good idea of these relations.

Placenta circumvallata appears to be due to the fact that a smaller part than usual of the periphery of the early ovum becomes converted into the chorion frondosum, with the result that the chorionic plate of the placenta is so small that further growth of the organ can be effected only by the proliferating villi invading the surrounding decidua. As the resulting extrachorionic, or subdecidual, portion of the placenta develops, it becomes covered by the fetal membranes after they have become folded at the margins of the chorionic plate. Various writers hold the condition responsible for all kinds of clinical manifestations, but in our experience it has very slight, if any, effect upon the course of pregnancy or labor. Consequently it should be regarded solely as an interesting abnormality, the production of which could not be explained satisfactorily until our ideas concerning the development and growth of the placenta had attained a certain degree of finality. Hobbs and Price, studying 150 cases of placenta circumvallata, found an increased incidence of abortion associated with this condition.

Placenta Previa. Once in several hundred cases the placenta, instead of being inserted upon the anterior or posterior wall or the fundus of the uterus, is implanted upon the lower uterine segment in such a manner as to overlap more or less completely the internal os. As this condition, known as *placenta previa,* is unavoidably associated with hemorrhage during the first stage of labor and is a most serious complication, it will be dealt with in a separate section.

DISEASES OF THE PLACENTA

The most frequent abnormalities of the placenta are a group of lesions which, though of diverse origins, unfortunately have come to be included in the common term, "placental infarcts." This fallacy has led to a maze of misconception concerning their formation and significance to such an extent that no further purpose can possibly be attained by continuing its use. For this reason we shall speak of etiologic factors and pathologic processes in the hope that nomenclature may adjust itself with sufficient clarity.

There is a considerable group of changes in the placenta which may be considered as physiologic inasmuch as they are by-products of its usual mode of development, growth and senescence but which often have pathologic significance. It may be well to enumerate them as they arise in different locations.

About the edge of nearly every term placenta there is a more or less dense yellowish-white fibrous ring which represents a zone of degeneration which is usually termed a "marginal infarct." It may be quite superficial in places, but occasionally extends a centimeter or two into the substance of the placenta. Likewise underneath the covering plate, careful observation of a cross section nearly always reveals similar processes more or less pyramidal in shape, ranging from 0.2 cm. to 2 or even 3 cm. across the base, extending downward, with their apices in the intervillous spaces (subchorionic infarcts). Not infrequently also one can demonstrate proliferations of a similar sort about the intercotyledonous septa. In this case the broadest portion rests upon the maternal surface and the apex points toward the covering plate. Occasionally these degenerative processes may meet and form a column of cartilage-like material extending from the maternal to the fetal surfaces. In addition there are found isolated round or oval islands of this same sort of tissue occupying the central portions of the placenta but these are somewhat less frequently seen. Collectively these degenerative growths have been termed "white infarcts" by many writers. But as a matter of fact this term has come to include any similar white body found in the placenta whether of the same origin or not. So the term is meaningless and should be discarded. Fibrinoid degeneration would be a more suitable term for this particular process. These lesions have a similar origin in that they are produced by the degeneration of trophoblastic remnants. These remnants represent, for the most part, a surplus of chorionic epithelium which is not utilized during the growth of the placenta in the process of lining the villi, the covering plate and the maternal tissues, but they may

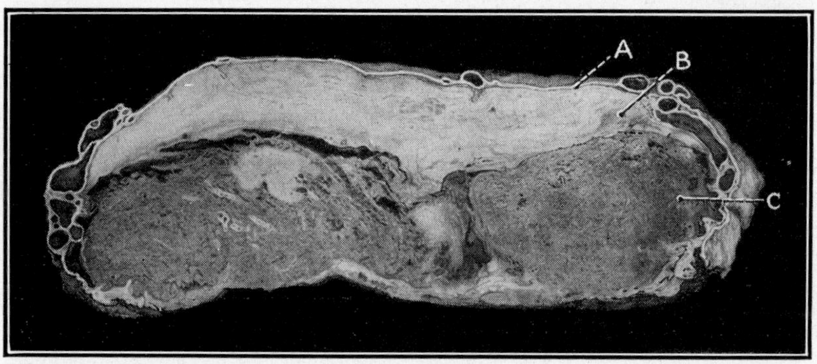

FIG. 341.—DEGENERATION OF THE PLACENTA. × ⅔.

A, amnion and chorionic membrane; *B*, fibrinoid degeneration localized beneath the chorionic plate; *C*, unchanged placental tissue. (In this instance the infarct was unusually extensive and led to the death of the fetus.)

form from the degeneration of the differentiated syncytium. In early placentas they may be identified as islands or knots of trophoblast and are located principally on the maternal side of the chorion plate, over the decidua, particularly in the vicinity of septa and at the margins of the placenta. Small patches may be observed about the tips of growing villi. Later on they will have proliferated to form a larger mass of large pale staining cells, while those about the periphery will show marked signs

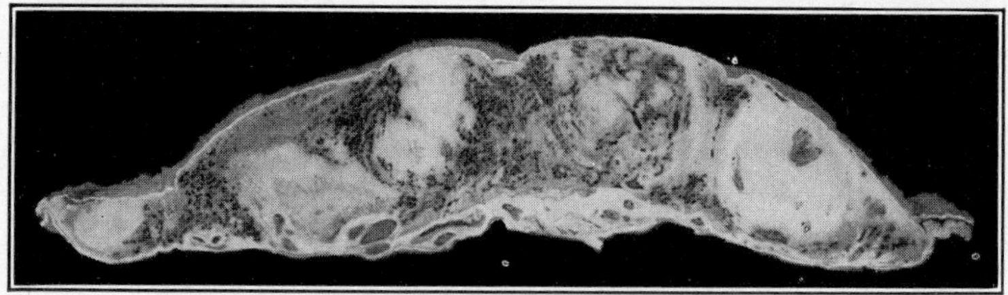

FIG. 342.—DEGENERATION OF THE PLACENTA. × ⅔.

Generalized fibrinoid involvement with little remaining normal tissue.

of degeneration. At term, practically all cells are dead, most of the material hyalinized, and the remaining structure arranged in a manner suggestive of, but not identical to, organized blood fibrin. For this reason they have been termed "fibrinoid" or more correctly "fibrinoid degenerations."

The degeneration of these cells is but a part of the picture of degeneration that is characteristic of every normal placenta. The chorion, including the mesodermal and the epithelial portions, has a definite life cycle which has a temporal duration similar to the duration of pregnancy. The placenta is presumably in active growth only during the first seven months of pregnancy. Thereafter it is senescent and at term quite senile. Therefore, these surplus islands of trophoblastic tissue merely reflect the characteristic life span of human chorionic tissue with the exception that they must depend upon the intervillous maternal blood for nourishment since they have no organized vascular system. Inasmuch as they form a considerable mass of cells, this circulation proves inadequate and degeneration commences earlier and progresses more rapidly than in other parts of the placenta where there is an adequate vascular

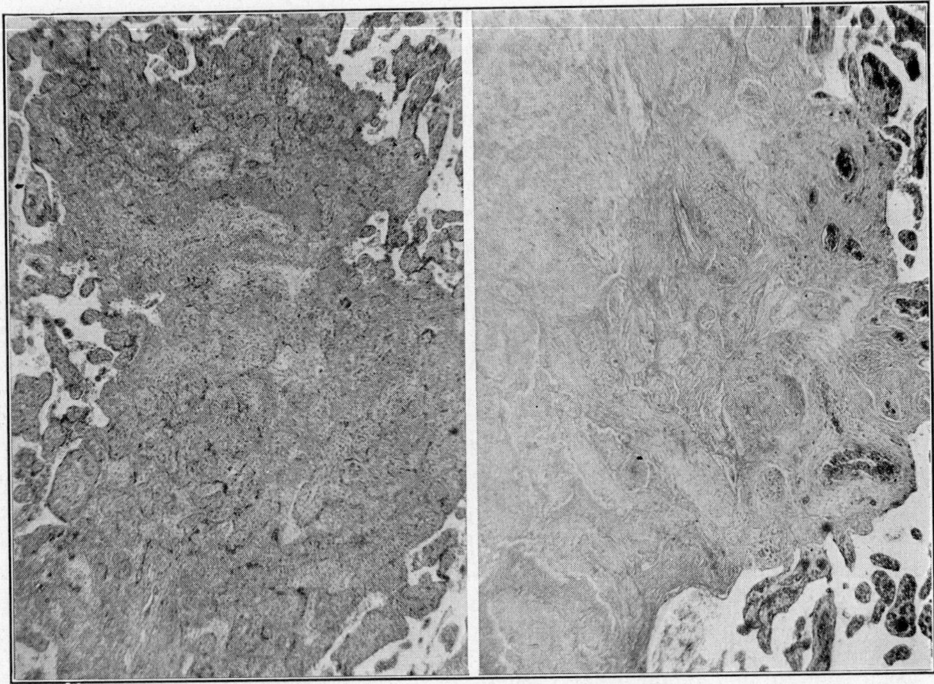

FIG. 343.—HEMOVILLOUS DEGENERATION OF PLACENTA. × 45.

FIG. 344.—FIBRINOID DEGENERATION OF PLACENTA. × 45.

system. Minute subchorionic and marginal areas of degeneration are present in every placenta. Williams found similar areas measuring 1 cm. in diameter in 63 per cent of 500 consecutive placentas. These lesions are of clinical significance only when they are of large size and abundant, in which case they may, by mechanical means, throw out of function so great a portion of the placenta as to seriously interfere with the nutrition of the fetus, and sometimes in rare instances cause its death.

In keeping with the senescent changes occurring in every placenta, the oxygen consumption of this organ, as recently reported by Wang and Hellman, decreases gradually with the advancement of pregnancy.

There is a different type of lesion which has also been termed a "white infarct" in its older forms, while in its earlier stages it has been termed a "red infarct." It is formed as a result of the senescence of the syncytium. During the latter half of pregnancy when the syncytium commences to degenerate, it is thrown up into many layers of cells which are known as syncytial knots; at the same time the villous connective tissue beneath them usually shows evidences of hyalinization. The syncytium then breaks away or floats off and the connective tissue beneath is exposed directly to maternal blood. As a result clotting occurs and thus is started a process which may propagate itself over a considerable space, incorporating into its substance other villi as it grows. In the gross, a section through such an area appears quite like an organized red blood clot but if not seen until it has become thoroughly organized, a section through it will reveal a firm white island of tissue which to the unaided eye is similar to that seen in fibrinoid degeneration. However, under the microscope the difference is at once apparent for in this hemovillous degeneration true organized fibrin is seen enmeshing many villi. In the central or older portions the villi may have been so completely hyalinized that they can be recognized as such only with difficulty, whereas, at the edges the villous elements will be seen in a much better state of preservation.

Placental Changes Resulting from the Type of Maternal Blood Supply. Much light has been thrown upon the degenerative phenomena of the placenta through Grosser's studies upon its biologic development. As a result of his work it seems likely that the placenta, in a manner similar to other organs of the human body, has been undergoing a process of evolution. It also seems probable that some of its present characteristics are the result of orthogenetic influences, by which is meant that some of the evolutionary trends have gained sufficient momentum so that they continue to develop in a given direction even though it is deleterious or somewhat harmful to the race.

The hemochorial placenta of man and the primates is a simplified type of organ as compared to the placentas of other viviparae, whereas that of many of the monkeys occupies an intermediate position. Grosser has presented evidence which indicates that the human placenta has evolved into its present simple form from more complicated ones. These more complex organs are different, chiefly, with respect to the manner in which respiratory gases and simple sugars and salts are transmitted on the one hand, and in which larger molecules such as colloids and proteins are prepared for transmission on the other. As an example, the endotheliochorial placenta of carnivora has a separate and supplementary arrangement for splitting proteins to amino acids and for absorbing these simplified products through a membrane into the nutrient vessels of the fetus. It has at the same time a labyrinth similar to the human placenta for the rapid exchange of the simpler substances. The reason apparently for this double type of placenta is that the splitting of proteins and similar substances by enzymes is a slow process, whereas the mere passage of gases and salts through a membrane by diffusion and osmosis is relatively rapid.

When, therefore, in the process of evolution these two types of activity combined in the hemochorial placenta with a common cavity, definite modifications were also necessary with regard to the time relationships of the processes involved. In the human this has taken the form of a retardation of the rate of flow of the maternal blood through the intervillous spaces. This stagnation, for it practically amounts to that, is an advantage in that it allows time for enzymatic digestive activities, but it is also a distinct disadvantage because it tends to promote the clotting of blood within the placenta, and progressive degenerative changes in the trophoblastic elements with the formation of fibrinoid degeneration and hemovillous degeneration, all of which augment a vicious cycle in further retarding the maternal blood flow.

It has been suggested that the digestion of the maternal proteins and their decomposition may be carried too far so that albuminoid substances may re-enter the maternal blood stream and lead to undesirable results such as the so-called toxemias of pregnancy. As stated earlier, such a view is without foundation at the present time.

Pathologic Conditions Resulting from Accidents to the Maternal Vessels. The arteries and veins of the decidua basalis have extraordinarily thin walls composed of endothelium and a scant layer of connective tissue so that they not infrequently suffer damage. This damage is usually a tear or rupture which is followed by extravasation of blood into the decidua forming a hematoma. We speak of them, therefore, as retroplacental hematomas. When they are small in amount, they serve to detach a small area of the placenta from the uterine wall and so do little harm to the fetus. By examining the maternal surface of the placenta, they may not infrequently be recognized as a depressed area which sometimes contains a bolus of clotted blood. If they have existed for a considerable time before delivery of the placenta there is usually, in addition to the above, an extensive area of fibrinoid or hemovillous degeneration extending up into the substance of the placenta.

When, however, the blood loss is extensive and its accumulation in the decidua basalis causes a larger detachment of the placenta, we term the process taking place, *abruptio placentae*. Of this more will be said in another section. It is mentioned here because the processes are similar in many respects. To account for the rupture of decidual vessels many theories have been advanced. Montgomery speaks of the trauma of fetal movements, others have stressed the effect of toxins circulating in the maternal blood with a degenerative effect on the endothelium, and James Young emphasizes the importance of thrombosis of maternal veins with resultant back pressure upon the thin arterial walls which they are not adapted to withstand. The fact is, we do not know the ultimate causes, but from the clinical point of view it is important to note that many of these retroplacental accidents occur in women suffering with elevated blood pressure associated with preeclampsia or nephritis.

Pathologic Conditions Resulting from Accidents or Changes in the Fetal Vessels. Ackermann was the first to call attention to "endarteritis" of the fetal vessels of the placenta. Eden, Williams and many others confirmed his findings and for a time at least considered that this process was responsible for more or less occlusion of the large vessels of the covering plate and of the larger trunk villi, which, in turn, produced an ischemia followed by degeneration of the villi, fibrin proliferation and "infarct formation." This point of view is no longer generally accepted for two reasons. In the first place, this proliferation of the medial wall with occlusion of fetal vessels is commonly seen without the formation of any form of pathologic process other than hyalinization of the villous connective tissue; and, in the second, many placentas are seen in which extensive fibrinoid and hemovillous degeneration has built up a widespread process in the placental spaces without the least sign of reduced caliber being demonstrable in the chorionic blood supply.

That occlusion of the fetal vessels does occur is well known but it seems to be due to the general senility so characteristic of chorionic tissue near term. There is every reason to believe that the villi receive their nourishment from the maternal blood stream and are thus little influenced by processes which occlude their own vascular system. In advanced syphilis of the placenta all, or nearly all, of the villous vessels have undergone extensive obliteration and yet the connective tissue and epithelium survive in a state of good preservation until the villi are so overgrown that there is insufficient circulation of maternal blood to supply them with the required nourishment.

Occasionally placentas are seen in which there has been a rupture of the large fetal vessels coursing beneath the amnion on the inner aspect of the placenta. This is associated with subamniotic hematoma formation which seldom reaches large dimensions but becomes organized and forms a small tumor.

Bartholomew and Kracke used their theory of traumatic injury to the large fetal vessels to account not only for infarct formation but also for the production of some of the toxemias of pregnancy. Bartholomew and Colvin have recently suggested that the hypercholesteremia of pregnancy is associated with the vascular changes in the placental arteries resulting in infarction. While ingenious, their hypothesis is not particularly convincing for, with the possible exception of essential hypertension, we do not find "infarction" of the placenta as a predominant characteristic of the toxemias. Indeed, in preeclampsia and eclampsia these forms of degeneration are seldom seen.

Clinical Significance of the Various Forms of Degeneration in the Placenta. There is little clinical importance to be ascribed to the so-called "infarcts of the placenta." In the past many attempts have been made to establish some association between these lesions and the clinical course of the patient. With the exception of chronic nephritis there has been no agreement among authors either as to what effect these lesions produced in the mother and fetus or as to the mode of their development. There are two fundamental reasons for this failure. On the one hand, the placenta is endowed with such an ample margin of physiologic capacity that it can withstand destruction of at least one-half its substance and still support the life of the fetus. On the other hand, as we have attempted to show, most of these lesions are the result of a long-standing evolutionary process and while nature has seemed to have encumbered the human placenta to its detriment, at the same time it has probably endowed the woman with mechanisms to overcome the handicap, which she does satisfactorily unless her kidneys are embarrassed by chronic disease.

Cysts of the Placenta. Cystic structures are frequently observed upon the fetal surface and occasionally in the depths of the placenta. Small cysts a few millimeters in diameter were noted in 56 per cent of the placentas studied by Kermauner. Larger ones, occasionally attaining the size of a lemon, are observed but rarely. In one of Williams' specimens five cysts varying from 3 to 5 cm. in diameter projected from the fetal surface of the placenta.

Such cysts are derived from the chorionic membrane, as is shown by the fact that the amnion can be readily stripped off from them. Their contents are usually clear and transparent, but sometimes are bloody or grumous. The walls, especially the portions adjacent to the intervillous spaces, are lined in great part by a dull whitish membrane, while occasionally a portion is occupied by an area of fibrinoid degeneration.

On microscopic examination the lining membrane is found to be made up of one or more layers of relatively large epithelial cells with round vesicular nuclei, which frequently present various degrees of degeneration. Here and there, depending upon the degree of organization, the cells are absent and the wall consists of fibrinoid materials. It is generally believed that the cells in question are trophoblastic in origin, and that the cysts result from their degeneration.

The cysts occurring in the depths of the placenta rarely exceed 1 cm. in diameter.

They frequently occupy the center of an area of degeneration, are filled with grumous contents, and were mistaken by the older writers for abscesses. In other cases the contents are clear, and in this event the walls of the cysts are lined by cells identical with those composing the trophoblastic or "decidual" septa of the placenta; the fluid contents are clearly derived from their degeneration.

So far as present experience goes, cystic formations, whether occurring upon the fetal surface or in the depths of the placenta, are of interest purely from a pathologic point of view and exert little or no influence upon the course of pregnancy or labor.

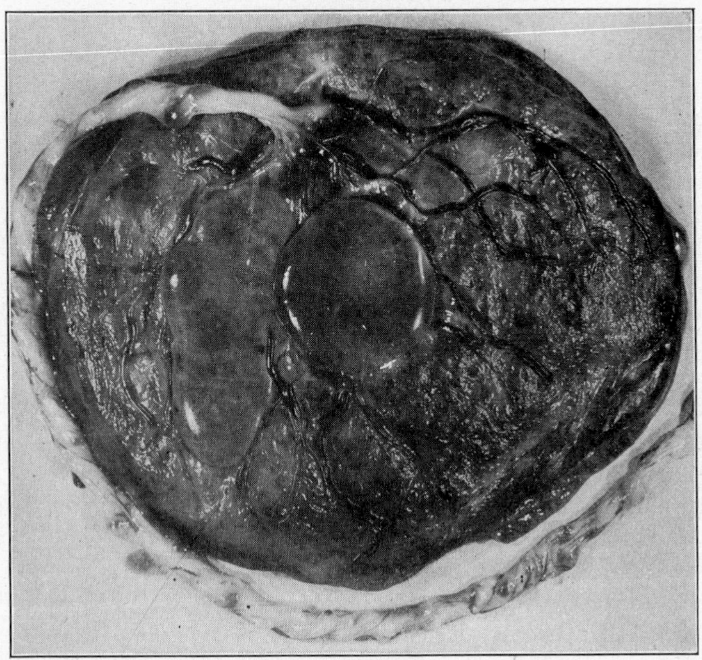

Fig. 345.—Chorionic Cyst of Placenta.

Tumors of the Placenta. John Clarke in 1798 described a solid tumor about the size of a man's fist which made up a large part of the placenta. In recent years a number of tumors varying in size from that of a pea to that of a man's fist have been described. In our experience careful routine examination shows that such tumors, from the size of a small pea upward, occur about once in every 3,500 placentas.

The work of all recent investigators, which has been well summarized by Marchetti, shows that they are practically all of one origin, and because of the resemblance of the components of the tumors to the blood vessels and stroma of the normally developing chorionic villus, the term chorio-angioma appears to be the best suited designation.

Various theories have been advanced as to their mode of origin, but none of them appears to be satisfactory. According to the most generally accepted theory, groups of blood vessels and stroma originating in the chorionic mesenchyme proliferate and grow outside of the regular arrangement of the normally developing chorionic villi.

Marchetti collected 209 cases of chorio-angioma from the literature up to 1939 and reported eight additional cases which had occurred in the New York Hospital. From a microscopic study of these eight cases he was able to differentiate three types, the most common being the vascular or mature type characterized by a loose groundwork of chorionic cells supporting many small blood vessels and capillaries which are usually dilated and filled with red blood corpuscles. The other two types are the immature or cellular, and the degenerative.

As the chorio-angiomata do not affect the surrounding placental tissue, they do no harm unless they involve so considerable an area as to throw a large part of the placenta out of function. As an interesting curiosity, Emge's case is mentioned, in which a pedunculated hemangiomatous tumor offered mechanical obstacle to the descent of the head, which could not be delivered until the tumor had been pushed up above it.

Inflammation of the Placenta. Under the term placentitis many of the older writers described changes which we now recognize as various forms of degeneration. Moreover, as has already been said, small placental cysts filled with grumous contents were formerly thought to be abscesses. Hence it follows that most of the statements in the abundant early literature upon inflammatory lesions of the placenta must be received with the greatest caution. At the same time acute inflammation of the placenta is occasionally encountered. It is not a primary condition but is usually due to the extension of a similar process from the decidua, resulting from an exacerbation of a pre-existing chronic gonorrhea, or from an acute infection due to pyogenic bacteria. Sometimes abscess formation may be a manifestation of a general infection originating in any portion of the body.

In cases of prolonged labor, as will be elaborated in a later section, Slemons has shown that as the result of intrapartum infection pyogenic bacteria may invade the fetal surface of the placenta and, after gaining access to the chorionic vessels, give rise to general infection of the fetus.

Frequently upon examining sections of placental tissue under the microscope, we have found the decidua basalis and the inferior surface of the chorionic covering plate infiltrated with leukocytes presenting the characteristic picture of an acute inflammation, while the adjacent intervillous spaces are crowded with leukocytes.

Tuberculosis of the Placenta. Tubercle formation in the fetal portion of the placenta is extremely infrequent. Whitman and Greene in 1922 collected 44 cases from the literature. Schaeffer in 1939 reported that in 150 consecutive placentas of tuberculous women he was able to find only one with tuberculous lesions and acid-fast bacilli present.

Calcification of the Placenta. Small calcareous nodules, sometimes occurring in the form of flat plaques, are frequently observed upon the maternal surface of the placenta, and are occasionally so abundant as to give to the finger the same sensation as when feeling a piece of coarse sandpaper. Schönig showed that the chalky material was usually deposited in the necrotic tissue surrounding the ends of the "fastening" villi, as well as in the superficial layers of the decidua basalis.

When the widely spread occurrence of degenerative changes in the placenta is remembered, it should be a matter of surprise not that calcification occasionally occurs, but rather that it is not encountered in almost every placenta, inasmuch as apparently ideal conditions for its formation are constantly present in the later months of pregnancy. Fleming, in a recent x-ray study of the placenta, observed a moderate degree of calcification in about half of his cases.

Variations in Insertion. The umbilical cord is usually inserted eccentrically upon the fetal surface of the placenta somewhere between its center and periphery. A central insertion is less common, while in a still smaller number of cases the junction has taken place near the margin giving rise to a condition known as *battledore placenta.* In a series of 2,000 placentas which were studied in this regard the insertion was eccentric in 73 per cent, central in 18 per cent, and marginal in 7 per cent. These variations possess no clinical significance. On the other hand, the so-called *velamentous insertion of the cord,* or *insertio velamentosa,* is of considerable practical importance. In this condition the vessels of the cord separate some distance from the placental margin and make their way to the latter in a fold of amnion. This mode of insertion

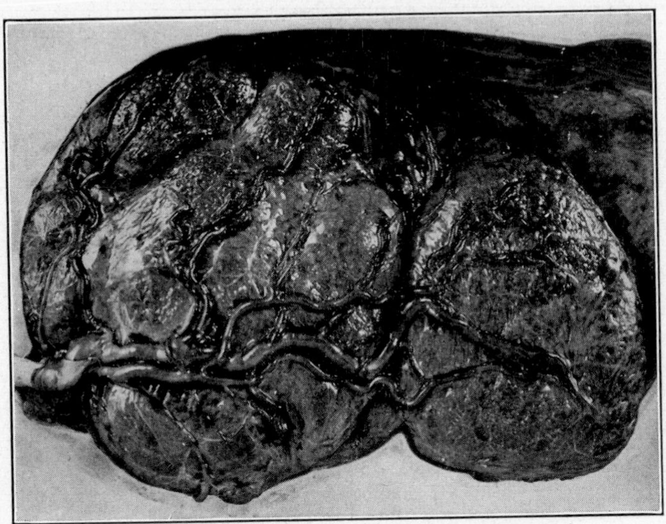

FIG. 346.—MARGINAL INSERTION OF CORD, BATTLEDORE PLACENTA, SUCCENTURIATE LOBE.

was noted in 0.84 per cent of 15,891 placentas examined by Lefèvre, and in 1.25 per cent of our cases. It has been stated that it occurs nine times more frequently in twin than in single pregnancies, being noted in 5 and 0.57 per cent of the cases respectively. (See Figs. 347 and 348.)

According to Franqué, the abdominal pedicle ordinarily extends to the fetus from that portion of the chorion which is in contact with the most richly vascularized portion of the decidua, usually the decidua basalis, so that the cord becomes inserted upon the placenta. Occasionally, however, during the first few days of pregnancy, the area of greatest vascularization may be in the decidua capsularis, and in such circumstances the abdominal pedicle originates at that location. With the advance of pregnancy, however, the area of vascularization eventually shifts to the decidua basalis, the site of the future placenta, while the abdominal pedicle retains its original position, and from its maternal end the vessels extend to the placental margin.

When the placenta is inserted low down in the uterus, the velamentous vessels may extend partially across the internal os—*vasa praevia*—and as dilatation progresses may be pressed upon by the presenting part, the interference with the circulation causing asphyxia of the fetus. In rare cases such vessels are torn through when the membranes rupture, and the fetus bleeds to death.

Figure 348 represents an unusual case of vasa praevia. In this instance the umbilical cord arose from the most dependent portion of the membranes instead of from the fetal surface of the placenta. Rupture of the membrane and escape of the child occurred in the V-shaped space between the vessels at the lower right side of the specimen, but did not involve them.

Variations in Length of Cord. Normally the umbilical cord averages about 55 cm. in length, though it may present marked variations from 0.5 to 198 cm. In rare instances it may be so short that the abdomen of the fetus is in contact with the placenta, but under such circumstances a congenital umbilical hernia is always present.

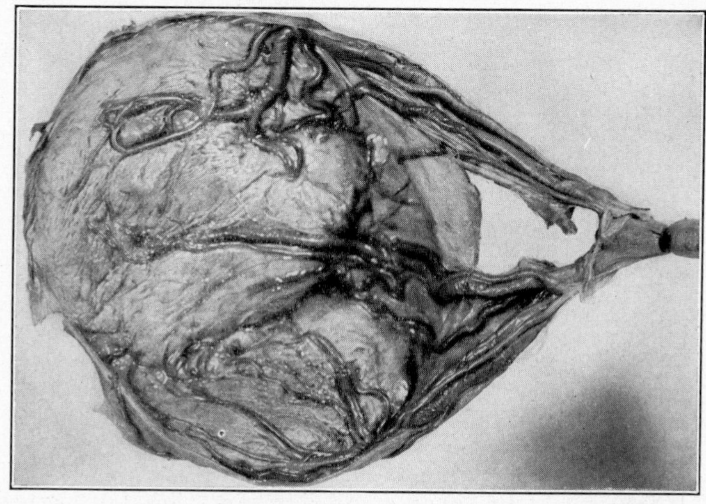

Fig. 347.—Velamentous Insertion of Cord.

It would seem obvious that the cord must be a certain length in order to permit delivery of the child; that is, it must be sufficiently long to reach from its placental insertion to the vulva, 35 cm. when the placenta is inserted high up, and 20 cm. when low down. Gardiner places the limit at 32 cm. On the other hand, it sometimes happens that cords which exceed the normal length may be so twisted about the child as to become practically too short. When a coil encircles the neck, Gardiner estimates that the cord must measure 76 to 101 cm. in length in vertex and breech presentations, respectively, if it is not to exert traction upon the placenta. Accordingly, one distinguishes between absolute and relative shortness of the cord. Either of these conditions may give rise to dystocia. Brickner states that delivery cannot occur under such circumstances unless one of the following accidents occurs: separation of the placenta, inversion of the uterus, umbilical hernia of the fetus, or rupture of the cord, the last two being of infrequent occurrence.

Rupture of the Cord may result from absolute or accidental shortness, being due to the former in Dyhrenfurth's case and to the latter in Ahlfeld's case, in which the cord measured 44 cm., but was tightly twisted about the fetus. Ordinarily an excessively long cord exerts no deleterious influence, although it predisposes to the formation of loops during pregnancy and to prolapse at the time of labor.

Knots of the Cord. It is customary to distinguish between false and true knots, the former being due to developmental anomalies in the cord, while the latter result from the active movements of the child. True knots occur very infrequently and occasionally are of the most complicated character. Ordinarily they are of no clinical importance, but occasionally they may be pulled so taut as to compress the vessels and lead to asphyxia of the fetus.

Loops of Cord. The cord frequently becomes wrapped around portions of the fetus, and in every third or fourth case of labor the child's neck will be found loosely encircled by one or more loops. In rare instances these may produce strangulation. Most of these accidents are not due to any drawing taut of the loop, but rather to the fact that it does not become looser in proportion as the neck of the child increases in size. In other cases loops of the cord may so tightly encircle the body or one of the extremities of the child as to give rise to deep depressions, which in extreme cases may eventuate in the strangulation or gangrene of the affected part.

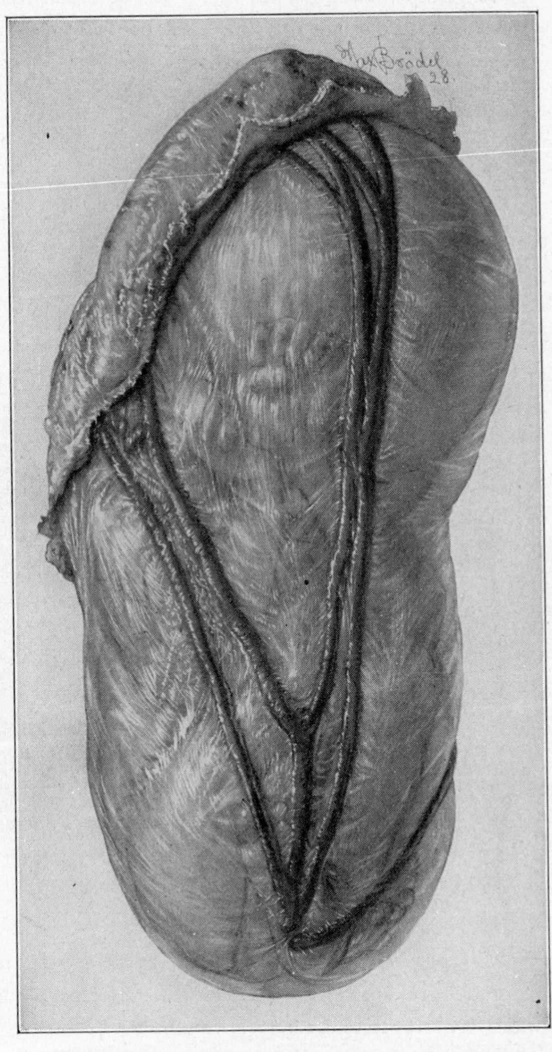

FIG. 348.—VASA PRAEVIA WITH BREECH PRESENTATION. $\times \frac{1}{3}$.

Note that cord arises from lowermost portion of fetal membranes.

In single-ovum twins in which the amniotic partition wall has already been broken through, it sometimes happens that the cord of one fetus may become wrapped around some portion of the other so tightly as to cause its death. A number of cases of this character have been collected by Hermann.

Torsion of the Cord. As the result of movements on the part of the fetus, the cord may become more or less twisted. Occasionally the torsion is so marked as to interfere seriously with the circulation. The most extreme degrees occur only after the death of the fetus. In rare instances separation of the cord is produced, though this is possible only after fetal death early in pregnancy.

Inflammation of the Cord. As long as the child is alive inflammatory conditions are rarely noted, but after its death the whartonian jelly may be found infiltrated with leukocytes. Obliterative changes may occur in the vessels, the lumens becoming almost completely occluded, with leukocytic infiltration of the spaces between the muscle fibers in the adventitia as well as in the adjacent whartonian jelly. Such changes may be due to syphilis; but this is by no means always the case, as Siddall was able to demonstrate their presence in 60 out of 1,000 cords from the children of women who presented no evidence of the existence of that disease. Furthermore, as most of the cases occurred when the labor was prolonged or complicated by premature rupture of the membranes or by intrapartum infection, he held that the condition was due to pyogenic bacteria.

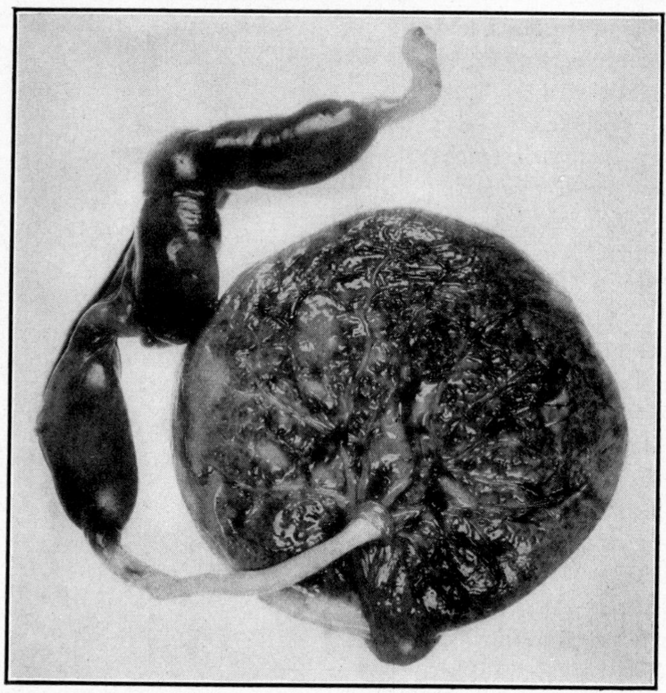

FIG. 349.—HEMATOMA OF THE UMBILICAL CORD.

Varices of the Cord. In rare instances varices of the cord may rupture as the result of undue pressure. Meier has reported a case in which the death of the fetus was attributable to such an accident.

Tumors of the Cord. Tumor formations implicating the cord are rarely seen. Hematomas occasionally result from the rupture of a varix with subsequent effusion of blood into the cord. In one instance we observed such a tumor, 5 cm. in diameter, at the fetal end of the cord. Dippel found hematoma of the cord to occur once in every 5,505 deliveries at or near term, and states that the hemorrhage usually comes from rupture of the wall of the umbilical vein. He observed that about one half of all fetuses with hematoma of the cord are stillborn. Myxomata and myxosarcomata have also been described. Winckel has reported two cases of sarcoma of the cord, while Budin has described a typical dermoid. The cases of Meyer and Haendly were of peculiar interest. In both instances a typical teratoma the size of a child's head, containing derivatives of all three germ layers, originated from the cord 10 cm. beyond its fetal insertion.

Cystic structures occasionally occur in the course of the cord and are designated as true and false cysts respectively according to their mode of origin. The former are always quite small and, according to Kleinwächter, may be derived from remnants of the umbilical stalk or of the allantois, while the latter may attain a considerable size and result from liquefaction of the whartonian jelly. As a rule such cysts are only apparent and result from the liquefaction of the myxomatous tissue of the cord.

Edema of the Cord. This condition is rarely noted by itself, but is frequently associated with edematous conditions of the fetus. It is very common in dead and macerated children. In one of our cases, in which the child was born alive at full term, the cord was 3 cm. in diameter. Microscopic examination showed that the condition was simply due to an increase in the amount of whartonian jelly.

BIBLIOGRAPHY

Abrams, A. A., and Abrams, S. B. Successful Treatment of Hydramnios with Ammonium Chloride. Am. J. Obst. & Gynec., 1946, 52:299.

Ackermann. Der weisse Infarct der Placenta. Arch. f. path. Anat., 1884, 96:439.

Acosta-Sison, H., and Espaniola, N. A. Clinicopathologic Study from Thirty-two Cases of Chorioepithelioma. Am. J. Obst. & Gynec., 1941, 42:878.

Ahlfeld, F. Die Verwachsungen des Amnion mit der Oberfläche der Frucht. Ber. u. Arbeiten, 1887, Bd. III, ff. 158.

——— Zerreissung der Nabelschnur eines reifen Kindes während der Geburt. Ztschr. f. Geburtsh. u. Gynäk., Stuttg., 1897, 36:467.

Anspach, B. M., and Hoffman, J. Perforating Chorionepithelioma of the Uterus with Free Intraperitoneal Hemorrhage. Am. J. Obst. & Gynec., 1931, 22:239.

Bartholomew, R. A. Pathology of the Placenta. With Special Reference to Infarcts and Their Relation to Toxemia of Pregnancy. J.A.M.A., 1938, 111:2276.

Bartholomew, R. A., and Colvin, E. D. Diagnosis of the Occurrence of Toxemia of Pregnancy by Examination of the Unknown Placenta. Am. J. Obst. & Gynec., 1938, 36:909.

Bartholomew, R. A., and Kracke, R. R. The Relation of Placenta Infarcts to Eclamptic Toxemia. Am. J. Obst. & Gynec., 1932, 24:797.

Brews, A. Hydatidiform Mole and Chorionepithelioma. J. Obst. & Gynaec. Brit. Emp., 1939, 46:813.

Brickner, S. M. A New Symptom in the Diagnosis of Dystocia Due to a Short Umbilical Cord. Am. J. Obst., 1902, 45:512.

Dietrich, H. A. Anatomie und Physiologie des Fetus und Biologie der Placenta Halban-Seitz. Biologie und Pathologie des Weibes, 1925, 6:163.

Dippel, A. L. Hematomas of the Umbilical Cord. Surg., Gynec. & Obst., 1940, 70:51.

Dyhrenfurth, O. Inversio Uteri Bedingt Durch zu Kurzen Nabelstrang. Zentralbl. f. Gynäk., 9:801, 804.

Eden, T. W. A Study of the Human Placenta. J. Path. & Bac., 1897, 8:265.

Emge, L. A. Dystocia Caused by an Hemangioma of the Placenta. Am. J. Obst. & Gynec., 1927, 14:35.

Fleming, A. M. Clinical Significance of the Degree of Calcification of the Placenta as Demonstrated by X-ray Photography. J. Obst. & Gynaec. Brit. Emp., 1943, 50:135.

Forssell, O. H. Zur Kenntnis des Amnionepithels in normalem und pathologischem Zustande. Arch. f. Gynäk., 1912, 96:436.

Franqué. Anat. und klin. Beobachtungen über Placentarerkrankungen. Ztschr. f. Geburtsh. u. Gynäk., 1894, 28:293.

Gardiner, J. P. The Umbilical Cord. Normal Length; Length in Cord Complications; Etiology and Frequency of Coiling. Surg., Gynec. & Obst., 1922, 34:252.

Goodall, J. R. Circumcrescent and Circumvallate Placentas. Am. J. Obst. & Gynec., 1934, 28:707.

——— Morgan, G., and Power, R. H. A Study of a Cause of Hydramnios. Am. J. Obst. & Gynec., 1939, 38:494.

Grosser, O. Frühentwicklung, Eihautbildung und Placentation des Menschen und der Säugetiere. München, 1927.

——— Human and Comparative Placentation, Lancet, 1933, 1:199.

GUTTMACHER, A. F. An Analysis of 521 Cases of Twin Pregnancy. I. Differences in Single and Double Twinning. Am. J. Obst. & Gynec., 1937, 34:76.

——— An Analysis of 573 Cases of Twin Pregnancy. II. The Hazards of Pregnancy Itself. Am. J. Obst. & Gynec., 1939, 38:277.

HASHIMOTO. See SCHULZE reference.

HERMANN, A. Ueber Verschlingung der Nabelschnüre bei Zwillingen. Arch. f. Gynäk., 1891, 40:253.

HERTIG, A. T., and EDMONDS, H. W. Genesis of Hydatidiform Mole. Arch. Path., 1940, 30:260.

——— and SHELDON, W. H. Hydatidiform Mole—A Pathologico-Clinical Correlation of 200 Cases. Am. J. Obst. & Gynec., 1947, 53:1.

HOBBS, J. E., and PRICE, C. N. Placenta Circumvallata. Am. J. Obst. & Gynec., 1940, 39:39.

HYRTL. Die Blutgefässe der menschlichen Nachgeburt. Wien, 1870.

KERMAUNER, F. Zur Lehre von der Entwickelung der Cysten u. der Infarcte in der menschlichen Placenta. Ztschr. f. Heilk., 1900, 21:1.

KLEIN, P. Das Chorionepithelioma malignum der Tube nach Extrauteringravidität. Arch. f. Gynäk., 1927, 129:662.

KÜSTNER, O. Ueber eine noch nicht bekannte Entstehungsursache amputierender amniotischer Fäden und Stränge. Ztschr. f. Geburtsh. u. Gynäk., 1890, 20:445.

LEFÈVRE, Gaston. De l'insertion vélamenteuse du cordon. Thèse de Paris, 1896.

LEHN, C. Ueber die Veranderungen des Körpergewichtes während der Normalen Geburt, nebst Bemerkungen über die Fruchtwassermenge. Ztschr. f. Geburtsh. u. Gynäk., 1916, 78:671.

MAHFOUZ, N. P., and ISMAIL, M. Chorionepithelioma. J. Obst. & Gynaec. Brit. Emp., 1940, 47:1.

MARCHAND, F. Ueber die sogenannten "decidualen" Geschwülste, etc. Monatschr. f. Geburtsh, u. Gynäk., 1895, 1:419, 513.

——— Ueber den Bau der Blasenmole. Ztschr. f. Geburtsh. u. Gynäk., 1895, 32:405.

——— Die Blasenmole. Ztschr. f. Geburtsh. u. Gynäk., 1898, 39:206.

——— Ueber das maligne Chorionepitheliom, nebst Mittheilung von 2 neuen Fälle. Ztschr. f. Geburtsh. u. Gynäk., 1898, 39:173.

MARCHETTI, A. A. A Consideration of Certain Types of Benign Tumors of the Placenta. Surg., Gynec. & Obst., 1939, 68:733.

MATHIEU, A. Hydatidiform Mole and Chorio-Epithelioma: Collective Review of Literature for Years 1935, 1936 and 1937. Internat. Abstr. Surg., 1939, 68:52. (Surg., Gynec. & Obst., Jan., 1939); and Internat. Abstr. Surg., 1939, 68:181 (Surg., Gynec. & Obst., Feb., 1939).

——— Recent Developments in the Diagnosis and Treatment of Hydatidiform Mole and Chorionepithelioma. Am. J. Obst. & Gynec., 1939, 37:654.

MCNALLEY, F. P., and DIECKMANN, W. J. Hemorrhagic Lesions of Placenta and Their Relation to White Infarct Formation. Am. J. Obst. & Gynec., 1923, 5:55.

MEYER, A. W. Teratom der Nabelschnur. Verhandl. d. deutsch. path. Gesellsch., 1914 ff. 582.

——— Hydatidiform Degeneration. Am. J. Obst., 1918, 78:641.

MEYER, R. Beitrage zur Path. u. Klinik des Chorionepithelioma uterimalignum. Ztschr. f. Geburtsh. u. Gynäk., 1927, 92:259.

MONTGOMERY. On the Spontaneous Amputation of the Foetal Limbs in Utero. An Exposition of the Signs and Symptoms of Pregnancy, 2d Ed. (reprinted), 1863, p. 625.

MONTGOMERY, T. L. Fibrosis of Placenta; Its Significance in the Normal and in the Syphilitic Organ. Am. J. Obst. & Gynec., 1936, 31:253.

MUELLER, P. F. Acute Hydramnios. Am. J. Obst. & Gynec., 1948, 56:1069.

NEEDHAM, J. Chemical Embryology. 1931, Cambridge University Press.

NOVAK, E. Hydatidiform Mole and Chorionepithelioma. Am. J. Surg., 1948, 76:352.

PADDOCK, R., and GREER, E. D. The Origin of the Common Cystic Structures of the Human Placenta Am. J. Obst. & Gynec., 1927, 13:164.

PAGE, Ernest W. The Relation Between Hydatid Moles, Relative Ischemia of the Gravid Uterus, and the Placental Origin of Eclampsia. Am. J. Obst. & Gynec., 1939, 37:291.

PALMER. See SCHULZE reference.

PETTIT, M. DeW. Hydatidiform Mole Following Tubal Pregnancy. Am. J. Obst. & Gynec., 1941, 42:1057.

RHAMY, B. W. Chorio-angiofibroma of the Placenta. J. Lab. & Clin. Med., 1937, 22:899.

ROSENBLOOM, D. Penetrating Chorionepithelioma with Rupture of Uterus and Fatal Intra-Abdominal Hemorrhage. Am. J. Obst. & Gynec., 1942, 43:133.

SÄNGER. Deciduoma malignum. Verhandl. d. deutsch. Gesellsch. f. Gynäk., 1892, 4:333.

——— Sarcoma uteri deciduo-cellulare, etc. Arch. f. Gynäk., 1893, 44:89.

SCHAEFFER, G. Tuberculosis of the Placenta. Quart. Bull., Sea View Hosp., 1939, 4:457.

SCHOENECK, F. J. Diagnostic Friedman Test in Hydatidiform Mole and Chorionepithelioma. Am. J. Obst. & Gynec., 1940, 39:485.

SCHONIG, A. Ueber den Kalktransport von Mutter zu Kind, etc. Ztschr. f. Geburtsh. u. Gynäk., 1929, 94:451.

SCHULZE, M. Hydatidiform Mole and Chorionepithelioma. Calif. & West. Med., 1942, 57:292.

SCHUMANN, E. Observations upon the Pathology and Treatment of Hydatidiform Mole. Tr. Am. Gynec. Soc., 1922, 47:193.

SCHUMANN, E. A., and VOEGELIN, A. W. Chorionepithelioma with Especial Reference to Its Relative Frequency. Am. J. Obst. & Gynec., 1937, 33:473.

SEITZ, L. Ueber das primäre Chorionepitheliom des Ovariums. Ztschr. f. Geburtsh. u. Gynäk., 1916, 78:244.

SIDDALL, R. S., and HARTMAN, F. W. Infarcts of the Placenta. A Study of 700 Consecutive Placentas. Am. J. Obst. & Gynec., 1926, 12:683.

SLEMONS, J. M. Placental Bacteremia. J.A.M.A., 1915, 65:1265.

STREETER, G. Focal Degenerations in Foetal Tissues and Their Relation to Intrauterine Amputation. Contributions to Embryology, Carnegie Institution of Washington, 1930, Vol. 22.

TAUSSIG, F. J. The Amniotic Fluid and Its Quantitative Variability. Am. J. Obst. & Gynec., 1927, 14:505.

THOMS, Herbert. A Roentgenographic Study of Placental Infarcts. Am. J. Obst. & Gynec., 1929, 17:176.

TRAUT, H. F., and KUDER, A. The Lesions of Fifteen Hundred Placentas Considered from a Clinical Point of View. Am. J. Obst. & Gynec., 1934, 27:552.

WANG, H. W., and HELLMAN, L. M. Studies in the Metabolism of the Human Placenta. Johns Hopkins Hosp. Bull., 1943, 73:31.

WHITMAN and GREENE. A Case of Disseminated Miliary Tuberculosis in a Foetus, etc. Arch. Int. Med., 1922, 29:261.

WIELOCH, J. Ueber Messungen des Druckes im normal graviden und hydramniotischen Uterus. Zentralbl. f. Gynäk., 1927, 51:129.

WILLIAMS, J. W. Deciduoma malignum. Johns Hopkins Hosp. Rep., 1895, 51:461.

——— The Frequency and Significance of Infarcts of the Placenta. Am. J. Obst., N. Y., 1900, 41:775.

——— Placenta Circumvallata. Am. J. Obst. & Gynec., 1927, 13:1.

WILSON, K. Chorioepithelioma. A Clinical and Pathological Study. Am. J. Obst. & Gynec., 1939, 38:824.

23

PLACENTA PREVIA AND ABRUPTIO PLACENTAE

In the three previous chapters the most frequent causes of bleeding in the first half of pregnancy were discussed, namely, abortion, ectopic pregnancy, and (a less common cause) hydatidiform mole. In the present chapter the two most common causes of hemorrhage in the last half of pregnancy will be reviewed, namely, placenta previa and abruptio placentae.

PLACENTA PREVIA

In placenta previa, the placenta, instead of being implanted high up on the anterior or posterior wall of the uterus, is implanted low in the uterus and either overlies or reaches to the vicinity of the internal os. Three degrees of the condition are recognized:

Total Placenta Previa. The internal os is totally covered by placenta.

Partial Placenta Previa. The internal os is partially covered by placenta.

Low Implantation of Placenta. The region of the internal os is encroached upon by the placenta so that the placental edge can be palpated by the examining finger when introduced through the cervix, but the placenta does not extend beyond the margin of the internal os.

These several degrees of placenta previa may be better visualized by inspecting Figs. 350, 351 and 355. A moment's consideration of these illustrations will make it plain that the degree of placenta previa, as defined above, will depend in large measure on the cervical dilatation at the time the examination is made. Thus, a low implanted placenta previa at 2 cm. dilatation may become partial at 8 cm. because the dilating cervix has uncovered placenta. Similarly, a placenta previa which appears to be total at 3 cm. dilatation may become partial at full dilatation because the dilating cervix has uncovered successively the edge of the placenta and membranes. Since extensive exploration of the region of the internal os in placenta previa is one of the most dangerous undertakings in obstetrics, it is impractical, at least with any precision, to ascertain these changing relationships between the edge of the placenta and the internal os as the cervix dilates; as a consequence, the diagnosis of the degree of the previa existing in a given case is established on the grounds of the conditions existent at the first examination after the complication has made itself manifest. In other words, these several varieties of placenta previa are only relative and provide simply an approximate picture of the extent to which the placenta has encroached upon the region of the cervix.

In both the total and partial varieties, a certain degree of separation of the placenta is an inevitable consequence of the formation of the lower uterine segment and the dilatation of the cervix. This is always associated with the tearing through of blood vessels which cannot become constricted until after the uterus has been emptied; the resulting hemorrhage was appropriately designated by Rigby as *unavoidable*.

Frequency. Placenta previa is fortunately a comparatively uncommon complication, although the statements as to its frequency vary considerably. Thus Green-Army-

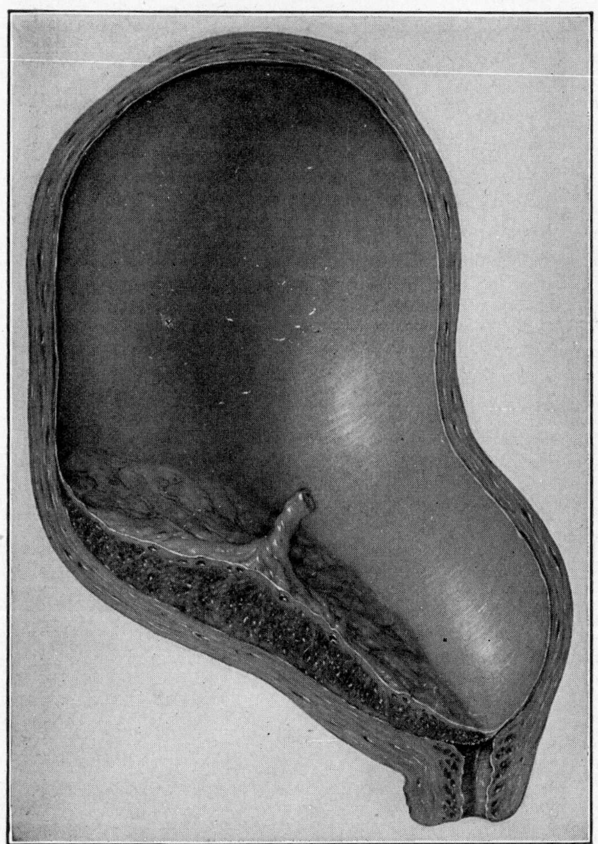

FIG. 350.—PARTIAL PLACENTA PREVIA.

tage and Dutta report an incidence in the tropics of 1 in 300, while Berkeley, in a series of over 500,000 cases collected from 17 British maternity hospitals, records a frequency of 1 in 98. The incidence of 1 in 206 labors noted in the New York Lying-In Hospital during a 12-year period is lower than that reported by Berkeley. Chakraverti, in five large maternity hospitals in India, found an incidence of 1 in 100 labors and Caldera reports a frequency of 1 in 104 labors. Pagliari noted the condition once in every 183 deliveries in the Royal Maternity Hospital in Turin, Italy. The incidence at the Johns Hopkins Hospital is 1 in 200 deliveries.

The statistics on the incidence of the various degrees of placenta previa are contradictory—the inevitable result of the fact that these varieties are not precise entities. In 304 cases of the complication studied at the Johns Hopkins Hospital by Gutierrez-

Yepes and Eastman, the total type was found in 23 per cent, the partial in 29 per cent, and low insertion in 48 per cent.

Etiology. Concerning the etiology of placenta previa comparatively little is known. Two factors, however, appear to favor its occurrence—multiparity and atrophic changes in the endometrium.

The abnormality occurs comparatively rarely in primigravidae and increases in frequency with the number of children which the individual has borne. This point is strikingly illustrated by the following figures of Doranth, which were based upon 30,796 labors occurring in Chrobak's clinic. In these the incidence of placenta previa was 0.17, 0.48, 1.37, 1.28, 3.39, and 5.51 per cent, according as the patients had given birth to 0, 1, 2, 3, 4, 5, or more children, respectively.

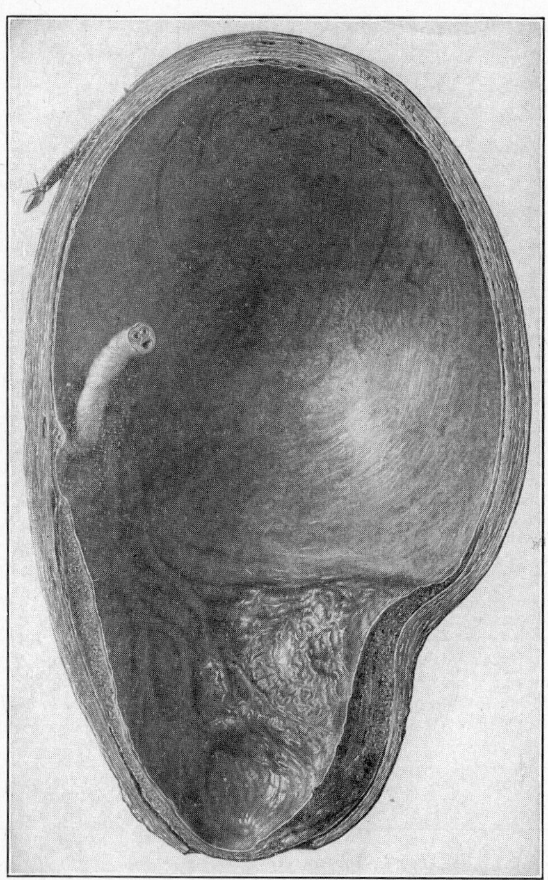

Fig. 351.—Total Placenta Previa and Velamentous Insertion of Cord.

Note the cuplike form of the placenta and its varying thickness. × 2/5.

The occurrence of placenta previa is not only favored by the absolute number of children, but also by the rapidity with which the labors have followed one another, Strassmann finding that the average age of his patients was 32.9 years and that the average number of labors was 6.38. In 80 multiparous women with placenta previa Stander found that they had averaged 4.2 children each in the 10 years following the first delivery.

Strassmann also pointed out that one of the most important factors in its development was to be found in defective vascularization of the decidua, the result of inflammatory or atrophic changes, the latter being favored by repeated and closely following pregnancies. Such conditions, he maintained, limit the amount of blood going to the placenta, so that, in order to obtain the requisite supply of nutriment, it becomes necessary for the placenta to spread over a larger area of attachment; in so doing its lower portion occasionally approaches the region of the internal os, completely or partially overlapping it, as the case may be. Plausibility is lent to such a view by the fact that the placenta in this abnormality is attached over a greater area of the uterus than usual, while at the same time it is often considerably thinner. Thus, in one of Williams' cases which came to autopsy, the placenta was almost membranous and its site occupied nearly four fifths of the interior of the uterus. Morton has recently given an excellent anatomic description of a case of low implantation of the placenta. He observed marked scarcity of decidua beneath the placenta, while the decidual reaction in the cervix and lower uterine segment was relatively profuse. He further noted a circular sinus at the level of the internal os and regards it as dividing the upper and lower segments late in labor, which leads him to suggest that only the cervix enters into the formation of the lower uterine segment. He is of the opinion that the cervix often becomes a part of the lower segment before the onset of labor and this may explain the production of antepartum bleeding due to placenta previa both before and after the onset of parturition.

Hofmeier and Kaltenbach advanced the theory that a part of the chorion laeve continued to grow instead of undergoing involution early in pregnancy, with the result that a part of the placenta developed in contact with the decidua capsularis. As pregnancy advanced, this *capsularis placenta* gradually bridged over the internal os and eventually came in contact and fused with the decidua vera, after which vascular connections with the uterine wall became established.

In view, therefore, of our present knowledge concerning the normal implantation of the ovum, as well as Strassmann's theoretical deductions, it appears probable that placenta previa results either from the primary implantation of the ovum in the lower portion of the uterus, associated with such extensive cleavage of the decidua vera that the extension of the placenta to the region of the internal os is facilitated, or that it results from the development of a part of the placenta upon the internal surface of the decidua capsularis.

Very exceptionally, a part of the placenta is developed upon the upper portion of the cervix—cervical pregnancy, discussed on page 525.

Symptoms. The most characteristic symptom of placenta previa is painless hemorrhage, which usually does not appear until after the seventh month of pregnancy. At the same time it is probable that many abortions are due to this abnormality, although the true state of affairs usually escapes observation. We have seen abortions in the third month which were clearly due to it. In such instances, hormonal and vitamin therapy would be useless.

The hemorrhage frequently comes on without warning in a pregnant woman who had previously considered herself in perfect health. Occasionally it makes its first appearance while the patient is asleep, so that on awakening and feeling the bedclothes moist, she is surprised to find that she is lying in a pool of blood. The initial bleeding is rarely, if ever, so profuse as to prove fatal and ceases spontaneously, to recur again when least expected. In other cases, the bleeding does not cease entirely, there being a continuous discharge of small quantities of bloodstained fluid which eventually so weakens the woman that a comparatively slight, additional, acute hemorrhage may be sufficient to cause death. In a certain proportion of cases, particularly when the insertion is low, the bleeding does not appear until the time of labor, when it may vary from a slight, bloodstained discharge to a profuse hemorrhage.

The mode of production of the hemorrhage is readily understood when one recalls the changes which take place in the later weeks of pregnancy and at the time of labor. When the placenta is inserted over the internal os, it is evident that, as the formation of the lower uterine segment and the dilatation of the internal os progress, its attachments must inevitably be torn through, the rupture being necessarily followed by a hemorrhage from the maternal vessels. Furthermore, the bleeding is favored by the fact that it is impossible for the stretched fibers of the lower uterine segment to compress the torn vessels, as is the case when the normally implanted placenta becomes separated during the third stage of labor. Moreover, when the placenta has developed in the capsularis, it is apparent that the thin tissue is devoid of all support where it bridges over the region of the internal os, and consequently a slight trauma will open up the intervillous space.

As the placenta previa occupies the lower portion of the uterine cavity, it interferes with the accommodation of the fetal head, and consequently abnormal presentations are unusually frequent, Müller having noted 272 transverse and 107 breech presentations in 1,148 cases. Greenhill found that fetal monsters and deformities occur more frequently; he ascribes this to poorly developed decidual reaction in the isthmus of the uterus.

As a result of abnormal adhesions or an excessively large area of attachment, the process of placental separation is sometimes interfered with, so that profuse hemorrhage frequently occurs after the birth of the child, and exceptionally continues even after the manual removal of the placenta. In other cases hemorrhage is due to the fact that the overstretched lower segment, which normally retracts but poorly, is unable to compress the vessels traversing its walls. In still others it is due to lacerations in the very friable cervix and lower uterine segment.

Diagnosis. In patients suffering from uterine hemorrhage during the last third of pregnancy, placenta previa or abruptio placentae should always be suspected, and the possibility of the existence of the former should not be dismissed until careful examination has demonstrated its absence, in which event the latter condition should be diagnosticated. Prior to this examination a suitable donor should be at hand and the procedure conducted in an operating room where preparations have been made for vaginal or abdominal treatment. In the great majority of cases of placenta previa the cervix is softer and more succulent than usual, and its canal more patulous, so that but little difficulty is experienced in carrying the finger through the internal os and feeling the characteristic sponge-like placental tissue, or at least making out a soggy, thick substance lying between the finger and the presenting part. When, however, the cervix is not patulous it becomes more difficult to establish a diagnosis, as we are not justified in dilating the cervix for this purpose. In such cases palpation of the lower uterine segment around the cervix is helpful. If the fetal skull with suture lines can be plainly felt, placenta previa is unlikely. On the other hand, the palpation of a boggy mass between the lower uterine segment and the presenting part is presumptive evidence of placenta previa. The head is usually high in placenta previa and the great frequency of transverse presentation makes this finding additional evidence in favor of the diagnosis.

Several roentgenological diagnostic procedures for localization of the placenta in utero have recently been proposed. Certain of these depend upon the injection of radiopaque substances either intravenously or directly into the amniotic sac by puncture through the abdominal and uterine walls. As such procedures may not be wholly safe to either mother or child, Snow and Powell, in 1934, suggested a soft-tissue technic, by which they were able to outline the placenta in the majority of cases. In the same year, Ude, Weum and Urner injected sodium iodine solution into the bladder and by cystogram determined the relationship of the fetal head to the bladder wall. Normally, the fetal head is separated from the upper margin of the bladder by a distance of 1 cm. which should be uniformly maintained throughout the entire length of the upper bladder margin. With this method Beck and Light obtained a high degree of accuracy in diagnosis but emphasize that, while definitely positive findings are usually accurate, negative results do not exclude the possibility of placenta previa. Prentiss and Tucker favored air cystograms, believing that these provide a clearer and simpler method than do those made with liquid media. They, furthermore, recommended the combination of semilateral and semi-erect anteroposterior positions as offering greater accuracy than the anteroposterior position alone.

We employ the soft-tissue technic, as outlined by Carty, and procure a lateral 14 by 17 inch film, the patient being placed on her right side and the x-ray tube centered at the iliac crest. From such a film it is possible, in the majority of cases, to localize the placenta. It should be pointed out that, with only one lateral film, it is often necessary, as recommended by Brown and Dippel, to view overexposed areas with a 200-watt frosted bulb in a gooseneck lamp with a shade.

Demonstration of placental location by the soft-tissue technic is based on visualization of an area of thickening of the structures between the fetal soft parts and the outer uterine wall. It is not possible to distinguish placenta from uterine wall because, except in rare instances of placental calcification, the radio-opacity of these organs is so similar that the shadows merge into one another. As shown by Moir, the subcutaneous tissues of the fetus yield a dark band demarcating the periphery of the fetal soft parts. This is shown in the upper right quadrant of Fig. 352. If now, beginning a short distance above the iliac crest in this figure, the dark line is followed upward and if at the same time the shadow demarcating the posterior aspect of the uterus is traced upward, it will be seen that the two lines diverge. In other words, the structures lying between the two surfaces mentioned reveal a thickening. This thickening represents the placenta. The same dark line surrounding the fetus can be seen faintly in Fig. 352 close to the anterior femur. Here it is clear that the structures surrounding the fetus present a thickness which is only a fraction of that shown in the upper right quadrant of the figure.

It must be emphasized that soft-tissue roentgenography of the placenta has its limitations: (1) It is not possible to visualize the placenta in all cases. Thus, in hydramnios and in multiple pregnancy (presumably because of the resultant thinning of the placenta) it is particularly difficult to identify the organ. (2) If the placenta is seen extending down into the lower uterine segment, it is usually impossible, on the basis of the x-ray film, to be certain just how far down it goes, because the placental shadow in this location becomes obliterated by that of the ilium; and in such a case vaginal examination is necessary to establish the diagnosis. Hence, the value of the method lies simply in its ability to rule out placenta previa in a substantial proportion of patients who bleed in the last trimester, thus sparing them vaginal and cervical exploration.

In an extensive experience with the soft-tissue technic of placental roentgenography, our results have been generally satisfactory. Provided the film is made by a thoroughly trained and meticulous technician and is read by a person experienced in the interpretation of such films, it is possible to visualize the placenta in 85 per cent or more of the cases. In a recent review of the experience of the Boston Lying-In Hospital with this method, Stevenson reports a higher degree of success; his group

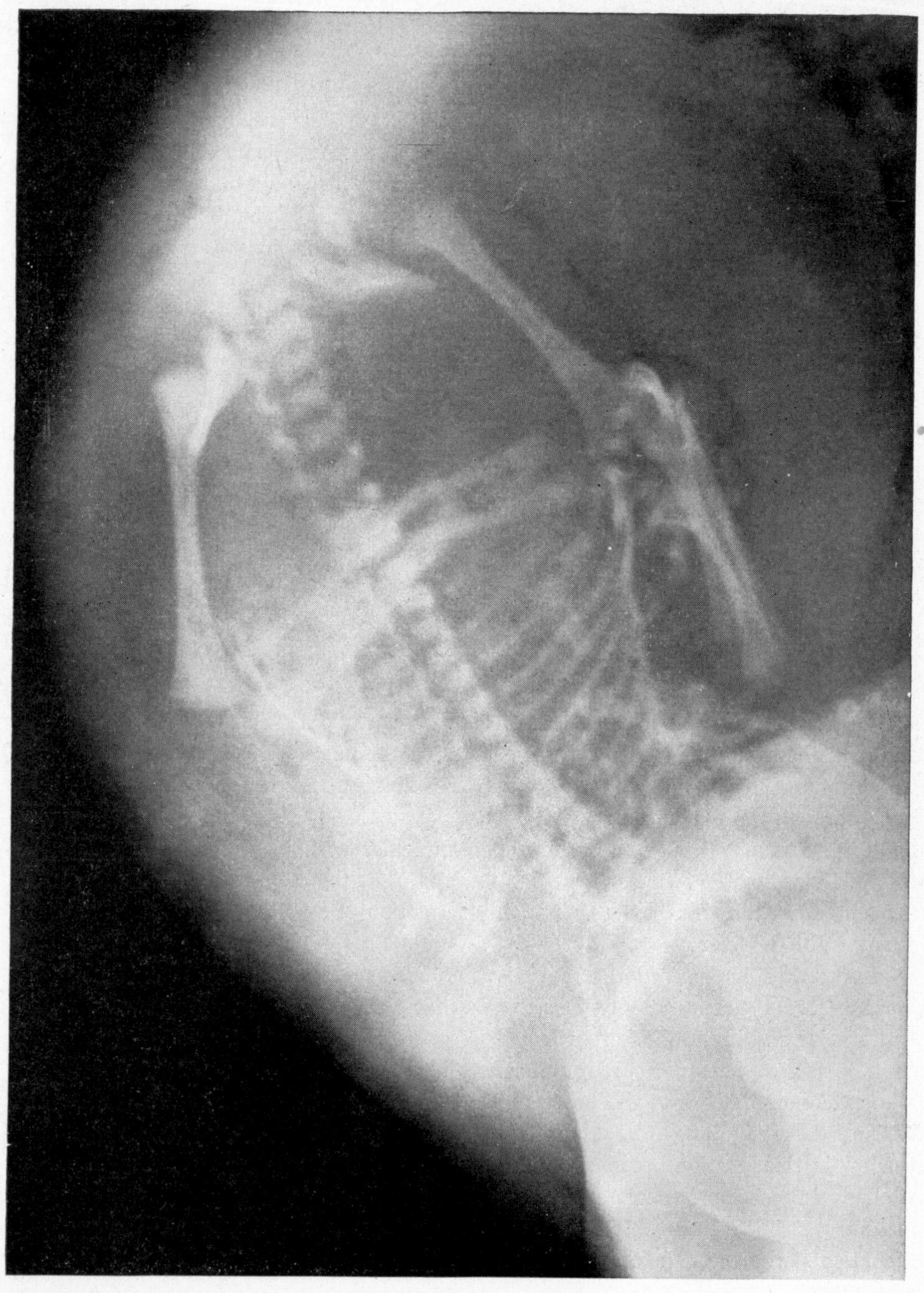

Fig. 352.—Soft Tissue Roentgenogram Showing Placenta on Upper Posterior Surface of Uterus.

(Courtesy of Dr. A. L. Dippel and Dr. W. H. Brown.)

was able to establish or refute the diagnosis of placenta previa in 95.3 per cent of 488 cases.

Prognosis. A marked improvement in the end-results of treatment has been noted in the past 10 years, as evidenced by reports from numerous large clinics. Irving, at the Boston Lying-In Hospital, gives a maternal mortality of 11.6 per cent for the period of 1924 to 1930, and one of 2 per cent for the years 1930 to 1934; Davis, at the Chicago Lying-In Hospital, for the years 1927 to 1936 records no maternal mortality; and Siegel, at the University of Maryland Hospital, reports a maternal mortality of 5.22 per cent prior to 1931 as compared to 0.99 per cent since. Wilson reported 102 cases of placenta previa with a maternal mortality of 1.96 per cent. In the New York Lying-In Hospital, in 155 cases of placenta previa occurring during the period 1932 to 1943, there was one maternal death, a mortality rate of 0.64 per cent. In 162 cases of placenta previa observed at the Johns Hopkins Hospital between 1935 and 1949, there was, likewise, only one maternal death.

In hospital practice, where many patients are admitted after inefficient treatment by poorly trained practitioners, in addition to acute anemia, puerperal infection plays a large part in increasing the maternal mortality. The prognosis is much more serious in total placenta previa than in the other varieties. Furthermore, the mortality depends upon the condition of the patient when first seen, it being evident that women who have suffered from profuse and repeated bleeding have far less chance of recovery than those who come under observation after the first slight hemorrhage.

The fetal mortality, although showing some decrease in recent years, remains high. Findley, in an analysis of 47,828 cases of placenta previa collected from the literature, finds a gross fetal mortality of 55.61 per cent for the period prior to 1922, and 50.84 per cent for the years 1922 to 1937. Liepelt reports a fetal death rate of 33.25; Siegel, 24.75; and Irving, 20.3 per cent. During the 12-year period of 1932–1944, the fetal mortality, including neonatal deaths, in the New York Lying-In Hospital was 25.1 per cent.

Treatment of Placenta Previa

General Considerations. Every patient who bleeds in the last half of pregnancy to an extent substantially greater than "show," should be sent to a hospital *without either vaginal or rectal examination.* This statement holds true even though the hospital be 50 miles away. Any digital manipulation of the region of the cervix in placenta previa is likely to precipitate sudden, massive and even fatal hemorrhage; and it should be a rigid rule that local examination should never be done in the home, and even in the hospital it must be carried out only in the operating room after all preparations are in readiness for either vaginal or abdominal surgery as well as blood transfusion. Not only is it dangerous to rush in on cases of placenta previa but it is altogether unnecessary, since it is very rare for a woman with placenta previa to bleed to death from the initial hemorrhage, provided no vaginal or rectal examinations have been done. This general principle has been especially emphasized by Herman Johnson who, in a vast experience, has never seen or heard of a fatality from the initial bleeding of placenta previa, in the absence of digital manipulation of the cervix. Nor in our experience with placenta previa at the Johns Hopkins Hospital, which extends far back to before transfusion days and which comprises over

375 cases, is there such a death on record. Likewise in Macafee's extensive experience, a severe initial hemorrhage rarely occurs in this complication.

These two basic facts, (a) that the initial hemorrhage in placenta previa is rarely, if ever, fatal and (b) that vaginal or rectal examination often precipitates severe hemorrhage, constitute the basis for certain general principles in the management of these cases as follows: (1) As stated, vaginal or rectal examination should not be done in suspected cases, except in an operating room where all facilities are in readiness to combat massive hemorrhage. (2) Vaginal packing (as a supposed prophylactic measure while the patient is en route to the hospital) is dangerous since it may only cause more bleeding and introduce infection; moreover, it is unnecessary and usually futile. (3) After admission to the hospital, there is ample time to arrange for blood transfusion, to prepare the operating room, and to collect one's thoughts in regard to the most judicious type of management for the case. (4) Vaginal examination should be carried out gently in order, if possible, not to precipitate fresh bleeding. The maternal surface of the placenta has a characteristic gritty feel, even to the gloved finger. A common error is to mistake a blood clot in the cervix for placenta. The latter does not have a gritty feel. (5) In selected cases in which the baby is quite premature, it is justifiable, with certain reservations, to postpone delivery until the infant has a better chance of survival. This expectant treatment of placenta previa will be discussed in more detail subsequently.

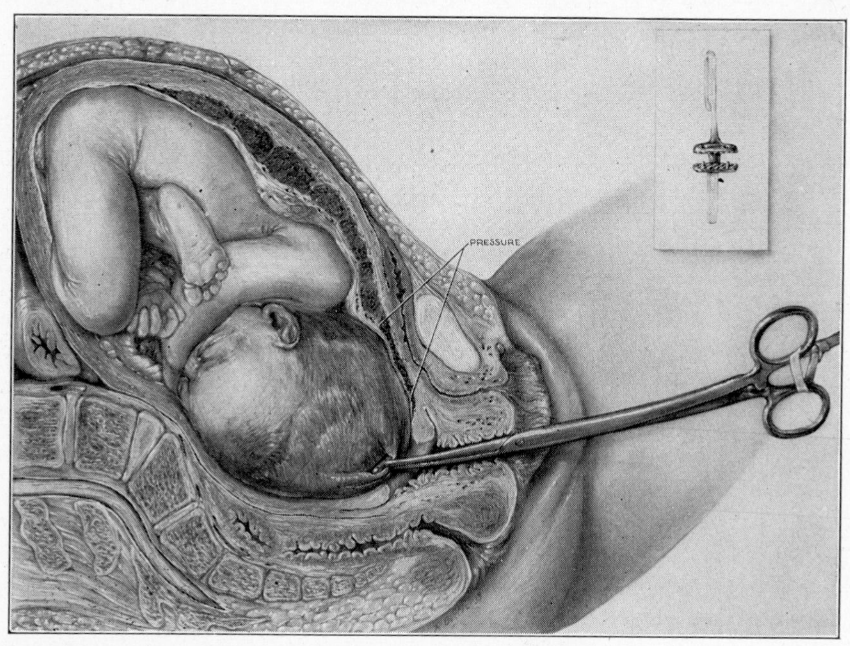

Fig. 353.—The Willett Forceps in a Case of Low Insertion of the Placenta.

In placenta previa, as in other major hemorrhagic complications of obstetrics, blood transfusion is lifesaving and in many cases plays a larger role in the outcome than does the particular method used to combat bleeding. It should be the physician's first thought in every such case.

Methods Employed. The procedures available for the treatment of placenta previa fall into two main categories: (1) vaginal methods, the rationale of which is to exert pressure against the placenta and placental site and thereby occlude the bleeding vessels, and (2) cesarean section, the rationale of which is twofold—first, through immediate delivery to allow the uterus to retract and so stop the bleeding, and second, to forestall the possibility of cervical lacerations, a frequent complication of vaginal delivery in total and partial placenta previa.

Vaginal Methods. The vaginal or "compression" methods are four in number: (1) simple rupture of the membranes, (2) Willett's forceps, (3) insertion of a bag, and (4) Braxton Hicks version.

1. Rupture of the membranes allows the head to drop down against the placenta and is often an efficacious procedure in multiparae with low implantation of the placenta. It has its greatest usefulness in multiparae with this milder variety of placenta previa which does not start to bleed until labor has set in. After rupture of the membranes, fundal pressure should be exerted to force the head as tightly as possible against the placenta and lower uterine segment.

2. If simple rupture of the membranes does not suffice to control bleeding, additional pressure of the head against the placenta may be effected by Willett's forceps. This instrument, as shown in Fig. 353, is a forceps of the T-shaped clip type, the grasping bars being one-half inch long, narrow enough to pass where a finger will, and rigid enough to maintain the requisite weight when fixed on the fetal scalp. The holding teeth are rounded. The application of the forceps is easy and it can be applied as soon as the os will admit a finger. After rupturing the membranes, the forceps, with the blades closed, is passed through the cervix until the head is reached. The blades are then separated, and pressing on the scalp, closed, when a grip on the scalp will be obtained. A weight, attached to the forceps by means of a tape, is allowed to hang over the edge of the bed. Although Willett originally suggested that the weight be from one to two pounds, subsequent observations indicate that the weight for use on a living child should not exceed one pound. Even with one pound some degree of scalp injury with subsequent necrosis of the area embraced by the forceps, occurs in about one third of the cases, but in our experience this has never been serious. If bleeding continues, despite the use of the Willett's clamp, it means that an error has been made in the type of case selected for this kind of treatment. Rupture of the membranes and Willett's forceps should not be employed in primigravidae, in total or partial placenta previa, nor in cases in which, before labor or early in labor, hemorrhage is massive. These severer grades of placenta previa are most safely managed by cesarean section.

3. Although, in our opinion, the more advanced degrees of placenta previa are best treated by abdominal delivery, this attitude is not unanimous, and both the bag and Braxton Hicks version are still employed in many clinics in the partial variety of this complication, as well as in low implantation. Today, few, if any, obstetricians would take exception to the statement that total placenta previa always demands cesarean section. The technic of inserting the bag in placenta previa is illustrated in Figs. 354A and 354B. A 10 cm. bag is employed. After it has been placed in the uterus it is filled tightly with sterile water, the tube clamped or shut off with a stopcock, and a tape attached to the tube. The tape is hung over the edge of the bed and sufficient weight attached to control bleeding, usually about two or three

pounds. The patient must be watched constantly because at complete dilatation the bag is naturally expelled from the uterus and falls into the upper vagina. With the compression which has been exerted by the bag thus released, bleeding from the placental site may be profuse and immediate version and extraction are often necessary.

We have virtually abandoned the use of the bag in placenta previa and in our last 162 cases, treated between 1935 and 1949, it was employed only 11 times, for the most part during the early years of this period. The only maternal death in

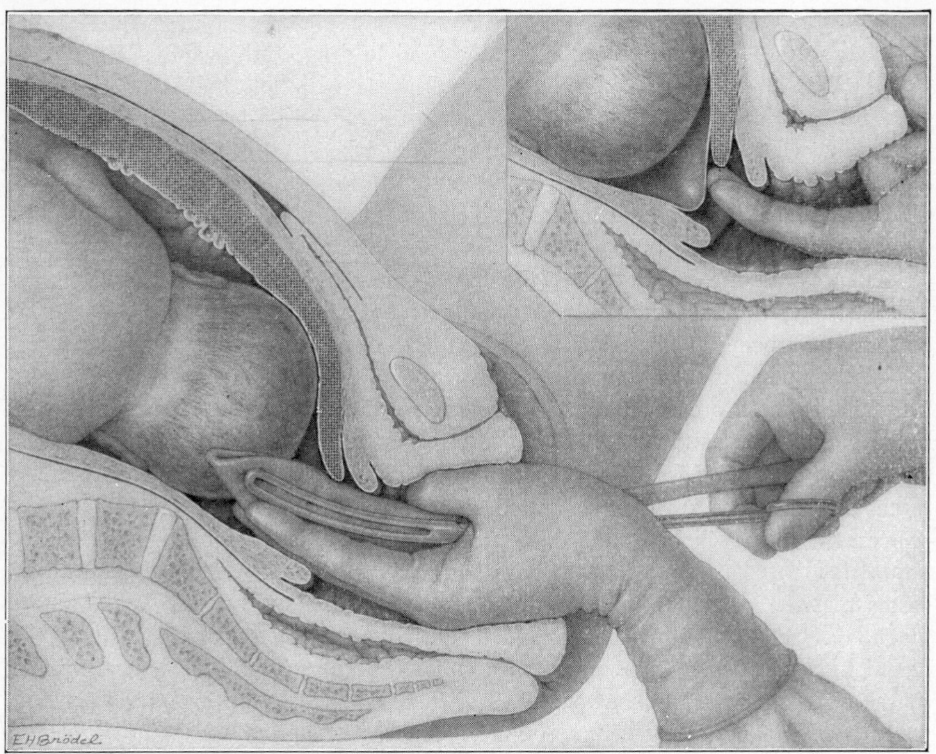

Fig. 354A.—Insertion of Voorhees Bag.

these 162 cases was due to rupture of the uterus produced in the course of inserting a bag. Our experience with the bag prior to 1935 was extensive and can leave little doubt that the bag has many disadvantages: (1) in the manipulations necessary, the cervix and lower uterine segment, especially friable and vascular in placenta previa, may be traumatized, as exemplified by the fatality mentioned; (2) bleeding may be profuse between expulsion of the bag and delivery of the infant; (3) if the bag is expelled before the cervix is quite fully dilated, as often happens, version and extraction may produce extensive cervical lacerations; (4) the bag is conducive to infection through blockage of uterine drainage; and (5) a bag not infrequently leaks and another has to be inserted at the cost of blood loss.

4. The Braxton Hicks procedure is not directed at immediate delivery but has as its objective the utilization of the fetal buttocks and thigh as a tamponade to

compress the placenta. It differs from the full operation of version and extraction in several other important respects: two fingers and not the whole hand are inserted into the uterus to grasp a foot; Braxton Hicks version is done at 4 to 8 cm. dilatation; and, after a foot has been delivered, no further effort at extraction is made but simply enough traction exerted on the leg to control bleeding. Only with complete dilatation is extraction effected.

Braxton Hicks version is a difficult operation to perform unless the baby is very small; and the manipulations necessary to grasp a foot and turn the baby are

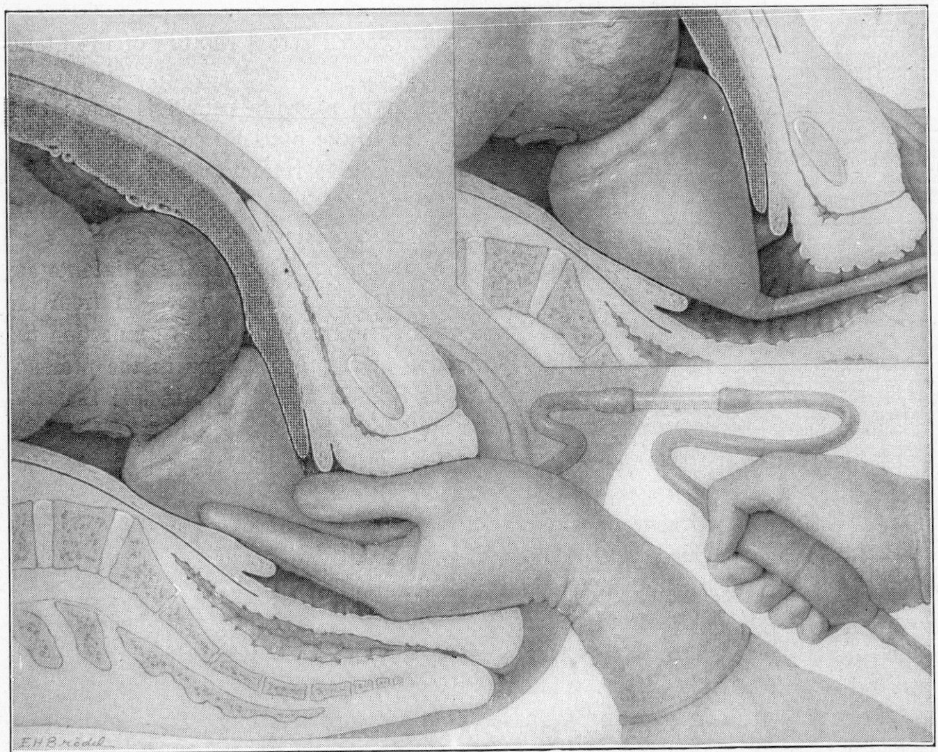

FIG. 354B.—DISTENTION OF BAG RESULTING IN COMPRESSION OF THE PLACENTA.

likely to produce extensive cervical and lower segment lacerations. Moreover, the fetal mortality is high and, all in all, it is our opinion that this operation has little or no place in modern obstetrics. Occasionally, however, the principle of bringing down a foot may be employed to advantage in cases of placenta previa in which a small (especially if dead) infant presents as a footling breech.

Cesarean Section. In the foregoing paragraphs, repeated reference has been made to the likelihood of cervical and lower segment lacerations in the vaginal management of placenta previa. Because of the extreme vascularity of the placental site, the cervix and lower uterine segment are so succulent and friable in placenta previa that they tear like wet blotting paper. This is especially true of the total and partial varieties. Herein, in large measure, lies the rationale of cesarean section in this complication. In an extensive statistical study of placenta previa carried out by Hitschmann in 1921, among 242 women whose death from placenta previa was the direct result of hemorrhage, the fatal outcome in 80, or 34.3 per cent, was ascribable to bleeding from lacerations of the cervix and the lower uterine segment. Of the women dying from hemorrhage due to lacerations, 80 per cent had total placenta previa. Hitschmann's observations, as well as those of others, indicate that bleeding from cervical and lower segment lacerations may even be a more frequent cause of maternal death than hemorrhage from the placental separation; it is frequently, moreover, the determining factor in death since, when superimposed on antepartum hemorrhage, it may constitute the final death blow. Thus, in 11 autopsies performed at the Johns Hopkins Hospital between 1896 and 1944, in cases of placenta previa in which death was due to exsanguination, six revealed actual rupture of the uterus or extensive cervical lacerations.

The rationale of performing cesarean section in placenta previa is hence twofold: (1) it abbreviates antepartum bleeding due to the partially separated placenta by effecting immediate delivery and subsequent uterine retraction and (2) it forestalls the possibility of cervical and lower segment lacerations. It is directed primarily, therefore, at safeguarding the life of the mother. Abdominal delivery yields an additional reward in a better infant mortality, but, since about half the infants are premature when bleeding first occurs, the advantages of cesarean section from the viewpoint of the infant must be evaluated with some reserve. In this connection the question sometimes arises as to the justification of cesarean section in the presence of a dead baby. Here again it is necessary to bear in mind the principle that abdominal delivery is done primarily for the mother and that the delivery of a dead baby by vaginal methods can cause lacerations just as readily as can delivery of a living infant. Therefore, repellent though it may be, cesarean section may be the most judicious method of treatment even though the infant has succumbed, especially in all total placenta previa and in all total and partial varieties in primigravidae. On the other hand, in less difficult cases, the presence of a dead baby may well cause one to veer toward vaginal procedures (preferably just rupture of the membranes with or without the Willett's clamp) although abdominal delivery might have been preferable with a living infant.

Summary of Methodology. In selecting the best treatment for a given case of placenta previa, numerous factors must be given consideration. First, is any sign of infection present? If so, as evidenced by fever, foul discharge, or history of vaginal manipulations, the case falls in an especially dire category which will be discussed shortly. Otherwise, the following factors and their significance must be reviewed. What is the degree of the previa? In all cases of total placenta previa, regardless of other factors, cesarean section is the procedure of choice. What is the parity? In all primigravidae, both total and partial placenta previa are indications for abdominal delivery, regardless of other factors. This is also true of most cases of marginal placenta previa. In primigravidae cervical dilatation is slower and lacerations more likely to occur and, with few exceptions, the primigravida with this complication is always best treated by abdominal delivery. Has bleeding been massive? If it has, this circumstance suggests either a more advanced degree of placenta previa than examination may show, or extreme vascularity of the cervix and lower uterine segment; massive bleeding points to the desirability of section, regardless of other factors. At the other extreme, multiparae with low insertion of the placenta, especially if they are already in labor with 4 cm. dilatation or more, are best handled by rupture of the membranes with or without the Willett's clamp. This last mentioned group will comprise numerically a large proportion, perhaps one half of any given series. If a vaginal method is used, the simpler it is, the better, since prolonged and complicated manipulations greatly increase the risk to both mother and child. If cesarean section is done, the classical type is preferable, in my opinion, since trauma to the friable and vascular placental site is avoided.

If outright intra-uterine infection is present in addition to placenta previa, the outlook at once becomes grave and many of the above generalizations do not apply. Intensive penicillin therapy should be started immediately and blood transfusions given to replace blood loss. In this type of case, abdominal delivery is contraindicated and vaginal methods of treatment, with all their drawbacks, must be relied upon. Finally, in all cases of placenta previa, let it be emphasized again that liberal blood transfusions (more blood than the patient has lost!) are frequently more decisive in life-saving than is the type of local treatment employed.

Expectant Treatment. Until recent years there has been general agreement that placenta previa demands prompt delivery and that temporizing for any purpose is rarely, if ever, indicated. As the result of the important observations of Herman Johnson, Macafee, J. Tiffany Williams, and others, it is now clear that a waiting policy is justifiable in certain cases, in order to minimize the high neonatal mortality which is levied by prematurity in this complication. These authors base their contention on the circumstance that the initial hemorrhage in placenta previa is rarely, if ever, fatal in the absence of vaginal manipulation, and that subsequent hemorrhages are rarely, if ever, fatal in the absence of vaginal manipulation, provided the hemoglobin is normal at the onset of the hemorrhage. As already indicated, these general facts, which underlie the justification of the expectant treatment, are well documented. Since the sole purpose in this type of therapy is to allow small premature babies opportunity for longer intra-uterine development, it does not concern itself with patients who are near term or in whom the infant is plainly of a size of 2,500 gm. or more. In the event that the child seems so small that the likelihood of its survival is poor, and if labor has not begun, an expectant attitude may be adopted. A gentle vaginal examination is done and inspection of the vagina and cervix carried out to eliminate the possibility of some infrequent cause of bleeding such as ruptured varices or cervical tumors, but the cervical canal should not be explored. However, the lower segment surrounding the cervix is carefully palpated; when the presenting part cannot be readily felt through the tissues lateral to the cervix, it suggests the presence of placental tissue in the lower segment. A presumptive diagnosis of placenta previa is then made. These patients should be kept under close observation, preferably in the hospital, although J. Tiffany Williams has permitted some of them to return home, with instructions to abstain from sexual intercourse, to permit no vaginal examination, and to return to the hospital with the first recurrence of bleeding. It is essential that the mother's blood picture be followed carefully; this, and not an alarming history derived from a lay estimate of the amount of blood lost, must be the criterion for interruption of pregnancy before the fetus has reached easy viability. Forty-one patients have been treated in this manner by J. Tiffany Williams for periods of time varying from two days to three months in an effort to obtain a child which would survive. Fourteen of these patients had two or more periods of hospitalization for recurrent episodes of bleeding. Among these 41 patients, 5 babies (12 per cent) were lost. This fetal mortality of 12 per cent with expectant treatment is considerably better than that usually reported for placenta previa, which, as already stated, ranges in excess of 25 per cent. There were no maternal deaths in this group of cases handled expectantly. Likewise, Macafee has reported 174 cases treated by this regime with but one maternal death and a gross fetal mortality of 23.5 per cent. Herman W. Johnson has reported 79 cases managed similarly with no maternal death and a fetal mortality of 22.5 per cent. This program demands an intelligent patient, vigilant supervision in respect to hemoglobin levels and the evaluation of blood losses, and astute judgment, but, provided it does not lead to callousness toward hemorrhage, it is a justifiable undertaking in carefully selected cases.

ABRUPTIO PLACENTAE

Nomenclature. Whenever the normally located placenta undergoes separation from its uterine attachment between the twentieth week of pregnancy and the birth of the infant, the condition is known as *abruptio placentae.* Frequently employed synonyms are: "premature separation of the normally implanted placenta," "ablatio placentae," and "accidental hemorrhage." As already discussed, detachment of the

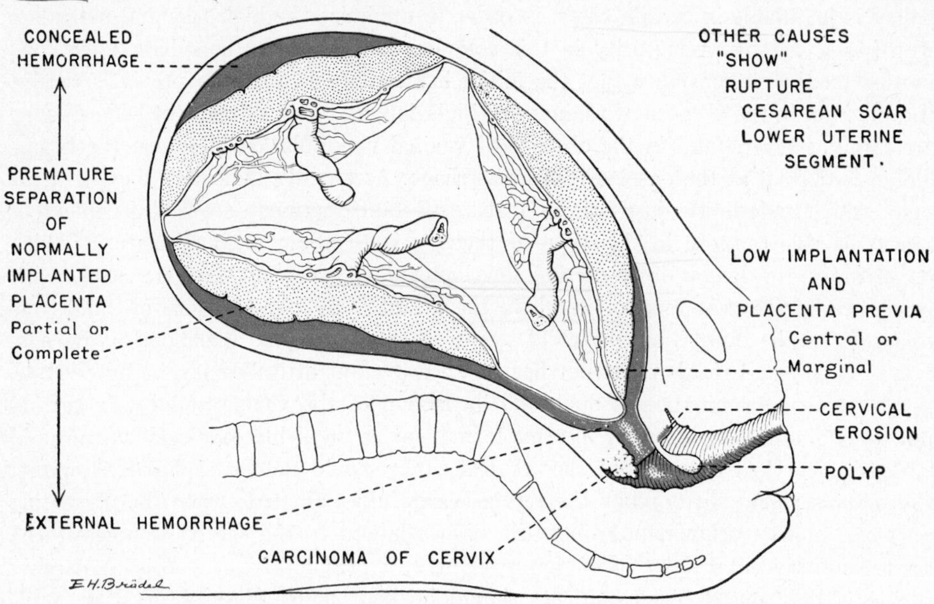

Fig. 355.—Causes of Bleeding in the Third Trimester.

placenta prior to the twentieth week is abortion. The reason for regarding placental separation early in pregnancy and late in pregnancy as two different entities is that the clinical and pathological picture produced by the accident at these two times is quite different. However, the earlier in pregnancy abruptio placentae occurs, the more it resembles an abortion; thus, between the twentieth and twenty-eighth week the picture is frequently very similar to that of an abortion, not only in signs, symptoms, and prognosis, but also in the treatment required.

The Latin word *abruptio* means a rending asunder and also carries with it the connotation of a sudden accident, a clinical characteristic of most cases of this complication. Throughout the previous editions of this book, "premature separation of the normally implanted placenta" was the phrase employed to designate this condition. While this is a most descriptive term, it is so long as to be somewhat cumbersome for either written or oral use. "Ablatio placentae" means a carrying

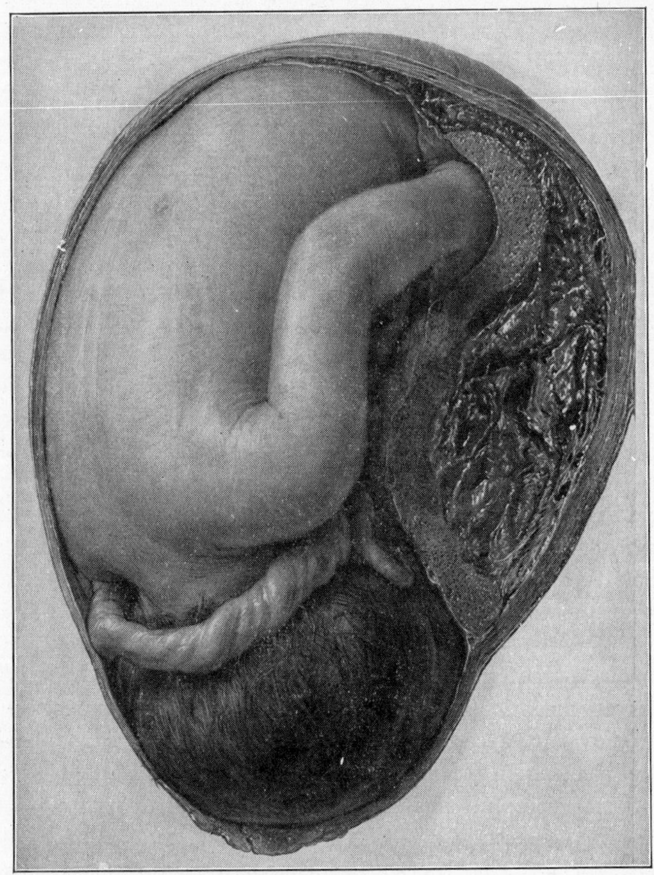

FIG. 356.—ABRUPTIO PLACENTAE WITH CONCEALED HEMORRHAGE.

away of the placenta, finds an analogy in "ablatio retinae," but, while preferred by some authors, is not extensively used. The term employed for this condition in Great Britain is "accidental hemorrhage." The rationale of its use is that the condition is an "accident" in the sense of an event that takes place without expectation in contrast to the *unavoidable* hemorrhage of placenta previa in which hemorrhage is to be anticipated because of the anatomical relationships. However, since the term "accidental hemorrhage" may suggest to some the element of trauma (which is rarely a factor in these cases), it is sometimes misleading to students and is rarely employed in the United States.

The bleeding of abruptio placentae usually insinuates itself between the membranes and uterus, escapes through the cervix, and appears externally, in which case it is called *external hemorrhage*. Less often, the effused blood does not escape externally but is retained between the detached placenta and the uterus, in which case it is designated as *concealed hemorrhage* or *internal hemorrhage*. Abruptio placentae with concealed hemorrhage is characterized by a more catastrophic picture than is seen in abruptio placentae with external hemorrhage and carries with it much greater maternal hazards. Other important differences between abruptio placentae with external hemorrhage and with concealed hemorrhage are: in the former, detachment of the placenta is generally incomplete, whereas in the latter it is usually complete; furthermore, concealed hemorrhage (a term sometimes used separately to indicate this type of abruptio placentae) is associated with hypertensive toxemia in a substantial proportion of cases, whereas this is less frequently true in cases with external bleeding. In about 80 per cent of cases of abruptio placentae the bleeding is external and in about 20 per cent concealed.

All degrees of premature separation of the placenta may occur, from an area only a few millimeters in diameter to the entire placenta, with all gradations of signs and symptoms. As a consequence, abruptio placentae is not a sharply circumscribed entity. Moreover, the marginal sinus of the placenta (Fig. 120) occasionally ruptures and gives rise to signs and symptoms which simulate exactly abruptio placentae with external hemorrhage. In these cases, some slight marginal detachment of the placenta may also occur. Cases of marginal sinus rupture are usually grouped with abruptio placentae since it is often impossible to distinguish them clinically or pathologically. In this connection, it should be noted that of all cases of antepartum hemorrhage in the last trimester of pregnancy, less than one third can be ascribed positively either to placenta previa or abruptio. Of the remaining two thirds, some are due to cervical erosions or polyps, but most are probably examples of very minute marginal separation of the placenta which it is impossible to demonstrate either clinically or pathologically.

Because of the great variability in the clinical as well as in the pathological manifestations of abruptio placentae, the classification of these cases is sometimes uncertain. In the main, a case is considered as one of abruptio placentae only if, in addition to bleeding, there are definite clinical manifestations of the condition, such as abdominal pain, uterine tenderness and/or rigidity, and fetal distress or death, or if clear-cut placental evidence is found, such as clots and a depressed area on the maternal surface. The reported incidence of abruptio ranges between one in 85 deliveries to one in 250, depending upon the diagnostic criteria used.

Etiology. Unfortunately, the primary cause of premature separation of the placenta is imperfectly understood, and the following conditions have been invoked as etiologic factors: traumatism, shortness of the umbilical cord, chronic hypertension, acute toxemia, and histamine intoxication. Formerly it was held that a fall or a blow upon the abdomen might cause it, and traumatism was noted in 67 of the cases collected by Holmes, but was mentioned less frequently in the statistics of subsequent writers and is demonstrable in less than 5 per cent of cases. Its influence has doubtless been exaggerated, and, while it may occasionally be concerned with, it cannot be regarded as the cause of the complication. Picardi, in 104 cases of premature separation of the placenta, noted no instance of trauma as a precipitating cause. In the classical specimen of Pinard and Varnier, the accident was clearly due to traction exerted upon the placenta by an abnormally short umbilical cord. Gardiner has laid great stress upon its importance, but as such an abnormality is almost always lacking, it is evident that it can only exceptionally be an etiologic factor.

It has long been believed that some relationship exists between toxemia of pregnancy and abruptio placentae, a few observers even believing that abruptio placentae is actually a form of toxemia loosely akin to eclampsia. The frequency with which abruptio placentae is preceded by hypertension has been variously reported as being from 25 to 60 per cent. In 200 cases of abruptio placentae, studied in our clinic by Delfs, in which the data permitted evaluation of this question, 94 cases, or 47 per cent, gave evidence of hypertension prior to the placental separation. In 1.5 per cent of the cases the accident occurred in association with eclampsia, in 21.0 per cent with preeclampsia, in 14.5 per cent with chronic hypertensive vascular disease, and in 10.0 per cent with some unclassified type of non-convulsive toxemia. Since the frequency of toxemia in our clinic population as a whole is approximately 17 per cent, it is clear that in our experience, abruptio placentae is associated with hypertension almost three times more often than would ordinarily be expected. Goethals found toxemia present in 24.2 per cent of his cases, Dieckmann in 30 per cent, and Bartholomew in 52.5 per cent. The last named author has advanced extensive evidence, especially the occurrence of hemorrhagic placental infarcts both in eclampsia and abruptio placentae, to demonstrate a toxemic origin for all cases of abruptio placentae. However, most students of the question would not go so far, and, although it is true that abruptio placentae is very frequently preceded by hypertension, the exact relationship which exists between the toxemias and abruptio placentae is a moot question.

In 1915, Williams observed peculiar degenerative lesions in the intima of the smaller uterine arteries and suggested that the condition may be due to some type of toxemia producing such vascular changes. McKelvey recently described lesions, in the arterioles of the upper part of the decidua basalis, which he frequently observed in normal gestation. He believes that abruptio placentae is an extension of such arteriolar changes, occurring in probably all human placentas, which in turn are associated with the modified arteriovenous aneurysm effect of the intervillous spaces.

Most of the conditions just mentioned may come into play either during pregnancy or at the time of labor. On the other hand, certain other etiologic factors cannot become operative until labor has set in. Among these may be mentioned traction exerted by an abnormally short umbilical cord, as well as a sudden diminution in the bulk of the uterine contents following the birth of the first child in a twin pregnancy, or the too rapid expulsion of a large amount of amniotic fluid in hydramnios.

Hofbauer, in 1926, by the injection of weak solutions of histamine, produced highly suggestive lesions in experimental animals and believes that the same agent may be operative in women; he holds that histamine may be produced by degenerative changes occurring in the chorionic tissues of the placenta. While his theory is suggestive and interesting, it should not be accepted until further evidence is adduced in its support.

We may thus conclude this discussion with the statement that at present the underlying cause of premature separation of the normally implanted placenta is unknown.

Pathology. Abruptio placentae is inaugurated by an effusion of blood into the decidua basalis, which sometimes appears to come from areas of hemorrhage within the placenta itself—red infarcts—and at other times from alterations in the permeability of the smaller uterine vessels. The decidua then splits so that a thin layer remains in contact with the maternal surface of the placenta while a thicker layer adjoins the muscularis. Consequently, the process in its earliest stages consists in the development of a decidual hematoma which leads to separation, compression, and ultimate throwing out of function of the portion of the placenta adjacent to it. In its early stage there are no clinical symptoms, and the condition is discovered only upon examination of the freshly delivered organ, which will present on its maternal surface a sharply circumscribed depression, measuring a few centimeters in diameter and containing dark and partially disorganized, clotted blood. In most instances the decidual hemorrhage is more profuse, so that the area of separation becomes more extensive, and gradually extends to the margin of the placenta. As the uterus is still distended by the product of conception, it is unable to contract and compress the torn vessels in the decidua basalis; consequently, the escaping blood makes its way between the membranes and the uterine wall and eventually appears externally, but, as stated, may be retained within the uterus. This is liable to occur (1) when there is an effusion of blood behind the placenta, its margins still remaining adherent; (2) when the placenta is completely separated while the membranes retain their attachment to the uterine wall; (3) when the blood gains access to the amniotic cavity after breaking through the membranes; and (4) when the head is so accurately applied to the lower uterine segment that the blood cannot make its way past it. In the majority of such cases, however, the membranes are gradually dissected off from the uterine wall, and part of the blood eventually escapes from the cervix.

Formerly, in considering the pathology of the condition, attention was centered upon the extent of the separation—partial or total—and whether the hemorrhage was external or concealed. It is now recognized that, in certain cases at least, characteristic lesions occur in the uterine wall, which serve to explain not only the mode of origin of the separation, but also the failure of the organ to contract after being emptied of its contents. The uterus, and occasionally the tubes and ovaries as well, take on a bluish, purplish, coppery coloration and resemble an ovarian cyst with a twisted pedicle (Fig. 357). The process may likewise invoke one or even both broad ligaments, as well as the tubes and ovaries which are then gorged with blood. In some instances the uterus fails to contract and retract following cesarean section, and, as it remains soft and flabby, one is forced to amputate it supravaginally in order to prevent death from hemorrhage. In such cases, microscopic examination shows extensive intramuscular hemorrhage which has so dissociated the muscle fibers as to destroy completely their contractile properties (Fig. 358). Furthermore, similar hemorrhagic changes in the decidua basalis afford a ready explanation for the inauguration of the process of separation. In most specimens the hemorrhagic discoloration is greatest in the area corresponding to the placental site, and the muscular dissociation is most pronounced in the outer and inner layers of the uterine wall.

Couvelaire has designated the condition as *uteroplacental apoplexy*. Its mode of production is not yet clear, but, as has already been indicated, it appears to be associated with a toxemic process. In several of the uteri which Williams examined endarteritic changes and lesions of continuity in the smaller vessels afforded a satisfactory explanation for the production of the intramuscular hemorrhage. The utero-

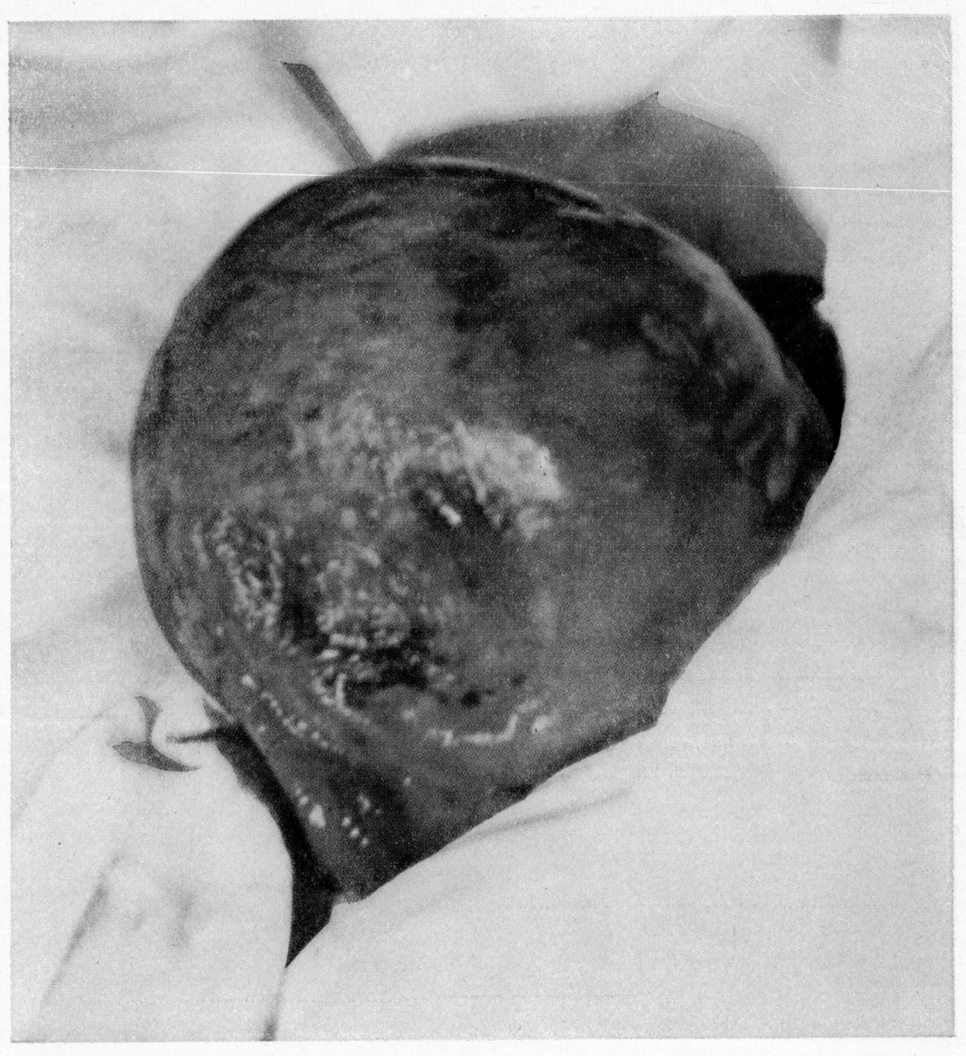

Fig. 357.—Couvelaire Uterus at Cesarean Section.

placental apoplexy of Couvelaire occurs only in the severer forms of abruptio placentae and is especially likely to develop in cases of concealed hemorrhage. In the course of 83 cesarean sections, performed in our clinic for abruptio placentae, uteroplacental apoplexy was present in sufficient degree to warrant hysterectomy in five cases, or once in every 16 cases of the abruptios managed abdominally. Furthermore, in an additional 49 cases, ecchymotic areas of greater or less extent were observed, so that of our abruptios treated by cesarean section, Couvelaire changes were found in 65 per cent. These 54 known cases of Couvelaire uterus occurred in a total series

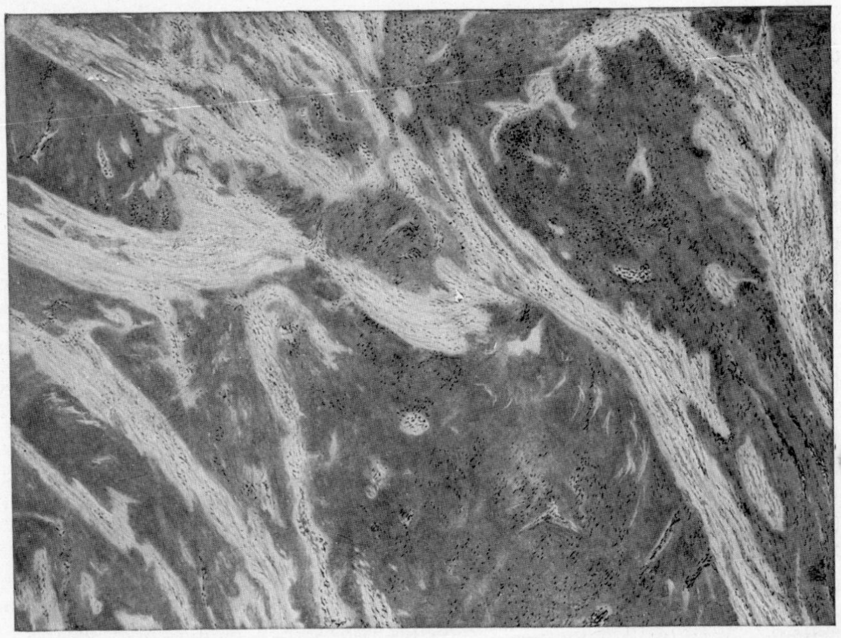

Fig. 358.—Section through Uterine Wall from a Case of Abruptio Placentae Showing Dissociation of the Muscle Fibers by Hemorrhage.

Light areas represent muscle; dark areas, effused blood. × 40.

of 241 patients with abruptio placentae. The figure cited for the incidence of Couvelaire uterus at cesarean section for abruptio placentae is higher than usually reported, Goethals finding only one in three, approximately. However, despite the rather high frequency of Couvelaire uterus in our series, it should be noted that hysterectomy was deemed necessary in only some 6 per cent of the cases of abruptio placentae managed abdominally.

Occasionally, superficial longitudinal fissures develop upon the surface of the uterus. These are usually multiple, a few centimeters in length, and extend only a slight distance into the muscularis. It is not yet known whether they are due to excessive distention of the organ or to the rupture of the superficial hemorrhagic areas. Whatever their mode of production, they occasionally lead to fatal intraperitoneal hemorrhage, as recorded by McNair, Oldfield, and Shaw.

Clinical History. Abruptio placentae may occur during the later months of pregnancy or at the time of labor. In the former case the resulting external or concealed hemorrhage is soon followed by the onset of uterine contractions. Fortunately, in most cases the loss of blood is moderate, but if it is marked, the patient presents signs of acute anemia and passes into a condition of profound shock which may end fatally if delivery is not effected promptly. In many instances, the degree of shock is out of proportion to the amount of blood lost and, consequently, appears to be the result of some unknown factor, perhaps a type of intoxication, rather than of hemorrhage. For example, in the patient from whom Fig. 356 was obtained, the retroplacental hematoma did not contain more than 500 cc. of blood, yet the pulse was 140 when she was admitted to the service.

In concealed hemorrhage the first symptom often consists in intense, colic-like abdominal pain, and, on palpation, the uterus presents a board-like, almost ligneous consistency and no longer alternates between contraction and relaxation; consequently, the outlines of the child cannot be distinguished. Because the child is dead, auscultation gives negative results. Occasionally, the uterus gradually enlarges and eventually attains a size considerably larger than would normally correspond to the duration of the pregnancy. Particular attention should be paid to the pain and to the consistency of the uterus; signs of shock do not usually appear until later. Ligneus consistency of the uterus does not always develop, but in our experience its presence is pathognomonic. On the other hand, when the hemorrhage is external, the pain is less severe; there is little enlargement of the uterus, whose consistency may or may not be changed. In concealed hemorrhage the pain and shock are often attributed to other conditions, and the patient sometimes dies before the condition is diagnosed.

When abruptio placentae occurs at the time of labor—as the result of traction upon an abnormally short cord, or of the sudden partial emptying of the uterine cavity in twin pregnancy or hydramnios—the hemorrhage is usually external and the fetal heart sounds suddenly become imperceptible.

Diagnosis. In the absence of external bleeding, the occurrence of sharp abdominal pain associated with a uterus of ligneous consistency in a patient in the later months of pregnancy, is almost pathognomonic of concealed hemorrhage; the diagnosis becomes more definitely assured when the patient develops clinical signs of acute anemia with manifestations of shock. While the last-mentioned symptoms may follow the rupture of an advanced extra-uterine pregnancy, or the very exceptional spontaneous rupture of the uterus, such conditions can be excluded if the uterus presents the characteristic boardlike consistency.

When, however, the hemorrhage is external, the diagnosis is rendered practically positive by the failure to demonstrate the presence of a placenta previa on vaginal examination. It is, of course, sometimes impossible to exclude such rare accidents as rupture of the cord, or velamentous vessels, or the still more infrequent tear of the circular or marginal sinus of the placenta.

There is a group of patients with partial separation of the placenta, in whom the above mentioned characteristic findings are not so prominent and may even be lacking; in these the diagnosis may be extremely difficult. In certain of these patients it is not until after delivery that the diagnosis becomes clear, as shown by inspection of the placenta. This organ, in such cases, will usually be seen to have undergone detachment of a small area. As a general rule, where the placenta is implanted high in the uterus the area of separation is situated in the central portion, while in low implantation of the placenta the detachment takes place at or near the margin of the organ.

Prognosis. The prognosis depends in large measure upon the type of bleeding, whether external or internal, the degree of shock, and the amount of blood loss. That the type of bleeding is an important factor is brought out by numerous statistical studies, well exemplified by that of Irving who reported 234 cases with external, and 119 with internal hemorrhage, and a maternal death rate of only 1.7 per cent in the former as against 11.8 per cent in the latter. In the New York Lying-In Hospital, during the past 12 years the maternal mortality in those with external hemorrhage was 1.1 per cent, while in those with internal bleeding it was 9.1 per cent.

When the hemorrhage is external, the prognosis is dependent upon the amount of blood lost. It should always be remembered that in many cases the loss of blood is very moderate and the area of separation not great enough to interfere with the life of the child. Indeed, in not a few cases, the first intimation of the existence of the condition is the discovery of a depressed area upon the maternal surface of the placenta when examined after its extrusion. Not all cases, however, end so satisfactorily; in some the external hemorrhage indicates that blood has escaped from a large retroplacental hematoma which has slowly separated the membranes from the uterine wall.

Treatment. In the more serious forms, the life of the mother can be saved only by prompt evacuation of the uterus; only after the evacuation can the organ contract down and check the bleeding. On the other hand, when the separation is partial and the loss of blood but slight, the accident may be without serious significance. In the latter class of cases an expectant treatment should pursued, and labor allowed to take its natural course, interference being indicated only when the symptoms become urgent.

On the other hand, if the patient presents signs of acute hemorrhage, whether of the concealed or external variety, the uterus should be emptied with the least possible delay. If labor has not yet set in, abdominal cesarean section should be performed and the uterus retained or removed, according as it contracts satisfactorily or remains atonic. The same applies even if labor is already in progress, unless the cervix is partially dilated and an early vaginal delivery may be expected. Radical operative treatment is the more justified, for the reason that no one can predict to what extent the uterine muscle may be disorganized by hemorrhage; in some cases only the amputation of the uterus can prevent death from postpartum hemorrhage. At the same time it should be remembered that after cesarean section the great majority of uteri retract sufficiently rigorously to justify their retention without any danger of postpartum hemorrhage.

It should be stated, however, that conservative treatment, even in the concealed hemorrhage type, has given good results in the hands of several writers, particularly Irving and Couvelaire. The former reports a maternal mortality of only 2.9 per cent with conservative treatment, as compared with 14.5 per cent with cesarean section in premature separation of the normally implanted placenta with internal hemorrhage. Such conservative treatment consists mainly in rupture of the membranes, the use of a tight cervical and vaginal pack, and the application of an abdominal binder. Many authors advocate the use of multiple small doses of pituitrin because of its oxytocic properties.

No one treatment is applicable to all cases. As previously stated, we believe that cesarean section is the procedure of choice in the treatment of patients with uteroplacental apoplexy in the presence of a tetanically contracted uterus showing no signs of relaxation with the cervix not dilated to any appreciable extent. On the other hand, conservative methods are indicated in partial separation with slight or controllable bleeding. The extent to which labor has progressed is a determining factor in the type of treatment for all cases of abruptio placentae.

In 122 cases of abruptio managed in our clinic between 1935 and 1946 under the above policy, the incidence of cesarean section was 37.7 per cent. There was only one maternal death, in a patient who was admitted in extremis and who died undelivered.

In severely shocked patients, the state of shock should be treated by one or more blood transfusions before the cesarean section is performed. The operation should be done under local anesthesia if possible; sodium pentothal or cyclopropane are preferable to ether or chloroform. In any event, unless the condition of the patient is unusually satisfactory, blood should be transfused during and after the section. A certain number of women have been lost by failure to observe such precautions.

In some instances, following delivery through the natural passages, the tonicity of the uterus has been so impaired by the dissociation of its fibers by intramuscular hemorrhage that it fails to contract and retract during the third stage of labor and, as a result, profuse postpartum hemorrhage may follow. This possibility should always be borne in mind, and the operator should have in readiness the necessary materials for meeting the situation at a moment's notice. If, however, bleeding continues in spite of the usual treatment of postpartum hemorrhage, no time should be wasted in palliative expedients, but the abdomen should be opened at once and the uterus amputated. In such cases, the outlook is not so promising as if the uterus had been removed primarily.

The value of transfusion cannot be overemphasized. As soon as a patient is admitted to the hospital because of the history of bleeding or symptoms and signs suggesting premature separation of the placenta, one of the very first procedures should be to procure a suitable donor or blood from the blood bank. This procedure is of the first importance, irrespective of whether the obstetrical treatment to be followed is vaginal delivery or cesarean section.

In addition to shock and hemorrhage, one of the most feared complications of abruptio placentae is complete or partial anuria. Batizfalvy encountered it in 2.8 per cent of his cases and Goethals in 4 per cent. Its occurrence is restricted almost entirely to cases of concealed hemorrhage, and in 20 patients with abruptio placentae of this type, James Young found it in five patients, or 25 per cent. It may occur without antecedent toxemia of pregnancy, without antecedent blood transfusion, and without shock; these possible etiological factors play little or no role. Two types of renal lesions are found in these anuric cases of abruptio placentae. The first and less frequent is bilateral cortical necrosis. The other and more common is a lower nephron lesion affecting the second convoluted and collecting tubules associated with the generation of the epithelium and frequently causing the deposit of crystals of blood pigment in the tubules. This lower nephron lesion is similar to that encountered in fatal cases of crush injury, and, since in both abruptio placentae and crush injury there may be massive destruction of muscle, it is conceivable that the anuria occasionally seen in abruptio placentae may be due to toxic metabolites of tissue origin. It is an exceedingly grave complication with a maternal mortality in excess of 50 per cent. In the treatment chief reliance is placed on intravenous injections of hypertonic glucose solutions, but not infrequently all therapeutic measures fail.

BIBLIOGRAPHY

Aldridge, A. H., and Parks, T. J. End Results in 400 Cases of Placenta Previa. Am. J. Obst. & Gynec., 1938, 36:859.

Arnell, R. E., and Guerriero, W. F. The Management of Placenta Previa. With an Analysis of 260 Consecutive Cases. Am. J. Obst. & Gynec., 1940, 39:32.

Ball, R. P., and Golden, R. A Roentgenologic Sign for the Detection of Placenta Previa. Am. J. Obst. & Gynec., 1941, 42:530.

Bartholomew, R. A., Colvin, E. D., Grimes, W. H. Jr., and Fish, J. S. Facts Pertinent to a Rational Concept of Abruptio Placentae. Am. J. Obst. & Gynec., 1949, 57:69.

Batizfalvy, J. Pathologie und Chirurgische Therapie der mit uteroplacentarer Apoplexie einhergehenden vorzeitigen Placentalösung. Arch. f. Gynäk., 1937, 163:552.

Beck, Alfred C., and Light, Frank P. The Use of the X-ray in the Diagnosis of Placenta Previa. New York State J. Med., 1939, 39:1678.

Berkeley, C. Unavoidable Hemorrhage. J. Obst. & Gynaec. Brit. Emp., 1936, 43:393.

Bill, A. The Treatment of Placenta Previa by Prophylactic Blood Transfusion and Cesarean Section. Am. J. Obst. & Gynec., 1927, 14:523.

Bjerre, Hans. On the Roentgenological Diagnosis of Placenta Praevia. Acta obst. et gynec. Scandinavica, 1940, 20:47.

Brown, W. H., and Dippel, A. L. The Uses and Limitations of Soft Tissue Roentgenography in Placenta Previa and in Certain Other Obstetrical Conditions. Bull. Johns Hopkins Hosp., 1940, 66:90.

Browne, F. J., and Dodds, G. H. Further Experimental Observations on the Etiology of Accidental Hemorrhage and Placental Infarction. J. Obst. & Gynaec. Brit. Emp., 1928, 35:661.

Caldera, R. Placenta Praevia. A Review of 251 Cases. J. Obst. & Gynaec. Brit. Emp., 1939, 46:531.

Carvalho, M. A. A Study of 111 Cystograms for Diagnosis of Placenta Previa. Am. J. Obst. & Gynec., 1940, 39:306.

Chakraverti, J. Placenta Previa and Its Management in Indian Conditions. Ind. Med. Gaz., 1937, 72:9.

Couvelaire. Deux nouvelles observations d'apopléxie utéro-placentaire. Ann. de gynéc. et d'obst., 1912, 9:416.

Couvelaire, A., and Couvelaire, R. Apoplexies Utero-Placentaires. Gynéc. et Obst., 1937, 36:143.

Davis, M. Edward. Placenta Previa; Present-day Treatment. Collective Review. Surg., Gynec. & Obst., 1939, 68:504.

Dieckmann, W. J. Blood Chemistry and Renal Function in Abruptio Placentae. Am. J. Obst. & Gynec., 1936, 31:734.

Dippel, A. L., and Brown, W. H. Roentgen Visualization of the Placenta by Soft Tissue Technique. Am. J. Obst. & Gynec., 1940, 40:986.

Doranth, K. Statistiches über Placenta Previa. Ber. a. d. 2. geburtsh.-gynakol. Klin. in Wien, 1897, 1:77.

Eastman, N. J. Obstetric Hemorrhage. Internat. Clin., 1939, 3:264.

Essen-Möller, E. L'hémorrhage rétroplacentaire. Arch. mens. d'obst. et de gynéc., 1913, 4:145.

——— Quelques remarques sur le traitement du placenta praevia. Acta obst. et gynec. Scandinav., 1921, 1:1.

Findley, David. Management of Placenta Previa. An Analysis of 47,828 cases. Am. J. Obst. & Gynec., 1938, 36:267.

Gardiner, J. P. The Umbilical Cord. Surg., Gynec. & Obst., 1922, 34:252.

Goethals, T. R. Premature Separation of the Placenta. Am. J. Obst. & Gynec., 1928, 15:627.

Goodell, W. Concealed Accidental Hemorrhage of the Gravid Uterus. Am. J. Obst., 1870, 2:281.

Green-Armytage, V. B., and Dutta, H. K. Textbook of Midwifery in the Tropics. Calcutta, 1936, page 274.

Greenhill, J. P. The Increased Incidence of Fetal Abnormalities in Cases of Placenta Previa. Am. J. Obst. & Gynec., 1939, 37:624.

Gutierrez-Yepes, L., and Eastman, N. J. The Management of Placenta Previa. South. Med. Jour. 1946, 39:291.

HALL, S. C., CURRIN, F. W., and LYNCH, J. F. The Diagnostic Value of the X-ray in Placenta Previa. Am. J. Obst. & Gynec., 1937, 33:625.

HITSCHMANN, F. Die Therapie der Placenta Previa. S. Karger, Berlin, 1921.

HOFBAUER, J. Experimental Studies on the Toxemias of Pregnancy. Am. J. Obst. & Gynec., 1926, 12:159.

HOFMEIER, M. Ueber Placenta praevia. Verhandl. d. deutsch. Gesellsch. f. Gynäk., 1888, ii. 159-163.

——— Zur Entstehung der Placenta praevia. Ztschr. f. Geburtsh. u. Gynäk., 1894, 29:1.

HOLMES. Inversio Uteri Complicating Placental Praevia. Obstetrics, N. Y., 1899, 1:297.

——— Ablatio Placentae. Am. J. Obst., 1901, 44:753.

IRVING, F. C. Problems in Placenta Praevia. Surg., Gynec. & Obst., 1927, 45:834.

——— The Conservative Treatment of Premature Separation of the Normally Implanted Placenta. Am. J. Obst. & Gynec., 1937, 34:881.

——— Premature Separation of the Normally Implanted Placenta. Collective Review. Surg., Gyn., & Obst., 1938, 67:56.

JARCHO, J. Placenta Previa. Roentgen Diagnosis, Treatment and a Technic for Induction of Premature Labor. Am. J. Surg., 1940, 48:485.

JOHNSON, H. W. The Conservative Management of Some Varieties of Placenta Previa. Am. J. Obst. & Gynec., 1945, 50:248.

KALTENBACH, R. Zur Pathogenese der Placenta praevia. Ztschr. f. Geburtsh. u. Gynäk., 1890, 18:1.

KING, G., and CHUNG, D. The Treatment of Placenta Previa with Special Reference to the Use of Willett's Forceps, a Report on 134 Cases. Brit. M. J., 1945, 1:9.

LEY, G. Utero-placental (Accidental) Hemorrhage. J. Obst. & Gynaec. Brit. Emp., 1921, 28:69.

LIEPELT, M. Kritische Betrachtungen zur Frage der besten Placenta-praevia-Therapie. Arch. f. Gynäk., 1938, 167:52.

MACAFEE, C. H. G. Placenta Praevia—A Study of 174 Cases. J. Obst. & Gynaec. Brit. Emp., 1945, 52:313.

McDOWELL, J. F. Cystographic Diagnosis of Placenta Previa. Am. J. Obst. & Gynec., 1937, 33:436.

McKELVEY, John L. Vascular Lesions in the Decidua Basalis. Am. J. Obst. & Gynec., 1939, 38:815.

McNAIR, A. J. Concealed Accidental Hemorrhage with Intraperitoneal Bleeding. Proc. Roy. Soc. Med., 1917, 10:13.

MOIR, Chassar. Fallacies in Soft Tissue Placentography. Am. J. Obst. & Gynec., 1944, 47:198.

MORSE, A. H. Premature Separation of the Normally Implanted Placenta. Surg., Gynec. & Obst., 1918, 26:133.

MORTON, Daniel G. Anatomic Description of a Case of Marginal Placenta Previa. With a Discussion of the Etiologic Implications. Am. J. Obst. & Gynec., 1937, 33:547.

MÜLLER, W. Placenta Previa. Stuttgart, 1877.

NEUMANN, H. O. Zur Pathologie u. Klinik der Placentarverwachsung bei Placenta Praevia. Arch. f. Gynaek., 1923, 119:320.

PAGLIARI, M. Considerazioni Cliniche sur una Centuria di Casi di Placenta Previa Centrale e Marginale, Ginecologia, 1935, 1:537.

PICARDI, M. Sulla Patogenesi del distacco intempestivo della placenta normalmente inserta con speciale riguardo alla intossicazione da solfuro di carbonio. Ginecologia, Torino, 1936, 2:1039.

PINARD, A. De la rupture prématurée, dite spontanée, des membranes, etc. Ann. d'obst. et de gynéc., 1886, 25:171, 321.

——— et VARNIER, H. Décollement prématuré par brièvete du cordon du placenta normalement inséré. Études d'anat., obst., 1892, p. 57.

PORTES, L. Contribution à l'Étude de l'Apoplexie Utéro-Placentaire. Gynéc. et obst., 1923, 7:56.

PRENTISS, R. J., and TUCKER, W. W. Cystography in the Diagnosis of Placenta Previa. Am. J. Obst. & Gynec., 1939, 37:777.

REYCRAFT, J. L., and PLATZ, C. P. Incidence of Placenta Previa During a Ten-year Period at Cleveland Maternity Hospital. Am. J. Obst. & Gynec., 1942, 44:509.

RIGBY. An Essay on the Uterine Haemorrhage which Precedes the Delivery of the Full-grown Foetus. London, 1776.

SIEGEL, I. A. A Study of Results in 332 Consecutive Cases of Placenta Previa. Am. J. Obst. & Gynec., 1940, 39:301.

SNOW, W., and POWELL, C. B. Roentgen Visualization of the Placenta. Am. J. Roentgenol., 1934, 31:37.

SNOW, W., and ROSENSOHN, M. Roentgenologic Visualization of the Soft Tissues in Pregnancy. Am. J. Roentgen. & Radium Therapy, 1939, 42:709.

STEVENSON, C. S. X-ray Visualization of the Placenta: Experiences with Soft-tissue and Cystographic Techniques in the Diagnosis of Placenta Previa. Am. J. Obst. & Gynec., 1949, 58:15.

STRASSMANN, P. Placenta Previa. Arch. f. Gynäk., 1902, 67:112.

TARNIER et BUDIN, P. Hémorrhagie par insertion vicieuse du placenta. Traité de l'art des accouchements, 1898, T. III, pp. 571-659.

UDE, W. H., WEUM, T. W., and URNER, J. A. Roentgenologic Diagnosis of Placenta Previa; Report of Case. Am. J. Roentgenol., 1934, 31:230.

UDE, W. H., and URNER, J. A. Roentgenologic Diagnosis of Placenta Previa. Am. J. Obst. & Gynec., 1935, 29:667.

WATSON, B. P., and GUSBERG, S. B. The Treatment of Placenta Previa, Bagging versus Cesarean Section. Am. J. Obst. & Gynec., 1943, 46:524.

WILLETT, J. A. The Treatment of Placenta Praevia by Continuous Weight Traction—A Report of Seven Cases. Proc. Roy. Soc. Med., 1925, 18:90.

WILLIAMS, J. T. The Expectant Management of Placenta Previa. Am. J. Obst. & Gynec., 1948, 55:169.

WILLIAMS, J. W. Premature Separation of the Normally Implanted Placenta. Surg., Gynec. & Obst., 1915, 21:541-554.

——— Further Observations Concerning Premature Separation of the Normally Implanted Placenta. J. Obst. & Gynaec. Brit. Emp., 1925, 32:259-279.

WILSON, R. A. Placenta Previa. The Results of the Treatment of 102 Cases Occurring in 16,310 Consecutive Deliveries. Am. J. Obst. and Gynec., 1934, 27:713.

YOUNG, J. Discussion on the Pathological Features of Cortical Necrosis of the Kidney and Allied Conditions Associated with Pregnancy. Proc. Roy. Soc. Med. Sect. Obst. & Gynaec., 1949, 42:375.

24

COMPLICATIONS DUE TO DISEASES AND ABNORMALITIES OF THE GENERATIVE TRACT

DISEASES OF THE VULVA, VAGINA AND CERVIX

Varices. Varicose veins sometimes appear in the lower part of the vagina but are more common around the vulva, where they may attain considerable proportions and give rise to a sensation of weight and discomfort. Treatment has practically no effect upon the local condition. In rare instances the varices may rupture during pregnancy, although this accident is more frequently observed at the time of labor when, especially in vaginal varicosities, profuse and sometimes fatal hemorrhage may result if appropriate surgical treatment is not available.

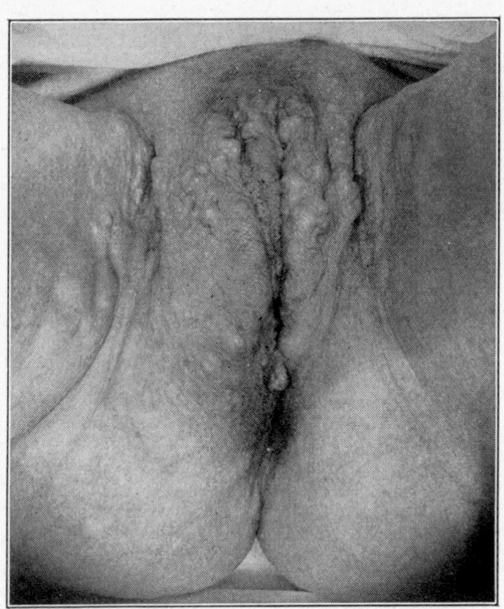

Fig. 359.—Varicosities of Vulva.

Inflammation of Bartholin's Glands. The gonococcus may gain access to Bartholin's glands and give rise to abscess formation. In this event the labium majus on the side affected becomes swollen and painful and incloses a collection of pus. Most often the infection is gonorrheal in origin, although other bacteria are sometimes secondarily associated with the gonococcus. Aside from the pain and discomfort, this complication may be the starting-point of a puerperal infection. For these reasons, whenever a labial abscess develops during pregnancy it should be opened and drained, or, better still, in the first seven months of pregnancy the entire pus sac should be excised. Owing to the increased vascularity incident to the inflammatory process, as well as pregnancy, enucleation is sometimes accompanied by considerable loss of blood and is not always easy.

The treatment of Bartholin's duct cysts, which are frequently the sequels to abscesses, is best left until after delivery. They are usually of small size and therefore are not the cause of dystocia. Occasionally a large labial cyst is seen, of sufficient size to be the source of trouble at delivery; in this case aspiration with syringe and small needle will suffice as a temporary measure, while operative removal, if necessary, may be postponed till later.

Condylomata. As the result of gonorrhea, syphilis, or other irritation, condylomata are sometimes observed on the vulva or about the introitus. Condylomata lata (Fig. 361) are small, flat, and highly infectious; the treponema pallidum of syphilis is usually present on darkfield examination. Occasionally, the condylomata acuminata attain immense proportions, as shown in Fig. 360, but rarely cause serious dystocia.

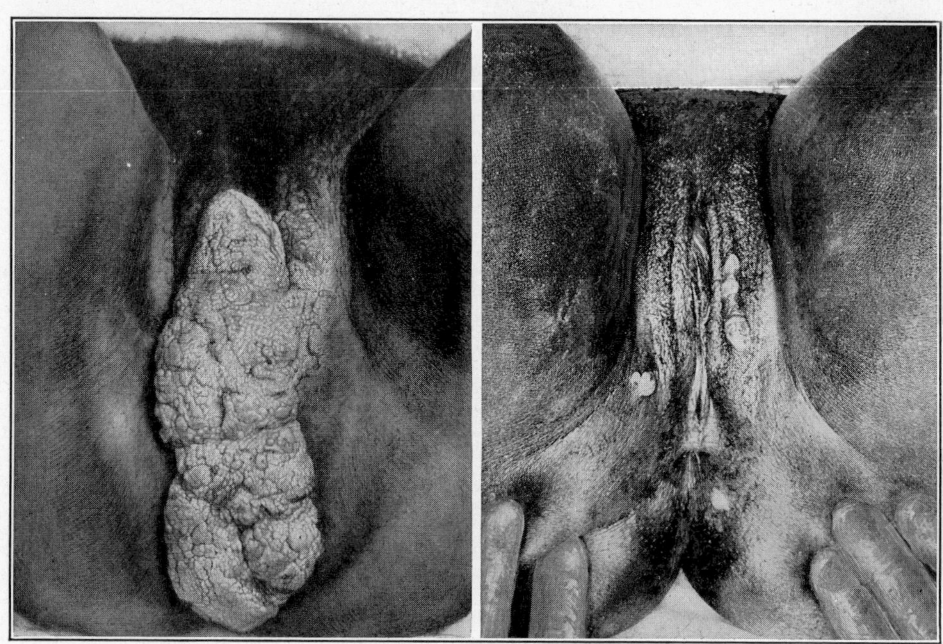

FIG. 360. FIG. 361.

FIG. 360.—CONDYLOMATA OF VULVA, TREATED BY FULGURATION AND EXCISION DURING PREGNANCY, NORMAL LABOR.

FIG. 361.—CONDYLOMATA LATA, ANNULAR LESIONS OF SECONDARY SYPHILIS.

If the patient is seen several months prior to the end of pregnancy they should be removed by excision and fulguration. If not seen until the time of labor, hemorrhage from tears in the base of the condylomata may be anticipated, but often the vulva is pushed aside by the descending head and no difficulty develops. Cesarean section is not indicated unless there is extensive scar formation.

Relaxation of the Vaginal Outlet. Even in nulliparous women the congestion incident to pregnancy frequently causes the anterior or posterior vaginal wall to protrude through the vulva as a redundant mass, while in multiparous women, particularly when the outlet is torn or relaxed, a distinct cystocele or rectocele may result. This condition is generally associated with dragging pains in the back and lower abdomen, and may interfere with locomotion. It is not amenable to treatment during pregnancy although the symptoms may be temporarily relieved by rest in bed.

Vaginitis. This complication will be considered in a later section under the heading of gonorrhea and other infections.

Vaginal Tumors. Vaginal cysts, the most frequent of benign vaginal tumors, may be discovered during a pregnancy or sometimes not until the time of labor. Such cysts, usually of the inclusion or the rest (Gartner's or müllerian) types, may be of sufficient size to cause serious dystocia. Treatment depends upon the size and location of the cyst as well as the time at which the tumor is first recognized. Drainage or excision may be necessary; in other cases it may be more advisable to postpone treatment until after delivery and the puerperium. The treatment of vaginal cysts, as well as other vaginal tumors, is discussed in a subsequent section on dystocia.

Endocervicitis. Gonorrheal infection of the cervical canal is frequently observed during pregnancy, the most prominent symptom being a profuse and persistent leukorrhea. The treatment will be considered in Chapter 28.

Carcinoma. Carcinoma of the cervix in pregnancy is sufficiently uncommon that statistics on its incidence vary widely. In 41,457 pregnancies observed at the New York Hospital cervical carcinoma occurred 3 times, or once in every 14,000 cases. The incidence of the condition at the Chicago Lying-In Hospital, as reported by Willson, is once in every 6,620 deliveries. A survey of the literature by W. C. Danforth, however, indicated a higher frequency, namely, once in every 3,100 pregnancies. The actual incidence of the complication probably lies somewhere between the two extremes cited, possibly once in every 7,000 pregnancies or so. It is most common in gravidae between the thirtieth and fortieth years of life, about two thirds of the cases occurring within this decade. Most of the patients have had previous pregnancies. It is extremely rare to observe carcinoma of the cervix in a primigravida, while on the other hand the greatest incidence is in those who have given birth four or five times.

In the majority of instances the condition has existed before conception, but it may make its appearance during pregnancy. A bloody, foul-smelling vaginal discharge is suggestive of malignant disease, but unfortunately the early stages are often unaccompanied by symptoms and may escape detection unless a vaginal examination is made for some other reason; an indurated and excavated ulceration of the cervix is discovered.

It is common experience that this malignant disease influences pregnancy very unfavorably, abortion being noted in 30 to 40 per cent of the cases. Furthermore, if the patient reaches full term the dangers of labor are greatly increased. In the first place, the presence of the ulcerating crater affords opportunity for the access of pyogenic bacteria to the uterine cavity, while the cervix may be so indurated by carcinomatous infiltration that dilatation becomes impossible and spontaneous rupture of the lower uterine segment becomes imminent, unless suitable operative measures are undertaken to prevent it. In other instances, the cervix may be lacerated and give rise to profuse hemorrhage. It should be noted also that the general mortality in the second half of pregnancy is markedly higher and the relative cures over a five-year period of time are fewer in this group of patients. The explanation of these results seems to lie in the fact that the majority of these lesions existed before the onset of pregnancy and were overlooked.

Although it used to be believed that pregnancy accelerates the growth of cervical carcinoma, the more recent evidence refutes this old idea. Thus, Peller, after demonstrating that the relative number of carcinomas occurring during pregnancy was significantly less than the number occurring in similar age groups in the nonpregnant, concluded that pregnancy not only increases the resistance to cancer, but raises the average age of its occurrence and retards its progress. Experimental evidence advanced by Emge likewise indicates that pregnancy does not favor the growth of genital carcinoma.

In regard to diagnosis, any persistent bleeding in pregnancy should call to mind the possibility of cervical carcinoma. While the vast majority of such cases of bleeding are due to threatened abortion, it must be emphasized that the prolonged management of bleeding gravidae on this assumption and without palpation and inspection of the cervix is dangerous and may sooner or later lead to an overlooked cancer. Upon inspection of the cervix, any suspicious area of induration or any lesion which bleeds should be biopsied. An extensive experience in our clinic with cervical biopsy in pregnancy, as well as the reports of many others, shows that this procedure does not cause abortion. An accurate pathological diagnosis by an observer who is familiar with the microscopic picture of the normal cervix in gestation is essential. This has become especially true since attention has been focused on the significance of *carcinoma in situ,* or "non-invasive carcinoma" of the cervix. Not infrequently the physiologic changes which the cervix undergoes in pregnancy simulate those of carcinoma in situ; and, in general, a positive diagnosis in gravidae should only be made in the presence of a clearly invasive process.

The prognosis of carcinoma of the cervix in pregnancy, when properly treated, appears to be about the same as that in the nonpregnant. Five of Emge's 6 cases and 3 of the 4 cases reported by Richman and Goodfriend, survived more than 5 years. Maino and Mussey reported a 30 per cent 5-year survival rate in 20 cases treated at the Mayo Clinic.

The treatment of carcinoma of the cervix in a pregnant woman is essentially the same as that employed in the nonpregnant individual with this condition. If the diagnosis is made in the first half of pregnancy, x-ray radiation followed by radium is the method of treatment pursued. As abortion almost inevitably follows as a result of this treatment, no serious consideration need be given to the fetus. If, however, for some reason or other abortion does not occur within three or four weeks after completion of the radiation therapy, it becomes necessary that the pregnancy be terminated by miniature section, because of the unfavorable effects of the x-ray radiation on the fetus. These effects are in the form of brain damage which sometimes results in microcephaly. As emphasized by Jones and Neill, however, such injuries are much more frequent when the irradiation is administered before the twentieth week of gestation. Thus, in 3 cases of carcinoma of the cervix complicating pregnancy in which these authors applied radium to the cervix before the end of the fifth month, 2 yielded microcephalic infants, whereas in 5 cases treated similarly after the fifth month, no infants developed microcephaly. Goldstein and Murphy, nevertheless, have reported 1 case in which the application of radium to the cervix at the sixth month resulted in a microcephalic child. Therefore, to prevent the birth of a microcephalic infant, it would seem advisable to carry out abdominal hysterotomy in all cases of cervical cancer in pregnancy in which irradiation has been given before the twenty-fourth week and in which spontaneous abortion has not occurred after several weeks.

Should the pregnancy be advanced beyond the sixth month and the offspring, though alive, be still nonviable, it would appear that the best treatment consists of radium application, in adequate dosage, to the cervix as soon as the diagnosis is established, followed at an appropriate time after viability has been reached, by cesarean section. Further irradiation, in the form of deep x-ray, may then be given soon after delivery. Danforth, on the other hand, recommends moderate radium dosage to check the growth of the carcinoma in order that the child may attain viability with less chance of injury and then be delivered by cesarean section. He prefers, following the section, a radical or subtotal hysterectomy with irradiation of the cervical stump. Maino and Mussey found that in cases with operable lesions total abdominal hysterectomy gave the best results.

Finally, if the malignancy of the cervix is not recognized until the last month or two of gestation, cesarean section may be performed, a procedure which need not necessitate delay in radium and x-ray treatment to the cervical lesion. It should be stressed that under no circumstances should the patient with carcinoma of the cervix be allowed to deliver a viable or full-term child per vaginam; the dilatation of the cervix occurring with labor is contraindicated because of the danger of trauma, hemorrhage, or extension of the growth.

DEVELOPMENTAL ABNORMALITIES OF THE UTERUS

Abnormalities in the development or fusion of one or both müllerian ducts may result in malformations which sometimes possess an obstetrical significance. Various degrees of malformation—from an almost total absence of the uterus on the one hand to its duplication on the other (uterus didelphys)—are encountered. The accompanying diagrams (Figs. 362 and 363) give an idea of the nature of the more important varieties.

Pregnancy may be associated with any one of these malformations, provided an ovum is cast off from the ovaries and no serious obstacle be opposed to the upward passage of the spermatozoa and their subsequent union with it.

Pregnancy in the Rudimentary Horn of a Double Uterus. In this condition the course of pregnancy is exposed to serious deviations from the normal. In 78 per cent of the 84 cases collected from the literature by Kehrer in 1900, the proximal end of the rudimentary horn did not communicate with the uterine cavity so that pregnancy must have followed external migration of the spermatozoa or of the fertilized ovum.

The development of pregnancy in a rudimentary horn is associated with the formation of a decidua in the nonpregnant horn, as well as by a marked increase in size. Unless there is free communication between the two horns, which is but rarely the case, a pregnancy in this situation is a very serious occurrence since normal delivery is impossible. If the muscular tissue of the rudimentary horn is poorly developed, as is usually the case, spontaneous rupture occurs within the first four months and may lead to the death of the patient from intraperitoneal hemorrhage. This result was noted in 87, 47.6, and 5.5 per cent of the cases collected by Sänger, Kehrer, and Beckmann, respectively, in 1884, 1900, and 1911. The marked improvement is attributable to greater accuracy in diagnosis and more frequent recourse to operative interference. On the other hand, if the muscular tissue is abundant, the pregnant horn may hypertrophy normally and the pregnancy go on to term. In such cases, the fetus, if not removed by operative means, may be gradually eliminated by suppurative processes or be converted into a lithopedion.

The existence of pregnancy in a rudimentary horn can occasionally be recognized during the early months, a positive diagnosis having been made in 20 per cent of Kehrer's cases. When a tumor corresponding in size to the duration of pregnancy can be detected alongside of what appears to be the slightly enlarged uterus, this condi-

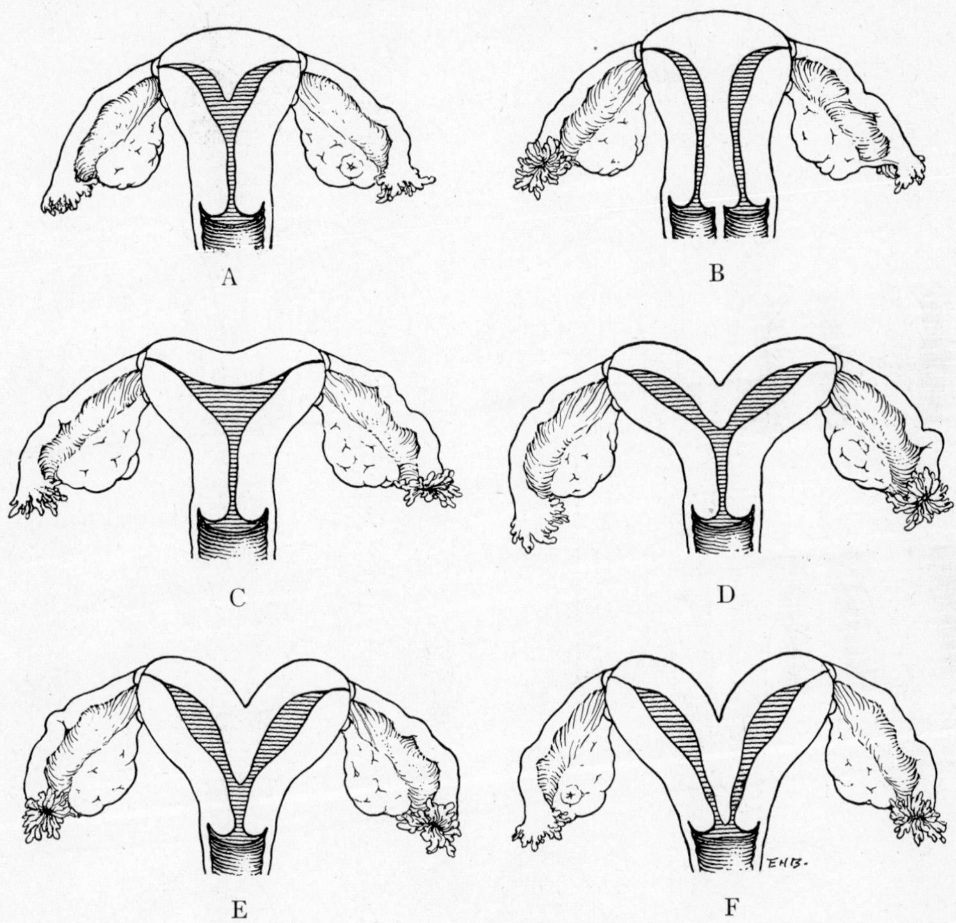

Fig. 362.—Developmental Abnormalities of the Uterus.

A. Uterus subseptus unicollis.
B. Uterus septus duplex, double vagina.
C. Uterus arcuatus.
D. Uterus bicornis unicollis.
E. Uterus bicornis subseptus.
F. Uterus bicornis septus.

tion should always be thought of. In differentiating it from a tubal pregnancy, it is important to remember that the round ligament is felt coming off from the distal side of the tumor instead of from its proximal or uterine portion, as in the latter condition. In the later months, a diagnosis is usually not made until false labor sets in at term. In other cases this does not occur and the child dies, but, in either event, no abnormality is suspected until one attempts to empty the uterus, when it is found that its cavity is empty and that the child lies in a sac to one side of it, which must represent

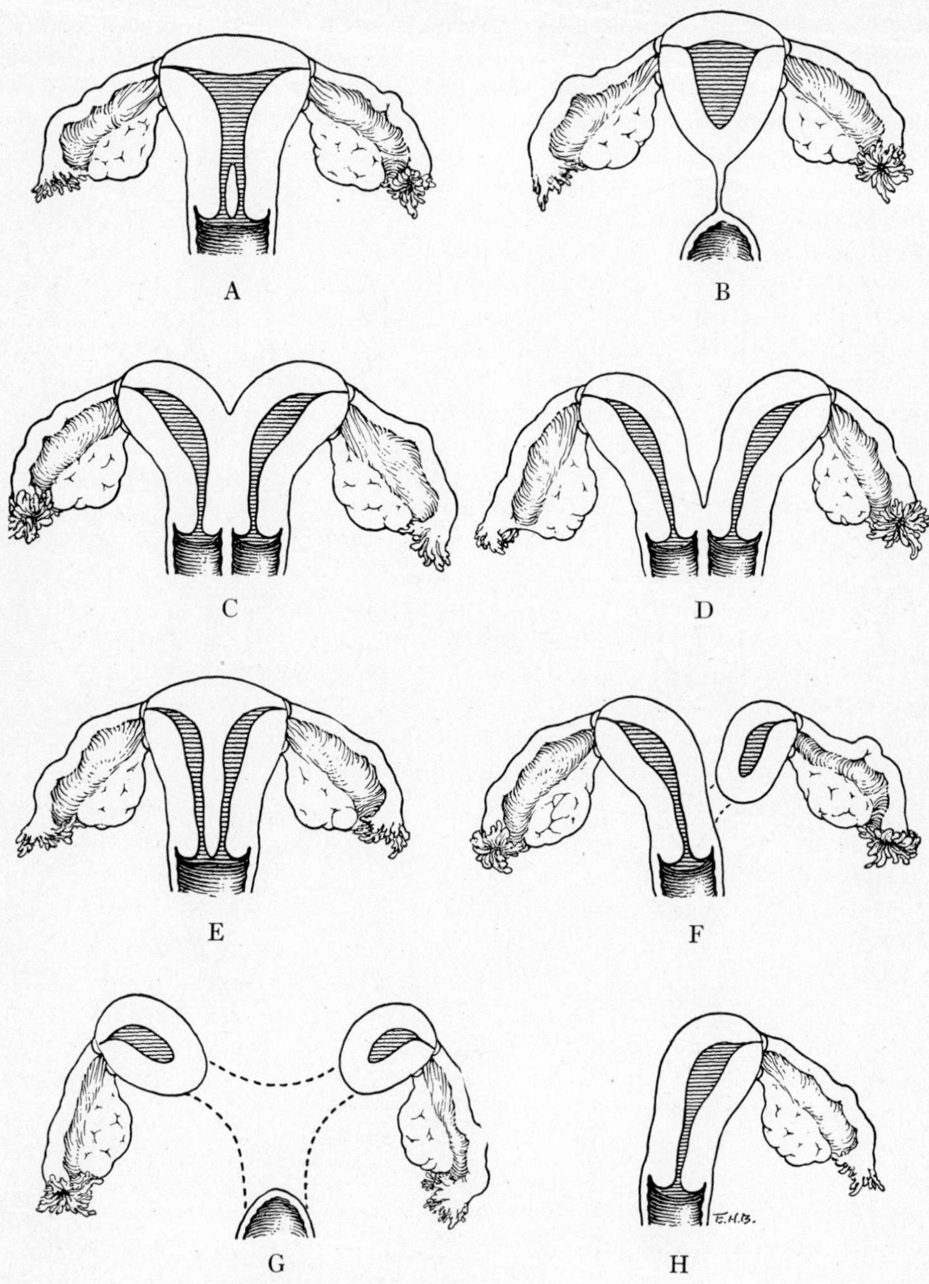

FIG. 363.—DEVELOPMENTAL ABNORMALITIES OF THE UTERUS.

A. Uterus biforis supra simplex.
B. Partial gynatresia.
C. Uteris bicornis duplex, double vagina.
D. Uterus didelphys, double vagina.
E. Uterus septus duplex.
F. Uterus bicornis unicollis, one rudimentary horn.
G. Uterus didelphys, two rudimentary horns; gynatresia.
H. Uterus unicornis.

either a pregnant tube or a rudimentary horn. A satisfactory differentiation can frequently be made by determining the location of the round ligament as just described.

Treatment. When the condition is diagnosed, treatment consists in promptly opening the abdomen and amputating the pregnant horn. This operation was first performed by Sänger, in 1884, and has since been repeated on many occasions with constantly improving results; Kehrer and Wells reported 44 cases up to 1900, and Beckmann a large series in 1911, with mortalities of 13.4 and 4.3 per cent, respectively. Too frequently, however, the first suggestion of the existence of the abnormality is afforded by the symptoms of intraperitoneal hemorrhage, when the operation is undertaken in the expectation of finding a ruptured extra-uterine pregnancy.

Pregnancy in Uterus Unicornis. Occasionally only one horn of the uterus is developed, the opposite tube and ovary being lacking or arising from the lower portion of the uterus. In such cases pregnancy usually pursues an uneventful course and the abnormality is only accidentally recognized at the operating or autopsy table.

Pregnancy in Uterus Bicornis. When the two horns of the uterus are well developed but no connection exists between them, as in uterus didelphys, or when they are partly fused, as in the various varieties of uterus bicornis, pregnancy may occur in either horn. In the very rare instances in which a twin pregnancy is observed, the two products of conception may occupy the same horn, although now and again a fetus may be found in each, as in several of our cases.

When pregnancy occurs in one horn of a bicornuate uterus, the other horn undergoes sympathetic hypertrophy and a distinct decidua is formed in its cavity. Ordinarily there is no interference with the course of pregnancy, and spontaneous labor may be looked for. Much more rarely, the nonpregnant horn may block the pelvic cavity and give rise to dystocia similar to that produced by tumors of other origin. In a case reported by Bettman, the nonpregnant horn obstructed the pelvic cavity and gave rise to rupture of the uterus.

Miller, in 1922, analyzed the clinical histories of 54 cases reported in the literature. That the abnormality does not interfere with the possibility of conception is shown by the fact that 31 of the 34 married women conceived and had 67 pregnancies. It does, however, predispose toward the occurrence of abortion and premature labor; only 61 per cent of the pregnancies went to term. When difficulty was encountered at the time of labor, it was usually due to mechanical interference by the enlarged nonpregnant horn. Uterine inertia is also common.

The diagnosis is usually not made; the uneventful course of pregnancy affords no indication for careful exploration and in most patients spontaneous labor occurs at term. Sometimes the existence of a double vagina or a double cervix puts one on the alert. The former may occur with a normal uterus, whereas the latter condition almost invariably indicates the existence of a double uterus. When there is only a single cervix, as in uterus bicornis unicollis, the condition always escapes observation, unless the patient is subjected to examination at an early period of pregnancy and the depression noted between the two halves of the uterus gives a clue to the true state of affairs.

Falls has recently emphasized the increased incidence of complications accompanying pregnancy in a uterus arcuatus, a form of bicornuate uterus in which normal fusion is almost complete. He finds this type of bicornuate uterus to be associated with increased frequency of prematurity, postmaturity, prolonged first stage of labor, abnormal presentations, intra-uterine death of the fetus and retained placenta.

The occurrence of abortion is definitely increased in patients with uterine malformations, Findley reporting an incidence of 39.6 per cent and Schauffler one of 53 per cent. Taylor, in a recent review of the literature, places the incidence at about 25 per cent.

Diverticulum from Uterine Cavity. Freund and Schickele have reported instances in which the pregnancy developed in a diverticulum from the uterine cavity, so that the fetus lay in a sac surrounded by uterine muscle, and connected with the main uterine cavity only by a narrow passage. It is apparent that such a condition would escape clinical recognition, unless the fingers were introduced into the uterine cavity, and also that it might give rise to serious complications at the time of labor.

A much more common complication is due to a sacculation or to a considerable variation in the thickness and consistency of the uterine walls. In such circumstances, the sacculation may be mistaken for a tumor of ovarian or other origin and the abdomen opened for its removal.

DISPLACEMENT OF THE UTERUS

Anteflexion. Exaggerated degrees of anteflexion are frequently observed in the early months of pregnancy but are usually without significance. In the later months, particularly when the pelvis is markedly contracted or the abdominal walls are very lax, the uterus may fall forward; the sagging occasionally is so exaggerated that the fundus lies considerably below the lower margin of the symphysis pubis. Even in less marked instances of the so-called *pendulous abdomen,* the patient may complain of various annoyances, more especially of exhaustion on exertion and dragging pains in the back and lower abdomen. Amelioration of symptoms frequently follows the wearing of a properly fitting abdominal support.

Anteversion. Anteversion of the pregnant uterus is occasionally observed in patients who have previously been subjected to operative procedures for the relief of symptoms incident to retroflexion of the uterus, particularly after vaginal fixation, less frequently after an improperly performed ventrosuspension, and now and again after shortening of the round ligaments. The condition is accompanied by marked discomfort during pregnancy and at the time of labor may give rise to serious dystocia, which will be considered in the section on Dystocia Due to Abnormalities of the Generative Tract.

Retrodisplacement of the Pregnant Uterus. Retroflexion and retroversion of the uterus are frequently observed in nonpregnant women, and may exist for years without any abnormal manifestation. In pregnancy several eventualities are possible: the displacement may undergo spontaneous reduction without any interruption of pregnancy, the outcome in the vast majority of cases; abortion may occur; or, if neither of the preceding takes place, the uterus may become incarcerated in the pelvic cavity and serious consequences follow.

If the displaced uterus is not adherent, spontaneous reduction usually occurs during the third month. This is rendered possible by an eccentric hypertrophy, as a result of which the anterior wall undergoes more rapid distention than does the posterior and, emerging above the superior strait, eventually draws up the rest of the organ. After the fundus has passed the promontory of the sacrum there is no fear of a recurrence of the condition. Moreover, spontaneous reduction is not wholly out of the question even when adhesions exist, since they often become stretched and occasionally disappear without treatment.

In rare instances when the fundus is firmly adherent, pregnancy may remain uninterrupted for a long while. This prolongation is rendered possible by the hypertrophy occurring almost entirely in the anterior wall of the uterus, while the posterior wall fills out the pelvic cavity and forms a sac in which one pole of the fetus is re-

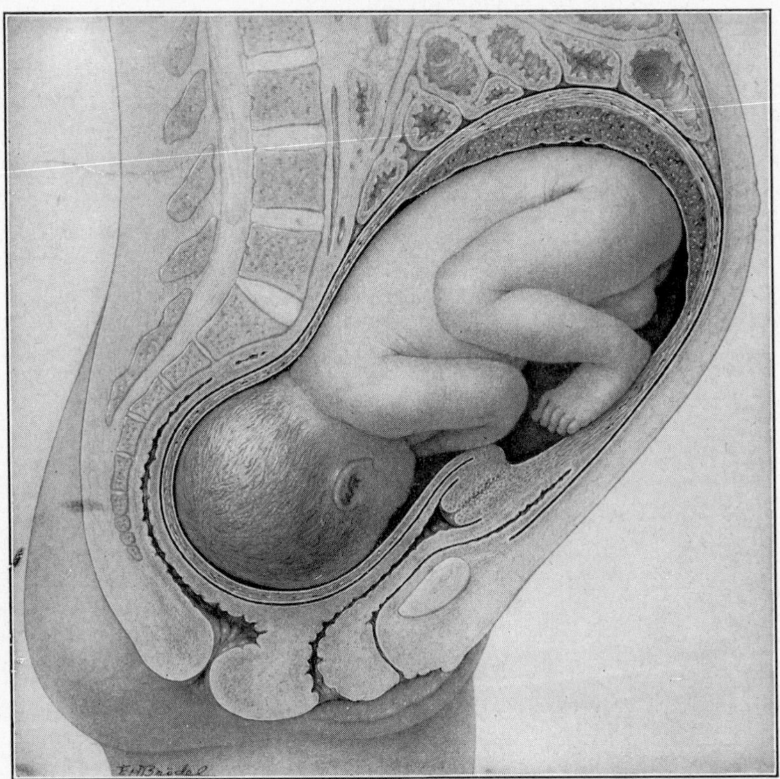

Fig. 364.—Posterior Sacculation of a Retroflexed Pregnant Uterus.

tained. This so-called *sacculation of the uterus* has been described in detail by Oldham, Dührssen, and others. Owing to the abnormal position of the cervix and the fact that the presenting part lies far below it, serious difficulties are to be expected at the time of labor; these will be considered in Chapter 32. (See Figs. 364 and 365.)

Since abortion occurs in 10 per cent of all pregnancies and since retroversion is also an extremely common condition, the mathematical chances of the former occurring now and then in the presence of the latter are very good. That any causal relationship exists between retroversion and abortion, however, is most dubious. Thus, Brackett has studied 54 cases in which retroversion of the uterus was demonstrable before the fourth month and has compared their courses with 325 cases in which the uterus was in normal position at the fourth month. The incidence of abortion in the women with retroverted uteri was 11.6 per cent; in the control group it was 13.6 per cent. In none of the 54 cases of retroversion did incarceration occur.

If pregnancy continues and the displacement is not reduced in the natural course of events, or as the result of manipulations on the part of the physician, the uterus will continue to increase in size until it completely fills the pelvic cavity and, being unable to free itself, becomes impacted, and we have what is known as *incarceration.* If this occurs, it does not take place until the thirteenth to the seventeenth week; it is, moreover, a rare complication, being observed perhaps once in every two or three thousand pregnancies. Incarceration is accompanied by characteristic symptoms; the

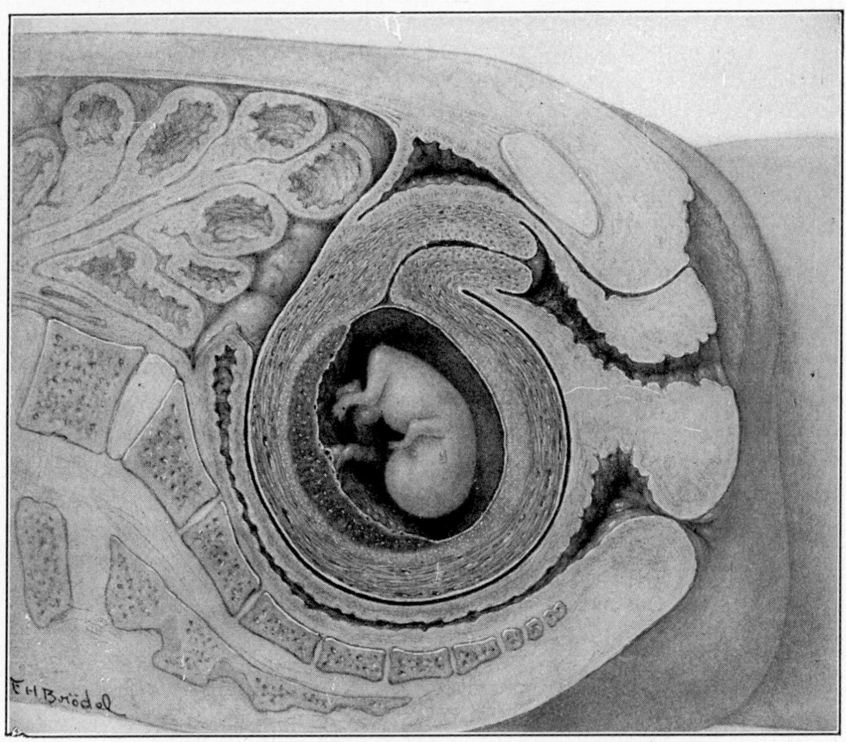

Fig. 365.—Incarceration of Retroflexed Pregnant Uterus.

woman complains of pain in the lower portion of the abdomen and back, and of disturbances in the functions of the urethra, bladder, and rectum. As the pelvis becomes more and more filled by the growing uterus, the pressure upon the neck of the bladder and urethra becomes so pronounced as to cause retention of the urine with consequent overdistention. When the retention has reached a certain limit, the overstretched viscus squeezes out small amounts of urine at frequent intervals, but never empties itself—*paradoxical incontinence.* If the condition is not soon relieved, the symptoms become more intense, cystitis develops, the bladder walls become thick and edematous, the urine becomes bloody, and eventually gangrene may result, necrotic portions of the lining membrane of the bladder being cast off and finally expelled through the urethra with severe cramplike pains. In other cases the weakened walls of the bladder are unable to withstand the distention and rupture occurs, followed by a fatal peritonitis.

Occasionally, as the result of the pressure to which the organ is subjected, the nutrition of the uterus may so suffer that the organ offers little resistance to bacterial invasion, after which it becomes densely adherent to the surrounding parts. Now and again the organ may be forced down and out of the pelvic cavity and emerge through the vulva or anus. In some cases the rectum is compressed to such an extent that defecation becomes impossible and gangrene results. Ileus, however, is an exceedingly rare complication.

Gottschalk found that the following were the most frequent causes of death in 67 cases reported in the literature:

Peritonitis of vesical origin	17
Uremia	16
Rupture of the bladder	11
Septicemia of vesical origin	4
Gangrene of the bladder	3

The possibility of a retroflexed pregnant uterus should always be suspected when a woman in the early months of pregnancy complains for any length of time of frequent micturition or retention, especially if there is a history of antecedent uterine trouble. Incontinence of urine during the first half of pregnancy is a most suggestive sign and always calls for a thorough vaginal examination. With the bimanual method, the soft body of the uterus will be found occupying the pelvic cavity, while the cervix is forced up against the symphysis or lies above it, according as one has to deal with a retroflexion or retroversion. It should be remembered that a pregnant tube lying behind the uterus may give somewhat similar signs, and this possibility should be borne in mind until careful examination has shown that the enlarged uterus does not lie in front of the soft mass.

Treatment. Since (1) the retroverted pregnant uterus almost always undergoes spontaneous restitution before the twelfth week, (2) this condition rarely causes abortion, (3) there is no danger of incarceration before the thirteenth to the seventeenth week, the presence of retroversion in the first trimester of pregnancy is a matter of no concern. No treatment is indicated; however the recommendation is made that the patient assume the knee-chest position night and morning. In the rare instance in which the retroposition persists until after the twelfth week, an attempt may be made to replace the uterus with the patient in knee-chest position and, if necessary, with the aid of traction on the cervix with a vulsellum forceps. If the procedure is successful, the uterus, because of its size at this stage of pregnancy, will usually be held up by the promontory of the sacrum and remain there. To test this, however, the patient should be examined again in a day or two; if the uterus has fallen back, it should be kept in position for a few weeks by a pessary. If the attempt at reposition is not successful the patient is advised to assume the knee-chest position for ten minutes four times daily, to report at once any slight bladder symptoms, and to return again in a week for examination and another attempt at reposition. In the absence of bladder symptoms, attempts at reposition under anesthesia or operative interference are not recommended because of the great likelihood of restitution taking place in ample time, either spontaneous or manipulative.

In the presence of incarceration, hospitalization and prompt treatment are imperative. The bladder should be catheterized immediately and the catheter allowed to remain in place. Because of the elongation and displacement of the urethra and neck of the bladder, a flexible rubber catheter should be used; if difficulty is encountered, its introduction may be facilitated by traction on the cervix with a tenaculum. With the patient in knee-chest position, an attempt at reposition is then made. If unsuccessful, there is no hurry about operative intervention (with the catheter in place). The knee-chest position is assumed by the patient for ten minutes every two or three hours for three or four days with daily attempts at reposition. If at the end of this time, the position is still uncorrected (a very rare contingency), abdominal operation is indicated. This consists of freeing any adhesions about the uterus and of lifting the uterus out of the pelvis into proper position.

Lateral Displacement of the Pregnant Uterus. Slight degrees of lateral displacement of the uterus during pregnancy are relatively frequent but usually have no effect upon its course and do not give rise to symptoms. It should, however, be borne in mind that in the early months similar conditions are sometimes mistaken for tubal pregnancy.

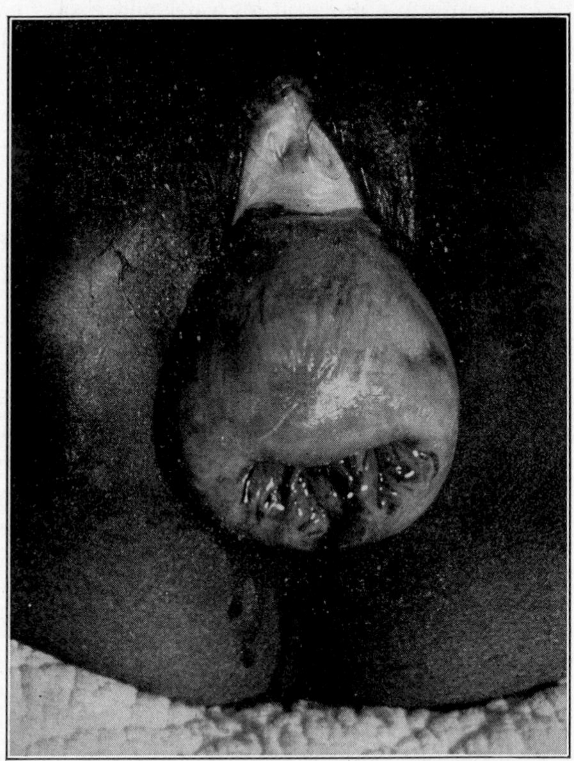

Fig. 366.—Prolapse of Cervix in Pregnancy.

Note extreme edema.

Prolapse of the Pregnant Uterus. Impregnation in a totally prolapsed uterus is very rare because of the difficulties attending a successful coitus, but impregnation is comparatively frequent if the prolapse is only partial. In such cases the cervix, and occasionally a portion of the corpus, may protrude, to a greater or lesser extent, from the vulva during the early months, but as pregnancy progresses the body of the uterus gradually rises up in the pelvis and draws the cervix up with it, so that as soon as the former has passed above the superior strait, prolapse is no longer possible. On the other hand, if the uterus retains its abnormal position, symptoms of incarceration appear during the third or fourth month and abortion is the inevitable result, there being no cases on record in which pregnancy has progressed to term with the uterus outside of the body.

If there is a tendency toward prolapse during pregnancy, the uterus should be replaced and held in position by a suitable pessary. If, however, the pelvic floor is too relaxed to permit its retention, the patient should be kept in a recumbent position as much as possible until after the fourth month. When the cervix reaches to or slightly protrudes from the vulva, the greatest cleanliness is necessary; instances of fatal infection have been reported as occurring even without any internal examination. If the uterus persistently lies outside of the vulva and cannot be replaced, it should be emptied of its contents.

When the vaginal outlet is markedly relaxed, the congested anterior or posterior vaginal walls sometimes prolapse during pregnancy, although the uterus may still retain its normal position. This condition may give rise to considerable discomfort and interfere with locomotion. It is not amenable to treatment until after delivery. At the time of labor these structures may be forced down in front of the presenting part and interfere with its descent. When this occurs they should be carefully cleansed and pushed back over it.

In rare instances a hernial protrusion may occur through the vagina, the anterior or posterior wall forming part of the sac. Such a *vaginal enterocele* may form a tumor of considerable size filled with intestines. Hirst collected 27 instances from the literature. If the condition occurs during pregnancy, the protrusion should be replaced and the patient kept in the recumbent position. At the time of labor it may seriously interfere with the advance of the head. In such cases, the mass should be pushed up if possible, and, when this cannot be done, it should be held as well out of the way as possible, and the head delivered past it.

Torsion of the Pregnant Uterus. Torsion of the pregnant uterus of sufficient degree to arrest the uterine circulation and produce an acute abdominal calamity is one of the rarest accidents of human gestation. In 1931, Robinson and Duvall made a study of this complication and could find in the literature only 25 such cases; in the opinion of these authors, moreover, certain of the reported cases were not true examples of this disorder, so that the number of genuine cases on record is probably even less than the above figure would indicate.

While torsion of the uterus is a rare complication of human pregnancy, it is not uncommon in cattle. Indeed, the complication was first described by an Italian veterinarian, Hippiaper Columbi, in 1662, and since that time it has received much attention in veterinary literature. Fleming, in his "Veterinary Obstetrics," devotes no less than 18 pages to the diagnosis and treatment of this complication of bovine labor. From the viewpoint of etiology, the rather frequent occurrence of this accident in cattle is of considerable importance, because it calls attention to one of the chief predisposing causes of the condition, namely, the bicornuate uterus, as noted by Manahan. Whereas the normal human uterus is stayed on both sides by ligaments which reciprocally prevent excessive motion and rotation, the pregnant horn of a bicornuate uterus, due to the absence of the round and broad ligaments on one side, is subject to no such restraint and is permitted a wide range of movement. When it is further recalled that these unilateral uteri are longer and narrower than normal, with peritoneal and muscular attachments which are often defective, their tendency to torsion is readily understood. Among the cases of torsion of the pregnant uterus reviewed by Robinson and Duvall, three occurred in women with bicornuate uteri. The only case of a torsion of a pregnant uterus which I have seen likewise occurred in a woman with a double uterus (uterus duplex, bicornis, cum vagina septa). The clinical picture resembles that of abruptio placentae but there is no vaginal bleeding. The treatment is hysterectomy.

Hypertrophic Elongation of the Cervix. An abnormally elongated cervix seriously interferes with the occurrence of conception but, as a rule, does not complicate the course of pregnancy or labor. The canal usually becomes shorter and more dilatable as term is approached. In one of our patients the vaginal portion of the cervix in the early months was 5 cm. in length and the external os protruded from the vulva; later it had undergone marked softening and become reduced to normal dimensions so that labor occurred spontaneously.

Acute Edema of the Cervix. In very rare instances the cervix, particularly its anterior lip, may become so acutely edematous during pregnancy and attain such proportions as to protrude from the vulva. This condition is referable to an angioneurosis and, if not associated with pre-existing hypertrophy, may, on rest in bed, disappear almost as suddenly as it developed. Jolly was able to collect, from the literature, 10 cases which were increased to 24 by Hunter in 1927.

Hernia. Pregnancy occurring in women suffering from *inguinal hernia* is not influenced by the condition, although, owing to the increased intra-abdominal pressure, the defect may become aggravated. Generally speaking, the hernia should be treated palliatively by rest and the use of a truss, operative treatment being deferred until after delivery. Very exceptionally, the uterus may form part of the contents of an inguinal hernia, and, indeed, several cases are on record in which conception has occurred under such circumstances. Full literature upon the subject will be found in the articles of Adams and Eisenhart, the latter having reported a case in which one horn of a five months' pregnant bicornuate uterus occupied the right inguinal canal.

Umbilical hernias are frequently noted during pregnancy, but are usually without effect upon the condition. During the early months the uterus is not in the neighborhood of the hernial opening; later, when the fundus reaches the level of the umbilicus, it is usually too large to gain access to the hernial opening, but when the abdomen is markedly pendulous, such an occurrence is not beyond the range of possibility, and several such instances are on record. Much more common are the cases in which the cicatrix of an abdominal incision yields to the increased intra-abdominal pressure incident to pregnancy, and along the linea alba is formed a hernial sac into which the pregnant uterus often makes its way, being then covered merely by a thin layer of skin, fascia, and peritoneum.

A similar condition is occasionally observed in women suffering from extensive *diastasis of the recti muscles*. Ordinarily, such hernias have no effect upon pregnancy, although they may add markedly to the discomfort of the patient. Temporary relief is frequently obtained by holding the uterus in its normal position by a properly fitting binder. At the time of labor, owing to the loss of muscular tone in the abdominal walls, the second stage is liable to be prolonged, and the employment of forceps is often called for.

Hydrorrhea Gravidarum. Occasionally, marked hyperplasia of the glandular structures of the decidua is present, usually associated with persistence of the glandular ducts. It is believed by some that this affection manifests itself by a profuse secretion of clear fluid, which may dribble away as rapidly as it is produced, or be retained in the uterus to be suddenly discharged in large quantities at variable intervals. The amount of fluid expelled varies considerably; Ahlfeld has reported a case in which it exceeded 500 cc. on several occasions. This condition precludes the fusion of the

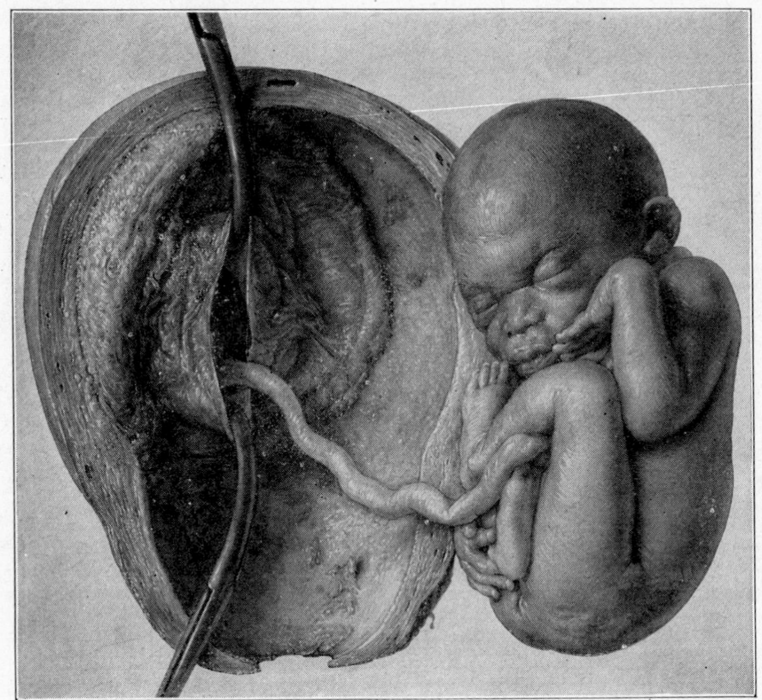

Fig. 367.—Extramembranous Pregnancy (Hofbauer). × ⅗.
Note collapsed fetal membranes held apart by clamps. (Drawing by Max Brödel.)

decidua vera and capsularis, and, therefore, in the occasional instances in which it continued throughout pregnancy it must be assumed that these structures had failed to unite as usual.

Considerable discussion has arisen concerning the nature of hydrorrhea gravidarum. Stoeckel, Meyer-Ruegg, and other authorities believe that it does not result from changes in the decidua but is due to premature rupture of the fetal membranes, which then collapse upon the fetal surface of the placenta so that the child comes to lie free in the uterine cavity—in other words, the pregnancy becomes extramembranous, while amniotic fluid continues to be secreted and escapes in an intermittent trickle. Figure 367 is an excellent illustration of the condition and shows that the amniotic cavity has retracted to such an extent as to become almost negligible. In other cases, the membranes may develop a small defect but still surround the fetus.

Decidual Endometritis. Acute inflammatory lesions of the decidua frequently follow prolonged rupture of the membranes and attempts at criminal abortion. In many instances it is possible to demonstrate the presence of cocci or bacilli in sections and occasionally in cultures. In these cases the decidua vera and basalis are thickened and their external surface covered by a yellowish, purulent exudate. Under the microscope the tissue is found to be infiltrated with leukocytes and plasma cells, and presents the typical picture of acute inflammation, with here and there areas of acute necrosis. Clinically, an elevation in temperature usually gives evidence of the intrapartum infection, as discussed on page 845.

Meyer-Ruegg, in 1904, was able to collect from the literature 15 cases of hydrorrhea in which a period varying from 50 to 120 days had elapsed between the rupture of the membranes and the termination of pregnancy. Van der Hoeven inclines to the

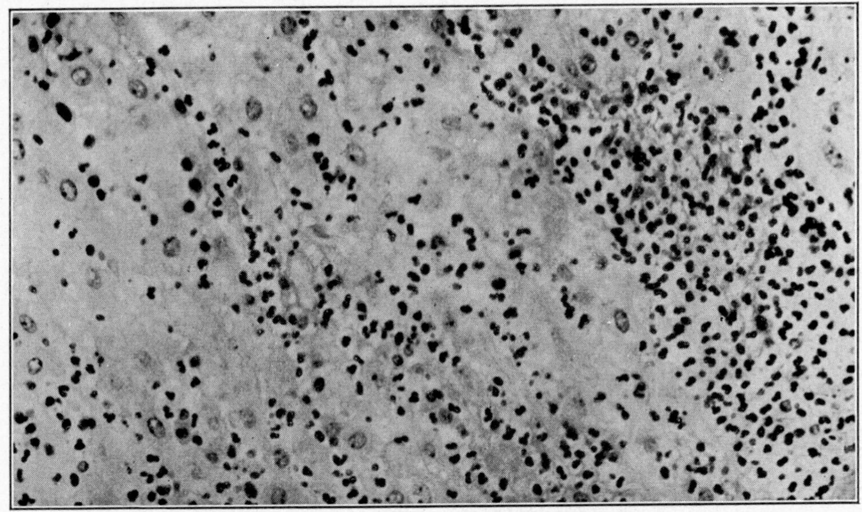

FIG. 368.—DECIDUAL ENDOMETRITIS. × 280.

older view and bases his belief upon the chemical analysis of the fluid expelled. Where the fluid escapes in sufficient quantity to be collected, its amniotic origin can be demonstrated by finding lanugo hairs on microscopic examination after centrifugalization.

Chronic Pelvic Inflammatory Disease. In the rare instances where pregnancy occurs in women suffering from an old inflammatory process considerable discomfort may at times result from the stretching of adhesions. It is surprising, however, to note how frequently patients with extensive pelvic adhesions have no symptoms during gestation, and, moreover, it is very unusual for such patients to have exacerbations of the process at this time.

Pregnancy Complicated by Pelvic Tumors. Pregnancy is occasionally complicated by ovarian or uterine tumors. Although, as a rule, they do not materially affect its course, they sometimes give rise to serious dystocia at the time of labor and will therefore be considered in detail in Chapter 32.

Endometriosis. Since endometriosis is frequently associated with sterility, it is an uncommon complication of pregnancy. As emphasized in Scott's extensive study of the subject, however, patients suffering from endometriosis occasionally do become pregnant and, in the course of gestation, sometimes exhibit bizarre and vexing clinical pictures. In 12 cases of internal endometriosis associated with pregnancy (adenomyoma or adenomyosis) which Scott was able to collect from the literature, 5 were complicated by uterine rupture, 3 by postpartum hemorrhage and 2 by dystocia as the result of the adenomyoma. Rectovaginal endometriosis may present symptoms simulating threatened abortion and has been reported in the literature 11 times. Ovarian endometriosis is perhaps less frequently seen, 7 cases having been published. Scott reports from our clinic a very rare complication of ovarian endometriosis in pregnancy, namely, rupture of an endometrial cyst, the clinical syndrome suggesting acute appendicitis. While many cases of unrecognized endometriosis doubtless go through pregnancy and labor without complication, it is apparent that the condition may occasionally produce grave as well as puzzling pictures.

BIBLIOGRAPHY

ADAMS, S. S. Hernia of the Pregnant Uterus. Am. J. Obst., 1889, 22:225.

AHLFELD. Ueber Endometritis decidualis tuberoso-polyposa. Arch. f. Gynäk., 1876, 10:168.

——— Hydrorrhoea gravidarum. Endometritis atrophicans. Lehrbuch der Geburtshülfe, II. Aufl. 1898, f. 253.

BECKMANN, W. Weiterer Beitrag zur Gravidität im rudimentären Uterushorn. Ztschr. f. Geburtsh. u. Gynäk., 1911, 68:600.

BENJAMIN, E. L., and DANFORTH, W. C. Bipartite Uterus. Am. J. Obst. & Gynec., 1940, 39:704.

BETTMANN, R. B. A Case of Labor in a Bicornuate Uterus. Bull. Johns Hopkins Hosp., 1902, 13:56.

BRACKETT, E. S. Retroversion of the Uterus. Am. J. Obst. & Gynec., 1948, 55:184.

BREUS, C. Ueber cytöse Degeneration der Decidua vera. Arch. f. Gynaek., 1882, 19:483.

BULIUS, G. Ueber Endometritis decidua polyposa et tuberosa. München. med. Wchnschr., 1896, Nr. 28.

DANFORTH, W. C. Carcinoma of the Cervix During Pregnancy. Am. J. Obst. & Gynec., 1937, 34:365.

——— and GALLOWAY, C. E. Retrodisplacement of the Uterus during Pregnancy and the Puerperium —Analysis of 1,000 cases. J.A.M.A., 1926, 87:826.

DÜHRSSEN, A. Ueber Aussackungen, etc., der schwangeren Gebärmutter. Arch. f. Gynäk., 1899, 57:70.

EASTMAN, N. J. Torsion of the Pregnant Uterus. Chinese M. J., 1934, 48:745.

EISENHART, H. Fall von Hernia Inguinalis Cornu Dextri Uteri Gravidi. Arch. f. Gynäk., 1885, 26:439.

EMGE, L. A. The Influence of Pregnancy on Tumor Growth. Am. J. Obst. & Gynec., 1934, 28:682.

FALLS, Frederick H. The Uterus Arcuatus. Am. J. Obst. & Gynec., 1939, 38:661.

FALLS, F. H. Study of Pregnancy with Parturition in Primipara with Bicornuate Uteri. Am. J. Obst. & Gynec., 1928, 15:399-405.

FINDLEY, P. Pregnancy in Uterus Didelphys. Am. J. Obst. & Gynec., 1926, 12:318.

GOLDSTEIN, L., and MURPHY, D. P. Microcephalic Idiocy following Radium Therapy for Uterine Cancer during Pregnancy. Am. J. Obst. & Gynec., 1929, 18:189.

GOTTSCHALK, S. Zur Lehre von der Retroversio uteri gravidi. Arch. f. Gynäk., 1894, 46:358.

HIRST, J. Vaginal Enterocele in Pregnancy and Labor. Tr. Am. Gynec. Soc., 1893, 18:351.

HUNTER, J. W. A. Acute Postpartum Oedema of the Cervix Uteri. J. Obst. & Gynaec. Brit. Emp., 1927, 34:72.

JOLLY, R. Ueber acutes Oedem der Portio vaginalis in der Schwangerschaft. Ztschr. f. Geburtsh. u. Gynäk., 1904, 52:396.

JONES, Howard W., Jr., and NEILL, W., Jr. The Treatment of Carcinoma of the Cervix During Pregnancy. Am. J. Obst. & Gynec., 1944, 48:447.

KEHRER. Das Nebenhorn des doppelten Uterus. Heidelberg, 1900.

KEITLER, H. Ein Beitrag zur Retroflexion und Retroversion der schwangeren Gebärmutter. Monatschr. f. Geburtsh. u. Gynäk., 1901, 13:285.

LOBENSTINE, R. W. Incarceration of the Pregnant Uterus. Am. J. Obst., 1909, 160:1003-1016.

MAINO, C. R., and MUSSEY, R. D. Carcinoma of the Cervix Coincident with Pregnancy. Am. J. Obst. & Gynec., 1944, 47:229.

MANAHAN, C. P., and CORONADO, J. Axial Torsion of the Uterus. J. Philippine M. A., 1946, 22:233.

MEYER-RUEGG, H. Eihautberstung ohne Unterbrechung der Schwangerschaft. Ztschr. f. Geburtsh. u. Gynäk., 1904, 51:419-468.

MILLER, N. F. Clinical Aspects of Uterus Didelphys. Am. J. Obst. & Gynec., 1922, 4:378-408.

MUNDE, P. F. Seven Unusual Cases of Congenital Malformation of the Female Genital Organs. Am. J. Obst., 1893, 27:329.

NEWTON, F. C. Uterus Didelphys. Notes on its Developmental Etiology and Clinical Significance. Am. J. Surg., 1924, 79:102.

OLDHAM. Case of Retroflexion of the Gravid Uterus. Tr. Obst. Soc., London, 1860, 1:317.

PELLER, S. Die Sterblichkeit der Schwangeren und Wöchnerinnen an Krebs. Ztschr. f. Krebsforsch., 1931, 34:394.

REED, C. B. The Aetiology of Ischuria in Retroflexion of the Gravid Uterus. Am. J. Obst., 1904, 49:145.

RICHMAN, S., and GOODFRIEND, M. J. Cancer of the Cervix Uteri Associated with Pregnancy. Am. J. Roentgenol., 1942, 48:677.

ROBINSON, A. L., and DUVALL, H. M. Torsion of the Pregnant Uterus. J. Obst. & Gynaec. Brit. Emp., 1931, 38:55.

SANGER. Ueber Schwangerschaft in rudimentären Nebenhorn bei Uterus duplex. Zentralbl. f. Gynäk., 1883, 7:324.

SCHAUFFLER, G. C. Double Uterus with Pregnancy. J.A.M.A., 1941, 117:1516.

SCHICKELE, G. Die Schwangerschaft in einem Uterusdivertikel. Beitr. z. Geburtsh. u. Gynäk., 1904, 8:267.

SCOTT, R. B. Endometriosis and Pregnancy. Am. J. Obst. & Gynec., 1944, 47:608.

STOEKEL, W. Beitrag zur Lehre von der Hydrorrhoea uteri gravidi. Zentralbl. f. Gynäk., 1899, 2:1353.

TAYLOR, HOYT C. Pregnancy and the Double Uterus. Am. J. Obst. & Gynec., 1943, 46:388.

VAN DER HOEVEN, P. C. T. Hydrorrhoea Gravidarum. Monatschr. f. Geburtsh. u. Gynäk., 1899, 10:329.

WILLSON, J. R. Carcinoma of the Cervix Complicated by Pregnancy. Am. J. Obst. & Gynec., 1945, 50:275.

25

MULTIPLE PREGNANCY

The number of young ordinarily resulting from a single pregnancy is an inherited characteristic which is fixed for each species. In mammals, multiple offspring represent a more primitive condition than single offspring. The average litter size for the various mammals is loosely related to several other characteristics. The number of young is inversely proportional to the adult size of the species: the larger the animal, the fewer her young. Animals with gestation periods exceeding 150 days rarely have multiple young. Two breasts usually mean one offspring at a birth and many breasts, many young. Most animals with a simplex or unicornuate uterus have single young, while animals with a bicornuate uterus may or may not have more than one. Finally, the life span of the species is also related to the matter under discussion. Those mammalian species which live longest produce the fewest young at a single birth.

The catarrhine primates, of which man is the most distinguished member, ordinarily have but one young at a birth, but all of the members of this mammalian order occasionally have two or more.

Miraculous litter size has been imputed to man, the most extravagant recorded being for the haughty Countess of Hagenau. Mauriceau discusses the events in his textbook of 1668: "But I esteem it either a miracle, or a fable, what is related in the history of the Lady Margaret, Countess of Holland, who in the year 1313 was brought to bed of 365 children at one and the same time." It is likely some mathematically minded midwife counted each vesicle of a hydatid mole as an embryo.

In a borderline between fancy and fact lies the birth of seven children at one time, the famous septuplets of Hameln Town, more famous for its thirteenth century Pied Piper. A tablet erected at the supposed spot more than two centuries later is all there is to authenticate this birth. In part it reads: "It came about in the year 1600, as man reckons time, at 3 o'clock in the morning on the ninth of January, she was delivered of two small boys and five small girls. . . . All peacefully died by 12 o'clock of the twentieth of January."

Several valid births of sextuplets have been reported. A South African case in 1903 was investigated by two English medical officers. Their report contains a photograph of the children, five boys and one girl. Four placentas were involved. An earlier case published by Vassali is equally well established. The total weight of the six fetuses born on the 115th day of pregnancy was 1,739 gm. The four boys and two girls had a single fused placenta.

The birth of the Dionne quintuplets in May, 1934 stimulated great interest in multiple births of this magnitude. MacArthur and Ford have summarized 45 cases from the world literature, 1694 to 1936. Thirty-four were published in the last 100 years and 11 during the previous century and a half. This in no way signifies that quintuplets are becoming increasingly common, simply a greater proportion are being reported. Several additional cases have been reported since 1936.

The Dionne quintuplets, largely because of the early skillful medical care they received, have shattered all previous records for both group and individual survival. Previously no single quintuplet had survived more than 50 days and no entire set more than 15 days.

FREQUENCY OF MULTIPLE BIRTHS

Two striking biological verities have been claimed in respect to the frequency of human multiple births. First, in a large population a mathematical relationship exists between the occurrence of twins, triplets, and quadruplets. Second, there is a consistent and significant variation in the frequency of multiple births among different racial stocks.

The existence of the mathematical relationship between the various orders of multiple births was first stated by Hellin in 1895 when he claimed that twins occurred once in 89 births, triplets once in 89^2, and quadruplets once in 89^3. Zeleny, to take into account the variation in frequency between one racial stock and another, generalized Hellin's law: "If 1:N is the ratio of twin births to all births in a large population during any period, then the ratio of triplet births during the same period is very near $1:N^2$. . . . The expected number of quadruplets is $1:N^3$."

Strandskov analyzed 28 million deliveries, the total number of births occurring in the U. S. Birth Registration area from 1922 to 1936. The mean frequency of twinning for the 15-year period was 1.161 per cent or one in 86.13 deliveries. Applying Hellin's rule, triplets would be expected to occur with the frequency of .01348 per cent and quadruplets .000156 per cent. However, the actual incidence was .01189 per cent and .000203 per cent respectively. His conclusion is that there is no close agreement with Hellin's law. Hamlett did a similar study on a smaller sample 10 years earlier and his conclusion was: "We must conclude that the 1:N to $1:N^2$ ratio between twin and triplet births is only an approximation, and not a very close one at that."

There is marked variation in the frequency of plural births among different racial stocks. This can be most clearly demonstrated by considering the three most diverse ethnic groups: Caucasians, Negroes, and Mongols. Strandskov showed that the white twin frequency in the United States is 1.129 per cent, the colored 1.415 per cent, the incidence for triplets .01089 per cent and .01970 per cent, and quadruplets .000175 per cent and .000420 per cent respectively. Hamlett demonstrated that this difference between whites and blacks was racial rather than environmental or climatic, for he found an equal difference between the two races in the northern and southern states. Twinning in Japan is about half as common as it is in the United States. Komai and Fukuoka found that this is due to the fact that the incidence of two-egg twin births "in the Japanese is only one-fourth to one-third times that in the Caucasians or Negroes," while one-egg twin births occur with the same frequency in all three races. All magnitudes of plural birth are most frequent among Negroes and least frequent among Mongols, with whites occupying an intermediate position.

Some marriages appear to be destined to have an inordinately high frequency of multiple births. Greulich reports with careful accuracy the superior fecundity of a couple from Putnam, Connecticut. In nine births the 35-year-old mother delivered six pairs of two-egg twins and three single children. In some instances this ability seems to have no hereditary background but in many there is a family history for plural gestations. Davenport has shown that this hereditary trait may be carried by either the female or male line and has no tendency to skip a generation as the laity confidently assumes. Guttmacher, in a study of 521 cases of twinning, concludes that single-ovum twinning is a matter of chance, while double-ovum twinning, on the other hand, is influenced by heredity, age, and parity.

Twin pregnancy may result either from the fertilization of two separate ova or of a single ovum; the first gives rise to double-ovum, dizygotic, or fraternal, and the second to single-ovum, monozygotic, or identical twins. In the former case the ova may be from the same ovary, or one from each ovary; in the latter case only a single ovum is involved. It is interesting to note that Allen and his associates, in their first communication upon the recovery of human ova from the fallopian tubes, state that in one of their cases a normal ovum was found in each tube on the fifteenth day after the onset of menstruation and would have given rise to double-ovum twins had each egg been fertilized.

Fraternal twins may or may not be of the same sex, and do not necessarily resemble one another more than other children of the same parents; identical twins are necessarily of the same sex and resemble one another closely. Approximately one out of three sets of twins born in the United States belong in the latter category, as based upon the 1946 publication of Strandskov and Edelen. They state that 33 per cent of all twins born in this country are monozygotic, the group comprising 34 per cent of the white twins and 29 per cent of the colored. Their respective colored and white dizygotic incidence was 1.01 per cent and 0.74 per cent, while the monozygotic frequency was 0.41 per cent and 0.39 per cent. This reported 33 per cent incidence of identical twins is greater than other authorities admit. Most place the figure at about 25 per cent, making three out of four pairs fraternal or dizygotic.

According to Hellin, Patellani, and Larger, multiple pregnancy should be regarded as a sign of atavistic reversion analogous to the litters of many domestic animals. Hellin states that the ovaries of women who have had a number of multiple pregnancies contain an excessive quantity of ova. According to this view, which can apply only to double-ovum twins, we have to deal with the maturation and fertilization of several ova at a single ovulation period.

Biologically, double-ovum twins are not twins at all, but are due to the maturation and fertilization of two ova at a single ovulation period. Such ova may come from two different follicles situated either in one ovary or in both ovaries. On the other hand, Greulich has directed attention to two possible ways by which fraternal or dizygotic twins may be derived from the contents of one follicle: (1) the follicle may have two ova (polyovular follicles in human ovaries have been described by Stockard, Bumm, and others); and (2) the fertilization, by separate spermatozoa, of the definitive ovum and the second polar body, or a cell homologous to it. In the second hypothesis, certain spermatozoa may have the ability, upon penetrating the ovum, to cause it to form two cells, each of which is susceptible to fertilization by different spermatozoa. He believes this hypothesis may explain how heredity of the father could influence the formation of fraternal twins.

Single-ovum twins, on the other hand, represent twins par excellence, as is well expressed by Newman—"Strictly speaking, twinning is twaining or two-ing—the division of an individual into two equivalent and more or less completely separate individuals." Their mode of production has given rise to a considerable literature, to which American investigators have made important contributions.

Recent biologic investigations have shown that single-ovum twinning occurs frequently in many species of animals and can be produced experimentally and at will in several varieties of fish, and also that it is fundamentally associated with the production of monstrosities—the normal twins representing the complete, and the monstrosities an imperfect form of the same process.

Stockard has shown that retardation in the growth of the egg, at what he calls critical periods of development, is the essential factor concerned; he has demonstrated that it may be brought about either by exposing the egg to cold or by diminishing its supply of oxygen. When exposed to such retarding influences, just as it is about to undergo gastrulation, the egg may die, or its development rate may be arrested or slowed down for a time, with the result that when growth is resumed two embryonic areas will develop instead of one. If these are far apart two separate individuals will be formed, whereas if the two areas are partially in contact double monsters presenting varying degrees of fusion will result.

Furthermore, Stockard showed that one can alter at will the degree of duplicity by changing the time at which the retarding influences are brought into play. In other words, he adduced experimental proof of the closest relationship between single-ovum twins and double monsters. In human beings one can readily follow all gradations between typical identical twins and the well-known Siamese twins on the one hand, and double-bodied, double-headed, or four-legged monsters downward to monsters by inclusion, and finally to teratomata, on the other.

The most striking example of the development of multiple pregnancy from a single egg is afforded by the nine-banded armadillo. As is well known, this animal gives birth to four young at a time, which are always of the same sex and are all enclosed within a common chorion. The details of the process have been exhaustively worked out by Newman and Paterson; it would appear that the key to it lies in the fact that the fertilized ovum lies quiescent in the uterine cavity for three weeks before placental attachments are formed, and the resulting retardation in growth during this period of quiescence causes a partial loss of polarity, so that when growth is resumed four embryonic areas result instead of one.

Newman in his two monographs—*The Biology of Twins* and *The Physiology of Twinning*—has considered in detail the problems concerned in human beings. He states that single-ovum twins may be due to (1) fission of the blastoderm, (2) double gastrulation, or (3) fission of the bilateral halves of a single embryonic axis. In each instance some retarding factor must come into play, and he considers that any one of the following three possibilities may be concerned: (a) understimulation of the egg due to some defect in the development-stimulating mechanism of the sperm, (b) belated placentation due to a failure of the corpus luteum to stimulate the uterine mucosa, and (c) that twinning is a hereditary character dependent upon a recessive gene.

While such explanations may not be entirely satisfactory, enough has been said to indicate that single-ovum twinning is a well-recognized biologic phenomenon, and that it does not necessarily represent an inherent attribute of the ovum but may be attributable to conditions which affect its rate of growth after fertilization. Accordingly, in human beings at least, its cause may sometimes be sought in environmental conditions with which we are as yet unacquainted. That some fundamental difference exists between single-ovum and double-ovum twins is shown by the fact that, in the material of the Johns Hopkins Hospital, in the two groups 42.2 and 19.1 per cent of the mothers were primiparae respectively.

Triplet pregnancy may be derived from one, two or three ova, so that one has to deal with single-ovum, double-ovum, or treble-ovum triplets. The first are the least frequent, and, according to Sasse, who has described two cases of his own and collected 32 one-egg triplets from the literature, the order of incidence of the three varieties is as one to six to three. In the only case of quadruplets which we have seen, each child was derived from a single ovum. In the quintuplet pregnancy described by Blécourt and Nijhoff, three of the children were connected with a single placenta, while each of the other two had separate placentas, thus indicating that three ova had been fertilized, one giving rise to triplets, and the other two to single children. The Dionne quintuplets, according to the study of MacArthur, were derived from a single ovum.

SEX OF CHILDREN AND SEX RATIO

It has been estimated that in 63.1 per cent of twin deliveries only one sex is represented and in 36.9 per cent both sexes are represented. In the 717,907 observations collected by Nichols, both children were males in 234,497, both females in 219,312, and of different sex in 264,098 cases.

The sex ratio of multiple births has been studied extensively, the most recent survey by Strandskov and Siemens confirming the earlier findings of Nichols and Knibbs. The percentage of males in the human species decreases with each increase in the number of children per pregnancy. The sex ratio, that is percentage of males, for 31 million United States single births was 51.59 per cent, while for three quarters of a million twins, 50.85 per cent. The figure for triplets was 49.54 per cent, and for quadruplets 46.48 per cent. Two explanations have been suggested. It is well known that a differential mortality exists between the sexes for the fetus in utero, for the infant during its delivery, and for the child and adult during the postnatal period. The mortality is always in favor of the female and against the male. It may be that the population pressure of a multiple pregnancy exaggerates this biological tendency noted in single pregnancies. A second theory is that the female-producing egg has a greater tendency to divide into twins, triplets, or quadruplets. If so, the sex ratio of monozygotic pregnancies should be lower than dizygotic pregnancies. This has not been analyzed.

ANATOMICAL CONSIDERATIONS

Relation of the Placentas and Membranes. The development of one child in either horn of a bicornuate uterus, or of one twin in the uterus and the other in a fallopian tube, affords indubitable evidence of their origin from two ova; in uterine twin pregnancy the examination of the placenta and fetal membranes frequently enables one to determine the mode of origin of the twins. When they are derived from a single ovum, there is generally a single large placenta from which the two umbilical cords come off, but when they are developed from two ova there are usually two separate placentas, although, when these are originally inserted near one another, their contiguous margins may fuse, thus giving rise to an apparently single large placenta.

In double-ovum twins, no matter whether the placentas are separate or fused together, there are always two chorions and two amnions, each child being enveloped in its own membranes. Single-ovum twins, as a rule, possess only a single chorion, but two amnions; this occurs because the chorion represents the wall of the original blastodermic vesicle, while the amnion is more directly connected with the embryo itself. In rare instances a single amnion may be found. Hertig and his co-workers have

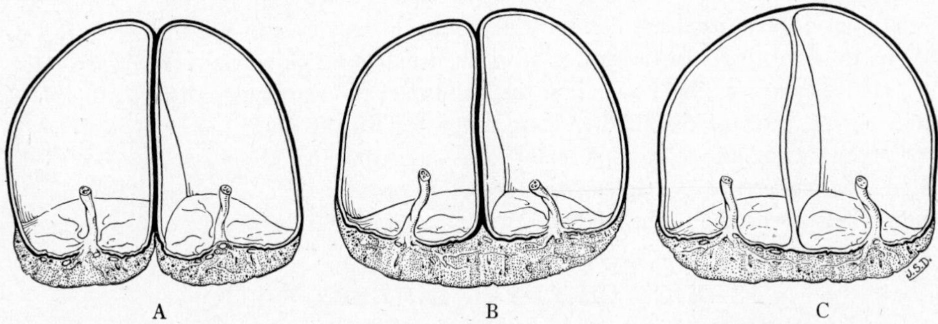

Fig. 369.—Diagram Showing Relation of Placenta and Membranes in Double and Single Twin Pregnancy.

A, double-ovum twins; B, double-ovum twins, double membranes, single placenta; C, single-ovum twins, one chorion, two amnions and one placenta.

summarized the literature on this topic up to 1947. They collected a total of 116 cases. The condition carries with it a tragically high fetal mortality due to knotting of the intertwining cords, since there is no partitioning membrane to prevent this. In 21 cases both twins were born alive and in another 21 one twin was live born and the other stillborn; in the remaining 74 cases both twins were stillborn. Schatz writes of a primary and a secondary form of monamniotic twinning; in the former no partitional wall ever existed and in the latter it is supposed to have disappeared early in pregnancy. The more recent investigators feel that in all monamniotic twin pregnancies we are dealing with an original single amnion, that there never were two. If the germ disc splits before the formation of the amnion two amnions arise in response to the presence of the 2 embryos. In monamniotic twins the germ disc splits late, after the amnion has already formed, and, therefore, the two embryos are surrounded by a single amnion. Hertig thinks that, in ordinary monozygotic twinning, the split of the germ disc occurs before the seventh day post-fertilization. If the split occurs between the seventh and the thirteenth days monamniotic twins are likely to result. If the split is very late, after the thirteenth day, conjoined twins and other double monstrosities appear.

In recent years Siemens, Curtius, Lassen, and others have questioned our ability to determine the origin of twins from the relations between the placenta and its membranes, and therefore lay more stress upon the similarity or dissimilarity of the children, particularly when they had advanced beyond babyhood. There is full agreement that twins presenting heart increases rapidly in size, while that of the weak and eventually atrophies. In this theory is to be found a known as acardia. In such cases almost the entire plac the normal embryo, while the deformed twin receives its lower extremities; occasionally it is represented only —*acardius amorphus*.

Schatz stated that in other instances a difference in leads to the production of hydramnios in the larger ov that the stronger heart appropriates an ever-increasin

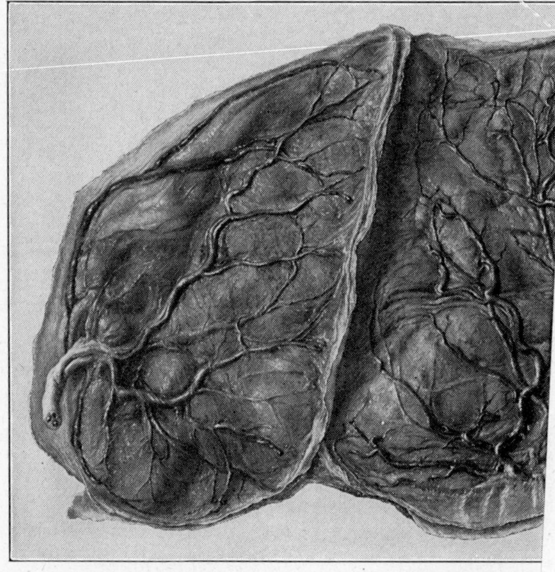

FIG. 372.—FUSED THREE-EGG PLACENTA FROM A Q

One child from a single placenta not shown in the drawi placenta.

placenta and undergoes hypertrophy, which in tur the kidneys which leads to increased urinary secr the quantity of amniotic fluid.

Ordinarily, in twin pregnancies, whether derive occupies, roughly speaking, one-half of the uterus, cally. Occasionally, however, they run transversel lie above the other. In such circumstances, the pl child must be expelled from the uterus before th the latter can make its way past them.

Generally speaking, twins are smaller and wei single pregnancies, although their combined weigh single child. The smaller size may be considere partly to be explained by the fact that the excess premature labor so that the twins are born several observed that viable twin pregnancies terminate, single pregnancies. He was unable to note any

two amnions and no chorion in the partition wall are from a single egg. If, however, there are two separate placentas, or one placenta with two amnions and two chorions in the partition wall, we may, in a small percentage of cases, yet be dealing with single ovum or one-egg twins. It appears that if the cells divide into two eggs at a very early stage, say in the 8-cell to 12-cell stage, each new ovum thus formed will develop independently. As at this stage there is as yet no embryo or anlage of a placenta, the separation is quite complete with the result that two embryos (single-ovum but dichorionic twins), each with a distinct and

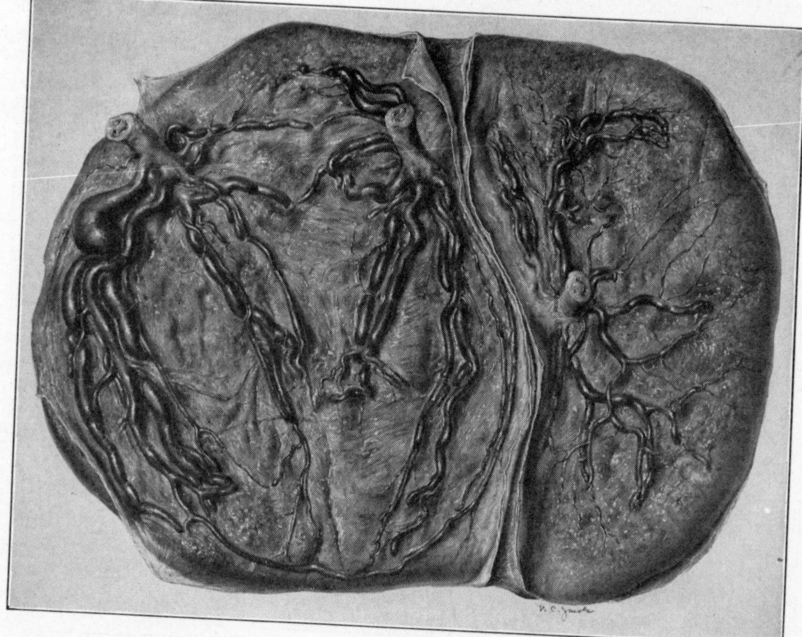

FIG. 370.—TRIPLET PREGNANCY FROM TWO EGGS. × ⅓.

One child from the right side of the fused placenta, and single-ovum twins from the larger left side.

separate placenta, are formed. On the other hand, if separation into two eggs occurs later, when the cells which are to be the embryo have been differentiated and are surrounded by trophoblast, division of the embryonic area will form one placenta and the partition wall will consist only of two amnions, no chorions. Biologists are generally agreed that the only absolute way of determining whether or not twins are from one or two eggs is by physical comparison from the age of two until adolescence, the period when they are most alike.

Essen-Möller in 1941 summarized the data on this topic by collecting 498 cases of like-sexed twins in whom both the anthropologic status and the status of the placenta and membranes were known. Of these, 127 were monochorionic and therefore monozygotic, that is, indisputably of one-egg origin. Three hundred and seventy-one were like-sexed dichorionic and, therefore, of either two-egg or one-egg origin. Physical resemblance tests proved that 17 per cent of the dichorionic pairs were identical and from one egg, while 83 per cent were of two-egg origin, that is, fraternal twins. In other words, 33 per cent or one-third of 190 pairs of one-egg twins have dichorionic placentas, while 17 per cent or one-sixth of the 308 dichorionic placentas from like-sexed twins were from one-egg pregnancies. Since theoretically there are as many fraternal twins of opposite sex as there are fraternal twins of the same sex, we may assume that in 1 out of 12 instances of dichorionic twin placentas a single egg is involved, while in 11 out of 12 two eggs are implicated.

In one-egg, or single-ovum twins, if division occurs early, both children are right or left handed; if division takes place later, when the embryonic area has already oriented a right

and left side, one child will be left handed while tl
twins, which evidently are the latest to divide, th
member of the pair.

In summary, the placental and membrane
whether the twins are from one or two eggs. The
ovum divides so early that the placental rela
seen in a two-egg pregnancy.

In triplet pregnancy, the conditions are st
is concerned, one may find a single large placen

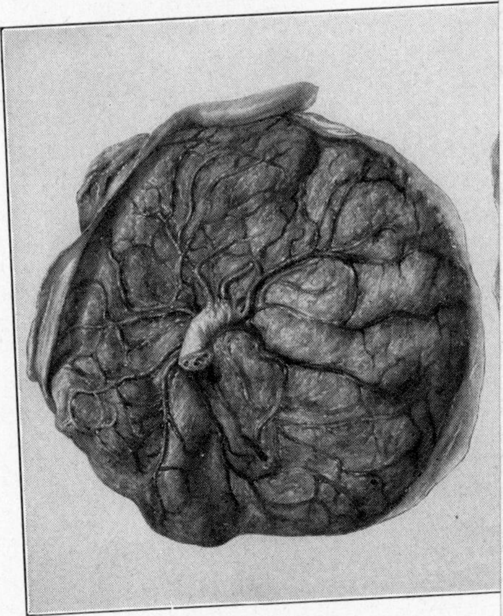

FIG. 371.—TRIPLET PREGNANCY
One child from the smaller placenta, and dou

or with a chorion as well as an amnion in on
upon the stage of division. In two-egg tripl
single large placenta, which has resulted fr
another belonging to single-ovum twins (th
from one of our specimens); or (2) the tw
the other hand, if three ova are concerned,
separate placentas, each with its own chorio
one single and the other fused, the latter be
in Fig. 371; and (3) a huge single placen
amnion, as shown in Fig. 372. In quadruple
may be still more complicated.

In single-ovum twins there is always a
is anastomosis between the two vascular
four per cent of the fused placenta of dou
degree. Schatz advanced the theory that if
is considerably stronger than that of the
communicating portion of the placenta is

pregnancy and parity. Slightly more than one third of his primiparae had twins of term weight, while more than half of the multiparae had term babies. He considers a twin pregnancy as having reached full term if either of the twins weighs 2,500 gm. or more.

It is not unusual for twins to differ considerably in size and weight, especially when derived from a single ovum. Ahlfeld has reported cases in which living twins weighed, respectively, 2,320 and 1,120, and 1,920 and 790 gm.

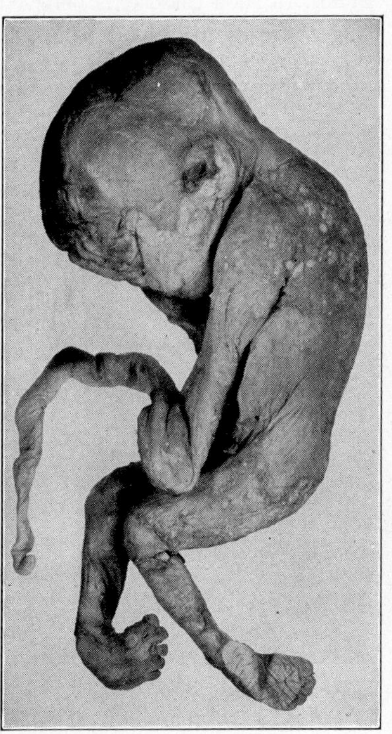

FIG. 373.—FETUS PAPYRACEUS. × ½.

Probably due to germinal defect, growth arrested in twentieth week. Twin pregnancy at term; other infant was normal. (Carnegie Col. 4159A.)

In double-ovum twin pregnancy one child may die at an early period and be expelled from the uterus soon afterward, while the other may go on to full development. More frequently, however, the dead fetus is retained until the end of pregnancy and, being compressed between the uterine wall and the membranes of the living child, becomes flattened and partially mummified—*fetus papyraceus* or *compressus* (Fig. 373).

Superfecundation and Superfetation. The consideration of the difference in the weight of twins, and the possibility of one's being aborted while the other develops until full term, lead up to the question of superfecundation and superfetation. By superfecundation, we understand the fertilization of two ova within a short period of one another, but not at the same coitus; in superfetation several months may intervene.

Superfecundation is a well-recognized occurrence in the lower animals and undoubtedly occurs in human beings, although it is impossible to determine its frequency. It is probable that in many cases the two ova are not fertilized at the same coitus, but this can be demonstrated only under exceptional circumstances. It is interesting to note that John Archer, who was the first physician to receive a medical degree in America, related in 1810 that he had observed a white woman who had had connection with a white and a colored man, respectively, within a short period, and who was delivered of twins, one of which was white and the other a mulatto. Since that time many instances of superfecundation have been reported and in 1917 a most convincing case was recorded by Robertson. In this instance a mare was covered by a horse and 10 minutes later by a jackass, and gave birth to twins, one being a horse and the other a mule.

The occurrence of superfetation has never yet been demonstrated, although its theoretical possibility must be admitted, as long as the uterine cavity has not become obliterated by the fusion of the decidua vera and reflexa. As this occurs at the end of the third month of pregnancy, superfetation is out of the question after that time but prior to that there is no theoretical objection to supposing that, should ovulation occur, a second ovum might find its way into the uterine cavity after fertilization. Still more favorable conditions would be afforded by a duplex uterus.

Certain French authorities consider that such an event has been conclusively demonstrated, and many of the arguments which have been advanced in its favor are given by Tarnier. On the other hand, most English and German authors are skeptical and believe that the majority of instances put under this category have been due either to the abortion of one twin or to marked inequality of development. Moreover, the fact that ovulation is usually in abeyance during pregnancy still further diminishes the probability of such an occurrence. The arguments against the occurrence of superfetation in the human, as well as in the lower animals, were well reviewed by A. W. Meyer in 1919. Studdiford, in 1936, stated that he could find in the literature no proved case of superfetation in the human, although a few reported cases suggest that such an occurrence is possible. He, furthermore, presented complete histologic studies on two cases which superficially suggest superfetation. In each instance he was able to disprove the occurrence of superfetation, the explanation being ordinary twinning with the early death of one fetus and the continued growth of the co-twin. He concludes that superfetation seems most unlikely because of the marked inhibition of ovulation during pregnancy.

Cases occasionally occur which, at first glance, appear to bear out the possibility of superfetation but, upon closer study, fail to do so. Thus, a physician sent Williams two fetuses which he thought afforded conclusive evidence in favor of such an occurrence. They had been expelled spontaneously by a healthy multipara who thought herself 4½ months pregnant. One fetus measured 18 cm., and the other 4 cm. in length. The former was perfectly fresh, while the latter showed signs of atrophy and had evidently been dead for some time, so that there was but little doubt that each had begun development at about the same period. Even had both fetuses been alive, the evidence would not have been unassailable unless both placentas presented identical conditions upon examination; it is conceivable that some lesion might have been present in the placenta corresponding to the smaller child, which would seriously interfere with growth without, however, causing death.

In this connection a word may be said concerning telegony, by which is meant the possibility that, at the time of the first conception, something is added to the mother which will be transmitted to later offspring, even though by another mate. Some veterinarians hold that the breeding qualities of a highly bred mare or bitch inevitably suffer if she is ever covered by a male of inferior breed. The article of Tcherepoff shows that many physicians hold similar views, but all scientific biologists contend that they entirely lack foundation.

Conjoined Twins. In this country such united twins are commonly termed Siamese twins, after Chang and Eng Bunker who were displayed to the whole civilized world for more than three decades by P. T. Barnum. Actually, they were three quarters Chinese and one quarter Siamese. Double monsters have been known and recorded since antiquity. It was assumed until the nineteenth century that the phenomenon was caused by the intra-uterine collision and fusion of two early twin embryos. It is now generally assumed that the etiology is failure of the germ disc to split into two in its entirety, leaving portions of tissue in common to both embryos. Most conjoined twins are pygopagus, that is, joined back to back with part of the buttocks, sacrum, rectum, and perineum in common. The females usually have a single vagina but separate uteri and cervices. Conjoined twins are of several other types, designation being by the portion of their anatomy which is single. One of the common varieties is omphalopagus, a common abdominal wall. This is the only type for which surgical separation has succeeded; there are three authentic cases in which surgical separation has been accomplished with the survival of one twin and the death of the other. No case has been reported with the separation and survival of both. Dystocia is rare in the birth of conjoined twins, since most of the union is pliable soft tissue. If any bone is shared, it is usually insufficiently ossified at the time of birth to prevent one twin from sliding ahead of the other in the birth canal; the elastic bond being greatly stretched in the birth process. One pair of Siamese twins, the Blazek sisters, had a child of their own; the birth was very easy.

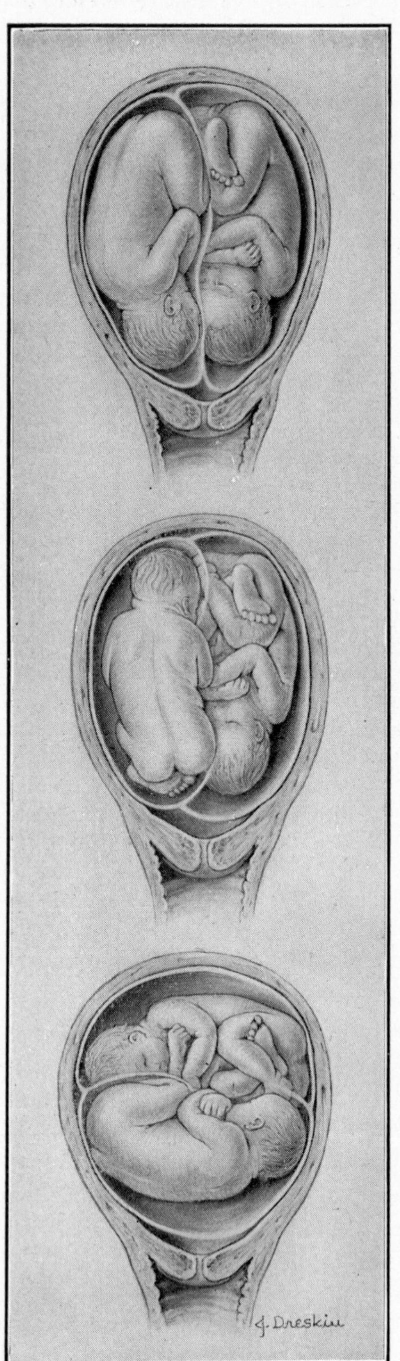

Fig. 374.—Position of Twins in Utero.

DIAGNOSIS

It sometimes happens that the first intimation which the physician has of the presence of twins is afforded by the unusually large size of the uterus after the expulsion of the first child. Guttmacher, in his analysis of 573 cases of twin pregnancy, found that a correct diagnosis was made in only 50 per cent of the cases when both infants weighed less than 2,500 gm., and in slightly more than 70 per cent when the larger twin was 2,500 gm. or more.

Excessive size of the abdomen during pregnancy frequently causes one to suspect the presence of twins, although usually it will be found to be due to some other condition. Thus, owing to the relaxation of the abdominal walls and the resulting forward protrusion of the uterus following the birth of a first child, women pregnant for the second time often think that they will give birth to twins, although, as a matter of fact, their fears are generally without foundation.

The diagnostic methods are palpation, auscultation, vaginal examination, and the x-ray. If a multiplicity of small parts is encountered on palpation, the possibility of a twin pregnancy should always be suspected. Positive evidence is afforded by the palpation of two heads, two breeches, and two backs, or at least of one back and four fetal poles. The detection of three fetal poles is not conclusive; in rare instances a subperitoneal or intramural myoma may simulate the head of a child.

Auscultation frequently gives most valuable information, and if one can distinguish two areas, considerably removed from one another, in which a fetal heart can be heard, twins should be suspected, but a positive diagnosis should not be made unless there is a difference of at

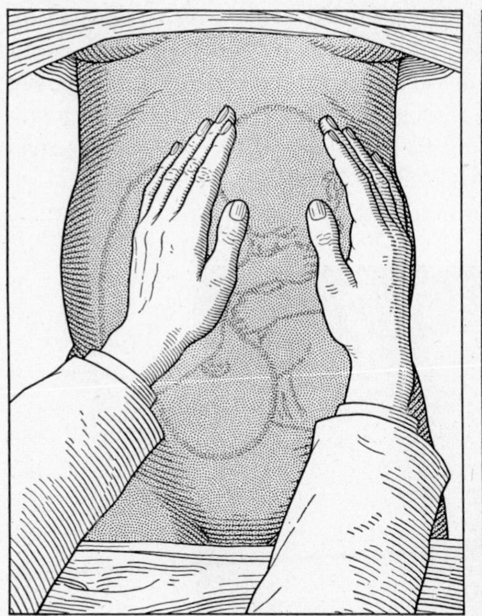

First Maneuver.

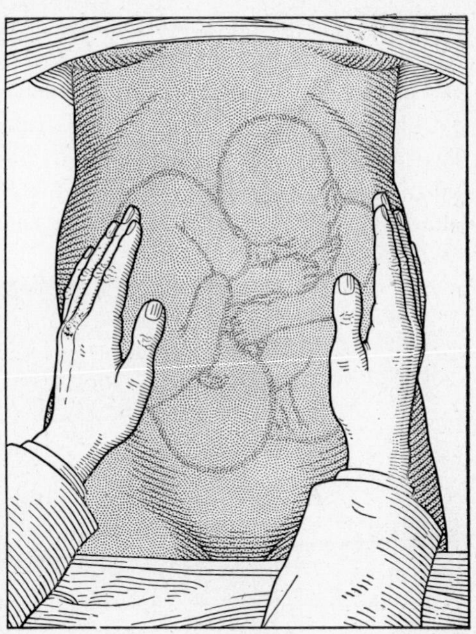

Second Maneuver.

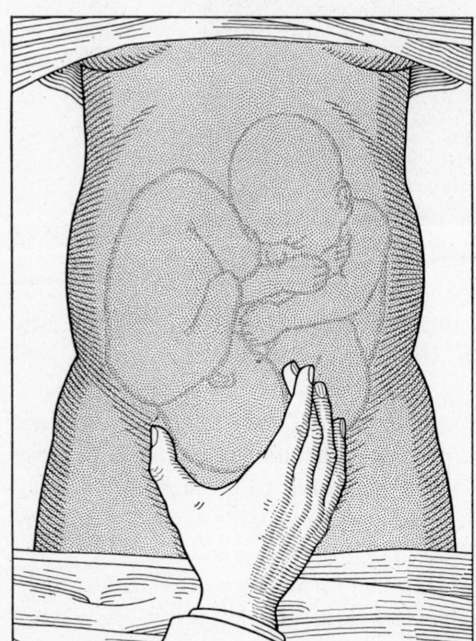

Third Maneuver.

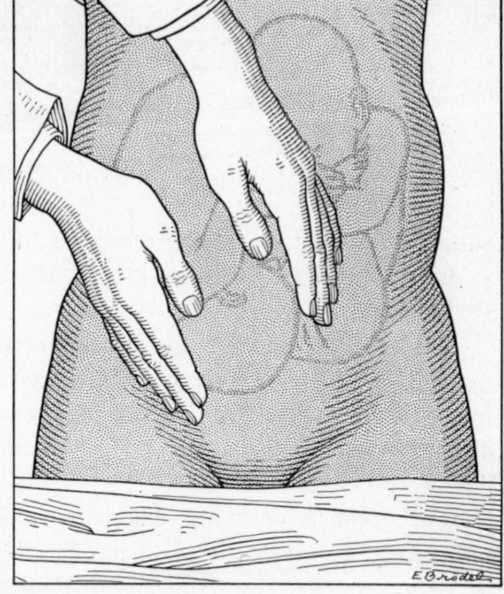

Fourth Maneuver.

Fig. 375.—Palpation in Twin Pregnancy.

Twin at left in ROA position; twin at right in LSP position.

least 10 beats per minute in the rate of the two hearts, the sounds being counted for at least a minute in each location.

In rare instances vaginal touch may reveal important findings; it is sometimes possible to distinguish a macerated head through the intact membranes, or a prolapsed and pulseless cord may be felt through the cervix, while auscultation gives positive evidence of the presence of a living child. Moreover, the discovery of an effaced cervix, 2 cm. or more dilated, before the onset of labor, may give grounds to

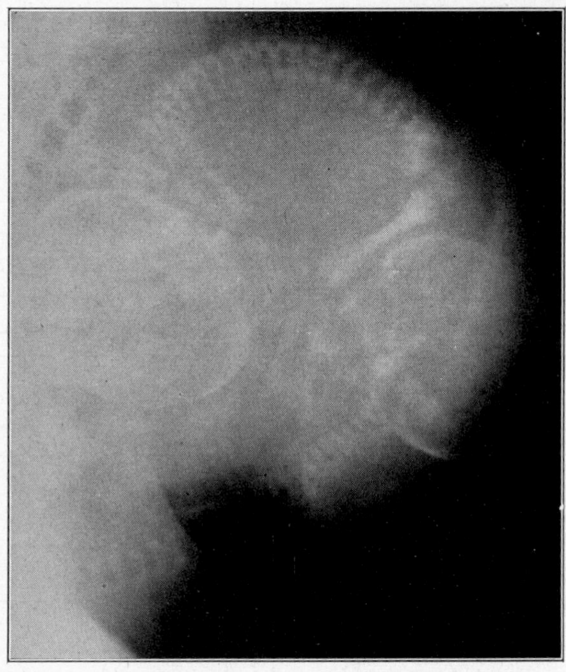

FIG. 376.—ROENTGENOGRAM OF TWINS IN UTERO.

suspect twins. In truth, the diagnosis of a multiple pregnancy is not difficult. The reason it is missed so frequently is because the examiner forgot to keep the possibility in mind.

In doubtful cases, the use of x-ray usually enables one to make a positive diagnosis by detecting the skeletons of two children in the plate. On the other hand, a negative finding does not preclude the possibility of twins, as, owing to the unfavorable conditions under which the picture may be taken, the presence of the second child may not be revealed.

The presence of more than two children can be predicted with certainty only under very exceptional and favorable circumstances, although Ribemont-Dessaignes, in 1894, reported the diagnosis of triplets during pregnancy, and its confirmation at the time of labor. When such a suspicion arises, certainty is sometimes secured by means of the x-ray. R. A. Johnston made a correct diagnosis by that means, while Marcus, Wilson, and others have reported similar successes.

Multiple pregnancy is frequently associated with hydramnios. Guttmacher was unable to determine exactly the incidence of this complication, although it had been clinically diagnosed in 7 per cent of the twin pregnancies in his series. Potter and Fuller report a little less than 5 per cent incidence of hydramnios. They found this complication to be associated with a significant increase in fetal mortality, mainly because of the frequent occurrence of very premature labors. Both Guttmacher

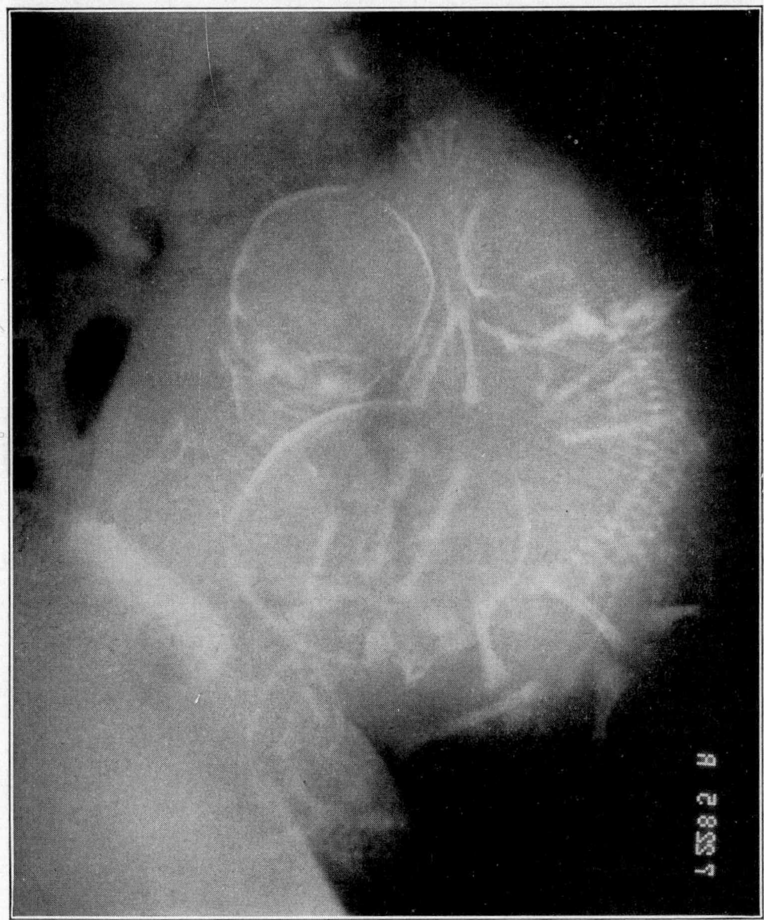

Fig. 377.—Roentgenogram of Triplets in Utero.
(Courtesy of Dr. Karl M. Wilson.)

and Potter found all forms of hypertensive toxemia, most notably eclampsia and preeclampsia, far more frequent in twin than in single pregnancies. Their observations are in accord with those of other writers.

It is also frequently seen that the distention of the uterus incidental to multiple pregnancy leads to greater discomfort on the part of the patient. Nausea and vomiting may be more frequent, although Guttmacher found no increased incidence of severe or toxemic vomiting. It is stated that relaxation of the pelvic joints may be more marked than in single gestations, resulting in more difficult locomotion. If the multiple pregnancy is further complicated by hydramnios, interference with the circulatory and respiratory systems may result, as shown by such symptoms as marked dyspnea, extreme edema, or huge varicosities, of the legs and vulva.

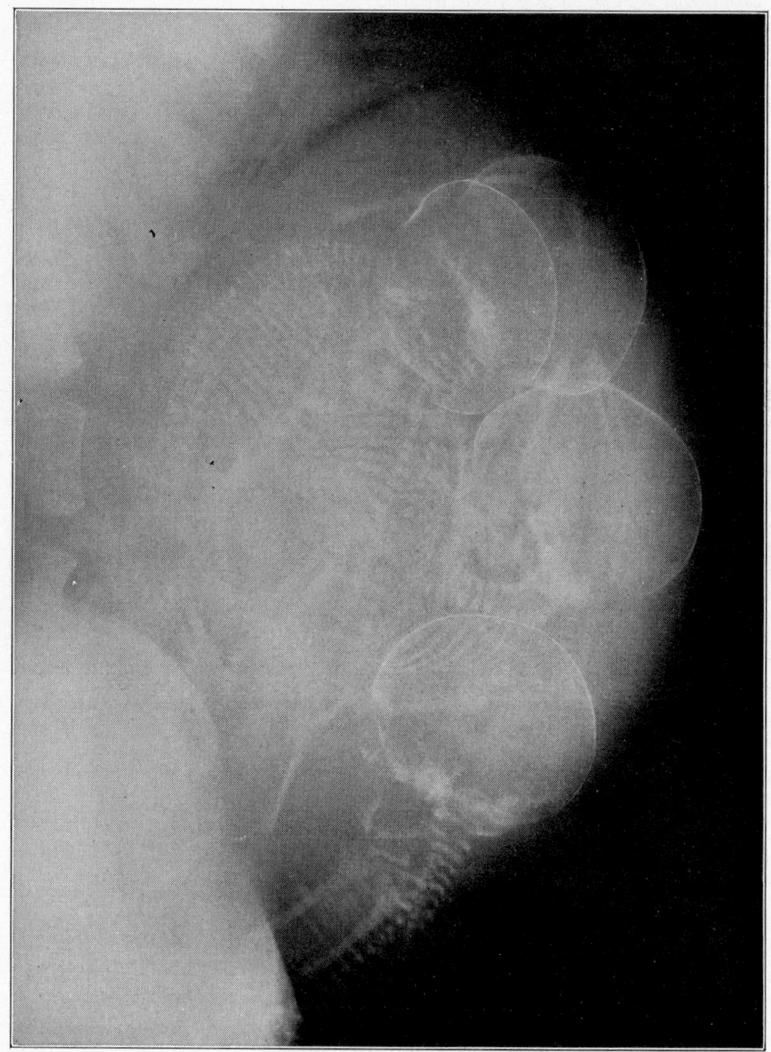

Fig. 378.—Roentgenogram of Quadruplets in Utero.
(Courtesy of Drs. John C. Ullery, Norris W. Vaux and Paul Bishop, Philadelphia.)

Anemia is encountered more frequently than in single pregnancies. Guttmacher found anemia to be not only more frequent but also more pronounced in twin pregnancies. Reference has already been made to the increased tendency to premature labor, due, probably, to the overdistention of the uterus. Potter and Crunden found the average duration of pregnancy to be 256 days in twin pregnancies as compared with 281 days in all other cases; in Guttmacher's series the average twin pregnancy was carried 258 days.

At any time from the twentieth week on, physical examination may create a strong suspicion of multiple pregnancy. If this possibility can be neither confirmed nor refuted, a flat plate of the abdomen should be taken. It is probably best to wait until about the twenty-eighth week for the x-ray.

As soon as the diagnosis is made the patient should be given especially careful prenatal supervision, with visits every week.

Iron should be prescribed forthwith to forestall the development of anemia. The patient should eliminate free salt in the diet because of the excessive tendency to develop edema and hypertensive toxemia. A maternity girdle should be advised to relieve backache or abdominal pressure; since varicose veins are made rapidly worse, elastic stockings or ace bandages are indicated for many. Because premature labor is so common a complication, coitus should be eliminated the last 10 weeks. For the same reason, the patient should be advised to remain in the vicinity where she is to be delivered. Trips are forbidden during her last trimester. Again, since premature labor is so common a complication, it may be advisable to put the patient on oral vitamin K daily, beginning with the twenty-eighth week. Since transfusions during labor or the early puerperium are more frequently used and more urgently needed in multiple pregnancies, every patient with such a diagnosis should be grouped and have her Rh type established before labor begins. As soon as she enters the hospital in labor, a bottle of blood should be matched and reserved until all possibility of its use in the case is eliminated.

Presentation. In twins we find all possible combinations of position for two fetuses, either or both of which may be a vertex, breech, or transverse presentation. The range of incidence of these combinations, as gathered from several sources, is as follows:

Both vertex	31—47 per cent
Vertex plus breech	34—40 per cent
Both breech	8—12 per cent
Longitudinal plus transverse	4—12 per cent
Both transverse	0.3—10 per cent

In approximately 70 per cent of vertex-breech combinations, the first twin is the vertex presentation. In about 90 per cent of the longitudinal-transverse pairs, the longitudinal child is the first. Compound, face and brow, are relatively common because of the small size of the fetuses and the frequent excess of amniotic fluid.

Labor. The conduct of labor in multiple pregnancy is an excellent test of the obstretician's acumen, skill, judgment, and patience, for many complications—uterine inertia, abnormal presentations, prolapse of the cord, and postpartum hemorrhage—are significantly increased. Every statistical analysis demonstrates the twofold or threefold death hazard that the woman faces with a plural delivery as compared with the single birth. To meet this challenge the obstetrician must be especially vigilant. Whenever possible, he should conduct the case in an obstetrical hospital where complications can be more effectively handled.

Length of Labor. There is a difference of opinion concerning the effects of multiple pregnancy on the length of labor. On the basis of the study of the literature and the statistical analysis of 418 births at the Johns Hopkins Hospital, Guttmacher came to the following conclusions: (1) The majority of twin labors are satisfactory.

Because of the small size of the fetuses and the fact that the cervix is frequently obliterated before labor actually begins, the ordinary plural labor is shorter than the ordinary single labor. (2) There is a greater proportion of unsatisfactory dilatory labors among plural pregnancies than among single pregnancies. These in the main are due to primary inertia. (3) False labor is more common in multiple pregnancy.

In 100 primiparous twin labors Guttmacher calculated that the mean length of labor was 17.2 hours and the median, 11.8 hours. This is in comparison to Busby's findings of 14 and 11.5 hours for single primiparous labors. In 318 multiparous twin deliveries the mean length of labor was 11.0 hours and the median, 7.1 hours, in comparison to a mean length of labor for single multiparous births of 9 and 6.7 hours.

Delivery. In the ideal case, labor begins after the fetuses are fully viable. In such a situation the first stage is conducted as usual. However, if labor begins several weeks prematurely or if the fetuses are judged to be very small when at term, one may either reduce markedly the amount of analgesic drugs used or even entirely withhold them. Under such conditions the labor is conducted similarly to that with a single premature fetus.

A spontaneous delivery is especially sought in twins because their birth is so commonly followed by an increase in puerperal morbidity and blood loss. Furthermore, if the twins are small, a spontaneous delivery gives greater chance for fetal salvage. As soon as the first twin is delivered the obstetrician ruptures the sac of the second twin. Then, by combined vaginal and abdominal manipulation, he attempts to adjust the fetus into a longitudinal presentation, either vertex or breech. If he succeeds in doing this, pressure on the fundus, usually best administered by an assistant, will engage the presenting part and rapidly propel it downward through the birth canal which has been so recently dilated. Such pressure is continued until either spontaneous delivery of the second twin eventuates or an easy forceps or breech extraction is carried out. If it is impossible to manipulate the second fetus into a longitudinal position, or if pressure does not engage it in the pelvis, version and extraction should then be carried out on the second twin. In this day of modern obstetrics when anesthesia is a routine procedure, it is impractical to wait for any length of time between the delivery of the two fetuses and therefore the delivery of the second twin follows within a few minutes the birth of the first.

As soon as the first twin is delivered its cord is carefully clamped by two clamps and cut between. It is particularly important that the placental end of the cord be thoroughly clamped since it is possible for the intra-uterine twin to bleed to death through the leaking end of its co-twin's cord. It is usually undesirable and unnecessary to deliver the placenta of the first twin until after the second twin has been delivered.

Immediately after the delivery of the second twin an oxytocic is given and the fundus carefully observed to make sure that it is not being distended by an accumulation of blood. As soon as the placentas give evidence of separation they are expressed. Vigilant observation of the fundus for at least one hour after delivery of the placentas is particularly important since uterine atony is such a common complication after the delivery of twins. A prophylactic therapeutic measure to prevent atony is the administration of intravenous glucose during the delivery, and, as soon as the placentas have been delivered, one cc. of pitocin added to the glucose and a pitocin-glucose drip given during the first hour. This keeps the uterus well contracted and in large measure prevents atony hemorrhage.

Interval Between Infants. Surprising intervals have been reported between the births of twins and triplets. Uthmöller records an interval of four days and eight hours between the births of the first and second triplets, each weighing 4 pounds. In this case labor was re-initiated only after the obstetrician himself had ruptured the membranes of the second sac. Jahreiss gives the complete details of a twin birth in which there was an interval of 11 days and seven hours. These two cases in no way establish a record; we read in Strassmann's textbook a report of cases in which the two births were supposedly separated by 35 and 44 days respectively.

Cesarean section is rarely necessary in multiple pregnancy, except for the rapid termination of pregnancy in the face of a fulminating preeclamptic toxemia or some grave antepartum bleeding complication. In rare instances, when the first twin lies in transverse presentation, cesarean section may offer the best solution, since manipulation of the fetus is likely to induce rupture of the membranes, with prolapse of the cord. Cesarean section may also be necessary in the case of a separate twin pregnancy in each horn of a bicornuate uterus. In such case, the delivered contracted horn may block the pelvic inlet and cause insuperable dystocia for the undelivered fetus. Cesarean section is also indicated if the patient has had a previous delivery by cesarean section. The over-distention of the uterus attendant upon multiple pregnancy may very well rupture the scar of a previous section and therefore a repeat section is more or less mandatory in the presence of a multiple pregnancy.

Collision or the entrance of a fetal pole of each fetus into the pelvis at the same time is most likely when the fetuses are small or the pelvis of a justo major type. The upper displacement of the presenting part of the less well-engaged fetus usually solves the problem. A second and somewhat similar complication is locking. In order for locking to occur the first child must present by the breech and the second by vertex. With the descent of the breech the chin of the breech child locks in the neck and chin of its cephalic co-twin. If unlocking cannot be done, either cesarean section or decapitation must be resorted to. The locking of twins is said to occur about once in 90,000 deliveries which would be approximately once in 1,000 twin births.

Anesthesia for Delivery. Gas-oxygen-ether is most frequently used as the anesthetic of choice in plural births. However, this has several disadvantages. First, the fetuses are usually small and inhalation anesthesia may present a risk to them and second, ether promotes atony of the uterus post-delivery. Therefore, conduction anesthesia is being more and more commonly used for the delivery of twins. In such an instance either saddle block or caudal anesthesia is given as in a single pregnancy. This is entirely satisfactory unless a version has to be done on the second twin. If the uterus is tight and version would be difficult, then an ether-oxygen anesthetic is superimposed on the conduction anesthetic. The advantages, of course, are that conduction anesthesia is best for the small fetus and also that it in no way interferes with the contraction of the post-delivery uterus.

Antepartum and Intrapartum Hemorrhage Complications. Placenta previa has been reported in 0.5 to 3.5 per cent of twin pregnancies. Strassmann claims that the frequency of placenta previa in twin gestations is one in 41. Spirito reported three cases of placenta previa in 81 twin deliveries and three cases of twins in 70 instances of placenta previa. In current articles Hawker and Allen report a 2.1 per cent incidence from the St. Louis City Hospital and Potter reports 1.2 per cent from the Chicago Lying-In Hospital. The increased incidence of placenta previa in multiple pregnancies is no doubt due to the greater surface area of the uterus covered by the twin placentas. The course and treatment of placenta previa in multiple pregnancy does not differ from that in single pregnancy. Premature separation of the placenta is no more frequent before the birth of the first child than it is in single pregnancies; it is due to the same etiologic factors in both cases. However, premature separation of the placenta is not infrequent between the births of a first and second twin. It may involve either the placenta of the first twin already born, or the second twin, or both. It is due, of course, to a diminished area of attachment caused by the reduction in size of the uterus following the expulsion of the first child. It causes external and concealed hemorrhage, with distress of the fetal heart if the placenta of the second twin is involved. Occasionally, one or both placentas are born before the birth of the second infant. The treatment of premature separation between a first and second twin is immediate vaginal delivery. Because of the prevalence of velamentous insertion of the cord in multiple pregnancy, vasa previa is naturally also more frequent than in single pregnancies. The diagnosis of its rupture depends on the contemporaneous appearance of the bleeding with either the spontaneous or artificial rupture of the membranes. Prompt delivery, when possible, is essential, not only to the twin from whom the blood is coming, but to the co-twin as well, if the "third circulation" is well developed.

Prolapsed Cord. A multiple pregnancy presents the ideal background for prolapsed cord, an excess of amniotic fluid, and small fetuses. The incidence at the Hopkins hospital was 1.1 per cent. Treatment of the prolapse is not materially altered by a plural gestation, but the prognosis is usually more favorable since the infants are smaller and compression is ordinarily not so complete.

Constriction Ring. This complication may be encountered while doing a version on the second twin. In our experience, it had no relationship to a protracted labor but in each instance followed the operative delivery of the first twin in a term pregnancy. The complication was met in 0.9 per cent of the cases at the Johns Hopkins Hospital.

Postpartum Hemmorhage. The ordinary hazards of the third stage—the unwelcome trinity, postpartum hemorrhage, adherent placenta, and post-delivery shock—are exaggerated in multiple pregnancy. The unusual frequency of these complications arises from the increased area of placental attachment, the abnormal uterine distention with resultant atony, and the sudden release of intra-abdominal pressure. In view of this, the value of having intravenous fluids running during the delivery and the ability to add an oxytocic agent to the intravenous fluid immediately after the delivery of the placentas becomes obvious. The additional safety factor of having properly matched blood readily available needs little comment. Manual removal of the placenta becomes necessary twice as often after twins as after single infants. This necessity is increased by operative twin deliveries and by an excessively long interval between the births of the two children. The increased incidence of post-delivery shock after twins has been stressed by several authors. It therefore becomes important in plural deliveries to hold blood loss to a minimum, to eliminate, whenever possible, traumatizing procedures such as manual dilatation of the cervix, and to have in readiness therapeutic agents to treat shock.

Among the white patients of the Johns Hopkins Hospital the average viable—that is, term and premature—single fetus weighed 3,350 gm. and among the colored patients the average weighed 3,100 gm. The average for viable white twins was 2,649 gm., and 2,446 gm. for colored. In other words, the average white child when born singly weighed about 700 gm. or one pound and 9 ounces more than the average white twin at birth. Among the colored patients the difference was slightly less, about 650 gm. One important factor is the commonly abbreviated duration of twin pregnancies; in addition, as Stehle has proved in material gathered from the University Clinic at Freiburg, the twin fetus weighs and measures less per unit time of intra-uterine residence than does the single child. Stehle compared the weight and length of twins born during various weeks of pregnancy with Ahlfeld's Tables of Weights and Lengths arranged in the same way for single fetuses. From the thirtieth to the fortieth weeks of gestation he found a mean difference of 536 gm. in weight, and 2 cm. in length between single fetuses and twins of equal intra-uterine age. In explanation, Stehle quotes Strassmann: "One gets the impression that the body, that is, the mother's body, cannot furnish enough nutritive material for the proper growth of the multiple fetuses." Because of the parasitic nature of the fetus in relationship to its mother one doubts whether the explanation is as simple as this. It is likely that the smaller twin fetus finds its analogy with the child born to a mother with a chronic hypertensive toxemia. It is probable that in both instances there is an interference with adequate placental nutrition. When compared to a single fetus, twins probably have a relatively diminished placental bed which curtails nutritional interchange.

There is less relative difference in length than in weight between the single and twin fetus. This means that the twin is a thin child at birth. Further, it is a child which is viscerally more mature than the weight would indicate. Englehorn believes that a twin does as well at birth and in the neonatal period as does a single fetus 500 grams heavier.

Guttmacher noted a steady rise in the weight of the average newborn twin with increasing parity. This rise was progressive up to the sixth pregnancy; from then on no further weight progression occurred. Of 684 twins analyzed 21, that is 3 per cent, exceeded 3,600 gm. at birth and 3.4 per cent 4,000 gm. The three largest weighed 4,060, 4,080, and 4,115 gm. The heaviest pair in 346 sets totaled 7,680 gm. The heavier twins listed above by no means establish a weight record. Holzapfel in 1935 reports the birth to a woman in her third pregnancy of twin boys weighing 4,670 gm. and 4,510 gm. Both infants survived. The placenta weighed 1,300 gm. and this with an estimated 3 liters of amniotic fluid amounted to 13.5 kg. of intra-uterine contents. According to several German authorities, there is a greater intra-pair weight and length difference between one-egg than between two-egg twins. This is true when comparing groups of like sex as well as opposite sex twins. The male twin is ordinarily larger than the female. In both single-egg and double-egg births, the heavier twin usually presents first and is born first.

It is generally believed that congenital malformations are more common in twins than in singly born children. It is further believed that malformations are probably commoner in the one-egg than in the two-egg varieties. If a one-egg twin has an abnormality it is almost certain that the co-twin will have a similar defect. It may be on the same side or opposite side owing to mirror imaging. MacFarland and Meade think that the following generalization seems justified: "Heterologous (two-egg) twins never suffer from identical malformations, nor does one of homologous (one-egg) twins ever suffer from a malformation not shared by its fellow." The reported minor exceptions to the latter half of the above law include: cryptorchidism, congenital inguinal hernia, hydrocele, dislocation of the optic lens, and perhaps rare instances of clubfoot. All other congenital malformations appear in both of a pair of identical twins.

FETAL AND MATERNAL MORTALITY

Fetal Mortality. W. L. Williams in his text, *Veterinary Obstetrics,* states that, because of the reproductive wastage involved, many breeders of horses and cattle consider it an undesirable trait when the stock is prone to multiple births. More of the animal mothers die, more pregnancies terminate in abortion, and a higher percentage of young succumb. If human multiple births were viewed in this way, the same conclusion would be reached. Yerushalmy and Sheerar compared the stillbirth rate of twins to single-born infants. In studying the stillbirth rate for a quarter of a million twins born in the United States from 1931 to 1935, they found a rate of 77.5 per 1,000 twins. This was more than twice the stillbirth rate of 35.6 per 1,000 for all births during the same period. The stillbirth rate for triplets was 152.2 per 1,000. All authorities are in agreement that the total fetal mortality for twins is two to three times that for single births. In her recent study at the Chicago Lying-In Hospital, Potter found an uncorrected mortality for a series of twins of 15.6 per cent. If the abortions and fetuses weighing less than 1,000 gm. are excluded, the mortality is 8.2 per cent; if those of less than 1,500 gm. are excluded it falls to 4.4 per cent. This latter figure was twice the total hospital mortality of 2 per cent which existed during the same period for all infants weighing more than 1,500 gm. A predominant cause, of course, is prematurity. However, when one realizes the many complications—prolapsed cord, placenta previa, premature separation of the second placenta, contraction ring, malformations, etc.—which beset twins, there is little reason to be surprised at the differential mortality between multiple and single infants. The chief way to reduce fetal mortality in multiple pregnancy is to combat the effects of prematurity.

Maternal Mortality. By combining the viable twin deliveries reported by six authors, Guttmacher noted that 43 women died in 1,645 plural pregnancies and labor. This gives a rate of 261.4 deaths per 10,000. At the Johns Hopkins Hospital there have been 11 women who have died with a multiple pregnancy. In each instance the patients had hypertensive toxemia plus excessive postpartum blood loss. If either condition existed without the other the patient survived; that is, if she had hypertension without postpartum hemorrhage or postpartum hemorrhage without hypertension, death did not occur. However, when combined the two seemed singularly lethal. More recent studies of multiple pregnancy have shown the anticipated decrease in maternal mortality. This is probably due in large measure to the greater use of adequate transfusions. The best way to protect the mother's life in a plural pregnancy is through punctilious, intelligent, prenatal care with the prompt recognition and treatment of a hypertensive toxemia; spontaneous delivery of the infants when possible; and complete readiness to replace immediately postpartum blood loss of more than an average amount.

BIBLIOGRAPHY

Allen, Edgar, and others. Recovery of Human Ova from the Uterine Tubes. J.A.M.A., 1928, 91:1018.

Archer. Observations Showing That a White Woman, by Intercourse with a White Man and a Negro, May Conceive Twins, One of Which Shall Be White and the Other a Mulatto. Medical Respiratory, 1810, 3rd Hexade, 1:319.

Barfuth. Ein Zeugniss für eine Geburt von Siebenlingen beim Menschen. Anat. Anz., 1895, 10:330.

de Blécourt, J. J., and Nijhoff, G. C. Fünflingsgeburten. Wolters. Groningen. 1904.

Busby, T. The Duration of Labor, Mean, Median and Mode. Am. J. Obst. & Gynec., 1948, 55:846.

Coulton, D., Hertig, A., and Long, W. N. Monoamniotic Twins. Am. J. Obst. & Gynec., 1947, 54:119.

Curtius, F. Nachgeburtsbefunde bei Zeillingen und Ahnlichkeitsdiagnose. Arch. f. Gynäk., 1930, 140:361.

——— and Korkhaus, G. Klinische Zwillingsstudien. Ztschr. f. d. ges. Anat., 1930, 15:229.

Dafoe, A. R. Dionne Quintuplets. J.A.M.A., 1934, 103:673.

——— Further History of Care and Feeding of the Dionne Quintuplets. Canad. M. A. J., 1936, 34:26.

——— and Dafoe, W. A. Physical Welfare of the Dionne Quintuplets. Canad. M. A. J., 1937, 37:415.

Davenport. Is There an Inheritance of Twinning Tendency through the Father? Ztschr. f. indukt. Abstammungs- u. Verebungsl., 1928, Suppl. Bd. 1, 595.

Essen-Möller, E. Empirische ähnlichkeitsdiagnose bei zwillingen. Hereditas., 1941, 27:1.

Greulich, W. W. The Birth of Six Pairs of Fraternal Twins to the Same Parents. A Discussion of the Possible Significance of Such Cases in the Light of Some Recent Observations. J.A.M.A., 1938, 110:559.

Guttmacher, A. F. An Analysis of 521 Cases of Twin Pregnancy. I. Differences in Single and Double Ovum Twinning. Am. J. Obst. & Gynec., 1937, 34:76.

——— An Analysis of 573 Cases of Twin Pregnancy. II. The Hazards of Pregnancy Itself. Am. J. Obst. & Gynec., 1939, 38:277.

——— Clinical Aspects of Twin Pregnancy. M. Clin. North America, 1939, 23:427.

——— Life in the Making. The Viking Press, New York, 1933.

Hamblen, E. C., Baker, R. D., and Derieux, G. D. Roentgenographic Diagnosis and Anatomic Studies of a Quintuple Pregnancy. J.A.M.A., 1937, 109:10.

Hamlett, G. W. Human Twinning in the United States. Genetics, 1935, 20:250.

Hawker, W. D., and Allen, M. A Study of 145 Consecutive Twin Pregnancies. Am. J. Obst. & Gynec., 1949, 57:996.

Hellin, D. Die Ursache der Multiparität der uniparen Tiere überhaupt und der Zwillingschwangerschaft beim menschen. Seitz and Schauer, Munich, 1895.

Holzapfel, K. Gemini permagni. Monatschr. f. Geburtsh. u. Gynäk., 1935, 98:30.

Johnston. Triplets Diagnosed by X-ray, etc. Texas State J. Med., 1925, 20:570.

Kerr, J. W., and Cookman, H. A remarkable case of multiple pregnancy. M. Press & Circular., 1903, N. S., 75:537.

Komai, T., and Fukuoka, G. Frequency of Multiple Births among the Japanese and Related Peoples. Am. J. Phys. Anthropol., 1936, 21:433.

MacArthur, J. Genetics of Quintuplets: Diagnosis of the Dionne Quintuplets as a Monozygotic Set. J. Hered., 1938, 29:323.

——— and Ford, N. Collected Studies on the Dionne Quintuplets. Univ. Toronto Press, 1937.

Marcus, H. Grossesse triple diagnostiquée par les rayons. Röntgen. Gynéc. et obst., 1928, 17:315.

Meyer, A. W. The Occurrence of Superfetation. J.A.M.A., 1919, 72:769.

Newman, H. H. The Biology of Twins. 1923, Chicago.

——— The Physiology of Twinning, 1917. Chicago.

——— Methods of Diagnosing Monozygotic and Dizygotic Twins. Biol. Bull., Boston, 1928, 55:283.

Nichols. Sex Ratio of Twins. Mem. Am. Anthropol. Ass., 1907, 1.

Patellani, S. Die mehrfachen Schwangerschaften, etc. Ztschr. f. Geburtsh. u. Gynäk., 1896, 35:373.

Paterson and Newman. The Development of the Nine-banded Armadillo, etc. J. Morphol., 1910, 21.

Potter, E. L., and Crunden, A. B. Twin Pregnancies in the Service of the Chicago Lying-In Hospital. Am. J. Obst. & Gynec., 1941, 42:870.

POTTER, E. L., and FULLER, H. Multiple Pregnancies at the Chicago Lying-In Hospital, 1941-1947. Am. J. Obst. & Gynec., 1949, 58:139.

RIBEMONT-DESSAIGNES et LEPAGE. Précis d'obstétrique, 1894, 864-897. (Grossesse gémellaire).

SASSE, A. Beitrag zum Stumium der eineifigen Drillinge. Acta obst. et gynec. Scandinav., 1926, 4:79.

SCHATZ, F. Die Gefässverbindungen der Placentakreisläufe eineiiger Zwillinge, ihre Entwickelung und ihre Folgen. Arch. f. Gynäk., 1882-1900, Bde. 19, 24, 27, 29, 30, 53, 55, 58, 60.

SCHULTZ, A. The Number of Young at a Birth and the Number of Nipples in Primates. Am. J. Phys. Anthropol., 1948, 6:1.

SIEMENS, H. W. Die diagnose der eineiigkeit. Arch. f. Gynäk., 1925, 126:623.

SPIRITO. Placenta Previa in Twin Pregnancy. Abstract in J. Obst. & Gynaec. Brit. Emp., 1924, 31:116.

STOCKARD, C. R. An Experimental Study of Twins, Double Monsters and Single Deformities. Am. J. Anat., 1921, 28:115.

STRANDSKOV, H. H. Plural Birth Frequencies in the Total, the "White" and the "Colored" U. S. Populations. Am. J. Phys. Anthropol., N. S., 1945, 3:49.

——— and EDELEN, E. W. Monozygotic and Dizygotic Twin Birth Frequencies in the Total White and Colored U. S. Population. Genetics, 1946, 31:438.

——— and SIEMANS, G. J. An Analysis of the Sex Ratios among Single and Plural Births in the Total "White" and "Colored" U. S. Populations. Am. J. Phys. Anthropol., 1946, N. S., 4:491.

STREETER, G. L. Formation of Single Ovum Twins. Bull. Johns Hopkins Hosp., 1919, 30:235.

——— Single Ovum Twins in the Pig. Am. J. Anat., 1924, 34:183.

STUDDIFORD, W. E. Is Superfetation Possible in the Human Being? Am. J. Obst. & Gynec., 1936, 31:845.

SZENDI, B. The Significance of the Structure of the Ovular Membranes and of the Vascular Network of the Placenta: on the Basis of 112 Twin Births. Arch. f. Gynäk., 1938, 167:108.

VASSALI. Gazetta med. Ital. Lombardia, 1888. Reported under Miscellany. Boston Med. & Surg. J., 1895, 132:243.

WEINSTEIN. Beiträge zur Physiol. u. Pathologie der Mehrlingsgeburten beim Menschen. Arch. f. d. ges. Physiol., 1901, 88:346.

WILLIAMS, J. W. Note on Placentation in Quadruplet and Triplet Pregnancy. Bull. Johns Hopkins Hosp., 1926, 39:271.

WILLIAMS, W. L. Veterinary Obstetrics. 2nd ed. 1931, Ithaca, New York.

WILSON, K. M. Practitioners Library of Medicine and Surgery. D. Appleton-Century Company, 1934, 6:135.

YERUSHALMY, J., and SHEERAR. Studies on Twins. Part II. On the Early Mortality of Like Sexed and Unlike Sexed Twins. Human Biol., 1940, 12:247.

ZELENY, C. L. The Relative Numbers of Twins and Triplets. Science. N. S. 1921, 53:262.

26

VOMITING OF PREGNANCY

The mild type of nausea and vomiting which is frequently noted in the early weeks of gestation has already been mentioned. This occurs in approximately one half of all pregnant women, usually appearing at about the sixth week and disappearing spontaneously six or eight weeks later. In such circumstances the patient suffers from nausea, or even vomits, shortly after arising, whence the term "morning sickness." In other cases the vomiting occurs at other times and at more frequent intervals, occasionally lasting for a longer period; exceptionally it becomes so frequent and severe as to put the life of the patient in danger. In the latter circumstances, it is designated as pernicious vomiting, or *hyperemesis gravidarum*.

Ordinarily, the so-called "morning sickness" is attended by no more serious results than the actual discomfort connected with it, and many women consider it so natural an accompaniment of pregnancy that they do not complain of it. Others, however, soon demand relief from the physician, and the mere enumeration of some of the many remedies recommended affords conclusive evidence that a specific cure has not yet been discovered. In some instances the first remedy administered is followed by immediate relief, while in other cases various drugs may be employed in succession without result.

Drugs are rarely required, except for the relief of constipation, and the condition can usually be cured, or at least greatly ameliorated, by suggestion, the adoption of more hygienic methods of living, and regulation of the diet. The physician should not make light of the condition, but he should impress upon the patient that vomiting is not a necessary accompaniment of pregnancy, as is shown by the fact that less than one-half of all pregnant women suffer from it, and, furthermore, that it can be controlled by exercise of the will and the adoption of suitable and dietetic measures. He should then inquire carefully into her mode of life, and see that proper exercise, occupation, amusement, and rest are obtained. The diet should be carefully regulated. We lay great stress, particularly on account of its suggestive influence, upon the patient's eating a hard dry biscuit the moment she awakens, before raising her head from the pillow. Afterward, breakfast may be taken in bed, or not, according to her habit. The important point, however, is to arrange that food be taken at frequent intervals throughout the day, so that the patient gets six small meals instead of three larger ones. It is not sufficient to prescribe this in general terms, but precise directions should be given as to exactly what should be eaten at definitely appointed hours. If the patient is impressed with the necessity of following these minutiae implicitly, the condition will usually pass off within a few days and the employment of drugs will be unnecessary.

While all gradations of nausea and vomiting may occur, a patient is considered to suffer from hyperemesis rather than the milder and more common phases of the disorder when the condition has advanced to such a degree that hospital admission is necessary; in turn, hospital admission is usually desirable whenever the patient exhibits acetone or diacetic acid in the urine, and/or shows a weight loss of 5 per cent or more. On the basis of these criteria one obstetrical admission to our clinic in every 143 is because of hyperemesis.

Etiology. Since pernicious vomiting is always preceded by the so-called morning sickness, and, as the latter occurs in approximately every other pregnant woman, it may be assumed that the cause of vomiting in general may lie in some factor commonly present in normal pregnancy and that pernicious vomiting is due to an increase in the amount or in the potency of that factor, or to decreased resistance to its action on the part of the woman. Harding, Titus and his associates, Dieckmann and Crossen, and other writers attribute it to depletion of the glycogen stores of the liver. On the other hand, the constant entrance into the maternal circulation of fragments of chorionic villi (deportation), the increased amounts of estrogenic substances, as well as the other endocrine changes discussed in an earlier section, and the metabolic changes of normal gestation, all indicate the existence of conditions which, by slight aberration, might give rise to clinical symptoms. Roughly speaking, alterations in any one of these factors, as well as a decrease in the resistance on the part of the mother to their action, afford a theoretic basis for a "toxemic" origin, which we believe is concerned in all cases of vomiting of pregnancy, whether mild or severe. Unfortunately, however, our knowledge along such lines is still so defective that any theory concerning the etiology of the condition must be regarded as tentative.

Further evidence suggesting an organic basis for hyperemesis is the diminished motility of the stomach, which is a constant physiologic concomitant of gestation. According to the studies of Hansen, the emptying time of the stomach during pregnancy is prolonged 50 to 130 minutes beyond the two-hour period considered to be normal for nonpregnant persons. In a few gravid women Hansen found that the stomach never emptied itself completely. These studies have been confirmed by N. H. Williams. In general, gastric motility is proportional to the acid content of the stomach; from what has been said it is not surprising that hypochlorhydria is common in pregnancy. Stanley Way has shown that the acid content of the stomach is inversely proportional to the urinary gonadotrophin concentration. Since the latter reaches its highest levels in the first trimester of gestation, just when nausea and vomiting are most common, there may well be some relationship between chorionic gonadotrophin levels, hypochlorhydria, diminished gastric motility, and nausea and vomiting.

It has long been thought that nausea and vomiting in pregnancy are in large measure a neurosis, that is, a functional disturbance of the patient's psyche. In all life's encounters there are probably few experiences which are at first more upsetting, mentally and emotionally, than the realization by a young woman that she is pregnant. At the outset, there are several weeks of anxious uncertainty before she can be sure of the diagnosis. Then, numerous adjustments may have to be made and plans changed. Emotionally, the implications of pregnancy extend far back into the past when she met her husband, while its future ramifications are endless. The responsibilities entailed are plain enough also, and may seem on first thought more than can be assumed. These, and many other thoughts, crowd themselves into the mind and, in women who cannot adjust themselves to all these new circumstances, it is understandable that the groundwork for a neurosis is laid. Beyond question, there is an important neurotic element in most of these cases, a factor which looms large in the treatment of the condition.

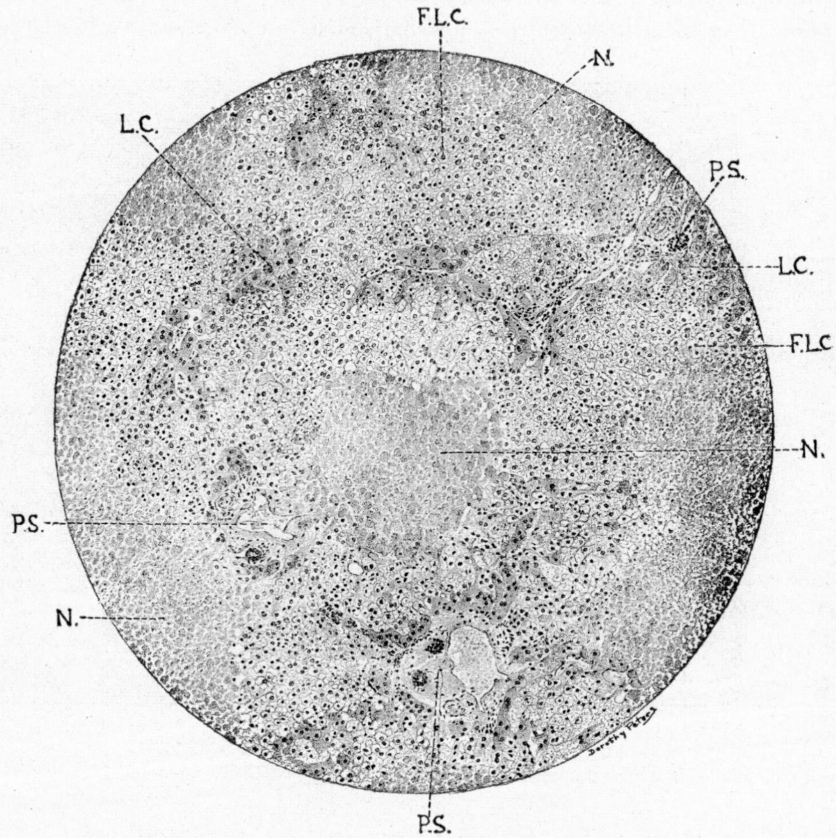

Fig. 379.—Liver from Vomiting of Pregnancy Showing Central Necrosis. × 50.

F.L.C., liver cells showing fatty degeneration; *L.C.*, unchanged liver cells; *N.*, areas of necrosis; *P.S.*, portal space.

The neurotic factor, on the other hand, is not the whole cause of nausea and vomiting, nor, in all probability, even the basic cause. In every case an important underlying organic process is also at work—either the dissemination of toxins into the maternal organism, some maladjustment of the maternal metabolism to the changes wrought by the growing fetus, or alterations in gastric motility. It is this toxic or organic element which is doubtless the fundamental cause of the disease. To what extent the patient reacts to this underlying process by vomiting seems to be determined in large measure by neurotic factors, that is, by her psyche, emotional stability, and by the mental stress and strain which pregnancy has imposed.

Pernicious vomiting is sometimes associated with serious hepatic lesions. In such cases there is profound necrosis of the central portion of the lobules, while the periphery remains intact. In several of Williams' specimens the destruction of tissue was so great that practically nine-tenths of the organ was thrown out of function (Fig. 379). In other fatal cases, the characteristic necrosis is absent, but the liver has undergone such marked fatty degeneration that upon staining frozen sections with sudan the entire specimen seems to be filled with fat. All these hepatic lesions may be noted in women dying after a long illness and are probably a manifestation of starvation rather than of acute toxemia. The renal lesions are degenerative in character

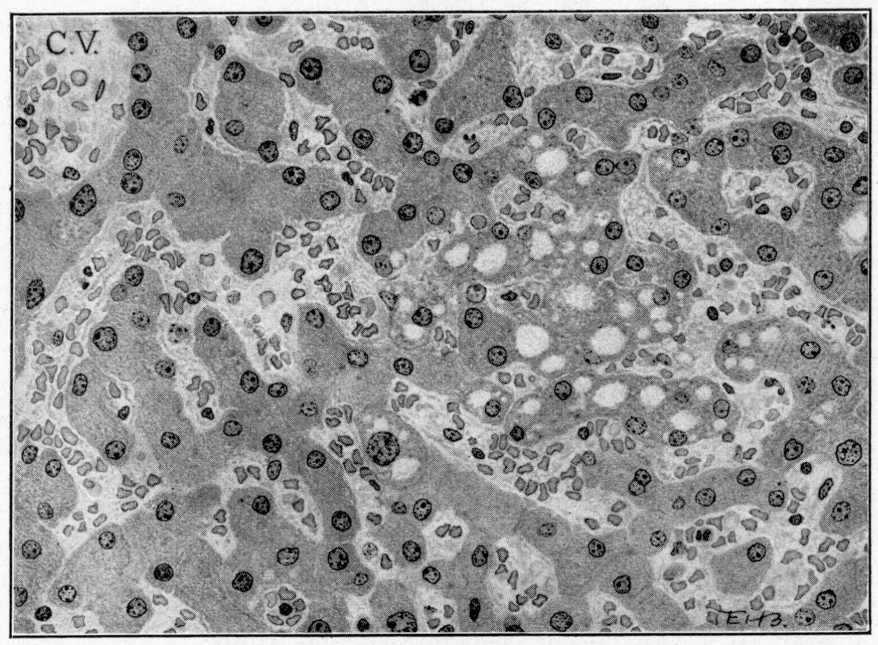

FIG. 380.—LIVER DAMAGE IN VOMITING OF PREGNANCY. × 480.
Portion of lobule showing vacuolization and necrosis of liver cells in vicinity of central vein, *C.V.*

and are practically limited to the convoluted tubules whose epithelium in many cases is necrotic and whose lumina are filled with debris.

As the hepatic necrosis is altogether different from that observed in eclampsia, in which the process begins in the periportal spaces and is primarily due to thrombosis, toxemic vomiting is an entirely distinct process and has only three points in common with eclampsia, namely, that both occur in pregnant women, are manifestations of disturbed metabolism, and are accompanied by hepatic lesions.

Dieckmann and Crossen reported no marked disturbances in the urine, except a decrease in chlorides. Our findings are similar. The urea excretion in the urine is within normal limits. The ammonia coefficient of the urine may be elevated, so that instead of 3 or 4 per cent of the total nitrogen being excreted in the form of ammonia, the figure might rise to 10, 20, or even 40 per cent. The high ammonia coefficient is undoubtedly the result of starvation and not necessarily indicative of serious hepatic lesions; consequently it gives no specific information as to the severity of the disease, except in so far as it reveals increased ammonia formation in the kidneys, which is an essential part of the mechanism for neutralizing such acids as are brought to them for excretion.

Numerous investigators have studied the blood chemistry in severe vomiting in the hope of learning more about the changes in metabolism and possibly of obtaining a clue as to the treatment to be pursued. In general, it may be said that there is little change in the mild, but that considerable changes occur in the severe cases. In the latter there is a definite increase in the nonprotein nitrogen, uric acid, and urea, a moderate decrease in the chlorides and little alteration in the carbon dioxide combining power. These changes appear to be associated with starvation, dehydration, and incomplete oxidation of fatty acids, rather than with the etiology of the actual vomiting of pregnancy.

The polyneuritis which occasionally develops in women suffering from severe vomiting of pregnancy is undoubtedly due to a vitamin B deficiency; with adequate vitamin therapy this condition usually improves. This observation suggests that the etiology of vomiting may be related to a vitamin B deficiency. However, the evidence to date indicates that vomiting of pregnancy may lead to a vitamin deficiency, which in turn results in such complications as polyneuritis.

Symptoms. The disease varies in degree of severity from nausea and morning sickness to the severe or pernicious type of vomiting which may have a fatal outcome.

Morning sickness starts with a feeling of nausea upon rising in the morning. Although the patient is unable to retain her breakfast, by noon she has completely recovered and remains so till the next morning. In many patients, however, the time relationships are not so definite and the nausea and vomiting may persist throughout the day and even be worse in the afternoon. This state of affairs continues from one to three weeks and then suddenly ceases. It is self-limited and associated with only a slight loss of body weight and with no other signs or symptoms of toxemia. The majority of patients suffering from vomiting of pregnancy fall in this group.

A smaller number of these patients develop persistent vomiting, lasting four to eight weeks or longer and resulting in a loss of body weight of 10 to 20 pounds or more. These patients vomit two, three, or more times a day and may be unable to retain any nourishment by mouth. There may be dryness of the skin accompanied sometimes by jaundice. The severe type of vomiting may occur in either acute or chronic form. In the former the disease pursues a rapid course, and the patient, after a few days of ordinary vomiting, may begin to eject coffee-ground vomitus and soon passes into a somnolent or comatose condition, and dies within a week or 10 days without marked emaciation. In the latter and more frequent variety, persistent vomiting may continue for weeks, the patient becoming markedly emaciated before the seriousness of the condition is appreciated. Later she begins to vomit coffee-ground-like material in large quantities and without apparent effort. At this time symptoms indicative of toxemia appear, the patient becoming torpid or violently excited and finally passing into a condition of coma. In some instances, slight jaundice may develop, and, toward the terminal stage of the disease, the urine becomes greatly diminished in amount and contains albumin, casts, and even blood. Even in patients who ultimately recover, great emaciation may occur, so that losses of 20 to 30 pounds are not unusual.

In the later stages of the disease—rarely seen today—a low-grade fever frequently develops. This seldom exceeds 101° F. but may persist despite adequate hydration. The behavior of the pulse is not constant but in the severer forms of hyperemesis it is almost always accelerated, often above 130.

The **diagnosis** of hyperemesis rarely presents any difficulties although in rare instances coincidental diseases of the gastro-intestinal tract, including catarrhal jaundice, may simulate it, at least for a few days. With prompt, persistent, and intelligent therapy, the **prognosis** of nausea and vomiting in pregnancy, including hyperemesis, is excellent. Thus, in 150 cases of hyperemesis admitted to our clinic in the past decade, there has been no maternal death and only one therapeutic abortion. As indicated, the gravity of the situation from day to day is best judged by the presence or absence of acetone and diacetic acid in the urine and by the body weight.

Treatment. The principles underlying the treatment of hyperemesis gravidarum are: (1) combat the dehydration by liberal administration of parenteral fluids; (2) combat the starvation by administration of glucose intravenously and thiamine chloride subcutaneously and, if necessary, by feeding a high caloric, high vitamin, fluid diet through a nasal tube; and (3) combat the neurosis by psychotherapy, sedatives, and isolation.

Although it may be necessary on occasion to treat cases of hyperemesis in the home, hospitalization is desirable because isolation from relatives, change of atmosphere, and better facilities for intravenous medication confer unusual benefits in this condition. During the first 24 hours in the hospital it is customary to withhold all food and fluids by mouth in order to give the gastro-intestinal tract as complete a rest as possible. Glucose solution, usually in 10 per cent concentration, is administered intravenously; in addition, normal saline solutions are given subcutaneously or intravenously. The total fluid intake should approximate or exceed 3,000 cc. in the 24 hours. A careful record must be kept of the exact quantity of fluids given, the amount of urine excreted, and the quantity of the vomitus. Sedation is accomplished either by sodium luminal hypodermically in dosage of 1 or 2 grains every 4 hours, or by the rectal instillation of some barbiturate drug such as sodium amytal, 3 grains every 6 hours. Thiamine hydrochloride, 50 mg. daily hypodermically, supplies the most urgent vitamin needs during the first 24 hours. All visitors are excluded during this period, including husband and relatives.

After such a regimen for 24 hours, dry toast, crackers, or cereal is given by mouth in small quantities every two or three hours. Fluids are given on alternate hours in small amounts (not over 100 cc. at a time); hot tea and ginger ale usually are tolerated better than plain water. If no vomiting occurs, the amounts and variety of the food are gradually increased until the patient is on a regular soft, high vitamin diet. The intravenous administration of fluids may have to be continued for several days, depending on the oral intake.

The success of the treatment will depend in large measure on the tact, understanding, and attitude of the attendants. While optimism must be the keynote of the approach to the patient, this must be coupled with a plainly avowed determination to conquer the complication. The patient must gradually be led to understand that, in the treatment of vomiting, the physician knows no such word as "failure." Not a few of these patients are in psychologic conflict because of family, financial, or social difficulties; many are averse to the whole idea of pregnancy. If one can only get to the root of these difficulties in a tactful, sympathetic way, and by suitable readjustments reconcile the patient to becoming a mother, a great deal will have been accomplished.

Great care must be exercised in preparing and serving trays for patients suffering from hyperemesis. The portions should be extremely small and attractively arranged. Cold liquids such as ginger ale or lemonade must be ice-cold; hot foods, such as soups, cocoa, and tea, must be steaming hot, since lukewarm liquids may be nauseating. It is best not to discuss food with the patient, but simply assume that she will enjoy it and talk about other matters. At all times keep the emesis basin out of view; the sight of it may be enough to start vomiting. Likewise, the smell of food may be nauseating and, accordingly, the patient's room should be kept well aired and be as far from the kitchen as possible.

If vomiting continues despite these measures (as it rarely does), nasal feeding may be instituted. A small rubber tube (Levin tube) is inserted through a nostril and on down into the stomach; the tube is strapped to the patient's cheek, connected with an overhanging bottle, and left in place. By this means, large amounts of vitamin-rich liquid foods may be administered. The secret of success with nasal feeding lies in very slow but constant introduction of food into the stomach. The apparatus should be so arranged that the number of drops per minute passing through the tube can be counted. This should not exceed 50 per minute. Even this slow rate, it may be noted, yields about 200 cc. per hour.

Even the most severe cases of hyperemesis will usually respond favorably to the treatment described if patience and persistence are exercised, but, in rare instances, the patient may continue to vomit despite all efforts, and such grave signs may develop that the physician is forced to the conclusion that further continuation of pregnancy will be at the cost of the woman's life. The following signs are grave omens and, especially when several are present, may call for therapeutic abortion: (1) jaundice; (2) delirium; (3) steadily rising pulse rate to levels of 130 or above; (4) fever of 101° F. or above which persists despite liberal fluid intake; and (5) hemorrhages in the retina.

Countless hormones and vitamins have been employed in the treatment of vomiting of pregnancy, including suprarenal cortical hormone, estrogens, parathyroid extract, testosterone propionate, Lugol's solution, vitamin B complex, ascorbic acid and liver extract. When it is recalled that the proponents of each of these substances reported gratifying results, there is reason to suspect that the effects were due to psychotherapy rather than to any specific action of the agent used; and, in general, there is justified skepticism about the intrinsic value of such medication in this condition. The present trend is toward vitamin B complex, and various reports would seem to indicate that this form of treatment may have considerable value. Thus, Weinstein, Mitchell, and Sustendal have reported complete or considerable relief from nausea and vomiting of pregnancy in 68 patients treated with oral administration of pyridoxine hydrochloride (vitamin B_6). Other authors report success with the use of thiamin (vitamin B_1), pyridoxine, and ascorbic acid (vitamin C). Hart, McConnell, and Pickett found thiamin hydrochloride and pyridoxine hydrochloride, combined in doses of 100 mg. each, to give better results than pyridoxine alone.

It is, of course, essential that any vitamin deficiency should be corrected in patients suffering from vomiting of pregnancy, particularly if polyneuritic symptoms should develop. Prolonged vomiting is frequently accompanied by such vitamin deficiencies and thus the parenteral administration of the B complex fractions and of vitamin C is recommended as part of the routine therapy outlined above.

In the severe type of vomiting of pregnancy, where there is great loss of body weight, marked dehydration, and jaundice, it is imperative that the patient receive an adequate amount of fluid in order to restore the water balance of her body. To this end we employ 10 per cent glucose solution intravenously. Very occasionally the patient suffering from such severe vomiting and starvation may develop an acidosis, as indicated by a sharp fall in the CO_2 combining power of the blood to values below 30 volumes per cent. In such an event it is, of course, necessary that the acidosis be treated. This may be accomplished by administering molar sodium lactate solution intravenously. Utilizing the following modification of Hartmann and Senn of the Palmer and Van Slyke formula, we can accurately calculate the amount of sodium lactate required to raise the CO_2 combining power to any given volumes per cent:

$$\begin{matrix}\text{Desired increase in } CO_2 \\ \text{(volumes per cent)}\end{matrix} = \frac{2.24 \times \text{ml. sodium lactate}}{\text{Body wt. in kg.} \times 0.67}$$

In 1932 Stander reported hemorrhagic retinitis in two patients suffering from severe vomiting of pregnancy. He advised routine and repeated eyeground examinations in all patients with vomiting of pregnancy and advocated the interruption of pregnancy should hemorrhagic retinitis develop. Since then Tillman and others have reported fatal cases of hyperemesis gravidarum with retinal hemorrhages. The character of such hemorrhages makes it probable that the cause is a change in the permeability of the capillary walls, although it has been suggested that it may be due to a vitamin B deficiency. The appearance of retinal hemorrhages in vomiting of pregnancy must be regarded as a definite indication for termination of the pregnancy. Ballantyne recently emphasized the ocular changes, such as slight dimness of vision to varying degrees of involvement of the visual fields which may precede gross hemorrhages and optic neuritis, and pointed out that the early recognition of these ocular complications may be of substantial aid in determining whether or not the pregnancy should be interrupted.

BIBLIOGRAPHY

Ballantyne, A. J. Ocular Complications in Hyperemesis Gravidarum. J. Obst. & Gynaec. Brit. Emp., 1941, 48:206.

Bokelmann, O., and Bock, A. Analysis of Blood and Urine for Acetone Bodies in Hyperemesis Gravidarum. Ztschr. f. Geburtsh. u. Gynäk., 1927, 92:184.

Brindeau, A., Lantuéjoul, and Hinglais, H. The Pathogenesis of the Vomiting of Pregnancy. Gynec. et Obst., 1937, 35:5.

Dieckmann, W. J., and Crossen, R. J. Changes in the Metabolism and Their Relation to the Treatment of Vomiting of Pregnancy. Am. J. Obst. & Gynec., 1927, 14:3.

Duncan and Harding. A Report on the Effect of High Carbohydrate Feeding on the Nausea and Vomiting of Pregnancy. Canad. M. A. J., 1918, 8:1057.

Finch, J. W. The Etiology of Nausea and Vomiting of Pregnancy. J.A.M.A., 1938, 111:1368.

Hansen, R. Zur Physiologie des Magens in der Schwangerschaft. Zentralbl. f. Gynäk., 1937, 61:2306.

Harding, V. J. Nausea and Vomiting in Pregnancy. Lancet, 1921, 2:327.

Hart, B. F., McConnell, W. T., and Pickett, A. N. Vitamin and Endocrine Therapy in Nausea and Vomiting of Pregnancy. Am. J. Obst. & Gynec., 1944, 48:251.

Hartman, A. F., and Senn, M. J. E. Studies in the Metabolism of Racemic Sodium Lactate. J. Clin. Investigation, 1932, 11:345.

Jones, O. H. Polyneuritis of Pregnancy. Am. J. Obst. & Gynec., 1943, 45:869.

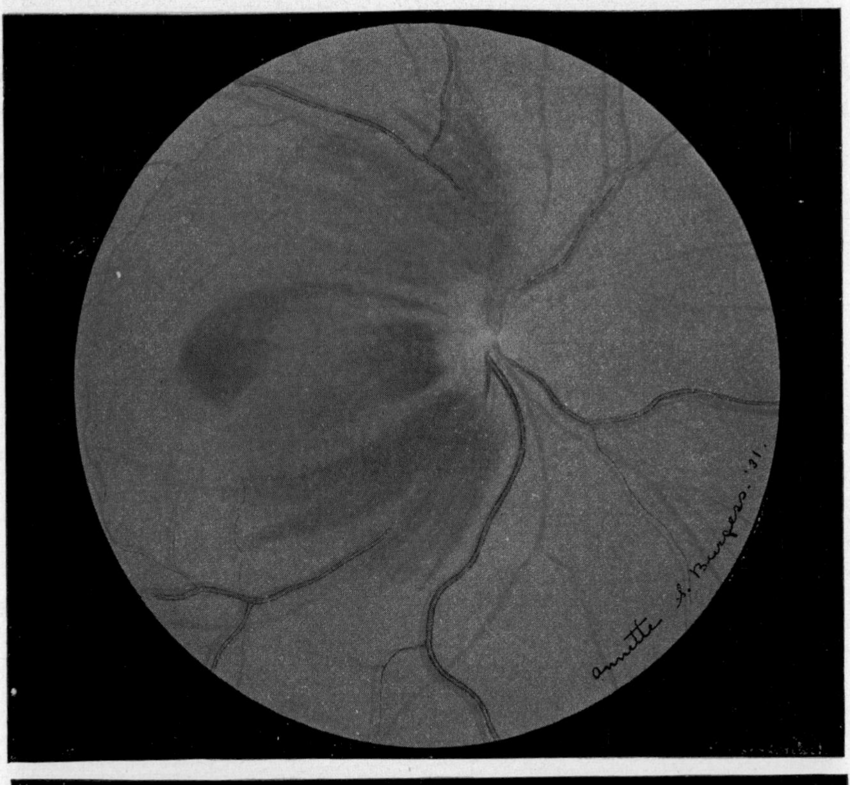

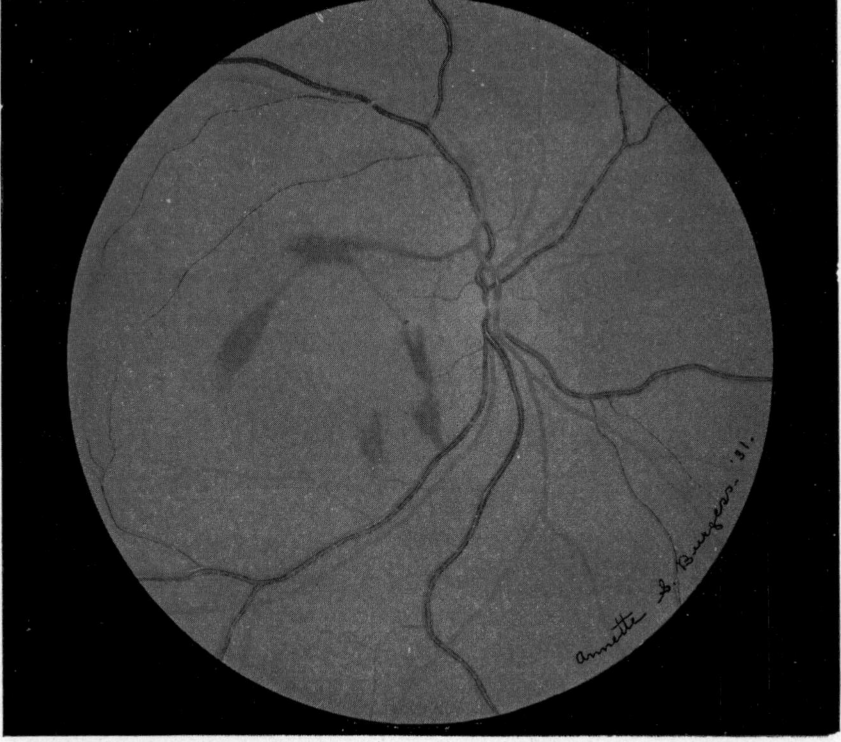

Fig. 381.—Hemorrhagic Retinitis in Vomiting of Pregnancy.
(From Stander. By permission of *Surgery, Gynecology and Obstetrics.*)

Kotz, J., and Kaufman, M. S. Adrenal Cortex in the Treatment of Nausea and Vomiting in Pregnancy. Am. J. Obst. & Gynec., 1940, 39:449.

McGoogan, L. S. Severe Polyneuritis due to Vitamin B Deficiency in Pregnancy. Am. J. Obst. & Gynec., 1942, 43:752.

Peckham, C. H. Observations on 60 Cases of Hyperemesis Gravidarum. Am. J. Obst. & Gynec., 1929, 17:776.

Schjott-Rivers, E. Historical and Critical Review of the Problems Concerning Hyperemesis Gravidarum. Acta Obst. et Gynec. Scandinav., 1938, 18:1. (Supp. 1).

——— Hyperemesis Gravidarum. Acta obst. & gynec. Scandinav., 1939, 19:290.

Sheehan, H. L. The Pathology of Hyperemesis and Vomiting of Late Pregnancy. J. Obst. & Gynaec. Brit. Emp., 1939, 46:685.

Stander, H. J. Hemorrhagic Retinitis in Vomiting of Pregnancy. Surg., Gynec. & Obst., 1932, 54:129.

Tillman, A. J. B. Two Fatal Cases of Hyperemesis Gravidarum with Retinal Hemorrhages. Am. J. Obst. & Gynec., 1934, 27:240.

Titus, P., and Dodds, P. The Etiologic Significance of Lowered Blood Sugar Values in Vomiting of Pregnancy. Am. J. Obst. & Gynec., 1928, 16:90.

Watt, L. O. Hyperemesis Gravidarum and High Vitamin Therapy. J. Obst. & Gynaec. Brit. Emp., 1941, 48:619.

Way, S. Relation between Gastric Acidity and the Anterior-Pituitary-Like Hormone Content of Urine in Pregnant Women. Brit. M. J., 1945, 2:182.

Weinstein, B. B., Mitchell, G. J., and Sustendal, G. F. Clinical Experiences with Pyridoxine Hydrochloride in the Treatment of Nausea and Vomiting of Pregnancy. Am. J. Obst. & Gynec., 1943, 46:283.

——— Wohl, Z., Mitchell, G. J., and Sustendal, G. F. Oral Administration of Pyridoxine Hydrochloride in the Treatment of Nausea and Vomiting of Pregnancy. Am. J. Obst. & Gynec., 1944, 47:389.

Williams, N. H. Variable Significance of Heartburn. Am. J. Obst. & Gynec., 1941, 42:814.

27

THE TOXEMIAS OF PREGNANCY

ORIENTATION

The toxemias of pregnancy are a group of diseases which are encountered frequently during gestation, or in the early puerperium, and are characterized by one or more of the following signs: hypertension, edema, proteinuria, and in certain severe cases, convulsions and coma.

As described in Chapter 8 the alterations which take place in the maternal organism as the result of pregnancy are many and extensive. They include such changes as a great enlargement in uterine size, a concomitant augmentation of its blood supply, a decided increase in blood volume and cardiac output, a substantial hydration of the blood with an increased retention of fluid in all tissues, and in addition, many morphological alterations in the thyroid, parathyroid, ovaries and pituitary body. Moreover, a new and complex organ, the placenta, is added to the maternal organism; and as pregnancy progresses this structure, as well as other endocrine organs, exhibits secretory activities which have no parallel in the nonpregnant woman.

In view of the number and extent of these alterations, it is understandable that some of them occasionally go awry. To the best of our knowledge the toxemias of pregnancy are the result of pathologic deviations in these physiologic changes, but the precise nature of the underlying mechanism is quite unknown. Indeed, the cause of the toxemias of pregnancy, despite decades of intensive research, remains the great enigma of obstetrics and constitutes one of the most important unsolved problems in the whole field of human reproduction.

The toxemias of pregnancy are very common complications of gestation, being seen in 6 or 7 per cent of all gravidae. They constitute, together with hemorrhage and puerperal infection, the great triad of diseases responsible for the vast majority of maternal deaths and themselves account for some 1,000 maternal fatalities in the United States each year. As a cause of fetal death, they are even more important and it can be estimated conservatively that at least 30,000 stillbirths and neonatal deaths each year in this country are the result of toxemia of pregnancy. The great majority of these deaths are due to prematurity of the infant.

This huge toll of maternal and infant lives taken by the toxemias of pregnancy is in large measure preventable. Assiduous and astute prenatal supervision, particularly the early detection of signs and symptoms of oncoming toxemia and appropriate treatment, will prevent many cases and so ameliorate others that the outcome for baby and mother is usually satisfactory.

above, and second, evidence of the superimposition of an acute process as demonstrated by an elevation of systolic pressure of 30 mm. Hg or more and/or an elevation in diastolic pressure of 15 mm. Hg or more, and/or the development of a significant degree of proteinuria.

The simple classification of the toxemias of pregnancy presented above differs in several ways from some which are currently employed. The main differences and the reasons therefor are as follows:

1. The term "acute toxemia" is used to connote the disease entity of preeclampsia and eclampsia by way of emphasizing the unity of this morbid process. A word is urgently needed which embraces this whole syndrome and "acute toxemia" has been chosen for this purpose because it is the one most commonly used in clinical parlance.

2. Mild and severe preeclampsia are not differentiated. Although the blood pressure level of 160/100 has been widely employed as a dividing line between so-called "preeclampsia mild" and "preeclampsia severe," this criterion has proved generally unsatisfactory and sometimes misleading to a dangerous degree. The outlook in any given case (as connoted by these adjectives) cannot be so easily established. Blood pressure alone is not a dependable indication of severity since a young girl with a pressure of 135/85 may develop convulsions while many patients with pressures of 180/120 do not. The whole ensemble of the patient, the blood pressure, edema, facies, proteinuria, urinary output, age, eye signs and headache, must all be evaluated in estimating prognosis; and a clinical picture of such infinite variety cannot be accurately classified into mild and severe types by any one or any two criteria.

3. Acute toxemia, that is preeclampsia and eclampsia, is listed first because this is the toxemia of pregnancy par excellence. Moreover, in presenting the subject to students, an understanding of preeclampsia and eclampsia is a prerequisite to any intelligent survey of chronic hypertensive vascular disease in pregnancy. For instance, the most common complication of hypertensive vascular disease in gestation is superimposed preeclampsia.

4. Hyperemesis is omitted. The toxemias included in the above classification possess the unifying factor in common that they are all primarily vascular disorders. Whatever the underlying mechanism of hyperemesis may be, it is clearly not a vascular disturbance. Moreover, it bears no resemblance whatsoever to the conditions described above, either in pathologic anatomy, pathologic biochemistry or a clinical picture. Hence to include it in the toxemias is not only illogical but serves only to confuse further a confusing enough group of diseases. Dieckmann has already expressed the same opinion.

5. Acute nephritis, chronic glomerulonephritis, nephrosis and other renal conditions which stem from inflammatory or metabolic etiology, are not included but are discussed elsewhere as coincidental disorders of pregnancy. These rare complications of gestation may occasionally simulate preeclampsia but can usually be differentiated in a short time and, from an etiological viewpoint, are quite different entities from the vascular disorders included in the above classification.

Type	Number of Cases	Per Cent of Total Cases of Toxemia
Preeclampsia	1,708	78.1
Eclampsia	27	1.2
Chronic hypertensive vascular disease	365	16.7
Preeclampsia superimposed on chronic vascular disease	87	4.0
Total	2,187	100.0

TABLE 15. INCIDENCE OF VARIOUS TYPES OF TOXEMIA BASED ON 2,187 CASES. (J.H.H.)

An approximate idea of the relative incidence of the several types of toxemia, based upon the criteria given above, may be had from Table 15. Because of differences in the standards of classification employed in various clinics, the reported figures on the relative frequency of preeclampsia and chronic hypertensive vascular disease show great discrepancies. For instance, both Dieckmann and Mengert find the latter more common than the former; on the other hand, the statistics of Stander and Kellogg are more in keeping with those in Table 15. As explained on page 686, these differences are to be attributed for the most part to the moot question as to whether preeclampsia actually causes chronic hypertensive vascular disease.

PREECLAMPSIA

Preeclampsia is characterized by the development of hypertension, proteinuria and edema in a gravida who has previously been normal in these respects. It is a disease of the last two or three months of gestation for the most part and rarely occurs prior to the twenty-fourth week; it is most often seen in young primigravidae. Preeclampsia is the forerunner or prodromal stage of eclampsia; in other words, unless the preeclamptic process is checked by treatment or by delivery, it is more or less likely that eclampsia (convulsions and coma) will ensue.

Clinical Course. The earliest and most dependable warning sign of preeclampsia, in most cases, is suddenly developing hypertension. Although a systolic blood pressure of 140 mm. and/or a diastolic of 90 mm. is usually taken as the borderline between normal and toxemic levels, absolute figures are sometimes of less clinical significance than the relationship they bear to previous determinations and to the age of the patient. For example, a rise from 105/70 to 135/85 is a definite danger signal despite the fact that the levels reached are below those cited as borderline; and in a young woman in her teens such an increase in pressure becomes especially significant. Indeed any increase in the systolic pressure of 30 mm. or more which persists for several days is a cause for concern even though the highest level attained is less than 140 mm. By and large, the diastolic pressure is a more reliable prognostic sign than the systolic and any persisting diastolic pressure of 90 mm. or more is absolute evidence of preeclampsia provided it develops after the twenty-fourth week in a patient without prior hypertension. In the severer gradations of preeclampsia the systolic pressure frequently reaches 180 mm. and the diastolic 110, but systolic levels in excess of 200 mm. are rarely seen. When the systolic blood pressure exceeds 200 it usually will be found that the underlying cause of the hypertension is either chronic hypertensive vascular disease or preeclampsia superimposed upon chronic hypertensive vascular disease.

The next most important sign of preeclampsia is sudden and excessive weight gain. Indeed in many cases this is the first sign. Weight increments of 1 pound a week or so may be regarded as normal, but when they reach 2 pounds in any given week, or as much as 6 pounds in a month, preeclampsia is to be suspected. Evans has reported that 63 per cent of his patients who gained over 7 pounds in one month developed toxemia, whereas only 0.9 per cent of those who gained less than 4 pounds were so affected. An abnormal weight gain was the first sign in 65 per cent of his preeclamptic patients and it appeared on the average one month before the proteinuria and, as a rule, before hypertension.

Sudden and excessive weight gains in gestation are due almost entirely to abnormal water retention by the tissues and are demonstrable, as a rule, long before visible signs of edema, such as swollen eyelids and puffiness of the fingers, become manifest. In cases of fulminating preeclampsia waterlogging of the body may be extreme, and in such patients increments of 10 pounds or more in a week are not unusual. It should be noted that it is the suddenness of the excessive weight gain that is especially pathognomonic of preeclampsia rather than any overall increase distributed throughout gestation.

Proteinuria is a very common finding in preeclampsia but varies greatly not only from case to case but also in the same patient from hour to hour. This fluctuating nature of proteinuria in preeclampsia, as well as in eclampsia, has been studied especially by Chesley and his associates who believe that the variability points to a functional (vasospasm) rather than to an organic cause. In the milder examples of preeclampsia proteinuria may be entirely lacking or limited to a trace; on the other hand, in the severer grades, proteinuria is demonstrable in the majority of cases and is often as much as 6 or 8 gm. per liter, but the exact figure and its significance will depend somewhat upon the concentration of the urine specimen examined. Proteinuria usually develops later than the hypertension and weight gain and for this reason must be regarded as a serious omen when superimposed on the two other findings.

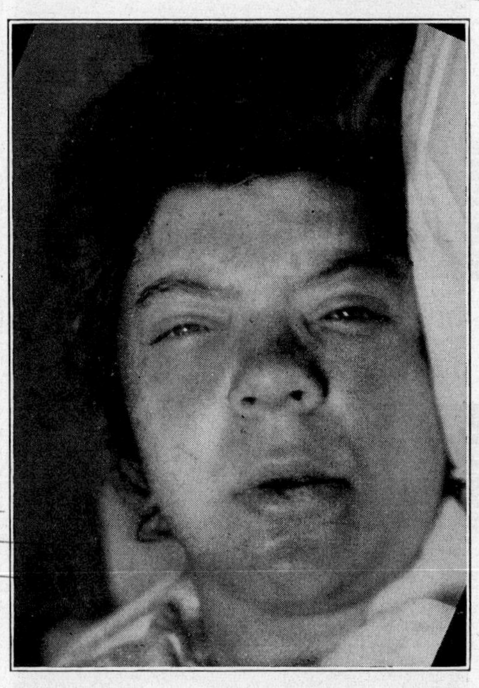

FIG. 382.—FACIES IN FULMINATING PREECLAMPSIA.

Note edema of eyelids, general puffiness of entire face, coarseness of features and acromegalic appearance of this 16-year-old girl.

It should be emphasized that these three early and important signs of preeclampsia, namely, hypertension, weight gain and proteinuria, are changes of which the patient is usually in no wise aware: all three may be present in substantial degree, and yet she may feel quite well. Only by regular and careful prenatal examinations can these warning signs be detected. Hence, the transcendent importance of prenatal care in the early detection and early management of this complication. By the time a preeclamptic patient has developed symptoms and signs which she herself can detect, such as headache, visual disturbances, puffiness of the eyelids and fingers, she is usually in an advanced stage of the disease and much ground has been lost.

Headache is rarely observed in the milder cases but is encountered with increasing frequency as the more severe grades are met. In general its incidence parallels the severity of the process; thus in patients who actually develop eclampsia, severe headache is a frequent forerunner of the first convulsion. It is most often frontal but may be occipital and is resistant to ordinary therapy. Epigastric pain is another late symptom in preeclampsia, so late a one indeed, that its presence indicates that convulsions

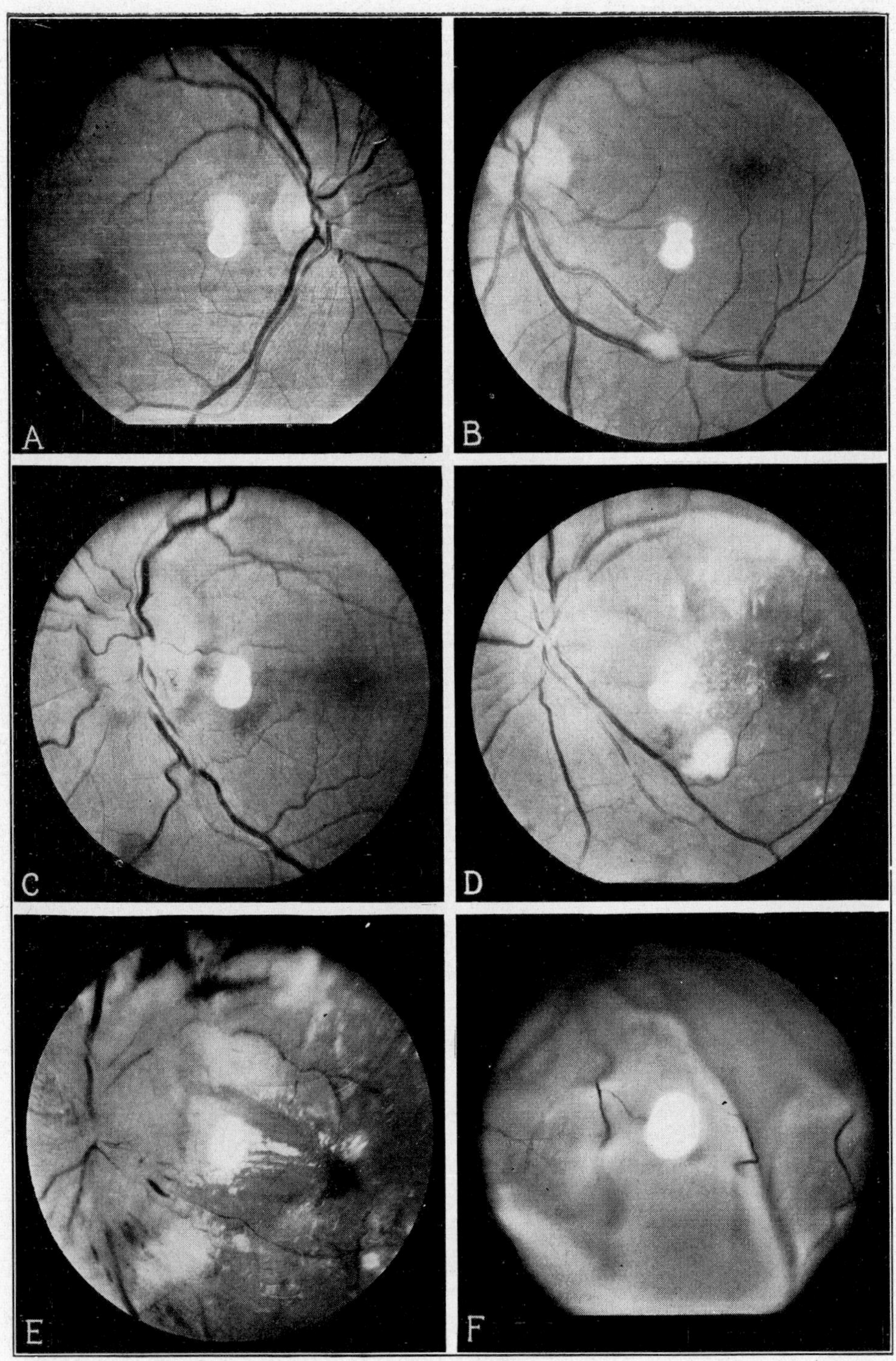

Fig. 383.—The Retinal Changes in Various Types of Toxemia.
(Courtesy of Dr. A. J. Bedell.)

See description on opposite page.

are immediately imminent. It may be due to stretching of the liver capsule by hemorrhage, although it is thought by some to be of central origin.

Visual disturbances ranging from a slight blurring of vision to various degrees of temporary blindness are frequent accompaniments of preeclampsia, being demonstrable in more or less degree in one third to one half of cases. Although they are thought by some to be of central origin, they are more likely attributable to certain pathologic changes which the retina is known to undergo in preeclampsia, namely, arteriolar spasm, ischemia, edema and, in rare cases, actual retinal detachment.

Retinal Changes. The most common retinal findings in preeclampsia are spasm of the retinal arterioles and, with lesser frequency, retinal edema. On the basis of an extensive study of the retinal arterioles in the hypertensive toxemias of pregnancy, Hallum points out that the first change observed in the normal retinal arterioles during preeclampsia is constriction of the lumen. This constriction may be localized to a single point resembling a sausage-link constriction or there may be a series of these localized constrictions, some elongated and spindle-shaped, and usually limited to the first half of the retinal arteriole. This is the portion of the arteriole nearest the optic disc and the constrictions are seen more frequently in the nasal branches. These elongated, spindle-shaped constrictions appear as uniformly symmetrical indentations of both sides of the arteriole, and resemble the constriction that would be produced by stretching a glass tube, the middle section of which has been heated almost to the melting point. In other patients the first change observed may be a generalized arteriolar constriction, so that instead of the diameter ratio of vein to arteriole being the normal 3 to 2, the arterioles may be constricted so that the ratio is 2 to 1. As the severity of the toxemia progresses the arterioles are usually seen to become more constricted until the ratio increases to 3 to 1, or more. As the retinal arterioles become more and more constricted in preeclampsia there may be signs of retinal ischemia such as edema of the retina. Edema of the retina is ordinarily the first sign of its involvement and usually makes its appearance at the upper and lower poles of the disc, and progresses away from the disc along the course of the retinal vessels, which is likewise the general course of the nerve fibers of the retina. In the earlier stage of edema of the retina the portion involved appears milky, and on close examination with the very best focus of the ophthalmoscope, while doing a very gentle and slow to and fro rotation of the hand holding the ophthalmoscope, the surface shows faint striations running in the direction of the nerve fiber layers. Retinal edema is illustrated in

---

A. Retinal vessel spasm, showing unequal caliber of inferior temporal artery near disc as sometimes seen in preeclampsia.

B. Early hypertensive retinitis. Cotton wool exudate forms the fluffy mass overlying the junction of the inferior temporal artery and vein.

C. Papilledema with hypertension, showing rounded, elevated disc, distended veins, and unevenly contracted arteries. Deep, dark, granular hemorrhages appear as black smudges.

D. Advanced hypertensive retinitis (malignant nephrosclerosis). Terminal stage characterized by very marked constrictions in the inferior temporal artery, thick cotton wool spot, several hemorrhages and an irregularly outlined macular star of exudate with widespread edema of the retina obscuring the disc.

E. Terminal nephritis. Immense swelling of the disc with loss of outline. Striate and deep hemorrhages, massive exudates, macular star. Marked variation in the caliber of both veins and arteries.

F. Detachment of retina, showing the retinal folds forming ridges over which the vessels are clearly outlined. Usually transitory in eclampsia.

Carbon arc forms figure 8 image.

Fig. 383. In rare instances retinal edema may go on to detachment of the retina but in general the prognosis of such detachments is good, the retina re-attaching within a few weeks, as a rule, after delivery. Hemorrhages and exudates are extremely rare in preeclampsia and when present usually indicate an underlying chronic hypertensive vascular disease.

Etiology and Pathologic Anatomy. The etiology of preeclampsia, whatever it may be, is doubtless identical with that of eclampsia and is discussed under the latter heading. What little is known about the causation of this disease complex is, at the present writing, of theoretical importance only and has no bearing on the diagnosis, prognosis and management of preeclampsia. Since patients rarely die in the preeclamptic stage of the process, few data are available on pathologic anatomy, but it is assumed that organic alterations in preeclampsia are similar to those observed in eclampsia but of lesser degree. The most characteristic pathologic lesions of eclampsia at autopsy, themselves inconstant, are hemorrhagic necrosis of the periphery of the liver lobule, narrowing of the glomerular capillaries caused usually by increased thickness of the basement membrane, and cerebral edema; these changes, together with other anatomical alterations, are discussed on page 666. The deviations from normal physiology and biochemistry which are of greatest importance in preeclampsia are generalized spasm of the smaller arterioles and water retention. Since much of the evidence relating to these changes is to be found in observations made on eclamptic patients (in addition to preeclamptic), these important underlying mechanisms are discussed in detail in connection with the pathologic physiology and pathologic biochemistry of eclampsia (page 672).

Diagnosis. If a gravida who is known to have been normal in respect to blood pressure, weight gain and urine examinations prior to the twenty-fourth week, subsequently manifests hypertension, edema, and/or proteinuria, the diagnosis of preeclampsia can be definitely established almost without exception. In rare instances, acute glomerulonephritis developing at this time may be confused, but this complication is rather rare (page 752) and can usually be differentiated by the hematuria commonly present, the history of a prior streptococcal infection which can often be elicited and the greater likelihood of nitrogenous retention. Lipoid nephrosis in pregnancy is also very uncommon, but when encountered can be recognized as a rule by the massive proteinuria, edema, hypoproteinemia, increase in blood cholesterol and the doubly refractive bodies in the urine, all in the presence of a normal blood pressure. The eventual outcome of this disease is usually nephritis.

Great difficulty, however, may be met in establishing clearly the diagnosis of preeclampsia in gravidae first seen in the last trimester of pregnancy and who are already manifesting hypertension, edema and/or proteinuria. In many of these cases it is impossible to know whether the picture is one of preeclampsia or chronic hypertensive vascular disease until four to six months postpartum. In general, the following findings suggest chronic hypertensive vascular disease rather than preeclampsia: (1) systolic blood pressure over 200; (2) retinal exudate and hemorrhages as well as narrowing and tortuosity of the retinal vessels; (3) cardiac enlargement; (4) less definitely, parity of five or more, especially if the patient is 30 years or more of age; and (5) still less dependably, absence of edema and proteinuria.

In view of the difficulties which are occasionally encountered in differentiating preeclampsia and chronic hypertensive vascular disease, various tests have been recommended for the purpose. The most widely studied of these is the cold pressor test which was proposed by Hines and Brown and measures the response of the blood pressure to the immersion of one hand in ice water. Prehypertensive patients are believed to show an exaggerated rise in response to the test, thus enabling the clinician to predict their eventual hypertension. On the same basis, it has been hoped that this procedure might permit forecasting which women will and which women will not develop hypertensive toxemia in pregnancy. In regard to the differentiation of preeclampsia and chronic hypertensive vascular disease, pregnant women with the latter disorder appear to have a vascular system which is more labile, together with a nervous system which is more irritable than normal, and hence give an exaggerated response. Contrariwise, relatively small increases in pressure are manifested in preeclamptic and eclamptic patients possibly because the vascular spasm has reached its maximum in this group. The results reported on this test, whether as a means of predicting or differentiating the toxemias, have been contradictory, some authors (Reid and Teel, Chesley) concluding that the procedure is inconstant and without value, while others (Dieckmann, Randall, Murray and Mussey, Krieger and Weiden) consider that it possesses some merit. Since the injection of pituitary extract (½ to 2 minims) into preeclamptic and eclamptic patients usually causes an abrupt rise in pressure with urinary suppression, whereas in chronic hypertensive vascular disease it does not, this procedure has been suggested as a differentiating test, but it is too hazardous to be recommended. Combinations of the latter procedure and the cold pressor test have also been employed. In the main, however, these various tests have not received widespread endorsement and are not established clinical methods.

Immediate Prognosis. The immediate prognosis for the mother depends almost entirely on whether or not eclampsia supervenes. In 2,418 cases of preeclampsia under our surveillance at the Johns Hopkins Hospital between 1924 and 1943, 92 patients, or 3.8 per cent, developed eclampsia. As the result of improvements in prenatal care, this percentage has been lowered in the last decade to 1.4 (0.4 per cent in white preeclamptics and 2.3 in colored). If eclampsia ensues, the prognosis becomes immediately grave, the death rate from eclampsia in this country being 10 to 15 per cent.

The outlook for the infant in preeclampsia is generally diminished, but will depend largely upon the stage of pregnancy when the disease appears and its severity. In the 2,418 cases of preeclampsia mentioned above, the total infant loss was 7.4 per cent. In the severer grades of preeclampsia, the fetal mortality approximates 20 per cent. Thus, in 137 cases of severe preeclampsia recently reported by McLane, the gross fetal mortality was 17.3 per cent. Most of these infant deaths in preeclampsia are due to prematurity consequent upon the frequent necessity of terminating pregnancy at an early date.

Ultimate Prognosis. Within 10 days or so after delivery, the majority of patients with preeclampsia enjoy a complete return to normal in respect to blood pressure, urine and edema. In a certain proportion of cases, however, the hypertension persists indefinitely and in another fraction, although the patients apparently return to normal and remain so when not pregnant, they suffer recurrence of the toxemia in subsequent pregnancies. The frequency with which these unfortunate sequels occur has been the subject of countless statistical investigations, one of the earliest of which was carried out in this clinic in 1924 by Harris. He examined 55 women who had suffered from preeclampsia one year previously and found that the appalling number of 33, or

60 per cent, showed signs of chronic hypertensive vascular disease. He was able to show, moreover, that the length of time the toxemia symptoms persisted was an important determining factor in the occurrence of permanent vascular damage.

These studies of Harris have been confirmed and amplified by many subsequent observers. The investigations of Chesley in this field are especially authoritative because of the large number of cases studied, the thoroughness with which they have been analyzed and the meticulous statistical methods employed. He and his group have studied from various viewpoints 267 cases of mild preeclampsia and 52 of severe preeclampsia three and one-half to five and one-half years after the toxemic pregnancy. Employing as a standard for hypertension any pressure greater than 140 mm. in the systolic *or* 90 mm. in the diastolic readings, they found that 37.5 per cent of the mild preeclamptic group and 42.3 per cent of the severe preeclamptic patients manifested hypertension at follow-up. If the patients at follow-up who showed *either* a systolic *or* a diastolic level of the figures cited, but not both, were excluded, the corresponding figures become 32.6 and 36.5 respectively. Among 134 mild preeclamptic patients who became pregnant again, the incidence of recurrent toxemia was 32.8 per cent, while the corresponding figure in 21 patients who had previously had severe preeclampsia was 66.7 per cent. In addition to these statistical studies Chesley and his associates have investigated the renal hemodynamics in posttoxemic hypertensive women and find: (a) diminished plasma flow (usually); (b) diminished filtration (usually); and (c) normal filtration fraction. These findings point to the glomerular capillaries as the site of obstruction to the blood flow. Either there are fewer glomeruli than normal, or the lumens of the capillaries are narrowed. It is just such capillary narrowing which Bell, and Page and Cox have described as persisting after toxemia of pregnancy.

Duration of Preeclampsia (weeks)	Total Patients	Residual Hypertension	Per Cent
1 — 2	115	19	16.5
3 — 4	47	9	19.2
5 — 6	18	7	38.9
7 — 8	11	7	63.6
9 — 12	24	17	70.8

TABLE 16. INCIDENCE OF RESIDUAL HYPERTENSION FOLLOWING PREECLAMPSIA IN 215 PRIMIPARAE ACCORDING TO TIME ELAPSING BETWEEN ONSET OF TOXEMIA AND DELIVERY. (Peckham.)

In individual cases of preeclampsia the most important determining factor in the development of subsequent hypertension is the duration of the preeclamptic attack. This fact is brought out very clearly by Table 16 which shows the results observed by Peckham in 215 preeclamptic primigravidous pregnancies studied by him in this clinic. These figures make it plain that when the duration of preeclampsia has not exceeded four weeks the incidence of residual hypertension reaches about 20 per cent, and in cases in which the preeclamptic attack lasted longer than six weeks, the corresponding figure soars to over 60 per cent. The severity of the preeclamptic attack also has a bearing on the ultimate prognosis since the more severe the degree of hypertension during the toxic pregnancy, the greater the incidence of later hypertension and of toxemia recurrence. The same unfavorable prognosis holds when proteinuria increases concomitantly with hypertension. Moreover, the older the patient is at follow-up, the more often hypertension is to be found. This, of course, is to be expected from the fact that the incidence of hypertension rises with age in the population as a whole. Patients who are over 30 years of age and who have had a prior attack of preeclampsia face a likelihood of repetition which is over 50 per cent. In connection with this factor of age and directly dependent upon it is the circumstance that recurrence of toxemia is greater in proportion to the length of the interval since the preeclamptic pregnancy; from a practical viewpoint this means that these patients have nothing to gain by waiting or "resting" for several years before attempting another pregnancy since their most favorable outlook insofar as toxemia is concerned depends on having a pregnancy within the next year or two, that is, before the effect of age becomes pronounced. Obesity is always an unfavorable factor in pregnancy and especially so in patients with toxemia or in those with a history of previous toxemia. Chesley and his associates have put this on a quantitative basis by showing that the greater the body weight relative to the height, the greater the incidence of high blood pressure at follow-up, and the greater the likelihood of toxemia recurrence. When the weight in pounds divided by the height in inches is 2.2 or less the probability of hypertension at follow-up is of the order of 15 to 20 per cent, but when it exceeds 2.2 the incidence of permanent hypertension climbs to 40 per cent and above, while the likelihood of recurrence of toxemia also augments greatly.

Finally, it must be recalled that repeated toxemias have an additive bearing on prognosis for future childbearing. Thus if a patient has had two previous attacks of preeclampsia of severe degree, or three of moderate degree, the likelihood of permanent hypertension or recurrence in subsequent pregnancies is probably greater than 75 per cent.

In evaluating the above statistics on the ultimate prognosis of preeclampsia, it must be recalled that the criterion for diagnosis of permanent hypertension or recurrence in a subsequent pregnancy has been for the most part a blood pressure which exceeds 140 systolic *or* 90 diastolic. While actual experience bears out the contention of these figures in general, it also shows that many of the recurrent toxemias which follow preeclampsia are exceedingly mild in degree and are not alarming either from the viewpoint of the mother or the child. In my opinion this should give the physician greater optimism in discussing future pregnancies with posttoxemic patients than the above figures would seem to justify.

Treatment. *Prophylaxis.* Since in its early stages preeclampsia rarely gives rise to signs or symptoms which the patient herself will notice, the early detection of this disease demands meticulous prenatal observation. Therefore let it be emphasized again that every gravida should be examined by her obstetrician every week during the last month of pregnancy, and every fortnight during the two previous months. At these visits, careful blood pressure readings, weighing of the patient and urine analyses must be routine. Furthermore all patients should be advised either verbally or, better, by means of suitable printed instructions to report between visits any of the well-known symptoms of preeclampsia such as persistent headache, visual disturbances and puffiness of the hands or face. The reporting of any such symptoms of course calls for an immediate examination to confirm or rule out preeclampsia.

The most promising prophylaxis of the disease lies in reduction of salt intake and curtailing weight gain in all gravidae. Water retention, which is inherently part of the disease process of acute toxemia, is inseparably linked with sodium retention and experience has shown that it is exceptional for patients on a minimal salt intake to develop the disease. Accordingly restriction of salt is desirable in all gravidae, especially during the last trimester and they should be so advised. This is especially necessary in certain groups of patients who are known to be predisposed to preeclampsia such as women with chronic hypertension, diabetics, obese patients and those with twin pregnancies. Curtailment of weight gain to 20 pounds during the whole of gestation also reduces the likelihood of preeclampsia. The attainment of these objectives, however, requires the utmost vigilance on the part of the obstetrician as well as the patient.

Objectives of Treatment. If a case of preeclampsia is to be managed with complete success, a number of objectives must be attained. Among these are: (1) prevention of convulsions; (2) prevention of residual hypertension; (3) delivery of a child which survives; and (4) delivery with minimum trauma, yet in a manner which will not handicap the patient in future pregnancies as would cesarean section.

In certain cases of preeclampsia, especially in patients near term, all four of these objectives may be served equally well by the same treatment, namely, prompt induction of labor; and no question of conflict between any two of them arises. In other instances, however, the attainment of certain of these desiderata may so conflict with the realization of another as to make it virtually impossible to gain all four objectives. For instance, if a patient develops severe preeclampsia two or three months before her expected date of confinement, prompt termination of her pregnancy may seem indicated if objectives (1) and (2) are to be realized, but this course may well result in the delivery of a nonviable premature infant and consequent failure to attain objective (3). Again, when preeclampsia develops at such an early date, a long closed cervix may make induction of labor extremely hazardous; and if in this case convulsions seem imminent, cesarean section may become almost mandatory. While it may therefore be impossible to attain all four of these objectives in every case, the extent to which we are able to do so is a rough gauge of our success in the management of this complication.

Foremost of these objectives is the first named, prevention of eclampsia, because the development of convulsions in a case of preeclampsia under observation is a grave catastrophe and represents a grievous failure of prenatal care. As already noted, in 2,418 cases of preeclampsia under our surveillance at the Johns Hopkins Hospital between 1924 and 1943, eclampsia developed despite the fact that the patients were under our care, in 92 instances or in 3.8 per cent. Quite obviously these 92 cases represented failures on our part to achieve this important objective. Just how costly these failures were is made plain by the fact that 7 of the 92 mothers and 20 of the infants died, giving mortality rates of 7.6 and 21.7 per cent respectively. By contrast, in the 2,326 cases of preeclampsia in which convulsions did not develop, only 4 mothers (0.2 per cent) and 158 infants (6.8 per cent) succumbed. A total of 398 convulsions were suffered by these 92 eclamptic patients, an average of 4.3 each. Some of the more common causes, on retrospect, of our failure to prevent eclampsia in these 92 cases of preeclampsia, were as follows: in 16 cases failure to evaluate gravity of sudden weight gain; in 15 cases failure to evaluate gravity of moderate deviations from normal (BP, albuminuria, edema) in young primigravidae; in 10 cases failure to see patients every week in last month; in 6 cases failure to evaluate gravity of symptoms (headache, epigastric pain, vomiting); in 3 cases failure to evaluate gravity of moderate deviations from normal (BP, albuminuria, edema) in twin pregnancy; and in 3 cases failure to evaluate gravity of high diastolic pressure. These are all common potential sources of failure in the prevention of eclampsia and should be borne in mind in the management of every case of preeclampsia.

Ambulatory Treatment. An even more common cause of failure to forestall convulsions in the 92 cases of preeclampsia just discussed was tardiness in hospitalization, a lapse which was responsible for the outbreak of convulsions in 19 cases. Ambulatory treatment has no place in the management of preeclampsia as defined. Some patients, however, whose systolic blood pressure does not exceed 135 mm. and whose diastolic pressure does not exceed 85 mm. and in whom edema and proteinuria are absent or minimal, may be handled tentatively at home pending the aggravation or abatement of signs and symptoms. The activities of such a patient should be confined to one floor; she should be instructed to add no salt to her food in the kitchen and none at the table; she should be given written instructions with a list of salt-containing foods to avoid, and should also be cautioned not to use baking soda for the relief of heartburn; magnesium sulfate, 15 gm., or citrate of magnesium, 200 cc., should be prescribed every other morning and bed rest encouraged throughout the greater part of the day. Such patients, moreover, should be examined twice a week rather than once and especially instructed about the reporting of symptoms. In minor elevations of blood pressure the response to a regime such as the above is often immediate and gratifying but the patient must be cooperative and the obstetrician wary.

Hospital Management. The indications for hospitalization in preeclampsia are: a systolic blood pressure of 140 mm. or above, or a diastolic of 90 mm. or above; or significant proteinuria (2 + in a catheterized specimen); or repeated weight gains of 3 pounds a week or more. In most cases the first and third of these indications will combine to emphasize the urgent desirability of hospitalization.

For an intelligent appraisal of the present severity of the case, a systematic method of study should be instituted upon admission to the hospital, such as the following: a general physical examination and history, followed by daily watchout for the development of such symptoms as headache, visual disturbances and edema of the fingers and eyelids; weight on admission and every other day; blood pressure readings every 4 hours (except between midnight and morning unless the midnight pressure has risen); daily fluid intake and urinary output record; daily quantitative analysis of the urine for protein and microscopic examination for casts; retinal examination on admission and every second or third day depending on findings. Blood chemical determinations in preeclampsia have yielded very little practical information in my experience but if they can be readily obtained, the most informative are: total serum protein, uric acid and carbon dioxide content. Hematocrit determinations are helpful in following hemoconcentration.

Complete bed rest is essential. The most important dietary specification is a salt-poor diet, 3 gm. per day or less of sodium chloride. Ample proteins should be included in the diet in the form of lean meats, eggs and one quart of milk daily. Since a quart of milk itself contains about 1.25 gm. of sodium chloride, any drastic attempt to approach an actual salt-free diet entails use of dialyzed milk or one of the commercial sodium-free milk powders. Such radical dietary measures may occasionally prove worth while in preeclampsia, but I do not recommend them, since my own (admittedly limited) experience with sodium-free milk in this disease has not shown any dramatic effects over the ordinary salt-poor diet containing 2 to 3 gm. of sodium chloride; moreover, the milk preparations of this type which have come to my attention are most unacceptable to patients. The fluid intake should be neither limited nor forced and is best set at 2,500 cc. except in hot weather when 3,000 cc. is permissible. Even in milder cases minimal doses of a sedative drug are helpful, such as phenobarbital (Luminal) 0.03 gm. (0.5 grain) four times daily, or twice this dosage in cases of moderate severity. Magnesium sulfate, 15 gm., or citrate of magnesia, 200 cc., every second or third day has been a routine in our clinic for many years and in our opinion it is helpful in ridding the body of excess water.

If clinical edema is present ammonium chloride may prove helpful but it must be used with full realization of its acidotic action and never for more than three days at a time. Ammonium chloride, after absorption from the gastrointestinal tract, is converted by the liver into urea and an excess of chloride ions. The latter reduce the alkaline reserve and this alteration, in turn, lowers the capacity of the proteins in the tissues to bind water; consequently, fluid moves from the tissues to the blood and diuresis ensues. In other words, ammonium chloride promotes diuresis by inducing acidosis and should not be used if there is any suspicion of renal insufficiency. Ammonium chloride is given in enteric-coated capsules or tablets of 0.5 gm. each and the official U. S. P. dose of 4 gm. per day is recommended. As indicated, it should be discontinued after three days, but may be given again after a two or three day rest period.

The further management of a case of preeclampsia will depend upon its severity as demonstrated by the course in the hospital, upon the condition of the cervix and upon other factors. Fortunately the great majority of cases prove to be sufficiently mild, and near enough to term, so that they can be handled under the above regime until labor starts spontaneously or the cervix is suitable for the induction of labor. Complete abatement of all signs and symptoms, however, is uncommon until after delivery unless the infant succumbs in the uterus.

Occasionally the picture presented by a preeclamptic patient may be fulminating as evidenced by blood pressure in excess of 160/110, massive edema, heavy proteinuria and by a general nervous ensemble, indicating that convulsions are imminent. Such severe preeclampsia demands immediate and intensive medicinal therapy for at least 24 hours. Sedation is of the first importance in order to forestall convulsions. Whatever drug is used for this purpose the objective should be to produce drowsiness, or sleep from which the patient can be easily awakened, but not coma. Dosages should be regulated accordingly. Sedation may well be initiated by a hypodermic injection of morphine sulfate 0.016 gm. (0.25 grain), followed either by paraldehyde per rectum, or one of the barbiturates.

If paraldehyde is employed, the dose should be about 10 cc. for a woman weighing under 160 lbs. or 15 cc. if she appears to weigh over 160 lbs.; in either event it is administered in 30 cc. of olive oil. This dosage may be repeated every 6 to 10 hours depending on restlessness and blood pressure levels. Paraldehyde usually produces a gratifying fall in blood pressure, is a dependable prophylactic against convulsions, has no effect on urinary excretion since a very small fraction is excreted by the kidneys and has a wide margin of safety. We much prefer it to the barbiturates both in severe preeclampsia and in eclampsia.

If the paraldehyde is expelled, or if a barbiturate is preferred, one of the longer acting of the latter compounds should be used such as: phenobarbital sodium (Luminal sodium) 0.1 gm. (1.5 grains) orally every 6 to 8 hours; or sodium amytal 0.2 gm. (3 grains) intramuscularly every 8 to 12 hours.

In fulminating preeclampsia (as well as in eclampsia) magnesium sulfate, intramuscularly or intravenously, is a most valuable agent as attested by the experience of many clinics over many years. The efficacy of magnesium sulfate as a central nervous system depressant and as a vasodilator is well known, and is substantiated by a large amount of experimental and clinical evidence. Thus it is widely considered the most efficient drug in allaying the convulsions of tetanus. As a vasodilator it has been employed extensively in the treatment of hypertension and uremia. In 1925 Blackfan and Hamilton observed that intravenous injections of magnesium sulfate produced a favorable influence by lowering the blood pressure and increasing the flow of urine in children suffering from hemorrhagic nephritis. These observations have been confirmed by numerous workers and more recently Haury has shown that intravenous injection of magnesium sulfate produces a marked dilatation of the splanchnic organs, including the kidneys. Since both sedative and vasodilator effects of magnesium sulfate are urgently to be desired in the treatment of preeclampsia and eclampsia, it is not surprising that this drug has been widely employed in the management of these conditions over the past 20 years. In the main, however, the dosages used have been very small, the total amount administered intramuscularly being limited as a rule to 10 gm. per day. It has been shown by many workers that such dosage is not adequate to produce the full therapeutic action of this agent. The question then arises: what effect can be expected from magnesium sulfate by the parenteral route in dosages which are considerably larger than those usually employed? More important is the question: how large a dosage of this drug may be employed with complete safety?

In evaluating the safety of magnesium sulfate it is important to recall that toxic signs and symptoms do not develop until the serum magnesium reaches 10 to 12 mg. per 100 cc. At or near this level the knee jerks disappear. Between 12 and 15 mg. per 100 cc. respirations are likely to cease and when the serum magnesium concentrations reach 15 mg. per 100 cc., cardiac action may stop and death ensue. We have now employed this drug in over 400 cases with rather large total dosages and believe it is possible to administer magnesium sulfate intramuscularly in several times the dosage usually employed without approaching hazardous levels of serum magnesium. On the basis of our experience, which includes more than 300 serum magnesium determinations done at various times after the administration of the drug, we feel in the first place that it is entirely safe to administer 10 gm. intramuscularly as an initial dose, followed by 5 gm. every six hours. We have continued this for as long as two to three days with total dosages reaching 60 to 110 gm. and never have observed a serum magnesium level above 7 mg. per 100 cc. Usually the range obtained by such dosage is between 4 and 6 mg. per 100 cc. In the second place, it is our impression that such levels of magnesium contribute substantially to a lowering of the blood pressure and prevention of convulsions. The main place of this drug in the management of preeclampsia, in our opinion, is in protecting patients with this complication against convulsions during labor. If labor is to be induced magnesium sulfate injections are often started several hours before the procedure is carried out. Although we feel certain that the use of magnesium sulfate intramuscularly in the dosages cited is generally safe, the following precautionary measures are recommended: (a) the knee jerks should be tested before each injection and the drug administered only if they are active; (b) the respirations should be counted before each injection and the drug administered only if they are 16 or more per minute; (c) the drug should not be continued for more than 24 hours if the urinary output is less than 600 cc. daily since the kidneys are the only route of excretion; and (d) as a further precautionary measure an intravenous calcium preparation (calcium gluconate, 1 gm. in 10 cc.) should always be by the bedside, for it is an immediate antidote. The technic of administration is important. The injection is made in the upper outer gluteal quadrant, the skin having been prepared with ether, iodine and alcohol as for a surgical operation. A 50 per cent solution of magnesium sulfate is employed in which a 1 per cent concentration of procaine has been introduced in order to reduce discomfort from the injection. The needle is moved about while the solution is being introduced in order to obtain even dispersion and, after withdrawal of the needle, the area is massaged with a dry, warm pack, the pack being then affixed to the site of injection by adhesive tape.

Although we prefer the intramuscular route of administration to the intravenous, the latter technic of giving magnesium sulfate, especially in actual eclampsia, is probably more widely employed in this country than the intramuscular method. In severe preeclampsia Page uses magnesium sulfate, 2 gm. (20 cc. of 10 per cent solution) injected very slowly (one minute) intravenously. If it seems advisable this can be repeated every two or three hours provided the precautionary measures cited above are followed.

In severe preeclampsia associated with oliguria (urinary output of less than 400 cc. during the 12 hours of observation, let us say), intravenous glucose is indicated; and in many clinics, this procedure is routine in all severe cases for the purpose of stimulating diuresis. It is usually administered in 200 cc. quantities of a 20 per cent cc. solution in distilled water, this amount to be run in within about 30 minutes. While this measure is often helpful, dramatic effects are not to be expected and my own experience has led me to place less reliance upon it in preeclampsia than many authorities do. In the main, oliguria of any substantial degree in preeclampsia is an indication for termination of pregnancy rather than for continued attempts to effect diuresis.

Termination of Pregnancy. The treatment of preeclampsia par excellence is termination of the pregnancy. There are two main reasons why prompt delivery is desirable, namely, prevention of convulsions and prevention of residual hypertension. As already explained, the longer a preeclamptic patient is carried the more likely she is to have residual hypertension. However, because the baby may be premature, the tendency is widespread to temporize in many of these cases in the hope that a few more weeks of intra-uterine life will give the infant a better chance. In the milder varieties of preeclampsia such a policy is often justifiable, at least up until the thirty-fifth week of gestation. On the other hand, in severe preeclampsia, the opinion is growing, as McLane has recently emphasized, that even for the sake of the baby such a waiting policy may be ill-advised since preeclampsia itself may kill the child and that, even in the lower weight brackets, the likelihood of its survival in severe preeclampsia may be better outside than inside the uterus.

Whether or not to terminate pregnancy in preeclampsia resolves itself into a problem of balancing risks. Which course carries the greater hazard: on the one hand, allowing the pregnancy to continue with the hazards of convulsions, residual hypertension and possible fetal death in utero, or, on the other, termination of the pregnancy with the hazards attendant upon operative interference plus the possibility of a premature baby which succumbs? In a patient near term with a soft, open and partially effaced cervix, even the mildest degrees of preeclampsia probably carry more risk to the mother and her infant than does induction of labor by simple rupture of the membranes. On the other hand, if the preeclampsia is mild but the cervix is firm and closed (indicating the necessity of abdominal delivery if pregnancy is to be terminated), the hazard of cesarean section is usually greater than allowing the pregnancy to continue for a few weeks under treatment, at the end of which time the cervix may be suitable for induction. If severe preeclampsia, as judged by the general ensemble of the patient, does not improve with medicinal therapy after one or two days, termination of pregnancy is usually advisable from the viewpoint both of the mother and the infant. If the cervix is favorable for induction, rupture of the membranes should be carried out but if it is not favorable, cesarean section is the procedure of choice. In balancing the relative advantages of induction of labor and cesarean section in fulminating preeclampsia, it must be recalled that the hours consumed by labor are themselves a drawback and, moreover, that the blood pressure can be counted upon to rise 20 mm. or more in the course of labor. As indicated above, however, it is our experience that even in rather fulminating preeclampsia it it possible to forestall convulsions in labor by maintaining a suitable level of serum magnesium.

The termination of pregnancy in preeclampsia should rarely be carried out, either by the induction of labor or cesarean section, until at least 24 hours of intensive hospital therapy have elapsed. As the result of this treatment the patient will invariably be a much better operative risk for either procedure than she was on admission. If cesarean section is to be done the anesthesia of choice is probably local infiltration anesthesia provided the patient has been protected against convulsions by magnesium sulfate or some dependable type of sedation. Ether anesthesia should not be used because it is conducive to edema of the lungs in the mother and narcosis in the infant, and the infant under these circumstances is often premature.

ECLAMPSIA

Eclampsia is an acute disease peculiar to gravid and puerperal women which is characterized by clonic and tonic convulsions during which there is loss of consciousness followed by more or less prolonged coma. It frequently results in death. The word "eclampsia" is derived from the Greek word "ἐκλάμπειν," used by Hippocrates to designate a fever of sudden onset. The word means a flash or shining forth and is indicative of the fulminating character of the disease which has come to be generally known as eclampsia. Convulsions and eclampsia are usually considered as synonymous terms, but such a view is not altogether correct inasmuch as a few well-authenticated cases of "eclampsia without convulsions" are recorded; contrariwise, convulsions without eclampsia are occasionally seen in obstetrical practice as, for instance, in epilepsy.

Incidence. Eclampsia is becoming rarer each year as more and more women receive better prenatal care. The incidence throughout the country is probably one in every 500 to 800 deliveries, but there are wide deviations from this figure in different localities and countries. These variations appear to depend on economic, dietary and social conditions and especially upon the availability of good prenatal care. Owing to the interaction of these factors, eclampsia is encountered more commonly in this country in the nonwhite races. Thus, in 1944, there were 800 deaths attributed to the disease in the United States, of which 245, or 31 per cent, were in nonwhites. Since the percentage of nonwhite births is only about 13 per cent, it becomes apparent that fatal eclampsia is almost two and one-half times more frequent among nonwhites.

Eclampsia occurs more often in primigravidae than in multiparae, the ratio being approximately 3 to 1. Its frequency appears to vary greatly at different times and in many hospitals it is observed that months elapse without the occurrence of a single case, when suddenly a number are observed in quick succession. This circumstance has suggested that eclampsia may be related to climatic conditions but efforts to establish any such correlation have met with little success. The incidence of the disease appears to be greatest in the late winter months, reaching a maximum perhaps in March and April.

According as the disorder first appears before, or during labor, or in the puerperium, it is designated as *antepartum*, *intrapartum* or *postpartum* eclampsia. Roughly speaking, about one-half of the cases develop antepartum, approximately one-quarter intrapartum and another quarter postpartum. The vast majority of cases of postpartum eclampsia make their appearance within 24 hours after delivery and cases in which the first convulsion is observed more than 48 hours postpartum should be regarded with some skepticism. Nevertheless, in rare instances, cases are said to have begun as late as six days after delivery. Convulsions which begin more than one week after delivery may be confidently attributed to some other origin. Eclampsia occurs almost exclusively in the last third of pregnancy and becomes more frequent the nearer term is approached.

The disease is noted four times more often in twin than in single pregnancies, and four or five times more frequently when the pregnancy is complicated by hydramnios. Eclampsia may occur during the course of advanced extra-uterine pregnancy, and Pride and Rucker have recently reported a case occurring in a woman with an ovarian pregnancy. Falk, Sitzenfrey and others have reported cases occurring in association with hydatidiform mole and, indeed, the disease is thought to be more frequent and more severe in that condition than in normal pregnancy. Of 30 women with hydatid mole observed by Ernest W. Page, 10 developed preeclampsia, in contrast to a 9 per cent incidence of preeclampsia in his clinic population in general. Three of these 10 cases were graded as severe preeclampsia, while the remainder were mild. The cases were arbitrarily divided into early stages (less than four months' amenorrhea, or a tumor below the level of the umbilicus), and late stages (from four to seven months' amenorrhea, or a tumor above the level of the umbilicus). Of the 16 early cases, there were no instances of preeclamptic toxemia. All 10 of the toxemias were found among 14 hydatid moles which were of four to seven months' duration, an incidence of 71 per cent. In a study of 57 consecutive cases of hydatidiform mole by Chesley, Cosgrove and Preece, it was found that one of the patients developed eclampsia between the fourth and fifth month. This case was of extraordinary interest in that the patient had developed severe preeclampsia in a previous molar pregnancy but had manifested no evidence of toxemia in three intervening normal pregnancies without mole. These authors found in the literature 35 cases of probable or alleged eclampsia occurring in association with hydatidiform mole, or with partial hydatidiform degeneration of the placenta. In practically all these cases eclampsia was said to have occurred extremely early, that is, between the third and sixth months.

Clinical Course. Almost without exception, the outbreak of convulsions is preceded for a longer or shorter time by premonitory symptoms indicative of preeclampsia. Isolated cases are now and then cited in which an eclamptic convulsion is said to have occurred without warning like a "bolt from a clear sky," in women who were apparently in good health. Careful inquiry into such cases will usually show that the patient had not been examined by her physician for some days or weeks previously and that she had neglected to report symptoms of preeclampsia. Occasionally the onset is preceded by a distinct aura, but this is usually lacking. Severe epigastric pain, or a sensation as if the thorax were encircled by a tight girdle, is a frequent precursor of a seizure and is a sign which should excite grave concern.

The attack may come on at any time, sometimes while the patient is sleeping. If she is awake, the first sign of the impending convulsion is a fixed expression of the eyes and a tense turning of the head to one side. The pupils are usually dilated, less often contracted. The convulsive movements begin first about the mouth in the form of facial twitchings. This is the *stage of invasion* of the convulsion and lasts only a few seconds.

The whole body then becomes rigid in a generalized muscular contraction; the face is distorted, the eyes protrude, the arms are flexed, the hands are clenched and the legs inverted. Since all the muscles of the body are now in a state of tonic contraction, this phase may be regarded as the *stage of contraction*, and lasts 15 or 20 seconds.

Suddenly the jaws begin to open and close violently, and forthwith the eyelids also. The other facial muscles and then all the muscles of the body alternately contract and relax in rapid succession. So forceful are the muscular movements that the patient may throw herself out of bed and, almost invariably unless protected, the tongue is bitten by the violent jaw action. Foam, often blood-tinged, exudes from the mouth; the face is congested and purple, and the eyes bloodshot. Few clinical pictures are so terrifying. This phase in which the muscles alternately contract and relax is called the *stage of convulsion*, and may last a minute or so. Gradually, the muscular movements become milder and farther apart, and finally the patient lies motionless.

Throughout the seizure the diaphragm has been fixed with respiration halted. Still no breathing occurs. For a few seconds the woman appears to be dying from respiratory arrest, but just when this outcome seems almost inevitable, she takes a long, deep, stertorous inhalation, and breathing is resumed. Then coma ensues. The patient will remember nothing whatsoever of the convulsion or, in all probability, events immediately before and afterward.

When the disorder appears in the latter part of labor or during the puerperium, a single convulsion only may be observed. Oftener, however, the first is the forerunner of other convulsions, which may vary in number from one or two in mild, to 10 to 20 or even 100 or more in severe cases, the intervals between them becoming shorter in inverse proportion to the number. In rare instances they follow one another so rapidly that the patient appears to be in a prolonged, almost continuous convulsion.

The duration of the coma is quite variable. When the convulsions are infrequent, the patient usually recovers consciousness after each attack, while in severe cases the coma persists from one convulsion to another, and death may result without any awakening from it. In rare instances a single convulsion may be followed by profound coma from which the patient never emerges though, as a rule, death does not occur until after a frequent repetition of the convulsive attacks. The immediate cause of death is usually edema of the lungs, apoplexy or an acidosis, though if the fatal issue is postponed for several days it may be attributable to aspiration pneumonia or marked liver injury.

While the convulsions are by far the most striking clinical manifestation of eclampsia, instances are occasionally met in which they are absent, with the patient dying in coma and presenting at autopsy the hepatic and renal lesions characteristic of the affection. For instance, Dieckmann and Wegner have reported a case without convulsions in which the liver pathology was absolutely typical of eclampsia. Moreover, Reis and Bernick have reported a case, which they refer to as eclampsia, in which there occurred neither convulsions, hypertension nor coma. It seems to me that a clearer and more logical concept of the whole disease process of acute toxemia would be afforded if cases of eclampsia without convulsions or coma, and possibly also cases of eclampsia without convulsions, were regarded as exceedingly severe cases of preeclampsia. This would serve to bring more forcibly to our attention the fact that preeclampsia and eclampsia constitute one disease process in which all gradations of pathological changes may be encountered and in which the clinical picture, in rare instances, may show wide variations. In some cases the absence of convulsive attacks has led to an erroneous clinical diagnosis, the condition having been regarded as uremic coma, phosphorus poisoning, fulminating bacterial infection, Weil's disease, or acute yellow atrophy of the liver.

In almost all cases of eclampsia the arterial pressure is markedly augmented, the systolic pressure averaging about 180 mm. and the diastolic about 110. Very exceptionally, little or no increase is observed above levels which are accepted as normal and on occasions patients go through the eclamptic attack with a maximal systolic pressure of 140 mm. or less. Careful study of these patients, however, will usually reveal that they are young girls in whom the usual pressure had been of the order of 105 systolic and 70 diastolic; in them, in other words, an elevation to 135 systolic and 90 diastolic would represent hypertension. The pulse is usually full and bounding, but in very severe cases it is weak and rapid, becoming more compressible and filiform with each succeeding convulsion. The temperature remains normal in the majority of the cases, but rises to 101° F. or above in a third or more of cases. Temperatures of 103 and 104 are not unusual in severe cases but such a finding is of very grave prognostic import. The cause of the fever is probably a disturbance of the thermal centers due to cerebral edema.

Respiration in eclampsia is usually increased in rate and stertorous in character.

The rate may reach 50 or more per minute, a circumstance which may have profound effects on the acid-base equilibrium of the blood. Cyanosis may be observed in severe cases.

Proteinuria is almost constantly present, and frequently is so pronounced that it is necessary to dilute the urine to several times its volume before an accurate determination can be made by means of the Esbach tube. In the majority of cases this test shows the presence of at least 4 gm. of albumin per liter during the acute stage of the disease, while in many instances much larger quantities are noted—sometimes as high as 30 or 40 gm. The urinary protein excreted in eclampsia has a high globulin content, the urinary albumin to globulin ratio being 2 to 1 according to Willis and 3 to 1 on the basis of my own studies. The high globulin content of the urine in this disease is probably the direct result of increased capillary permeability in the glomerulus. The urine is invariably diminished in amount and occasionally entirely suppressed. On microscopic examination various types of casts are found in great abundance, although the hyaline and granular varieties predominate. Epithelial casts also occur, as well as isolated renal cells, while blood is nearly always present. Hemoglobinuria may also be observed.

Edema is probably present in 100 per cent of eclamptic patients, but in 10 or 15 per cent it is latent and not demonstrable on superficial examination. Often it is massive and occasionally eclamptic patients are encountered whose histories show that they have gained 70 or more pounds during the course of gestation. Most of this gain represents, of course, extreme waterlogging of all the body tissues.

In antepartum eclampsia, as a rule, labor sets in after a short while, and often progresses rapidly to completion, sometimes before the attendants are even aware that the patient is having contractions. If the attack occurs during labor, the pains usually increase in frequency and severity so that the child is born somewhat sooner than usual. Following delivery, improvement with subsidence of convulsions may be anticipated provided proper treatment has been instituted. Not infrequently labor does not supervene but the patient improves greatly, convulsions cease, the coma disappears and the patient becomes completely oriented. This improved state may continue for several days or longer, a condition known as *intercurrent eclampsia*. It has been claimed in the past that such patients may often return entirely to normal with complete subsidence of the hypertension and albuminuria, but such a gratifying course of events has been extremely rare in my experience. It is true that convulsions and coma, that is, the eclamptic state, may entirely subside and that the blood pressure and albuminuria may decrease to a certain extent. As a rule, however, such patients continue to show substantial hypertension and demonstrable albuminuria and have in actuality only returned to the preeclamptic state. It is not uncommon for such patients, after a few days of apparent improvement, to develop convulsions again and this second attack may be exceedingly severe, even fatal. Accordingly, one must be wary about these cases of so-called intercurrent eclampsia for unless delivery has taken place, return of convulsions is always a threat.

Improvement is most likely to be observed 12 to 24 hours after delivery, when the convulsions usually decrease in frequency and then subside altogether. The duration of coma prior to complete mental orientation varies from a few hours to several days. As the patient arouses from her coma there often ensues a semiconscious, combative state which may last for as long as a day. The first sign of improvement is usually an increase in urinary output. The proteinuria and edema ordinarily disappear within four or five days. The hypertension is likely to persist for 7 to 10 days, but in most cases the blood pressure has returned to normal two weeks after delivery. However, as will be discussed later (page 685), a substantial minority of patients are left with a residuum of chronic hypertension.

In fatal cases pulmonary edema is a conspicuous feature of the clinical picture, especially during the terminal hours. It may be present as well in patients who survive but if of substantial degree, is a grave prognostic sign. Other signs of heart failure make their appearance in the terminal stage of fatal eclampsia, especially cyanosis, a rising pulse rate and a falling blood pressure. As the cardiovascular system fails, convulsions usually cease and may not occur at all during the last six or eight hours of life. On the other hand, in some cases of eclampsia death occurs suddenly, synchronously with or shortly after a convulsion, as the result of massive brain hemorrhage.

In about every twentieth case, eclampsia is followed by an acute psychosis in which the patient may become very violent. The psychotic condition usually manifests itself on the second or third day after delivery, or about the time that the patient is coming out of coma, and ordinarily lasts for about four weeks. The prognosis in general is good, except when the patient possesses a psychopathic tendency, as evidenced by past history or mental disease in the immediate family. In rare instances hemiplegia may ensue as the result of a sublethal brain hemorrhage. I saw such a case some time ago in which four and one-half years after the eclamptic seizure the patient's right arm remained sufficiently paralyzed to be of no practical use and there was a detectable slur in her speech. Parks and Pearson, and also Abbott, have reported similar cases.

In one or two per cent of cases, an amaurosis makes itself manifest as soon as the patient begins to arouse from her coma. Most frequently the disturbed vision which sometimes precedes the attack is due to edema of the retina which usually disappears spontaneously. It is sometimes central in origin being caused by some disturbance in the optic nerve or in the visual centers in the occipital lobe, the most logical explanation being edema of these structures. The blindness may persist for a few hours or for several weeks. Usually, however, the vision returns to normal within a week and the prognosis for sight is good. Occasionally, hemorrhagic retinitis or detachment of the retina is observed. In an ophthalmologic study of 132 eclamptic patients, Schiotz found seven cases of retinal detachment, in two of whom the detachment persisted for years. Clapp reported six cases of detachment with complete recovery in all of them. Doggart stresses four points of distinction in retinal detachment in eclampsia: rapidity of onset, subretinal fluid, no hemorrhage or exudate with extensive bilateral detachment, and the generally good prognosis. As indicated, the prognosis of ocular lesions accompanying eclampsia is surprisingly good and most cases of incomplete detachment of the retina and many cases of complete detachment result in no permanent impairment of vision.

Pathologic Anatomy. The most common postmortem alterations in eclampsia are found in the liver, kidneys, brain, lungs and heart.

The characteristic *liver* lesion is hemorrhagic necrosis of the periphery of the hepatic lobule. This may make itself manifest grossly as irregularly shaped reddish areas both beneath the capsule and on the cut surface, giving the liver a mottled

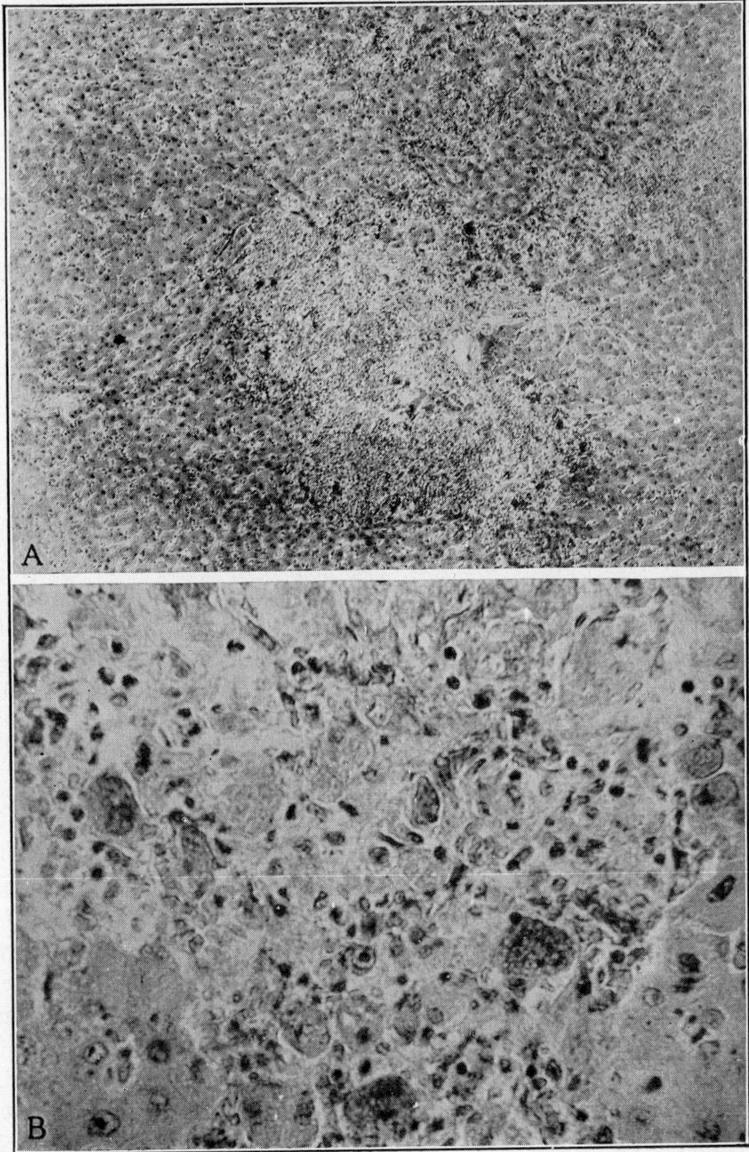

FIG. 384.—LIVER FROM ECLAMPSIA.

A, section showing periportal necrosis (× 70); B, area of same section showing damage of liver cells (× 480).

appearance. The hemorrhages are most commonly found in the right lobe of the liver. Upon microscopic examination the areas of hemorrhagic necrosis begin about a periportal space and are usually associated with extensive thrombosis in the smallest vessels in the periportal connective tissue. In the opinion of Dieckmann, as well as earlier authors, this lesion is the result primarily of a marked dilatation or ectasia of the capillaries about the portal space. Rupture of the capillary walls occurs and thrombosis then follows with the result that the liver cells about these hemorrhages are compressed, with interference to their blood supply. Although hemorrhage is usually present in these necrotic areas, this is not always the case and sometimes simply a focal hyaline or fibrinoid necrosis of the periportal spaces presents itself. In all probability the latter type of lesion represents a late stage in the process of hemorrhagic necrosis, the hemoglobin being now dissolved out and the fibrin having contracted into a solid necrotic mass.

Although the characteristic hepatic necrosis of eclampsia is periportal in location, the lesion may sometimes extend into the center of the liver lobule, as has been described by Acosta-Sison, Way and others. As Dieckmann has pointed out, it is barely possible that this central and midzonal necrosis is the result of the relative starvation which most eclamptic patients undergo, rather than of any specific disease process. The most characteristic aspect of the hepatic lesion in eclampsia is its variability in extent and severity. Many cases have been reported in which it has been impossible to demonstrate any hepatic necrosis whatsoever, and in Acosta-Sison's series of cases the hepatic necrosis was so variable and bizarre in distribution that she was unable to confirm the prevalent view that focal necrosis around the portal areas is the characteristic lesion of eclampsia. In addition, Bell, Theobald and Davidson are of the opinion that peripheral necrosis is not always the typical or frequent liver lesion in this disease. Davidson, in a study of 19 cases, found three types of liver lesions, peripheral necrosis, widespread necrosis of the cells in the central and midzones and lastly, cases where no gross hepatic lesions were found, but only small zones of focal necrosis. Theobald studied the liver in 44 women who died from eclampsia and found that peripheral necrosis was not a constant finding. He observed hemorrhagic necrosis in 70 per cent of his cases whereas fibrinothrombotic lesions appeared in only 40 per cent. Moreover, all observers agree that there is no correlation between the clinical severity of a case of eclampsia and the extent of the hepatic lesion. In view of these circumstances it is generally agreed that the liver lesions of eclampsia are the result and not the cause of the disease process.

Hepatic biopsy studies have been made on five cases of eclampsia by Ingerslev and Teilum. The liver was apparently quite normal in two cases but in two other cases showed changes characteristic of eclampsia as known from autopsy material. In one of these cases even the fresh specimen was grossly flecked, presenting small red spots and streaks in contrast to the grayish-brown color of the tissue in general. Sections from this specimen showed scattered areas of coagulation necrosis which were extensive. These changes were localized especially in the periphery of the lobules where the capillaries in several places were filled with large or small thrombi of fibrin often appearing as an anastomosing network enveloping granular necrotic liver cells. The necrotic areas as well as the hemorrhages are presumably attributable to blocking of the peripheral capillaries with fibrin thrombi. These fibrinous precipitates are regarded by the authors as the essential histological feature of the hepatic lesion in eclampsia. It is informative to note that their two patients with the severest hepatic changes survived quite satisfactorily. Prior to these observations such changes in the liver have been known to exist only in fatal cases.

In rare instances hemorrhage beneath the liver capsule may be so extensive as to cause rupture of the capsule with massive hemorrhage into the peritoneal cavity. Sanes and Kaminski have reported a case of their own and have abstracted five additional cases from the literature of this accident. All of the five cases of rupture of the liver in pregnancy with hemorrhage into the peritoneal cavity occurred in eclampsia. No patient had a definite history of abdominal trauma. In two cases the clinical picture of rupture and hemorrhage appeared after transportation of the patient. Five of the six patients died.

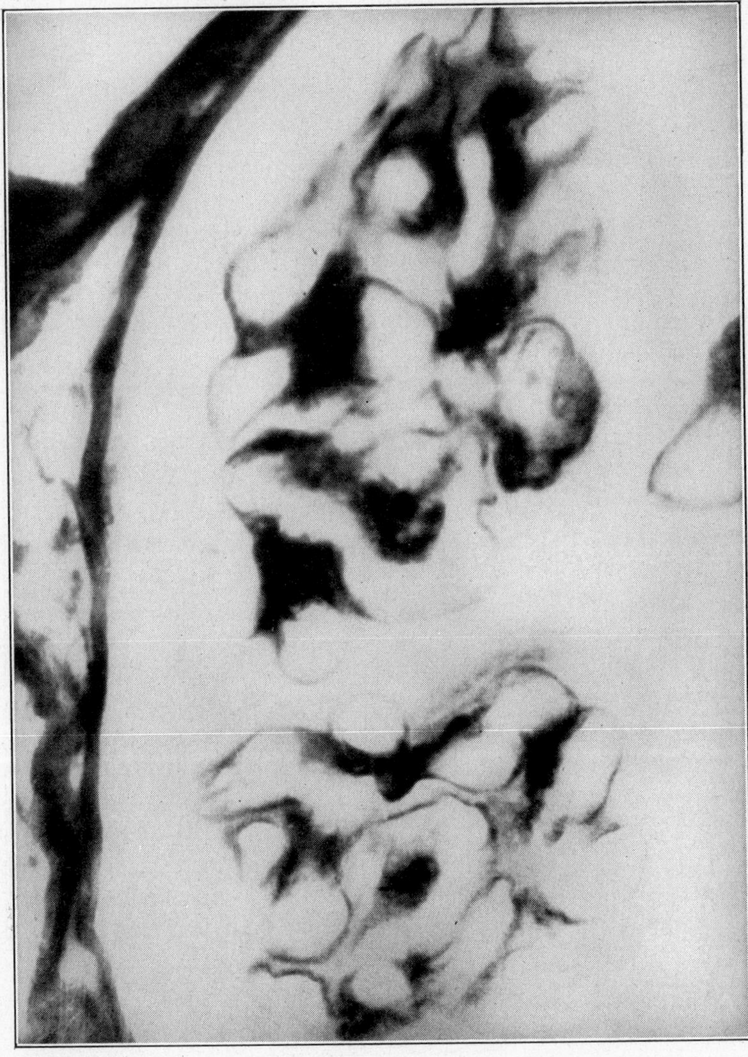

FIG. 385.—GLOMERULAR BASEMENT MEMBRANE OF THE NORMAL KIDNEY, CONSISTING OF A SINGLE THIN LAYER. (From Dexter and Weiss, *Preeclamptic and Eclamptic Toxemia of Pregnancy*, Williams and Wilkins Company, Baltimore.)

The most characteristic *renal* lesion in fatal cases of eclampsia is a marked narrowing of the glomerular capillaries caused usually by an increase in the thickness of the basement membrane, although occasionally brought about by increased endothelial cells, as indicated by the increase in nuclei present. The glomeruli are usually avascular and devoid of erythrocytes. The typical picture of the glomerular basement membrane in eclampsia is a characteristic splitting or lamination as shown in Fig. 386. These changes differ from those of acute glomerulonephritis in that in eclampsia there is absence of polymorphonuclear leukocytes, intracapillary fibers and epithelial crescents; moreover, in eclampsia the glomeruli are smaller and the basement membrane thicker. These characteristic changes in glomeruli in cases of fatal eclampsia were first described by Bell in 1932. Baird and Dunn likewise state that the common lesion in the kidneys of women dying from eclampsia is glomerular,

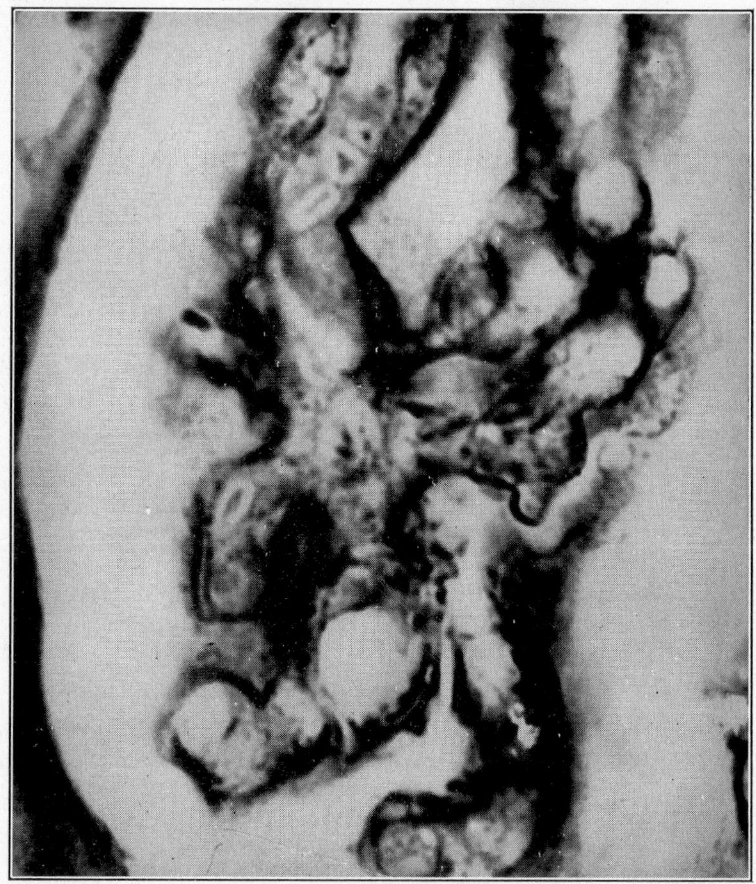

Fig. 386.—Glomerular Basement Membrane of the Kidney in Eclampsia Showing Marked Degree of Thickening and Duplication. (From Dexter and Weiss, *Preeclamptic and Eclamptic Toxemia of Pregnancy,* Williams and Wilkins Company, Baltimore.)

being thickening of the capillary walls and of the endothelium, resulting in partial obstruction to the blood flow. In an extensive study of fatal eclampsia by Way, based on 33 necropsies, the author notes that all the changes in the glomerulus in eclampsia are quantitative in nature and represent progressions of the same pathologic process.

Tubular lesions are also very common in eclampsia. These are essentially those of nephrosis, that is, they consist of degenerative changes of varying intensity in the epithelium of the convoluted tubules. There are usually no signs of inflammatory or atrophic change unless the process has been engrafted upon a pre-existing disease. Although tubular changes have long been regarded as the outstanding renal lesion in eclampsia, most modern students of the subject consider them less constant and less important than the glomerular changes.

In rare cases the major portion of the cortex of both kidneys undergoes complete necrosis. This is the result of thrombosis of the intralobular arteries with extension in both cases into the glomerular capillaries. Infarction and necrosis ensue. The condition is probably due to a spasm of the renal arteries with resultant thrombosis and anemic infarcts. Although cortical necrosis of the kidney is known to have occurred in nonpregnant persons, including men, the majority of cases have been associated with pregnancy. In a group of 45 authentic and 16 questionable cases collected by Dieckmann from the literature, 9 were encountered in the course of autopsies on eclamptic patients. The disease is characterized clinically by oliguria, or anuria, and rapid increase in the nonprotein elements of the blood (see page 765).

The main postmortem lesions encountered in the *brain* in eclampsia are edema, hyperemia, anemia, thrombosis and hemorrhage. Prutz noted edema in 42 per cent, hyperemia in 35 per cent and hemorrhage in 13 per cent, while the brain was apparently normal in only 10 per cent of his cases. Schmorl, in 58 out of 65 autopsies, noted the presence of thrombi in the smaller cerebral vessels, and regarded them as the cause of the small areas of necrosis which are so often observed. In Way's more recent study of 33 eclamptic autopsies, cerebral hemorrhage was present in three cases, in two of which it was massive. These two cases also demonstrated cerebral arteritis and arteriolitis with necrosis of the vessel walls.

In most cases of eclampsia the *heart* is more or less involved, and was perfectly normal in only 8 out of 102 autopsies analyzed by Polak. According to Schmorl, the changes usually consist in degenerative processes in the myocardium. Disregarding cloudy swelling and fatty degeneration, which were very frequently present, he found hemorrhage and necrosis in the myocardium in 43 of 73 autopsies. In the neighborhood of the hemorrhages the muscle fibers were disintegrated into hyaline layers, usually with the nucleus gone and the transverse striations no longer recognizable. In Way's 33 cases, the heart was the site of hemorrhage in 12 patients. Four of these showed focal necrosis of the myocardium with slight cellular reaction. There were two cases of myocarditis, one characterized by the focal aggregation of polymorphonuclear leukocytes, and the other by a diffuse scattering of round cells.

The *lungs* show varying degrees of pulmonary edema, often extreme, while in about half the cases bronchopneumonia is demonstrable as the result of aspiration of infectious material during coma. Owing to the same mechanism, a few cases of pulmonary abscess have been known to follow eclampsia.

Lesions in the *adrenal glands* are frequent and consist essentially of necrosis and hemorrhage of varying degrees. Eleven, or one-third, of Way's cases showed this pathologic change in the adrenal glands. Of these, 45 per cent were classified as severe in that practically no functional adrenal cortical tissue remained. The other 55 per cent showed involvement of approximately half of the cortical tissue. There were no cases with minimal lesions. In Way's opinion, adrenal insufficiency secondary to recent widespread injury may be a contributory factor in the terminal shock-like syndrome in eclampsia and in the death of certain patients.

The Common Denominator in the Pathology of Eclampsia. Although pathologic changes in eclampsia, as described above, are widespread and varied, a factor common to all of them may be found in the abnormal behavior of the vascular tree, especially its terminal branches. The thrombosis of the hepatic arteries with rupture and hemorrhage, the glomerular changes, the brain, heart and adrenal hemorrhages, all attest this fact. Accordingly, the belief is growing that eclampsia is not a disease of the liver, or of the kidneys, or indeed of any special organ, but of all the smaller arterioles. Hertig believes that the essential lesion exists in the precapillary arteriole and that the nature of the change is an arteriolitis. In the present state of our knowledge, the best explanation of this vascular process is that it is initiated by widespread vasospasm. As the result, hypertension ensues and also hypoxia of the capillaries and arterioles distal to the spasm with consequent injury to their walls. These vascular changes, together with local tissue hypoxia, are presumably the cause of the hemorrhages, the necroses and most of the other disturbances observed in this disease.

Placental Changes. The frequency of so-called *infarcts of the placenta* is increased somewhat in toxemic cases over the 60 per cent incidence observed in the placentas of normal cases (page 549). Tenney and Parker believe that the characteristic placental lesion consists primarily of a premature aging of the placenta. As has been known for many years, the full term placenta shows a certain amount of syncytial degeneration. This is normal and physiologic. On further investigation Tenney and Parker found that this involves from 10 to 50 per cent of the small terminal villi. They note that in toxemia the majority of the villi are involved and in severe preeclamptics and eclamptics all of the small villi may be affected. The type of syncytial degeneration is quite characteristic. In its first stages it consists of the clumping together and autolysis of the nuclei in the syncytial cytoplasm (not the syncytial buds), leaving clumps of darkly staining masses with no cell outlines and wide areas of syncytial cytoplasm without nuclei. The final stage is the disappearance of all nuclei from the syncytial layer, leaving the villus surrounded by a thin irregular layer of hyaline material. They observe also a marked congestion of the villous blood vessels in toxemic cases.

Pathologic Physiology. As noted previously, a 25 per cent increase in the minute output of the heart is an invariable accompaniment of normal pregnancy. This increment in the amount of blood coursing through the vascular tree per minute requires, of course, certain adjustments by the vessels, especially those in the pelvis. The natural elasticity of normal vessels permits accommodation to this augmented blood flow without difficulty, but in a small minority of cases the response of the vascular tree to this new load is abnormal and, for this or other reasons, vasospasm ensues. Some plausibility is given to this concept by the reaction to pregnancy of women with chronic hypertensive vascular disease, a condition characterized by more or less sclerosis of the smaller arterioles. Some 25 per cent of these women develop preeclampsia in the course of gestation. In other words, they are three or four times more vulnerable to the changes of pregnancy than normal women. Some authorities, notably Dieckmann, believe that even apparently normal women, who have never shown evidence of hypertension, develop preeclampsia and eclampsia because they possess an inherently abnormal vascular tree which has been made manifest for the first time by pregnancy. Although this reasoning may explain certain cases of preeclampsia and eclampsia, especially those in which the hypertension continues throughout life, or recurs in future pregnancies, I do not agree that it is generally applicable. As will be pointed out when prognosis is considered, the majority of women who experience eclampsia in one pregnancy, go through subsequent gestations without return of hypertension. This fact is difficult to understand on the basis that an intrinsically abnormal vascular tree was responsible for the previous eclamptic attack. Another, and to me more logical, way of looking at this problem is that certain gravidae in certain pregnancies are hampered by transitory circumstances, perhaps dietary, perhaps endocrine, perhaps of unknown etiology, which render their vascular trees at that time more vulnerable to the alterations of pregnancy. Certainly the much higher incidence of eclampsia in the nonwhite races is explicable only on the grounds that environmental factors do play an important role in the etiology of this disease.

Although there may be grave doubt in regard to the etiology of vasospasm in preeclampsia and eclampsia (a question, after all, which hangs on the unknown cause of eclampsia), there is agreement that vessel spasm looms large in the mechanism of this whole disease process. This concept was first advanced by Volhard in 1918 and has been widely accepted. It is based on evidence obtained from nail folds, ocular fundi, and specimens of muscle taken for biopsy, as well as from autopsy studies on various organs including the kidney, liver, brain and heart muscle. Hinselmann, Linzemeier, Hynemann, Baer and Reis, and others, have noted in preeclampsia changes in the smaller vessels of the nail fold consisting of alterations in the size of the arterioles, with evidence of spasm producing alternate regions of contraction and dilatation, together with elongation of the capillary loops and more or less capillary stasis. Similar capillary changes were found in a large number of eclamptic patients. Several observers, including Mussey of the Mayo Clinic, have studied histologically small sections of muscle taken from preeclamptic patients and have found alterations in the arterioles identical with those which we have just described in the small vessels of the nail fold.

Further evidence that vascular changes play an important role in preeclampsia and eclampsia is afforded by the constancy with which spasms of the retinal arterioles are met in these disorders. Mylius, in 1928, demonstrated that in toxemias of pregnancy associated with rise of blood pressure, the primary and most commonly observed lesions of the fundus were spasms and tonic constrictions of the retinal arteries. In the opinion of Wagener and of Hallum also (page 651), the first visible sign in the retina of preeclamptic patients is a narrowing of the arterioles because of spastic contraction and increased tonus of the walls of the arterioles. This change in the arterioles, the former points out, may disappear entirely if there is an early and permanent fall in blood pressure. If, however, the toxemia continues, at some stage of the spastic process permanent sclerotic changes occur in the walls of the arterioles. This is apparently brought about by an ischemia of the vessel walls due to the continual compression of the vasa vasorum by the spastic contractions. The findings of these ophthalmologists indicate, then, that during the acute toxemias of pregnancy, spasms of the arterioles develop which in time cause permanent changes in the walls of the small vessels. Their observations afford some basis for the fact that eclampsia and preeclampsia are frequently followed by chronic hypertensive vascular disease and indicate that the common factor which links the acute toxemias with their chronic sequels is not the kidney, but the vascular system.

But the question arises as to how vasospasm can cause the whole eclamptic syndrome including proteinuria, edema and convulsions. Abundance of evidence indicates that any constriction of the renal blood flow causes immediate proteinuria whether the constriction be caused by mechanical clamping of the renal vessel, vasoconstrictor drugs such as adrenalin or ephedrine, or by swimming in cold water. After reviewing the literature on the subject, Chesley, Markowitz and Wetchler demonstrated that the cold pressor test (page 653) caused proteinuria whenever it caused a blood pressure rise of 16/16 mm. or more, that is, whenever vasoconstriction ensued. These authors conclude from the promptness of the reaction, independence of venous return from the chilled hand and from calculations of the renal tubular volume capacity, that the proteinuria begins with the release of the vascular spasm. If vasospasm can cause such leaks in the glomerular capillaries, presumably as the result of transient anoxia, it would seem reasonable to believe that the capillaries throughout the body are similarly affected. Theoretically, at least, this would be expected to permit protein to pass through the capillaries, disturb osmotic pressure relationships and so cause edema. Proof that the capillaries of the general circulation are actually more permeable in preeclampsia and eclampsia, however, is lacking. As for eclamptic convulsions, they are probably produced either as the direct result of anoxia consequent upon the vasospasm, or by cerebral edema, or through a combined action of these two disturbances.

Renal function tests in preeclampsia and eclampsia yield normal figures. Thus, in a study of 79 eclamptic and 237 preeclamptic patients, Chesley found that the urea clearance does not differ significantly from values observed in normal women. It has been shown also by Chesley and his coworkers that in preeclampsia and eclampsia the renal blood flow, as measured by the diodrast clearance, is characteristically normal. The studies of kidney function in preeclampsia and eclampsia carried out by Taylor, Wellen and Welsh, by Dill, Isenhour, Cadden and Schaffer and others, have likewise revealed no extensive kidney damage. The glomerular filtration rate is only slightly reduced, the renal blood flow is normal or slightly increased, the filtration fraction is decreased, and the Tm * is normal. In patients who recover clinically after delivery the glomerular filtration rate rises slightly, the renal blood flow falls slightly and the filtration fraction rises slightly. The Tm remains normal. In patients in whom the hypertension persists after delivery the filtration rate rises and the renal blood flow falls about one-third. This results in a high filtration fraction. These changes are similar to those found in essential hypertension. Taylor has concluded, from such observations, that "The high effective renal blood flow found in association with the increased arterial blood pressure of the acute phase of toxemia is evidence against the view that renal ischemia is the primary cause of hypertension."

Clinically, the frequency of pulmonary edema and cyanosis in severe eclampsia suggests heart failure. Moreover, autopsy findings in this disease, as described in the discussion of pathologic anatomy, indicate that cardiac damage is not uncommon. Stroganoff, as the result of a vast experience, has been so impressed with the important role played by heart failure in eclampsia that he included digitalis in his regime of therapy. Paul White, in his well-known book "Heart Disease," writes: "Associated with acute hypertension in the toxemias of pregnancy (eclampsia) there

* When the plasma level of diodrast is raised to the point where the tubule cells become saturated, the excretion of this substance reaches a maximum rate. This is constant under standard conditions and serves as a measure of the total functioning tubular tissue. It is referred to as the *tubular excretory mass* or diodrast *Tm*.

may be serious toxic myocardial dilatation with acute heart failure and pulmonary edema." In 1946 Wallace, Katz, Langendorf and Buxbaum examined the electrocardiographic records of 12 patients suffering from toxemia and found significant changes in six, with actual left ventricular failure in two of these. They felt that the alterations simulated those occasionally seen in acute nephritis and attributed them to focal myocardial necrosis, infiltration or edema rather than to myocardial infarction secondary to occlusion of the coronary artery. In a similar study Szekely and Snaith made detailed observations on the heart in 19 unselected cases of toxemia of pregnancy and found that seven cases showed significant clinical and/or cardiographic changes. Left ventricular failure was observed in three and the first of these also showed T wave changes similar to those seen in anterior myocardial infarction. Significant cardiographic changes were seen in five, these changes consisting of transient alterations of the T waves usually in both standard and chest leads. On the other side of the question, Burton E. Hamilton, on the basis of a large experience with heart disease in pregnancy, takes a very strong stand, stating: "Our present opinion is that uncomplicated preeclampsia or eclampsia causes neither heart failure nor significant acute myocarditis." Over the years he has carried out a searching study of this problem and is still looking for a case where undoubted myocarditis of clinical importance appears during uncomplicated eclampsia or preeclampsia. In regard to edema of the lungs, he believes that this is due to causes other than cardiac weakness. There is thus a decided difference of opinion among cardiologists in regard to the role which cardiac alterations play in the pathologic physiology of this disease. This is most regrettable since the question has to do with such important problems as the justification of digitalization in preeclampsia and eclampsia. Despite Hamilton's opinion I cannot help but be impressed by the abundant evidence documenting the contrary point of view and for some years have digitalized all eclamptic patients.

Pathologic Biochemistry. The outstanding biochemical alteration in preeclampsia and eclampsia is water retention over and above that found in a normal pregnancy. Indeed, the edema of the eclamptic syndrome may be regarded as an exaggeration of that often seen in normal pregnancy and whatever causes the one is probably responsible also for the other. The accumulation of tissue fluid seen in eclampsia, in other words, represents simply a physiologic process gone awry. Water retention and sodium retention are so inseparably connected that it is not possible to state whether the edema seen in acute toxemia, as well as in normal pregnancy, represents a primary disorder of water or of sodium metabolism.

The evidence that sodium chloride is retained in the toxemias is severalfold. Rupp fed 5 gm. of sodium chloride to normal nonpregnant women, to normal pregnant women, and to women suffering from the toxemias of pregnancy, and then investigated the resultant changes in the chlorides of the blood and urine in order to deduce the fate of the salt. In normal nonpregnant individuals the ingestion of this amount of sodium chloride was followed by a marked rise in the blood chlorides together with a simultaneous increase in the urinary output of sodium chloride. In normal pregnant women, on the other hand, the blood chlorides augmented only slightly after feeding, while the urinary excretion of chlorides was delayed. In cases of toxemia with edema this effect was still more marked, the ingestion of sodium chloride having no effect on either the blood or the urinary chlorides, all of the ingested salt being held by the tissues. Finally, Rupp analyzed the edema fluid of these patients and showed that in cases of toxemia with edema, the ingestion of salt caused a characteristic increase in the sodium chloride content of this fluid. The observations of Harding and Van Wyck made some years ago are also pertinent to this problem. These authors gave several patients, who were suffering from various grades of toxemia of pregnancy, intravenous injections of 300 cc. of 6 per cent sodium chloride solution, in the belief that this might be a valuable therapeutic measure. The results were well-nigh disastrous. One patient who had received two such injections within 24 hours, developed a fulminating preeclampsia with dramatic suddenness and, worse still, went shortly into actual eclampsia and had three typical convulsions; meanwhile the blood pressure had risen from 128/100 to 200/140 and the albuminuria had more than doubled in intensity. The patient recovered, but the authors write that they have no wish to continue their observations in this direction. They believe firmly that a high intake of salt, ingested at the right moment in a developing toxemia, will produce albuminuria, increase the blood pressure and even cause convulsions in a short period of time. Renal function studies indicate a decreased ability to concentrate sodium chloride during pregnancy, an impairment which is intensified in toxemic patients. Thus, Dieckmann recalls that the normal kidney can concentrate sodium chloride to 1.3 per cent. He finds that the maximum concentration in normal pregnant patients is 0.9 per cent, with an average of 0.5 per cent. In regard to eclampsia he found that all specimens of urine obtained on admission from 26 patients with eclampsia were highly colored but contained an average concentration of sodium chloride of only 0.185 per cent. In 12 patients with preeclampsia, the average concentration of sodium chloride was 0.169 per cent.

Another important biochemical alteration in eclampsia is blood concentration, a change which has been studied and emphasized especially by Dieckmann. In Table 7 in his exhaustive monograph, "The Toxemias of Pregnancy," he shows that during the two days before the eclamptic attack the serum proteins usually rise from a level of about 5.7 per cent to one of 6.7 per cent; meanwhile the cell volume increases from 41 to 45 per cent on the average, while hemoglobin augments from 87 to 108 per cent, (using 13.8 gm. of hemoglobin as equivalent to 100 per cent hemoglobin). The hemoconcentration, which is seen both in severe preeclampsia and eclampsia, is associated with a decrease in both blood and plasma volumes. Dieckmann has emphasized especially the fact that clinical improvement in eclampsia is associated with blood dilution and that failure of the blood to dilute with usual treatment indicates that eclampsia is of a very severe type.

Eclampsia is seldom accompanied by any significant degree of nitrogenous retention but an increased uric acid concentration of the blood is almost constantly observed. Although it was originally thought that the elevated uric acid seen in eclampsia and severe preeclampsia was the result of a liver injury and hence might be regarded as a valuable prognostic sign, Chesley and Bonsnes have both shown that this phenomenon is related simply to a decreased ability of the kidney to excrete uric acid as evidenced by a diminution in uric acid clearance. Starvation, which most eclamptics undergo more or less, may also play a role since there is general agreement that starvation usually reduces the daily excretion of uric acid. Hoeffel and Moriarity noted in children a rise of blood uric acid to 10–12 mg. per 100 cc. at the end of a four day fast.

The CO_2 combining power of the blood is usually reduced in eclampsia and it is not uncommon to see values below 30 volumes per cent. In 1929 Stander, Eastman, Harrison and Cadden demonstrated that the period immediately after an eclamptic convulsion is associated with a true acidosis, due to an uncompensated alkali deficit, as shown by a definite increase in the hydrogen-ion concentration of the blood. They concluded that usually the eclamptic patient overcomes the true acidosis by such means as lowering the carbonic acid through deepened breathing, but when she is unable to overcome the acidosis, death may result. These authors conclude from their previous work on lactic and other organic acids in the blood that it is probable that the periods of acidosis result from accumulations of these acids following the muscular work incident to the convulsion.

Although many attempts have been made to establish a relationship between the serum proteins and eclampsia, especially the albumin-globulin ratio, no correlation has been demonstrated, except as mentioned above, namely, that there is some elevation in total serum proteins in eclampsia as the result of hemoconcentration. The albumin-globulin ratio is slightly reduced from a normal of 1.6 to 1.3 perhaps, and while this may play an auxiliary role in the production of edema in some cases of preeclampsia and eclampsia, there is general agreement that neither reversal of the albumin-globulin ratio nor hypoproteinemia plays an important role in the causation of either eclampsia or preeclampsia. The inorganic elements are within normal limits, except for a slightly increased phosphorus, resulting in an elevation of the P/Ca ratio. The blood sugar is not greatly disturbed except that occasionally a definite hyperglycemia follows the eclamptic fit, due perhaps to muscular activity. Blood thioneine, gluthathione and nucleotide nitrogen are within normal limits. Blood lactic acid is usually not elevated except after convulsions but in severe cases of eclampsia the total organic acids are definitely elevated. Blood chlorides are lowered when there is marked edema present.

Etiology. So many theories have been advanced concerning the etiology of eclampsia that it has aptly been called "the disease of theories." Unfortunately, exact knowledge is still lacking. Any theory, to be regarded as acceptable, must explain certain clinical and pathologic facts, a few of which are as follows: (1) the predisposing influence of primiparity, multiple pregnancy, hydatidiform mole and hydramnios; (2) the fact that the disease is more common in certain localities and among the indigent; (3) its increasing incidence as term approaches; (4) the fact that repeated eclampsia is rare; (5) the improvement which usually ensues after death of the fetus; (6) the characteristic accompaniments of the disease, that is, hypertension, edema, proteinuria, convulsions and coma; (7) the rather characteristic hepatic and renal lesions.

Some idea of the scope of the investigations which have been carried out on the cause of eclampsia, may be gained by considering the following theories.

1. *Uremia* (Nineteenth century theory). Objection: no significant increase in nonprotein nitrogen of the blood occurs.

2. *Infection.* Objection: no bacteria are demonstrable in the blood tissues or urine. In regard to focal infections in tonsils, teeth, etc., no convincing evidence has been adduced.

3. *Autointoxication.* Some heaping up of a noxious agent in the maternal organism such as might ensue, for instance, from constipation, has been postulated. Objection: no toxin has been demonstrated; blood from eclamptic patients has been transfused into normal pregnant women without the slightest effect of any kind (page 682).

4. *Biological Reactions.* (a) Incompatibility between maternal and fetal blood has been suggested as a cause. This theory further postulates escape of fetal red cells into the maternal circulation, followed by their agglutination and resultant periportal thrombosis. Objection: incompatibility of maternal and fetal blood is just as frequent in normal gravidae as in eclamptic patients (Allen). The Rh factor is not involved.

(b) *Anaphylaxis.* The belief that the mother becomes sensitized to small quantities of fetal protein and later reacts to this protein, has been advanced by many investigators (Egorow; Jegorow). Objection: although not disproved, this theory has no convincing evidence to support it.

5. *Mammary Toxemia; Hypocalcemia.* This is based on the suspicion that a convulsive disorder seen in puerperal cows, parturient paresis, may be identical with eclampsia. Objection: it is now known that parturient paresis is due to hypocalcemia and is quite a different disease. Hypocalcemia of significant degree is not seen in eclampsia; and conversely, osteomalacic patients with extreme hypocalcemia show no increased incidence of eclampsia.

6. *Increased Abdominal Pressure.* Both Paramore and Theobald have advanced the theory that increased abdominal pressure brings about diminution in the blood flow to the placenta, kidneys and liver, resulting in pathological changes in those organs which are responsible for eclampsia. Circumstantial evidence in support of this concept is afforded by these facts: eclampsia occurs oftenest in primigravidae, whose abdominal walls are stronger than those of multiparae and hence effect greater abdominal pressure; eclampsia is more common in twin pregnancies; it is more frequent as term approaches; the disease does not occur in lower animals whose dependent abdomen predisposes to lower abdominal pressure than develops in humans in whom the erect posture favors increased pressure. Objections: eclampsia occurs with special frequency in hydatidiform mole at periods when pressure of the uterus on surrounding organs is negligible. Strauss and Maddock have shown experimentally that increased abdominal pressure does not produce liver necrosis. But see theory of uterine ischemia (page 679).

7. *Fetal Metabolic Products.* Objection: eclampsia occurs with especial frequency in hydatidiform mole in which there is no fetus. It is true that preeclampsia and eclampsia often improve after fetal death but not always. Serum gonadotrophin studies indicate that when this improvement does occur, it is paralleled by diminution and cessation of placental function, and that, contrariwise, when such improvement does not ensue, the placenta continues to live and function.

8. *Pyelitis.* Reviewing 320 cases of toxemia of pregnancy, Peters and his co-workers noted that 41, or 13 per cent, of the patients suffered at one time or another from pyelitis or pyelonephritis. Among 93 patients with pyelitis complicating pregnancy, these authors noted that 25 had hypertension or edema or both before pregnancy was terminated. Peters and his associates therefore regard pyelitis as an important etiological factor in preeclampsia and eclampsia. Objection: the high frequency of pyelitis in patients with toxemias of pregnancy cannot be confirmed by other observers. Thus, Dieckmann finds that the incidence of pyelitis in toxemic patients is only 1 per cent; moreover, Mussey and Lovelady report that acute hypertensive toxemia was present in but 3 of 117 cases of pyelitis complicating pregnancy. Only 6 out of 163 patients with preeclampsia or eclampsia had pyelitis in the puerperium. Theobald has pointed out that eclampsia is very rare in the natives of Siam, where involvement of the urinary tract is prevalent. In 38 cases of eclampsia which came to autopsy Acosta-Sison found evidence of pyelonephritis in only one instance. In sum, observers other than Peters have found the incidence of pyelitis in preeclampsia and eclampsia about the same as that observed in nontoxemic gravidae, namely, about 2 per cent.

9. *Placental Decomposition Products.* While it is very easy to theorize concerning the part which the placenta may play in the etiology of preeclampsia and eclampsia, it is extraordinarily difficult to adduce conclusive proof.

(a) *Placental Endotoxins.* Countless placental extracts have been injected into lower animals and claims made that convulsions and/or liver lesions were produced. Objection: the same results ensue with extracts of other organs. Furthermore, Lichtenstein has demonstrated that the results achieved by placental extract have been in great part mechanical, and that large quantities of such preparations can be injected with impunity provided all suspended particles have been previously removed by filtration. As subsequent writers have confirmed his observations, it may be stated that there is no evidence to indicate that eclampsia can be produced by normal placental tissue, provided suitable precautions have been taken in the preparation of the material used for experimentation.

(b) *Placental Infarcts.* So-called infarcts of the placenta of a diameter of 1 cm. or more, are present in about 60 per cent of all placentas (page 549). All types of infarcts are somewhat more frequent in placentas associated with toxemia of pregnancy, as is also the extent of the process. Following the original suggestion by Fehling in 1886, that a connection existed between infarction and albuminuria of pregnancy, many authors down to the present day have claimed that autolysis of placental infarcts is the cause of preeclampsia and eclampsia. In modern times the main proponents of this theory have been James Young in England and Bartholomew and Kracke in this country. The former laid especial emphasis on the red infarct (early stage of white infarct) as an etiological factor and even claimed to have produced eclampsia experimentally by injecting autolyzed infarcts. Bartholomew and Kracke likewise believe that it is in the acute and subacute stages of infarct development that poisonous protein-split products enter into the maternal circulation, causing eclampsia. They also state that autolysis of these acute, purplish or brownish infarcts yields a substance which passes a Berkefeld filter and yields clinically and pathologically a condition in rabbits which closely resembles eclampsia. Bartholomew and Kracke suggest also that the hypercholesteremia of pregnancy may play a role in the production of certain vascular changes in the placenta which result in infarction and that the amount and location of such infarction determine whether eclampsia, preeclampsia or premature separation of the placenta will develop. Objection: lifelong students of the placenta have been unable to discover any correlation between infarct formation and toxemias of pregnancy and regard any increased incidence of infarction in toxemic cases as the result rather than the cause of the disease. Thus, Williams wrote: "For years it has been my custom to cut into one centimeter strips all placentae coming from toxemic and eclamptic patients, and while their study reveals the presence of all types of infarcts somewhat more frequently than in normal pregnancy, I have not been able to convince myself that any characteristic change occurs, so that whatever gross lesions one may detect should be regarded as accidental or coincidental, but in no way connected with the causation of eclampsia." Likewise Traut and Kuder, in a study of 1,500 placentas, found no evidence to support the view that obliterative lesions of the placenta are responsible, either wholly or in part, for the development of the toxemias of pregnancy. Although Dieckmann finds the incidence of infarction to be highest in placentas from toxemic patients, he states: "The presence of extensive infarcts in placentae from normal pregnant patients indistinguishable from those found in placentae of eclamptic patients indicates that the infarcts are not the cause of the toxemia." He cites, moreover, the frequent occurrence of toxemia in patients with hydatidiform mole, in which there are no fetal vessels to thrombose and where infarcts, such as are found in the placenta, do not occur, as further evidence against placental infarcts as the cause of toxemia. Likewise Siddall and Hartman regard the higher incidence of infarct formation in the toxemias as a consequence rather than a cause.

10. *Uterine Ischemia.* During pregnancy the uterus and its contents demand an augmented supply of blood which must flow in constantly; otherwise the fetus would not be provided with oxygen. As was noted on page 219, late gestation is accompanied by an increase of approximately 1,500 cc. in the total blood volume (32 per cent) as well as an increase of 1,500 cc. in the cardiac output. Inasmuch as the volume of blood flowing through the kidneys, the liver, an arm, or the brain, has been shown to be the same in pregnancy as in nonpregnant women, it follows that the volume of blood flowing through the gravid uterus approximates 1.5 liters per minute. In adjustment to this great increase, a parallel

enlargement in the capacity of the vascular system in and around the uterus occurs as well as a doubling in the caliber of the arterial tree.

The uterine ischemia theory of eclampsia (first advanced in clear-cut fashion in 1914 by James Young and subsequently sponsored, in one connection or another, by Beker of Holland, Dexter and Weiss, Ernest W. Page, Dieckmann and many other authorities) postulates that this large blood supply which the uterus in pregnancy normally receives may become impaired as the result of a number of factors. These factors fall into three main groups: (1) mechanical conditions in or about the uterus militating against adequate blood flow; (2) nervous factors which influence blood flow through the autonomic nervous system; and (3) deficient adaptation of the general circulation to the requirements of the uterus in pregnancy and labor.

As examples of mechanical conditions in the uterus which may militate against satisfactory blood flow, may be cited multiple pregnancy, hydramnios, hydatidiform mole and approach to term. In the first two of these conditions, overstretching of the uterine wall with a resultant increase in tension of its muscular lamellae may offer increased resistance to the circulation of blood within the uterine wall. The greatly increased incidence of eclampsia in twin pregnancy and in hydramnios is well established (page 662). Hydatidiform mole may result in impaired blood supply because the more rapid growth of the vesicular placenta demands a greater blood supply than does the normal placenta of the same age. The increased incidence of preeclampsia and eclampsia in hydatidiform mole, especially after the fourth month when the necessity of augmented blood supply mounts rapidly, is stressed on page 662.

Although the role played by the autonomic nervous system in vasomotor function is well known, the part it plays in the hypertension of the toxemias, if any, is not established. In the opinion of Brust, Assali and Ferris, based on studies with tetra-ethyl-ammonium chloride, the neurogenic factor is much less important than the humoral.

Deficient adaptation of the general circulation to the requirements of the uterus in pregnancy might conceivably ensue from a number of causes. In chronic hypertensive vascular disease, the generalized sclerosis of the arterioles might well hinder the vasodilatation necessary for adequate blood supply to the uterus. The fact that about a quarter of the patients with chronic hypertensive vascular disease develop preeclampsia fits in well with this theory. Also in keeping with this concept is the demonstration by Priscilla White that in women with longstanding diabetes the uterine arteries are often calcified and that such diabetics are especially prone to develop preeclampsia in pregnancy. In addition, one might speculate that hormonal imbalance and dietary deficiencies may exert deleterious effects on the circulation and thus handicap the uterine blood flow.

But how can uterine ischemia cause hypertension and the other phenomena characteristic of preeclampsia and eclampsia? As the result of the studies of Goldblatt it is well known that renal ischemia causes hypertension as the result of a vasopressor substance, renin, manufactured by the ischemic kidney as a compensatory mechanism to obtain more blood flow. The uterine ischemia theory of eclampsia postulates that in a similar manner a placental pressor substance (a protein breakdown product of syncytial degeneration) is produced as a result of faulty blood supply and that this substance causes the vasospasm and hypertension characteristic of the disease. However, at the present writing, no such placental pressor substance has been isolated and the actual mechanism by which the hypertension is caused remains unexplained.

As a corollary to this theory, Ernest W. Page believes that the liberation of thromboplastin from the ischemic placenta (along with other catabolic products of syncytial degeneration probably) plays an important role in the causation of eclampsia. Substance is lent to this viewpoint by the fact that Schneider has identified the lethal factor of human placental extracts (when such extracts are injected into the tail veins of mice) as thromboplastin. In these animals the liver appears to be the primary site of fibrin deposition and capillary thrombosis, just as in human eclampsia. The production of similar lesions was effected by Dieckmann in dogs and although he called his injected material "tissue fibrinogen," it is possible that he was dealing with tissue thromboplastin. The whole idea that some thromboplastin-like substance is active in eclampsia is not new since the concept that thrombokinase (*i.e.*, thromboplastin in the presence of calcium ions) may play a role in the production of certain eclamptic lesions was discussed in 1924 by Hinselmann in his monograph and credited to Dienst, and the general hypothesis was advanced in the nineteenth century by Wooldridge (1888) and Schmorl (1893). As shown by Chargaff's studies, the placenta is the richest source of thromboplastin in the body. As the result of injury from ischemia and hypoxia, cytolysis of the syncytial epithelium would be expected, followed by entry of thromboplastin into the maternal circulation. This would explain the high incidence of "infarcts" in toxemic placentas and also some of the hepatic changes.

The uterine ischemic theory of eclampsia is probably more widely held today than any other explanation because it fits in well with many known facts about eclampsia: (1) The lower incidence in multiparae is explained on the grounds that once the uterine vessels have undergone gestational hypertrophy, they might be expected to do so again without difficulty. In the opinion of Beker, the arteries in the multiparous uterus, before as well as during pregnancy, are of a distinctly larger caliber than in the primigravidous uterus. As explained under theory 6, moreover, the greater tone of the abdominal walls in primigravidae might conceivably play a role in uterine ischemia and correlate this theory with that of Paramore and Theobald. (2) The higher incidence in multiple pregnancy, twin pregnancy and hydatidiform mole becomes readily understandable as explained above. (3) The aggravation of preeclampsia in labor, as well as the increased incidence of convulsions at that time, is explained by the ischemic effect exerted by uterine contractions. (4) The increased incidence of eclampsia as pregnancy approaches term becomes readily understandable. (5) The fact that eclampsia is not known to occur in lower animals is explained on two grounds. In the first place, as stressed by Beker, the uterine artery in the human enters the cervix and then the main branches bend immediately upwards. They are thus working around a hairpin angle. Secondly, with the woman in the upright position, they are working against gravity and are hence functioning at a handicap although anastomosis with the ovarian artery makes the circulation more plentiful. The erect posture may therefore be said to be a deterrent to optimal uterine circulation. (6) With the inclusion of the thromboplastin concept, the hepatic and placental lesions may possibly be explained. In hypertensive toxemia of long standing the infant is often small, a circumstance which might be expected in the presence of uterine ischemia.

Although the theory of uterine ischemia has much in its favor, let it be understood that it has not yet been proved. Thus, as indicated, no placental pressor substance has yet been demonstrated. In some unique experiments reported recently, Chesley and McFaul have kept placental cotyledons alive by organ perfusion for as long as four weeks, and could render them artificially ischemic at will. While no pressor substance was elaborated, the "ischemic" surviving placentas regularly produced an antidiuretic substance which did not appear when the perfusion was maintained at normal rates. The experimental evidence that constriction of the uterine arteries does cause hypertension is fragmentary and not altogether convincing, as Page himself has pointed out. Moreover why, in the light of this theory, is the incidence of eclampsia so high in certain areas, such as the southeastern states and in the Philippines? Why is it so high in nonwhites? How is salt retention explained? Valid answers to these questions may well be forthcoming in the future but meanwhile the theory, appealing though it may be, must be held *sub judice*.

11. *Endocrine Disturbances.* Since the *thyroid* gland normally undergoes hypertrophy in pregnancy, failure of such hypertrophy to occur with consequent hypothyroidism has been suggested as a cause of toxemia. According to Dexter and Weiss this hypothesis is extremely unlikely since the clinical picture does not suggest hypothyroidism, the basal metabolic rate is not at myxedematous levels and the protein content of the edema fluid is very low. Nor is there any valid evidence which points to hyperthyroidism as a cause.

Hofbauer postulated in 1908 that eclampsia is due to *hyperfunction of the posterior lobe of the pituitary body*. Along similar lines but more recently, Hoffman and Anselmino attempted to show that preeclampsia and eclampsia are dependent upon an increased amount of pituitary antidiuretic and vasopressor hormones circulating in the blood stream. These authors prepared from the blood of eclamptic patients a substance which produced decreased urinary output and hypertension in rabbits. Objection: subsequent work by several investigators indicates that the antidiuretic principle is not increased, certainly not to the extent indicated by Hoffman and Anselmino; nor has their idea regarding the pressor principle of the posterior pituitary been corroborated. Page tested the effect of eclamptic blood upon the urinary output and blood pressure and was unable to demonstrate the existence of an antidiuretic or a pressor substance in eclamptic blood. Krieger and Kilvington have reviewed the conflicting literature concerning the antidiuretic property of blood and toxemia and tested the blood of 303 women. They found blood antidiuretic activity in 29 to 41 per cent of the groups of patients studied and that the activity in both normal and toxemic cases was related to labor and the early puerperium. In their opinion the contrary results in the literature might be explained if considered in relation to labor. On the other hand, according to Teel and Reid, the urine of eclamptic patients regularly contains an antidiuretic substance which is not present in the urine of normal gravidae. Since hypersecretion of the posterior pituitary might, through its antidiuretic principle, produce edema and, through its pressor principle, bring about hypertension, this general theory is intriguing since it would account for two of the most frequent disturbances encountered in preeclampsia and eclampsia. Factual proof, however, is lacking.

Excessive chorionic gonadotrophic hormone in the blood and urine of patients with toxemia was first reported by Smith and Smith who demonstrated also that the placentas of toxemic patients contained more of this hormone than could be recovered from the placentas of normal pregnancy. They showed, furthermore, that this high gonadotrophic titer of blood and placenta was not accountable to pituitary gonadotrophes. Browne, Henry and Venning, however, could find no correlation between elevated chorionic gonadotrophin and toxemia. Taylor and Scadron as well as Cohen, Wilson and Brenan, found only a slight correlation. Moreover, as the Smiths point out, increased chorionic gonadotrophin is not demonstrable in all cases, bears no direct relationship to the severity of the disease and is associated also with stillbirth and premature delivery in the absence of toxic signs. The significance of any rise which may occur in chorionic gonadotrophin in preeclampsia and eclampsia is hence a moot question.

Smith and Smith find also a progressive *deficiency of progesterone and estrogen before* and *during toxemia.* They do not, however, consider this deficiency of estrogen and progesterone as the final precipitating cause of toxemia, but rather as an intermediary and contributing factor. In their opinion the evidence at hand appears to establish premature senility of the placental syncytium and premature withdrawal of the placental steroid hormones as the final intermediary pathology. They believe that these disturbances must be brought about by the working of the primary etiology which probably involves either an intrinsic metabolic abnormality or a decrease in blood supply to the placenta or both. In the latter connection, Smith and Smith have shown that decreased blood supply to the placenta results in a decrease in the secretory activity of this organ as far as estrogen and progesterone are concerned. Since, conversely, an adequate vascular supply to the placenta is contingent upon an adequate production of estrogen and progesterone, they picture here a vicious circle in which vascular and hormonal deficiencies are augmenting each other.

12. *Dietary Alterations.* During World War I there was a startling reduction in the incidence of eclampsia in Central Europe, with return to the prewar frequency after its conclusion. Some years ago this was attributed to the food blockade and since the food lack was greatest in meats and fats, the deduction has been drawn that a diet rich in meat is conducive to the development of preeclampsia and eclampsia. This decreased occurrence of eclampsia during World War I has more recently been shown to be the result of quite other causes, namely, a great decrease in marriages during the war with a consequent diminution in the percentage of primigravidae among childbearing women. After the war the number of marriages increased and concomitantly the incidence of eclampsia rose. As a matter of actual fact, moreover, the drop in the frequency of eclampsia began in 1915, before there was any lack of food, and the great return in incidence began at once in 1919, reaching a maximum in 1921, when the condition of nutrition as far as the majority of the population was concerned, had not changed materially from its war status. Nor has any subsequent evidence been advanced that the inclusion of large amounts of meat in the diet plays any role whatsoever in the causation of the toxemias.

The geographical variation in the incidence of eclampsia, such as its high incidence in the southeastern states of this country, in the Philippines and in China, has suggested the possibility of dietary deficiency of one kind or another as a cause. Thus, the geographical distribution of eclampsia in this country shows a striking relationship to the distribution of the *vitamin B complex deficiencies.* For instance, in the southeastern quadrant of the country where eclampsia is notoriously common, occurs almost all the pellagra in the United States. This circumstance has been emphasized especially by Siddall who points out that the highest incidence of pellagra is among adult married women, which suggests a relationship between pellagra and pregnancy and lactation. No other vitamin deficiency is so localized in the southeastern states. Siddall adduces other evidence to show that in countries where pellagra is rare, eclampsia is also uncommon. More recently Hobson has presented evidence also that nicotinic acid deficiency, or at least some deficiency of the B complex, may be responsible.

On the basis of extensive experience with eclampsia in China, the Philippines and the midsouth, Whitacre believes that the disease increases in proportion to indigency and is of the opinion that dietary deficiencies play an important role in the etiology of the condition, especially *deficiency in first-class proteins, vitamins and essential minerals.* Among Chinese in the lower economic groups, animal protein is almost entirely lacking in their diet, their source of protein being chiefly soy bean and other grains; at the same time their foods are very highly seasoned with salt. The same criticisms would apply to the diet of American Negresses of the indigent group. Bertha S. Burke has shown, on the basis of prenatal dietary ratings, that there was no toxemia among the women she studied whose diets were fair and in 44 per cent of those with the poorest diets. The great decrease in the incidence of eclampsia in most areas of the United States during recent years has caused many obstetricians to suspect that the improved dietary status of the populace at large may be responsible in part at least. Although the evidence suggests that dietary deficiencies may well have something to do with the etiology of eclampsia, this hypothesis must be regarded as suggestive only and far from proven.

Diagnosis. Except for the possibility of confusion with purely uremic conditions, the recognition of eclampsia usually offers no difficulty. It might be confounded with acute poisoning from strychnine, phosphorus or nitrobenzol as in certain cases which have been reported. However such instances are extremely rare, and careful inquiry into the history of the patient should prevent error. Generally speaking one is much more likely to make a diagnosis of eclampsia too frequently than to overlook the disease, because epilepsy, encephalitis, meningitis, brain tumor, acute yellow atrophy of the liver, and even hysteria may simulate it. Consequently such conditions should be borne in mind whenever convulsions or coma occurs during pregnancy, labor or the puerperium, and must be excluded before a positive diagnosis is made. As noted previously, it is unusual for eclampsia to develop after the first 24 hours postpartum, although a few authentic cases have been reported as late as the sixth day. Convulsions developing later than one week postpartum are probably never due to eclampsia.

Prognosis. The prognosis is always serious, eclampsia being one of the most dangerous conditions with which the obstetrician has to deal. The maternal mortality in the United States probably lies between 10 and 15 per cent, being higher in the nonwhite races. The mortality for the child approaches 45 per cent.

Although the bearing of parity on prognosis has been a matter of dispute, it is the consensus that the outlook is worse in multiparae. This is well brought out by Way's study of 33 eclamptic fatalities. His ratio of primigravidous patients to multiparae in this series was 1.1 to 1. Since in eclampsia in general the ratio of primigravidous women to multigravidae is about 3 to 1, his findings suggest that when the disease does occur in multiparae it is more likely to be fatal. The increased gravity of eclampsia in multiparous women (if actual) is probably due to the fact that many of them have an underlying hypertensive vascular disease of a chronic nature and hence are handicapped by pre-existing pathological changes in their vascular, cardiac and renal systems. In this connection the age factor also plays a role and, in general, the prognosis is much graver in women over 35. Formerly the outlook was thought to be more serious in ante- and intrapartum eclampsia than in the postpartum variety, but with the adoption of medicinal methods of treatment the death rate in the former has become materially diminished, while it has remained relatively stationary in the latter. Present day figures indicate that the mortality rates in these varieties of eclampsia do not differ greatly. This historical observation carries with it important practical implications since it shows that the high death rate which obtained in ante- and intrapartum eclampsia in former years was the result of injudicious operative interference. Naturally the prognosis will depend also upon the type of patient, being much more favorable when she is seen immediately after the first convulsion than in neglected cases which are sent to the hospital only as the last resort. By the same token the outlook is better in women who have had good prenatal care.

In individual cases the single most important prognostic sign is urinary output. Thus, eclamptic patients who excrete urine at the rate of 800 cc. or more per 24 hours (or 200 cc. or more every six hours) may be regarded as having a favorable prognosis, whereas extreme degrees of oliguria or complete anuria indicate a grave outlook. The transcendent importance of urinary output as a prognostic sign in eclampsia is, of course, the basis of the commonly used hypertonic glucose treatment of eclampsia to produce diuresis.

Other signs pointing to a grave prognosis in individual cases of eclampsia were worked out by Eden as the result of an extensive statistical study of the disease in England and are known as Eden's criteria. They are: (1) prolonged coma; (2) pulse rate above 120; (3) temperature 103° F. or higher; (4) blood pressure above 200 mm.; (5) more than 10 convulsions; (6) 10 gm. or more of albumin in the urine; and (7) absence of edema. If none, or only one, of these signs was present, he classified the case as "mild"; if two or more were observed, he called it "severe." In 706 of his cases, which could be so classified, the mortality was 6.6 and 37.2 per cent in the mild and severe groups, respectively. Using the same criteria, Peckham analyzed 129 cases of eclampsia, observed at the Johns Hopkins Hospital between 1924 and 1933, and found that the maternal mortality in the mild cases (as defined by Eden) was 2.86 per cent and in the severe ones 21.05 per cent. By amending these criteria slightly (by omitting albuminuria, changing blood pressure figure to 180 and the number of convulsions to 20), Peckham was able to demonstrate further and quite convincingly that the maternal death rate increases progressively according to the number of these phenomena exhibited. While it is, of course, impossible to set any fixed standards by which the prognosis in eclampsia can be established with precision, the criteria of Eden are often helpful and at least permit the obstetrician to differentiate between very mild and very severe cases of this disorder. A graver prognostic sign than any of those mentioned by Eden is edema of the lungs. If pronounced, this is a forerunner of death in the majority of cases. Likewise apoplexy and paralysis are serious complications and usually end fatally. If eclampsia comes on during pregnancy the prognosis is favorably affected, as a rule, by the death of the fetus, the convulsions usually ceasing soon afterwards.

In general, the maternal prognosis in eclampsia must always be guarded since extremely severe cases sometimes terminate happily, whereas apparently mild ones occasionally become severe and go on to death. Some patients survive after a huge number of convulsions, Jardine reporting a recovery after 200.

Ultimate Prognosis. As in preeclampsia, a certain proportion of eclamptic women suffer vascular damage as a result of this acute hypertensive toxemia and manifest either lifelong hypertension or blood pressure elevations in subsequent pregnancies. Because of the catastrophic implications of convulsions, patients who have suffered them, and especially their families, are often loath to consider subsequent pregnancies. Moreover, the literature in general presents a rather gloomy forecast for these women in later childbearing, the recurrence rate of toxemia (not necessarily eclampsia) in some series running as high as 80.0 and 94.5 per cent (Browne and Dodds, Peters), the average for all recent reports being near 45 per cent. Because of these several circumstances the actual outlook which posteclamptic women face in subsequent pregnancies assumes great practical importance.

No. of Pregnancies Per Patient Subsequent to Eclampsia	Number of Patients	Total Subsequent Pregnancies	Toxemia		Fetal Loss		Abruptio
			Cases	Per Cent	Cases	Per Cent	
1	24	24	5	20.8	0	0	0
2	8	16	4	25.0	0	0	0
4	1	4	0	0	0	0	0
Therapeutic Abortions	4	4	3	75.0	4	100.0	0
Total	37	48	12	25.0	4	8.3	0

Table 17. Outcome of 48 Pregnancies Subsequent to Eclampsia.

All of these cases were followed at the Johns Hopkins Hospital and in all of them the prior eclamptic attack was also observed in that institution. In addition to the gestations listed, 5 pregnancies occurred in these posteclamptic women which terminated in spontaneous abortion before the twelfth week, about the usual incidence. One of the four therapeutic abortions was done because of rheumatic heart disease in a patient without evidence of hypertension or renal pathology. The other 3 were performed because of advanced chronic hypertensive vascular disease.

Our results at the Johns Hopkins Hospital have been better in posteclamptic pregnancies than those commonly reported and I am inclined to be rather sanguine about the outlook for these patients provided they have neither hypertension nor proteinuria at the time of the subsequent conception. In 48 posteclamptic pregnancies in 37 patients followed during the past 12 years in our clinic and in which the prior eclamptic attack was also observed in this institution, the recurrence of some form of toxemia was seen in 25 per cent (Table 17), but the picture was usually mild. Eclampsia was not repeated. In only 3 of the 37 patients was advanced hypertensive vascular disease present. No fetal loss occurred in patients who went beyond viability, and abruptio was never observed. In addition, 84 patients have been studied who were said to have had eclampsia in other institutions. In 245 subsequent pregnancies in this group there were two instances in which eclampsia recurred, or less than one per cent. In pregnancies which went to viability, the fetal loss was 6.4 per cent. There were no maternal deaths in either of these two series and the impression we derived from reviewing them is that the likelihood of recurrence of toxemia after eclampsia, including even the mildest examples, is not more than 30 per cent, that the chance of eclampsia repeating itself under good management is less than one per cent, that the probability of permanent hypertensive vascular disease resulting is about 10 per cent, while the outlook for a living infant is better than 80 per cent. If the patient has no hypertension or proteinuria at the time of the subsequent conception, the outlook for a living infant is probably better than 90 per cent. On the other hand, if the same patient has experienced a toxemic pregnancy since the eclampsia, the prognosis for subsequent pregnancies is less good but not altogether discouraging.

In individual cases there are a number of circumstances which must be evaluated in establishing ultimate prognosis. In a study carried out in this clinic by Peckham some years ago, he found that chronic hypertensive vascular disease was more likely to follow if the eclamptic attack had been severe (*i.e.*, blood pressure high) rather than mild, particularly when it was of the antepartum type and when a prolonged period intervened between the first convulsion and delivery. Its development was found to be favored also if any of the following circumstances was present at the time of the eclamptic attack: age over 30; multiparity; blood pressure over 200; and albuminuria exceeding 10 gm. On the other hand, the ultimate prognosis did not seem to be influenced by the number of convulsions or the duration of the coma. Chesley and his associates have confirmed these findings and have enunciated other important factors which bear on ultimate prognosis. Among these are the following: the greater the weight-height ratio at follow-up (when the patient asks about another pregnancy) the higher is the incidence of toxemia in later pregnancies. When the weight in pounds divided by the height in inches is less than 2.2, they find the incidence of recurrence of toxemia to be about 25 per cent; on the other hand, when this ratio is 2.2 or above, the frequency of recurrence soars to over 70 per cent. In other words, obesity is a bad prognostic sign. Failure of the blood pressure and urine to return to normal by the tenth postpartum day is another unfavorable portent for the future, according to this group.

Do Preeclampsia and Eclampsia Cause Chronic Hypertension? As stated above, there appears to be a correlation between the duration and severity of a preeclamptic or eclamptic attack and the development of permanent hypertension. Whether, however, these acute toxemias actually *cause* the ensuing chronic hypertensive process is a subject of debate with two opposing schools of thought.

It is the opinion of Dieckmann that a posttoxemic patient who still shows hypertension, proteinuria or impaired renal function six months or more after delivery, represents, and did represent in her hypertensive pregnancy, a case of chronic hypertensive vascular disease or vascular-renal disease. He believes that such a patient "either had hypertensive disease before pregnancy or a predisposition to it by inheritance or by physical or mental instability (nervous and high-strung) and the pregnancy was the exciting factor."

The other point of view on this question, which is shared by Chesley, myself and others, is that preeclampsia and eclampsia represent an acute vascular process in the form of muscle spasm which, if allowed to continue for several weeks or so, results in a permanent structural injury to the vessel wall through anoxia. This injury makes itself manifest by arteriolar fibrosis, consequent hypertension and possible renal vascular damage. As shown in Table 16, the way in which the incidence of permanent hypertension following toxemia parallels the duration of that toxemia seems difficult to explain on any basis other than cause and effect. Chesley's comparable statistics are even more convincing in their correlation between duration of eclampsia and later evidence of hypertension. Cogent arguments, however, may be advanced on both sides of this question and in the present state of our knowledge it seems difficult to prove or disprove either contention. In any event, it is largely an academic problem since there is general agreement that, from the viewpoint of managing individual cases, the outlook both for mother and infant is improved if the acute toxemic process can be abbreviated.

Treatment. *Prophylactic.* Since eclampsia is preceded in the vast majority of cases by premonitory symptoms, its prophylaxis is in many ways more important than its cure, and is identical with the treatment of preeclampsia. Indeed, the chief aim in treating the latter condition is to prevent the possible outbreak of eclampsia. Hence the necessity of regular and frequent blood pressure determinations, weighings, examinations of the urine and the immediate institution of appropriate dietary and medical treatment just as soon as the earliest signs and symptoms appear. By the employment of these precautionary measures, and by promptly terminating pregnancy in those cases which do not improve, or which become progressively worse under treatment, the frequency of eclampsia will be greatly diminished and many lives saved. On the other hand, we have become convinced that prophylactic treatment, while productive of untold good, is not invariably successful; and that those who teach that eclampsia is wholly preventable, and that its occurrence always indicates neglect on the part of the obstetrician, take too extreme a view and have been led astray by their enthusiasm.

General Rationale of Curative Therapy. Williams used to speculate occasionally on the prognosis of the more serious obstetric complications when they occurred in women who were without benefit of medical counsel and who were forced to deliver themselves as best they could. He felt that the gravest outcome under such circumstances awaited patients with advanced degrees of contracted pelvis, while a fate almost as ominous would obtain in the severer forms of placenta previa and premature separation of the normally implanted placenta. The condition in which patients would suffer the least from lack of medical attention was, in his opinion, eclampsia.

As a result of special circumstances existing in China, I had the opportunity of following, throughout their course, several cases of eclampsia in which the patients' relatives, for reasons of their own, refused all forms of treatment. I have seen these Chinese women lie for days in coma, suffer an untold number of convulsions, and finally deliver themselves spontaneously after the head had been in sight for hours; meanwhile, let it be remembered, these women were virtually untouched. I have followed four such cases and have seen all four mothers survive. (Among 73 cases of eclampsia in Chinese women treated over the same period at the Peiping Union Medical College by a modified Stroganoff regime and with all the refinements of modern obstetrics, there were 13 maternal deaths, a mortality of 17.8 per cent.)

By citing these facts, I do not mean to advocate a policy of therapeutic nihilism in eclampsia, but wish simply to recall that *this disease, like many others, shows a strong tendency to spontaneous abatement, provided the patient is not killed by obstetric trauma or overtreatment.*

Since eclampsia occurs only in association with pregnancy, it might seem logical to reason that pregnancy must be the cause of the disease and that the best treatment would be to remove the cause as quickly as possible, that is, terminate the pregnancy by some rapid means such as cesarean section. The objection to this theoretical reasoning is that the trauma inflicted on these sick women by any extensive operative procedure far outweighs any good that may be achieved. This fact was learned by sorry experience in the early years of this century when rapid delivery was the usual method of treating eclampsia. During the first two decades of this century, when the maternal mortality from this disorder ranged between 25 and 30 per cent, the cause of half the deaths was obstetric trauma, either in the form of accouchement forcé or cesarean section. It has been shown by Peterson that the mortality from eclampsia in the United States, when treated by cesarean section, was 26 per cent, and by Holland that the mortality in Great Britain was 32 per cent. But it may be objected that this high mortality is partly attributable to the fact that many of the operations were performed on severe cases which had failed to respond to medical treatment. That this is not the case is demonstrated by a collective investigation made in Great Britain, in which the cases were grouped according to their severity. As may be seen in Table 18, which reproduces the results of this study, radical methods of delivery increase the maternal mortality both in mild and in severe cases of eclampsia.

	Mild Cases Mortality Per Cent	*Severe Cases* Mortality Per Cent
Natural delivery, assisted delivery or induction of labor	5	34
Cesarean section	11	46
Accouchement forcé	18	63

TABLE 18. SHOWING THAT RADICAL METHODS OF DELIVERY INCREASE THE MATERNAL MORTALITY IN ECLAMPSIA, WHETHER THE CASES BE MILD OR SEVERE. (Eden.)

Similarly, the results obtained over a long period of time at the Johns Hopkins Hospital attest plainly the danger of radical interference in eclampsia. In the early days of this clinic major surgical procedures were employed in this disease, and among 85 patients treated for ante- and intrapartum eclampsia between 1896 and 1911, only two escaped operative delivery, the methods of choice being accouchement forcé and vaginal, and abdominal cesarean section. Among a total of 110 eclamptic patients treated during this period, the maternal mortality was 22.8 per cent. Beginning in 1912 these measures were gradually abandoned and were supplanted by more conservative methods which did not aim at the immediate delivery of the patient. A transition period thus followed, but between 1924 and 1935 all eclamptic patients were treated in exactly the same manner, by a modified Stroganoff regime. Among 127 cases so handled, the maternal mortality was 11 per cent, or just one half what it had been during the "radical era." In the ensuing interval between 1935 and 1949, with greater individualization of treatment and the use of magnesium sulfate, there have been 3 deaths in 63 cases, a mortality rate in this small series of 4.9 per cent.

The immediate treatment of eclampsia today, then, is not concerned with the question of obstetric interference, but is simply a matter of determining the particular form of conservative therapy which is to be employed.

First Steps in Management. Because of its sedative effect, quick action and ready availability, morphine sulfate offers obvious advantages as an initial therapeutic agent in eclampsia. It is the drug most often given at the patient's home to allay convulsions during transport to the hospital, or in the admitting room of a hospital pending the institution of other types of medication. When given as an initial dose, the amount administered should be between 0.016 and 0.032 gm. (0.25 and 0.5 grain), depending on the size of the patient. The 0.016 gm. dose may be administered intravenously if desired. Morphine may be given also in the subsequent course of the treatment, but it is advisable to rely largely on other drugs for the main sedative program since, when administered repeatedly in large amounts, morphine reduces urinary output, increases intracranial pressure and tends to cause acidosis because of decreased elimination of carbon dioxide from the lungs.

All eclamptic patients should be hospitalized and placed as soon as possible in a somewhat darkened, quiet room. The room, however, should not be darkened to the extent that cyanosis and the earliest twitchings of an oncoming convulsion can not be detected. If the patient is comatose, the foot of the bed should be elevated about 4 inches to expedite drainage of any bronchial or pharyngeal secretions. Constant and expert nursing care is of paramount importance. The eclamptic patient should never be left alone for a second. When in the throes of a convulsion she may strike her head against a bedpost or throw herself onto the floor; or she may bite her tongue violently. To prevent the latter injury some device should be kept within easy reach which the nurse or physician can insert between the jaws at the very onset of a convulsion. A piece of very heavy rubber tubing, a rolled towel or a padded clothespin may be employed. Eclamptic patients must never be given fluids by mouth unless thoroughly conscious. Failure to adhere to this rule may result in aspiration of fluid and consequent pneumonia. Meanwhile every effort should be made to keep the room quiet and to shield the patient's face from any bright light because any form of stimulation may provoke a convulsion.

The physician now evaluates the patient's general condition as evidenced by her pulse, rate and character of respiration, blood pressure, degree of coma, and the presence or absence of cyanosis. In addition, the fetal heart tones are listened for. The time required for carrying out the arrangements recommended in the above paragraph, together with the physician's general survey of the picture, is usually sufficient to allow the initial dose of morphine to give the patient some degree of protection against convulsions, and only then should more stimulating manipulations, such as catheterization, intramuscular or intravenous therapy be considered. The first of these to be carried out is catheterization. The catheter should be left in place, secured to the patient's thigh with adhesive and connected with a bottle under the bed so that urinary output may be estimated every three or four hours.

One or another of the following programs of treatment should now be instituted with four main objectives in mind: (1) to provide sedation and thereby allay convulsions; (2) to promote vasodilatation and so combat vasospasm; (3) to promote diuresis; and (4) to correct hemoconcentration. It is not necessary, and indeed rarely advisable, to place reliance on just one drug or just one procedure and two or more of the methods of therapy listed below may often be used to advantage. For instance, the intravenous administration of glucose is often a valuable adjunct to the use of any of the sedative drugs. It should be remembered at all times, however, that continual bedeviling of the patient with needles and other disturbing procedures may do more harm than good.

Magnesium Sulfate. As was discussed on page 659, intramuscular or intravenous magnesium sulfate is an especially valuable drug in both fulminating preeclampsia and eclampsia, because of its dual action, that is, central nervous system depression and vasodilatation. We employ intramuscular magnesium sulfate in the treatment of eclampsia as follows: as an initial injection, 10 cc. of a 50 per cent solution are injected deep into the gluteal muscles on *each* side, making a beginning dose of 10 gm.; this is then repeated in one half this dosage, namely 10 cc. of a 50 per cent solution, or 5 gm., into only one gluteal region, every four hours for the first 24-hour period. Provided the urinary output has exceeded 600 cc. in this period, the magnesium sulfate injections are continued every six hours for the next 24 hours. In some cases we have employed the latter dosage for as long as three days. In order to obtain the full therapeutic effect of magnesium sulfate we believe that the rather large dosages cited above are necessary and, as already indicated, in over 300 cases in which they have been so used we have never seen a single alarming reaction. It is generally agreed that respiratory depression from magnesium sulfate occurs only after disappearance of tendon reflexes. Accordingly, the knee jerks are always tested before each injection and if they are absent the medication should be withheld, but in over 300 cases in which this drug has been used as described, we have never observed absence of knee jerks in a single case.

We prefer intramuscular to intravenous magnesium sulfate in the belief that it is just as efficacious, is safer from the viewpoint of sudden respiratory depression and, in restless patients, is easier to administer. Dieckmann also prefers intramuscular administration of this drug but uses it in smaller doses as follows: 10 cc. of a 50 per cent solution are injected into the gluteal muscles on admission and repeated in 6 cc. doses after each convulsion until they cease or the maximum amount of 20 cc. per 24 hours has been given. Nevertheless, several authorities have had gratifying results from the intravenous use of magnesium sulfate, one of the most widely employed regimes being that recommended by Lazard. He gives 20 cc. of a 10 per cent solution intravenously and repeats it every hour until the convulsions are under control. Subsequent dosage is based on a recurrence of convulsions, elevation of blood pressure and other signs. McNeile, using intravenous injections of magnesium sulfate, reported that the maternal mortality in 259 cases of eclampsia was 13 per cent. The fatality rate for the period prior to the use of magnesium sulfate had been 36 per cent. Dorsett and Dieckmann, using intramuscular injections of this drug, reported in 1929 a mortality of 7 per cent in 186 cases of eclampsia. Stroganoff and Davidovitch have used magnesium sulfate intramuscularly along with other measures in the treatment of 201 cases of eclampsia with a mortality rate of only 3 per cent. They recommend that the total amount of magnesium sulfate administered in 24 hours be limited to 24 gm. As may be calculated from the figures given above, we have pushed this to 35 gm. in the first 24 hours without any evidence of deleterious effects. Nevertheless, when using magnesium sulfate in any dosage, it is prudent to have on hand as an antidote either calcium chloride in 10 per cent solution or calcium gluconate in the same concentration for administration in the remote event that respiratory depression should be evidenced. If the patient has been digitalized, calcium salts should be given very slowly.

Barbiturates. Many barbituric derivatives are available for sedation in eclampsia but in general they have similar effects. They differ mainly in their effective dosage, persistence of action, speed of action and untoward side reactions. They are all capable of preventing or suppressing convulsions. The most commonly employed barbiturates in eclampsia are perhaps luminal sodium and sodium amytal. The former may be given subcutaneously in a dosage of 0.3 gm. and repeated in 12 hours. This is a valuable adjunct to the magnesium sulfate therapy reviewed above and may be started if desired shortly after the initial dose of morphine. Dieckmann prefers sodium amytal subcutaneously to other varieties of barbiturate compounds. If convulsions prove very difficult to control, sodium amytal intravenously is a valuable agent in a dose between 0.3 and 0.6 gm., care being taken to administer it slowly over a period of three or four minutes. When sodium luminal or any other barbiturate is employed intravenously, however, the blood pressure must be carefully watched since precipitous falls occasionally occur. These can usually be corrected without difficulty by the administration of ephedrine sulfate. Lewis has treated 45 eclamptic patients by means of sodium amytal, with a maternal mortality of 9 per cent and a fetal mortality of 34 per cent. Pentobarbital sodium (Sodium Nembutal) and other barbiturate derivatives have also been used to control convulsions in eclampsia and have proved generally satisfactory.

Paraldehyde. Paraldehyde is one of the safest and most efficacious drugs to combat convulsions and we have employed it extensively prior to and in conjunction with magnesium sulfate therapy. It is almost always given per rectum diluted with an equal amount of olive oil. If the patient is estimated to weigh around 150 pounds, 30 cc. paraldehyde are administered, while if she is thought to weight near 200 pounds or more, 40 cc. One half or one third this amount may be repeated as may be indicated by continuation of convulsions, restlessness and rising blood pressure. An especial advantage of paraldehyde, according to a recent study by Brown, Bradbury and Kraushaar, is that it exerts no antidiuretic effect, whereas morphine and some barbiturates do.

In the opinion of Douglass and Linn, paraldehyde in sufficient dosage, and repeated often enough, will, without exception, prevent convulsions, keep the patient quiet, and lower the blood pressure. The latter effect may not be pronounced and is never precipitous, but there is usually a drop of 30 to 40 mm. Hg in the systolic and 10 to 20 mm. Hg in the diastolic pressures with continuation of such levels for several hours. The initial dose of paraldehyde recommended by Douglass and Linn is 40 cc. per rectum in 20 or 25 cc. of olive or mineral oil. In 48 cases of eclampsia which they treated with paraldehyde, there was only one maternal death, or 2 per cent mortality. In contrast, a control series of 49 cases, comparable in every respect except for paraldehyde, showed 7 maternal deaths, or 14 per cent mortality.

Chloral Hydrate. This drug, together with morphine, is an integral part of the famous regime of therapy for eclampsia recommended by Stroganoff in the early years of this century. A modified Stroganoff regime was employed rather rigidly at the

Johns Hopkins Hospital over a 10-year period ending in 1935, with results that were generally satisfactory, namely, a maternal mortality of slightly less than 10 per cent.

Chloral hydrate has been superseded to a great extent in the treatment of eclampsia by paraldehyde and barbiturate compounds, largely because it is such a powerful depressant. Thus, Stander stated that although he had seen no untoward results from the use of chloral hydrate in the treatment of eclampsia, he had recently substituted barbiturates.

Intravenous Glucose. The administration of glucose solutions intravenously is an extremely valuable measure in eclampsia, especially in the presence of oliguria. It serves two main purposes: hypertonic solutions promote diuresis, while isotonic solutions supply caloric and fluid needs in patients who have been in prolonged coma. To promote diuresis 500 cc. of a 20 per cent solution are given intravenously over a period of from 30 to 60 minutes and this is repeated every six to eight hours. In many clinics this therapy is started shortly after admission regardless of urinary output. It has been our custom to wait three or four hours in order to ascertain urinary output; if the rate of excretion is less than 800 cc. for 24 hours, it is given; but if the rate is of this order or more, it is withheld. In the presence of a rapid pulse (120 or over), cyanosis, edema of the lungs, or other evidence of heart failure, intravenous fluids must be administered cautiously—only 200 cc. of a 30 per cent solution over a 60-minute period. In addition to promoting diuresis the intravenous administration of hypertonic glucose solutions seems to restore the blood to a more normal state. Thus, hemoconcentration is corrected and the blood chlorides, and probably sodium, are reduced.

In patients who have been in coma more than 12 hours, 5 or 10 per cent glucose may be given to provide fluid and caloric needs, to assist in overcoming uncompensated acidosis and as an added protection to the liver. It should be noted at this point, however, that there is such a thing as giving an eclamptic or preeclamptic patient too much fluid and to my knowledge a number of eclamptic deaths have occurred which have been plainly due to forcing intravenous fluids to the extent of 5,000 or 6,000 cc. in 24 hours. Mengert has sounded the same warning. The total amount given in any 24-hour period should not exceed 3,000 cc. and had best be kept close to 2,500 cc.

The therapeutic measures discussed above, namely morphine, magnesium sulfate, barbiturates, paraldehyde, chloral hydrate and intravenous glucose, are generally accepted procedures in eclampsia and have been widely employed. There are a number of other methods of treatment which have given gratifying results in certain clinics but which at the present time have not achieved universal endorsement. Among these are veratrum viride, the dehydration regime of Arnold and Fay, venesection and caudal anesthesia.

Veratrum Viride. During the latter years of the nineteenth century and first decade or two of this, veratrum viride was one of the most widely employed drugs in the treatment of eclampsia, but it was largely abandoned because of the grave and unpredictable blood pressure falls which often attended its administration. Its use has been revived by Bryant and Fleming who employ a purified preparation known as "Veratrone." They report a gross maternal mortality of 1.6 per cent in 186 cases in which Veratrone was used together with sedation, glucose, magnesium sulfate and the induction of labor. Actually, two of the three maternal deaths in their series were due to sepsis and not to eclampsia, so that the death rate from eclampsia itself was only 0.54 per cent, a superlatively good record. Irving has also reported favorably on the use of veratrum viride in eclampsia at the Boston Lying-In Hospital. Using this agent in conjunction with morphine, paraldehyde, magnesium sulfate and intravenous glucose, he reports two deaths in 32 cases of eclampsia observed between 1940 and 1946; both were neglected emergency cases, were moribund on entrance and died soon afterwards. Irving's use of Veratrone entails the hypodermic injection of 5 minims on admission. It is repeated as is necessary in 5 to 10 minim doses at 20-minute intervals to keep the blood pressure between 120 and 150 systolic and the pulse below 80, or if there is a convulsion. In view of the danger of circulatory collapse, Veratrone must be employed with great caution and, despite the excellent results achieved by Bryant and Fleming and their group, it is the general consensus that equally good results can probably be obtained without its use and that tentatively it should be held *sub judice*. As far as I am aware, no one has used *only* Veratrone in the treatment of eclampsia.

Venesection. Since the days of Hunter, bloodletting has been a favorite therapeutic procedure in a wide range of circulatory disorders, including eclampsia. The outstanding modern proponent of venesection in eclampsia is Beck who has employed it in 129 cases of eclampsia with a maternal mortality of 7.7 per cent. In 70 per cent no convulsions were observed after the completion of the phlebotomy. Soon after the initial injection of morphine has been given, a large-bore, paraffin-coated needle is inserted into the median basilic vein and 1,000 cc. of blood are withdrawn. By noting the pulse and blood pressure, the loss of too much blood is avoided. Only rarely is it necessary to discontinue the procedure before the desired 1,000 cc. are removed. In Beck's experience, venesection of less than 600 cc. is seldom of value.

With the tendency to circulatory collapse and shock in eclampsia, venesection should be used with discrimination and, in my opinion, only with specific indications. Otherwise, it can be responsible for grave consequences. The chief indications are congestion within the pulmonary circulation as shown by pulmonary edema and congestion in the peripheral circulation as manifested by cyanosis.

Lumbar Puncture. Lumbar puncture followed by drainage of various quantities of spinal fluid has been used here and there in the treatment of eclampsia since 1904. From 20 to 30 cc. is the amount which has been most often removed, but as much as 101 cc. has been withdrawn at one time with recovery. The objective is to reduce cerebral edema through lowering of the spinal fluid pressure.

This subject was reviewed in 1922 by Spillman who reported on 70 cases collected from the literature. The spinal fluid pressure appeared to be increased in about half the cases and in two instances was 600 and 540 mm. of water, respectively. The procedure was not notably beneficial in stopping the convulsions, the average per patient after spinal drainage being eight. The maternal mortality was 27 per cent.

Lumbar puncture with drainage of as much spinal fluid as possible is an important part of the Temple University program of treatment in which this procedure is combined with limitation of fluid intake, hypertonic glucose intravenously and purgation by magnesium sulfate. The results reported from this regime by Arnold and Fay were good, but in general, spinal drainage is believed to be of little value and is not without harmful potentialities.

Conduction Anesthesia. Continuous catheter caudal or spinal anesthesia is the most recent addition to our therapeutic armamentarium in eclampsia. Its rationale is based on the following effects of conduction anesthesia: (1) a maximum vasodilatation of the lower extremities enormously increasing the capacity of the vascular bed and exceeding the vasodilator effects of veratrum viride; (2) a lowered blood pressure which can be maintained constantly for hours; (3) a block of the vasoconstricting elements of the kidney, thereby increasing the flow of urine in these potentially anuric patients; and (4) a temporary denervation of the suprarenal gland with a corresponding diminution in the manufacture of the endocrine vasospastic substance. Hingson, Whitacre and Turner have reported 74 cases of eclampsia treated by conduction anesthesia with or without magnesium sulfate with three maternal deaths, a mortality rate of only 3.9 per cent. Although this series is obviously too small to carry appreciable statistical significance, the results in individual cases were most gratifying. Thus, the blood pressure was regularly reduced, convulsions were controlled, urinary excretion augmented and in many instances patients aroused promptly out of coma.

Conduction anesthesia is therefore a measure which carries much promise but which must await further study before final evaluation can be made. Meanwhile, it must be stressed that this method should be attempted only by the expert anesthesiologist or by the obstetrician who has had special training and experience in these technics.

Adjuvant Measures. As discussed on page 671, it seems probable that a weakness of the myocardium exists at times in association with eclampsia. For this reason it has been our custom for a number of years to digitalize all eclamptic patients. Whether this measure is necessary as a routine procedure remains a moot question, but there is general agreement that digitalization is always indicated in the presence of pulmonary edema associated with evidence of circulatory collapse. Oxygen therapy should be instituted in all patients who show the slightest evidence of cyanosis or in whom the respiratory rate exceeds 30 per minute. Inhalations of oxygen should also be administered after each convulsion and continued until the respiration is normal. Many obstetricians believe that oxygen therapy should be routine in this disease as long as convulsions and coma persist. In very severe cases in which convulsions follow one another in rapid succession, light ether anesthesia may be necessary in order to control them. In general, however, the administration of one or another of the barbiturate compounds, as previously discussed, is preferable since the irritating effects of ether on the mucous membrane of the pulmonary alveoli are undesirable.

The Question of Delivery. As long as either convulsions or coma persists, no thought should be given to delivery. It is true that some authorities consider that in patients who become worse under medicinal therapy, cesarean section may be indicated as a sort of last resort measure. This policy is ill advised in my opinion for two reasons: (1) some of the worst cases of eclampsia to all appearances go on to recovery without operative interference; (2) any major operative trauma, such as an abdominal delivery, may well be the blow which turns the tide to death in these critically ill women. Over a span of more than 25 years we have never performed a single cesarean section on patients who were either having convulsions or were in coma; and we have seen no reason to regret this general tenet.

Intercurrent Eclampsia. As soon as the patient has exhibited neither convulsions nor coma for 24 hours, delivery should be considered. She is now no longer suffering from actual eclampsia but corresponds to a very severe preeclamptic patient. If the cervix is unfavorable for delivery, cesarean section should be done. If the cervix is favorable or "ripe," that is, if it is soft, dilated 1 cm. or more and well effaced, induction of labor by rupture of the membranes is the preferable procedure. Whether delivery is carried out abdominally or vaginally, local infiltration anesthesia is the method of choice provided the patient has been protected against convulsions with magnesium sulfate or some effective sedative.

CHRONIC HYPERTENSIVE VASCULAR DISEASE

As its name implies, chronic hypertensive vascular disease is a chronic disorder of the vascular system characterized by persistent hypertension. It is frequently referred to also as "essential hypertension" and is seen of course in males as well as in nonpregnant women. Hence it is not a condition restricted to gravidae but for reasons already stated (page 646), it is desirable to include it under the general category of the toxemias. A diagnosis of chronic hypertensive disease is made in association with pregnancy whenever the evidence points to chronicity of the process. This evidence may be of two kinds: (1) a well-authenticated history of elevated blood pressure (140 systolic or above and/or 90 diastolic or above) prior to the present pregnancy; (2) the presence of such a hypertension prior to the twenty-fourth week, that is, before the time in gestation when preeclampsia develops. This finding of hypertension before the twenty-fourth week is taken as indicating that the pressure had been elevated prior to pregnancy and, by the same token, is high whether the patient is pregnant or not. As in preeclampsia, the blood pressure reading is not considered valid unless it can be demonstrated on two occasions six or more hours apart.

In addition to the instances of outright chronic hypertension as specified above, there are many cases in which successive pregnancies are associated with hypertension but in which the pressure is normal between pregnancies. Many authors, notably Dieckmann, regard these so-called "repeat toxemias" as invariable evidence of chronic hypertensive vascular disease. Many such patients, it is true, end up finally as chronic hypertensives, but on the other hand, I have seen so many cases in which two or even three pregnancies were associated with hypertension, only to be followed by a perfectly normal gestation with no subsequent evidence of vascular disease, that I question the wisdom of dogmatically classifying these "repeat" cases in this category without further evidence. After all, preeclampsia, especially in its milder forms, is such a common complication of gestation that, according to the law of probability, occasional women will be likely to have repeated attacks of preeclampsia without necessarily implying any chronic vascular process.

In the great majority of cases of chronic hypertensive vascular disease, hypertension is the only demonstrable finding. However, a certain minority of patients show secondary alterations which are often of grave import not only in relation to pregnancy, but also in regard to life expectancy. These include hypertensive heart disease, arteriolosclerotic kidney disease and various retinal manifestations such as hemorrhages and exudate. The blood pressure, moreover, may vary from levels scarcely above normal to extreme heights of 300 or more systolic, and 160 or more diastolic. In other words, it is a disease in which all gradations of vascular pathology may be encountered with or without secondary changes in the heart, kidney, retina and brain.

Hypertensive vascular disease in pregnancy is met most frequently in women in the older age group and in multiparae. The average age of patients suffering from this condition is about 33 years, while about 80 per cent of the cases occur in multiparae. In addition to age, obesity seems to be an important predisposing factor to chronic hypertension; more than 25 per cent of gravidae weighing over 200 pounds show elevated blood pressures. Heredity also seems to play a role in the development of this condition. Frequently many members of one family show hypertension, and upon questioning, patients will often reveal the fact that a sister or mother suffered from this disease.

Aside from persisting hypertension, signs and symptoms may be negligible or absent altogether. Ranking next to hypertension among physical findings are retinal changes which are demonstrable in the severer cases in more than 75 per cent of patients. These comprise irregular tortuosity of the smaller vessels, variations in their caliber, visibility of the walls of the smaller macular arterioles and arteriovenous compression. Retinal hemorrhages and exudates are often encountered in advanced stages of the disease, especially if there is renal involvement. Usually these patients feel well and are often annoyed by the discovery of the high blood pressure and by the examinations incident to its study. Except for advanced cases headache is about the only symptom which is at all common and even this may be completely absent. Albuminuria and abnormalities of the urinary sediment are usually lacking; the renal function is usually normal; and edema is minimal or altogether absent. It is not uncommon in these patients for the blood pressure to manifest a decided fall during the second trimester but this improvement is usually temporary since it is followed in the majority of cases by a rise in hypertension during the last trimester to levels somewhat above those observed early in pregnancy. It has been observed repeatedly that the babies in these cases, as palpated in utero, tend to be smaller than the gestational age would suggest and seem to grow less rapidly than the average infant. It is possible in some cases to correlate these small babies with placental infarcts and consequent later interference with fetal nutrition, but in many cases no clear-cut explanation for the phenomenon is at hand. The incidence of abruptio placentae is decidedly increased in these chronic hypertensive gravidae and approximates 3 per cent.

	No Superimposed Toxemia	Superimposed Toxemia	All Cases
Fetal loss	18.5	50.0	38.2
Abruptio placentae	3.8	10.0	5.6
Eclampsia	0	10.0	3.0
Immediate maternal mortality	0	6.7	2.0
Late puerperal deaths (1 to 4 mo.)	0.9	5.5	2.3

TABLE 19. HAZARDS RESULTING FROM SUPERIMPOSITION OF TOXEMIA ON HYPERTENSIVE DISEASE. (Cosgrove and Chesley.)

Superimposed Acute Toxemia. The most common hazard faced by gravidae with chronic hypertensive vascular disease is the superimposition of preeclampsia which occurs in about 25 per cent of cases. When preeclampsia becomes superimposed on chronic hypertensive disease it makes itself manifest by a more or less sudden rise in blood pressure of 30 or more mm. Hg and is almost always associated with the appearance of substantial amounts of protein in the urine. Meanwhile edema, often massive, makes its appearance. Not infrequently the picture is explosive and is characterized by extreme hypertension (systolic, 280–300; diastolic, 140–160), oliguria and nitrogenous retention; it is in this type of case that the retinae may show extensive hemorrhages and many old and new cotton-wool exudates. In one or two per cent of cases of chronic hypertensive vascular disease in pregnancy, actual eclampsia, at least convulsions and coma, is superimposed and here, in its full-blown form, the resultant syndrome is very similar to hypertensive encephalopathy. With the superimposition of preeclampsia the outlook, both for the infant and for the mother, becomes much more grave. About one half the babies are lost and the maternal mortality is of the order of 5 or 10 per cent.

Prognosis. Fully one half, possibly 60 per cent, of women with chronic hypertensive vascular disease may be expected to go through pregnancy successfully and with fairly constant blood pressure levels. In approximately one quarter or one third, as already noted, preeclampsia of varying degrees becomes superimposed. When preeclampsia does develop in such patients it is prone to occur earlier than it does in normal gravidae and in some 10 per cent of cases appears toward the end of the second trimester. In the latter circumstance the outlook for the baby is extremely grave: if gestation is allowed to continue fetal death in utero is common, whereas if delivery is decided upon, prematurity takes a large toll. With superimposed preeclampsia, moreover, the incidence of abruptio placentae rises. In sum, the over-all fetal mortality for cases of preeclampsia superimposed on chronic hypertensive vascular disease is about 50 per cent. The hazards which have resulted in Cosgrove and Chesley's experience from the superimposition of acute toxemia on hypertensive disease, are shown in Table 19.

With certain important exceptions, women with chronic hypertensive vascular disease can go through pregnancy without great hazard as far as their own outlook is concerned. As has been emphasized, the great threat is the likelihood of superimposed preeclampsia, but even if this contingency develops, prompt and astute management (usually termination of pregnancy) will safeguard her life as a rule. As for the ultimate effect of pregnancy on the vascular disease, it ordinarily leaves no residua provided acute toxemia is not superimposed; if it is superimposed but cut short by appropriate treatment, the same prognosis holds true.

But let it be emphasized that there are certain important exceptions to the relatively sanguine forecast given in the preceding paragraph. These exceptions are:

(1) Patients with hypertensive heart disease as evidenced by cardiac enlargement and/or electrocardiographic changes, face a grave outlook in pregnancy. Both in pregnant and in nonpregnant persons, heart failure is the most common cause of death in hypertensive vascular disease. In Chesley's 35 remote deaths following pregnancy in chronic hypertensives, 9 were due to heart failure.

(2) If renal function is markedly impaired the life expectancy of the mother is poor, of course, regardless of pregnancy, but even moderate diminution in renal function augurs ill for the success of gestation. In a study by Chesley among 82 patients who failed to concentrate as high as 1.022, there were 36 fetal deaths, or 43.9 per cent. Urea clearances were done in the patients who failed to concentrate to 1.022. There were 11 pregnancies in 11 patients, where the clearances were less than 70 per cent. Nine of the babies were lost, a mortality rate of 81.8 per cent.

(3) Patients with old retinal exudates or fresh hemorrhages will usually show evidence of renal disease also or of superimposed preeclampsia, but whatever the

etiology, the presence of these advanced retinal changes is of such grave import as to deserve especial mention.

(4) Patients with initial blood pressure of 200 systolic or above, and/or 120 diastolic or above, face a fetal mortality rate in excess of 50 per cent and a higher incidence of maternal complications than milder chronic hypertensives.

(5) If in a previous pregnancy acute toxemia was superimposed on chronic hypertensive disease, the chances of repetition are so great as to render another pregnancy hazardous and usually futile. Chesley notes a 71 per cent rate of recurrence of superimposed preeclampsia in this group.

Management. All gravidae with chronic hypertensive vascular disease should be admitted to the hospital for evaluation of their blood pressure levels at rest, cardiac assay, including if possible teleoroentgenographic study of heart size, urine and renal function investigations and a careful survey of the retinal picture. Upon the basis of this evidence an impression is gained about the degree of the hypertension at rest, the presence or absence of secondary alterations in the heart, kidney and retina, and about the general hazard which pregnancy will possibly impose.

In patients who fall in the five categories just mentioned, fortunately a small minority, pregnancy is a sufficient threat to the life of the mother and sufficiently futile from the fetal viewpoint that interruption of gestation, combined with tubal sterilization, is often the best management of the problem. This is especially true of the first three categories. As Cosgrove has said, "If there is any legitimate indication for therapeutic abortion it is in that type of case (fixed hypertension)." During the past decade 11.5 per cent of our patients with chronic hypertensive vascular disease have undergone therapeutic abortion and, with a few exceptions, the operation was combined with tubal ligation. Since many of these patients were referred to us in advanced stages of the disease, our incidence of therapeutic abortion is undoubtedly higher than should obtain in unselected chronic hypertensives in whom the necessity for interrupting pregnancy prior to viability should probably not exceed 5 per cent.

The treatment of hypertensive disease, per se, in pregnancy is the same as in the nonpregnant person. Abundant rest with curtailment of any strenuous activity, a salt-poor diet, sharp curtailment of weight gain and mild sedation as may be indicated, are the main injunctions. These patients should be seen not less frequently than every two weeks and warned especially about reporting headache, visual disturbances, scanty urine and other signs of preeclampsia. Provided preeclampsia is not superimposed, the patients are carried to term and delivered vaginally. In many of them, however, puerperal tubal ligation is warranted.

In the event clear-cut evidence of superimposed preeclampsia becomes manifest, hospitalization and intensive treatment of the preeclampsia are of course indicated. If, after 24 or 48 hours, the signs and symptoms of the acute process continue, interruption of pregnancy is usually desirable, sometimes imperative. This decision is often a disturbing one to make since the infant is usually premature, but the mother will unquestionably benefit by such interference and, as for the baby, its chances under these circumstances are usually better outside than inside the uterus. In most such cases, cesarean section under local infiltration anesthesia is the procedure of choice.

A number of successful pregnancies have been reported following the Smithwick operation for hypertension (lumbodorsal splanchnicectomy). Kellogg and Hertig have reported 10 such cases followed through 11 pregnancies. Blood pressure averaging

190/92 mm. Hg. prior to operation, averaged 125/92 mm. Hg. afterwards and remained within normal limits throughout pregnancy in five cases; in these there was no albuminuria. Four showed moderate hypertension up to 160/90 mm. Hg., and two had systolic pressures of 180. The pregnancy of one of the latter had to be interrupted at eight and one half months. There were 9 normal deliveries and two cesarean sections; one a repeat section and one done for fulminating preeclampsia. Ten babies were born alive. Newell and Smithwick reported a study of 14 cases with blood pressures averaging 196/130 mm. Hg. prior to the surgical procedure. Following operation and before the pregnancies the blood pressures averaged 135/87 mm. Hg.; only two had persistent albuminuria. In 9 cases the blood pressure remained within normal limits during pregnancy without albuminuria. In the other five there was little change in blood pressure until the third trimester; in one of these a 4 + albuminuria necessitated interruption of the pregnancy at eight and one half months. Austin and Frymire have also reported a successful case. This experience indicates that the Smithwick operation in carefully selected hypertensive women, may be of sufficient benefit to permit them to go through pregnancy without much difficulty.

BIBLIOGRAPHY

Acosta-Sison, H. Clinicopathologic Study of Eclampsia Based Upon 38 Autopsied Cases. Am. J. Obst. & Gynec., 1931, *22*:35.

Allen, W. M. Interagglutination of Maternal and Fetal Blood in the Late Toxemia of Pregnancy. Bull. Johns Hopkins Hospital, 1926, 38:217.

Anselmino, K. J., and Hoffmann, F. Uber die Ausscheidung von hypophysär gebildeten, gonadotropen Hormonein der normalen Schwangerschaft und bei den Schwangerschaftstoxikosen. Ztschr. f. Geburtsh. u. Gynäk., 1937, 114:52.

Arnold, J. O., and Fay, T. Eclampsia; Its Prevention and Control by Means of Fluid Limitation and Dehydration. Surg., Gynec. & Obst., 1932, 55:129.

Austin, B. R., and Frymire, L. J. Pregnancy Following the Smithwick Operation for Hypertension. Am. J. Obst. & Gynec., 1948, 56:805.

Baird, D., and Dunn, J. S. Renal Lesions in Eclampsia and Nephritis of Pregnancy. J. Path. and Bact., 1933, 37:291.

Bartholomew, R. A., and Kracke, R. R. The Probable Role of the Hypercholesteremia of Pregnancy in Producing Vascular Changes in the Placenta, Predisposing to Placental Infarction and Eclampsia. Am. J. Obst. & Gynec., 1936, 31:549.

Beker, J. C. The Effects of Pregnancy on Blood Circulation in their Relation to So-called Toxemia. Am. J. Obst. & Gynec., 1929, 18:368.

——— Aetiology of Eclampsia. J. Obst. & Gynaec. Brit. Emp., 1948, 55:756.

Bell, E. T. Renal Lesions in the Toxemias of Pregnancy. Am. J. Path., 1932, 8:1.

Bell, J. Warren. Postmortem Findings in Ten Cases of Toxemia of Pregnancy. Am. J. Obst. and Gynec., 1926, 12:792.

Bonsnes, R. W., and Stander, H. J. Blood Nucleotides in Pregnancy and in the Toxemias of Pregnancy. Am. J. Obst. & Gynec., 1943, 45:827.

Boyd, E. M. Blood Lipids in the Puerperium. Am. J. Obst. and Gynec., 1935, 29:797.

—— Blood Lipids in Preeclampsia. Am. J. Obst. & Gynec., 1936, 32:937.

Brown, W. E., Bradbury, J. T., and Kraushaar, O. F. Effect of Sedatives on Urinary Volume of Pregnant Women. J. Lab. & Clin. Med., 1948, 33:1465.

Browne, F. J., and Dodds, G. H. Remote Prognosis of Toxaemias of Pregnancy Based on Follow-up Study of 400 Patients in 589 Pregnancies for Periods Varying from 6 Months to 12 Years. J. Obst. & Gynaec. Brit. Emp., 1939, 46:443.

Browne, J. S. L., Henry, J. S., and Venning, E. H. The Urinary Excretion of Prolan, Estrin and Pregnanediol in Normal Pregnancy and in Early and Late Pregnancy Toxemias. J. Clin. Investigation, 1938, 17:503.

Brust, A. A., Assali, N. S., and Ferris, E. B. Evaluation of Neurogenic and Humoral Factors in Blood Pressure Maintenance in Normal and Toxemic Pregnancy Using Tetra-Ethyl-Ammonium Chloride. J. Lab. & Clin. Med., 1948, 33:1466.

BRYANT, R. D., and FLEMING, J. G. Veratrum Viride in the Treatment of Eclampsia. J.A.M.A., 1940, 115:1333.

CANTAROW, A., STUCKERT, H., and GARTMAN, E. Studies of Function. IV. Hepatic Function during Pregnancy. Am. J. Obst. and Gynec., 1935, 29:36.

CHESLEY, L. C. Certain Laboratory Findings and Interpretations in Eclampsia. Am. J. Obst. & Gynec., 1939, 38:430.

——— The Variability of Proteinuria in the Hypertensive Complications of Pregnancy. J. Clin. Investigation, 1939, 18:617.

——— Weight Changes and Water Balance in Normal and Toxic Pregnancy. Am. J. Obst. & Gynec., 1944, 48:565.

——— Does Eclamptogenic Toxemia Cause Chronic Hypertension? Bull. Margaret Hague Mater. Hosp., 1948, 1:81.

——— and ANNITTO, J. E. A Study of Salt Restriction and of Fluid Intake in Prophylaxis against Preeclampsia in Patients with Water Retention. Am. J. Obst. & Gynec., 1943, 45:961.

——— and ANNITTO, J. E. Pregnancy in the Patient with Hypertensive Disease. Am. J. Obst. & Gynec., 1947, 53:372.

——— ANNITTO, J. E., and JARVIS, D. G. A Study of the Interaction of Pregnancy and Hypertensive Disease. Am. J. Obst. & Gynec., 1947, 53:851.

——— and CHESLEY, E. R. The Cold Pressor Test in Pregnancy. Surg., Gynec. & Obst., 1939, 69:436.

——— Renal Blood Flow in Women with Hypertension and Renal Impairment. J. Clin. Invest., 1940, 19:475.

——— An Analysis of Some Factors Associated with the Development of Preeclampsia. Am. J. Obst. & Gynec., 1943, 45:748.

——— CONNELL, CHESLEY, KATZ, and GLISSEN. The Diodrast Clearance and Renal Blood Flow in Toxemias of Pregnancy. J. Clin. Invest., 1940, 19:219.

——— COSGROVE, S. A., and PREECE, J. Hydatidiform Mole with Special Reference to Recurrence and Associated Eclampsia. Am. J. Obst. & Gynec., 1946, 52:311.

——— and MCFAUL, I. E. Studies on Surviving Human Placental Tissues. I. A Search for Pressor and Antidiuretic Factors. Am. J. Obst. & Gynec., 1949, 58:159.

——— MARKOWITZ, I., and WETCHLER, B. B. Proteinuria Following Momentary Vascular Constriction. J. Clin. Investigation, 1939, 18:51.

——— and SOMERS, W. H. Eclampsia and Posteclamptic Hypertension. Surg., Gynec. & Obst., 1941, 72:872.

——— and VANN, F. H. The Effect of Sodium Lactate in Raising the CO_2 Combining Power in the Toxemias of Pregnancy. Am. J. Obst. and Gynec., 1938, 36:660.

COLVIN, E. D., BARTHOLOMEW, R. A., and GRIMES, W. H. A Comparison of Thyroid Extract and Iodine Therapy in the Prevention of Toxemia of Pregnancy. Am. J. Obst. & Gynec., 1942, 43:183.

CORCORAN, A. C., and PAGE, I. H. Arterial Hypertension. Correlation of Clinical and Experimental Observations. J.A.M.A., 1941, 116:690.

COSGROVE, S. A., and CHESLEY, L. C. The Clinical Management of the Late Toxemias of Pregnancy. Obst. & Gynec. Surv., 1948, 3:769.

CRAWFORD, M. D. Changes in Blood Concentration in Normal and Toxaemic Pregnancy. J. Obst. & Gynaec. Brit. Emp., 1940, 47:63.

DAVIDSON, J. Eclampsia and Puerperal Toxaemia: Study of Histological Changes Occurring in Liver and Kidneys. Edinburgh M. J., April, 1931. Tr. Edinburgh Obst. Soc. 1930-31, p. 24.

DAVIS, J. A., and SNOOK, L. O. The "Pressure Theory" of Eclampsia. Surg., Gynec. & Obst., 1941, 73:336.

DEALVAREZ, R. The Use of the Neutral Diet and Hydration in the Treatment of Toxemias of Pregnancy. Am. J. Obst. & Gynec., 1940, 39:476.

DESNOO, K. The Prevention of Eclampsia. Am. J. Obst. & Gynec., 1937, 34:911.

DEXTER, L., and WEISS, S. Preeclamptic and Eclamptic Toxemia of Pregnancy. Williams and Wilkins Co., Baltimore, 1941.

——— HAYNES, F. W., and SISE, H. S. Hypertensive Toxemia of Pregnancy. J.A.M.A., 1943, 122:145.

DIECKMANN, W. J. The Hepatic Lesion in Eclampsia. Am. J. Obst. & Gynec., 1929, 17:454.

——— Further observations on the Hepatic Lesion in Eclampsia. Am. J. Obst. & Gynec., 1929, 18:757.

——— Acute Nephritis and Pregnancy. Am. J. Obst. & Gynec., 1936, 32:227.

——— Blood and Plasma Volume Changes in Eclampsia. Am. J. Obst. & Gynec., 1936, 32:927.

——— The Geographic Distribution and Effect of Climate on Eclampsia, Toxemia of Pregnancy, Hyperemesis Gravidarum and Abruptio Placenta. Am. J. Obst. & Gynec., 1938, 36:623.

DIECKMANN, W. J. The Prevention and Treatment of Eclampsia. Am. J. Surg., 1940, 48:101.
——— The Toxemias of Pregnancy, St. Louis, 1941.
——— and BROWN, I. Do Eclampsia and Preeclampsia Cause Permanent Vascular Renal Pathology? Am. J. Obst. & Gynec., 1939, 37:762.
——— and CROSSEN, R. J. Changes in the Metabolism and Their Relation to the Treatment of Vomiting of Pregnancy. Am. J. Obst. and Gynec., 1927, 14:3.
——— and KRAMER, S. Proteinuria in Toxemia of Pregnancy. Am. J. Obst. & Gynec., 1944, 47:285.
——— and MICHEL, H. L. A Thermal Study of Vasomotor Lability in Pregnancy. Arch. Int. Med., 1935, 55:420.
——— and WEGNER, C. R. Eclampsia without Convulsions or Coma. Am. J. Obst. & Gynec., 1932, 23:657.
DILL, L. V., ISENHOUR, C. E., CADDEN, J. F., and ROBINSON, C. E. Glomerular Filtration and Renal Blood Flow in "Normal" Patients Following Toxemias of Pregnancy. Am. J. Obst. & Gynec., 1942, 44:66.
——— ISENHOUR, C. E., CADDEN, J. F., and SCHAFFER, N. K. Glomerular Filtration and Renal Blood Flow in the Toxemias of Pregnancy. Am. J. Obst. & Gynec., 1942, 43:32.
DOGGART, J. H. Eclamptic Detachment of Retina. Proc. Roy. Soc. Med., 1936, 29:753.
DOUGLASS, L. H., and LINN, R. F. Paraldehyde in Obstetrics, with Particular Reference to Its Use in Eclampsia. Am. J. Obst. & Gynec., 1942, 43:844.
EASTMAN, N. J. Puerperal Hemiplegia. Am. J. Obst. & Gynec., 1928, 15:758.
——— The Serum Proteins in the Toxemias of Pregnancy. Am. J. Obst. & Gynec., 1930, 19:343.
——— The Vascular Factor in the Toxemias of Pregnancy. Am. J. Obst. & Gynec., 1937, 34:549.
——— and STEPTOE, P. P. The Management of Preeclampsia. Canad. M. A. J., 1945, 52:562.
——— and WHITRIDGE, J. Jr. The Prevention of Toxemia of Pregnancy. J.A.M.A., 1942, 120:729.
EDEN, T. W. A Commentary on the Reports Presented to the British Congress of Obstetrics and Gynecology, June 29, 1922. J. Obst. & Gynaec. Brit. Emp., 1922, 29:386.
FALKINER, N. M., and APTHORP, J. O. E. The Placenta in Eclampsia and Nephritic Toxaemia. J. Obst. & Gynaec. Brit. Emp., 1944, 51:30.
GARBER, S. T., and ASSALI, N. S. Toxemia of Pregnancy. J. Indiana M. A., 1947, 40:979.
GIBBS, F. A., and REID, D. E. The Electroencephalogram in Pregnancy. Am. J. Obst. & Gynec., 1942, 44:672.
GOLDBLATT, H., LANDIS, E. M., ADSON, A. W. Hypertension. Univ. Penn. Press, Phila., 1941.
HALLUM, A. V. Eye Changes in Hypertensive Toxemia of Pregnancy, a Study of 300 Cases. J.A.M.A., 1936, 106:1649.
HAMILTON, B. E., and THOMSON, K. J. The Heart in Pregnancy and the Childbearing Age. Little, Brown & Co., Boston, 1941.
HARDING, V. J., and VAN WYCK, H. B. Effects of Hypertonic Saline in the Toxaemias of Later Pregnancy. Brit. M. J., 1930, 2:589.
HARRIS, J. W. The After-Effects of Late Toxemias of Pregnancy. Bull. Johns Hopkins Hosp., 1924, 35:103.
HELLMAN, L. M., REID, D. E., and MOORE, R. A. The Lipid Amino-Nitrogen in Eclampsia and Preeclampsia. Am. J. Obst. & Gynec., 1939, 38:631.
HELLMUTH, K. Beitrage zur Biologie des Neugeborenen. Archiv. f. Gynäk., 1926, 127:293.
HERRICK, W. W., and TILLMAN, A. J. B. Toxemia of Pregnancy; Its Relation to Cardiovascular and Renal Disease; Clinical and Necropsy Observations with a Long Follow-up. Arch. Int. Med., 1935, 55:643.
HINGSON, R. A., WHITACRE, F. E., and TURNER, H. B. The Treatment of Eclampsia by Means of Regional Nerve Block. Obst. & Gynec. Surv., 1949, 4:350.
HINSELMANN, H. Die Eklampsie. Bonn, 1924.
HOEFFEL, G., and MORIARITY, M. The Effect of Fasting on the Metabolism of Epileptic Children. Am. J. Dis. Child., 1924, 28:16.
HOFBAUER, J. Zur Klärung der Eklampsiefrage, Zentralbl. f. Gynak., 1921, 41:1797.
——— Graviditäts-toxikosen. Ztschr. f. Geburtsh. u. Gynäk., 1908, 61:258.
——— Experimental Studies on the Toxemias of Pregnancy. Can Histamine Poisoning Be Regarded as the Etiologic Factor? Am. J. Obst. & Gynec., 1926, 12:159.
HOFFMANN, F., and ANSELMINO, K. J. Machweis der antidiuretischen Komponente des Hypophysehinterlappenhormons und einer blutdruck-steigernden Substanz im Blute bei Nephropathie und Eclampsie. Arch. f. Gynäk., 1931, 147:604-620.
HUNT, A. B., and WAKEFIELD, E. G. Concentration of Serum Sulfate during Pregnancy and in Preeclamptic Toxemia. Am. J. Obst. & Gynec., 1939, 38:498.
INGERSLEV, M., and TEILUM, G. Biopsy Studies of the Liver in Pregnancy. Acta. Obstet. et Gynec. Scandinav., 1946, 25:339.

Irving, F. C. A Study of Five Hundred Consecutive Cases of Preeclampsia. Canad. M. A. J., 1939, 40:137.

Jardine, R., and Kennedy, A. M. Symmetrical Necrosis of the Cortex of the Kidney Associated with Puerperal Eclampsia. Tr. Edinb. Obst. Soc., 1912-1913, 38:158.

Kapeller-Adler, R. The Histidine Metabolism in Normal and Toxemic Pregnancy. J. Obst. & Gynaec. Brit. Emp., 1941, 48:141.

——— The Significance of the Isolation of Histamine from the Urine in the Toxemia of Pregnancy. J. Obst. & Gynaec. Brit. Emp., 1941, 48:155.

——— and Cartwright, J. A. Vitamin B_1 and Toxemia of Pregnancy, Am. J. Obst. & Gynec., 1944, 47:575.

Kellar, R. J., Arnott, W. M., and Matthew, G. D. Observations on the Morbid Histology of the Kidney in Eclampsia and other Toxemias of Pregnancy. J. Obst. & Gynec. Brit. Emp., 1937, 44:320.

Kellogg, F. S. Toxemias of Pregnancy. Clinics, 1945, 4:585.

——— and Reid, D. E. Group Incidence of Hypertensive-Albuminuric Pregnancy under the New Classification. Am. J. Obst. & Gynec., 1943, 45:651.

Krieger, V. I. The Guanidine, Glucose and Calcium Contents in the Blood in Eclampsia. M. J. Australia, 1934, 2:746-749.

——— and Kilvington, T. B. Antidiuretic Substance in Urine in Relation to Normal and Toxaemic Pregnancy. M. J. Australia, 1940, 1:575.

Lamport, H. The Effects on Renal Resistance to Blood Flow of Renin, Angiotonin, Pitressin and Atropine, Hypertension, and Toxemia of Pregnancy. J. Clin. Investigation, 1942, 21:685.

La Vake, R. T. The Cause of Toxemias of Pregnancy. Journal-Lancet, 1943, 63:51.

Lazard, E. M. Analysis of 575 Cases of Eclamptic and Preeclamptic Toxemias Treated by Intravenous Injections of Magnesium Sulphate. Am. J. Obst. and Gynec., 1933, 26:647.

Lazard, E. M., Irwing, J. C., and Vruwink, J. The Intravenous Magnesium Sulphate Treatment of Eclampsia. Am. J. Obst. & Gynec., 1926, 12:104.

Lichtenstein. Zur Klinik, Therapie und Aetiologie der Eklampsie, nach einer neuen Statitik bearbeitet auf Grund von 400 Fallen. Arch. f. Gynäk., 1912, 95:183.

McClellan, G. S., Strayhorn, W. D., and Densen, P. M. A Review of Seventy-five Cases of Eclampsia. With Particular Reference to Late Cardiovascular Renal Effects. Am. J. Obst. & Gynec., 1942, 43:493.

McKelvey, J. L., and MacMahon, H. E. A Study of the Lesions in the Vascular System in Fatal Cases of Chronic Nephritic Toxaemia of Pregnancy. Malignant Nephrosclerosis. Surg. Gynec., & Obst., 1935, 60:1.

McLane, C. M. Results in the Treatment of Severe Preeclampsia. M. Rec. & Ann., 1948, 42:669. Abstract in Obst. & Gynec. Surv., 1949, 4:36.

——— and Kuder, K. Severe Preeclampsia. Am. J. Obst. & Gynec., 1943, 46:549.

McLennan, C. E. Antecubital and Femoral Venous Pressure in Normal and Toxemic Pregnancy. Am. J. Obst. & Gynec., 1943, 45:568.

——— The Rate of Filtration Through the Capillary Walls in Pregnancy. Am. J. Obst. & Gynec., 1943, 46:63.

McNalley, F. P., and Dieckmann, W. J. Hemorrhagic Lesions of the Placenta and Their Relation to White Infarct Formation. Am. J. Obst. & Gynec., 1923, 5:55.

Mengert, W. F., Jennett, R. J., and Brown, W. W., Jr. The Physiopathology of Eclampsia. Am. J. Obst. & Gynec., 1949, 57:97.

Minot, A. S., and Cutler, J. T. Increase in Guanidine-like Substances in Acute Liver Injury and Eclampsia. Proc. Soc. Exper. Biol. and Med., 1929, 26:607.

Mudaliar, A. L., Nayar, A. S. M., and Menon, M. K. K. Eclampsia; A Clinical and Biochemical Study. Inter. Abst. Surg. (Surg., Gynec. & Obst.), 1941, 72:367.

Mussey, R. D. The Relation of Retinal Changes to the Severity of the Acute Hypertensive Syndrome of Pregnancy. Am. J. Obst. & Gynec., 1936, 31:938.

——— Hunt, A. B., and Sluder, F. S. Hypertension and Pregnancy. Am. J. Obst. & Gynec., 1943, 45:224.

——— and Lovelady, Sim B. Is There a Clinical Relationship Between Pyelitis of Pregnancy and Preeclamptic Toxemia. Am. J. Obst. & Gynec., 1940, 39:236.

Mylius, K. Spastische und tetanische Netzhautveränderungen bei der Eklampsie. Ber. u. d. Versamml. d. deutsch. ophth. Gesellsch. 1929, 47:379.

Newell, J. L., and Smithwick, R. H. Pregnancy following Lumbodorsal Splanchnicectomy for Essential and Malignant Hypertension, etc. New England J. Med., 1947, 236:851.

Nichol, R. W. The Etiology of Pregnancy Toxemia. J. Obst. & Gynaec. Brit. Emp., 1938, 45:609.

NICHOLAS, H. O., JOHNSON, H. W., and JOHNSTON, R. A. Diffusible Serum Calcium in Pregnancy. Am. J. Obst. & Gynec., 1934, 27:504.

NICODEMUS, R. E. Oxygen Tent Therapy in the Treatment of Eclampsia. J.A.M.A., 1941, 117:1238.

NIXON, W. C. W., WRIGHT, M. D., and FIELLER, E. C. Vitamin B_1 in the Urine and Placenta in Toxemia of Pregnancy. Int. Abst. Surg. (Surg., Gynec. & Obst.), 1942, 75:369.

OARD, H. C., and PETERS, J. P. Concentration of Acid and Base in Serum in Normal Pregnancy. J. Biol. Chem., 1929, 81:9.

OBERST, F. W., and PLASS, E. D. Blood Changes Induced by Venesection in Women with Toxemia of Late Pregnancy. J. Clin. Invest., 1940, 19:493.

PAGE, E. W. The Effect of Eclamptic Blood Upon the Urinary Output and Blood Pressure of Human Recipients. J. Clin. Invest., 1938, 17:207.

——— The Relation between Hydatid Moles, Relative Ischemia of the Gravid Uterus, and the Placental Origin of Eclampsia. Am. J. Obst. & Gynec., 1939, 37:291.

——— Placental Dysfunction in Eclamptogenic Toxemias. Obst. & Gynec. Surv., 1948, 3:615.

——— and COX, A. J. Renal Changes Following Toxemias of Late Pregnancy. West. J. Surg., 1938, 46:463.

——— PATTON, H. S., and OGDEN, E. The Effect of Pregnancy on Experimental Hypertension. Am. J. Obst. & Gynec., 1941, 41:53.

PAGE, I. H. Studies on the Mechanism of Arterial Hypertension. J.A.M.A., 1942, 120:757.

PARAMORE, R. H. An Introduction to the Mechanistic Conception of Eclampsia. Lancet, 1928, 2:914.

PARKS, J., and PEARSON, J. W., Jr. Cerebral Complications Occurring in the Toxemias of Pregnancy. Am. J. Obst. & Gynec., 1943, 45:774.

PECKHAM, C. H. Chronic Nephritis Following Eclampsia. Bull. Johns Hopkins Hosp., 1929, 45:176-188.

——— The Fetal Mortality in the Toxemias of Pregnancy. J.A.M.A., 1933, 101:1608.

PETERS, J. P. The Nature of the Toxemias of Pregnancy. J.A.M.A., 1938, 110:329.

PLASS, E. D. The Significance of the Noncoagulable Nitrogen Coefficient of the Blood Serum in Pregnancy and the Toxemias of Pregnancy. Am. J. Obst., 1915, 71:608.

——— Variations in the Distribution of the Nonprotein Nitrogenous Constituents of Whole Blood and Plasma During Acute Retention and Elimination. J. Biol. Chem., 1923, 56:17.

——— Nonprotein Nitrogen Constituents of Blood in Eclampsia and Allied Conditions. J.A.M.A., 1924, 84:266.

——— and MATTHEW, C. W. Plasma Protein Fractions in Normal Pregnancy. Am. J. Obst. & Gynec., 1926, 12:346.

POSATTI, F., and BEIGLBÖCK, W. Potassium and Sodium Content of Serum in Preeclamptic Conditions and Its Modification by Insulin Hypoglycemia. Monatschr. f. Geburtsh. u. Gynäk., 1938, 108:237.

PRIDE, C. B., and RUCKER, M. P. Eclampsia and Ovarian Pregnancy. Am. J. Obst. & Gynec., 1942, 44:575.

PRUTZ, W. Ueber das. anat. Verhalten der Nieren bei der Puerpereklampsie. Ztschr. f. Geburtsh. u. Gynäk., 1892, 23:1.

REID, D. E., and TEEL, H. M. Nonconvulsive Pregnancy Toxemias. Am. J. Obst. & Gynec., 1939, 37:886.

REIS, R. A., and BERNICK, E. A. Eclampsia without Convulsions, Hypertension or Coma. Am. J. Obst. & Gynec., 1944, 48:257.

ROBINSON, C. E., DILL, L. V., CADDEN, J. F., and ISENHOUR, C. E. Glomerular Filtration and Renal Blood Flow in the Hypertensive Woman and in Posttoxemic Hypertension. Am. J. Obst. & Gynec., 1942, 44:616.

ROSENBAUM, M., and MALTBY, G. L. The Relation of Cerebral Dysrhythmia to Eclampsia. Am. J. Obst. & Gynec., 1943, 45:992.

ROSS, J. W. Nembutal in the Treatment of Preeclampsia and Eclampsia. Am. J. Obst. & Gynec., 1936, 31:120.

ROSS, R. A., PERLZWEIG, W. A., TAYLOR, H. M., MCBRYDE, A., YATES, A., and KONDRITZER, A. A. A Study of Certain Dietary Factors of Possible Etiologic Significance in Toxemias of Pregnancy. Am. J. Obst. & Gynec., 1938, 35:426.

RUPP, H. Salt Metabolism in Pregnancy. Ztschr. f. Geburtsh. u. Gynäk., 1929, 95:383.

SANES, S., and KAMINSKI, C. A. Spontaneous Rupture of the Liver in Eclampsia with Fatal Hemoperitoneum. Am. J. Obst. & Gynec., 1946, 52:325.

SCHAFFER, N. K., BARKER, S. B., SUMMERSON, W. H., and STANDER, H. J. Relation of Blood Lactic Acid and Acetone Bodies to Uric Acid in Pre-Eclampsia and Eclampsia. Proc. Soc. for Exper. Biol. & Med., 1941, 48:237.

SCHAFFER, N. K., DILL, L. V., and CADDEN, J. F. Uric Acid Clearance in Normal Pregnancy and Preeclampsia. J. Clin. Invest., 1943, 22:201.

SCHMORL, G. Path. anat. Untersuchungen über Puerperal-eklampsie. Leipzig, 1893. Zur Lehre von der Eklampsie. Arch. f. Gynaek., 1902, 65:504.

SCHWARZ, O. H., and DORSETT, E. L. Further Observations on Conservative Treatment of Eclampsia, South. Med. J., 1930, 23:288.

——— SOULE, S. D., and DUNIE, B. Blood Lipids in Pregnancy. Am. J. Obst. & Gynec., 1940, 39:203.

SIDDALL, A. C. Vitamin B_1 Deficiency as an Etiologic Factor in Pregnancy Toxemias. Am. J. Obst. & Gynec., 1938, 35:662.

SIDDALL, A. C., and OBERLIN, O. Vitamin B_1 Deficiency as an Etiologic Factor in Pregnancy Toxemias. Am. J. Obst. & Gynec., 1940, 39:818.

SIEGLER, S. L. Estrogenic and Chorionic Gonadotropic Hormone in Normal Pregnancy and in Toxemia of Pregnancy. J. Lab. & Clin. Med., 1939, 24:1277.

SIOLL. Eklamptische u. posteklamptische Psychosen Hinselmann. Die. Eklampsie, Bonn, 1924, p. 597.

SITZENFREY, A. Eklampsie im 6sten Schwangerschaftsmonat bei Blasenmole, etc. Zentralbl. f. Gynäk., 1911, 35:343.

SLEMONS, J. M. Eclampsia without Convulsions. Bull. Johns Hopkins Hosp., 1907, 18:448.

SMITH, J. A. The Phenoltetrachlorphthalein Test of Liver Function in the Toxemias of Pregnancy. Am. J. Obst. and Gynec., 1924, 8:298.

SMITH, G. V., and SMITH, O. W. Estrogen and Progestin Metabolism in Pregnant Women. With Especial Reference to Preeclamptic Toxemia and the Effect of Hormone Administration. Am. J. Obst. & Gynec., 1940, 39:405.

——— The Anterior Pituitary-like Hormone in Late Pregnancy Toxemia. A Summary of Results since 1932. Am. J. Obst. & Gynec., 1939, 38:618.

SPILLMAN, R. S. Lumbar Puncture in the Treatment of Eclampsia. Collective Review. Am. J. Obst. & Gynec., 1922, 4:568.

STANDER, H. J. Effect of the Intravenous Administration of Magnesium Sulphate. J.A.M.A., 1927, 92:631-636.

——— The Toxemias of Pregnancy. Baltimore, 1929.

——— Blood Guanidine Base Concentration in Eclampsia. Am. J. Obst. and Gynec., 1932, 23:373.

——— Hemorrhagic Retinitis in Vomiting of Pregnancy. Surg., Gynec., and Obst., 1932, 54:129-132.

——— and CADDEN, J. F. Acute Yellow Atrophy of the Liver in Pregnancy. Am. J. Obst. and Gynec., 1934, 28:61.

——— Blood Chemistry in Preeclampsia and Eclampsia. Am. J. Obst. and Gynec., 1934, 28:856.

——— DUNCAN, E. E., and SISSON, W. E. Chemical Studies on the Toxemias of Pregnancy. Bull. Johns Hopkins Hospital, 1925, 36:411.

——— EASTMAN, N. J., and others. The Acid-base Equilibrium of the Blood in Eclampsia. J. Biol. Chem., 1929, 85:233.

——— and KUDER, K. Low Reserve Kidney. Am. J. Obst. & Gynec., 1938, 35:1.

——— and PECKHAM, C. H. A Classification of the Toxemias of the Latter Half of Pregnancy. Am. J. Obst. & Gynec., 1926, 11:583.

STRAUSS, M. B. Observations on the Etiology of the Toxemias of Pregnancy. The Relationship of Nutritional Deficiency. Hypoproteinemia, and Elevated Venous Pressure to Water Retention in Pregnancy. Am. J. M. Sc., 1935, 190:811.

——— Observations on the Etiology of the Toxemias of Pregnancy. Am. J. M. Sc., 1938, 196:188.

STROGANOFF, W. Results Obtained in the Treatment of Eclampsia by the Improved Prophylactic Method. Tr. Edinburgh Obst. Soc., 1927, p. 161.

——— Über die Behandlung der Eklampsie. Zentralbl. f. Gynäk., 1901, 25:1309.

——— and DAVIDOVITCH, O. Two Hundred Cases of Eclampsia Treated with Magnesium Sulphate. J. Obst. & Gynaec. Brit. Emp., 1937, 44:289.

SZEKELY, P., and SNAITH, L. The Heart in Toxemia of Pregnancy. Brit. Heart J., 1947, 9:128.

TAYLOR, H. C., Jr. Relationship of the Hormones to the Toxemias of Pregnancy. J.A.M.A., 1942, 120:595.

——— and SCADRON, E. N. Hormone Factors in the Toxemias of Pregnancy. Am. J. Obst. & Gynec., 1939, 37:963.

——— WARNER, R. C., and WELSH, C. A. The Relationship of the Estrogens and other Placental Hormones to Sodium and Potassium Balance at the End of Pregnancy and in the Puerperium. Am. J. Obst. & Gynec., 1939, 38:748.

——— WELLEN, I., and WELSH, C. A. Renal Function Studies in Normal Pregnancy and in Toxemia Based on Clearances of Inulin, Phenol Red and Diodrast. Am. J. Obst. & Gynec., 1942, 43:567.

TEEL, H. M., and REID, D. E. Observations Upon the Occurrence of an Antidiuretic Substance in the Urine of Patients with Preeclampsia and Eclampsia. Endocrinology, 1939, 24:297.

TENNEY, B., JR., and PARKER, F., JR. The Placenta in Toxemia of Pregnancy. Am. J. Bost. & Gynec., 1940, 39:1000.

THEOBALD, G. W. Effect of Calcium and Vitamins A and D on the Incidence of Pregnancy Toxemia. Lancet, 1937, 232:937.

——— Hepatic Lesions Associated with Eclampsia and Those Caused by Raising Intra-abdominal Pressure. J. Path. and Bact., 1932, 1:1397.

THOMPSON, K. J., REID, D. E., and COHEN, M. E. Studies on Circulation in Pregnancy. Venous Pressure Observations in Normal Pregnant Women, in Pregnant Women with Compensated and Decompensated Heart Disease and in the Pregnancy "Toxemias." Am. J. M. Sc., 1939, 198:665.

TILLMAN, A. J. B. Two Fatal Cases of Hyperemesis Gravidarum with Retinal Hemorrhages. Am. J. Obst. and Gynec., 1934, 27:240.

——— Classification and Medical Relationships of Hypertensive Albuminuric Pregnancy, J.A.M.A., 1942, 120:587.

TITUS, P., and DODDS, P. The Etiologic Significance of Lowered Blood Sugar Values in Vomiting of Pregnancy. Am. J. Obst. & Gynec., 1928, 16:90.

——— DODDS, P., and WILLETTS, E. W. The Fluctuation in Blood Sugar during Eclampsia and Its Relation to the Convulsions. Am. J. Obst. & Gynec., 1928, 15:303.

TORPIN, R., and COPPEDGE, W. W. Eclampsia: Review of 350 Cases Stressing Therapy. South. M. J., 1940, 33:673.

TRAUT, H. F., and KUDER, A. The Lesions of 1,500 Placentas Considered from a Clinical Point of View. Am. J. Obst. & Gynec., 1934, 27:552.

VOLHARD, F. Eclamptic and Uremic Convulsions. Monatschr. f. Geburtsh. u. Gynäk., 1924, 66:79.

WAGENER, H. P. Artericles of the Retina in Toxemias of Pregnancy. J.A.M.A., 1933, 101:1380.

——— and KEITH, N. M. Diffuse Arteriolar Disease with Hypertension and the Associated Retinal Lesions. Medicine, 1939, 18:317.

WALLACE, L., KATZ, L. N., LANGENDORF, R., and BUXBAUM, H. Electrocardiogram in Toxemias of Pregnancy. Arch. Int. Med., 1946, 77:405.

WAY, G. T. C. Fatal Eclampsia. A Clinical and Anatomic Correlative Study. Am. J. Obst. & Gynec., 1947, 54:928.

WEISS, S., and PARKER, F., Jr. Pyelonephritis: Its Relation to Vascular Lesions and to Arterial Hypertension. Medicine, 1939, 18:221.

WELSH, C. A., WELLEN, I., TAYLOR, H. C., Jr., and ROSENTHAL, A. The Filtration Rate, Effective-Renal Blood Flow, Tubular Excretory Mass and Phenol Red Clearance in Normal Pregnancy. J. Clin. Invest., 1942, 21:57.

WHITACRE, F. E., HINGSON, R. A., and TURNER, H. B. The Treatment of Eclampsia by Means of Regional Nerve Block. South. M. J., 1948, 41:920.

——— LOEB, W. M., and CHIN, H. A Contribution to the Study of Eclampsia. A Consideration of 200 Cases. J.A.M.A., 1947, 133:445.

WHITE, P. Pregnancy Complicating Diabetes of More than Twenty Years' Duration. M. Clin. North America, 1947, 31:395.

WIELOCH, J. Weiteres Material über die Eclampsie unter Berücksichtigung der Hirndrucktheorie. Arch. f. Gynaek., 1925, 123:337.

WILLIAMS, P. F., and WEISS, E. Application of the New Classification of Toxemias of Pregnancy in 318 Fatal Cases. Am. J. Obst. & Gynec., 1943, 45:2.

WILSON, P. A Contribution to the study of Eclampsia as a Toxemia of Possible Mammary Origin. Am. J. Obst., 1913, 67:1111.

YAMADA, K. A Study of the Relationship Between the Origin of Eclampsia and Allergy. Am. J. Obst. & Gynec., 1942, 43:540.

YOUNG, J. Recurrent Pregnancy Toxemia and Its Relation to Placental Damage. Tr. Edinb., Obst. Soc., 1927, 47:61.

——— Prognosis and Treatment of Eclampsia and Albuminuria of Pregnancy, with Special Reference to Risk of Recurrence in Subsequent Pregnancies. Brit. M. J., 1929, 1:91.

——— Renal Failure after Utero-Placental Damage. Am. J. Obst. & Gynec., 1944, 47:282.

ZIMMERMAN, H. M., and PETERS, J. P. Pathology of Pregnancy Toxemias. J. Clin. Investigation, 1937, 16:397.

Additional literature will be found in the monographs of Hinselmann, Die Eklampsie, 1924, Stander, The Toxemias of Pregnancy, 1929, and Dieckmann, The Toxemias of Pregnancy, 1941.

28

COINCIDENTAL COMPLICATIONS OF PREGNANCY

Gravid women are naturally subject to all the diseases from which nonpregnant persons suffer. Whenever such a coincidental condition is present, whether it antedated conception or developed in the course of gestation, certain important questions must be answered. Will pregnancy aggravate the disease process? Will it activate some latent condition? Conversely, will the disease conduce to abortion or premature labor? Will it injure the baby in any way? Will it interfere with the normal course of labor?

There are a few rather common diseases in which the superimposition of pregnancy may sometimes alter substantially the clinical course and prognosis of the pathological process. In certain other instances, the outlook for the pregnancy may be jeopardized by the coincidental disorder. In still other cases, fortunately few, both effects may be observed, a deleterious action being noted both on the disease and on the course of gestation. Among the diseases in which one or another or both of these adverse effects may sometimes (but by no means always) be observed are: rheumatic heart disease, diabetes mellitus, chronic hypertensive vascular disease, pyelonephritis, pneumonia, untreated syphilis, and rubella. With the exception of these diseases, and possibly a very few others, the questions asked in the first paragraph of this chapter, may all be answered in the negative. In other words, whenever a physician encounters some coincidental disease as a complication of pregnancy (perhaps some disease with which he has had no experience in gravid women) he can usually rest assured that the disease will not be aggravated by pregnancy and that the coincidental condition will not affect the normal course of gestation, with the possible exceptions noted.

ACUTE INFECTIOUS DISEASES

Smallpox. Smallpox complicating pregnancy carries with it a more serious prognosis than at other times. Thus Vinay reported a mortality of 36 per cent in 235 cases, as compared with 25 per cent in the nonpregnant condition. The hemorrhagic form of the disease is particularly fatal in pregnant women, Mayer having recorded the loss of 13 consecutive cases.

Moreover, smallpox exerts a deleterious influence upon the product of conception, although the incidence of abortion or premature labor varies with the severity of the disease, Queirel stating that it is almost universal in the hemorrhagic, and comparatively infrequent in the discrete, variety. This may be due to hemorrhagic changes in the decidua, or to the direct transmission of the disease to the fetus, with its subsequent death and expulsion. The occurrence of intra-uterine smallpox is well authenticated, children being occasionally born in the eruptive stage of the disease or with distinct pock-marks, as in the case reported by Puig y Roig, in which the mother presented no manifestations of the disease. Mauriceau is said to have been infected in this manner, and the condition was well known to John Hunter and Smellie. Moreover, in double-ovum twin pregnancy it sometimes happens that one child is definitely pock-marked while the other shows no signs of the disease.

German Measles (Rubella). As the results of observations made during an epidemic of German measles (Rubella) in Australia in 1941, it was established that pregnant women who suffer from this disease in the first trimester of pregnancy frequently give birth to infants afflicted with certain malformations, notably, cataracts, heart lesions, deaf-mutism, and microcephaly. The lens of the eye first appears during the fourth week and, in association with other structures of the eyeball, reaches its typical appearance during the third month. The appearance of the primordium of the internal ear has been observed in embryos of three to four weeks. Development continues until morphologic differentiation is practically complete in the third month. Partition of the primitive chambers of the heart begins between the fifth and sixth weeks. Development of the interatrial and interventricular septums is completed by the end of the seventh week. These early embryonic processes appear to be peculiarly vulnerable to the virus of rubella and in its presence the development of the structures mentioned may be grossly defective.

From a practical viewpoint the important question is: Among mothers who have suffered well authenticated attacks of rubella in the first trimester of pregnancy, what percentage of the infants will be defective? In 262 cases of rubella in pregnancy studied by Patrick in Australia, the incidence of seriously defective infants was 28 per cent; in a similar study carried out in Massachusetts by Ober, Horton, and Feemster, 49 women who had had rubella in gestation gave birth to six babies with serious congenital malformations, or 12.3 per cent. If, however, in the Massachusetts study, only cases of rubella which occurred in the first three months of pregnancy be considered, a more significant figure is obtained; in 22 such cases, five infants had serious defects, or 22.7 per cent. In view of these and other similar studies, it would appear that when a woman suffers from rubella in the first three months of pregnancy, the likelihood of the infant being afflicted with one or more serious developmental defects is 25 per cent or possibly greater. This raises the question as to the justification of performing therapeutic abortion in such cases. Opinion about this differs widely. However, it is my own feeling that if the attack of rubella has been observed by a dependable physician and if the validity of the diagnosis is beyond question, and provided that the disease occurred in the first three months of pregnancy, therapeutic abortion is justifiable if the mother and her husband do not want to assume the obvious risks involved. After the end of the third month the incidence of congenital malformations as the result of maternal rubella is decidedly less; from the fourth month the chances of the infant's being affected are almost nil.

Measles. Measles is not a frequent complication of pregnancy, but when it occurs is very prone to cause premature delivery, as was observed by Klotz in 9 out of 11 cases. According to Fellner, the prognosis is much more serious during the puerperium than during pregnancy. It is stated that intra-uterine transmission of the disease to the fetus is now and again noted, a number of observers having reported cases in which the child presented a characteristic eruption at birth.

Scarlet Fever. It is generally believed that the pregnant woman possesses a certain immunity to scarlet fever. The older authors on the subject considered that this was demonstrated by the fact that the disease occurs much less frequently during pregnancy than in the puerperium. Posch, in 1926, stated that less than 30 cases were recorded in the literature. It is quite possible that many of the puerperal cases were not examples of true scarlet fever, confusion having arisen on account of the somewhat similar rash which sometimes occurs in puerperal infection. The correctness of this latter supposition is supported by the fact that many authors believe in the intercommunicability of the two diseases; the demonstration by Dick, Dochez, and others that scarlatina is due to a specific hemolytic streptococcus certainly indicates that they are closely related. Certainly it appears well established that a streptococcus is the main etiologic agent causing scarlet fever.

When occurring in the early months of pregnancy, the disease sometimes causes abortion. This accident is usually attributed to the high temperature of the mother, although in very rare instances it is attributed to the direct transmission of the disease to the fetus. Ballantyne recorded a case in which the child presented a characteristic rash at birth, and Liddell and Tangye reported one in which they thought that desquamation and albuminuria proved the nature of the disease. This view, however, has never met with any general acceptance.

It is essential and of the utmost importance that rigid isolation technic be instituted and maintained in the treatment of a pregnant, parturient, or puerperal patient with scarlet fever. Two principles are here involved, first the prevention of transferring hemolytic streptococci from the nose or throat and other parts to the genital tract, and second the prevention of the transmission of the disease to other women. Chemotherapy has, of course, revolutionized the outlook for both mother and baby in scarlet fever.

Cholera. Pregnant women do not appear to be attacked by cholera more frequently than others, although they succumb more readily to the disease. Schütz states that the mortality among them in the Hamburg epidemic of 1892 was 57 per cent.

The disease exerts a very deleterious effect upon pregnancy, 54 per cent of the cases, according to Schütz, ending in abortion or premature labor. This may be due to various causes. One third of the women suffering from cholera have uterine hemorrhage, which, when occurring during pregnancy, must be associated with changes in the decidua, Slavjansky having described a peculiar form of hemorrhagic endometritis. Moreover, in nearly every instance, the disease causes uterine contractions supposed to result from the circulation of toxins in the blood.

Typhoid Fever. Typhoid fever is a serious, and often a dangerous, complication of pregnancy. Moreover, it increases largely the fetal mortality, abortion or premature labor occurring in from 40 to 60 per cent of the cases. Formerly it was held that the death of the fetus and its subsequent expulsion were due to the high temperature characterizing the disease; it is now known that it is usually due to the direct transmission through the placenta of toxins or of the bacilli themselves. Since F. W. Lynch demonstrated the bacilli in the organs of a fetus aborted by a woman suffering from typhoid fever, and Hicks and French stated that similar findings were noted in 10 out of 21 cases reported in the literature, it is generally admitted that the death of the fetus is frequently due to a typhoid septicemia. The literature upon the subject was collected by Wichels, in 1924.

Although typhoid fever is rarely seen today, the question sometimes arises as to the possible hazards involved in giving pregnant women inoculations to produce typhoid immunization. It is customary for Occidentals living in the Orient to take typhoid inoculations every two years and, especially at times of epidemics, a few pregnant women receive them. I know personally of two such cases in which abortion ensued promptly after either the first or second injection, and physicians who have practiced long in the Orient can tell of many more. Sauramo also finds that immunization against typhoid during the first half of pregnancy may lead to violent reactions and that it often results in abortion.

Pneumonia. The maternal mortality is materially augmented when pneumonia occurs during pregnancy, since the disease frequently leads to premature labor or abortion. This result is generally attributed to imperfect oxygenation of the fetal blood, though it is frequently due to the direct transmission of bacteria to the fetus, in whose organs pneumococci have often been demonstrated. At the New York Lying-In Hospital there were six deaths from pneumonia in 46,861 obstetrical discharges during the period 1932-1943. In other words, pneumonia accounted for 7.5 per cent of all the maternal deaths, being surpassed as a cause of death only by hemorrhage and puerperal infection. Premature labor is a very untoward complication in such cases as the exertion incident to it subjects the already weakened maternal organism suffering from the infection to so great an additional strain that death frequently results.

When pneumonia develops during the last days of pregnancy or early in the puerperium, it is not unusual for pneumococci to be transmitted, by means of the blood stream, to the uterus where they give rise to hematogenous puerperal infection. Nuckols and Hertig, in 1938, reviewed the literature and described three cases of pneumococcal puerperal infection, endogenous in origin, an incidence of one in 6,788 deliveries, which they believed is probably too low owing to failure to identify the organism.

With the massive use of antibiotic drugs, pneumonia in pregnancy is a less formidable condition than it was formerly. Not only has the outlook for the mother been immensely improved, but premature labor and abortion are much less common. The initial dose of penicillin should be 500,000 units followed by 200,000 units every three hours. Present trends indicate that aureomycin may be even more effective.

Influenza. Williams' experience in the pandemic of 1918 showed that, at that time, influenza constituted an unusually serious complication of pregnancy, more particularly when of the pneumonic type. J. W. Harris, in a statistical study based upon 1,350 cases, found that the gross maternal mortality was 27 per cent, which increased to 50 per cent when pneumonia developed. The disease also had a most deleterious effect upon the pregnancy, which was interrupted in 26 per cent of the uncomplicated cases, and in 52 per cent of those accompanied by pneumonia. Moreover, when the disease ended fatally, spontaneous termination of pregnancy before the death of the mother occurred in 62 per cent of the cases. Here again, the introduction of the sulfonamides and penicillin has revolutionized the prognosis of a disease. Although these agents may not be effective against the virus of influenza they do forestall the development of pneumonia and thereby give the gravida and her infant a vastly better outlook than obtained in the pandemic of 1918.

Common Cold. The pregnant woman appears to be slightly more susceptible to acute upper respiratory infections than is the nonpregnant woman. Considerably more than one half of the instances of pneumonia complicating pregnancy are preceded by an acute cold. Hemolytic streptococcic puerperal infections in patients who had an acute upper respiratory infection at the time of delivery are not infrequent. The incidence of hemolytic streptococci in the upper respiratory passages of such patients is much higher than it is in healthy women. In addition, the condition represents a contraindication to general anesthesia at the time of delivery. For these reasons, such infections should never be regarded lightly. Every effort should be made to prevent the expectant mother from coming in contact with infections of this kind and in the event that an infection does develop, it is essential that she be confined to bed and given the best of supportive measures until recovery is complete.

Erysipelas. Erysipelas is a very serious disease at any time, but is particularly dangerous when ocurring in pregnant women, because of the danger of the development of puerperal infection. The hemolytic streptococci associated with erysipelas may become more invasive, causing a septicemia, and so may pass through the placenta and produce a fetal septicemia and death of the child.

Of the utmost importance in the care of a pregnant, parturient, or puerperal patient suffering from erysipelas are the rigid and extraordinary precautions which must be exercised by the patient, the nurse, and the doctor, in order to prevent the transfer of hemolytic streptococci from the local lesion of the erysipelas to the genital tract. It is, furthermore, evident that, for the protection of other patients, segregation and strict isolation of women with erysipelas are absolutely essential. The disease should be actively treated, utilizing sulfadiazine and penicillin, irrespective of the duration of pregnancy. By this means the patient will usually be free of hemolytic streptococci in a relatively short period of time. In the event that delivery follows shortly thereafter, or the patient is suspected of still being a carrier of such organisms, sulfadiazine or penicillin should be administered prophylactically during the puerperium.

Gonorrhea. Gonorrhea may be acquired before, coincidental with, or at any time following conception. The incidence of this disease complicating pregnancy is very difficult to determine as it exists most frequently, at this time, in a latent form which may be asymptomatic or relatively so. The frequency undoubtedly varies considerably in different social, racial, and economic groups. Tucker, Trussell, and Plass, employing cultural methods, found an incidence of 4 per cent among 500 consecutive normal obstetrical patients. A basis of comparison is afforded by the fact that serologic evidence of syphilis was found in 2.7 per cent of the same group of patients. In general, during pregnancy, the disease remains confined to the lower genital tract and it appears quite evident that the pregnancy acts as a barrier against an ascending infection. Accordingly, the pregnancy is not affected but, naturally, such an individual may transmit the disease in the usual manner.

More important, however, are the consequences of gonorrheal infection following an abortion or during the puerperium, leaving out of consideration ophthalmia neonatorum, to which reference has already been made. After labor, the gonococci, which have remained limited to the cervical canal during pregnancy, may gain access to the uterine cavity and give rise to febrile phenomena. The condition, although rarely fatal, is always serious, and will be considered in detail in the section on puerperal infection. In rare instances the gonococcus may produce a general infection, Dabney and Harris, and J. T. Smith having reported fatal cases of gonorrheal endocarditis observed in women delivered at the Johns Hopkins Hospital.

Undoubtedly, many patients who are followed carefully during pregnancy, labor, and the puerperium actually have the disease and yet it is unrecognized. In many instances there may be no complication during the postabortal or postpartum period. Modern bacteriologic methods should be employed to facilitate the diagnosis whenever there is any reason to suggest the presence of the disease. Cultural means of identifying the organism have been shown by Carpenter, Douglas, and others to be much superior to the reliance on smears alone. Treatment should be instituted, as soon as possible after the diagnosis is made. Cure following the administration of 200,000 units of penicillin injected intramuscularly is usually established in six to eight hours.

Trichomonas Vaginalis. This organism is found in about 20 to 30 per cent of women presenting themselves for antenatal examination; however, symptoms are present in a much smaller percentage of patients. The condition is characterized by a bubbly leukorrhea with irritation and itching. Trichomonads are readily demonstrated in fresh vaginal secretions, appearing as pear-shaped organisms somewhat larger than leukocytes.

The general principles underlying the therapy of trichomonas vaginalis vaginitis are: (1) thorough cleansing of the vaginal surfaces; (2) maintenance of a low vaginal pH; and (3) application of antiseptic or trichomonicidal agents. The vaginal walls should first be cleansed with green soap and water, or with hydrogen peroxide, if the soap proves too irritating. In either event, the vaginal surfaces are then thoroughly dried with cotton swabs. The next step recommended is the introduction into the posterior fornix of two moistened *floraquin* tablets, as first suggested by Karnaky. *Floraquin* is the commercial name for a combination of diodoquin (N.N.R., an effective protozoacide) with lactose and dextrose. The patient is instructed to insert one moistened tablet into the posterior fornix night and morning for seven days thereafter, and finally one every other night for 10 days. The patient should then be instructed emphatically about douching in pregnancy. *Under no circumstances should a bulb type of syringe be used.* (To my knowledge two deaths have occurred in pregnant women as the result of inadvertent insertion of the nozzle of such a syringe into the external os of the cervix followed by air embolism.) The douche bag should be located no more than 18 inches above the hips and the nozzle inserted no more than three inches. With this clearly understood the patient should take morning douches of three tablespoonfuls of vinegar to two quarts of water, followed in the active stage by the insertion of one tablet of floraquin into the fornix.

One form of treatment may give good results in one patient and be entirely disappointing in the next; recurrences are common. Other forms of treatment which may be used after the initial cleansing of the vagina are: the application of a 10 per cent aqueous solution of mercurochrome; the application of about 5 gm. of a silver picrate solution, available commercially, containing 1 per cent silver picrate dispersed in kaolin. This may be blown into the vagina by a suitable insufflator but only with a speculum introduced, since, here again, the danger of air embolism in pregnant women is a real one. Still another method that may be tried to advantage in some cases is the instillation of a jelly containing 0.02 per cent phenylmercuric acetate and available commercially. From time to time countless other antiseptics have been recommended for this common and annoying condition, but at the present writing the most popular and probably the most effective is the floraquin program as described.

Monilia Albicans. By cultural methods yeast may be found in the vagina in about 25 per cent of women at term. The thorough investigation of women complaining of leukorrheal discharge during pregnancy will reveal the presence of monilia with desquamated epithelial cells and leukocytes in some instances. Both the mycelial and cellular forms may be present. An extremely profuse, irritating discharge results from the disease. Occasionally, quite extensive edema of the external genitalia may be seen. Gentian violet (2 per cent aqueous solution) has proved to be a valuable therapeutic agent. The vagina must be distended by means of a speculum and filled with the solution which should be allowed to remain *in situ* for fifteen minutes. The treatment at first should be carried out daily, the interval between treatments being gradually lengthened. Cure is indicated by subsidence of symptoms and absence of the organism in stained smears and in cultures. It is not necessary to treat patients in whom monilia are found in the absence of signs or symptoms.

Tetanus. Always a very dangerous disease, tetanus is fortunately a rare complication of pregnancy, nor does it appear to be more fatal than in nonpregnant women. Archambaud has reported a case which terminated favorably.

Anthrax. Anthrax, or malignant pustule, is rarely observed in human beings under any circumstances but is almost always fatal. Rostowzen met with three deaths in pregnant women and was able, in each case, to demonstrate anthrax bacilli in the tissues of the child. A similar observation was made by Paltauf. Moreover, in certain animals the placental transmission of anthrax can frequently be demonstrated experimentally. It is recently reported that streptomycin is effective in anthrax.

CHRONIC INFECTIOUS DISEASES

Tuberculosis. During the past century the pendulum has swung back and forth from conservatism to radicalism in the management of the tuberculous gravida, but over the last decade it has settled on a conservative policy in most cases. Prior to 1850, pregnancy was thought to exert a beneficial effect on tuberculosis—so much so that physicians were in the habit of advising marriage for tuberculous women in the hope that future pregnancies would benefit the disease. In 1850, Grisalles reported 27 cases and pointed out the deleterious effect of pregnancy on tuberculosis. Following this publication, the management of these patients veered sharply to interruption, even in arrested cases, until 1906 when Rosthorn emphasized the fact that pregnancy may be relatively harmless in tuberculous women in whom the condition is quiescent and who have been without fever and hemoptysis for one year.

In 1929 Klemperer made an extensive review of the statistics bearing on the subject, particularly the very gratifying ones from sanatoria, and reported his own experience. On the basis of this survey, he reached the following conclusions which represent, in succinct form, the policy which most obstetricians perhaps follow today: Interruption of pregnancy on account of tuberculosis is never justified unless there is positive sputum or hemoptysis. If hemoptysis is persistent the pregnancy, if early, should be ended. In the presence of positive sputum, the course depends on the social and economic condition of the patient. If she is able to avail herself of institutional treatment, interference is not necessary.

Certainly a host of statistics from various tuberculosis sanatoria attest the fact that pulmonary tuberculosis is not affected by pregnancy per se. Thus, in one of the largest series reported, Marshall and his associates compared a group of 309 nonpregnant with 303 pregnant women in various stages of tuberculosis. In the group of "dormant" or "healed" cases, 2 per cent of the nonpregnant and 1 per cent of the pregnant cases died the first year. In the advanced stages of the disease 46 per cent of the nonpregnant women died, compared with 37 per cent of the pregnant group. Similarly, Forssner found no difference in the mortality of 341 pregnant women and 396 nonpregnant women who came to the outpatient department with tuberculosis. One of the most carefully studied series is that reported by Ornstein and Kovnat. It comprised 85 pregnant women with tuberculosis, mostly advanced, observed at the Sea View Hospital, Staten Island, New York. The average duration of stay before confinement was 2.1 months and the average after delivery was three months. Of these 85 cases, 31, or 36 per cent, died; 15, or 18 per cent, were unimproved and progressed; and 39, or 46 per cent, improved. Therefore, 54 per cent died or did poorly. Comparing these cases with a large group of women with tuberculosis uncomplicated by pregnancy at the Sea View Hospital: among 5,470 cases, 1,805, or 33 per cent, died; 1,696, or 31 per cent, were unimproved; and 1,969, or 36 per cent, improved. In this group then, 64 per cent died or did poorly. Among the 85 pregnant women in the Sea View series, 51 had a cavity formation. Of these, 51, or 69 per cent, died within one year. This experience was almost identical with 700 caseous-pneumonia tuberculosis cases studied at the Metropolitan Hospital; in these the death rate was 68 per cent in the first year.

Collapse therapy is frequently helpful in pregnant women as in nonpregnant; gestation is in no wise a contraindication to this procedure. In a noteworthy clinical study of this question, Seeley, Siddall, and Balzer reviewed in detail the results obtained in 54 tuberculous pregnant women who were given collapse therapy. Collapse therapy caused no serious ill effects, regardless of the type and extent of the lesions; the majority of even their worst cases did well. Results were especially good when this type of treatment has been instituted before pregnancy, or not later than the first trimester. Bilateral collapse was well tolerated in four very ill patients. However, although results for the series were generally good, there were at least five patients who would probably have fared better, in the opinion of the authors, if early therapeutic abortion had been done.

In a subsequent paper the same authors have reported observations on 34 pregnancies in 31 women subsequent to thoracoplasty. Their findings indicate in general that the majority of women go through pregnancy safely after thoracoplasty. In only three instances was mention made of dyspnea during pregnancy or labor, but in one of these the dyspnea reached a serious degree during labor. One mother died and five others had serious exacerbations of the tuberculosis during pregnancy or within one year after delivery. It is noteworthy that thoracoplasty has been done successfully during pregnancy in at least four instances.

An important practical point, brought out in the first Seeley paper cited above, is that the tuberculous gravidae who had neither collapse nor hospital treatment during pregnancy suffered a very high mortality—36.4 per cent, as contrasted with 11.1 per cent in the group subjected to collapse therapy and 10 per cent in their hospitalized non-collapse cases.

This raises the important role played by social and economic factors in the management of tuberculosis complicated by pregnancy. It may be true that pregnancy itself has little or no effect on tuberculosis, but the things which pregnancy normally brings with it, unless controlled, do exert a most deleterious effect. Chief of these is increased work, both before and after delivery, and everyone agrees that this is harmful to tuberculous women. If this additional work can be completely circumvented by prolonged hospitalization, both prior and subsequent to birth, tuberculous gravidae seem to do about as well as the nonpregnant tuberculous woman. However, social and economic conditions sometimes make it virtually impossible to provide the institutional care which these women need; hence, therapeutic abortion may still be desirable in some of these cases, as indicated in Klemperer's dictum above.

As a rule, tuberculosis of the mother does not affect the child. On the other hand, the disease is occasionally transmitted in utero so that the child is born with congenital tuberculosis. Whitman and Greene, in 1922, were able to collect 38 cases with characteristic histologic findings, as well as 21 others in which bacilli could be demonstrated in the fetus and placenta, but without histologic lesions. White and Porter, in 1938, reported a case of miliary tuberculosis in a newborn infant and expressed the opinion that tuberculous involvement of the placenta, causing systemic disease in the offspring, just before or during labor was probably the mode of infection in this instance.

It appears, however, that in the vast majority of cases, the disease is not transmitted directly through the placenta to the fetus, but that the latter is born with a lessened resistance rather than with tuberculosis itself. Hence, it follows that such children should be brought up under the best hygienic surroundings and their mothers should not nurse them.

Following the description by Lehmann of the first cases of placental tuberculosis, the subject has been carefully studied by many investigators. Novak and Ranzel collected 39 such cases in 1910, while Whitman and Greene increased the number to 47 in 1922. As the former investigators found tubercle bacilli in 7 out of 10 placentas from women in various stages of the disease, it is apparent that the condition occurs more frequently than is generally believed, and the opinion of Baumgarten and Maffucci is confirmed that the incidence of congenital tuberculosis is generally underestimated. According to Lanz, tuberculous lesions of the placenta may occur in the following forms: (1) tubercles attached to the periphery of the chorionic villi but projecting in great part into the intervillous spaces; (2) tubercles in the stroma of the villi, which are due to bacilli which have penetrated the villous epithelium; (3) tuberculous changes in the chorionic membrane; and (4) caseous tuberculous deposits in the decidua basalis. Of these, (1) and (4) are the most frequent, while (2), which is the lesion most concerned in the production of congenital tuberculosis, has only occasionally been observed.

The possibility of germinal infection should also be borne in mind. Friedman, in experiments upon rabbits and guinea pigs, showed that tubercle bacilli may be carried to the ovum by means of the spermatozoa, while Sitzenfrey has demonstrated in women dying from tuberculosis the presence of bacilli in the interior of ova still within the graafian follicles. It is, of course, questionable whether such infected ova could go on to development, but should it occur, the supposition that the bacilli might lie dormant for some time would afford a plausible explanation for the cases in which the tuberculosis does not become manifest until some time after birth. Ehlinger and Künsch, investigating tuberculosis in 46 pairs of twins, found a greater similarity in the tuberculosis histories of single ovum than in those of double ovum or dizygotic twins; from this they conclude that there must be a hereditary predisposition for the development of this disease.

Pulmonary tuberculosis, just as cardiac disease, is often first recognized during routine antenatal care. Eisele and Mason, by means of routine roentgenologic examination carried out in 4,040 pregnant women, found 43 cases of unsuspected tuberculosis, an incidence of 1.06 per cent. Ianne and Muir, using the tuberculin test on 805 women, discovered that 252 gave a positive reaction and, of these, 12 proved to have tuberculosis. They recommended the tuberculin test, with x-rays of the reactors, as an addition to routine antenatal care, while Eisele and Mason believe that all pregnant women should have routine chest roentgenologic examination. There is much to be said in favor of such ideal antenatal care as it pertains to this disease.

Malaria. Goth has reported that 19 out of 46 cases of malaria in pregnancy resulted in premature labor. In spite of the fact that the fetal mortality is high in localities where pernicious malaria prevails, there is no very convincing evidence that placental transmission occurs. Blacklock and Gordon, in Sierra Leone, while able to demonstrate the presence of the characteristic parasites in the maternal blood of the placenta in 59 cases, never succeeded in finding them in the blood of the villous vessels nor in the umbilical cord. Schwartz examined 56 Negro women in central Africa and found malarial infection in the placenta in 74 per cent, in the cord blood in 6 per cent, and in the blood of the infant in only 3.6 per cent of his cases. In none of his patients did the placental infection appear to have a detrimental effect on the baby. He concludes that, although congenital malarial infection is possible even in children born of mothers who are healthy though infected, it is of very little practical importance, as most infections are acquired after birth. Wickramasuriya, on the other hand, although agreeing with Blacklock and Gordon, is convinced that fetal infection does occur and is more often the cause of fetal death than was formerly believed. Da Leas, from his large experience in Indo-China, comes to a similar conclusion.

There is a marked tendency toward recrudescence of the disease during pregnancy and the puerperium, just as is frequently observed after surgical operations.

Quinine should be administered unhesitatingly to women suffering from malaria during pregnancy, its oxytocic properties, if any, being ignored.

Leprosy. The disease is so rare in this country that information is somewhat lacking as to its effect on pregnancy. In 1934, Vigne and Guerin-Valmale reported a case where both parents were suffering from active cutaneous leprosy. Two healthy children were born, both without signs or serologic reactions of the disease.

Syphilis. Syphilis is one of the most important complications of pregnancy, and, before the institution of efficient prenatal care, it constituted the most frequent single cause of fetal death. In 1915, Williams reported that it was responsible for 26.4 per cent of the 705 fetal deaths occurring in 10,000 consecutive labors, including all deaths occurring after the period of viability had been reached, as well as during the first two weeks following labor. These figures, however, do not tell the whole story of the ravages of the disease, for many children who were discharged alive either died soon afterward or presented manifestations of hereditary syphilis later in life. Syphilis should be suspected whenever a satisfactory explanation for the occurrence of a premature or full-term, deadborn infant cannot be adduced. On the other hand, it plays little or no part in the causation of early abortion, although McCord has observed syphilis in the fetus as early as the fourth month. In 1920, Williams reported that a positive Wassermann reaction was present in 11.2 per cent of 4,547 consecutive women passing through the Johns Hopkins Hospital but was noted much less frequently in white than in black patients—2.5 and 16.3 per cent, respectively.

When infection occurs during pregnancy, owing to the vascularity of the parts the initial sore may assume larger proportions than under ordinary circumstances. The secondary lesions, however, are often but slightly marked and may be practically limited to the genitalia, where they appear as large, elevated areas which occasionally undergo ulcerative changes and sometimes lead to the destruction of superficial portions of the vulva. In most patients, however, no history of a primary sore or of a rash can be elicited, and the first intimation of the existence of the disease is afforded by the birth of a premature or macerated fetus, or by the demonstration of a positive Wassermann reaction. Indeed, it appears that syphilis, in general, runs a much less severe course in women than in men, and Warthin, in 1928, clearly pointed out the salient differences.

The syphilitic child is often dead when it comes into the world; less frequently, it is born alive with definite manifestations of the disease. Again, in a still smaller number of cases, it may be born without signs of the disease, which, however, make their appearance later; occasionally, particularly when the infection had occurred some years previously, the child may never manifest any signs of the disease. Moreover, syphilis is the actual cause of death in many children who were apparently normal at birth but succumbed some weeks later to what is usually designated as inanition or marasmus.

The influence of syphilis upon pregnancy varies materially, and three classes of cases are distinguished, according as infection has taken place: (1) before pregnancy, (2) at the time of conception, or (3) during pregnancy.

When inoculation with the *Treponema pallida* has occurred before conception and treatment is not instituted, the disease usually causes premature labor or the expulsion of a macerated fetus. Le Pileur obtained a striking illustration of the disastrous effects of syphilis from a study of the reproductive histories of 130 women before and after its inception; 3.8 per cent of the children were born dead before infection, as compared with 78 per cent after infection. When the mother is suffering from an acute infection at the time of conception, the offspring is always syphilitic, unless proper antenatal treatment is instituted. The same applies when the infection and conception occur at the same time. On the other hand, when syphilis is contracted during pregnancy, its effect upon the fetus varies. If infection occurs within the first months, the fetus, as a rule, likewise manifests signs of the disease, but when it occurs later the child may not be infected.

Congenital syphilis in only one of two twins has been reported from time to time. In a recent review of these cases, as well as of five cases of their own, Smith and Spence find this condition not so rare as might be expected. The twins in their series were all dizygotic. They believe that, as the fetus becomes infected by transmission of the spirochete through the placenta, the best explanation for the occurrence of congenital syphilis in only one of two dizygotic twins rests upon the circumstance of syphilitic inflammation—evidently necessary to transmission of the organism—of only one of the two placentas. Congenital syphilis in only one of two monozygotic twins has not been reported.

One of the most outstanding advances of obstetrics and one of the most important functions of prenatal care is the recognition and treatment of the syphilitic pregnant woman. As the great majority of women give no history of infection and present no visible manifestations of the disease, this can be accomplished only by routinely taking a sample of blood for a Wassermann test at the first visit. In New York, Illinois, and several other states, laws have been enacted which make a serologic test mandatory in the case of every pregnant woman. That the reliability of the Wassermann reaction is unaffected by pregnancy is shown by McCord in a careful 12-year follow-up study of 2,150 cases of syphilis in pregnancy.

The treatment of syphilis in pregnancy has been revolutionized as the result of the introduction of penicillin. In 580 cases from published reports analyzed by Ingraham, in which the infants had been followed sufficiently to permit valid conclusions, the results of penicillin therapy were much superior to those which had been achieved in previous years with arsenic and bismuth treatment. The women studied had primary, secondary, or early latent syphilis. A living syphilitic infant was born in only 2 per cent of the cases, in contrast to 5 to 7 per cent of syphilitic infants in the days when arsenic and bismuth were employed. Prior to the use of penicillin, a woman with primary or secondary syphilis in the last two months of pregnancy almost invariably gave birth to an infected child. Now treatment in the last few weeks of pregnancy results in a normal infant, occasionally seropositive at birth but reaching sustained negativity without additional therapy.

Since the average period required to reach seronegativity is 245 days and many mothers are treated only in the last months of pregnancy, a negative maternal blood test at the time of delivery is not a requisite for obtaining a healthy nonsyphilitic infant. Penicillin, in curing at least 70 per cent of the mothers, has accomplished more than any other form of therapy. A single course of penicillin treatment during pregnancy and monthly physical examinations and quantitative titered blood serological tests thereafter are usually sufficient to protect the fetus. Retreatment prior to delivery is to be considered if the mother fails to show a normal response.

The penicillin treatment is virtually reactionless. The whole treatment of the mother can be given during the pregnancy and can be completed in a few days. Penicillin permeates the placenta to the fetus in what appears to be therapeutically effective amounts.

Satisfactory dosage of penicillin to prevent congenital syphilis consists of 4.8 million units or more given over a period of seven days. There would seem to be little reason to add arsenic or bismuth to this regimen. There is not much choice between aqueous penicillin and penicillin in oil and bees' wax. A possible exception lies in the case of early syphilis occurring in late pregnancy when the fetus is likely to be infected already and it is necessary to maintain a sustained high level of penicillin in the mother. Here aqueous penicillin is most effective. A full dosage may be given from the start.

In the medical follow-up of the infant the serologic status at birth must be determined. However, Ingraham found that only 7.3 per cent of the seropositive infants had syphilis. The following criteria, in addition to positive darkfield examination of the skin lesions, may be used as indicative of actual syphilis of the newborn infant: (1) a titer of syphilitic reagin in the infant higher than that in the mother; (2) a high sustained or increasing titer during the first months of life; (3) a positive serologic test after three months; (4) unequivocal roentgenographic signs of osteochondritis or periostitis during the first three months. The infants while in the nursery should have a complete appraisal for syphilis. A seropositive infant should have the blood test repeated every two weeks and the roentgenogram repeated at six weeks. The seronegative infant should have blood tests at one, two, three, and six months. If no evidence of syphilis has been observed after six months no infantile congenital syphilis is present.

The question of retreatment in subsequent pregnancies in the woman who has had a standard course of penicillin for syphilis prior to conception is difficult to answer, according to Ingraham. However, various reports show that the number of syphilitic infants born in this group is extremely small, less than 1 per cent, when no treatment is given. If it is decided to withhold treatment it is necessary that the patient be followed carefully until term. A rational standard for withholding treatment has been suggested by Ingraham as follows: (1) the woman was treated for early symptomatic syphilis and had a normal clinical and serological response; (2) the woman was treated for late latent syphilis and maintained a negative spinal fluid and became seronegative and remained so; or (3) the woman was treated for symptomatic late syphilis and sustained a normal response.

The syphilitic child may be suckled with impunity by its own mother as she already has the disease. If, however, she is unable to nourish it, it should never be given to a wet-nurse but should be fed artificially.

Lymphopathia Venereum. This virus disease, which is rarely seen in white women but is relatively common in Negresses, is of great obstetrical importance because it frequently produces dense scarring of the soft tissues of the pelvis. As pointed out by Kaiser, the virus of lymphopathia venereum spreads from the vulva by the lymphatics to the perirectal lymph nodes and thence to the iliacs, leaving smouldering primary and secondary inflammatory changes in its wake. These produce varying degrees of rectal stricture which in some cases may be so extreme as to necessitate colostomy. In more severe cases the infection spreads to the bases of the broad ligaments and out laterally into the soft tissues of the pelvic wall. The rectovaginal septum is also involved with resultant fibrosis in the more advanced cases. With these extreme degrees of widespread pelvic scarring, it is understandable that labor may be impeded by this cicatrized and unyielding mass of tissues. As a further sequel, several cases of fatal rupture of the rectum into the peritoneal cavity have been reported but in these cases traumatic operative measures played an important role in addition to the condition of the tissues.

In 48 cases of rectal stricture complicating pregnancy, which have been managed in our clinic and which were analyzed by Kaiser, cesarean section was deemed necessary to meet the above difficulties in 10 per cent of the cases. There was one maternal death from rupture of the uterus; whether this accident was coincidental or was in some way related to the pelvic scarring is not clear. Kaiser reported a further study of 36 cases at the Charity Hospital in New Orleans, of rectal stricture complicating pregnancy in which three cesarean sections were performed—an incidence similar to ours—with no maternal deaths.

A careful vaginal examination is of the utmost importance in deciding upon the most suitable type of delivery. If there is widespread pelvic scarring, cesarean section is indicated. Marked perirectal fibrosis with cicatricial changes in the posterior rectovaginal septum is usually indicative of an extensive process and warrants abdominal delivery. It should be noted that it is these fibrotic changes and not the size of the rectal stricture which dictate cesarean section. As our statistics and those of the Charity Hospital demonstrate, 9 out of 10 patients with this condition can be delivered safely by the vaginal route. It is of the utmost importance, however, to avoid difficult vaginal delivery since most ruptures of the rectum reported in this complication have occurred in association with traumatic vaginal operations. Colostomy presents no special problems whether abdominal or vaginal delivery is carried out. Recent observations indicate that aureomycin will arrest lymphopathia venereum and clear up secondary infections, but of course no effect can be expected on already existing fibrotic changes. The literature on lymphopathia venereum as a complication of pregnancy and labor is reviewed extensively in Kaiser's two papers.

DISEASES OF THE JOINTS

Bierring in 1921, in a clinical study of the subject, reported more or less complete amelioration of symptoms in intermittent hydrarthrosis during pregnancy. The disease usually recurs about six weeks postpartum.

The effect of pregnancy on chronic atrophic arthritis is not so dramatic but, as Hench has pointed out in his study of the subject, 20 out of 22 women suffering from this disease experienced striking relief of their symptoms during pregnancy. These 20 patients were observed during 34 pregnancies and in only one pregnancy was the improvement not observed. According to Hench, relief usually occurs early in pregnancy and recurrence of symptoms returns within a month or two of delivery. It did not appear from his study that the subsequent course of the disease was adversely affected by the pregnancy.

Stander cared for a young woman 26 years of age when first seen in 1936. She was delivered spontaneously in May, 1937. The pregnancy and puerperium were uncomplicated. Six weeks after the delivery she developed an acute arthritis and was bedridden for six months. Symptomatically the patient then improved but had some residual disease. She became pregnant again early in 1939 and had minimal symptoms during pregnancy. Again she was delivered spontaneously, in November, 1939. Her arthritis again became severe to the extent of incapacitation about six weeks postpartum.

CIRCULATORY AND RESPIRATORY DISEASES

Valvular Lesions of the Heart. Organic heart disease, usually rheumatic, complicates pregnancy in about 1 per cent of gravidae. It is a serious complication as evidenced by the fact that it accounts for almost one tenth of all deaths from puerperal causes. Jensen estimates that in the United States about 1,000 maternal deaths from heart disease occur each year. Hamilton and Kellogg find heart disease to account for one quarter of their maternal deaths. In the country at large it is the fourth most prominent factor in maternal mortality, being exceeded only by hemorrhage, infection, and toxemia. Mackenzie holds that systolic murmurs without signs of heart failure are of little significance and that, while mitral stenosis is more serious, its prognosis is variable. If the process is stationary, the size of the heart normal, its rate regular, and the response good, the prognosis is good, whereas, if associated with enlargement of the heart, poor response, and fibrillation, it is very serious.

Functional cardiac murmurs are frequently heard in pregnancy, while serious organic lesions occur about once in every 100 cases. Lamb reported an incidence of cardiac murmurs in pregnant women of 6.1 per cent although only 2.7 per cent showed organic heart disease, the other 3.4 per cent being functional murmurs without lesions. The latter group showed no evidence of strain as pregnancy advanced; nearly all the functional murmurs disappeared after pregnancy. In 22,837 patients with full-term and premature deliveries in the New York Lying-In Hospital, 620 cases had organic heart disease and, of these, 26 or approximately 4 per cent developed congestive heart failure. Oppel, in a study of these 26 patients, found that the development of congestive heart failure depended upon the severity of cardiac damage as well as on extracardiac causes, particularly upper respiratory tract infection and anemia. He further observed that congestive heart failure developed during each of the last eight months of gestation, as well as during the first 24 hours after delivery; that its most frequent and important sign during pregnancy was congestion of the lungs; that it occurred in the older patients, showing that age, as previously emphasized by Hamilton, is an important guide to prognosis (Fig. 387); and that it almost always responded to proper management and treatment, even though pregnancy imposes a progressively increasing strain on the heart.

Generally speaking, the prognosis is most serious in mitral stenosis, either alone or in association with insufficiency. We agree, however, with most recent writers that, even with this lesion, the dangers are often exaggerated, provided the patient has been under observation during a considerable part of the pregnancy, and has received intelligent care. In such cases the prognosis depends less upon the character of the heart sounds and the area of cardiac dullness than upon the presence of myocardial or endocardial lesions, as manifested by the response of the heart rate and blood pressure to exercise.

Congenital heart disease is a rare accompaniment of pregnancy, occurring in only 1.9 per cent of a series of organic heart disease. Mendelson and Pardee, in a recent study of these patients, pointed out that with proper evaluation and management a low mortality will result. The various congenital cardiac lesions merit individual attention. In addition, adequate rest, digitalis, and appropriate obstetrical procedures will be required for those patients showing signs of cardiac insufficiency during pregnancy or labor.

While it is indisputable that mitral disease gives rise to the most untoward symptoms and is probably more serious than any other valvular disease of the heart, it is generally agreed that the prognosis fundamentally depends upon the cardiac function and not on any specific anatomical change. In the prognosis of cardiac patients, according to Hamilton and Thomson, emphasis should be given to signs or history of heart failure, auricular fibrillation, and complicating serious disease. Our own experience is in full agreement with theirs and we are most reluctant to allow pregnancy to continue in cardiac patients with auricular fibrillation or with a history of past failure. Age and the size of the heart are other influencing factors which must be given most serious consideration.

Grave heart lesions complicating pregnancy are generally believed to predispose to premature labor although the reported incidences of this accident vary greatly, as shown by Jensen (1938) in a comprehensive review of the literature. Congestive heart failure is probably associated with this tendency to premature labor. In addition to uterine congestion, insufficient oxidation or increased carbon dioxide content of the blood may play a role in the premature death or delivery of the fetus.

Classification of Patients. At present there is no accurate clinical test for measuring the functional capacity of the heart. Exercise tests are of some value in evaluating the functional ability of the heart but do not give complete information as to what the heart may do under such a strain as pregnancy. The best index of the functional capacity of the heart is obtained by grouping the patient according to the classification of the New York Heart Association. This classification depends upon an estimation of cardiac capacity derived from the patient's history of past and present disability and is not influenced by the presence or absence of physical signs. In 1939 the original functional classification, as proposed by Pardee in 1922, was modified as follows:

Class 1. Patients with cardiac disease and *no limitation of physical activity.* Ordinary physical activity does not cause discomfort. Patients in this class do not have symptoms of cardiac insufficiency, nor do they experience anginal pain.

Class 2 (formerly 2A). Patients with cardiac disease and *slight limitation of physical activity.* They are comfortable at rest. If ordinary physical activity is undertaken, discomfort results, in the form of undue fatigue, palpitation, dyspnea, or anginal pain.

Class 3 (formerly 2B). Patients with cardiac disease and *marked limitation of physical activity.* They are comfortable at rest. Discomfort, in the form of undue fatigue, palpitation, dyspnea, or anginal pain, is caused by less than ordinary activity.

Class 4 (formerly 3). Patients with cardiac disease who are *unable to carry on any physical activity without discomfort.* Symptoms of cardiac insufficiency, or of the anginal syndrome, are present, even at rest. If any physical activity is undertaken discomfort is increased.

As the functional capacity does not always determine the amount of physical activity which should be permitted, the New York Heart Association prepared the following "Therapeutic Classification" to serve as a guide in the management of patients:

Class A. Patients with cardiac disease whose physical activity need not be restricted.

Class B. Patients with cardiac disease whose ordinary physical activity need not be restricted, but who should be advised against unusually severe or competitive efforts.

Class C. Patients with cardiac disease whose ordinary physical activity should be moderately restricted, and whose more strenuous habitual efforts should be discontinued.

Class D. Patients with cardiac disease whose ordinary physical activity should be markedly restricted.

Class E. Patients with cardiac disease who should be at complete rest, confined to bed or chair.

The purpose of this therapeutic classification is to indicate the amount of activity which should be permitted in the individual case. In general, it may be said that in pregnancy the therapeutic classification would follow closely the functional capacity grading; in other words, patients in Class 1 would be given the therapeutic grouping B (Class 1B), those in Class 2, C; those in Class 3, D; and those in Class 4, E. The exception to the above is where activity (rheumatic) is present although the functional capacity may place the patient in Class 1; in such an event the proper grading may be Class 1E.

Treatment. The treatment of heart disease in pregnancy, like the prognosis, is dictated by the functional capacity of the heart. It is, accordingly, expedient in considering this subject to make use again of the functional classification of the New York Heart Association and to review separately the therapeutic problems presented by each group.

Classes 1 and 2. With rare exceptions, patients in these two classes may be allowed to go through pregnancy and the first stage of labor; if the second stage promises to be short spontaneous delivery may be permitted, but if it threatens to be long delivery by forceps is usually desirable.

The successful handling of these patients necessitates punctilious prenatal care and constant supervision during labor. It resolves itself into four chief considerations.

1. Adequate Rest. It is advisable that each patient be given a definite routine with specific instructions as to what she may and may not do. The rules laid down by Hamilton on this subject may be summarized as follows: The patient must be in bed 10 hours each night and, in addition, must lie down one half hour after each meal. Light housework and walking about on the level may be permitted; climbing hills and stairs should be restricted to the absolute practical minimum. The patient should do no washing, should not carry or lift heavy objects, or shake rugs. She should do no shopping; many women have developed congestive heart failure directly following and obviously as the result of a shopping trip to town. If it becomes necessary for the family to move to other quarters (as is so often the case when an addition to the family is expected), it is best to have the mother away from home during the whole process; moving has been the cause of many a failing heart. If possible, another woman should live in the house throughout the pregnancy, not only to help in the routine work and in the shopping, but also to enable the patient to go to bed at once should signs of a failing heart develop. If the gravity of the situation is made plain, a relative may sometimes be induced to serve in this capacity. The patient should, of course, take no exercise; she must learn to spare herself all unnecessary effort and must understand that she cannot have too much rest.

2. Avoidance of Infection. Upper respiratory infections are a particular menace to pregnant women with heart disease and constitute an important contributory cause of heart failure. These infections are, of course, largely unavoidable, but instructions should be given each patient to avoid contact with individuals who have colds or sore throats and to go to bed at once in case she herself develops even slight evidence of such an infection.

3. Recognition of Early Signs of Heart Failure. Every pregnant woman with genuine heart disease should be examined every two weeks. While in the majority of cases decompensation occurs suddenly and unexpectedly, in some instances its onset is slow and gradual and may be detected if attention is continually directed to certain particular signs. Hamilton concurs in the earlier observation of Mackenzie that the first warning sign of heart failure is likely to be persistent rales at the bases of the lungs. With this there is frequently a cough. To be significant, the rales must be persistent, that is, they must still be audible after the patient has taken two or three deep breaths; in this respect they differ from the rales sometimes heard in

normal pregnant women, which disappear, it will be recalled, after one or two deep inspirations. A sudden diminution in the patient's ability to carry out her household duties, increasing dyspnea on exertion, attacks of smothering with cough, and hemoptysis are other signals warning of heart failure.

It may be objected that the program outlined for the early detection of heart failure is scarcely applicable to patients belonging to Classes 1 and 2 since they rarely, if ever, become decompensated during pregnancy. If our prognosis in heart disease complicated by pregnancy were infallible such criticism might be valid. Mistakes, however, are made by the most experienced, and for all our efforts an occasional patient who really belongs to Class 3 will unwittingly be grouped in one of the better classes. In order to safeguard the interests of such a patient, it seems desirable to consider all cases of heart disease in pregnancy as potential subjects for decompensation and to carry out the fortnightly examinations as described.

4. Care during Labor. A period of rest in bed in the hospital, preferably for a week or two, is always a beneficial preparation for labor. For some patients in Class 1 this may be unnecessary; for patients in Class 2 it is extremely desirable; for patients in less favorable classes it is imperative. During the stay in the hospital the question often arises as to the advisability of digitalization as a prophylactic measure against heart failure during labor. While the question may be debatable, it seems more rational to withhold digitalis during pregnancy and labor until signs of cardiac embarrassment actually develop. This policy has at least the following advantage: in the event heart failure does become imminent during labor, digitalis may be administered in full doses and intravenously, whereas, if the patient has already been partly digitalized the drug must be employed cautiously and cannot be used intravenously without danger.

With active labor begun, the patient should be placed and kept in a semi-recumbent position with the head and shoulders well elevated by pillows. Observations on the pulse and respiration should be made every half hour during the first stage of labor and every 10 minutes during the second. A rise in the pulse rate above 115 or in the respirations above 28, particularly when associated with dyspnea, are signs of cardiac embarrassment which, unless checked, may become forerunners of heart failure. Only in the presence of a completely dilated cervix, however, may they be taken as indications for delivery. With the cervix only partially dilated and the patient showing evidence of cardiac embarrassment, there is no known method of delivery which will not tend to precipitate rather than to forestall heart failure. Under these circumstances the treatment is always morphine and digitalis. The latter may be most effectively administered by the intravenous route, advantage being taken of some of the modern preparations which are rapid in action. Under morphine, the labor pains usually cease for three or four hours and the patient is permitted an interval of rest and sleep. Under this therapy the signs of cardiac embarrassment usually disappear rapidly and when pains recur the patient may be allowed to continue in labor until complete dilatation is reached, when forceps may be applied.

Signs of cardiac embarrassment developing after complete dilatation of the cervix are indications for immediate forceps delivery, unless spontaneous birth may be expected within a few minutes. Of vital importance is the kind of anesthetic used. Chloroform is contraindicated for many reasons, chiefly because it is a cardiac depressant. Nitrous oxide is undesirable because of the attendant cyanosis. The anesthetic of choice is probably continuous caudal or ether, administered by the drop method on an open mask. Local infiltration anesthesia is also satisfactory.

Patients who have shown no evidence of cardiac distress during pregnancy and labor sometimes collapse suddenly immediately after the birth of the child. This is apparently the result of the sudden decrease in intra-abdominal pressure and the consequent engorgement of the splanchnic vessels. In order to prevent this accident, it should be a routine practice in cases of heart disease to apply a tight binder to the abdomen immediately after the delivery of the placenta. Some obstetricians apply sandbags to the abdomen for this purpose and believe them to be more effectual.

Even with the first day or two of the puerperium over, the danger of heart failure is not necessarily past, for sometimes following a latent period of two or three days there occurs an attack of decompensation on the fourth or fifth day of the puerperium. The cause of this delayed heart failure does not seem clear, but it may be associated with beginning diuresis. All patients with heart disease should be kept in bed two weeks or more following delivery and, upon discharge, should be given detailed advice concerning contraception.

Class 3. Patients whose cardiac reserve is so diminished that they have been grouped in Class 3 present difficult problems and sometimes demand such nicety of judgment and care in handling as to exhaust the combined resources of the cardiologist and the obstetrician. In the first place, the question arises: Should they become pregnant? Rationally the answer is "No." But considerations of sentiment sometimes outweigh in mothers' minds those of reason and many women will risk much for a baby. Provided that such patients appreciate the risk and are willing and able to cooperate with the physician to the fullest extent, it is probably the physician's duty to acquiesce. The husband and relatives must understand fully, of course, the contingencies which may develop. The rules for prenatal care which have already been laid down must be rigorously followed. In addition, it is advisable that patients in this group spend one full 24 hours out of every week in bed. Delivery is carried out vaginally as in Classes 1 and 2.

Should frank heart failure develop during the course of pregnancy, it should be an absolute rule that the patient remain in bed in the hospital throughout the remainder of the pregnancy. With rest in bed and digitalis, the signs and symptoms of decompensation often disappear rapidly. This must not, however, give rise to any permanent sense of security. Should the above rule be broken and the patient allowed to go home, the likelihood is that she will return to the hospital before many weeks with a severer grade of heart failure than she had before—possibly a fatal one.

Even though the patient has recently been in failure, or actually is in failure at the time of labor, delivery by the vaginal route is by far the safest. As for abdominal delivery, abundant evidence shows that these very sick women withstand major surgery poorly and that heart disease is never an indication for cesarean section—it is rather a contraindication.

As shown by the recent study of Bunim and Appel, of Class 3 cardiac patients who become pregnant, about one third suffer heart failure before the reproductive process is completed. Hence, provided such a patient presents herself in the first 12 weeks of pregnancy, the question of therapeutic abortion inevitably arises.

As already indicated, the desire of the patient for a child may be a determining factor in the decision. However, in most cases it is a decision which the obstetrician must make. The two factors which should carry the greatest weight in his reasoning are: a history of previous heart failure and the age of the patient. If there is a history of previous decompensation, whether or not it occurred in a previous pregnancy, the likelihood of heart failure in the present pregnancy is of the order of 65 per cent, according to Bunim and Appel's study as well as those of others. As I assess life's values, such a history is an urgent indication for therapeutic abortion. The other important factor which must be weighed in the balance is the age of the patient. As shown in Fig. 387, the incidence of failure rises sharply after the thirty-fifth year and reaches such levels that this age factor alone in a Class 3 patient may warrant interruption of pregnancy.

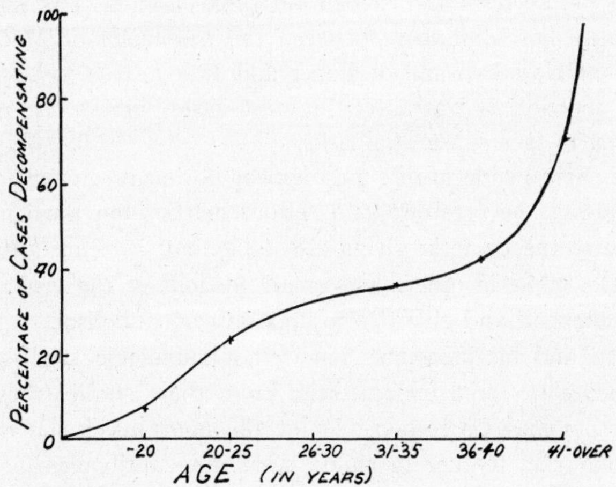

FIG. 387.—THE EFFECT OF INCREASING AGE ON THE FREQUENCY OF HEART FAILURE IN PREGNANCY. (Courtesy of Dr. Stanley Lesse.)

CLASS 4. The treatment of patients in Class 4 resolves itself, essentially, into the treatment of heart failure in pregnancy, labor, and the puerperium. A cardinal fact to be remembered in handling this type of patient is the following: *in the presence of heart failure, delivery by any known method carries with it a maternal mortality of more than 50 per cent.* Accordingly, the treatment of heart failure in the pregnant state becomes chiefly a medical one, the salient objective being to allay the decompensation. Only when this has been accomplished can one deliver the patient with any degree of safety.

Heart Block. Heart block is a very rare complication of pregnancy, Jensen being able to collect only 14 cases from the literature in 1938 and Hamilton having seen only two cases in 20 years as cardiologist to the Boston Lying-In Hospital. The infrequency of heart block in pregnancy is understandable when it is noted that the condition is twice as frequent in men as in women and that 90 per cent of the cases are seen in persons over 50. A number of women with complete heart block have gone through pregnancy satisfactorily, but if there is a history of repeated Stokes-Adams seizures, or other evidence of inadequate functional capacity of the heart, therapeutic abortion may be indicated.

Coarctation of the Aorta. Coarctation of the aorta is a rare but grave complication of pregnancy. In 29 cases reviewed from the literature by Mendelson, five patients died during pregnancy or soon after delivery. He found that the pregnancy had a deleterious effect on the condition in over half the cases and believes that therapeutic abortion is always indicated. On the basis of an extensive experience with heart disease in pregnancy, Hamilton gives a better prognosis but advises a regimen of restricted activity with careful guard against unnecessary strains. Baber and Daley are somewhat more sanguine about the outlook than is Mendelson. The one patient with coarctation of the aorta whom I have seen in pregnancy, a private patient, did very well, but there were definite signs of hypertensive encephalopathy in the last three months, especially severe headaches, dizziness, and arm numbness. Because of this she had to stay in bed the last six weeks. I delivered her by cesarean section two weeks before term and carried out tubal ligation. The way of wisdom in these cases probably lies somewhere between the pessimism of Mendelson and the relative optimism of Hamilton and of Baber and Daley. It is my opinion, however, that therapeutic abortion is warranted in most cases, unless the patient and her husband are willing to face substantial risks.

Endocarditis. Acute endocarditis may appear during pregnancy, just as at other times. It should always be regarded as a serious matter, but particularly so at this time, as occasionally the bacteria giving rise to it may be transmitted to the fetus and cause its death, while in other cases small portions of the vegetations upon the valves may be broken off and give rise to apoplexy or embolism.

In 1937 Felsen and his associates reported immunologic studies in a pregnant woman with subacute bacterial endocarditis. From these studies they reasoned that at least three factors may be responsible for the nontransmission of *Streptococcus viridans* bacteremia from mother to child: circulating antibodies, bactericidal properties of the placenta, and a protective filtration action on the part of the chorionic epithelium.

A careful review of the literature reveals only 18 authentic cases of subacute bacterial endocarditis in pregnancy. In a recent study of 200 cases of subacute bacterial endocarditis Wheeler was able to find evidence of a precipitating factor in 54. Nine of these cases were ascribable to delivery or abortion, such causes being second in incidence only to upper respiratory infections. It would seem reasonable that at the time of delivery the prophylactic use of sulfonamides and, particularly, penicillin would be of benefit in preventing the inception of subacute bacterial endocarditis in patients known to have had rheumatic heart disease or congenital heart disease. However, there are as yet no reliable published data in support of this belief.

Occasionally, cases of tachycardia for which no explanation can be given are observed during pregnancy.

Emphysema. When pregnancy occurs in women suffering from advanced emphysema, the dyspnea may become so intense as to demand its artificial interruption. In a certain number of cases premature labor occurs spontaneously, the untimely uterine contractions being attributed to insufficient aeration of the blood.

Asthma. The symptoms of asthma are sometimes markedly aggravated during pregnancy. However, complete or partial relief of symptoms at this time is encountered considerably more frequently. In rare instances the disease makes its appearance only during pregnancy or at the time of labor, disappearing spontaneously after childbirth.

Asthma should be investigated from an etiologic point of view, and, if the specific irritant is found by skin tests, its complete elimination will usually effect a cure. This is the experience in more than one-half the patients with this disease. The parenteral injection of 0.5 cc. of a 1:1000 solution of epinephrine hydrochloride, or 0.03 gm. of ephedrine sulfate administered orally, may be used several times a day with results comparable to those obtained in the nonpregnant state. Because of its action as a respiratory depressant, morphine should *not* be used. Local anesthesia at the time of delivery is best, but ether may be used if necessary. Asthma, save in exceptional circumstances, does not represent an indication for therapeutic abortion.

Dyspnea. Almost every woman in the last few weeks of pregnancy suffers more or less from shortness of breath resulting from interference with the motility of the diaphragm by the enlarged uterus. Dyspnea occurring in the earlier months of pregnancy is usually due to cardiac or renal disease, and demands a thorough physical examination. Occasionally it follows excessive distention of the uterus, as in hydramnios.

Bronchiectasis. Bronchiectasis is occasionally seen in pregnant women, the incidence in our hospital being 7 in 23,000 cases, or 0.03 per cent. In addition to the very productive cough, dyspnea becomes more marked as pregnancy advances, while sometimes cyanosis develops as term is approached. The treatment is essentially the same as in the nonpregnant individual. At the time of delivery special attention should be paid to the type of anesthesia employed; in our experience local infiltration has given very satisfactory results. Recently, continuous caudal anesthesia has been recommended as being well suited. Postural drainage, even during sleep, is of importance; patients with this disease have a decreased pharyngeal reflex and, often, other additional upper respiratory infections, with the result that constant reinfection occurs. As pulmonary tuberculosis may be associated with this condition, but more particularly because tuberculosis may be overlooked and diagnosed as bronchiectasis, a complete investigation to exclude an acid-fast infection should be carried out in all cases of bronchiectasis. In very advanced bronchiectasis it may be advisable that the mother not be allowed to suckle her offspring.

Varicosities. Owing to the pressure of the pregnant uterus upon the veins returning from the thighs and the resultant increase in venous pressure, abnormalities in the circulation are frequently observed in gestation and manifest themselves by the appearance of varicose veins. The condition is much more frequent in multiparae, especially in patients of great parity. The varicosities may assume considerable proportions in the legs and about the vulva, and in rare instances may develop in the vaginal mucosa. Varicose veins are a very common cause of discomfort in pregnancy and when vulvar in character may occasionally give rise to bothersome but rarely serious bleeding at the time of delivery. On the other hand, it has been reported that hemorrhage from rupture of a vaginal varix may give rise to such profuse hemorrhage as to be fatal.

The usual treatment of varicose veins in pregnancy comprises the use of elastic stockings or bandages. In addition, the patient should be urged to seize every opportunity to sit with her affected leg elevated in order to accelerate the return flow of blood. Moreover, for obvious reasons, she should be warned against prolonged standing, as in ironing, for instance. In regard to the justification of more active treatment of varicose veins in pregnancy by injection and/or ligation, there is difference of opinion. Hamilton, Pittam and Higgins have reported 591 cases of varicose veins in pregnancy treated with ligation and/or injection and obtained unsatisfactory results in only 4 per cent of their patients. No patient aborted or went into premature labor from treatment, nor was there any case of posttherapeutic embolism. Not one patient who had active therapy of her varicose veins during pregnancy had a postpartum phlebothrombosis or thrombophlebitis. Labial varicosities were treated in 58 multiparae with gratifying results; in this type of varicosity this is the only kind of therapy which offers consistent and substantial relief from symptoms. On the other hand, injection therapy and especially ligation are not without some slight hazard and a few isolated fatalities are on record. If the purpose of this active type of therapy is to forestall embolism in the puerperium, this would scarcely seem worth while because, as Mengert points out, the incidence of fatal pulmonary embolism in the puerperium is less than once in 7,000 cases and it is just as likely to occur in patients without external varicosities. If the main purpose is to relieve discomfort, this can usually be achieved, albeit less completely, by the simple methods mentioned above. In this connection it should be recalled that such varicosities always regress in the puerperium and often disappear entirely. Because of these several circumstances it is perhaps the consensus that ligation and/or injection therapy is infrequently indicated in pregnancy.

Estrogenic therapy in certain types of varicose veins complicating pregnancy has been recommended by McCausland and others. McCausland believes that estrogenic therapy is especially helpful in patients with telangiectatic areas unsuitable for injection or in patients who have symptoms from dilated veins which are not actually varicose. He reports relief from symptoms in 65 to 75 per cent of such cases by this method of management. Stilbestrol is the form in which estrogen is given for this purpose in dosages of 5 mg. three times daily. Although the estrogenic therapy of varicose veins in pregnancy is not a widely accepted method, it would seem worthy of trial.

Phlegmasia. Thrombosis of the veins of the thigh, or phlegmasia, is a very rare complication of pregnancy. Goldsborough, in 1904, reported a case and collected the literature upon the subject. Since 1932, Stander saw three cases in over 41,000 pregnancies. While there is no evidence that it is due to infection, as is the case with puerperal phlebitis, it should be regarded as a serious condition, particularly in view of the fact that incautious manipulations may lead to the detachment of small particles of a thrombus, which may then give rise to embolism of the pulmonary arteries. On the other hand, thrombosis of the superficial vessels of the leg is frequently observed in women suffering from varicose veins and is rarely serious.

Hemorrhoids. Hemorrhoidal varices may develop during the antenatal period and may produce rectal bleeding. On the other hand, they may become thrombosed or may protrude through the anal orifice thereby causing pain and discomfort. Protrusion of hemorrhoids is also seen during the second stage of labor when the patient is bearing down. A low-residue diet, mineral oil, cold applications, and anesthesan suppositories or ointment usually suffice for the average case. If bleeding is persistent, hemorrhoidectomy under local anesthesia may be required. The injection treatment is rarely employed during pregnancy.

Edema. Moderate edema of the ankles is a frequent accompaniment of late pregnancy, especially during warm weather. This is an understandable result of the increased venous pressure in the lower extremities during gestation (Fig. 160). While ankle edema should always prompt investigation to rule out toxemia, the condition is usually of no concern. On the other hand, finger and face edema may be an ominous sign and suggests preeclampsia.

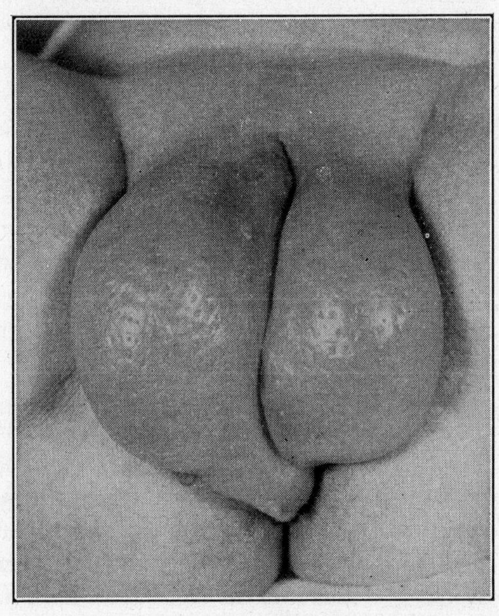

Fig. 388.—Edema of the Vulva in Pregnancy.

Edema of the vulva is occasionally seen in severe degree during late gestation, as illustrated in Fig. 388. As a rule it is encountered in association with either a twin pregnancy or preeclampsia or eclampsia, but may be observed in the absence of these conditions. It may also be seen after traumatic attempts at delivery. The treatment of edema of the vulva in pregnancy is bed rest, a salt-poor diet and temporizing, if possible, until delivery can be safely accomplished. Occasionally, the discomfort of the patient makes aspiration necessary. Because of the obvious danger of infection, meticulous sterile technic is mandatory and in addition it is well to accompany the procedure by an injection of penicillin. At the time of delivery, surprisingly enough, the swollen vulva usually rises away from the presenting part and seldom causes difficulty.

LIVER AND ALIMENTARY TRACT DISEASES

Icterus. Pregnancy is occasionally complicated by jaundice, which is usually due to an inflammatory process in the duodenum or to cholelithiasis. The catarrhal variety is generally without significance and undergoes spontaneous cure. At the same time, it should be borne in mind that jaundice may represent the onset of acute yellow atrophy of the liver, while its association with pernicious vomiting or eclampsia is indicative of profound lesions in the liver and adds greatly to the seriousness of the prognosis; for this reason simple icterus should not be diagnosed until a careful examination has excluded such possibilities.

Acute Yellow Atrophy of the Liver (Acute Infectious Hepatitis). Acute yellow atrophy of the liver, which has recently been shown to be an advanced form of acute infectious hepatitis, is an acute and widespread autolytic necrosis of the liver cells, characterized clinically by jaundice, a reduction in the size of the liver, and toxic disturbances of cerebration often leading to a fatal issue. Approximately 60 per cent of the reported cases have occurred in pregnant women. The explanation for this special predilection of pregnant women for the disease is not known. Acute yellow atrophy of the liver is ordinarily observed during the second half of pregnancy or early in the puerperium, although some authors have described cases at the sixth and eighth weeks of gestation approximately. Fortunately, the disease is a rare complication of pregnancy, being reported once in about every 10,000 pregnancies.

Etiology. As has been pointed out by Lucké and others, there can be little doubt that "idiopathic" acute yellow atrophy of the liver represents the end stage of epidemic hepatitis. In an outbreak of acute infectious hepatitis in Jerusalem, Zondek and Bromberg studied 29 cases in pregnant women, five of whom died from acute yellow atrophy. These authors believe that undernutrition is an important predisposing factor. A similar clinical and pathological picture can also be produced by certain chemical poisons, such as arsenic, chloroform, phosphorus, and cinchophen.

Pathology. In acute yellow atrophy the liver rapidly diminishes in weight; in a comparatively short time its weight may be reduced to less than one half of the normal. Its capsule assumes a wrinkled appearance and the entire organ becomes softened. On section it varies from dark red to almost chrome yellow in color, and upon closer examination each lobule is seen to present a reddish center surrounded by a yellowish periphery.

The histologic findings vary according to the severity of the disease. In mild cases the center of each lobule has undergone necrosis and the cells of the periphery present an almost normal appearance, while between the two is a thicker or thinner zone of cells presenting more or less advanced fatty degeneration. In other cases almost the entire parenchyma of each lobule is destroyed and is converted into a mass of necrotic débris, while about the periphery only an occasional well-preserved liver cell is seen; at the same time the interlobular spaces with their blood vessels and biliary canals are but little changed. The kidneys present signs of acute nephritis and the epithelial cells lining the convoluted tubules are in all stages of degeneration, and in extreme cases are entirely necrotic, while the lumens are filled with casts and débris. On the other hand, the glomeruli and the cells lining the collecting tubes are but little changed.

Symptoms. The symptoms are identical whether the disease occurs during pregnancy or the puerperium, and if convulsions appear it is usually mistaken for eclampsia. In acute cases the symptoms may come on so suddenly as to arouse a suspicion of phosphorus or some other form of poisoning. Thus it may happen that a woman, who previously was in apparently perfect health, may be seized with pains in the abdomen, intense headache, and possibly severe vomiting and purging. In a short time she becomes torpid or violently delirious and soon passes into a condition of coma which may be disturbed by convulsions. In most cases the coma continues for a few hours or days until death supervenes, but recovery may occasionally occur. There is generally a certain amount of jaundice, which may vary from a mere discoloration of the conjunctivae to pronounced general icterus. The vomited matter is frequently blood-stained and sometimes assumes a coffee-ground appearance. The urine is diminished in amount, very highly colored, and contains albumin, all varieties of casts, and frequently large quantities of blood. Fever is usually absent, or the temperature may be even subnormal until just before death when it may rise to a high point. The pulse and respiration tend to be rapid, and the blood pressure remains normal until renal insufficiency develops. Due to the concentration of the blood the red cells are slightly increased in number, and the leukocytes somewhat more so, while the hemoglobin content is diminished. In delayed chloroform poisoning the symptoms are very similar, and death usually occurs within a week following the anesthesia. Should the patient survive for a longer period, the chances for recovery are excellent. Sheehan recently reported the pathologic findings in a large series of cases to which reference is made in the section on delayed chloroform poisoning.

In other cases the course of the disease is less rapid, and in its early stages may in certain respects simulate preeclampsia. Slight jaundice, however, soon appears, the patient gradually becomes more and more apathetic and torpid, and eventually passes into a condition of coma, which often terminates in death. In this class of cases the diminution in the size of the liver may be traced by percussion, and in one of our patients the area of hepatic dullness became diminished by more than one half in the course of a week. If the disease occurs during pregnancy, the fetus usually dies as a result of the toxemia, and may be expelled from the uterus. In such cases, examinations of the fetal organs may reveal extensive hepatic and renal lesions, and thus aid in establishing the diagnosis before the death of the mother. When recovery ensues, the convalescence is sometimes tedious, not so much on account of the damage to the liver, which is relatively quickly repaired, but as a result of the renal insufficiency.

Chemical examination of the urine shows changes similar to those observed in acute phosphorus poisoning. The total nitrogen is usually increased, and its partition always presents marked changes, the urea being always diminished and the ammonia coefficient greatly elevated. Moreover, there is a marked increase in the amino acids, and crystals of leucine and tyrosine may occasionally be demonstrated by appropriate procedures. Acetonuria is usually present.

The blood chemistry has been studied in a few cases. In a patient studied by Stadie and Van Slyke, the urea nitrogen was within normal limits, but the amino acid nitrogen was so increased as to exceed it, while the total nonprotein nitrogen was not determined. The plasma-bicarbonate was at first above normal, but gradually fell, reaching 49 volumes per cent on the day of death. It would appear that a primary alkalosis had been replaced by an acidosis as the end approached. Examination of the liver showed that it contained three times the normal amount of amino acids. Such variations in the amino acid metabolism are satisfactorily explained by supposing that, as the result of cell destruction, the liver function had become so insufficient as to affect the normal mechanism for deaminizing the amino acids and for synthesizing urea. It is generally agreed that the increased amino acid content of the blood results from autolysis of the liver cells, rather than from the absorption of the products of intestinal digestion.

Stander and Cadden obtained several blood specimens, over a period of three days, from a patient who had developed acute yellow atrophy of the liver immediately following delivery. Their findings show remarkable changes in the blood chemistry, as indicated by the following values, obtained as soon as the diagnosis became apparent which was three days before death:

Nonprotein nitrogen	62.4 mg. per 100 cc. blood
Urea nitrogen	11.4 mg. per 100 cc. blood
Uric acid	5.7 mg. per 100 cc. blood
Amino acid nitrogen	9.9 mg. per 100 cc. blood
Creatinine	2.4 mg. per 100 cc. blood
Chlorides	480 mg. per 100 cc. blood
Sugar	47 mg. per 100 cc. blood
CO_2 combining power	34.3 volumes per cent.

It is fairly well established that urea is formed exclusively in the liver, that deaminization of amino acids depends on the liver and that the destruction of uric acid likewise takes place in the liver. We may then conclude that the above values, noted in acute yellow atrophy and showing an increase in amino and uric acid and a decrease in urea and sugar in the blood, may be adequately explained on a basis of liver damage. It has been well demonstrated by Mann and Magath that a decrease in blood sugar follows partial removal of or damage to the liver. The increase in nonprotein nitrogen, noted in the above case, is undoubted evidence of the effect of the disease on the kidneys, resulting in nitrogenous retention. The value for the CO_2 combining power indicates a relative or developing acidosis, dependent undoubtedly on the deranged carbohydrate metabolism and the accumulation of organic acids.

Diagnosis. The diagnosis can usually be made from the clinical findings and history. Although the occurrence of convulsions may lead to a suspicion of eclampsia, the appearance of jaundice should always be suggestive, in which case chemical examination of the blood and urine should confirm the diagnosis. When occurring in early pregnancy the condition sometimes cannot be differentiated from toxemic vomiting, since the lesions, symptoms, and urinary changes are almost identical. In rare cases of gas bacillus puerperal infection, the patient may present all of the clinical signs and chemical findings of acute yellow atrophy. In 1928, we made such a diagnosis, but autopsy showed that the liver did not present the characteristic lesions, but instead contained gas cysts, and that death was due to gas bacillus infection. Kohl has described a similar experience. The prognosis is always bad, the possibility of recovery depending upon the extent of the organic lesions; as this cannot be determined during life, one should be most cautious in stating the outlook.

The recent past history of the patient is important, as many drugs, taken for the relief of chronic pain, produce liver damage, especially cinchophen derivatives. Mercury, phosphorus, and arsenic, likewise, produce liver injury. Over 100 cases of acute yellow atrophy of the liver following salvarsan treatment have been reported in the literature.

Persistent vomiting, dizziness, and headache occurring in a pregnant woman, especially when near term, must be carefully investigated and, if not readily explained, the patient must be hospitalized in order that careful blood and urine examinations may be performed. Acute yellow atrophy of the liver must be considered in the differential diagnosis. If these symptoms are combined with jaundice and drowsiness, the diagnosis of liver damage is almost certain. Drowsiness is sometimes the outstanding early symptom.

In acute yellow atrophy the biphasic van den Bergh reaction is often observed, due to damage to liver cells and obstruction in the bile passages from cholangitis, the former giving the delayed and the latter the prompt direct reaction. The icteric index of the blood will also be very definitely raised, furnishing further evidence of clinical jaundice.

Treatment. If the condition occurs during pregnancy, the uterus should be emptied as rapidly as is consistent with the safety of the patient. General anesthesia, because of its effect on the liver cells, is contraindicated in any operative or delivery procedure in a patient suffering from acute yellow atrophy or in whom this disease is suspected.

Since the work of Whipple and his collaborators, the intravenous administration of glucose solutions has been recognized as most useful in protecting the liver from further damage and in stimulating its repair. When the diagnosis of acute yellow atrophy is definitely established, glucose should be administered immediately and in large amounts. A 20 to 25 per cent solution may be given intravenously in amounts ranging from 500 to 1,000 cc. In the case of the patient referred to above we gave a continuous 10 per cent glucose solution intravenously at the rate of 60 drops per minute. Careful and frequent estimation of the blood sugar and of acetone and diacetic acid in the urine should be made in order that a developing ketosis may be detected. When sugar is found to be passing through the kidneys, as shown by urinalysis, the amount of glucose administered by vein must be decreased. Should the alkali reserve decrease, resulting in an acidosis, as shown by a sharp drop in the CO_2 combining power, the patient should receive alkali in the form of sodium bicarbonate by mouth or per rectum, or molar solution of sodium lactate. It is of course essential that the CO_2 combining power of the blood be determined at intervals in order that one may detect and guard against an alkalosis following too vigorous an alkali therapy. With this form of therapy, that is, interruption of pregnancy if the disease occurs in the antenatal period, large amounts of glucose administered intravenously, and anti-acidosis treatment, Stander had three deaths in ten patients with acute yellow atrophy of the liver, or a mortality of 30 per cent.

Gallstones. The fact that cholelithiasis occurs more frequently (twice or three times more often) in women than in men would suggest a possible association with the increase in the amount of cholesterin in the blood which characterizes pregnancy. However, in a recent review of the literature Robertson and Dochat come to the conclusion that pregnancy cannot account to any great extent for the higher incidence of gallstones in women. Acute attacks may occur during pregnancy or the puerperium, and Peterson in 1910 collected 25 operations performed in the former, and 10 in the latter period. It is always a serious complication, and operation, if urgently demanded, should be undertaken without regard to the existence of pregnancy. In less urgent cases it is, of course, advisable to postpone interference until after the child has become viable or been delivered. In more than 40,000 pregnant women Stander encountered seven cases of gallbladder disease, four of which required operation, two suffering from acute and two from chronic cholecystitis and cholelithiasis. These operations were performed during the first four months of pregnancy. Of the four patients upon whom operation was performed, three were delivered at term of living children, while the outcome of the pregnancy in the fourth is not known, owing to unsuccessful follow-up.

Heartburn. Heartburn is one of the most common complaints of pregnant women. Gastric analyses in patients with heartburn show that in the majority of cases a relative anacidity exists. Hence, the old concept that heartburn is due to hyperacidity is not tenable in most cases. Heartburn, or the sensation of burning in the lower thorax, is essentially the manifestation of a neuromuscular disturbance consequent upon diminished gastric motility. The latter, as already explained, is a constant "physiological" accompaniment of pregnancy and results in reverse peristaltic waves and the regurgitation of stomach contents into the esophagus. It is this irritation of the esophageal mucosa which causes heartburn.

The most logical, and frequently the most effective treatment of the condition is the administration of prostigmine to stimulate gastric motility. N. H. Williams has found that a single injection of 0.5 mg. of prostigmine (neostigmine methylsulfate) intramuscularly will sometimes give relief for several days. Tablets of prostigmine for oral administration, in the form of neostigmine bromide, 15 mg., taken three times daily have been more helpful in my own experience. Designed also to improve gastric motility, dilute hydrochloric acid, U. S. P., 2 cc. in half a glass of water before meals, may also prove beneficial in some cases. The above measures are directed at the cause of heartburn. For immediate relief of the symptom, alkalis give the best results and are the most widely employed form of treatment. However, *sodium bicarbonate should not be used* because the sodium ion tends to promote water retention. Aluminum compounds are equally effective and may be given in several forms: aluminum hydroxide gel (colloidal aluminum hydrate), 4 cc. in water every two to four hours as needed; basic aluminum aminoacetate, in 0.5 gram tablets, three or four times daily as needed; and aluminum hydroxide gel with magnesium trisilicate in tablet form. The latter two preparations are manufactured for the purpose by pharmaceutical firms.

Constipation. Owing to distention by the growing uterus, the abdominal walls may become so impaired in tonicity that considerable difficulty is experienced in evacuating the bowels. Indeed, it may be said that the majority of pregnant women suffer from constipation. This condition should be carefully guarded against in order to avoid auto-intoxication and pyelitis. The association between the latter and constipation is discussed in the following section. Constipation is best overcome by appropriate diet, regularity in going to stool, and the occasional use of mild cathartic pills, the fluid extract of cascara, or compound licorice powder. Mineral oil by itself sometimes does not give satisfactory results, but when taken in combination with the milder laxatives, it enables one to decrease the dose of the latter. The stronger cathartics should be avoided on account of their tendency to cause abortion.

Salivation. In exceptional instances the salivary secretion becomes markedly increased during pregnancy. As a rule, this is not a serious complication, but now and again the amount of saliva is so great as to cause the patient great annoyance and sometimes even prevent her from sleeping. We have had several patients who expectorated between 500 and 600 cubic centimeters of fluid every day for several weeks, while some authors have reported cases in which the secretion in the 24 hours varied from 1,000 to 1,600 cc.

The condition is usually attributed to a reflex neurosis incident to pregnancy, but sometimes it is a manifestation of toxemia. In the first class of cases the treatment is very unsatisfactory, astringent mouth washes, and even comparatively large doses of atropine, being without effect.

It sometimes happens that the cloudy fluid which is supposed to be saliva in reality represents regurgitated gastric secretion. John G. Murray, Jr. had under his care a patient apparently suffering from salivation, who was daily excreting nearly a liter of fluid. Chemical examination in our laboratory revealed the surprising fact that the fluid presented an acid reaction, which was due to the presence of hydrochloric acid in the same proportion as in gastric juice.

That true salivation, amounting to 1,200 cc. or more a day, does occur during pregnancy is shown by the analysis of such secretion in a patient at the New York Hospital. The specific gravity of the secretion was 1.028 with a slightly alkaline reaction to litmus. It contained no free hydrochloric acid and no pepsin but gave a four plus reaction for amylase and contained a slight amount of mucin.

Gingivitis. Exceptionally, the gums of pregnant women become inflamed and spongy, and bleed upon the slightest touch. The condition is usually observed in run-down individuals and is very refractory to treatment, although in many cases it disappears almost immediately after delivery. It is best met by the employment of astringent mouth washes, especially those containing tincture of myrrh, combined with general tonic treatment and an abundant diet. Vitamin deficiencies, especially that of vitamin C, should be considered as possible etiologic factors and the appropriate tests made to prove or disprove such possibilities.

Dental Caries. Many women suffer during pregnancy from dental caries, which may be associated with more or less severe toothache. It is a popular belief that pregnancy predisposes to the condition, as is evidenced by the saying, "For every child a tooth." The literature on the subject is rather confusing in that some authorities believe pregnancy predisposes to dental caries while others hold the view that pregnancy per se plays no role in the condition. A unanimity of opinion probably cannot be reached until the etiology of dental caries is more thoroughly understood. It appears that hereditary, hormonal, dietary, and infectious factors as well as the acidity of the saliva and mineral metabolism may influence the condition. It is our belief that, if proper oral hygiene is maintained and the diet provides for an ample intake of vitamins and mineral elements, pregnancy exerts no deleterious effect on the teeth. Ziskin and Hotelling not only state that pregnancy is not a cause of dental caries but go so far as to say that some factors working during pregnancy actually prevent tooth decay to a significant extent.

It is our practice to advise our patients to consult their dentist more frequently during pregnancy than otherwise and to be sure of an ample supply of minerals and vitamins in their diet.

DISEASES OF THE NERVOUS SYSTEM

Paralysis. Paralysis of central origin sometimes occurs during pregnancy and is generally associated with toxemic or septic processes. Thus, in the toxemias of pregnancy and eclampsia serious disturbances may follow edema of the brain or apoplexy. In infectious processes thrombosis may occur in the cerebral vessels, and occasionally emboli may cut off the circulation of large areas of the brain and lead to various paralyses and even to death.

Paraplegia of spinal origin occasionally occurs but, except in rare cases of toxemia, is not directly dependent upon the existence of pregnancy. It does not appear that spinal paraplegias interfere with conception as women suffering from them frequently become pregnant. In this event, as well as in women with advanced tabes dorsalis, the course of pregnancy is usually uncomplicated and the labor easy and comparatively painless.

Multiple Sclerosis. This disease is a rare complication of pregnancy occurring in one out of every 2,258 patients admitted to the New York Lying-In Hospital. In the majority of cases pregnancy has no effect on the course of multiple sclerosis and it is rarely an indication for therapeutic abortion. It is true that many cases have been reported in which the condition seemed to have been aggravated by pregnancy;

but it must be borne in mind that multiple sclerosis in the nonpregnant state is characterized by unexplained exacerbations and alternating quiescent periods and that any change for the worse observed during gestation might well have developed just the same in the absence of pregnancy. The last four cases of multiple sclerosis complicated by pregnancy followed in our clinic have done very satisfactorily. Most of these patients, as is understandable, have less pain in labor than usual and in some the labors are almost painless.

Neuralgia. Neuralgic pains are frequent concomitants of pregnancy. In rare instances they are very obstinate and resist all treatment though they often disappear spontaneously after labor. During the later months of pregnancy the head of the child, after descending into the pelvis, may compress one or other sciatic nerve and give rise to severe pain along its course, which is sometimes accompanied by intense muscular spasm. Owing to its mode of origin this form of sciatica is not amenable to treatment.

Neuritis. Plass and Mengert, in 1934, reported 12 cases of polyneuritis of pregnancy. They advise prophylaxis with a high vitamin diet, as the etiology of the disease, although unknown, appears to be associated with a deficiency in the intake of vitamin B complex. Fouts, Gustafson and Zerfas advise the use of vitamin B complex for all patients with vomiting of pregnancy as a prophylaxis against the development of polyneuritis. Schultze states that about 7 per cent of all pregnant women show some signs of neuritis and reports good results in 60 patients treated with vitamin B_1. Theobald reported five cases of neuritis late in pregnancy, in four of which he obtained a complete cure with this vitamin.

In addition there is a traumatic neuritis appearing in the puerperium. Tillman reported 9 cases in 18,800 deliveries. In such cases delivery has usually been difficult and in about 75 per cent of them forceps had been employed. The neuritis is undoubtedly due to injury to the lumbosacral plexus, the peroneal portion of the sciatic nerve being most frequently affected according to Tillman. We have had four similar cases of foot-drop during the past two and one half years; and in each case delivery was performed with forceps. Treatment is designed to rest the affected member in proper position. Later passive and active exercises are instituted. The prognosis should be guarded as recovery, partial or complete, may extend over a period of years.

Poliomyelitis. Poliomyelitis occasionally develops in pregnancy but is generally regarded as not complicating the pregnancy or delivery save in an instance, such as Harmon and Hoyne report, of maternal respiratory paralysis resulting in maternal and fetal anoxemia. No evidence has been found that intra-uterine poliomyelitis occurs. Aycock was able to report 56 cases of poliomyelitis in pregnancy, 28 collected from the literature and 28 of his own. Recent reports have increased the number of cases to 75. In 1944 Weaver and Steiner presented experimental evidence suggesting that chorionic gonadotrophic hormone, or a related substance, might play a role in increasing resistance of the pregnant woman in the early months of gestation to the virus. In their experimental animals, cotton rats, they found no evidence of transmission of the virus from mother to fetus in utero or to the offspring through the secretions of the mammary glands.

In the rare instances where poliomyelitis is followed by maternal respiratory paralysis, the method of delivery will depend in great part on the extent and involvement of the paralysis. Where both the intercostal muscles and diaphragm are paralyzed, cesarean section under local anesthesia may be the procedure of choice. Satisfactory artificial respiration can be maintained through the use of a positive pressure closed system machine. We have seen only one patient with such complete respiratory paralysis and in her case a cesarean section under intratracheal positive pressure with cyclopropane anesthesia was performed with a satisfactory result to both mother and child.

Myasthenia Gravis. Myasthenia gravis is another rare complication of pregnancy. As in the nonpregnant it is characterized by exacerbations and remissions of an abnormal state of fatigability of certain voluntary muscles. It may become aggravated in pregnancy nothwithstanding adequate treatment with prostigmine and, as in a patient treated in our clinic, interruption may be required. On the other hand, Veits, Schwab and Brazier report improvement during pregnancy. An unusual case of myasthenia gravis occurring in an infant born of a myasthenic mother is reported by Strickroot, Schaeffer and Bergo.

Chorea. Patients who in the past have had rheumatic heart disease and who subsequently become pregnant may have a recurrent chorea. When choreic movements become so marked as to interfere with sleeping or the intake of food, the patient becomes maniacal and sedation may be necessary to prevent spontaneous abortion or premature labor. The occurrence of fever, indicating an associated active rheumatic infection, is of serious import and at autopsy evidences of malignant endocarditis are found in the majority of the cases. Apart from meningeal exudates the lesions noted in the central nervous system are variable.

The disease has been exhaustively studied by Buist in 1892, by Pineles in 1913, and by Willson in 1929, who collected 255, 426, and 906 cases, respectively. If the cases reported by Willson are all true Sydenham's chorea, chorea is preeminently a disease of young women, the average age in his tabulation being 22.4 years. With more rational treatment the mortality has slowly fallen from 25 to 30 per cent in the early reports to 14 per cent in Willson's series. In 34,569 pregnancies at the New York Lying-In Hospital, 12 patients were considered to have chorea, 1 of whom died from subacute bacterial endocarditis.

Many patients do very well upon simple medicinal treatment, the disease disappearing before delivery. On the other hand, the febrile cases, indicative of active rheumatic infection, do extremely badly no matter what is done. Willson believes that the induction of abortion is unnecessary in the milder cases and does no good in the severe ones.

Epilepsy. In Stander's experience the incidence of epilepsy complicating pregnancy is 0.14 per cent, or about 1 in every 725 pregnant women. He has had experience with a total of 37 cases of epilepsy in pregnancy. In only 6 of the 37 cases was there a familial history of the disease. Fertility does not appear to be affected as in this group there are 91 pregnancies. This disease appears to have no effect upon pregnancy though at the time of labor it may be mistaken for *eclampsia* by inexperienced observers. If the attacks are frequent the patient should be adjusted on suitable doses of phenobarbital or dilantin. As a rule it is not advisable to allow the mother to nurse her child, as lactation sometimes appears to aggravate the disease, while serious injury might possibly be done to the child during an attack. On the other hand, in occasional instances the mentality of the patient appears to undergo progressive deterioration with each succeeding pregnancy. In such circumstances pregnancy should not necessarily be interrupted, but the advisability of sterilization after delivery should be considered.

Tetany. Tetany is a clinical syndrome characterized by hyperexcitability of the nervous system which is manifested by painful, tonic spasms of the muscles of the arms and legs in the course of which consciousness is occasionally lost. It may result from a number of causes: (1) parathyroid deficiency due to trauma to the parathyroid gland at operation with resultant decrease in serum calcium levels and increase in inorganic phosphorus concentrations; (2) hypocalcemia due to inadequate intake or impaired absorption of calcium; (3) alkalosis due either to hyperventilation or to persistent vomiting with loss of chloride.

As pointed out in an extensive study of the subject by Anderson and Musselman, pregnant women are more prone to develop tetany than nonpregnant persons because of the calcium drain imposed by the fetus. Thus, women who have postoperative tetany are more likely to manifest the syndrome when they are pregnant, and osteomalacic patients usually develop tetany only during gestation. The condition may also make its appearance in cases of severe and persistent vomiting of pregnancy. Moreover, the leg cramps which pregnant women so often experience may possibly be due in certain instances to mild or latent tetany. In labor, tetany may occasionally develop as the result of hyperventilation.

Most cases of tetany encountered in pregnancy respond satisfactorily to calcium administered by mouth. From 2 to 5 gm. of calcium gluconate, dissolved in 30 parts of water, when given orally, will raise the serum calcium to a peak level within 4 hours and is the best initial medication in the majority of cases; after this dose, a calcium preparation should be continued in sufficient dosage to keep the serum calcium at a normal concentration. In tetany resulting from alkalosis the serum calcium and phosphorus are usually normal, but this condition likewise appears to respond favorably to calcium therapy. If the tetany is extremely severe, immediate relief may be had from intravenous calcium gluconate, 0.3 cc. of a 10 per cent solution per kilogram of body weight, but it must be given very slowly with full cognizance of the fact that some slight hazard is involved. Patients who are known to have chronic tetany of long standing are probably best treated with dihydrotachysterol, a synthetic derivative of irradiated ergosterol. Paradoxically enough, milk should be withheld from patients who suffer repeatedly from attacks of tetany and medicinal calcium substituted, because the rich phosphorus content of milk aggravates the condition.

METABOLIC CONDITIONS

Diabetes Mellitus. Prior to the advent of insulin in 1921, the great majority of diabetic women were sterile. At the London Hospital during the years 1893 to 1922, 190 married diabetic women up to the age of 46 years were admitted and of these four, or 2 per cent, were pregnant; from 1923 to 1931, 171 were admitted of whom 27, or 15 per cent, were pregnant, a seven-fold increase in the incidence of pregnancy (Skipper). In 1909 J. Whitridge Williams, after 13 years as Head of the Obstetrical Service of the Johns Hopkins Hospital and with a large consulting practice, had himself encountered but one case of diabetes complicated by pregnancy. During the past 10 years in that same hospital, among 227 married diabetic women between the ages of 15 and 45 who were admitted, 65, or 28.6 per cent, were pregnant. By coincidence this number of pregnant diabetics seen at the Johns Hopkins Hospital during the past decade, namely 65, happens to be the precise number which Williams was able to collect from the entire world's literature.

The underlying cause of the infertility in diabetes during the pre-insulin era was probably due to a number of factors, most of which are poorly understood. Structural changes have been observed in the reproductive organs of diabetics by a number of authors, including disappearance of the graafian follicles and uterine atrophy. Amenorrhea was common in diabetics of that period, its incidence having been placed as high as 50 per cent. Skipper has observed a diabetic patient in whom menstruation, absent for 10 years, returned when the patient was given insulin. This evidence of ovarian dysfunction suggests that the infertility of diabetic women in the pre-insulin era was in all probability hyper- or hypofunction of the "master clock" of the generative tract, the anterior pituitary gland. In addition to endocrine imbalance, nutritional deficiencies must have entered appreciably into the infertility of diabetics before the insulin era since the necessarily restricted diets doubtless entailed dire, if inadvertent, reduction in food elements essential for reproduction.

When diabetic women did occasionally became pregnant in the pre-insulin era, some 25 per cent of the mothers and about 50 per cent of the infants died. In 16 cases reported by Matthews Duncan (three his own, and 13 from the literature), four women died very shortly after delivery, that is, one quarter. In Williams' 66 cases, there was an immediate maternal mortality of 27 per cent. Most of these women died with the characteristic picture of acidosis and coma shortly after delivery. The infant mortality in the two series mentioned was 47 and 41 per cent respectively.

The experience of the pre-insulin era, as surveyed above, is not merely of historical interest but is of great clinical importance, because it shows that untreated diabetes and pregnancy are basically incompatible. On the one hand, the disease if uncontrolled so disrupts the reproductive mechanism as to make successful childbearing almost impossible. On the other hand, untreated diabetes is aggravated by pregnancy to a degree which is often fatal. This mutual incompatibility between neglected diabetes mellitus and pregnancy demands emphasis because only insofar as the disease process can be meticulously controlled and the associated metabolic disturbances curbed, can its baneful effects on the childbearing woman and her infant be forestalled.

Incidence. The frequency with which pregnancy complicated by diabetes is encountered has been variously reported between one in 500 and one in 1,000 pregnancies. The incidence of diabetes increases sharply with age and the maximum susceptibility to the development of the disease in women is not reached until the mid-fifties. Not only is diabetes much more common after the menopause, but its frequency in women between 35 and 44 is three times that seen in women between 25 and 34, and five times the incidence encountered in females between 15 and 24. These figures not only explain the relative infrequence of diabetes in pregnancy, but call to our attention an important clinical fact: when diabetes is encountered in pregnancy, the chances are greatly in favor of its being met in older women in whom various other complications are more frequent, particularly hypertension. The age factor, hence, will often itself contribute a count against diabetic gravidae.

Diagnosis. The presence of sugar in the urine of a pregnant woman may indicate one of three conditions or any combination of them: (1) lactosuria; (2) renal glycosuria; (3) diabetes.

Lactosuria of 100 mg. per cent or more, that is enough to give at least a faint Benedict reaction, is not common except for the last six weeks of pregnancy, being seen in only 1 or 2 per cent of gravidae prior to that time. During the last six weeks its incidence increases to 7 or 8 per cent and to 30 per cent or more on the day before delivery. Lactosuria is most frequent and most marked after delivery, the great majority of puerperae showing it on one day or another. At this time, moreover, the amount of lactose excreted in the urine is often large, reaching sometimes 1 per cent and more. This fact must be borne in mind when evaluating the significance of urinary sugar in diabetic patients in the puerperium.

As stated on page 216, a lowered renal threshold for sugar develops early in pregnancy. Some gravidae show glycosuria at blood sugar levels below 120 mg. per cent and as a consequence glucose may be encountered rather frequently in the urine shortly after meals. Since both diabetic and nondiabetic gravidae manifest this type of glycosuria occasionally, it is clear that, in the former, any reliance on urinary sugar in calculating insulin dosage may be very misleading.

It is an old rule that every patient who shows sugar in the urine should be regarded as a diabetic until proved otherwise. In pregnancy, of course, the frequency of renal glycosuria and lactosuria throws the odds somewhat against diabetes as the most probable diagnosis, particularly if the amount of sugar found is merely a trace. Nevertheless, the above rule should be observed in gravidae as in other patients because if it is not followed diabetics are certain to be overlooked through the erroneous assumption that any urinary sugar found is due either to lactosuria or a lowered renal threshold. This necessitates routine fermentation tests if urinary sugar is present and, if these are positive, routine fasting blood sugar determinations and/or tolerance tests in all pregnant women showing sugar in the urine. By general consensus the diagnosis of diabetes mellitus is established if the fasting blood sugar reaches 0.13 per cent or if, after a meal or during a glucose tolerance test, it reaches 0.17 per cent; if capillary blood is used the latter value is changed to 0.20, the former remaining the same. Since errors in chemical analyses do occur occasionally, all values indicative of diabetes should be confirmed on a second blood specimen.

Effect of Pregnancy on Diabetes. Pregnancy makes diabetes more difficult to control due to the interaction of a number of factors. These may be outlined as follows:

I. Changes in sugar tolerance.

(a) Sugar tolerance is often diminished (more insulin required) due presumably to increased activity of the anterior pituitary gland.

(b) Sugar tolerance is sometimes increased (less insulin required) due either to activity of fetal pancreas or to other factors.

(c) Vomiting, with loss of unknown amounts of carbohydrate food may simulate raised sugar tolerance, may provoke acidosis, and in any event confuses the dietary picture.

(d) During labor the muscular exertion entailed may so deplete the glycogen reserve that sharp alterations in carbohydrate and insulin requirements ensue.

(e) A gain in sugar tolerance often occurs after delivery and hypoglycemia in the puerperium is very common; it may be associated with sudden and extreme vacillations in blood sugar, due apparently to reconversion of bodily mechanisms to their nonpregnant states. Lactation, with conversion of certain amounts of blood glucose into lactose may also play a role. Puerperal infection, even though mild, may precipitate acidosis and coma with great rapidity.

II. Increased tendency to ketosis.

(a) The diminished carbon dioxide combining power of the blood in pregnancy makes gravidae less resistant to acidosis.

(b) The elevated basal metabolic rate in pregnancy increases the tendency toward acidosis.

The changes in sugar tolerance which diabetic women undergo in pregnancy are neither constant nor predictable; nor are they always in the same direction. In most instances they are in the form of a lowered sugar tolerance in the latter half of pregnancy. The four periods of a woman's life at which carbohydrate tolerance tends to be lowered, namely, puberty, menstruation, pregnancy and the menopause, are all, of course, times of intense endocrine change and all are associated with increased activity of the anterior lobe of the pituitary body. The hypertrophy which this gland undergoes in pregnancy, its well known cellular alterations and the acromegalic stigmata which gravidae often show, all attest the hyperactivity of this body in gestation. It is well established also that the anterior lobe of the pituitary secretes a hormone which elevates the blood sugar. On the basis of this and other evidence, the presumable explanation of the lowered carbohydrate tolerance shown in minor degree by many normal pregnant women, and in major degree by many diabetic gravidae, is overactivity of the anterior pituitary lobe. A substantial minority of diabetic gravidae show an increase in tolerance particularly in the latter part of gestation. Although the hypothesis has been suggested that this apparent improvement in diabetes in the latter part of gestation is due to the activity of the fetal pancreas, the evidence in support of this theory is contradictory and it is not generally accepted.

Ketosis and coma constitute the gravest complication which can befall the pregnant diabetic and her infant. Acidosis is probably more common than generally supposed for it may exist with few or no symptoms. Silent acidosis is the cause of many unexplained fetal deaths and, by general accord, acidotic coma is responsible for almost all maternal deaths in this complication. The inherent tendency of pregnant women toward ketosis, therefore, is still another count against them and still another reason why diabetes in pregnancy is more difficult to control.

The Effects of Diabetes on Pregnancy. The effects which diabetes exerts on pregnancy depend in great measure upon the extent to which the disease is controlled. If carefully regulated many of the deadly consequences to the fetus which neglected diabetes regularly imposes, can be eliminated. However, as all statistics show, the disease is potentially inimical to successful pregnancy and even with the best modern care the harmful influences of diabetes often make their appearance causing a greatly increased stillbirth and neonatal death rate. Pregnancy is affected by diabetes as follows:

(a) The incidence of spontaneous abortion and premature delivery is perhaps slightly increased, but very little.
(b) The frequency of toxemia of pregnancy is greatly augmented.
(c) Fetal death in utero before the onset of labor is much more common than in normal, nondiabetic gravidae.
(d) The incidence of excessive sized infants is many times that met in normal pregnancies with the result that mechanical difficulties in labor are more frequent and cesarean section more often necessary.
(e) Hydramnios is more common.
(f) Congenital malformations are more frequent.
(g) Lactation may be inhibited in some cases.
(h) The neonatal period is associated with especial hazards in the forms of hypoglycemia and anoxia.

All authors agree that the frequency of toxemia of pregnancy is greatly augmented. If 7 per cent is taken as the usual incidence of this complication, most reports show a several fold increase, the figures ranging from 25 to 50 per cent. Fetal death in utero prior to the onset of labor is also common. Kramer found that 60 of 238 cases collected from the literature, or about one quarter, resulted in stillborn infants. The incidence of babies weighing 10 or more pounds, born to diabetic mothers, ranges in the various series reported between 15 and 25 per cent. In the childbearing population at large the frequency of such large babies is approximately 3 per cent. The explanation usually given for the high frequency of large babies born to diabetic mothers is hyperglycemia. However, most authors agree that these infants are not just fat but are generally large and it is suspected that endocrine imbalance, particularly in relation to the growth hormone of the anterior pituitary of the fetus, may be a factor in addition to hyperglycemia.

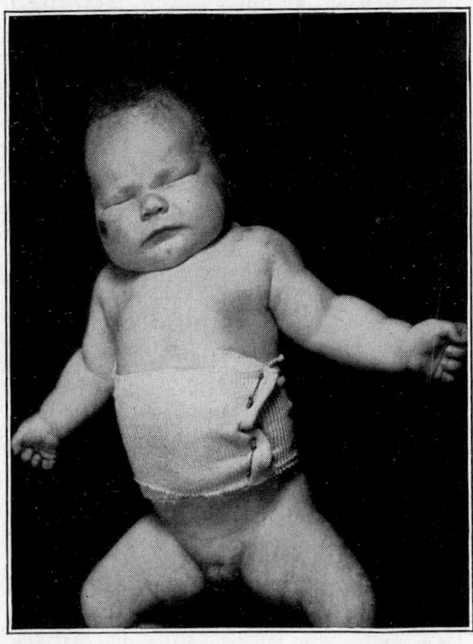

Fig. 389.—Characteristic Large Baby Weighing 5,200 gm., Born of Diabetic Mother.

Prognosis. In 1935 Kramer collected 238 cases from the literature with eight maternal deaths, that is, a maternal mortality rate of 3.0 per cent. *Almost all maternal deaths today from diabetes complicated by pregnancy are due to neglect.* Both the stillbirth and neonatal mortality rates are greatly increased. Although a few series have reported the percentage of infant loss as low as 15 per cent, the average figure recorded is in the neighborhood of 25 per cent. The prognosis for the infant becomes decidedly worse if the diabetes has been longstanding and in cases in which the disease is of 15 years' duration or more, more than half the infants are lost. This is presumably due to the frequency with which hypertensive vascular disease develops in diabetics who have had the disease for 10 years or more. In several such cases Priscilla White has been able to demonstrate the sclerosed uterine arteries by a flat plate of the abdomen and in the presence of such uterine vessels, it is understandable that the outlook for successful pregnancy would be precarious.

Management. The main objective in the management of diabetes complicated by pregnancy is *rigid control of the disease.* This is the responsibility of the internist, who should share jointly with the obstetrician the care of every such case. Once the diagnosis of diabetes is established the patient should be admitted to the hospital for careful evaluation of the diabetic status. She should be admitted again for the same purpose every other month throughout pregnancy and oftener if she shows evidence of a fluctuating carbohydrate tolerance. It is usually unnecessary for these hospital stays to exceed three days, but occasionally control of the disease proves so difficult that hospitalization is required for a fortnight or longer. In addition ambulatory visits to the internist and the obstetrician are made at two-week intervals and blood sugar determinations carried out, either fasting or postprandial. Three weeks before term the patient should again be admitted to the hospital to remain there until after the baby is born. The purpose of this admission is twofold: stabilization of the diabetic preparatory to delivery, and consideration of the desirability and possibility of early delivery.

As has been emphasized repeatedly in this section, blood sugar levels and not urinary sugar must determine the diet and insulin dosage recommended. Internists such as White and Sindoni agree that a rather liberal carbohydrate intake is desirable as a preventive against ketosis. White's recommendations are: 30 to 40 calories per kg., carbohydrate 150 to 250 gm., protein 2 gm. per kg. and fat to complete the caloric prescription. Sindoni finds that an average safe diet for the day is 60 gm. of protein, 80 to 90 gm. of fat and 150 to 180 gm. of carbohydrate; he advocates, however, an extra feeding upon retiring of 15 to 20 gm. of carbohydrate. The same author employs protamine zinc insulin in those patients requiring more than 40 units of plain insulin, but seldom alone, because of the dangers of hypoglycemic reactions during the interval between meals.

During the first trimester, nausea and vomiting may prevent the patient from adhering to her usual diet and insulin dosage. If vomiting is severe, acidosis may become extreme and control exceedingly difficult. During the last trimester vigilant observation must be maintained for evidence of shifting sugar tolerance and for signs of beginning preeclampsia. Changes in insulin dosage must be made cautiously since any sharp increases may subject the patient to hypoglycemic reactions. All authorities agree that if an error is to be made in insulin dosage it should be in the direction of a slight glycosuria. During labor, because of the glycogen demands on the liver, it is well to give the equivalent of 10 gm. of glucose every hour or so. Upon the patient's final admission to the hospital three weeks or so before term, two important obstetrical decisions must be made: when to effect delivery, and how. Because of the tendency of the fetus to succumb as term approaches, and for other reasons, there is a widespread but far from unanimous belief that pregnancy should be terminated by cesarean section before the last fortnight of gestation. Advocates of cesarean section point out that the infant is likely to be large (60 per cent over 8 pounds) with consequent mechanical difficulties in labor, that such babies with their inherent tendency to anoxia stand labor poorly and that this operation, performed a fortnight before term, forestalls the ever-present likelihood of fetal death in utero. Against this viewpoint is the contention that diabetics are poor operative risks and that the outlook is equally good with vaginal delivery provided the disease is well controlled.

It is our practice to admit all diabetic gravidae to the hospital three weeks or so before term not only for stabilization of the diabetes but for consideration of the whole problem of delivery. After it is established that the diabetes is well regulated, the size of the infant is estimated as accurately as possible by palpation and a sterile vaginal examination done. The purpose of the latter is to answer the question: Is the cervix favorable for the induction of labor? An affirmative answer is given to this query if (1) the head is at or below the spines, (2) the cervix admits easily one or more fingers and (3) the cervical canal is less than 1 cm. long. If all three of these criteria are present and provided the infant is thought to weigh between 3,000 and 3,500 gm., the membranes are stripped back and ruptured. In our last 600 inductions by artificial rupture of the membranes we have had no failures provided the cervix was favorable as indicated by the criteria mentioned. If the cervix is not wholly favorable for induction, the next question asked is: How urgent is immediate delivery? Three findings may indicate that it is very desirable: (1) the presence of an associated toxemia; (2) the presence of an obviously large child; and (3) inability to control the diabetes. In the presence of any of these conditions cesarean section is done. If they are not present and the cervix is unfavorable the patient is allowed to go to term in the hospital or until such time as the cervix is favorable. Naturally, such other factors as elderly primigravidity and previous infant loss would also argue for abdominal delivery; contrariwise, marked obesity might serve as a deterrent. Continuous spinal anesthesia is probably the anesthetic of choice if abdominal delivery is performed.

Diabetes may be more difficult to control in the early puerperium than at any other time. The wide and sudden fluctuations which the blood sugar sometimes undergoes during this period are presumably the result of a number of factors: endocrine and metabolic changes associated with the reconversion of bodily mechanisms to their nonpregnant state, slight degrees of puerperal infection, conversion of certain amounts of blood glucose into mammary lactose and possibly the sudden withdrawal of the fetal pancreas. Disturbances in sugar tolerance are most common during the first week postpartum after which the diabetes returns rapidly to its pre-pregnancy status. There is no evidence that pregnancy ever causes permanent aggravation of diabetes.

Two special problems present themselves in the management of the newborn infant of a diabetic mother: hypoglycemia and anoxia. In order to forestall the former Randall and Rynearson recommend the injection of 5 cc. of 10 per cent glucose into each buttock a few minutes after birth. Further such injections are given at intervals regulated by the value of the blood sugar as determined by the micromethod, by the behavior of the infant and by the ability of the infant to take feedings by mouth. The same authors attempt feeding within four hours, giving either 10 cc. of a 10 per cent solution of glucose or 7 cc. of a Karo syrup lactic acid mixture every two hours during the first two or three days. Whenever the feeding is taken poorly or whenever twitchings, convulsive movements or cyanosis indicates, in the opinion of the authors, the development of hypoglycemia, 10 cc. of a 10 per cent solution of glucose is given by mouth if possible; otherwise it is administered intramuscularly.

Although several authorities consider the administration of glucose to the infants to be unnecessary, it is customary to give them sugar, either by mouth or intramuscularly, at frequent intervals during the first three days. It can do no harm and may prove helpful in occasional cases. Obviously, because of the tendency of the newborn to hypoglycemia, insulin should not be given to the mother during the three hours immediately preceding delivery. During the first few days of life, the infants of diabetic mothers should be given the same treatment as premature babies receive in respect to oxygen and heat. This means placing them in an incubator with oxygen so regulated to provide a partial pressure of oxygen between 40 and 50 per cent. The temperature should be about 85° F. and sufficient nursing personnel available to permit constant observation during the first 72 hours. Their care, of course, should be the responsibility of a pediatrician.

Diseases of the Thyroid Gland. Simple colloid goiter, if not attended by hypothyroidism, probably has no influence on pregnancy or vice versa. Hypothyroidism, on the other hand, whether associated with colloid goiter or not, often results in miscarriage as well as in cretinism or congenital goiter in the child. Excellent results in these cases have been reported by Litzenberg and Carey with the use of thyroid extract.

While moderate degrees of exophthalmic goiter occur relatively frequently in women, there is little evidence that pregnancy plays any part in its production. Mussey, Plummer and Boothby reported in 1926 that pregnancy existed in 42 out of a series of 4,185 women of 40 years of age or less, who were treated at the Mayo Clinic for exophthalmic goiter, and stated that in general, pregnancy had little influence on the goiter, and vice versa. Furthermore, they stated that pregnant women stood thyroid operations well, and that there was little indication for interrupting the pregnancy. On the other hand, Seitz stated that in 60 per cent of the 112 cases which he collected from the literature, pregnancy led to exacerbation of the symptoms, with a fatal issue in seven cases. He held that serious consequences are to be apprehended especially when the condition is associated with a persistent thymus, and when death occurs it is usually due to circulatory conditions or to a general intoxication. The child is but little affected, although there is some evidence to indicate that the tendency toward spontaneous premature labor is increased.

Formerly the induction of premature labor was recommended whenever the symptoms became urgent, but with increasing surgical knowledge prompt operation upon the thyroid seems preferable. In 1931 Mussey and Plummer reported 29 cases of Graves' disease and 12 of toxic adenoma of the thyroid in pregnancy. Their statistics showed that with iodine treatment preparatory to surgery, the results are exceedingly good. In their series there was no maternal death, no miscarriage, and only one premature delivery and one stillbirth. In 1940 Javert reported 18 cases of hyperthyroidism in pregnancy at the New York Hospital and recorded an incidence of this complication of 0.07 per cent, in contrast to much higher incidences in the goiter areas. The frequency of toxemia of pregnancy was markedly increased in his cases of hyperthyroidism when compared with that in the entire obstetrical service.

In general, our treatment is in agreement with that of Mussey and his associates. Therapeutic abortion is rarely indicated, as women with hyperthyroidism may be followed safely during pregnancy; iodine therapy is of great value, both during and after pregnancy; thyroidectomy may be performed as part of the treatment regardless of the gestation, although it often is more advisable to postpone surgical procedures till three months or longer postpartum; and, at the time of labor and delivery, analgesia and local infiltration anesthesia are preferable to general inhalation anesthesia, especially nitrous oxide. Propylthiouracil therapy has superseded other methods in some cases of hyperthyroidism and it has been reported effective for control of hyperthyroidism in pregnant women. However, the drug crosses the placenta and may cause hyperplastic changes in the fetal thyroid. On this point available data in the human are meager; hence it may be wise at present to reduce dosage or discontinue the drug two to three weeks before term to allow recovery of the fetal thyroid.

Addison's Disease. Very rarely pregnancy may occur in women suffering from this disease, or it may first become manifest after the onset of pregnancy. In either event it is a very serious complication. Fitz-Patrick, who has collected 12 cases from the literature, reports that five of the women died before delivery, but in those who survived, pregnancy and labor appeared to have had no effect upon the underlying disease.

Obesity. Obesity is a handicap for pregnant women on several scores. The infants are likely to be excessive in size and in Matthews and Der Brucke's series of gravidae who weighed over 200 pounds, one half the babies weighed over 3,600 gm. (8 pounds). This was likewise true in 641 obese women (over 200 pounds) studied by Odell and Mengert; these authors found furthermore that in one in 20 of their cases, the infant weighed 4,500 gm. (10 pounds) or more. The incidence of chronic hypertensive disease is also increased and is manifest in over one quarter of such obese patients. Uterine inertia is encountered more often, due to the more frequent overdistention of the uterus by a large infant. Every effort should be made to control the weight of obese women in the course of prenatal care. Provided that careful dietary supervision is exercised so that the patient receives all the food essentials, the weight of such patients may actually be reduced as pregnancy proceeds with much benefit to the mother and without detriment to the child.

Disturbances of Vision. Disturbances of vision are largely observed during pregnancy, but inquiries should always be made and the patient cautioned concerning their diagnostic significance if they appear. Amaurosis or total blindness occurring at this time is generally due to albuminuric retinitis or to eclampsia. The significance of the eye changes in the various types of toxemia is discussed in the section dealing with these complications of pregnancy.

Finlay found that in the majority of cases normal pregnancy is associated with a bitemporal contraction of the visual fields with some tendency to limitation to a quadrant or intensification in a quadrant. It is possible that the pituitary gland, which normally hypertrophies during pregnancy, may produce pressure directly or indirectly through vascular changes, sufficient to bring about these defects of the visual fields, as observed by Finlay.

DISEASES OF THE BLOOD

Anemia. The anemias encountered in pregnancy are of three main types: (1) Anemia due to iron starvation. This may be normocytic or microcytic and is by far the most common form. (2) Macrocytic anemia, or the so-called "pernicious anemia of pregnancy." This is rarely seen in the United States but is a common and grave complication of pregnancy in India and other Oriental countries. (3) Sickle cell anemia, a disease found almost exclusively in the Negro race.

Since the physiologic blood dilution of pregnancy may cause a reduction of the hemoglobin to levels as low as 10.0 gm. per 100 cc. of blood, the diagnosis of anemia in pregnant women is not made unless the hemoglobin is less than 10.0 gm. (about 70 per cent), the red cell count less than 3.5 million, or the hematocrit reading less than 30 per cent, as discussed on page 220. On this basis, the incidence of anemia in pregnancy is approximately 10 per cent.

Almost all anemias in pregnancy encountered in this country are due to iron starvation. Although this condition is frequently referred to as "microcytic anemia," it is almost as likely to be normocytic as microcytic. The two factors which make anemia due to iron starvation in pregnancy especially frequent, according to traditional belief, have already been discussed on pages 218 and 224. These are, first, the drain imposed upon the maternal iron supply by the growing fetus, the enlarging uterus and the increased blood volume and, second, the tendency to hypochlorhydria which many gravidae show. In addition there are probably unknown factors which make it difficult for certain pregnant women to utilize post-absorptive iron to the best advantage; and it is possible that these unknown factors play a more important role in the causation of anemia in pregnancy than the two traditional explanations. The part played by hypochlorhydria is particularly open to question because little correlation appears to exist between the decreased gastric acidity and anemia (Watson); moreover, studies with radioactive substances in pregnancy indicate that iron is absorbed 2 to 10 times more rapidly than in nonpregnant persons (Balfour). In sum, the factors which enter into the causation of iron deficiency in pregnancy are not as clearly understood as we used to think; and current research suggests that our concept of the process may undergo considerable modification in the next few years.

Careful estimation of hemoglobin concentration constitutes an important part of prenatal care and this should be done every three months, including one determination four weeks before the expected date of confinement. For clinical purposes the best method of estimating the hemoglobin concentration is the hematocrit. It is more accurate than most methods of determining hemoglobin directly and is relatively simple. Since the blood of pregnant women sediments rapidly, however, care must be taken to mix the cells and plasma thoroughly just before they are introduced into the hematocrit tube. With a normocytic blood picture, division of the hematocrit reading by 3 gives the hemoglobin concentration in grams per 100 cc. of blood.

Prophylaxis of iron deficiency anemia in pregnancy is important and comprises stressing to prenatal patients the importance of daily ingestion of meat and eggs. The treatment will depend on the severity of the anemia and the patient's reaction to iron therapy. If the hemoglobin level is above 7.0 gm., therapy consists of increasing iron intake by (1) re-emphasis on the necessity of eating meat daily, with liver twice weekly and (2) the administration of some form of medicinal iron. The iron preparation most commonly employed is ferrous sulfate, 1.0 gm. daily. Not infrequently this is ineffectual and often causes annoying gastro-intestinal disturbances. As a consequence a large number of other iron compounds are on the market and it would appear that some of these provide greater absorption of iron and are less irritating than ferrous sulfate. As an example, Dieckmann and Priddle have reported very gratifying results with a molybdenum-iron complex. Of 49 anemic gravidae treated by them with this compound, 45 gained before delivery an average of 2.1 gm. of hemoglobin per 100 cc. of blood, the minimum being 0.6 and the maximum 5.5 gm. Only 4 patients showed no change; and but 1 of the 49 complained of gastro-intestinal disturbances.

If the hemoglobin level is below 7.0 gm., the patient should be hospitalized and, in most instances, given one or more blood transfusions. While such low hemoglobin levels sometimes respond to iron, they often do not and transfusion becomes essential if the hemoglobin is to be restored to normal levels. Likewise, in patients with lesser degrees of anemia who do not respond to iron, transfusion may be advisable.

The macrocytic anemia of pregnancy, as seen particularly in India, is a grave condition which resembles superficially Addisonian pernicious anemia. The hemoglobin concentration frequently falls to as low as 3.0 gm. per 100 cc., and the red cell count to one million or less. The stained smear shows the characteristic picture of pernicious anemia in relapse including macrocytosis, and much variation in size and shape of cells with many bizarre forms. Low grade fever, diarrhea, edema, dyspnea and weakness accompany the profound anemia and, under such circumstances, the patient becomes a ready prey to all types of infection. The maternal death rate is approximately 40 per cent. This macrocytic anemia of pregnancy differs from true pernicious anemia in that achlorhydria is not the rule and in that the response to liver therapy is poor; moreover, in patients who survive pregnancy and the puerperium, recovery is complete. The cause of the disease is not definitely known, but it is widely believed that it is due to some form of food deficiency, possibly to a lack of the extrinsic factor of Castle necessary for normal blood formation. The treatment is repeated, small blood transfusions, together with iron, liver and a diet rich in protein and vitamins. Recent observations suggest that folic acid may be of value.

Sickle cell anemia is a chronic anemia of unknown cause, which is confined almost entirely to the Negro race, is hereditary and is characterized by "sickling" of the red cells in association with a lowered hemoglobin level. Many Negroes have the sickle cell trait, but only some 7 per cent of these develop anemia and it is only to this last category that the term "sickle cell anemia" applies. Sickle cell anemia is generally believed to be a grave complication of pregnancy, a maternal mortality rate of 21 per cent having been reported in the literature. However, from a study of 11 cases seen in our clinic over the past 20 years, Anderson and Busby reach more sanguine conclusions, since no maternal death occurred in this series. The fetal mortality, however, was 21 per cent. The incidence of the complication was found to be once in every 1,296 pregnant Negresses.

The treatment of sickle cell anemia in pregnancy demands constant medical supervision and frequent hospitalization for investigation, blood transfusions, and treatment of concurrent toxemias and febrile states. The liberal use of blood transfusions and penicillin is needed to reduce both the maternal and fetal mortality rates. In the series of Anderson and Busby, the average number of transfusions per patient was 5.2, one patient requiring 10. The incidence of transfusion reactions in sickle cell patients is high, being 23 per cent in this series. For this reason it is prudent to give small transfusions frequently rather than large amounts of blood at any one time.

Leukemia. Leukemia is rarely found in pregnancy. Grier and Richter, in 1939, collected from the literature 61 cases of leukemia associated with pregnancy. To these they added one case of their own, and made the observation that the incidence of the acute and chronic forms is about the same, with the course of the latter being sometimes as long as six years, while that in the former is short, the patient usually dying during pregnancy, labor or the puerperium. All the chronic cases reported were of the myelogenous type, except one, which proved to be chronic lymphatic leukemia. The majority of the acute cases, according to Grier and Richter, were myelogenous.

In the chronic cases exacerbation usually occurs during pregnancy. Premature labor is less frequent in this type than in the acute form which accounts for the increased risk to the offspring in the latter. It has been noted that in the event of premature labor the symptoms sometimes undergo marked amelioration.

The diagnosis is rendered probable by the ordinary criteria by which leukemia is diagnosed, namely, enlarged spleen, enlarged lymph nodes, abnormal leukocytes in the peripheral blood and finally bone marrow study. Examination of the fetal blood indicates that the characteristic leukocytes are not transmitted to the fetus. None of the babies in the reported cases showed evidence of leukemia. In view of the good results which sometimes follow spontaneous premature labor, pregnancy may be terminated artificially in serious cases. In selected cases x-ray therapy may be given without harm to the fetus.

Purpura Hemorrhagica. Thrombocytopenic Purpura. Burnett and Klass reviewing the subject of purpura hemorrhagica in pregnancy were able to find 68 cases reported, four of which they regarded as true thrombocytopenic purpura. They believe, on the basis of the findings in these cases, including an additional one of their own, that thrombocytopenic purpura has periodic lapses which may coincide with pregnancy. As opposed to the opinion of Rushmore and Liebling, they find that thrombocytopenic purpura develops early in pregnancy and that it is equally common in primigravidae and multiparae. Hemorrhage at the time of delivery is uncommon. The treatment is symptomatic with blood transfusions as may be needed, unless one is prepared to extirpate the spleen. Stander had three cases of thrombocytopenic purpura, in two of whom splenectomy had been performed prior to any pregnancy, while in the third the spleen was extirpated between the second and third pregnancies. The findings in his cases are in agreement with those noted above: the lapses of the disease may coincide with pregnancy, postpartum hemorrhage is rare, and treatment in the form of transfusion, citrin pectin and a high vitamin diet is of great help. One baby of one of Stander's three patients with thrombocytopenic purpura died from congenital thrombocytopenic purpura. From an analysis of the seven cases reported in the literature and the three occurring in Stander's service, it would appear that the offspring has the best chance if a splenectomy had been done prior to pregnancy and if the disease is in a chronic phase during the gestation.

Asymptomatic or secondary purpura is much more common. It may develop from blood diseases, infections, intoxications, radiation, jaundice, chronic nephritis, food sensitivity, and vitamin deficiencies. The treatment in such instances is of course that of the causative process.

Lead Poisoning. C.Paul studied the histories of 141 pregnancies occurring in women suffering from chronic lead poisoning and found that 86 ended in abortion or premature labor. Moreover, a large number of the children which were born alive perished at an early period, only 10 per cent remaining alive at the tenth year. There is evidence suggesting that lead may be transmitted through the placenta, as in a premature child examined by Lewin, 16 per cent of the total weight of the liver was due to it. Aub, Fairhall, Minot and Reznikoff, on the other hand, firmly believe that lead is not transmitted through the placenta. They were unable to find lead in the young of "leaded" experimental animals. They are in agreement with Weller who found a direct effect on the male and female germ plasm. Fronga states that lead poisoning not only leads to abortion or premature labor, but is a potent cause of sterility; thus, in the vicinity of the lead works of Sardinia, 20 per cent of the married women are sterile, and an additional 23 per cent have only one child.

Experiments reported by Weller in 1915 indicate that the deleterious effect of lead poisoning may be traced to either parent. He found that sterility was common when normal female guinea pigs were mated with males suffering from chronic lead poisoning, and when pregnancy resulted the young were subnormal in weight and exhibited an increased mortality after birth. Likewise when normal males were united with poisoned females stillbirths occurred very frequently, and the living offsprings were undersized. In the light of his experiments Weller believes that lead exerts a direct unfavorable influence upon the sperm cells and the early ova.

SPLENIC CONDITIONS

Occasionally an enlarged spleen occupying the lower abdomen may be mistaken for the pregnant uterus. If pregnancy supervenes it is usually uninfluenced by the floating organ which is gradually forced into its normal position as the uterus enlarges. Occasionally, however, pronounced peritonitic symptoms may appear as the result of torsion of its pedicle, when splenectomy will be indicated.

Rupture of the spleen is a rare complication of gestation, Burnett and McMenemey finding only 15 cases in the literature up to 1930. Direct trauma was the main factor in most of the cases reported. Pain and tenderness over the splenic area, vomiting and weakness are the chief symptoms. Splenectomy is usually indicated.

Splenomegaly is very rarely a complication of pregnancy. Serbin states that Banti's disease is aggravated by pregnancy and advises transfusion and early splenectomy. Splenomegaly from chronic malaria may likewise demand splenectomy should the splenic tumor be large enough to interfere with the growing uterus. Moore and Pastore recently reported a case of erythroblastic splenomegaly occurring during pregnancy.

DISEASES OF THE SKIN

Impetigo Herpetiformis. Hebra was the first to call attention to the serious nature of this disease which occurs almost exclusively in pregnant or puerperal women, and is characterized by superficial pustules which are arranged in groups or clusters with inflammatory bases. New lesions appear on the borders of older and crusted confluent patches while recovery takes place in their centers. The lesions occur on the trunk, thighs, and in the neighborhood of the genitalia, but rarely upon the face. They are accompanied by itching and constitutional symptoms, chills and high fever. The recorded mortality is about 75 per cent. The disease as a rule does not lead to abortion or premature labor, and many of the women affected with it die undelivered. Treatment consists of local application of ammoniated mercury ointment, gentian violet or, more recently, penicillin, as well as sulfadiazine by mouth or penicillin intramuscularly.

Erythema Multiforme. This condition is at times aggravated by pregnancy. Treatment is the same as in the nonpregnant person.

Lupus Erythematosus. This disease is occasionally seen accompanying pregnancy. We have had experience with two such cases in the last two years. It would seem in many instances that pregnancy exerts a beneficial though perhaps transitory effect on the lesion.

Lupus Vulgaris. Plass has recently seen an unusual case of *lupus miliaris disseminatus* of the face in a pregnant woman of 36 years of age. Pulmonary tuberculosis was excluded and it was decided that interruption of the pregnancy was not indicated. Delivery was normal after an uneventful pregnancy and there was no exacerbation of the skin lesion.

Scleroderma. A case of pregnancy associated with scleroderma was reported by Guttmacher in 1943. He was unable to find any references on this subject; and on the basis of this and the parents' desire for the child, the pregnancy was allowed to continue. A premature infant was delivered per vaginam following an otherwise uneventful pregnancy of 34 weeks. It was felt that the scleroderma was little affected by the pregnancy; certainly it was not made worse and may have been temporarily arrested. Stander had two such cases and his experience is in agreement with that of Guttmacher.

Herpes Gestationis. This disease more frequently known as dermatitis herpetiformis is an inflammatory, superficially seated, multiform, herpetiform eruption, which is characterized by erythematous, vesicular, pustular, and bullous lesions. It occurs occasionally in pregnant women and is accompanied by marked burning and itching. It pursues a chronic course, is often attended with fever, and sometimes may even end in death.

Dühring believes that it is probably toxemic in origin though similar lesions sometimes occur during the course of sepsis. In view of its depressing character the patient should be placed upon tonic treatment, while the itching is best allayed by the use of ointments or lotions containing oil of cade, carbolic acid, or similar substances. Mueller and Lapp recently reviewed the literature and reported two cases. They found the disease to respond unsatisfactorily to any form of therapy and while the prognosis for the mother is good, that for the offspring is less so.

Pruritus. Itching may occasionally be a distressing complication. It may extend over the greater part of the body or be limited to the genitalia. It often gives rise to intense suffering, the itching sometimes being so constant that the patient is unable to sleep. In some patients the loss of rest and the nervous strain attendant upon it exert a marked influence upon the general condition. Such cases are best controlled by the administration of sedatives and general supportive treatment. A rigid milk diet is sometimes followed by excellent results. When the condition is not amenable to treatment and the patient shows objective signs of exhaustion the termination of pregnancy may be justifiable.

Genital pruritus (*pruritis vulvae*) may be due to several causes among which are irritating vaginal discharges, parasites or glycosuria. When due to the first-named cause, the vaginal secretions should be examined for the identification of trichomonas and monilia infestation or bacterial infection. Appropriate therapy may be instituted then and the condition alleviated by these measures as well as by the maintenance of absolute cleanliness. At the same time the itching may be allayed by the employment of ointment containing cocaine derivatives, menthol, or carbolic acid. Pruritus of diabetic origin is observed but rarely, but the possibility of its occurrence should always be borne in mind and the urine examined. If sugar is present, relief can be obtained only by adequate control of the diabetes, while at the same time appropriate ointments should be employed. Occasionally intense itching about the anus may be due to the presence of seatworms which are best destroyed by the use of rectal enemata of infusion of quassia. If local measures prove ineffectual a dose of 0.6 gm. of santonin on an empty stomach, followed by Rochelle salts or other saline cathartic an hour later, will often bring about the desired result. Estrogenic therapy has been advocated when no specific cause for the pruritus was found.

Abnormalities of Pigmentation. During pregnancy abnormalities in pigmentation are frequently noted which are particularly marked along the linea alba and about the breasts. In other cases unsightly, more or less symmetrical yellowish splotches (*cloasma*) appear upon the face. They are not amenable to treatment, but usually disappear promptly after childbirth.

Hematoma of the Abdominal Walls. Stoeckel has reported two cases of hematoma of the abdominal walls occurring during pregnancy. In one case the tumor was situated in the sheath of the right rectus muscle just above the symphysis, while in the other it appeared as a large mass in the right hypogastric region and was mistaken for the head of the child. The condition resulted from rupture of the inferior and superior epigastric arteries respectively.

DISEASES OF THE URINARY SYSTEM

Acute Nephritis. Acute glomerulonephritis, also known as acute hemorrhagic nephritis, can develop during gestation just as in the nonpregnant state. The incidence of this disease in 41,454 pregnant women admitted to the New York Lying-In Hospital during the past 12 years was 0.02 per cent.

Acute nephritis may occur suddenly during, or shortly after, an acute infectious process such as tonsillitis, scarlet fever or pneumonia. The hemolytic streptococcus is often the offending organism. The disease may also be caused by poisons such as lead, mercury or the arsenicals. The immediate past history of the patient is of importance in establishing a diagnosis. The clinical features of the disease although varying in extent are generally hematuria, oliguria or actual anuria, proteinuria, edema and hypertension. The urine usually has a relatively high specific gravity and may contain epithelial and coarsely granular casts.

Acute nephritis occurring during the latter half of pregnancy must be differentiated from preeclampsia which is discussed in Chapter 27. In the latter condition hematuria is a most uncommon and insignificant finding while in acute nephritis it is one of the most characteristic features of the disease.

The treatment of acute nephritis is the same in the pregnant as in the nonpregnant person, the main purpose being to prevent the disease from passing into a chronic stage. Spontaneous abortion may result. At times it may be advisable to consider interruption of the pregnancy although this has not been our general practice.

Chronic Nephritis. Acute glomerulonephritis may pass into a chronic form characterized by progressive decrease of renal function with resultant nitrogenous retention. In chronic glomerulonephritis there is gradual destruction of the glomeruli and tubules, accompanied by fibrous connective tissue infiltration, eventuating into the so-called "contracted kidney." Acute nephritis is not always the forerunner of chronic glomerulonephritis as the latter may have an insidious onset, sometimes apparently associated with no known cause, such as chronic lead poisoning. The condition is usually aggravated by pregnancy and therapeutic abortion is sometimes indicated.

Cystitis. Cystitis associated with pregnancy is predominantly a feature of the puerperium rather than the antenatal period. When it occurs before delivery it usually consists of a mild irritation of the trigone. Postpartum cystitis, on the other hand, is a different entity, occurs more frequently and often escapes recognition. The process of evacuation of the uterus is associated with stretching and trauma of the base of the bladder. Cystoscopic examination soon after delivery shows not only edema and hyperemia but frequently submucous extravasations of blood. At times the edema of the trigone is so marked as to be the cause of obstruction of the urethra and acute retention. In addition to these factors the puerperal bladder has an increased capacity and is not as sensitive to intravesical fluid tension as in the nonpregnant state, so that overdistention and incomplete emptying with the establishment of residual urine are common. The paralyzing effect of anesthesia and temporarily disturbed function of the nerve supply to the bladder are undoubtedly contributory factors.

Residual urine and the presence of bacteriuria in a traumatized bladder present the optimum conditions for the development of true bladder infection. Taussig found an incidence of cystitis of 3.8 per cent, while Prather reports 1.1 per cent.

The symptoms are often inability to urinate, frequent voiding in small amounts, dysuria, and a low grade fever which rarely rises above 101° F. The treatment is usually confined to intermittent catheterization of the bladder every eight hours, followed by the instillation of 15 cc. of a 3 per cent solution of strong silver proteinate or some other mild antiseptic irritant. This is continued until the patient voids spontaneously in satisfactory amounts and catheterization once in 24 hours fails to show a residual urine of over 30 cc. In more severe cases it is occasionally necessary to place an indwelling catheter in the bladder so that constant drainage is established. When this is done the bladder should be irrigated three or four times in each 24 hours with warm boric acid solution.

In view of the high incidence of bacteriuria, 11 per cent in the antepartum and 70 per cent in postpartum women, it is interesting to note the relatively small number of patients, approximately 3 per cent, who show an involvement of the bladder wall sufficiently severe to warrant the diagnosis of cystitis. Studies have shown the normal bladder to be very resistant to infection and that when inflammation of its tissues occurs it is due not only to the presence of infectious organisms, but also to stagnant urine or trauma. The diagnosis of cystitis, therefore, cannot be made upon the bacteriuria alone, but must involve the demonstration of pus cells associated with residual urine in the bladder. The treatment must therefore be concentrated upon the avoidance of accumulations of stagnant urine as well as trauma.

Pyelitis. The term pyelitis, although signifying inflammation of the renal pelvis, is generally employed to denote an inflammatory process involving both renal pelvis and ureter, or strictly speaking a pyelo-ureteritis. As it has been customary to speak of "pyelitis of pregnancy," we shall use the term pyelitis to denote a pyelo-ureteritis.

The incidence of pyelitis complicating pregnancy varies, as recorded by different authors, from 1 per cent (Crabtree and Prather) to 6 per cent (Falk). The incidence in the New York Lying-In Hospital, as reported by McLane in 1939, was 168 cases in 14,000 deliveries, or 1.2 per cent. There were 98 cases of antepartum, 62 of postpartum and 8 of intrapartum pyelitis. Since that time there has been a definite decrease in the incidence of pyelitis in that clinic, due probably to the prophylactic treatment which will be discussed below. The process is frequently bilateral, but is predominantly right-sided when unilateral. The disease most frequently appears in

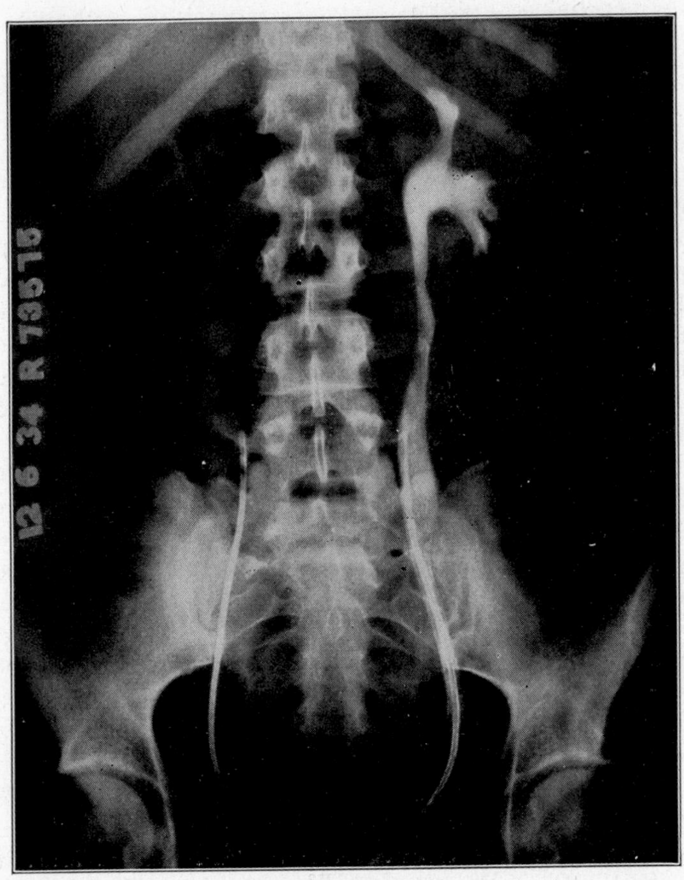

Fig. 390.—Retrograde Pyelogram Taken in the Seventh Month of Pregnancy Showing Moderate Hydronephrosis and Hydroureter.

This degree of dilatation is not at all uncommon.

the latter part of pregnancy, as shown in the series of 98 cases of antepartum pyelitis reported by McLane, where 3 occurred in the first, 35 in the second and 60 in the third trimester. The onset of the disease is usually acute; the patient who had been previously well, or who had complained of slight vesical irritation or hematuria, is suddenly seized with more or less severe paroxysmal pains usually in the right flank. This is accompanied by marked elevation of temperature usually running a hectic course. Palpation reveals a tender kidney and ureter with tenderness in the costovertebral angle. The urine sediment contains clumped pus cells and usually colon bacilli, although infrequently staphylococci and streptococci may be found. Urine culture of the catheter specimen removed from the pelvis of the kidney will reveal the B. coli as the predominant micro-organism in over 90 per cent of the patients suffering from this disease. If the inflammatory process is confined to the walls of the ureter and kidney pelvis, in which case true pyelitis and ureteritis are present, the temperature will fall rather promptly and the distressing symptoms disappear after a few days' rest in bed and treatment as outlined below. On the other hand,

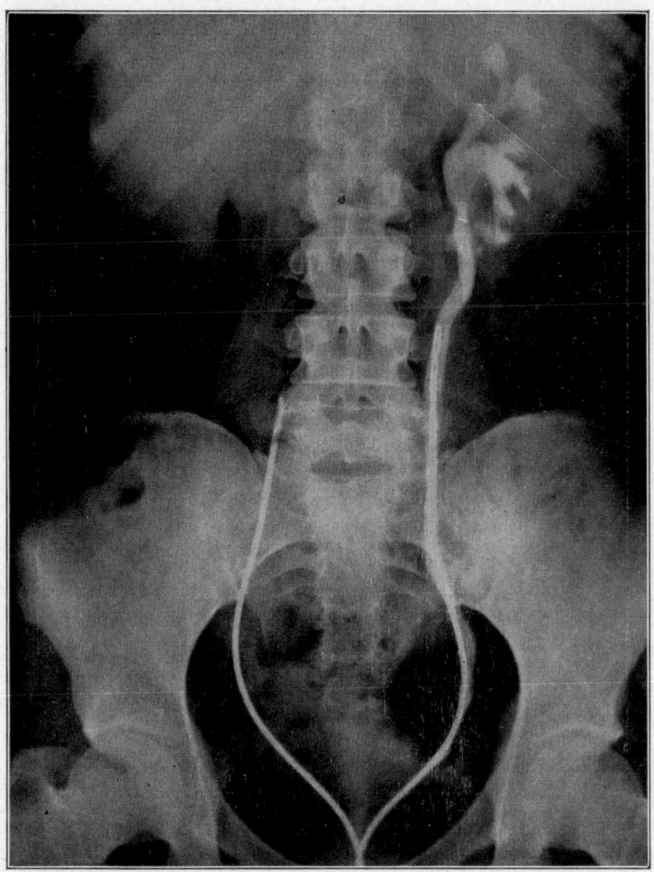

Fig. 391.—Three Weeks Postpartum, Illustrating Involution in the Ureter and Renal Pelvis.

Though not complete, the process has changed a marked hydronephrosis and hydroureter to nearly normal dimensions. This is what may be expected when infection does not produce edema and fibrosis.

when the infection has involved the peripelvic tissues or the parenchyma of the kidney, pyelonephritis is developed in which case the febrile course is much more prolonged, the disease more resistant to treatment and the significance to the patient more grave. The differentiation of the two stages of the disease is accompanied by much difficulty particularly in early and borderline cases. The advanced lesions of pyelonephritis are usually accompanied by some degree of nitrogenous retention and, when bilateral, may lead to uremia or to septic extension of the process.

Pyelitis is always due to bacterial infection, which is facilitated by the stasis of urine resulting from atony and distention of the ureters. The bacterial invasion may be due to an extension upward from the bladder, or to transmission of bacteria through the blood or lymph channels. The weight of evidence is against the theory of ascending infection as the cause of pyelitis since reflux and antiperistalsis apparently never occur except in marked pathologic states. Franke has demonstrated rather convincingly the passage of B. coli from various portions of the large bowel, which is often sluggish or atonic in pregnancy, through the lymphatics to those of the right

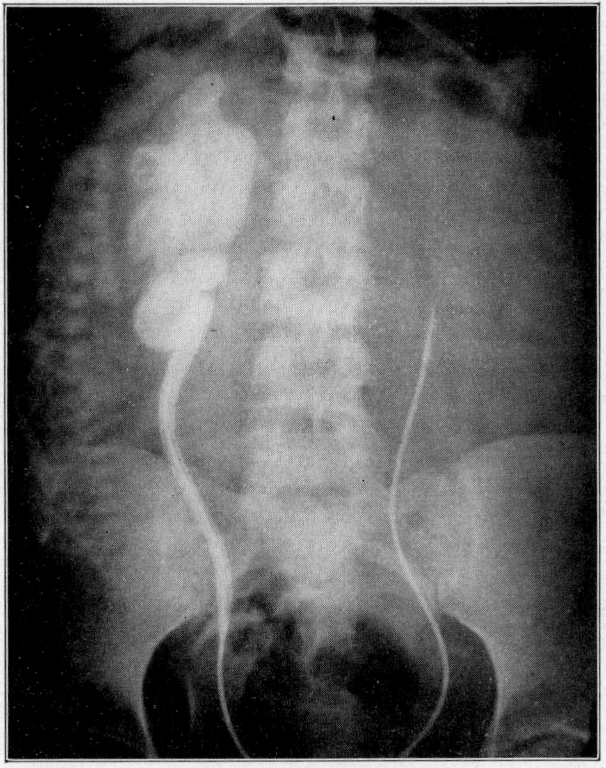

Fig. 392.—Retrograde Pyelogram Taken in the Eighth Month of Pregnancy.

The patient, a multipara, suffered from pyonephrosis which had its origin in hydronephrosis of pregnancy. This kidney and ureter had a capacity of 85 cc.

kidney region. Crabtree and Prather feel, on the contrary, that these infections are blood-borne despite the fact that blood culture almost uniformly fails to demonstrate the organism. From a consideration of all available evidence to date it appears that invasion of the urinary tract by way of the lymphatics is the most likely. Whatever the mode of entrance of the infective agent may be, the conclusion is unescapable that the pregnant woman with residual urine as a natural concomitant of the pregnant state is predisposed to the development of pyelitis. All that is necessary for the onset of the disease is the presence of the infective organism together with lowered immunity. Some claim that there is a definite group of patients whose acute pyelitis may be an exacerbation of a latent chronic form because they have had pyelitis in childhood or in a previous pregnancy. Still another possible etiologic factor seems to be foci of infection such as teeth, tonsils, gastro-intestinal tract, gallbladder or sinuses, from which organisms may be transmitted to the urinary tract through the lymphatic or blood channels. Paul and Galloway found the incidence of pyelitis greatly increased in patients in whom infected teeth were allowed to remain during gestation.

The pathologic changes in the ureter and kidney pelvis are quite simple. It is a well recognized pathologic principle that a distended organ is more vulnerable to pathogenic organisms than one in which a normal tonus exists, so that it is not at

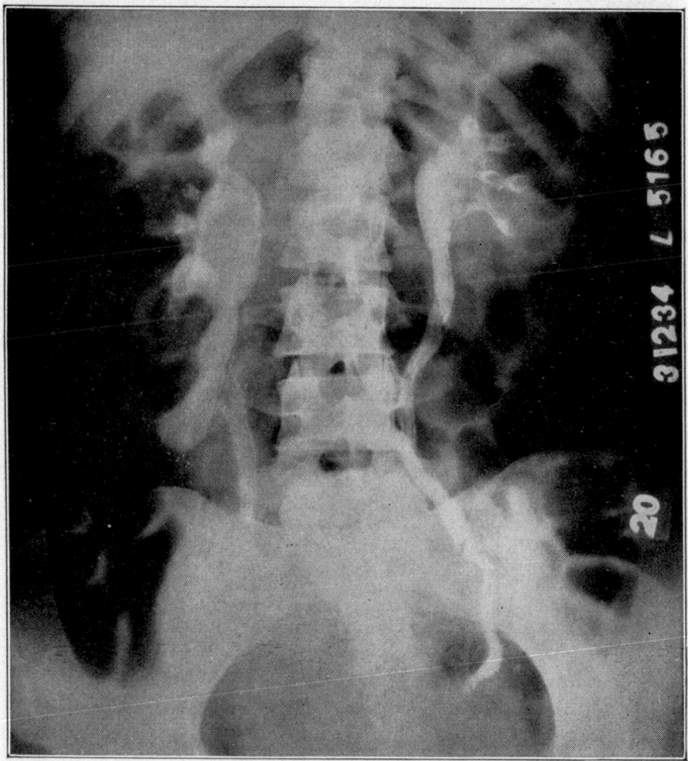

Fig. 393.—Postpartum Complication.

A persistent bilateral pyonephrosis in the puerperium, which had its origin in pyeloureteritis of pregnancy.

all remarkable that the distended ureter and kidney pelvis of pregnancy should frequently be invaded. The mucosa becomes congested with blood elements and lymph so that it has an edematous and sometimes a hemorrhagic appearance. This is followed by response on the part of blood and tissue wandering cells so that an exudate is formed and pus liberated as flakes of exudate become detached. As the process develops the deeper muscular and connective tissues become involved in the inflammatory reaction and the whole structure becomes turgid, while peristalsis completely disappears, increasing the stagnation of the column of urinary fluid. Some fibrosis is the inevitable sequel of any such inflammation as the condition becomes chronic or commences to heal, the degree depending upon the severity of the infection and its duration. This explains the reduced or absent motility of the ureter following longstanding pyelitis. In addition to the involvement of the walls of the pelvis and ureter there is frequently some extension of the process into the peripelvic tissues or into the parenchyma of the kidney itself. When this occurs we are dealing with pyelonephritis and we can expect the same connective tissue reactions with resulting fibrosis and permanent damage to the secretory elements of the kidney. Occasionally, in the absence of proper drainage of the tract, the ureter and kidney pelvis become con-

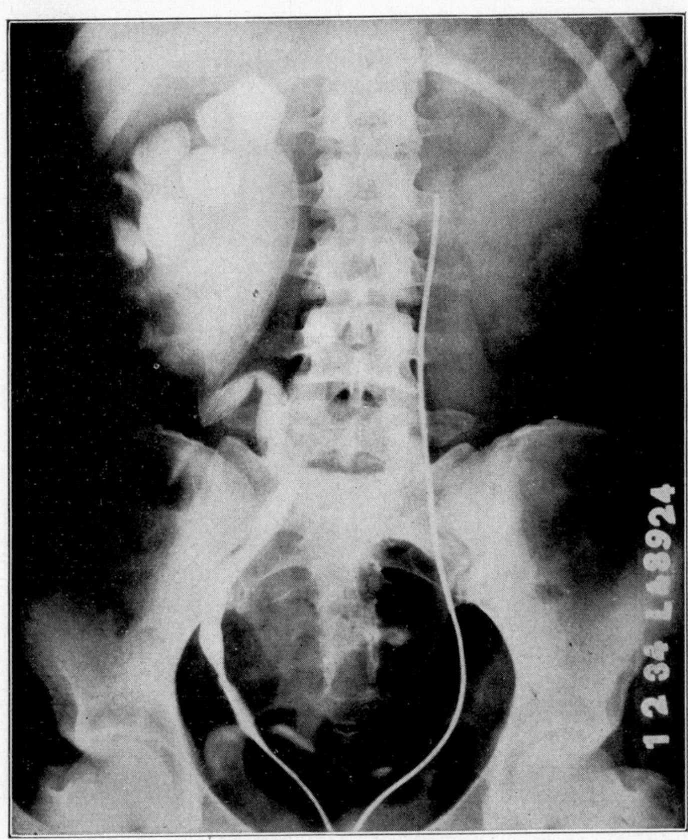

Fig. 394.—Postpartum Complication.

Longstanding hydronephrosis which had its origin during pregnancy. Despite the fact that months have elapsed since the termination of pregnancy this tract has failed to recover its normal function.

verted into a pus sac with metastatic abscesses in the cortex of the kidney with complete destruction.

Ordinarily, pain in one lumbar region, the palpation of an enlarged or tender kidney and the characteristic urinary findings, as well as the demonstration of fever, costovertebral tenderness and hydro-ureter should make the diagnosis clear. Yet the condition is frequently mistaken for appendicitis and, in the puerperium, for uterine infection. In the acute cases the severe pain, accompanying more or less complete blockage of the ureter with resultant distention of the ureter and renal pelvis, may cause vomiting and is occasionally associated with an ileus of the large bowel. In these cases intermittent high fever with chills, rapid pulse and sweating, are characteristic. In advanced pyelonephritis, especially when bilateral, examination of the blood may show nitrogenous retention as evidenced by the nonprotein and urea nitrogen values.

The most frequent complication of pyelitis gravidarum is probably secondary anemia due presumably to the general effects of toxic absorption, but more probably to the hemolytic effect of the colon bacillus upon the red blood cells. In addition to the anemia the resistance of the patient is lowered so that respiratory infections are

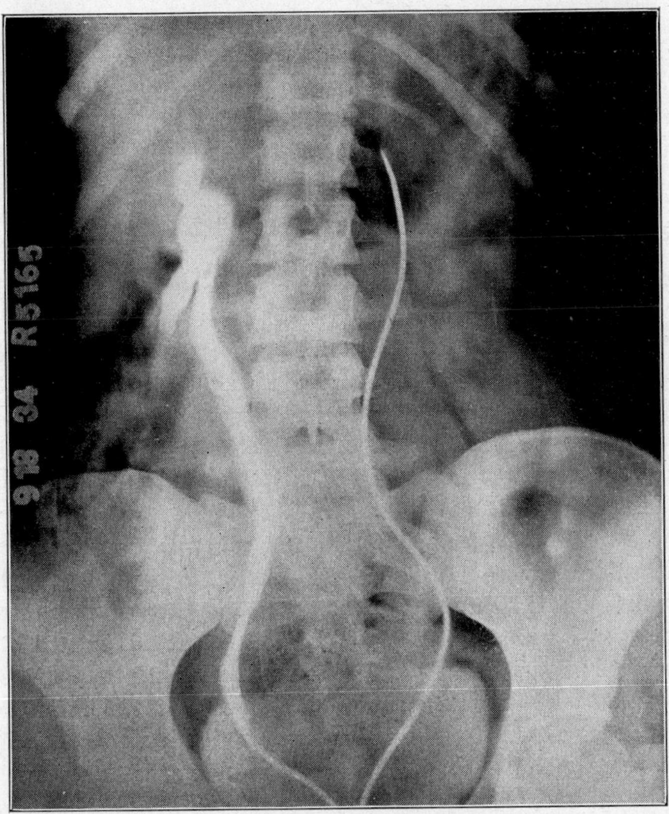

Fig. 395.—Postpartum Hydroureter Nine Months after Delivery, Showing a Partial but Incomplete Recovery of Contour and Function.

Probably this is the end of the process. Such a tract is prone to harbor the infection and to recrudescence in subsequent pregnancies.

prone to develop. By far the most serious complication is that resulting from the extension of the process into the glandular substance of the kidney. Occasionally ileus and hyperemesis may also complicate the disease. The pyelitis-ileus syndrome occurred in six of our severely ill patients. Treatment must be directed toward improvement of the pyelitis; however, should the patient not respond to conservative therapy, interruption of the pregnancy becomes imperative. In our experience operative treatment of the distention is ill-advised.

Treatment. The introduction of sulfonamides into clinical practice in 1935-1936 furnished us with a most efficient method of treating infections in the urinary system. Sulfanilamide, sulfapyridine and sulfathiazole were all employed in turn with increasing success. However, in our practice they have all been eliminated and replaced by sulfadiazine. Most of the urinary tract infections complicating pregnancy are initiated by the colon or the aerogenes bacillus. Sulfadiazine appears to be somewhat more specific in vitro and in vivo for these particular organisms. In severe infections 4 gm. of sulfadiazine as an initial dose followed by 1 gm. every four hours, usually provides an adequate concentration of the sulfonamides. It is absolutely essential that the urine be rendered alkaline prior to or very early in the treatment. This is best accomplished by an initial dose of 12 gm. of sodium bicarbonate followed by 4 gm. every four hours. In the event that there is serious nausea, vomiting, or other reason why the patient cannot tolerate the medication orally, the sulfadiazine may be given in the form of sodium salt, 2.5 gm. every 12 hours, intravenously. Alkalinization of the urine under such circumstances can be obtained by the repeated administration of 1/6 molar sodium lactate. The fluid intake should be maintained at at least 4,000 cc. per day in the hope that the urinary output will reach or exceed 1,500 cc. The urine should be examined grossly and microscopically at least twice each day for the presence of sulfadiazine crystals, red blood cells, pus cells and its hydrogen ion concentration determined. This latter test can be very quickly carried out by the employment of the nitrazine paper. The pH should, if possible, be maintained at 7.5 or higher. Catheterized specimens of urine from the bladder should be obtained every second day for culture. The nonprotein nitrogen, urea nitrogen and CO_2 combining power should be determined early in the course of therapy. If there are no signs of nitrogenous retention and the clinical course is satisfactory further blood chemistry studies are usually not indicated.

Under the above routine most infections respond with dramatic rapidity. Clinically, symptoms for the most part disappear during the first two days of therapy. The pyuria is eliminated often by the third or fourth day and the cultures usually become sterile by the fourth or fifth day. It is important to recall at this point that the physiologic changes in the urinary tract have not been altered by the treatment and, accordingly, a reinfection for the same reasons that cause the initial infection is always possible. For these reasons, if the urinary tract infection has developed during pregnancy its recurrence is always possible. A bacilluria always precedes the development of pyuria or clinical symptoms. Accordingly, if a positive culture is subsequently discovered, additional sulfadiazine is indicated. In this asymptomatic stage of the disease 1.5 to 2 gm. of the drug per day, while the patient is ambulatory, for a period of five days appear to be quite efficacious and safe. The urine should be rendered alkaline and maintained so during the course of therapy.

Occasionally, in longstanding infections, namely where pregnancy is complicating chronic pyelonephritis rather than a urinary tract infection complicating pregnancy, as was described above, nothing more than temporary relief is afforded by the sulfonamide drug. The acute stage of the disease can usually be controlled, but it may be necessary on some occasions to terminate the pregnancy to prevent irreparable and irreversible damage to the kidneys. During recent years we have catheterized the bladder and ureters less and less frequently with constant improvement in our end results. Following delivery the infection should be eradicated, if it recurs, by another course of sulfadiazine therapy. If this is not possible we may assume that we are dealing with some anatomical abnormality or a definite pathological entity which demands careful urological investigation and treatment.

In sulfonamide-resistant infections of the urinary tract and in sulfonamide-sensitized patients streptomycin has recently proved of great value, especially against gram-negative organisms. Intramuscular injections are given every three hours, the dosage ranging from 1 to 4 gm. per day, depending on the severity of the infection. The solution usually employed for intramuscular injection contains 1 gm. in 5 cc. of sterile water or physiologic salt solution or, better, 2 per cent procaine hydrochloride solution in order to minimize the pain of injection. Aureomycin promises to be an even more valuable agent in the treatment of urinary tract infections, but until further observations can be accumulated, its place must be held *sub judice*.

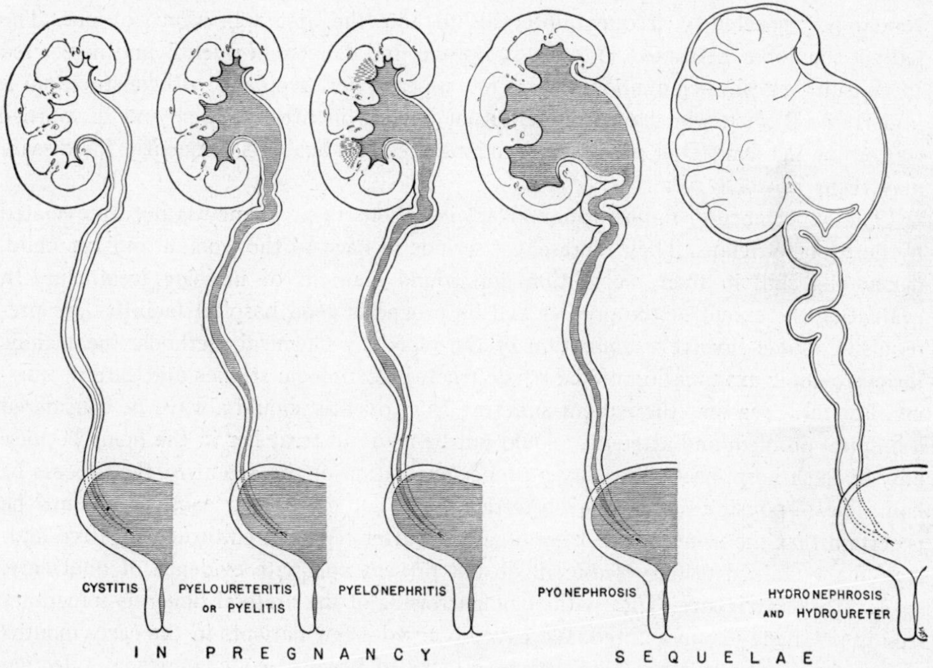

FIG. 396.—DIAGRAM SHOWING EXTENT OF URINARY TRACT INFECTIONS COMPLICATING PREGNANCY AND THE PUERPERIUM AND THEIR SEQUELAE.

(From Traut, *American Journal of Obstetrics and Gynecology.*)

The prognosis for those patients who suffer urinary infection of the upper tract in pregnancy depends upon several factors, such as duration and location of the infection. It should be clearly stated the pyelitis is not cured during pregnancy even though the symptoms subside completely and spontaneously unless specific therapy has been used and the urine is known to be sterile on repeated examination. The woman who is not treated harbors the infection for some time after delivery when, if drainage is satisfactory and immunity high, she will gradually heal the sites of infection in the ureter and renal pelvis. The time required for this result varies almost proportionately with the duration of the febrile reaction to the infection. Those who have been neglected and have extensive infiltrations of the upper tract will show pus cells and bacteria with some hydro-ureter and hydronephrosis for weeks or months. Some may never show normal peristaltic action of the ureter due to extensive fibrosis of the ureteral tube. Others will have deficient renal function as a result of the inflammatory infiltration of the cortex of the kidney. Fortunately the majority of patients show fever and symptoms for a few days or a week and then proceed to term with no acute exacerbations. With proper treatment this group of patients, if reinfection occurs, can usually be made bacteria-free by the end of the second week of the puerperium.

The serious results of pyelitis in pregnancy, together with the frequency of its occurrence, require that care should be exercised to obviate the incidence of the disease if this is possible, as well as to minimize its dangers if it does develop. This is definitely indicated as part of the antenatal care of pregnant women. The urine should be inspected at frequent intervals to note the first appearance of pus. The patient should be instructed as to the symptoms and dangers of pyelitis and instructed to consult her physician upon their first appearance. Avoidance of constipation is important. Women who have suffered from pyelitis in pregnancy should be warned concerning the dangers of promptly becoming pregnant again as frequently the disease may recur in worse form.

The importance of upper urinary tract infections in pregnancy is not appreciated by most obstetricians. They represent a serious menace to the woman and her child, demanding skill in their recognition and sound methods of urologic treatment. In evaluating the extent of the process and its prognosis good hospital facilities are prerequisite. These involve examination of the blood by chemical methods, the technic for cystoscopic examination of the whole tract, bacteriologic studies and careful nursing. For these reasons, the patient suffering from pyelitis should always be considered a hospital problem and attempts should not be made to treat her in the home because only by such hospital studies may a proper evaluation of the extent of the process be had. The responsibilities of the obstetrician are not discharged completely until he is certain that the urine is free from organisms after repeated cultures. Negative findings in the stained urinary sediment do not present adequate evidence of final cure.

Ureteral Stricture. That pathologic narrowing of the ureteral lumen is sometimes seen in pregnancy is undoubted. We have observed a few patients in the early months of pregnancy who suffered from severe attacks of ureteral colic, in whom infection played no immediate role and who were relieved and carried to term by dilatation of the ureter with wax bulbs. However, these cases are comparatively rare despite the work of Hunner who finds in ureteral stricture the cause not only of pyelitis of pregnancy, but also the chief etiologic factor in explaining repeated abortion.

Crabtree has reported cases in which he demonstrated rather satisfactorily that ureteral stricture was a sequel of severe pyelitis and ureteritis of pregnancy. Our own experience seems to indicate that recovery is markedly hastened in some postpartum patients under treatment for chronic pyelitis and ureteritis, especially the more resistant ones, by the passage of dilating wax bulbs through the whole length of the ureter. We have accounted for this result on the basis of improved drainage subsequent to the dilatation of constricted areas.

Dislocation of the Kidney. Minor downward displacements of a movable kidney tend to be rectified during pregnancy as the enlarging uterus pushes it upward toward its normal position. The older literature on the subject made much of the symptoms referable to the floating kidney and the alleviation of them during pregnancy. Recently, however, scant reference is made and we seldom see a patient who complains of the syndrome.

Marked malplacement, either congenital or acquired, however, may be the source of serious difficulty. Cragin has reported an instance in which a congenitally displaced kidney occupying the pelvic cavity led to symptoms of incarceration necessitating its removal. He collected five somewhat similar cases, while Stephans collected the literature upon the subject up to 1912. The condition usually escapes recognition until it gives rise to dystocia. However, with proper antenatal examination and care it would seem impossible to overlook a pelvic kidney. In one of our patients, in whom the condition had been discovered at a previous laparotomy, the displaced organ was gradually pushed out of the pelvic cavity by the enlarging uterus so that easy spontaneous labor occurred.

Renal Tuberculosis. Tuberculosis of the kidney is a most serious complication of pregnancy, though fortunately, somewhat infrequently seen. In a series of 41,454 pregnancies Traut observed it on 12 occasions; three patients were primigravidae and nine multiparae. In seven patients nephrectomy had been performed prior to pregnancy, while in three this operation was done during pregnancy and in the remaining two patients nephrectomy was not performed. Of the 10 patients with one remaining kidney, three had tubercle bacilli in the urine, as revealed by guinea-pig inoculation, while seven had negative urine. Phenolsulphonephthalein and urea clearance tests revealed satisfactory kidney function in all except one of the cases. Our treatment was conservative in nine patients, the pregnancy being allowed to proceed. Seven of these were delivered normally at term while two had a spontaneous abortion. Of the remaining three patients, two were delivered by cesarean section and one had a therapeutic abortion, the indication being a colon bacillus infection in the remaining kidney. A follow-up study of the patients showed that pregnancy evidently does not aggravate or cause an exacerbation of the disease in the remaining kidney unless the remaining kidney shows lowered function as indicated by the renal function tests and blood and urine chemical findings.

On the other hand, it has been generally thought that tuberculosis of the kidney pursues a rapidly unfavorable course, particularly during the latter months of pregnancy. For this reason, Marx feels that it is extremely dubious whether pregnancy should be allowed to continue in any case of proved renal tuberculosis and recommends interruption of pregnancy in all cases followed by nephrectomy when the lesion is unilateral. In view of our experience, as related above, we consider his view too radical and believe that a decision as to termination of pregnancy must be based upon the individual findings in each particular case.

Whether the patient who has had a nephrectomy for tuberculosis should be allowed to become pregnant is a practical question which sometimes arises. The consensus of opinion is that pregnancy should be interdicted until a period of two to four years has demonstrated not only no involvement, but also good function of the remaining kidney. It is usually found with this plan that the patient may then tolerate pregnancy quite as well as the woman with normal kidneys.

Urinary Calculi in Pregnancy. Renal and ureteral lithiasis is a comparatively rare complication of pregnancy. Prather and Crabtree report four kidney stones and eight ureteral stones in 9,823 deliveries. The reason for this low incidence would seem to be that renal lithiasis is distinctly a disease of middle life, whereas the vast majority of pregnancies occur before the age of 35. However, many pregnant women present some of the cardinal prerequisites for stone formation such as urinary stasis and infection, so that it would seem that the incidence ought to be higher unless there are other counteracting factors. One of these undoubtedly is the transiency of pregnancy. The stasis is usually of only nine months' duration and this would appear to be an insufficient period for the formation of stones. Contrary to Dozsa, who feels that endocrine or metabolic disturbances are definitely associated with stone formation in pregnancy, it would seem that their very rarity would indicate that there can be no very close association with any of the physiologic variations which we think of as characteristic of pregnancy.

The calculi are usually asymptomatic in pregnancy due to the reduced tonus of the musculature of the tract, only a few cases of ureteral colic having been reported. They are usually discovered in the roentgenogram or with the ureteral catheter during the study of the patient for urinary tract infection. Very rarely do they cause acute obstruction with the familiar train of symptoms.

Treatment is dependent upon the duration of pregnancy and the symptoms. If the symptoms are acute surgical removal is usually mandatory regardless of other considerations. Usually, however, one can choose the course to pursue. During the first five months of pregnancy surgical removal is frequently desirable. Operative procedures at this time need not interrupt the gestation, but a more important consideration is that the damage caused by the calculus will have a long duration and be proportionately more severe. Late in pregnancy it is usually found wiser to palliate the condition until term, reserving operative procedure until after delivery and late in the puerperium. However, each case requires individual consideration as to its proper therapy. It will be well to remind those contemplating surgery of the kidney or ureter during the latter half of pregnancy that the vessels of the organs are tremendously enlarged and that proper exposure of the lower ureter is almost impossible in the majority of cases.

Renal Tumors in Pregnancy. Pregnancy is occasionally a complicating factor in patients with congenitally malformed or polycystic kidneys. In both conditions the decision to allow pregnancy to continue depends almost entirely upon how well such organs can tolerate the additional strain. This must be determined in the individual case by observing the kidney function, the blood pressure curve formed by frequent readings, the appearance of edema, and the incidence of nitrogenous retention in the blood stream. Should these indicate renal decompensation of serious degree, interruption of pregnancy may be necessary to save the life of the woman. This is particularly true of those suffering from polycystic kidney where there is usually a very small margin of kidney reserve. Infrequently renal tumors of a malignant nature may complicate pregnancy. Inasmuch as these neoplasms are nearly always unilateral the treatment depends largely upon whether or not the other kidney is unimpaired.

Hematuria. The passage of bloody urine in pregnancy is always significant and calls for a careful urologic investigation. Chiaventone has described an idiopathic hematuria due to pregnancy and has collected 18 similar cases from the literature. He considers that the hemorrhage is probably due to histologic changes in the kidney which result from toxemia. However, the advent of more adequate diagnostic procedure has caused the idiopathic bleeding of pregnancy to seem relatively unimportant as an entity, because we have learned that by far the majority of patients with hematuria in pregnancy are bleeding from varicosities of the bladder mucosa, or because they have hydronephrosis or pyelitis. Other causes such as tuberculosis, stone, acute nephritis, tumor and occasionally, syphilis, must be ruled out.

Pregnancy after Removal of Kidney. With the extension of renal surgery it is not uncommon to have to consider what may be the outcome in women who have become pregnant after the removal of one kidney on account of tuberculosis, stone, pyelonephritis or other lesions. Large series of such cases, totaling about 365, have been reported by Bleynie, Matthews, Hartmann, Pousson and Prather. Some of these patients had been pregnant more than once following the nephrectomy. The predominant reasons for the nephrectomies were tuberculosis in 55 per cent, pyonephrosis in 10 per cent, and calculi in 9 per cent.

Owing to the fact that the potential renal function is much in excess of the needs of the individual, and that the surviving kidney undergoes definite parenchymatous hypertrophy with increased excretory capacity, such women do perfectly well, provided the remaining kidney is normal. On the other hand, if it is the seat of chronic nephritis irreparable damage may result from the additional strain incident to pregnancy, while the development of a toxemia or a urinary tract infection must be regarded as much more serious than in a patient with two kidneys. Accordingly, when consulted by a woman with one kidney as to the advisability of her becoming pregnant, we suggest a thorough evaluation of the capabilities of the remaining organ. Should it be found unsatisfactory we advise contraceptive practices; however, in the unintelligent sterilization may be justified. When the nephrectomy has been done for tuberculosis three or four years should be allowed to elapse without reappearance of the disease before pregnancy should be allowed to take place. Usually, however, pregnancy has commenced when the physician first sees the patient. In the absence of symptoms such individuals should be carefully watched and each month accurate chemical and kidney function tests made to ascertain that the single kidney is functioning satisfactorily, which is fortunately the case in most instances. On the other hand, if the patient is suffering from chronic nephritis abortion should be induced as soon as the diagnosis is made. Moreover, premature labor should be induced at the first sign of the development of a toxemia or pyelitis. In the 365 pregnancies in 296 nephrectomized women, as reported by Prather, who summarizes the literature up to 1934, the following complications occurred: miscarriage 8 per cent, toxemias 2.7 per cent, and death 4 times or 1.4 per cent, the cause being eclampsia in one and uremia in three patients. Interruption of pregnancy in these patients was deemed necessary in 11.5 per cent. The result to the product of conception is mentioned in connection with 135 of the series, and of this number, 115 were born alive and apparently healthy, while 20 or 14.9 per cent were lost through miscarriage or stillbirth.

Cortical Necrosis of the Kidney. Bilateral necrosis of the renal cortex, although rare, is a definite entity recognized as such since Jubel-Renoy's first description of it in 1886. Most of the cases reported occurred in pregnant women usually following such complications as retroplacental bleeding or premature separation of the placenta. The onset of the condition is insidious in that invariably it is not preceded by signs or symptoms of any toxemia or renal disease. Edema may be present and occasionally convulsions may appear. The characteristic finding is suppression of urine, often to complete anuria. Where some urine is being secreted albuminuria is always present and usually also erythrocytes.

In 1930 Scriver and Oertel reviewed the literature and reported three additional cases, two confirmed at autopsy and one in which recovery took place. These authors concluded that the condition is the result of "a terminal arterial segmentary collapse (vasoparalysis) with blood stasis and segmentary thrombosis with proximal extensions," and that these vascular changes in the kidneys may be related to a general abnormal vasomotor irritability of the pregnant state

The blood pressure may or may not be elevated. Kellogg reported a case in which the pressure rose to 200/120, while Crook recorded a case with a systolic pressure of 95. Davis recently reported a case of cortical necrosis associated with premature separation of the placenta in which the blood pressure rose within three days from 130/95 to 180/120. From a review of the literature and a consideration of his own patient he concludes that in most instances there is an association with preeclampsia or renal disease.

As a result of urinary suppression nitrogenous retention in the blood is the outstanding chemical finding. With improvement, the first evidence of which is increasing urinary secretion, the nitrogenous elements in the blood gradually return to normal. The prognosis is grave as is evidenced by the fact that most of the recorded cases in the literature had a fatal outcome. Treatment is mainly prophylactic in that the early signs or symptoms of toxemia or other abnormality, such as premature separation of the placenta, must be recognized and appropriate treatment instituted as outlined in the section on the toxemias of pregnancy. Once the condition has developed attempts should be made to stimulate urinary secretion. Intravenous administration of 15 to 20 per cent glucose solution is, in our opinion, preferable to other types of diuretic medication. Madding, Binger and Hunt recently reported a case of postpartum urinary suppression, resembling bilateral cortical necrosis of the kidneys, in which recovery took place following the administration of mild diuretics such as dextrose with aminophyllin intravenously. These authors stress the importance of treating acidosis and supplying fluids liberally, but not in excess.

Urologic Diagnostic Methods in Pregnancy. A consideration of diagnostic methods particularly applicable to the urinary complications of pregnancy may be helpful as frequently the symptoms of the patient are sufficiently vague so that one is in doubt as to the location and extent of the pathologic processes. To clarify the situation it is necessary to employ some of the procedures of the bacteriologist and urologist.

Bacteriologic Cultures of Urine, Blood and the Uterus. Not infrequently one must differentiate between postpartum fevers caused by uterine infections and those of the urinary tract. Culture of the lochia removed from the uterine cavity under sterile precautions is often helpful. The bacterial growth observed in patients with low grade febrile reactions due to uterine infection usually embraces the diphtheroids, anaerobic nonhemolytic streptococci and staphylococci. Such organisms seldom cause the high intermittent type of fever usually encountered in pyelitis. On the other hand, should the uterine culture disclose hemolytic types of streptococci or staphylococci one can expect much more marked excursions of temperature reaction. Culture of the bladder urine only occasionally discloses the same infective organism in both the urinary and genital tracts. The commonest cause of pyelitis is *B. coli.* But as it is found frequently in gravid women who do not develop cystitis or pyeloureteritis the positive culture alone is not sufficient evidence to clinch the diagnosis. If, however, one has in addition clumped pus cells in the urine, a hectic fever and a tender kidney, the diagnosis of pyelitis is usually justifiable. The presence of pus cells in specimens of urine obtained by ureteral catheterization, even though this procedure is rarely necessary, is even more significant than such microscopic and bacteriologic evidence obtained from bladder urine because the complicating factor of a possible cystitis has been obviated. Blood cultures done on patients with the thrombophlebitic type of puerperal infection are frequently positive, whereas those done on patients with pyelitis or pyelonephritis even when made at the height of a chill are usually negative.

Cystoscopy during Pregnancy. Previous to the eighth month of gestation cystoscopy is not greatly complicated by the proximity of the presenting part. During the last month, however, particularly in primigravidae, the vertex or breech descends and in doing so impinges upon the posterior surface of the bladder causing a marked elevation of the base and trigonum. Under such circumstances considerable difficulty may be encountered in inspection of the bladder, but more especially in locating the ureteral orifices. Occasionally it is practically impossible so that diagnostic and therapeutic procedures depending upon the passage of the ureteral catheter are attended by difficulty and uncertainty.

Kidney Function Tests. In the gravid state the kidneys are called upon to excrete a progressively increasing quantity of waste products. This burden in itself constitutes the best test of kidney function. However, inasmuch as the results of poor kidney function in pregnancy are difficult to evaluate and may be complicated by other factors, it is desirable to utilize tests designed to express the excretory ability of the kidney more specifically. Many have been devised but in our experience we have found the urea clearance test and the fractional phthalein test to be the most useful. The methods of doing these tests may be found in the section, The Toxemias of Pregnancy. Differentiation between the function of the two kidneys is obtained by placing a catheter in each ureter and collecting the specimens as indicated.

Visualization of the Urinary Tracts. Intravenous pyelography has proved to be a great aid in pregnancy. There are various modifications of the organic compound mono-iodo-methane sulfonate of sodium which are used by injection directly into the blood stream where they are broken down into iodine-bearing substances which are excreted almost entirely by the kidney. Because of this characteristic and the fact that they are opaque to the x-rays they can be used to visualize and outline the urinary tract. This method obviates the use of the cystoscope in a great many patients when it is undesirable or impossible to employ that procedure. There seems to be no contraindication as we have used it in a large number of patients with all manner of complications and in all stages of pregnancy. In fact it seems to give unusually good results in pregnancy because of the static condition of the urinary stream which allows a considerable accumulation of the material within the tract and for this reason gives clearly outlined structures. It has another advantage in that it visualizes both tracts simultaneously whereas we seldom feel justified in doing retrograde pyelograms on two sides at the same time. In addition it may be considered as a rough kidney function test. Failure to excrete any of the opaque substance in a 30-minute period nearly always indicates an extremely low kidney function, whereas clearly outlined tracts in a 15-minute plate can be assumed to mean a practically normal excretory ability. Retrograde pyelograms cannot be completely replaced by the use of intravenous contrast media because of the clearer shadows obtained by the former, and because in pregnancy the pelvic ureter is seldom outlined except by placing an opaque substance in the tract through the ureteral catheter. Therefore when we wish a complete and careful study we must resort to the retrograde method. This is usually done as part of a complete investigation in association with the kidney function test, bacteriologic culture, microscopic examination of urine specimen and the measurement of residual urine.

Interpretation of x-rays of the urinary tract of the pregnant woman requires a knowledge of the variations in the tract associated with pregnancy. We frequently see a widely dilated ureter and kidney pelvis during the period of gestation which we interpet as normal, whereas in the nonpregnant state a diagnosis of hydronephrosis and hydro-ureter would be justified. However, blunting of the shadows of the calyces always points to infection in our experience as do also fuzzy outlines in this region. Much has been written of ureteral "kinks" in the pyelo-ureterograms of pregnancy. These have been explained by the supposed sagging of the kidney particularly on the right side, by aberrant blood vessels causing obstruction, and by peristaltic waves in the ureter. It is well known that the ureter not only dilates in pregnancy but elongates as well. Sometimes this additional length is accommodated by a lateral displacement of the ureter. However, not infrequently it is too long to occupy the space between the bladder and kidney without some degree of convolution. These curves when viewed in the plane of curvature assume the appearance of "kinks"; however when seen at right angles they are recognized in their true character as curves. True kinking of the ureter, that is, actual angulation with some occlusion of the lumen is extremely rare in the pregnant woman. Presumably this is true because the tube is seldom empty and usually contains urine under slight pressure. Following delivery with the removal of the weight of the uterus from the pelvic brim, collapse of the ureter and kinking may occur, particularly when infection has caused delayed irritability and peristalsis of the musculature. In normal pregnancy, on the other hand, peristalsis and tonus return during the last month of pregnancy so that when the uterus is evacuated the ureter rapidly contracts. For these reasons kinking postpartum is rare except in those ureters that have suffered severe damage.

Inasmuch as it has been asserted that frequent exposure to the x-rays during pregnancy may be harmful to the fetus it is wise to observe caution in their use. A limit of three exposures with an interval of seven days has been accepted as an arbitrary standard. Under no circumstances should the fluoroscope be used for any but the briefest observation and then only at long intervals.

SURGICAL CONDITIONS IN PREGNANCY

Formerly it was believed that the performance of surgical operations during pregnancy would almost inevitably bring about abortion or premature labor, even the extraction of a tooth being considered a serious procedure. At present, however, thanks to anesthesia and a perfected surgical technic, many operations can be performed at this time with but little additional risk. Accordingly, whenever a condition arises in the pregnant woman which imperatively demands surgical treatment the necessary operation should be performed without hesitation. At the same time, if the indication is not pressing, it is advisable to defer interference until after delivery so as not to subject the patient to an added strain.

Considerable evidence appears to show that amputations are not more dangerous than at other times. Furthermore, Schmidt in 1915 collected from the literature 36 cases in which nephrectomy was performed, in 28 of which the operation had no effect upon the course of pregnancy. Numerous cases are on record in which paranephritic or broad-ligament abscesses have been opened. Tumors of the generative tract can likewise be excised without great risk of markedly increasing the danger of premature labor and are considered in the section, Complications Due to Diseases of the Generative Tract.

Appendicitis. Appendicitis probably occurs as frequently during pregnancy as at other times although it is quite impossible to substantiate such a statement by statistical data. Jerlov was able to collect 456 cases which had occurred in Scandinavia in the 20 years following 1900. Merger in 1939 reported 20 cases operated upon during the past twenty years in the Tarnier clinic in Paris, an incidence of 1:1,300 pregnancies. There were three maternal deaths and the author states that the complication becomes more serious as term is approached. In a recent review of the surgical complications occurring in 40,000 obstetrical patients admitted to the New York Lying-In Hospital, Child and Douglas found 40 cases of operative appendicitis. In agreement with other reports in the literature they noted that by far the greater number of cases of appendicitis occur during the early months of pregnancy, and when appendicitis does occur later it becomes a more serious complication. Of the entire group there were two maternal deaths, both with generalized peritonitis and occurring at or near term.

It should be regarded as a serious complication, as many women would die if not operated on, while the surgical procedures undertaken for its relief may, at times, be followed by abortion or premature labor. Pankow attributes its increased gravity at this time to the fact that the head of the cecum is displaced upward as pregnancy advances, being at the level of the iliac crest in the latter part of gestation, instead of at the level of the acetabulum as in nonpregnant women. On the other hand, Merger states that in his experience the site of the appendix was not appreciably modified by pregnancy. Our own observations lead us to believe that the appendix may be situated at a considerably higher level in some cases while in others it is found at the usual site. For this reason, as well as for other obvious reasons such as drainage if found advisable, we believe that a "high" McBurney incision has many advantages over midline or various types of right rectus incisions.

The symptoms do not differ from those observed in nonpregnant women but the condition is frequently not recognized as the pains are often considered as being due to the pregnancy itself, while the distention of the abdominal walls by the enlarged uterus makes difficult the appreciation of the rigidity and muscle-spasm which are usually valuable diagnostic aids. The relaxation of the abdominal walls also tends to make the spasm and rigidity a less prominent feature than it is in the nonpregnant woman. In addition there is a leukocytosis and increased sedimentation rate associated with pregnancy that may at times add to the difficulties of making a correct diagnosis.

One should always consider the possibility of appendicitis when a pregnant woman complains of pain in the right side of the abdomen associated with an elevation of temperature and pulse, provided some more satisfactory explanation for the condition cannot be found. It should, however, be remembered that pyelitis or inflammatory conditions of the appendages may give rise to identical symptoms. At the time of labor and during the puerperium its recognition is still more difficult and women have died from peritonitis with the diagnosis of puerperal infection.

If the diagnosis is not clear it is our practice to place the patient under close observation and to do a white blood count every four hours. During this period of time an ice cap over the affected region may be employed but the patient is permitted only clear fluids by mouth. Microscopic and bacteriologic examinations of catheterized specimens of bladder urine should also be carried out. In this connection it is important to note that sometimes the examination of the initial specimen of urine yields negative results while the examination of a second specimen a few hours later may reveal the presence of pus or other significant findings. At the same time, once the diagnosis is established with reasonable certainty, delay in operation will only add to the gravity of the situation. As previously stated we are convinced that the McBurney incision performed at a somewhat higher level, depending on the duration of pregnancy, is much superior to any other approach. At times it may be necessary to enlarge the incision to facilitate the procedure. If the operation is performed skillfully and proper sedation is employed postoperatively, including the use of morphine, we feel that there is but little danger of an abortion or premature labor following such a procedure.

Peptic Ulcer. Sandweiss, Podolsky, Saltzstein and Farbman recently reported a fatal case of perforation of a gastric ulcer in a six-months pregnant woman. In a review of the literature they were able to find 13 deaths attributable to a similar cause. It is felt that more deaths occur in pregnancy as a result of perforated peptic ulcer than is appreciated due to erroneous diagnoses. Pregnancy or the puerperium must not be considered a contraindication to surgery when this is indicated for peptic ulcer.

Ulcerative Colitis. Felsen and Wolarsky have analyzed the clinical courses of 34 women with ulcerative colitis in 50 pregnancies and find that in 30 per cent of the pregnancies the colitis was somewhat aggravated in the first trimester. The colitis was definitely ameliorated in 58 per cent and unchanged in 12 per cent. In cases of this disease which become worse in gestation, the causative factor may be of a psychogenic nature rather than any intrinsic effect of pregnancy itself. Thus, fear on the part of the patient that pregnancy will aggravate her disease may precipitate an exacerbation. Hence, reassurance is a most important part of management.

Colostomy. Patients with colostomies usually go through pregnancy without difficulty. Contrary to what one might expect, intestinal obstruction due to pressure of the enlarged uterus on the proximal loop of intestine concerned, rarely occurs. This complication, however, was observed in one of our patients near term, but was relieved immediately by cesarean section.

Intestinal Obstruction. This rare complication of pregnancy should be treated upon general surgical principles. Carcinoma of the colon complicating pregnancy is a rare association. We have had only one case and this was manifested by intestinal obstruction. In general we believe that, with the exception of the last two months, the pregnancy should be disregarded in the surgical treatment of the carcinoma.

Carcinoma of Breast. It is the consensus that carcinoma of the breast is aggravated by pregnancy, but opinion is by no means unanimous. Since estrogen is a specific growth hormone for mammary tissue, it might be expected theoretically that the saturation with estrogen which the pregnant organism undergoes would accelerate the growth of any malignant mammary cells present. In keeping with this concept is Geschickter's finding that the 5-year cure rate in 58 pregnant patients with mammary carcinoma was only 19 per cent, in contrast to 40 per cent in nonpregnant women with the disease. On the other hand, F. R. Smith, reporting from the Memorial Hospital in New York City, and Westberg, on the basis of an extensive statistical study in Sweden, believe that pregnancy is without influence on breast cancer. My own very small experience would lead me to believe that the growth of both primary mammary carcinoma and recurrence is accelerated by pregnancy and that therapeutic abortion is usually indicated.

Relaxation of the Pelvic Joints. In a previous section we referred to the action of the ovarian hormone (relaxin) on the pelvic joints. In addition to this hormonal change there is undoubtedly increased vascularity which may further favor increased mobility of the various pelvic joints. Occasionally, however, the softening of the interarticular cartilage at the symphysis pubis admits of such abnormal motion in the joint as to interfere seriously with the comfort of the patient who suffers from intense dragging pains in the pelvis and lower abdomen; while at the same time the gait may be so profoundly altered as to suggest the existence of cerebral or spinal trouble. In such cases the application of a tightly fitting bandage about the thighs is followed by marked improvement though occasionally the symptoms are so pronounced that the patient is obliged to take to her bed. The condition usually disappears spontaneously during the course of the puerperium but in exceptional instances it may persist and give rise to such great discomfort that it may become necessary to "wire" the joint.

Similar relaxation may involve the sacro-iliac joints and cause great suffering. Particular attention has been directed to its frequency and significance by Goldthwait and Osgood. In many instances great relief may be afforded by applying adhesive strips which extend outward from the posterior surface of the sacrum to the external portion of the thighs.

BIBLIOGRAPHY

Adler, L. u. Thaler, H. Exp. und klin. Studien über die Graviditäts-tetanie. Ztschr. f. Geburtsh. u. Gynäk., 1908, 62:194.

Albrecht, H. Zur Aetiologie der Chorea gravidarum. Ztschr. f. Geburtsh. u. Gynäk., 1915, 76:677.

Anderson, G. W., and Musselman, L. The Treatment of Tetany in Pregnancy with a Brief Review of the Literature. Am. J. Obst. & Gynec., 1942, 43:547.

Anderson, G. W., and Busby, T. Sickle Cell Anemia and Pregnancy. Am. J. Obst. & Gynec., 1949, 58:75.

Aub, J. C., Fairhall, L. T., Minot, A. S., and Reznikoff, Paul. Lead Poisoning. Medicine, 1925, 4:1.

Aycock, W. L. Frequency of Poliomyelitis in Pregnancy. New Eng. J. Med., 1941, 225:405.

Baber, M. D., and Daley, D. Coarctation of the Aorta in Association with Pregnancy (A Review of the Literature with Description of a Case). J. Obst. & Gynaec. Brit. Emp., 1947, 54:91.

Baird, D. Anatomy and Physiology of Upper Urinary Tract in Pregnancy: Relation to Pyelitis. J. Obst. & Gynaec., Brit. Emp., 1931, 38:516.

——— Upper Urinary Tract in Pregnancy. Lancet, 1932, 2:983.

——— A Study of Ureteral Tone during Pregnancy. J. Obst. & Gynaec., Brit. Emp., 1933, 40:472.

Balfour, W. M., and others. Radioactive Iron Absorption in Clinical Conditions; Normal Pregnancy, Anemia and Hemochromatosis. J. Exper. Med., 1942, 76:15.

Ballantyne, J. W., and Milligan, D. A Case of Scarlet Fever in Pregnancy, with Infection of the Foetus. Tr. Edinb. Obst. Soc., 1893, 18:177.

Barns, H. H. F. Diabetes Mellitus and Pregnancy. J. Obst. & Gynaec. Brit. Emp., 1941, 48:707.

Behm, C. Ueber intrauterine Vaccination. Ztschr. f. Geburtsh. u. Gynäk., 1882, 6:636.

Benensohn, S. J. Pregnancy in the Syphilitic Mother. A Study of 935 Pregnancies at the Cook County Hospital. Am. J. Obst. & Gynec., 1942, 43:508.

BIERRING, W. L. Intermittent Hydrarthrosis. J.A.M.A., 1921, 77:785.

BILL, A. H., and POSEY, F. M. Pregnancy and Diabetes. Am. J. Obst. & Gynec., 1944, 48:405.

BIX, H. The Relationship Between Maternal Diabetes and Giant Children. Am. J. Obst. & Gynec., 1935, 29:903.

BLACKLOCK, B., and GORDON, R. M. Malaria Infection as It Occurs in Late Pregnancy. Ann. Trop. M. & Parasitol., 1925, 19:326-364.

BRANDSTRUP, E., and OKKELS, H. Pregnancy Complicated with Diabetes. Acta Obst. et Gynec. Scandinav., 1938, 18:136.

BRIDGMAN, E. W., and NORWOOD, V. Pulmonary Tuberculosis and Pregnancy. Bull. Johns Hopkins Hosp., 1926, 38:83-111.

BRINDEAU, A. Indications and Methods for Terminating Pregnancy in Cases of Pulmonary Tuberculosis. Bruxelles Méd., 1937, 18:39.

BRINDEAU, A., KOURILSKY, R., and KOURILSKY, S. Pulmonary Tuberculosis in the Pregnant Woman. Bull. et mém. Soc. Méd. d. hôp. de Paris, 1935, 51:478.

BUNIM, J. J., and RUBRICIUS, J. The Determination of Prognosis of Pregnancy in Rheumatic Heart Disease. Am. Heart J., 1948, 35:282.

BUNIM, J. J., and APPEL, S. B. A Principle for Determining Prognosis of Pregnancy in Rheumatic Heart Disease. J.A.M.A. (in press).

BURKE, Hugh E. Pregnancy and Experimental Pulmonary Tuberculosis in Rabbits. Surg., Gynec. & Obst., 1940, 71:615.

BURNETT, C., and KLASS, I. A Review of the Problem of Purpura during Pregnancy. J. Obst. & Gynaec. Brit. Emp., 1943, 50:393.

BURNETT, E. C., and MCMENEMEY, W. H. Rupture of the Normal Spleen in Pregnancy. Brit. M. J. 1935, 1:1122.

CALMETTE, A., VALTIS, J. et LACOMME, M. Transmission Intrautérine du Virus Tuberculeux de la Mère à l'Enfant. Press méd., 1926, 34:1409.

CARPENTER, C. M., WILSON, K. M., and LEAHY, Alice D. Comparison of Results of Smear and Cultural Methods for Diagnosis of Gonococcal Infections in Adult Females. Am. J. Syph., Gonor., & Ven. Dis., 1938, 22:55.

CARR, F. Benjamin, and HAMILTON, Burton E. Five Hundred Women with Serious Heart Diseases Followed Through Pregnancy and Delivery. Am. J. Obst. & Gynec., 1933, 26:824.

CASTALLO, M. A., and RAKOFF, A. E. An Analysis of 259 Cases of Syphilis Complicating Pregnancy. Penn. M. J., 1935, 39:24.

CHEATHAM, G. R. Pyelonephritis of Pregnancy Due to Bacillus Dysenteriae. Am. J. Obst. & Gynec., 1934, 28:448.

CHILD, C. G., and DOUGLAS, R. G. Surgical Problems Arising during Pregnancy. Am. J. Obst. & Gynec., 1944, 47:213.

CORBUS, B. C., and DANFORTH, W. C. Pyelitis in Pregnancy. J. Urol., 1927, 18:543.

COSTELLO, M. J. Eruptions of Pregnancy. New York State J. Med., 1941, 41:849.

COUVELAIRE, A. Le Nouveau-né Issu de Mère Tuberculeuse. Gynéc. et Obst., 1927, 15:1-9.

CRABTREE, E. G. Nature and Significance of Renal Stasis. Surg., Gynec. & Obst., 1922, 35:733.

——— Stricture Formation in the Ureter Following Pyelonephritis of Pregnancy. J. Urol., 1927, 18:575.

——— Rate of Recovery after Pyelitis of Pregnancy. Tr. Am. Ass. Genito-Urin. Surg., 1929, 22:149.

——— Changes in the Urinary Tract in Women. The Result of Normal Pregnancy. New Eng. J. Med., 1931, 205:1048.

CRABTREE, E. G., and PRATHER, G. C. Clinical Aspects of Pyelonephritis in Pregnancy. New Eng. J. Med., 1930, 202:357.

——— Urinary Diseases in Pregnancy. A Consideration of Preventive and Therapeutic Measures in Treatment and Conservation Surgery. J. Urol., 1931, 26:499.

——— Urinary Tract Infections Associated with Pregnancy. Their Fate in Succeeding Pregnancies. J.A.M.A., 1933, 101:1928.

CRABTREE, E. G., and SHEDDEN, W. M. The Sagging Kidney as a Factor in the Persistence of Colon Bacillus Pyelitis. J. Urol., 1921, 6:207.

CRAGIN, E. B. Congenital Pelvic Kidneys Obstructing the Parturient Canal. Am. J. Obst., 1898, 38:36.

DABNEY, W. H., and HARRIS, N. M. Report of a Case of Gonorrheal Endocarditis in a Patient Dying in the Puerperium. Bull. Johns Hopkins Hosp., 1901, 12:68.

DALÉAS, P. Malaria and Pregnancy. Rev. franc. de gynéc. et d'obst., 1936, 31:232.

DANIEL, M., and ANTIS, M. Macrocytic Hyperchromic Anemia of Pregnancy. Am. J. Obst. & Gynec., 1942, 44:93.

DAUWE, O. Conservation of Pregnancy in Pulmonary Tuberculosis. Bruxelles Méd., 1937, 18:45.

Dieckmann, W. J., and Priddle, H. D. Anemia of Pregnancy Treated with Molybdenum-Iron Complex. Am. J. Obst. & Gynec., 1949, 57:541.

Dippel, A. L. The Relationship of Congenital Syphilis to Abortion and Miscarriage, and the Mechanism of Intrauterine Protection. Am. J. Obst. & Gynec., 1944, 47:369.

Douglas, R. G. Chemotherapy in Obstetrics and Gynecology. Am. J. Obst. & Gynec., 1940, 39:275.

Douglas, R. G., Davis, I. F., and Shandorf, J. F. Gonorrhea in the Female and Its Treatment with Sulfonamides. Am. J. Obst. & Gynec., 1942, 44:1026.

Eastman, N. J. Diabetes Mellitus in Pregnancy. Obst. & Gynec. Surv., 1946, 1:1.

Ehlinger, E., and Künsch, M. Tuberculosis in Twins: Investigations on Forty-Six Pairs. Beitr. z. Klin. d. Tuberk, 1938, 92:275.

Eisele, C. W., and Mason, E. W. Unsuspected Tuberculosis in Pregnant Women as Revealed by Routine Roentgenologic Examination. Am. J. Obst. & Gynec., 1938, 36:387.

Evans, R. S. The Use of Concentrated Red Cells as a Substitute for Whole Blood in Transfusion Therapy of Anemia. J.A.M.A., 1943, 122:793.

Felsen, J., and Wolarsky, W. Chronic Ulcerative Colitis and Pregnancy. Am. J. Obst. & Gynec., 1948, 56:751.

Fildes, P. The Prevalence of Congenital Syphilis Amongst the Newly Born of the East End of London. J. Obst. & Gynaec. Brit. Emp., 1915, 27:124.

Finlay, C. E. Visual Field Defects in Pregnancy. Arch. Ophthal., 1934, 12:207-219.

Finn, W. F. Thrombocytopenic Purpura in Pregnancy. Am. J. Obst. & Gynec., 1944, 48:497.

Fitz-Patrick, G. Addison's Disease Complicating Pregnancy. Surg., Gynec. & Obst., 1922, 35:72-76.

Forssner, H. Les Relations entre l'État de Gestation et la Tuberculose. Acta Gynec. Scandinav., 1925, 3:256-285.

Fouts, P. J., Gustafson, G. W., and Zerfas, L. G. Successful Treatment of a Case of Polyneuritis of Pregnancy. Am. J. Obst. & Gynec., 1934, 28:902.

Frey, W. Herz und Schwangerschaft. Leipzig, 1923.

Friedrich, H. Hormonbehandlung des Pruritus vulvae in der Gravidität. Zentralbl. f. Gynak., 1938, 62:1289.

Frisch, A. Pulmonary Tuberculosis and Pregnancy. Wien. klin. Wchnschr., 1936, 42:1287.

Gammeltoft, S. A. The Heart in Pregnancy. Surg., Gynec. et Obst., 1928, 46:382-390.

Geschickter, C. F. Diseases of the Breast. 2nd Ed., Lippincott, 1945.

Gilligan, D. R., Garb, S., Wheeler, C., and Plummer, N. Adjuvant Alkali Therapy in the Prevention of Renal Complications from Sulfadiazine. J.A.M.A., 1943, 122:1160.

Goldsborough, F. C. Thrombosis of the Internal Iliac Vein during Pregnancy. Bull. Johns Hopkins Hosp., 1904, 15:193-195.

Goodwin, M. S., and Moore, J. E. Penicillin in Prevention of Prenatal Syphilis. J.A.M.A., 1946, 130:688.

Grier, R. M., and Richter, H. A. Pregnancy with Leukemia. A Case Report and Review of the Literature. Am. J. Obst. & Gynec., 1939, 37:412.

Gustafson, G. W., and Garceau, G. J. Cerebral Spastic Paralysis. J.A.M.A., 1941, 116:374.

Guttmacher, A. F. A Case of Severe Scleroderma with Successful Delivery. Urol. & Cutaneous Rev., 1943, 47:107.

Hamilton, B. E., and Thomson, K. J. The Heart in Pregnancy and the Childbearing Age. Little, Brown and Company, Boston, 1941.

Hamilton, H. G., Pittam, R. F., and Higgins, R. S. Active Therapy of Varicose Veins in Pregnancy. South. M. J., 1949, 42:608.

Harmon, P. H., and Hoyne, A. Poliomyelitis and Pregnancy with Special Reference to the Failure of Fetal Infection. J.A.M.A., 1943, 123:185.

Harris, J. W. Influenza Occurring in Pregnant Women. J.A.M.A., 1919, 72:978-980.

Heath, C. W., and Patek, A. J. The Anemia of Iron Deficiency. Medicine, 1937, 16:267.

Hench, P. S. The Ameliorating Effect of Pregnancy on Chronic Atrophic (Infectious Rheumatoid) Arthritis, Fibrositis, and Intermittent Hydrarthrosis. Proc. Staff Meet. Mayo Clin., 1938, 13:161.

Herrick, W. W., and Tillman, A. J. B. Diabetes and Pregnancy. Surg., Gynec., & Obst., 1938, 66:37.

Hicks, H. T., and French, H. Typhoid Fever and Pregnancy, with Special Reference to Foetal Infection. Lancet, 1905, 1:1491-1493.

Hofbauer, J. Beiträge zur Ätiologie und Behandlung der Pyelitis gravidarum. Arch. f. Gynäk., 1928, 134:205.

——— Contributions to the Etiology of Pyelitis in Pregnancy. Bull. Johns Hopkins Hosp., 1928, 42:118-155.

Ianne, C. L., and Muir, J. C. Prevention of Tuberculosis Begins Before Birth. Tuberculin Testing during Pregnancy as a Fertile Field for Case Finding and Prevention. Am. J. Obst. & Gynec., 1939, 38:448.

INGRAHAM, N. R., Jr. Complications Due to Arsenical Therapy in Syphilitic Pregnant Women. Report of Seven Maternal Deaths. J.A.M.A., 1939, 112:1537.

——— Prenatal Management of Syphilis with Special Reference to Penicillin Therapy. M. Clin. North America, 1948, 32:1647.

IRVING, F. R. Anemia of Pregnancy. A Study of 60 Cases of the Hypochromatic Type. Am. J. Obst. & Gynec., 1935, 29:850.

JAVERT, C. T. Hyperthyroidism and Pregnancy. Am. J. Obst. & Gynec., 1940, 39:954.

JENSEN, F. G. Investigations on the Influence of Pregnancy and Parturition upon Organic Cardiac Disease. Acta obst. et gynec. Scandinav., 1927, 6:239-278.

JENSEN, J. The Heart in Pregnancy. The C. V. Mosby Company, St. Louis, Mo., 1938.

JERLOV, Emil. Ueber Appendicitis während der Gravidität und im Puerperium. Acta obst. et gynec. Scandinav., 1926, Bd. 4, Supplement 1-168.

KAISER, I. H. Rectal Stricture Complicating Labor. Am. J. Obst. & Gynec., 1943, 46:672.

——— and KING, E. L. Lymphopathia Venereum Complicating Labor. Am. J. Obst. & Gynec., 1947, 54:219.

KLEINBERG, S., and HORWITZ, T. The Obstetric Experiences of Women Paralyzed by Acute Anterior Poliomyelitis. Surg., Gynec., & Obst., 1941, 72:58.

KLEMPERER, F. Tuberkulose und Schwangerschaft. Ztschr. f. Geburtsh. u. Gynäk., 1929, 96:1.

KRAMER, D. W. Some Problems in Pregnancy and Diabetes. Am. J. Obst. & Gynec., 1935, 30:68.

KRAUS, J. Diabetes Mellitus and Pregnancy. Med. Klin., Berlin, 1936, 32:375.

KRETSCHMER, H. L. The Treatment of Pyelitis. Surg., Gynec. & Obst., 1921, 33:632.

——— Pyelitis of Pregnancy. J.A.M.A., 1923, 81:1585.

——— and HEANEY, N. S. Dilatation of the Ureter and Kidney Pelvis during Pregnancy. A Pyelographic Study. J.A.M.A., 1925, 85:406.

——— HEANY, N. S., and OCKULY, E. A. Dilatation of the Kidney Pelvis and Ureter during Pregnancy and the Puerperium. A Pyelographic Study in Normal Women. J.A.M.A., 1933, 101:2025.

KREUTZMANN, H. R. Studies in Normal Ureteral and Vesical Pressure. J. Urol., 1928, 19:517.

LABATE, J. S. Classification and Treatment of the Anemias of Pregnancy. Am. J. Obst. & Gynec., 1939, 38:48.

LAMB, A. E. Heart Disease in Pregnancy. Am. J. M. Sc., 1934, 187:177.

LANZ, W. Ueber einen Fall von Tuberkulose der Plazenta u. der Eihäute. Arch. f. Gynäk., 1915, 104:238.

LEE, H. P., and MENGERT, W. F. Effect of Pregnancy on Urinary Tract (pyelographic study). J.A.M.A., 1934, 102:102.

LESSE, S. The Prognosis of the Cardiac Patient in Pregnancy. Am. J. Obst. & Gynec., 1948, 56:477.

LIDDELL, R. M., and TANGYE, C. E. A Case of Intrauterine Scarlet Fever. Brit. M. J., 1916, 2:389.

LIEBLING, P. Purpura Haemorrhagica Complicating Pregnancy. Am. J. Obst. & Gynec., 1926, 11:847.

LITZENBERG, J. C., and CAREY, J. B. The Relation of Basal Metabolism to Gestation. Am. J. Obst. & Gynec., 1929, 17:550.

LUCKÉ, B. Pathology of Fatal Epidemic Hepatitis. Am. J. Path., 1944, 20:471.

——— and MALLORY, T. Fulminant Form of Epidemic Hepatitis. Am. J. Path., 1946, 22:867.

LYNCH, F. W. Placental Transmission, with Report of a Case during Typhoid Fever. Johns Hopkins Hosp. Rep., 1902, 10:283.

MACKENZIE. Heart Disease and Pregnancy. London, 1921.

MARSHALL, G., and others. Management of Pregnancy, Parturition, and Puerperium in Tuberculous Women. Brit. M. J., 1931, 1:140; Lancet, 1931, 1:186.

MATTHEWS, H. B. Pregnancy after Nephrectomy. J.A.M.A., 1921, 77:1634.

——— and DER BRUCKE, M. G. "Normal Expectancy" in the Extremely Obese Pregnant Woman. J.A.M.A., 1938, 110:554.

MAYER, A. Normales Schwangerschaftserum als Heilmittel gegen Schwangerschaftsdermatosen Zentralbl. f. Gynäk., 1911, 35:350.

MCCAUSLAND, A. M. The Influence of Hormones upon Varicose Veins in Pregnancy. West. J. Surg., 1943, 51:199.

MCCORD, J. R. Prenatal Treatment of Syphilis: Some Results of Antisyphilitic Treatment in a Series of 519 Pregnant Syphilitic Colored Women. Am. J. Syph., 1932, 16:78.

——— Syphilis of the Placenta. The Histologic Examination of 1,085 Placentas of Mothers with Strongly Positive Blood Wassermann Reactions. Am. J. Obst. & Gynec., 1934, 28:743.

——— Syphilis and Pregnancy. A Clinical Study of 2,150 Cases. J.A.M.A., 1935, 105:89.

MCKELVEY, J. L., and TURNER, T. B. Syphilis and Pregnancy. An Analysis of the Outcome of Pregnancy in Relation to Treatment in 943 Cases. J.A.M.A., 1934, 102:503.

MCLANE, C. M. Pyelitis of Pregnancy, 5 year Study. Am. J. Obst. & Gynec., 1939, 38:117.

McLaren, H. C., and McLeod, M. A Case of Diabetes Insipidus in Pregnancy. J. Obst. & Gynaec. Brit. Emp., 1942, 49:51.

Mendelson, C. L. Pregnancy and Coarctation of the Aorta. Am. J. Obst. & Gynec., 1940, 39:1014.

——— and Pardee, H. E. B. The Pulse and Respiratory Rates during Labor as a Guide to the Onset of Cardiac Failure in Women with Rheumatic Heart Disease. Am. J. Obst. & Gynec., 1942, 44:370.

Mengert, W. F. Venous Ligation in Obstetrics. Am. J. Obst. & Gynec., 1945, 50:467.

——— and Lee, H. P. Urinary Tract Changes during Late Pregnancy and Early Puerperium. Am. J. Obst. & Gynec., 1932, 24:205.

——— and Paul, W. D. Artificial Pyrexia in Four Pregnant Women. Am. J. Obst. & Gynec., 1942, 44:702.

Merger. Les Appendicites au Cours de la Grossesse et de la Puerpéralité à la Clinique Tarnier pendant les Douze Dernières Années (20 observations). Bull. de la Soc. gynéc. et d'obst., 1939, 28:314.

Meyer-Wedell, Lilli. Blood Examinations in Pregnancy. J. Obst. & Gynaec. Brit. Emp., 1943, 50:405.

Miller, Herbert C., Hurwitz, D., Kuder, K. Fetal and Neonatal Mortality in Pregnancies Complicated by Diabetes Mellitus. J.A.M.A., 1944, 124:271.

Moore, Robert A., and Pastore, J. B. Note on Erythroblastic Splenomegaly Occurring During Pregnancy. Am. J. M. Sc., 1939, 198:187.

Mueller, C. W., and Lapp, W. A. Herpes Gestationis. With a Report of Two Cases and a Survey of the Literature. Am. J. Obst. & Gynec., 1944, 48:170.

Mussey, R. D., and Plummer, W. A. Treatment of Goiter Complicating Pregnancy. J.A.M.A., 1931, 97:602.

Mussey, R. D., Plummer, W. A., and Boothby, W. M. Pregnancy Complicating Exophthalmic Goitre. J.A.M.A., 1926, 86:1009.

New York Heart Ass. Functional Capacity and Therapeutic Classification. Fourth Edition of Nomenclature and Criteria for Diagnosis of Diseases of the Heart. New York Heart Ass., 1939, N. Y.

Nuckols, H. H., and Hertig, A. T. Pneumococcus Infection of the Genital Tract in Women. Especially during Pregnancy and the Puerperium. Am. J. Obst. & Gynec., 1938, 35:782.

Ober, R. E., Horton, R. J. M., and Feemster, R. F. Congenital Defects in Year of Epidemic Rubella. Am. J. Pub. Health, 1947, 37:1328.

Odell, L. D., and Mengert, W. F. The Overweight Obstetric Patient. J.A.M.A., 1945, 128:87.

Oppel, T. W. Congestive Heart Failure in Pregnancy. Am. J. Obst. & Gynec., 1940, 39:24.

——— Pneumonia Associated with Pregnancy. Ann. Int. Med., 1939, 12:1983.

Ornstein, G. G., and Kovnat, M. Influence of Pregnancy on Pulmonary Tuberculosis. Am. Rev. Tuberc., 1935, 31:224.

Pardee, H. E. B. Treatment of Cardiac Failure in Pregnancy. Am. J. Obst. & Gynec., 1922, 3:620.

——— Treatment of Cardiac Failure during Pregnancy. Bull. Lying-In Hosp., N. Y., 1923, 12:207.

Patrick, P. R. Report of a Survey of Children Born in 1941 with Reference to Congenital Abnormalities Arising from Maternal Rubella. M. J. Australia, 1948, 1:421.

Paul, C. Étude sur l'Intoxication Lente par les Préparations de Plomb de son Influence sur le Produit de la Conception. Arch. gén. de méd., 1860, 1:513.

Peelen, J. Pregnancy Complicated by Acute Anterior Poliomyelitis. J. Mich. Med. Soc., 1943, 42:30.

Peterson, R. Gall Stones during Pregnancy. Tr. Am. Gynec. Soc., 1910, 35:84.

Pincus, G., and White, P. On the Inheritance of Diabetes Mellitus. II. Further Analysis of Family Histories. Am. J. M. Sc., 1934, 188:159.

Plass, E. D. Syphilis in Obstetrics. Am. J. Obst. & Gynec., 1942, 43:484.

Plass, E. D., and Mengert, W. E. Gestational Polyneuritis. J.A.M.A., 1934, 101:2020.

Plass, E. D., and Woods, E. B. Hemorrhagic Encephalitis (Neoarsphenamine) in Obstetric Patients. Am. J. Obst. & Gynec., 1935, 29:509.

Plummer, N., Liebmann, J., Solomon, S., Kammerer, W. H., Kalkstein, M., and Ensworth, H. K. Chemotherapy Versus Combined Chemotherapy and Serum in the Treatment of Pneumonia. A Study of 607 Alternated Cases. J.A.M.A., 1941, 116:2366.

Posch, W. Ueber Scharlach Wochenbett. Ztschr. f. Geburtsh. u. Gynäk., 1926, 90:609.

Posner, A. C. Purpura Hemorrhagica Complicating the Puerperium. Am. J. Obst. & Gynec., 1937, 34:155.

Prather, G. C. Postpartum Bladder Complications. Am. J. Obst. & Gynec., 1929, 17:215.

——— The Effect of Changes Due to Pregnancy on Urinary Tract Disease. New Eng. J. Med., 1931, 205:1051.

Prather, G. C., and Crabtree, E. G. Pyelitis in the Puerperium. New Eng. J. Med., 1930, 202:366.

PRATHER, G. C., and CRABTREE, E. G. The Lone Kidney in Pregnancy. Tr. Am. Ass. Genito-Urin. Surg., 1933, 26:313.

——— Impressions Relating to Urinary Tract Stone in Pregnancy. Urol & Cut. Rev., 1934, 38:17.

PRATHER, G. C., CRABTREE, E. G., and ROBINS, S. A. Intravenous Pyelography during Pregnancy. New Eng. J. Med., 1932, 206:62.

QUEIREL. Variole et grossesse. Ann. de gynéc. et d'obst., Paris, 1907, n. s., 4:137.

RANDALL, L. M., and RYNEARSON, E. H. Delivery and Care of the Newborn Infant of the Diabetic Mother. J.A.M.A., 1936, 107:919.

RAY, B. S. Study of Appendicitis; 1,500 Cases at the New York Hospital. New York State J. Med., 1938, 38:412.

REZNIKOFF, Paul. Treatment of Chronic Anemia. Med. Clin. North Am., 1944, 28:368.

ROBERTSON, H. E., and DOCHAT, G. R. Pregnancy and Gall-stones. Int. Abst. Surg. (Surg., Gynec. & Obst.), 1944, 78:193.

RONSHEIM, J. Diabetes and Pregnancy. Am. J. Obst. & Gynec., 1933, 25:710.

ROYSTON, G. D., JENSEN, J., and HAUPTMAN, H. Tuberculosis and Pregnancy. Am. J. Obst. & Gynec., 1937, 34:284.

RUSHMORE, S. Purpura Complicating Pregnancy. Am. J. Obst. & Gynec., 1925, 10:553-560.

SANDWEISS, D. J., PODOLSKY, H. M., SALTZSTEIN, H. C., and FARBMAN, A. A. Deaths from Perforation and Hemorrhage of Gastroducdenal Ulcer during Pregnancy and Puerperium. Am. J. Obst. & Gynec., 1943, 45:131.

SCHEUER, O. Zur frage der Aetiologie der Impetigo herpetiformis. Arch. f. Dermat. u. Syph., 1910, 103:285-304.

SCHULTZE, K. W. Schwangerschaftsneuritis und B_1-Vitamin. Zentralbl. f. Gynäk., 1938, 62:2533.

SCHUMACHER, P. Die Schwangerschaftsveränderungen der ableitenden Harnwege in Röntgenbild. Arch. f. Gynäk., 1930, 143:28.

——— Intravenöse Pyelographie bei Frauen in und ausserhalb der Gravidität. Zentralbl. f. Gynäk., 1930, 54:1474.

——— Kind and Causes of Changes in Upper Urinary Passages in Pyelitis during Pregnancy. Arch. f. Gynäk., 1931, 144:575.

——— Ergebnisse der intravenösen Pyelographie und röntgenologischen Suffizienzprüfung der vesicalen Ureterostien bei der Pyelitis gravidarum. Arch. f. Gynäk., 1931, 147:662.

——— Zur Differentialdiagnose zwischen Appendicitis und schmerzhafter Ureterstauung bzw. Pyelitis in graviditate. Zentralbl. f. Gynäk., 1932, 56:1120.

SCHÜTZ. Ueber den Einfluss der Cholera auf Menstruation. Schwangerschaft, Geburt u. Wochenbett. Zentralbl. f. Gynäk., 1894, 18:1138.

SCHWARTZ, J. Congenital Malaria and Placental Infections Amongst the Negroes of Central Africa. Riv. di malariol (sez I), 1934, 13:435.

SEELEY, W. F., SIDDALL, R. S., and BALZER, W. J. Collapse Therapy for Tuberculosis in Pregnancy. Am. J. Obst. & Gynec., 1939, 37:741.

SERBIN, W. B. Splenomegaly in Pregnancy. Am. J. Obst. & Gynec., 1937, 34:486.

SHEEHAN, H. L. The Pathology of Acute Yellow Atrophy and Delayed Chloroform Poisoning. J. Obst. & Gynaec. Brit. Emp., 1940, 47:49.

SKIPPER, E. Diabetes Mellitus and Pregnancy. Quart. J. M., 1933, 2:353.

SMITH, J. T., Jr. Severe Puerperal Sepsis Due to Gonococcus Infection. Cleveland M. J., 1911, 10:810.

SMITH, F. R. The Effect of Pregnancy on Malignant Tumors. Am. J. Obst. & Gynec., 1937, 34:616.

——— and SPENCE, John M., Jr. Congenital Syphilis in Only One of Twins. South. Med. J., 1941, 34:147.

SNOECK, J. A. Contribution to the Study of the Ptyalism of Pregnancy. Bruxelles méd., 1935, 15:390.

SPITZER, W. The Frequency and Obstetrical Significance of Rupture of Genital Varices. Zentralbl. f. Gynäk., 1933, 57:401.

STANDER, H. J. Heart Disease Complicating Pregnancy. Am. J. Obst. & Gynec., 1938, 36:413.

——— and CADDEN, J. F. The Cardiac Output in Pregnant Women. Am. J. Obst. & Gynec., 1932, 24:13.

——— and KUDER, K. The Treatment of Heart Disease Complicating Pregnancy. J.A.M.A., 1937, 108:2092.

STRAUSS, Maurice B. The Etiology and Treatment of Anemia in Pregnancy. J.A.M.A., 1934, 102:281.

STRICKROOT, F. L., SCHAEFFER, R. L., and BERGO, H. L., Myasthenia Gravis Occurring in an Infant Born of a Myasthenic Mother. J.A.M.A., 1942, 120:1207.

STRONG, R. P. Research in Some Aspects of Disease Associated with the Fields of Zoölogy, Entomology and Parasitology. Science, 1923, 57:513.

SUNDELIN, G. Diabetes and Pregnancy. Nord. med., 1938, 16:1239.

SWAN, C., TOSTEVIN, A. L., MOORE, B., MAYO, H., and BLACK, G. H. B. Congenital Defects in Infants Following Infectious Diseases during Pregnancy, with Special Reference to Relationship between German Measles and Cataract, Deafmutism, Heart Disease and Microcephaly, and to Period of Pregnancy in Which Occurrence of Rubella Is Followed by Congenital Abnormalities. Med. J. of Australia, Sydney, 1943, 2:201. Abstract. J.A.M.A., 1943, 123:1144.

THEOBALD, G. W. Neuritis in Pregnancy Successfully Treated with Vitamin B. Lancet, 1936, 1:834.

TILLMAN, A. J. B. Traumatic Neuritis in the Puerperium. Am. J. Obst. & Gynec., 1935, 29:660.

TISDALL, L. H. Pulmonary Tuberculosis in an Active Obstetric Service. With an Analysis of 15 Cases. Am. J. Obst. & Gynec., 1938, 36:472.

TRAUT, H. F., and MCLANE, C. M. Physiological Changes in the Ureter Associated with Pregnancy. Surg., Gynec. & Obst., 1936, 62:65.

TUCKER, W. W., TRUSSELL, R. E., and PLASS, E. D. Latent Gonorrhea in Obstetric Patients. Am. J. Obst. & Gynec., 1939, 38:1055.

URBANSKI, A., and HUTNER, C. Thrombopenic Purpura Complicating Pregnancy. J.A.M.A., 1942, 120:754.

VIETS, H. R., SCHWAB, R. S., and BRAZIER, M. A. B. The Effect of Pregnancy on the Course of Myasthenia Gravis. J.A.M.A., 1942, 119:236.

VIGNE, P., and GUÉRIN-VALMALE. Leprosy and Pregnancy. Bull. Soc. d'obst. et de gynec., 1934, 23:75.

WARTHIN, A. S. Sex Differences in the Pathologic Picture of Syphilis. Am. J. Obst. & Gynec., 1928, 15:595-611.

WATSON, H. G. The Blood Picture of Pregnancy. Am. J. Obst. & Gynec., 1938, 35:106.

WEAVER, H. M., and STEINER, G. Acute Anterior Poliomyelitis during Pregnancy. Am. J. Obst. & Gynec., 1944, 47:495.

WELLER, C. V. The Blastophthoric Effect of Chronic Lead Poisoning. J. Med. Research, 1915, 33:271-293.

WESTBERG, S. V. Prognosis of Breast Cancer for Pregnant and Nursing Women. Lund, 1946.

WHITE, G. M., and PORTER, D. F. W. Miliary Tuberculosis in Newborn Infants. Canad. M. A. J., 1938, 39:165.

WHITE, P. Pregnancy Complicating Diabetes of More than Twenty Years' Duration. M. Clin. North America, 1947, 31:395.

——— and HUNT, H. Prediction and Prevention of Pregnancy Accidents in Diabetes. J.A.M.A., 1940, 115:2039.

——— Pregnancy Complicating Diabetes: Report of Clinical Results. J. Clin. Endocrinol., 1943, 3:500.

WHITE, P., TITUS, R. S., JOSLIN, E. P., and HUNT, Hazel. Prediction and Prevention of Late Pregnancy Accidents in Diabetes. Am. J. M. Sc., 1939, 198:482.

WHITMAN, R. C., and GREENE, L. W. A Case of Disseminated Miliary Tuberculosis in a Foetus, etc. Arch. Int. Med., 1922, 29:261-273.

WHITNEY, L., and BARRITT, A. Spontaneous and Hereditary Thrombopenic Purpura in a Mother and Two Sons. Am. J. Dis. Child., 1942, 64:705.

WICHELS, P. Ein Beitrag zur Frage der intrauterinen Typhusinfektion, etc. Ztschr. f. u. ges. exper. Med., 1924, 41:452-461.

WICKRAMASURIYA, G. A. W. Some Observations on Malaria Occurring in Association with Pregnancy. With Special Reference to the Transplacental Passage of Parasites from the Maternal to the Fetal Circulation. J. Obst. & Gynaec. Brit. Emp., 1935, 42:816.

WILLIAMS, J. W. The Clinical Significance of Glycosuria in Pregnant Women. Am. J. M. Sc., 1909, 137:1.

——— The Limitations and Possibilities of Prenatal Care. J.A.M.A., 1915, 64:95-101.

——— The Value of the Wassermann Reaction in Obstetrics Based upon the Study of 4,547 Consecutive Cases. Bull. Johns Hopkins Hosp., 1920, 31:335-342.

——— The Influence of the Treatment of Syphilitic Pregnant Women upon the Incidence of Congenital Syphilis. Bull. Johns Hopkins Hosp., 1922, 33:383.

WILLIAMS, N. H. Variable Significance of Heartburn. Am. J. Obst. & Gynec., 1941, 42:814.

WILLSON, P., and PREECE, Alec A. Chorea Gravidarum. A Statistical Study of 951 Collected Cases, 846 from the Literature and 105 Previously Unreported. Arch. Int. Med., 1932, 49:471.

WILSON, C. L., and HESSELTINE, H. C. Effect of Lymphogranuloma Venereum on Pregnancy, Labor, and the Fetus. Am. J. Obst. & Gynec., 1942, 43:459.

WOODS, E. B. Complications of the Treatment of Syphilis in Pregnancy. Report of Three Cases of Arsenical Encephalitis Complicating such Treatment. J. M. A. Georgia, 1936, 25:23.

YOUNG, J. Pulmonary Tuberculosis and Pregnancy. Brit. M. J., 1936, 2:749.

ZISKIN, D. E. Effect of Hormonal Treatment on Gums and Oral Mucosa of Women, with Use of Estrogen; With Use of Gonadotropic Hormone of Pregnancy Urine. J. Dent. Research, 1937, 16:367.

ZONDEK, B., and BROMBERG, Y. M. Infectious Hepatitis in Pregnancy. J. Mt. Sinai Hosp., 1947, 14:222.

Section Seven: ABNORMALITIES OF LABOR

29

DYSTOCIA DUE TO ANOMALIES OF THE EXPULSIVE FORCES

Dystocia (difficult labor) may be defined as cessation of progress in parturition as the result of abnormalities in the mechanics involved. The causes of dystocia fall into three main groups:

1. Subnormal uterine or abdominal forces which are not sufficiently strong to overcome the natural resistance offered to the birth of the baby by the maternal soft parts and the bony birth canal. Weakness of uterine action is called "uterine inertia" and is by far the most common cause of dystocia.
2. Faulty presentation or abnormal development of the fetus of such a character that it cannot be extruded by the vis a tergo.
3. Abnormalities in the size or character of the birth canal which form an obstacle to the descent of the fetus.

It is true that certain accidental complications of labor such as eclampsia, abruptio placentae, placenta previa, and rupture of the uterus may lead to various irregularities which interfere with the normal progress of labor. The issues involved in these complications, however, are of quite a different nature from those in the three groups listed above; and it will lead to clearer thinking about dystocia if its connotation is limited to those conditions in which the mechanics of labor are at fault.

The expulsion of the fetus is brought about by the contractions of the uterus, reinforced during the second stage of labor by the action of the muscles of the abdominal wall. Either of these factors may be lacking in force or intensity, while occasionally they may be abnormally strong.

Unfortunately there is no absolute standard by which the character of the labor pains can be gauged. In an exceptional primigravidous woman a rapid and happy termination of labor may follow a few relatively slight pains which in the majority of normal primigravidae would prove quite inadequate to bring about the desired result. Clinically the efficiency of the uterine contractions may be measured by their effect upon the course and duration of labor, provided there is no serious mechanical obstacle to be overcome so that, other things being equal, prolonged labor, on the one hand, and precipitate labor, on the other, occur as a result of abnormalities in their frequency and intensity. Other than its effects, the best clinical index of the intensity of a labor pain is the degree to which the uterus can be indented by the palpating fingers at the acme of a contraction: if, at the height of a contraction the uterine wall can be appreciably indented, the contraction is not of the best quality. In this connection it should be emphasized that the complaints of the patient about her pains are not always indicative of the actual intensity of the contractions since, due to different pain thresholds and other unknown factors, patients occasionally complain bitterly of contractions which are of poor quality. This state of affairs is especially likely to be seen in posterior positions of the occiput.

UTERINE INERTIA

Normally, in the early stages of labor, the uterine contractions recur at infrequent intervals, and gradually increase in frequency, intensity and duration as its termination is approached. Moreover, a proper alternation between the contraction and relaxation of the uterus is a very important requisite for the successful accomplishment of delivery.

Anomalies are often noted in the first stage of labor. In many instances the pains recur at long intervals and are so feeble in character that dilatation of the cervix is unduly delayed with the result that labor, instead of being terminated within the usual period, may drag on for days. If the membranes are unruptured and the patient is in good condition the delay may be regarded with equanimity, since in the great majority of instances the pains eventually become stronger and more frequent so that the birth of the child is effected without interference. For this reason, in the absence of symptoms indicative of danger to the mother or child, mere prolongation of labor is not necessarily serious. It may happen that in a labor lasting 48 hours or longer one patient may suffer less and have actually fewer uterine contractions than another woman in whom the process is completed within the usual period. In such cases, the obstetrician should not interfere hastily, but should encourage the patient by a plain statement of the facts of the case and the assurance that a favorable outcome may be expected, not only for her but also for the child.

Again, labor sometimes begins in a perfectly typical manner and gives every promise of an ordinarily speedy termination, and yet after a certain lapse of time without any appreciable cause, the pains become less frequent and less intense, although giving rise to quite as much or even more suffering than previously. At the same time, the cervix, which was becoming obliterated and dilated in a satisfactory manner, ceases to make further progress, and labor apparently comes to a standstill. The former condition is attributed to **primary**, and the latter to **secondary** inertia uteri.

In other instances the contractions, although recurring at frequent intervals, are very painful and cramp-like in character, but exert very little influence upon the dilatation of the cervix. As a result obliteration of its canal is brought about very slowly, and the external os undergoes but little change. As a rule, such conditions do not give rise to serious complications since, with time, the pains usually assume a more normal character after which the termination of labor is speedily accomplished. Studies of such cases by means of Reynolds' tokodynamometer or Karlson's instrument (page 330) indicate that they are due to poorly co-ordinated uterine activity in which contractions in the mid and lower zones equal or even exceed those in the upper; in other words, the normal gradient of diminishing physiological activity from above downward is lacking (page 331).

In all these conditions the prolongation of labor is sometimes attributed to the imperfect dilatation of the cervix, which is supposed to be due to an abnormal rigidity of the tissues. Ordinarily, however, the converse is true and the tardy dilatation is the direct result of faulty uterine contractions. That this interpretation is correct is shown by the fact that the appearance of satisfactory contractions is promptly followed by rapid dilatation of the cervix and a happy termination of labor. On the other hand, however, especially in elderly primigravidae who have passed their thirty-fifth year, excessive rigidity of the cervix and its consequent tardy and imperfect dilatation may be the essential factor in the production of the dystocia.

Premature rupture of the membranes may occur before the onset of uterine contractions, and hours, days, and occasionally several weeks, may elapse between the escape of the amniotic fluid and the onset of uterine contractions. Consequently, it is unwise in such cases to express a definite opinion as to when labor will set in but in nine cases out of ten, one is safe in predicting that contractions will begin within 24 hours. In other cases the membranes may rupture early in labor and before any great degree of cervical dilatation has occurred. In either event we have to deal with what is designated as "dry labor." This, it was generally believed, tends to be unduly prolonged and more painful than usual but Schulze contends that in the absence of any other abnormality, the reverse is the case as, upon analyzing the course of 600 such cases, she found that the duration of labor was shorter than usual. Although recent evidence substantiates her conclusions, experience teaches that certain dry labors are unduly prolonged and in them the delay is attributable in great part to the fact that the presenting part is not well engaged and applied against the cervix. This complication occurs in about every tenth labor and is less serious in multiparae than in primigravidae, on account of the decreased resistance of the cervix in the former.

This accident also increases the probability of *intrapartum infection* even though vaginal examinations have not been made, as bacteria from the vulva and vagina may multiply in the capillary layer of fluid in the vagina and gain access to the open amniotic sac. Fortunately, such infections are not always serious, and all signs of them may disappear within 24 hours after delivery, but they may lead to *puerperal infection* of the patient and bacteria may be found in her blood before, but more frequently immediately after, the completion of delivery. Even when the mother escapes infection the condition is not devoid of danger, as it has long been known that in such cases the child may succumb from infection either in utero or a few days after birth. Hellendahl and others thought that it became infected by swallowing the contaminated amniotic fluid, but Slemons showed that in a certain proportion of cases the bacteria make their way through the amnion covering the fetal surface of the placenta, and, after invading the large vessels which lie just beneath it, gain access to the fetal circulation and give rise to general septicemia or to peritonitis. Slemons designated the process as placental bacteriemia and the confirmatory observations of Zangemeister, Williams and others indicate that it plays a considerable part in the production of late fetal mortality. Because of the threat of intrapartum infection whenever the membranes rupture prematurely, it is customary to administer penicillin and sulfadiazine in cases in which the membranes have been ruptured for 12 hours or more, or as clinical judgment may dictate.

Not uncommonly, obliteration of the cervical canal takes place without difficulty, while the external os alone appears to offer the obstacle to dilatation. In such cases its margins are often thin and sharp, and during a contraction may not exceed the thickness of a sheet of paper. On the other hand, especially when labor is unduly prolonged, they may become thick and edematous.

In the absence of any mechanical obstacle, prolongation of the second stage of labor is rarely due to abnormalities in the uterine contractions but rather to deficient action of the abdominal muscles. In primigravidous women especially, the tardy labor is often ascribed to the resistance offered by a rigid perineum and a small vaginal outlet, but ordinarily this is only apparent, the delay really being due to an insufficient vis a tergo or to the head descending with the occiput obliquely posterior, undergoing only partial rotation and being arrested in the deep transverse position.

Etiology. Uterine inertia is usually attributed to one of three causes: faulty development or diseased conditions of the uterine musculature, anomalies in its innervation, or mechanical interference with its contraction. The first factor is the one most often concerned in the causation of tardy labor, and is especially likely to be associated with imperfect general development, being frequently observed in patients possessing contracted pelves. It should, however, be remembered that uterine insufficiency is occasionally noted in apparently normal women and is relatively common in large, thick-set, and corpulent individuals.

Sometimes the faulty action of the uterine muscle is attributable to a loss of tonicity incident to excessive distention, and is therefore met with in women in whom the uterus has been subjected to acute distention, as in multiple pregnancy or hydramnios. As stated above, prolonged labor is associated with an increased incidence of intrapartum infection; furthermore, such infection often aggravates the inertia by direct involvement of the musculature or by gaseous distention of the uterus.

Apart from the fact that we know that the nerve supply of the uterus is derived from both the sympathetic and parasympathetic systems and that their action is generally antagonistic, we are almost entirely ignorant about the nervous control of the uterine contractions. Consequently direct proof of the existence of abnormalities in the innervation of the uterine musculature cannot be adduced; nevertheless, clinical observation indicates clearly that extraneous causes may interfere reflexly with the activity of the uterus. It is a matter of common experience that the entrance of the obstetrician into the lying-in chamber is frequently followed by a temporary cessation of the labor pains. Extreme nervousness, profound mental emotions, or excruciating pain may have a similar effect. In such cases the severe pain is often due to the irregular action of the uterus which in turn, by acting reflexly, interferes still further with its function, giving rise to a vicious circle. That reflex nervous influences are frequently responsible is shown by the fact that the administration of morphine and atropine may be followed by a return of satisfactory contractions. In addition to these intrinsic factors, it must be emphasized that **the most common cause of uterine inertia in modern obstetrics is the premature and injudicious administration of analgesic drugs and conduction anesthesia,** as discussed in Chapter 17.

Extensive observations by Murphy with the Lóránd tokograph indicate that primary uterine inertia (functional dystocia) is detectable early in labor. His recordings show that normal labor is characterized by contractions of definite magnitude and rhythmicity while in primary uterine inertia the contractions are of small magnitude and dissimilar in size and type and follow an arrhythmic pattern. The tonus of hardness of the uterus between contractions progressively increases as labor advances, according to Murphy. That the action of the uterus is occasionally influenced by mechanical conditions is shown by the frequent association of unsatisfactory contractions with the presence of multiple myomata in the uterine wall. Much the same effect is exerted when the organ sags markedly forward in a pendulous abdomen. Old adhesions about the uterus and appendages and fresh inflammatory areas in the same location may act in a similar manner.

In the *second stage* defective abdominal contractions may be due to a number of causes. The insufficiency may result from faulty development of the muscles themselves; more frequently it is due to a loss of muscular tone following excessive distention with the result that it is much more common in multiparous than in primigravidous women. In many instances the insufficiency is only apparent, and is due to the fact that for fear of increased pain the patient is unwilling to bring her abdominal muscles into full play, and accordingly makes voluntary efforts to restrain them. For this reason the obstetrician is sometimes obliged to terminate labor by means of low forceps, although he feels sure that a few minutes' effective use of the abdominal muscles would lead to spontaneous delivery. In many such cases the induction of light anesthesia is attended by happy results, since it dulls the sensations of pain sufficiently to enable the patient to bring her abdominal muscles into action.

Management of Primary Uterine Inertia. Before any type of therapy is instituted for uterine inertia it must first be established beyond all question that the patient is actually in true labor. Efforts to stimulate false labor are either completely futile or lead to a desultory type of uterine contractility which is most difficult to deal with. Hence, in any supposed case of inertia, the criteria of true labor must be fulfilled before any therapy is initiated, that is, there must have been evidence of progressive effacement and dilatation of the cervix despite the poor pains. If a primigravida with poor pains is less than 3 cm. dilated it is best to consider the case one of false labor and give no treatment until it can be proved otherwise; the same general rule applies to multiparae who are less than 4 cm. dilated.

The best treatment of primary uterine inertia is time. As Robert Gooch expressed it a century ago: "My remedy is tincture of time, the loss of which is the only thing to be regretted, for it at least produces no additional evils." In this connection it should be recalled that dystocia is defined as the *cessation* of progress in labor, not mere retardation, and that slow labors are not necessarily pathologic. Indeed, before the case is considered one of true uterine inertia, evidence of the pathologic state of affairs must be at hand in the form of poor pains and absence of progress for a substantial number of hours. Thus, we define uterine inertia as follows: in the first stage, sluggishness of the uterine contractions (after true labor has begun) of such a degree that (1) the cervix shows no change over an eight-hour period and (2) the uterine wall is easily indentable at the acme of each pain; in the second stage, sluggishness of uterine contractions of such a degree that the head neither rotates nor descends over a two-hour period with a uterine wall which is easily indentable at the acme of each pain.

Cases of slow labor in which four to six hours transpire without progress are best handled by repeated encouragement and reassurance of the patient and stimulation with enemas from time to time. Postural therapy directed to allow the presenting part to gravitate downward and press against the lower uterine segment is sometimes helpful. By this is meant the semi-recumbent position or, if the head is well engaged, walking about the room or corridor. Artificial rupture of the membranes to stimulate pains is not advisable unless (1) the cervix is dilated 5 cm. or more, and (2) a bag of forewaters is present in front of the head preventing it from making contact against the cervix. If these two conditions exist, artificial rupture of the membranes often results in a decided improvement in contractions. If these two conditions, especially the first, are not present, artificial rupture of the membranes may only aggravate the difficulties.

Cases of true uterine inertia, as defined above, should be treated initially as described in the foregoing paragraph, but occasionally the inertia is so refractory that the question arises as to the advisability of using a really effectual uterine stimulant such as pituitary extract. This is a powerful oxytocic agent which has killed many women through rupture of the uterus and many more babies through tumultuous uterine contractions with resultant anoxia and cerebral trauma. For this reason many authorities maintain that pituitary extract should never be given before the birth of the baby and they can document their claims by countless tragedies. On the other hand, advanced degrees of uterine inertia also impose serious hazards in the form of maternal exhaustion, intrapartum infection and traumatic operative delivery. Which is the greater risk: pituitary extract or prolonged uterine inertia? In my opinion, the balance lies slightly in favor of pituitary extract, but if serious accidents are to be minimized the following regulations must be rigidly enforced:

1. The case must be one of real uterine inertia as defined above, primary in character, with labor practically at a standstill and progress nil.

2. The patient must be actually in labor, not in false or prodromal labor. The only valid evidence of true labor is progressive effacement and dilatation of the cervix. Although this process may have come to a standstill, it must have progressed to the extent of 3 or 4 cm. dilatation. One of the most common mistakes in obstetrics is to try to "push" labor in patients who are not in labor at all. Pituitary extract will only lead to trouble in such cases.

3. There must be no mechanical obstruction to easy delivery as attested by every type of evidence possible, including x-ray study of the pelvis and fetal skull. Unless the latter is done an occasional instance of midpelvic contraction or of brow presentation may be overlooked. The agent should not be used in cases of breech presentation because it is impossible to rule out a certain element of mechanical obstruction, especially in frank breeches.

4. Pituitary extract should not be used in cases of obvious overdistention of the uterus, such as cases of twin pregnancy and those in which the infant appears to weigh in excess of 4,000 gm.

5. Patients of great parity (Paras IV and over, let us say) must not be given pituitary extract, because their uteri rupture more readily than those of women in the lower parity brackets; for the same reason it should be withheld in patients whose age is over 35 years.

6. The condition of the fetus must be good, as evidenced by regular heart rate and absence of meconium-stained liquor amnii. A dead fetus is of course no contraindication to pituitary extract.

7. The obstetrician must observe and time the first contraction after the administration of the drug, and give inhalations of ether if it lasts longer than three minutes.

8. The initial dose must not exceed 0.25 minim intramuscularly. This dosage should not be exceeded unless it is clear that no improvement in pains whatsoever ensues. In that event, it may be increased to 0.5 minim and then to 1 minim, but under no circumstances should more than 1 minim be given at a time. A period of 30 minutes must intervene between injections. These same regulations apply to pitocin (page 406).

9. When in doubt as to whether a given case meets the above criteria, do not give pituitary extract or pitocin.

A safer and more physiologic method of administering pituitary extract is the intravenous drip technic. Pitocin is usually employed for this purpose.

Intravenous Drip Pitocin. Five minims of pitocin are thoroughly mixed with 500 cc. of 5 per cent glucose solution. Hence, 50 cc. of the solution is equivalent to 0.5 minim of pitocin. If it is desired to give this amount of pitocin over 30 minutes, it is necessary to administer the solution at a rate of 1.7 cc. per minute. This is done in the following manner.

The glucose solution containing the pitocin is placed in an intravenous bottle with a Murphy drip apparatus interposed in the rubber tubing and an adjustable clamp placed on the tubing above the Murphy drip device. The particular Murphy drip apparatus should be tested beforehand in order that the number of drops which it gives per cubic centimeter is known. The needle with the flow entirely shut off is inserted into the arm vein and then the number of drops is very slowly increased to whatever number will yield 0.5 or 0.25 minim in one-half hour as previously determined. This usually runs 25 to 30 drops per minute if 0.5 minim of pitocin is desired and 12 to 14 drops in the latter instance. It is very important not to have the solution flowing when the needle is inserted because in this way dangerous amounts of pitocin may be given before the rate of flow is properly regulated. The number of drops should always be built up from zero.

Since the Murphy drip apparatus incorporated in the available commercial intravenous sets with glucose solutions included seems to be very well standardized in respect to size, it is very convenient to use. We employ one with 5 per cent glucose included and find that from set to set the number of drops per minute given is quite constant, namely, 28 drops to 1.7 cc. We are at present starting with 0.25 of a minim of pitocin over the first half-hour and find it surprising how often such a homeopathic dose may be effective. To administer 0.25 of a minim over 30 minutes, one starts with zero drops and gradually builds up to 14 drops per minute which gives the approximate rate of flow desired. It is desirable to have a clamp on the rubber tubing which permits precise adjustment.

The patient should never be left for a moment while the solution is running because the best of clamps sometimes slips and the rate of flow must be checked from time to time. Moreover, the uterine contractions must be observed continually and the clamp shut off immediately if they exceed two minutes in duration or if the fetal heart tones show any alterations. This has rarely happened in our experience but when it has occurred, we have found that immediate stopping of the flow corrects these disturbances at once and no harm has been done.

In 6,608 consecutive labors in our clinic between 1941 and 1945, intramuscular pituitary extract was used in 3.5 per cent of the cases and, in general, any appreciable employment of the agent in excess of this incidence represents abuse of the drug. In the great majority of cases improvement in labor is striking within a few minutes. If no benefit ensues despite repeated administration over a three-hour period, the drug should be abandoned as experience shows that if it is not successful in such an interval, continued administration is of no avail. Moreover, in cases in which the program outlined above fails, increasing the dosage above 1 minim is likewise futile as a rule and only adds to the dangers. Failure of pituitary extract to effect either a spontaneous or a low forceps delivery occurs in about 10 per cent of cases of uterine inertia. The management of such cases will depend upon several factors, as follows: the dilatation of the cervix, the station of the presenting part, the size of the baby, and the presence or absence of intrapartum infection. Provided the head is engaged and the cervix 6 cm. or more dilated. Dührssen's method of incisions and forceps delivery are generally the choice. If the head is high and/or the cervix less than 6 cm. dilated, cesarean section is usually indicated in the presence of a living infant, the extraperitoneal technic being employed if intrapartum infection is evident. Because of the likelihood of intrapartum infection in these cases, all patients who have been in labor 18 hours or more, or in whom membranes have been ruptured for 12 hours or more, should be given penicillin and sulfadiazine routinely. This prophylaxis against intra-uterine infection often makes it possible to perform low cervical cesarean section with safety in cases in which the extraperitoneal operation would otherwise have been necessary. In prolonged labor of all types, fluid intake must be watched carefully and maintained by 5 or 10 per cent intravenous glucose solutions if necessary.

Management of Secondary Uterine Inertia. To employ a homely simile, primary uterine inertia may be likened to a lazy horse which needs stimulation; secondary uterine inertia may be likened to an exhausted horse which needs rest. The therapy of the latter condition is morphine, 16 mg. (0.25 grain) and intravenous glucose, 700 to 1,000 cc. in 5 or 10 per cent concentration. After three or four hours' sleep which usually ensues, the pains often return to their previous intensity and the rest of labor is uneventful. Morphine is also helpful in occasional cases of primary uterine inertia in which it becomes desirable to give the patient an interval of rest between periods of stimulation. Not infrequently morphine exerts just the opposite effect than might be anticipated and is followed by rapid dilatation of the cervix.

Finally, it must be emphasized that manual dilatation of the cervix has no place in this or any other obstetrical condition. It is not only fraught with the danger of deep cervical lacerations but is rarely successful in achieving complete dilatation, so that any subsequent forceps operation is still confronted with the obstruction of an incompletely dilated cervix. If other measures have failed, Dührssen's incisions or cesarean section, as discussed above, are preferable.

PRECIPITATE LABOR

In certain multiparous women, and very rarely in primigravidae, precipitate labor may result from an abnormally slight degree of resistance offered by the soft parts, or from abnormally strong uterine and abdominal contractions, or very occasionally from the absence of painful sensations during labor. At the New York Lying-In Hospital Dixon found the incidence of precipitate labor, defined as lasting three hours or less, was 6.1 per cent.

Generally speaking precipitate labor is not attended by serious consequences, but the infant mortality is increased appreciably for several reasons. In the first place, the tumultuous uterine contractions, often with negligible intervals between, prevent proper oxygenation of the fetal blood; secondly, the rapid transit of the baby through the bony pelvis sometimes produces cerebral trauma; and thirdly, such babies are often born unattended and suffer from lack of proper care during the first few minutes of life. It sometimes happens that the woman is suddenly overtaken by intense labor pains and gives birth to the child before she can reach her bed. In such cases the child may fall to the ground and sustain severe or even fatal injuries. Occasionally the cord is torn through and it is generally believed that the child may bleed to death before aid is obtainable. This, however, is unlikely as experience shows that the jagged and irregular tear which must result in such circumstances will probably lead to coagulation of the blood and cessation of hemorrhage before a fatal issue ensues.

If tempestuous pains come on while the patient is under the observation of a physician, they should be controlled by the intravenous injection of 0.2 gm. (3 grains) of sodium pentobarbital and/or the administration of very light ether anesthesia. It is unwise, and may be actually harmful, to employ physical force to hold back an impending birth.

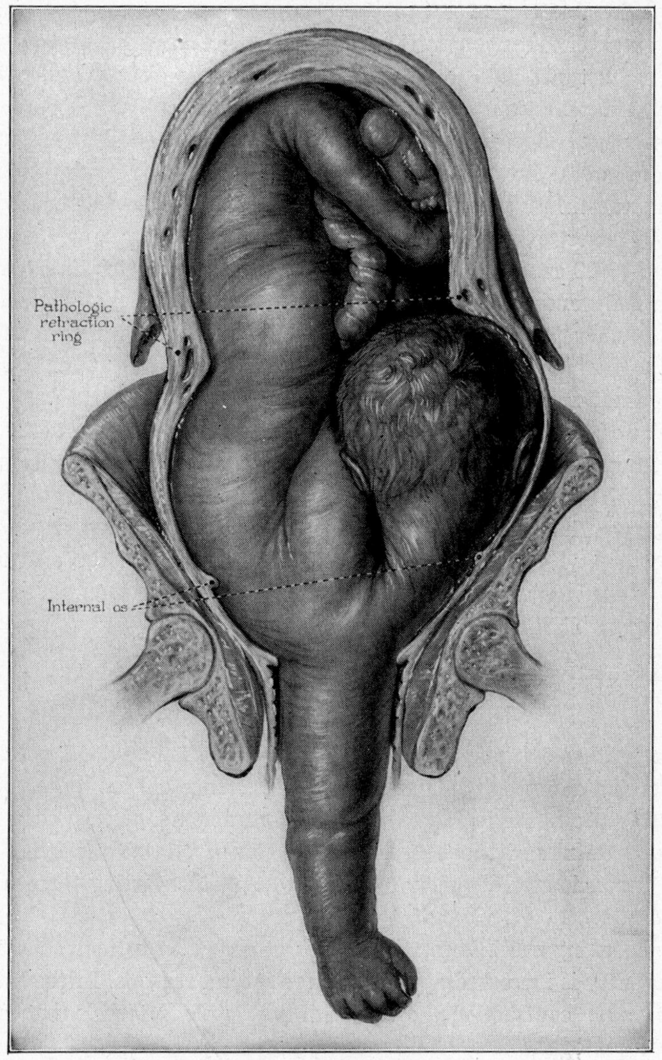

FIG. 397.—PATHOLOGIC RETRACTION RING IN CASE OF NEGLECTED TRANSVERSE PRESENTATION. (From Schroeder.)

LOCALIZED ABNORMALITIES OF UTERINE ACTION

Pathologic Retraction Ring. The physiologic retraction ring has been described on page 330. In prolonged labors in which a mechanical obstacle opposes the passage of the child, the process of retraction often progresses to an excessive degree and a marked exaggeration of the physiologic retraction ring results. Since this ring is present only in obstructed labors and is due to over-retraction, it has been designated by Rudolph as the "pathologic retraction ring." This type of ring was first described by Bandl, a German obstetrician, and is widely known as "Bandl's ring." The use of this synonym will doubtless continue, but in view of the general tendency to eliminate eponymy, it would seem desirable to give preferred usage to the more descriptive term suggested by Rudolph. An example of the pathologic retraction ring is shown in Fig. 397. Here it may be seen that the ring is in no way obstructing the passage of the baby; this type of ring never impedes the egress of the infant. On the contrary, it is the result of obstructed labor, and is pathologic also in the sense that it is invariably associated with extreme thinning of the lower uterine segment consequent upon the cephalward rise of the ring. The pathologic retraction ring may be seen abdominally in obstructed labor usually at about the level of the umbilicus, and is one of the classic signs of threatened rupture of the uterus.

The treatment will depend upon the cause of the obstruction, the condition of the child and that of the mother. Under certain circumstances cesarean section, either low cervical or extraperitoneal, may be indicated while in others, should the child be dead or the uterus infected, craniotomy may be the procedure of choice. Whatever operations are performed from below, deep anesthesia as well as great care in manipulation are most essential in order to forestall rupture of the lower segment.

Constriction Ring	*Pathologic Retraction Ring*
1. A localized thickening of the uterus due to the contraction of the circular fibers over a point of slight resistance, most frequently over a depression in the child's outline or below the presenting part.	1. Always located at junction of the thinned lower uterine segment with the thick retracted upper uterine segment.
2. The uterine wall at the site of the constriction ring will therefore be thicker than it is either above or below.	2. The uterine wall above the pathologic retraction ring is much thicker than it is below it.
3. The wall below is neither thinned nor overdistended.	3. The wall below a pathologic retraction ring is both thinned and overdistended.
4. The presenting part is not forcibly driven into the pelvis.	4. The presenting part is or has been jammed into the pelvis.
5. The child may be wholly or mainly above the constriction ring.	5. Part of the child must be below the pathologic retraction ring.
6. The body of the uterus above a constriction ring is usually relaxed and not tender.	6. The body above a pathologic retraction ring is tonically contracted and hard.
7. Round ligaments are not tense.	7. Round ligaments stand out.
8. A constriction ring may occur in the first, second or third stage of labor.	8. A pathologic retraction ring practically always occurs late in the second stage of labor.
9. A constriction ring does not vary in position as labor goes on.	9. A pathologic retraction ring gradually rises as retraction of the upper uterine segment proceeds.
10. A constriction ring is rarely felt on abdominal examination.	10. A pathologic retraction ring may frequently be felt per abdomen.
11. The patient's general condition is good.	11. The patient's general condition is poor.
12. Causation: premature rupture of the membranes; intra-uterine manipulations.	12. Causation: obstructed labor.

TABLE 20. DIFFERENTIAL DIAGNOSIS BETWEEN CONSTRICTION RING AND PATHOLOGIC RETRACTION RING. (Modified from Clifford White.)

Constriction Ring. In marked contrast to the retraction rings, both physiologic and pathologic, are the constriction rings which produce true spastic strictures of the uterine cavity because a zone of muscle goes into local tetanic contraction and forms a tight constriction about some part of the fetus. In vertex presentations the ring usually settles into the natural groove between the head and shoulder of the infant, or in breech presentation it is formed about the trunk or breech. Rudolph defines this term as "an annular contraction of the uterus which may occur theoretically at any

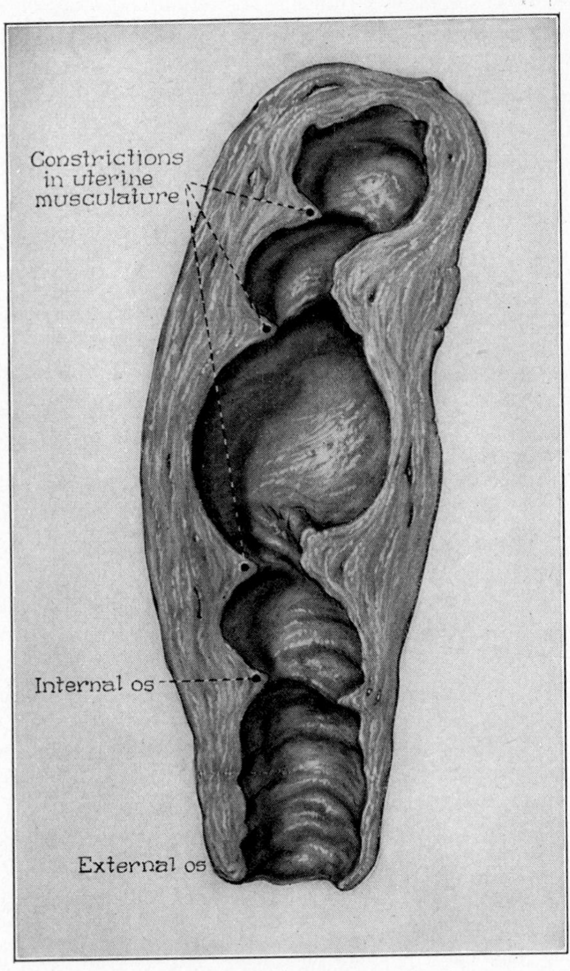

Fig. 398.—Multiple Constriction Rings in Postpartum Uterus.

Two definite constriction rings divide the upper uterine segment into three cavities. Below, two probable constriction rings are present: one at the junction of the upper and lower segments and another at the internal os (Blum and Blumreich).

level of the uterine musculature and cause dystocia per se in the presence of normal cephalopelvic relationships. It does not change position as labor continues. Rupture of the uterus has never been demonstrated unequivocally to result per se from a constriction ring. It is improbable that it would occur, because the segment below the ring is not excessively thinned or distended and the uterus above is often relaxed and the contractions are ineffective; that is, a constriction ring is associated with incoordination of uterine action." (See Fig. 398.)

We have, then, two types of pathologic rings: the pathologic retraction ring (Bandl's ring) and the constriction ring. An exceedingly clear differentiation of these two types of rings was published in 1913 by Clifford White of London and is shown in Table 20. Rudolph's terminology has been substituted for the older nomenclature used by White.

Rudolph summarized the literature on constriction rings up to 1935 and classified the 272 cases as follows:

(a) Palpable only internally, 248, or 91 per cent.
  1. About fetal neck at level of symphysis pubis, 186, or 75 per cent.
  2. Around other portions of the fetus and above the symphysis pubis, 39, or 14 per cent.
  3. Below the presenting part and still behind the symphysis, 23, or 9 per cent.

(b) Palpable externally and therefore above the symphysis pubis, 24, or 9 per cent.

This would seem to indicate the zone 7 to 8 cm. above the external os as a site of predilection.

One of the curious things about constriction rings is the wide discrepancy in their reported frequency. Herman W. Johnson encountered them 126 times in 10,000 private patients, or once in every 80 cases. On the other hand, Rudolph, who has likewise been on the lookout for them and has had a huge material at his disposal at the Cook County Hospital in addition to private practice, was able to report only 26 cases of his own in 1935, and could collect from the entire world's literature but 371 cases, or three times as many as Johnson has seen in private practice. At the Johns Hopkins Hospital we make this diagnosis once in every several thousand cases, and then usually put a question mark after it.

There are several possible explanations for this discrepancy. Through lack of awareness of constriction rings, many may be overlooked. A second possibility is that the great majority of constriction rings which have been described represent that type of uterine inertia which is described on page 779 and which is characterized by apparently vigorous contractions but no progress in cervical dilatation. Both these conditions may be examples of incoordinated muscular behavior in which the autonomic and sympathetic nervous systems act antagonistically so that the expulsive forces of the longitudinal muscle fibers of the fundus are resisted by the circular muscle bundles of the lower segment which, instead of relaxing as they are supposed to do, are continually contracting. Since the crux of the difficulty here would be the constricting action of the circular fibers of the lower segment, it would be possible to regard this in the light of ring formation even though the ring could not be actually palpated in most cases.

The treatment of constriction ring depends upon the stage to which labor has progressed. If the cervix is thick and insufficiently dilated to permit passage of the fetus, rest and the use of intravenous glucose (5 or 10 per cent) to provide available carbohydrate are indicated. Rest is the great need and narcotics must be used if necessary to insure it. This treatment will be found to suffice in the majority of cases of constriction ring. If, however, the cervix is fully dilated or nearly so, especially if the margins are thin and soft, it is better to treat the condition by administering deep anesthesia using open drop ether as the anesthetic of choice. No attempt should be made at delivery until the uterus is completely relaxed. When this has occurred, as may be determined by the examining hand, the fetus may be extracted by the simplest means indicated in the immediate circumstances. Rarely, even with the deepest anesthesia, relaxation of the ring may not occur, in which case laparotomy with incision of the uterus, including the constriction ring, is necessary to accomplish delivery. Rucker has recommended the hypodermic use of one third of a cc. of 1:1000 adrenalin solution, while others have suggested good results from amyl nitrite inhalations. Rudolph states that the adrenalin has sometimes proved successful, while on other occasions it has been of no avail. We cannot recommend either of the latter methods from personal experience, but in view of their simplicity they would seem to deserve a trial.

Missed Labor. In very exceptional instances uterine contractions come on at or near term and, after continuing for a variable time, disappear without leading to the birth of the child. The latter then dies, and may be retained in utero for months, undergoing mummification or putrefaction, according as the membranes have ruptured or not. This is known as missed labor. The term should not be applied to those cases in which a living child is born, as they are probably only examples of prolonged gestation.

Whereas missed labor, as described above, is a very rare condition, *fetal death in utero,* with retention of the dead fetus for periods as long as two months, is common. For fetal death in utero prior to the onset of labor, Dippel found an incidence of 1.2 per cent in 25,000 deliveries occurring on our service. In 25 per cent of the cases the period of retention exceeded two weeks; in his 306 cases the longest interval between fetal death and labor was 61 days. When the fetus dies in the course of pregnancy and a period appreciably longer than two months supervenes without expulsion, the chances are good that one is dealing with an abdominal pregnancy, and this possibility should always be kept in mind under such circumstances. In former times syphilis was by far the most common cause of fetal death in utero; today the toxemias of pregnancy, diabetes, and anomalies of the umbilical cord account for many cases, but in a large proportion no cause is demonstrable. The treatment is temporizing until labor ensues. It is general experience that the induction of labor is particularly hazardous in these cases and, although the family sometimes urges intervention, it is much safer to wait.

BIBLIOGRAPHY

Bandl, L. Ueber Ruptur der Gebärmutter. Wien, 1875.

Bell, W. B. The Pituitary Body, and the Therapeutic Value of the Infundibular Extract in Shock, Uterine Atony and Intestinal Paresis. Brit. M. J., 1909, 2:1609.

Dippel, A. L. Death of Fetus in Utero. Bull. Johns Hopkins Hosp., 1934, 54:24.

Eastman, N. J. Pituitary Extract in Uterine Inertia: Is It Justifiable? Am. J. Obst. & Gynec., 1947, 53:432.

Johnson, H. W. The Clinical Diagnosis of Varying Degrees of Uterine Contraction Rings. Am. J. Obst. & Gynec., 1946, 52:74.

Malpas, P. The Pattern of the Contractions of the Pregnant Uterus under Spinal Anesthesia and the Attendant Changes in the Reactivity of the Myometrium. J. Obst. & Gynaec. Brit. Emp., 1944, 51:112.

Mendenhall, A. M. Solution of Pituitary and Ruptured Uterus. J.A.M.A., 1929, 92:1341.

Murphy, D. P. The Pattern of Uterine Motility throughout Labor with Special Reference to Inertia. A Study of 105 Patients with the Lóránd Tocograph. Surg., Gynec. & Obst., 1943: 77:101.

Rucker, M. P. Treatment of Contraction Ring Dystocia with Adrenalin. Am. J. Obst. & Gynec., 1927, 14:609.

Rudolph, L. Constriction Ring Dystocia. J. Obst. & Gynaec. Brit. Emp., 1935, 42:992.

——— Constriction Ring Dystocia. J.A.M.A., 1937, 108:532.

——— The Prolonged First Stage of Labor. J. Arkansas M. Soc., 1939, 36:149.

Schulze, M. Dry Labor. Am. J. Obst. & Gynec., 1929, 17:20.

Slemons, J. M. Placental Bacteremia. J.A.M.A., 1915, 65:1265.

——— The Significance of Fever at the Time of Labor. Am. J. Obst., 1918, 78:321.

White, C. The Contraction Ring as a Cause of Dystocia. Lancet, 1913, 1:604.

Zangemeister, W., and Wieloch, J. Intrapartale Genitalinfektion. Halban and Seitz, 1925, 8:1815.

30

DYSTOCIA DUE TO ABNORMALITIES IN POSITION, PRESENTATION OR DEVELOPMENT OF THE FETUS

ABNORMALITIES OF POSITION OR PRESENTATION

Persistent Occiput Posterior Positions. In the great majority of cases, occiput posterior positions undergo spontaneous anterior rotation followed either by a spontaneous or an easy low forceps delivery. Since spontaneous outcome is the rule in these cases, labor with the occiput posterior should be regarded as simply a variation of normal labor, under which heading it has already been discussed. The duration of the second stage is often slightly prolonged, however, because more work by the expulsive forces is required to effect rotation through the greater arc. In at least a third of the cases, moreover, rotation does not take place until the vertex reaches the pelvic floor. These facts should be recalled in the management of these labors, since additional time and patience are sometimes required if spontaneous rotation is to be achieved. (See pages 363 to 368.)

In a small proportion of cases, estimated by Calkins to be about five per cent, rotation does not occur, and under such circumstances, the condition is referred to as a *persistent occiput posterior position.* The factors which cause the occiput to remain in posterior position are not clearly understood, but the condition is more frequent in anthropoid pelves, especially those of the high assimilation type (page 859). This is because the bulky occiput cannot find room in the narrow forepart of pelves of this type. It is also more common in android pelves and in cases of midpelvic contraction. Thus, Hanson found that persistent occiput posterior positions were 13 times more common when the interischial spinous diameter was shortened than when it was normal. Rotation of a posterior occiput is also less likely if the membranes have ruptured prematurely, if the head is poorly flexed, or, of course, if uterine inertia is present.

In a certain minority of cases of occiput posterior position, the occiput rotates posteriorly and spontaneous delivery ensues in this position, that is, with the face to the pubis. By taking these cases into consideration, it may be estimated that of all cases in which the initial position of the occiput was posterior, only about four per cent require operative interference. Some authors, however, cite a higher figure. The best type of operative procedure to be employed will depend on the experience and training of the operator, the type of pelvis, the degree of molding of the fetal head, and the size of the infant. If the head is considerably molded (as will often occur if patience has been exercised in allowing time for spontaneous rotation), delivery by forceps as an occiput posterior will usually prove the least traumatic measure both to mother and child. The same is true, in my opinion, if the pelvis is anthropoid or android in type or shows midpelvic contraction. Moreover, if the operator's experience with manual or forceps rotation is meager, delivery of the posterior occiput as such is usually the safest procedure. The decision to deliver the head as a posterior depends fundamentally on whether or not factors are present which threaten to make artificial rotation especially difficult. In order to ascertain whether such factors are present, some obstetricians attempt rotation gently, either by the hand or by forceps

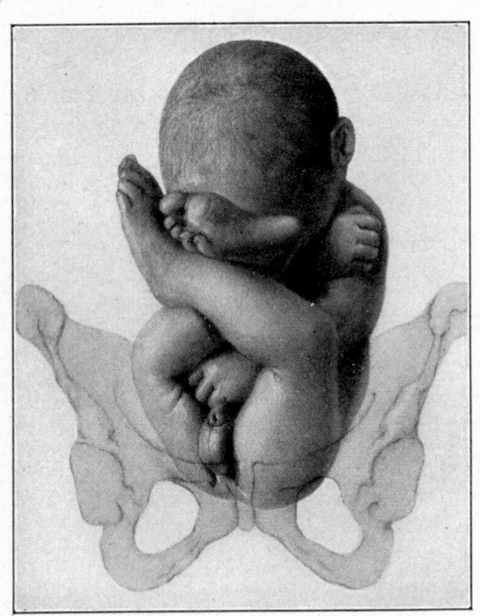

Fig. 399.—Frank Breech Presentation.

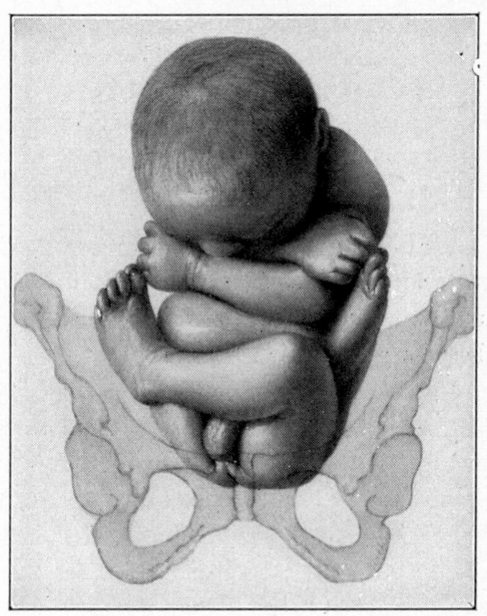

Fig. 400—Complete Breech Presentation.

rotation, and if it is easy, carry it out, but if a molded head is so wedged in the pelvis as to interfere with easy rotation, they deliver the infant as an occiput posterior. In general, operative rotation is preferred to delivery of the occiput posterior as such, provided it can be done readily. In two parallel series of cases in our clinic, studied by Whitridge, in one of which persistent occiput posterior positions were rotated either manually or by the Scanzoni maneuver (142 cases) and in the other of which forceps delivery was effected with the face to the pubis (216 cases), the total fetal mortality was about the same in both groups, namely, 4.2 and 5.1 per cent, respectively.

If delivery of the occiput posterior as such is decided upon, a deep mediolateral episiotomy should be made and the forceps extraction performed slowly. Considerably more traction is often required than usual and this should be spread over 10 or 15 minutes, with ample rest periods between pulls. Because of the longer duration of the operation, the baby should be spared the narcosis which might accrue from general anesthesia, and spinal or caudal anesthesia used. If it is elected to carry out operative rotation of a persistent occiput posterior, several procedures are available, namely, manual rotation followed by forceps extraction, rotation and delivery with the Kielland forceps, and the Scanzoni technic of rotation and extraction. These operations are described in Chapter 40.

Breech Presentations. As has already been pointed out, the relation between the lower extremities and buttocks of the child is not always the same in sacro-iliac presentations, and we therefore distinguish between frank breech, complete breech and incomplete breech (foot and knee) presentations (Figs. 399 to 401). Of these, the frank breech is the most common, at least in patients near term, in whom it can be demonstrated by x-ray in over 60 per cent of breech cases. In all these varieties, however, the mechanism of labor is essentially the same, so that they need not be considered separately. Usually the breech engages in such a manner that the sacrum is directed to the left side of the mother, and accordingly the left sacro-anterior or posterior is the position most frequently observed. In 100,000 cases of labor Pinard observed 3,301 breech presentations—about 3.30 per cent. These statistics include premature as well as full-term labors, but, if the latter alone were considered, the incidence would be somewhat less. Among 50,255 infants weighing 1,500 grams or more delivered in our clinic and studied by Moore and Steptoe, 1,444 presented by the breech, an incidence of 2.8 per cent. Breech presentations were more common in multiparae than in primigravidae, the incidence being 3.5 per cent and 2.5 per cent, respectively.

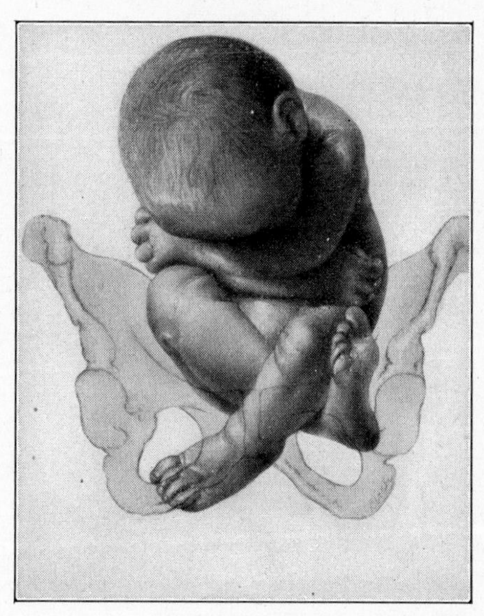

Fig. 401.—Incomplete Breech Presentation.

Diagnosis. On palpation, the first maneuver reveals a hard, round, readily ballottable body occupying the fundus of the uterus, and when the abdominal walls are very thin one can occasionally obtain a characteristic cracking sensation upon compressing the bones of the skull. By the second maneuver the back is found to occupy one side of the abdomen and the small parts the other, position and variety being determined by the location of the former. On the third maneuver, if engagement has not occurred, the irregular breech is freely movable above the superior strait, while, if it has already occurred, the fourth maneuver shows that the pelvis is filled by a soft mass which interferes with the penetration of the fingers (Fig. 403). Kautsky has made the interesting observation that in breech presentations a distinct slowing in the fetal pulse rate can be elicited by compressing the head at the fundus between the fingers.

In doubtful cases, the diagnosis may be facilitated by means of the x-ray, and in such circumstances it will usually be found that the head is less sharply flexed and that the arms occupy a much freer position than is generally taught.

On vaginal or rectal examination the diagnosis of a frank breech presentation is made by recognizing its characteristic portions. Usually one can feel both tubera ischii, the sacrum with its spinous processes, and the anus, and when further descent has occurred the external genitalia may be distinguished. Especially where labor is prolonged, the buttocks may become markedly swollen, so that differentiation between the face and breech may be rendered very difficult; the anus may be mistaken for the mouth, and the ischial tuberosities for the malar bones. Care in examination, however, should prevent this error, for when the finger is introduced into the anus it experiences a muscular resistance, whereas in the mouth the firmer more unyielding jaws are felt. Again, on removing the finger, it is sometimes found to be stained with meconium, which could never occur with a face presentation. The most accurate information, however, is obtained from the sacrum and its spinous processes; when these are felt the diagnosis of position and variety is established.

In complete breech presentations the feet may be felt alongside of the buttocks, and in footling presentations one or both feet may hang down into the vagina. In the

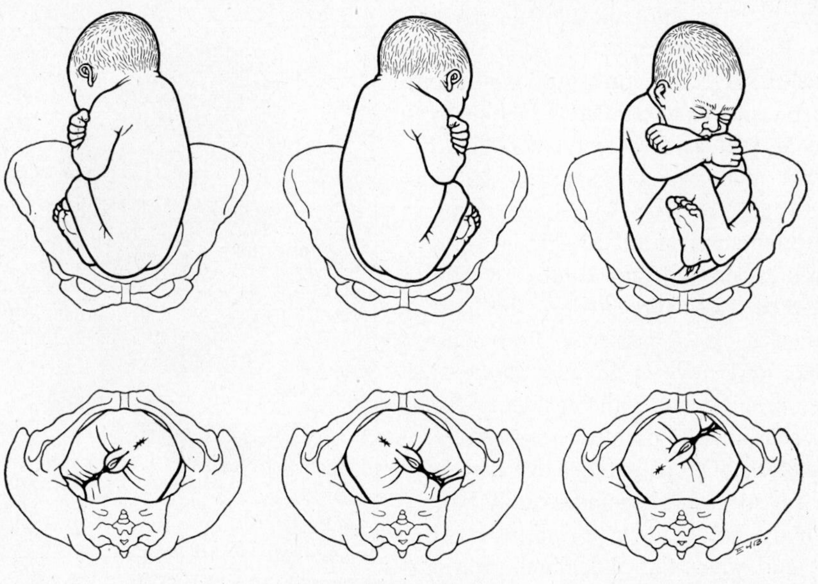

Fig. 402.—Showing Left and Right Positions of Breech Presentations.

latter case, one can readily determine with which foot one has to deal by bearing in mind the relation of the great toe. When the breech has descended deeper into the pelvic cavity, the genitalia may be felt, and if these are not deformed by an effusion of serum it is possible to determine the sex of the fetus. Only in such circumstances can we feel certain as to this point before delivery. The fetal heart sounds are heard through the back of the child, usually at the level of the umbilicus or slightly above it.

Etiology. In the later months of pregnancy head presentations result from a process of accommodation between the fetal ovoid and the uterus; accordingly, breech presentations are prone to occur when the process is interfered with. These factors do not so readily come into play in the earlier months, when breech presentations are much more common than at term. Thus, in 4,288 infants in our clinic who weighed between 1,500 and 2,499 gm., the incidence of breech presentation was 7.5 per cent. These factors are also frequently lacking in twin pregnancies and in cases of hydramnios, inasmuch as the increased distention of the uterus interferes with accommodation. According to Pinard's statistics, and in keeping with the observations of Moore and Steptoe, mentioned previously, 59 per cent of all breech presentations occur in multiparae in whom the flaccidity of the uterine and abdominal walls plays a part in their

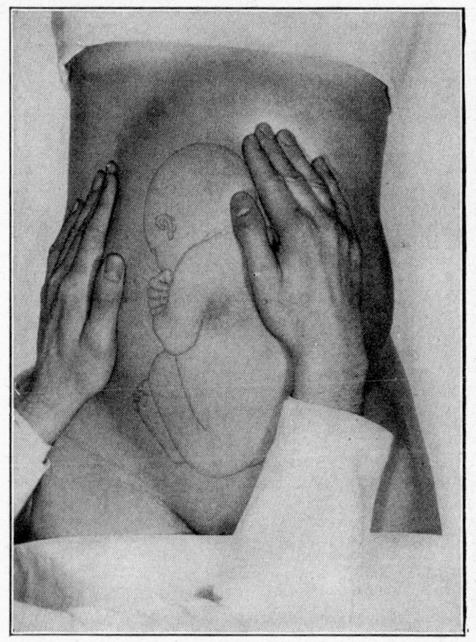

First Maneuver

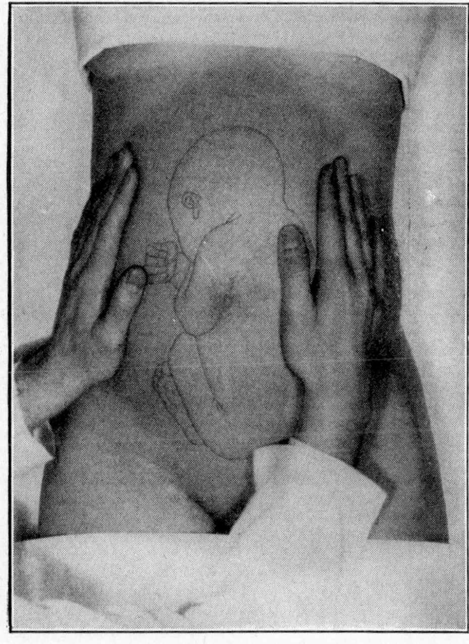

Second Maneuver

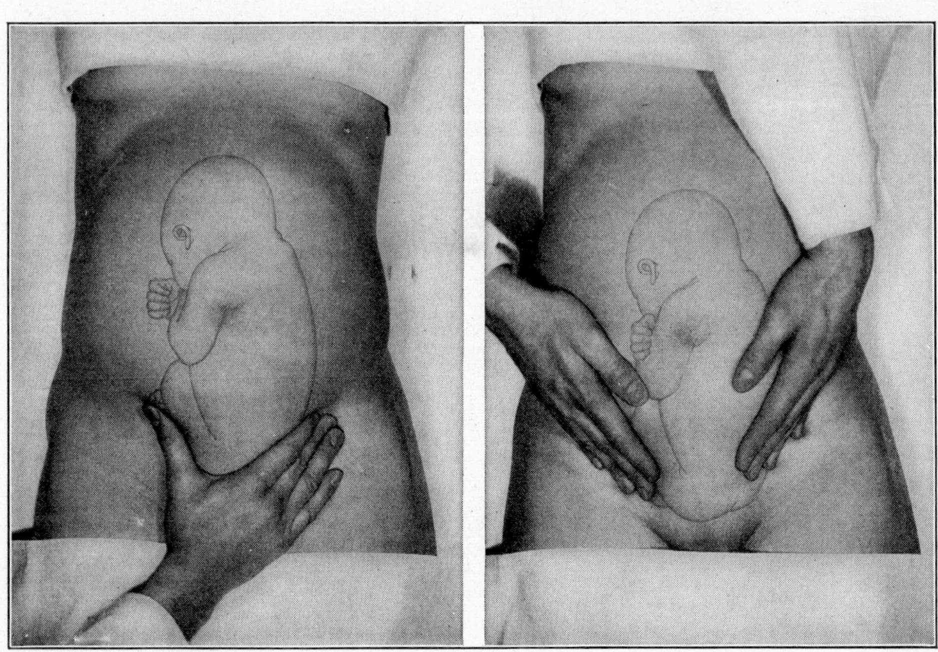

Third Maneuver

Fourth Maneuver

Fig. 403.—Palpation in Left Sacro-Anterior Position.

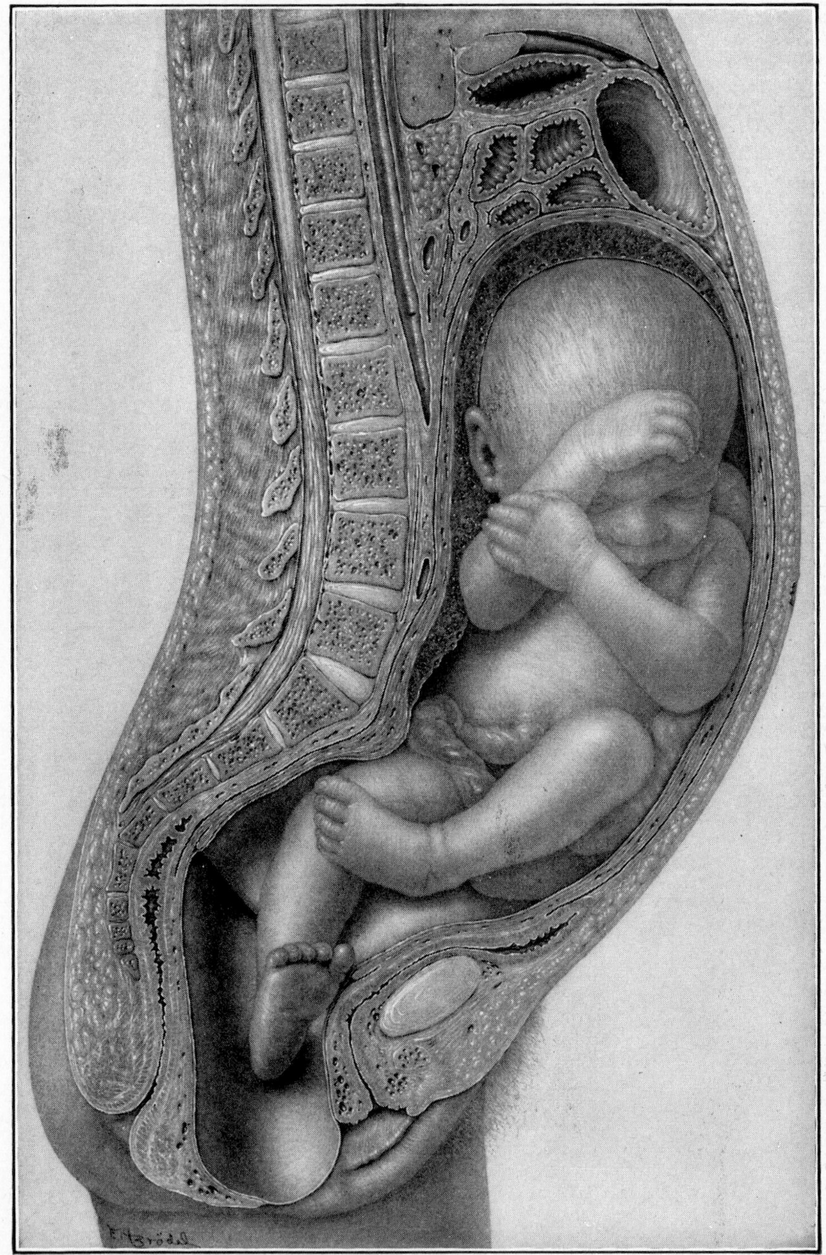

FIG. 404.—INCOMPLETE BREECH PRESENTATION (double footling). SECOND STAGE OF LABOR. FROZEN SECTION OF WILLIAMS' CASE.

production. Their occurrence is also favored by the presence of any gross obstacle which opposes the engagement of the vertex, such as placenta previa or hydrocephalus. However, contrary to usual statements, Moore and Steptoe were unable to show that pelvic contraction played any appreciable role in the causation of breech presentation.

Breech presentation is occasionally observed repeatedly in the same woman—

habitual breech presentation. Nandi, in an article on this subject, in which he discusses many of the factors responsible for breech presentation—such as pelvic contractions, abnormality of size and shape of the fetal head, abnormalities of the uterus, prematurity, and hydramnios—states that hereditary and individual tendency should be considered in certain instances of habitual breech presentation. Another cause of repeated breech presentation, as emphasized by Stanley Way, is partial fusion of the müllerian ducts with a resultant mid-line septum extending part way down into the uterine cavity.

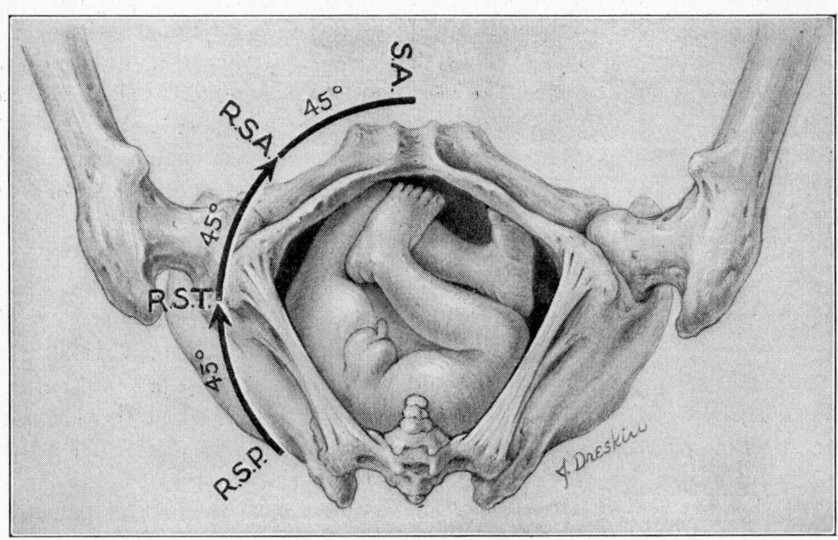

Fig. 405.—Direction of Internal Rotation in R. S. P. Position.

Mechanism. Unless there is some disproportion between the size of the child and the pelvis, engagement and descent readily occur in one of the oblique diameters of the pelvis, the anterior hip being directed toward one iliopectineal eminence, and the posterior hip toward the opposite sacro-iliac synchondrosis. The anterior hip usually descends more rapidly than the posterior, and, when it encounters the resistance of the pelvic floor, internal rotation usually occurs and brings the anterior hip to the pubic arch, the bitrochanteric diameter of the child coming into relation with the anteroposterior diameter of the pelvic outlet. Rotation usually takes place from the iliopectineal eminence to the pubis through an arc of 45 degrees. If, however, the posterior extremity is prolapsed it always rotates to the symphysis pubis, rotation ordinarily occurring through an arc of 135 degrees, but occasionally it will take place in the opposite direction, the prolapsed hip rotating past the sacrum and through the opposite half of the pelvis through an arc of 225 degrees. Sellheim explains the latter phenomenon by assuming that the retained leg acts as a splint to the corresponding side of the body, with the result that it cannot so readily undergo the lateral flexion necessary to delivery as the side which is not so splinted.

After rotation, descent continues until the perineum is distended by the advancing breech, while the anterior hip appears at the vulva and is stemmed against the pubic arch. By a movement of lateral flexion of the body, the posterior hip is then forced over the anterior margin of the perineum which retracts over the child, thus allowing its body to straighten out, when the anterior hip is born. The legs and feet follow the breech and may be born spontaneously, although the aid of the obstetrician is sometimes required. After the birth of the breech a slight movement of *external rotation* occurs, and the back usually turns somewhat to the front, as the result of the shoulders being brought into relation with one of the oblique diameters of the pelvis. They then descend rapidly and undergo internal rotation, the bisacromial diameter now corresponding with the anteroposterior diameter of the inferior strait. Immediately following the shoulders, the head, which is normally sharply flexed upon the thorax, enters the pelvis in one of the oblique diameters, and then rotates in such a manner as to bring the posterior portion of the neck under the symphysis pubis, after which the head is born in a position of flexion, the chin, mouth, nose, forehead, bregma, and occiput appearing in succession over the perineum. Not infrequently it happens that the breech engages in the transverse diameter of the pelvis, the sacrum being directed to the anterior or posterior side as the case may be. The mechanism of labor in the transverse position does not differ essentially from engagements in the oblique diameters, except that internal rotation occurs through an arc of 90 degrees.

Le Lorier has aptly directed attention to the fundamental difference between birth in vertex and breech presentations, respectively. In the former, after the extrusion of the voluminous head, the rest of the body follows without difficulty, whereas, in the latter, successively larger portions of the child are born, so that, for practical purposes, we have to deal with three births—that of the buttocks, of the shoulders, and finally of the head—each of which is preceded by a separate movement of internal rotation.

In a small number of cases rotation occurs in such a manner that the back of the child is directed toward the vertebral column, instead of toward the abdomen of the mother. In such circumstances the face appears under the symphysis pubis, the face, brow, and finally the occiput slipping down under it as the head is born. It is of the utmost importance to remember that if premature traction be employed the head may become extended; if this occurs its delivery can only be accomplished by the operation of extraction.

Prognosis. So far as the life of the mother is concerned, the prognosis differs but slightly in breech and vertex presentations, except that with the former, labor is slower, with higher morbidity, and in operative cases is more likely to be complicated by perineal tears which sometimes extend through the sphincter ani muscle. The prognosis for the child, on the other hand, is considerably worse, particularly so in the case of large infants in primigravidous women, than in vertex presentations.

The gross infantile mortality, including premature, full-term, and neonatal deaths, varies between 4 and 33 per cent. Goethals reported 25.7 per cent, Siegel and McNally 28.1 per cent, Macafee and McClure 33.8 per cent, Urnes and Timerman 19 per cent, and Caldwell and Studdiford 14 per cent. Goethals, in a careful review of 1,242 breech deliveries in the Boston Lying-In Hospital, found that, in 21.9 per cent of the total, pregnancy or labor was complicated with such conditions as toxemia, syphilis, diabetes, hydramnios, placenta previa, premature separation of the placenta, or prolapse of the cord. In his uncomplicated cases the gross fetal mortality was 18.5 per cent, but these included premature deliveries. He found that in full-term uncomplicated pregnancies, in the absence of accidents of labor from abnormalities of the placenta or cord, the fetal mortality was 6.9 per cent. Most of the other recent analyses of comparable series of breech deliveries are in close agreement with Goethals' deductions relating to the high incidence of prematurity and of abnormalities of pregnancy, labor, and offspring. Urnes and Timerman observed that of 346 babies born by breech, 65 were stillborn or died during the neonatal period, and that, of these, 43 or 64.6 per cent were nonviable, macerated, or monsters. Caldwell and Studdiford reported a gross fetal mortality (including neonatal deaths) of 8.3 per cent in primiparae and 20 per cent in multiparae, their total mortality being 14 per cent. Likewise, the figures of Macafee and McClure, as well as those from the New York Lying-In Hospital, show a higher incidence of fetal mortality in multiparae than in primiparae, Stander's gross, uncorrected infantile mortality being 14.8 per cent in multiparae and 12.01 in primiparae, with a combined rate of 12.1 per cent for all breech deliveries.

From the above statistics, it is evident that in breech presentation the uncorrected total infantile mortality (premature, full-term, and neonatal) is about 20 per cent. Gordon, from a comprehensive study of 3,301 breech deliveries, found a gross mortality of 20.3 per cent. It is also apparent that this high rate is mainly due to the increased incidence of prematurity, complications of gestation and labor, and abnormalities of the child, the presentation itself being responsible for only about one third of the deaths. Nevertheless, even in uncomplicated full-term breech deliveries, the risk to the offspring is more than twice that associated with vertex presentations.

The somber prognosis of the child is due to several factors. In the first place, after the breech is born as far as the umbilicus, the cord is exposed to a greater or lesser degree of compression between the head and the pelvic brim. It is usually stated that not more than eight minutes can elapse between the birth of the umbilicus and the delivery of the head, if the child is to be born alive. This is not correct, as a much longer time may elapse, especially if the mouth has appeared at the vulva and thereby affords the possibility for the establishment of pulmonary respiration.

Holland and Capon, in 1922, established the predominant cause of fetal death in breech presentations, by showing that the probability of the occurrence of tentorial tears and subsequent intracranial hemorrhage is twice as great as in head presentations; Crothers and Putnam have emphasized the part played by lesions of the spinal cord. The first-mentioned authors have also shown that when extraction is practiced, and especially when it is aided by suprapubic pressure upon the head, the medulla may protrude through the foramen magnum and actually become herniated into the spinal canal. It should also be remembered, when premature attempts at extraction are made, that descent of the head may be interfered with by the imperfectly dilated cervix, and great force may be required to overcome the resistance.

In complete and incomplete breech presentations, prolapse of the umbilical cord is a common complication. In Moore and Steptoe's total series of 1,444 breech cases, the incidence of this accident was 4.85 per cent. Since the incidence of prolapse of the cord in all presentations is usually reported as 0.5 per cent, it is apparent that this complication occurs nine times more frequently in breech presentations than may ordinarily be expected. The weight of the baby appears to have no effect on the incidence of prolapse of the cord, but the type of breech is all-important. The incidence of this complication in frank breech presentations was only 0.4 per cent in the above series, but in incomplete and complete breeches it was 22 and 12 times greater, respectively. The cause of the high frequency of prolapse of the cord in incomplete and complete breech cases is the failure in these cases of the presenting part to fill the lower uterine segment and cover the cervical os as do frank breech and vertex presentations. In Moore and Steptoe's series, prolapse of the cord was responsible for 53.3 per cent of the total deaths in incomplete breech presentations and none of the deaths in frank breech cases.

Treatment. In view of the serious fetal prognosis attending breech presentations, the obstetrician should aim to prevent their occurrence as far as possible; whenever they are recognized in the later weeks of pregnancy, an attempt may be made, by means of *external version,* to substitute a vertex presentation. This procedure, if properly and gently performed, carries little danger, although not as much is accomplished by it as might be supposed. In most series reported in which external version has been performed, the final incidence of breech presentation at delivery is not much less than would have resulted if nothing had been done. This circumstance is the result of several factors. In the first case, if nothing is done, spontaneous version occurs in many cases, especially in that type of case in which manual version is easiest to do. Second, although version may be temporarily successful, the breech presentation often recurs. Third, most breech presentations are of the frank variety in which version is especially difficult. However, a gentle attempt does no harm and many authorities recommend the procedure. Because of possible trauma, anesthesia should never be used. External version is readily accomplished in multiparae with lax abdominal walls, but is more difficult in primigravidae. If the head can be forced into the pelvis after the substitution has been effected, the new position becomes permanent, but if this is not possible, the child will not infrequently revert to its original position, notwithstanding the application of a properly fitting bandage or abdominal binder. Ryder found the optimum time for performing external cephalic version to be the sixth and seventh calendar months of gestation and advises that breech presentations should not be allowed to persist during the last two months without attempts at version. This procedure may also be attempted in the first stage of labor, provided the breech has not descended deeply into the pelvis; when it has once become fixed, all such efforts are unavailing. As a rule, the procedure is not advisable after rupture of the membranes, because of the possibility of prolapse of the umbilical cord. The fetal heart beat should be auscultated before and after the performance of this maneuver.

In most breech presentations spontaneous delivery occurs to the umbilicus, and the attitude of the obstetrician should be merely one of expectancy; nevertheless, he should always hold himself in readiness to intervene at a moment's notice. For this reason, as soon as the breech appears at the vulva, the patient should be prepared for delivery in order that not a moment may be lost in performing extraction should it become necessary. The breech should be allowed to advance spontaneously until the umbilicus has been born. It is most important to remember that the completion of labor is materially facilitated by the arms' retaining their normal crossed position over the thorax, as well as by sharp flexion of the head. This is best attained by avoiding traction as far as possible and also by avoiding any pressure on the fundus which, as Potter has emphasized, may push the head between the arms. Owing to the fact that the breech forms a less efficient dilating wedge than the head, premature rupture of the membranes occurs more frequently than in vertex presentation.

Generally speaking, the frank breech forms a better dilating wedge than the complete breech, inasmuch as it allows a closer application to the margins of the partially dilated os. On the other hand, if interference becomes necessary, the complete breech offers more satisfactory conditions for immediate delivery, as a foot can readily be brought down and used as a tractor, so that the question arises whether it might not be better in frank breech to make it a rule to bring down one or both feet prophylactically. Usually this is not advisable, unless some abnormality exists on the part of the mother or child which renders it probable that prompt delivery may be called for. In such cases, as soon as the cervix is fully dilated, the membranes should be ruptured and both feet brought down into the vagina so that extraction can be promptly effected when necessary. The technic of this manipulation, as well as the rules for extraction, will be considered in Chapter 41.

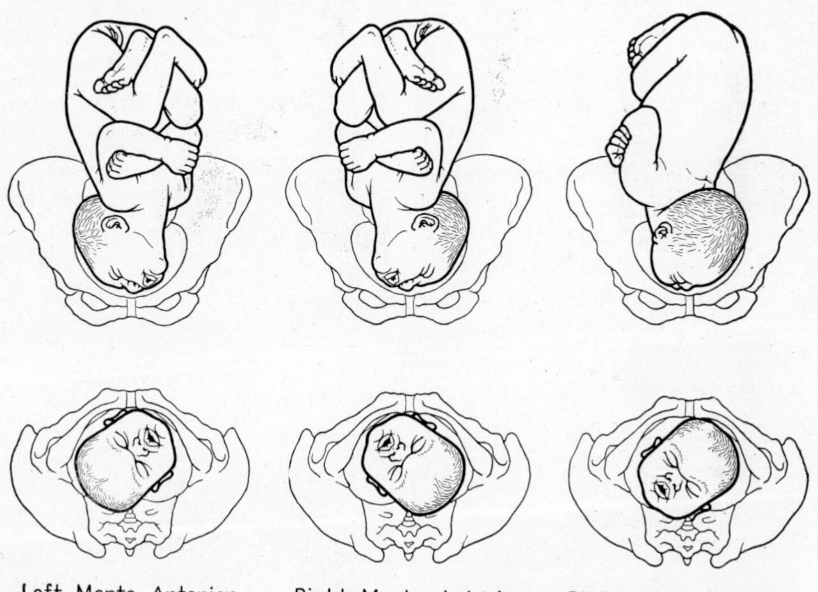

Fig. 406.—Showing Left and Right Positions in Face Presentations.

In view of the serious fetal mortality, many writers recommend a more radical policy, and Irving and Goethals advocate bringing down the feet as soon as the cervix has become fully dilated and eliminating the second stage by prompt extraction. Piper, on the other hand, held that many children are lost as the result of extraction, and advocated in its stead the application of forceps to the aftercoming head. The latter technic is becoming routine in the delivery of the aftercoming head as it offers many advantages. The former procedure, we feel, should not be resorted to until it becomes evident, after a satisfactory period of time in the second stage, that labor is going to be prolonged to the detriment of the mother or child. Such a practice will result in the spontaneous delivery of many frank breech presentations, and only in the exceptional case will it be necessary to break up the breech as suggested by Irving and Goethals.

Face Presentations. In face presentations the head is sharply extended so that the occiput is in contact with the back, while the face looks downward. An analysis of 31,000 consecutive cases of labor in the New York Lying-In Hospital revealed that the incidence of such presentations was 0.27 per cent—that is, 1 to every 369 labors. Posner and Buch recently reported an incidence of 1 in 529 deliveries.

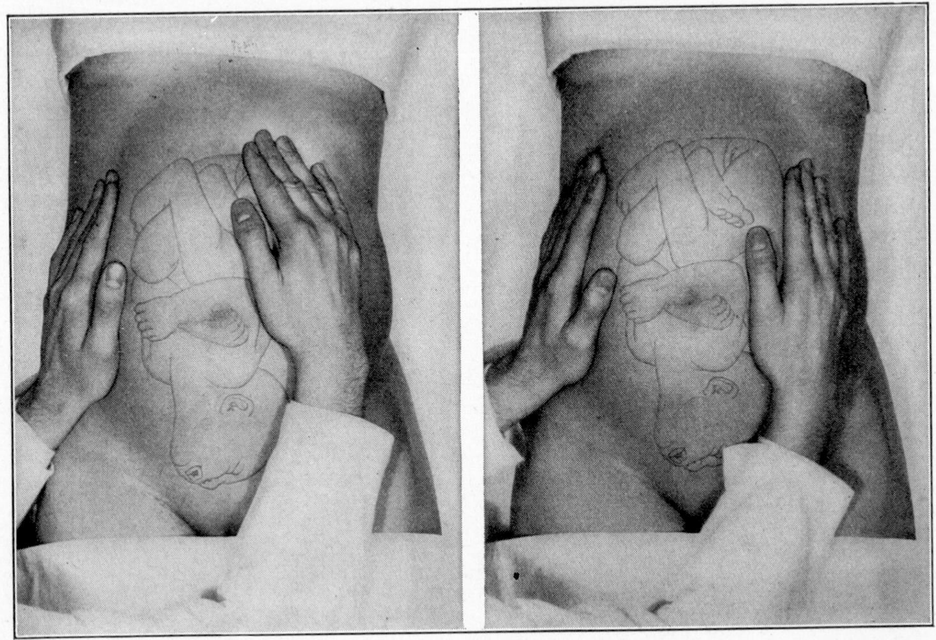

First Maneuver. Second Maneuver.

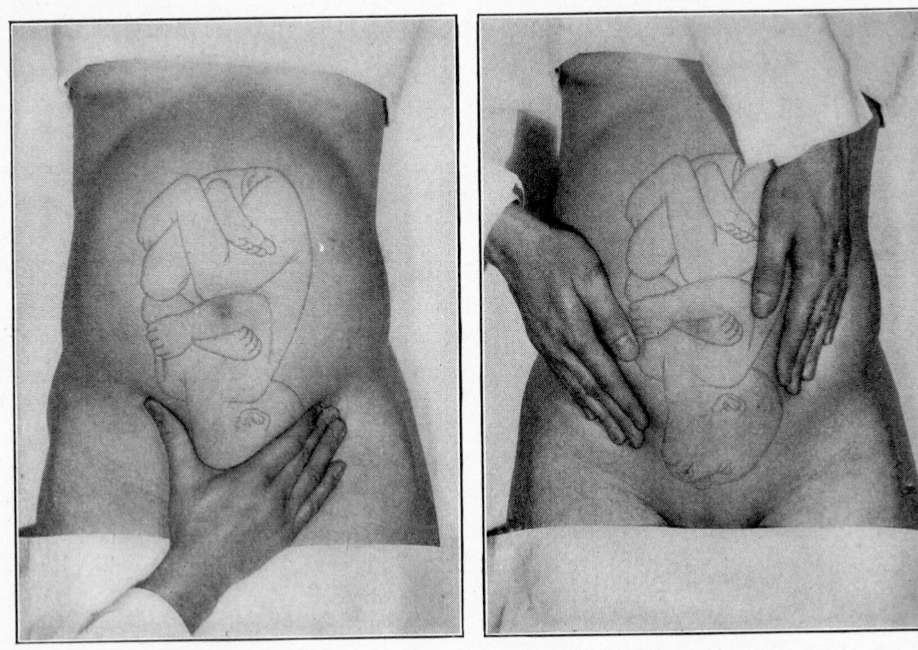

Third Maneuver. Fourth Maneuver.

Fig. 407.—Palpation in Right Mento-Anterior Position.

It is commonly stated that the face most frequently occupies the right oblique diameter of the pelvis, resulting in either L.M.A. or R.M.P. positions. Markoe found that these two varieties of face presentations constituted 62.4 per cent of his 250 cases, while they accounted for only 31.7 per cent of our cases, the right mental anterior variety being the most frequent (25 per cent). The initial position of the chin is posterior in about 30 per cent of cases.

Diagnosis. In the right mento-anterior variety, palpation gives the following data:

First maneuver:	Breech in fundus.
Second maneuver:	Back in the left and posterior portion of the abdomen, and distinctly felt only in its upper portion; small parts in right and anterior portion of the abdomen.
Third maneuver:	Head may be detected above superior strait.
Fourth maneuver:	Marked cephalic prominence on left side; fingers can be depressed deeply on right (Fig. 407).

The reverse holds good in the left posterior variety. With the less frequent engagements in the left oblique diameter, the various maneuvers give comparable findings. In the case of engagement in the transverse diameter, right and left mento-transverse, the findings differ from the corresponding anterior positions, only in that the back is directed to the lateral portion of the abdomen and the small parts are directed laterally on the opposite side. The characteristic sign is that the cephalic prominence is palpable on the same side as the back, instead of on the side of the small parts as in vertex presentations. The back is felt distinctly only in the neighborhood of the breech.

On vaginal or rectal touch the face is found in the birth canal, and the position is diagnosed by the differentiation of the various features, the mouth and nose, malar bones, and orbital ridges being the distinctive points. In the left anterior variety the chin occupies the anterior and the brow the posterior extremity of the right oblique diameter of the pelvis, while in right posterior position the reverse obtains.

The heart sounds are transmitted through the thorax; accordingly, they are heard through the side of the abdomen which contains the small parts, and generally below the umbilicus. The only other conditions in which auscultation gives similar results is in brow presentations and in the rare cases of occipitoposterior positions in which the head is partially extended.

It should be noted that the diagnosis of face presentation, based on the findings of abdominal palpation, is sometimes difficult and often not established until late in labor, by either rectal or vaginal examination. As disproportion is a frequent cause of face presentation, Posner and Buch advocate more extensive use of the x-rays in establishing early diagnosis of face as well as brow presentations.

Causation. The causes of face presentations are manifold and, generally speaking, are afforded by any factor tending to bring about extension or to prevent flexion of the head. Accordingly, they occur more frequently when the pelvis is contracted or the child very large. In a series of 141 face presentations, studied in our clinic by Hellman, Epperson, and Connally, the incidence of inlet contraction was 39.4 per cent. Similarly, in Posner and Buch's series of 87 face and 13 brow presentations, there were 29 instances of at least borderline disproportion, that is, either pelvic contraction or a baby in excess of eight and one-half pounds. Rudolf's series shows comparable figures. This high incidence of pelvic contraction and large infants is most important to bear in mind in the management of face presentation and dictates the necessity of x-ray pelvimetry before deciding on the program for delivery. Petitjean believes that the production of face presentation is favored by a low implantation of the placenta, which he has noted in two thirds of the cases observed in Pinard's clinic.

Matthews Duncan directed attention to a frequent causative factor concerned in the production of secondary face presentations—namely, an oblique position of the uterus, which permits the child's back to sag toward the side in which the vertex lies. He pointed out that in such circumstances the attitude of the fetus becomes abnormal,

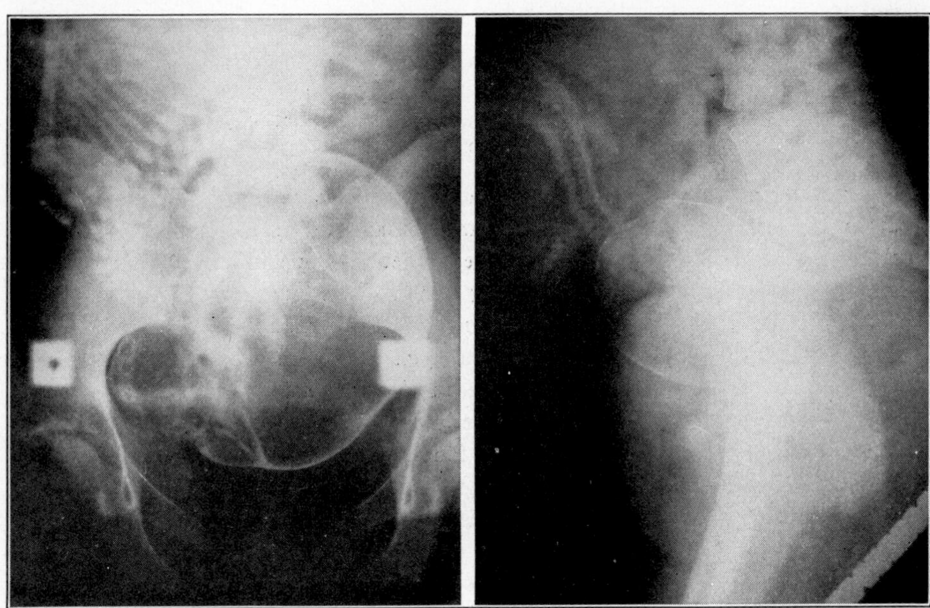

FIG. 408.—ROENTGENOGRAMS SHOWING FACE PRESENTATION.
Note spinal curvature of infant.

so that a slight obstacle to the descent of the posterior portion of the head will result in its extension. This occurs most frequently in right occipitoposterior positions, as is shown by the fact that, while left occipito-anterior are many times more frequent than right occipitoposterior positions, the same two varieties of face positions occur with almost equal frequency. That multiparity would naturally favor the production of this condition is evident, since lax abdominal walls allow the uterus to assume an oblique position. Hence, it is usually observed that some 60 per cent of the cases occurred in multiparous women.

In exceptional instances, marked enlargement of the neck or thorax, coils of cord about the neck, spastic contraction, or congenital shortening of the cervical muscles may cause extension (Morse). Again, it is well known that anencephalic children usually present by the face, as the result of the faulty development of the cranial vault.

Mechanism. As face are usually derived from vertex presentations, it is apparent that the former are but rarely observed in a fully developed state at the superior strait, where the brow generally engages, while the face descends only after further extension.

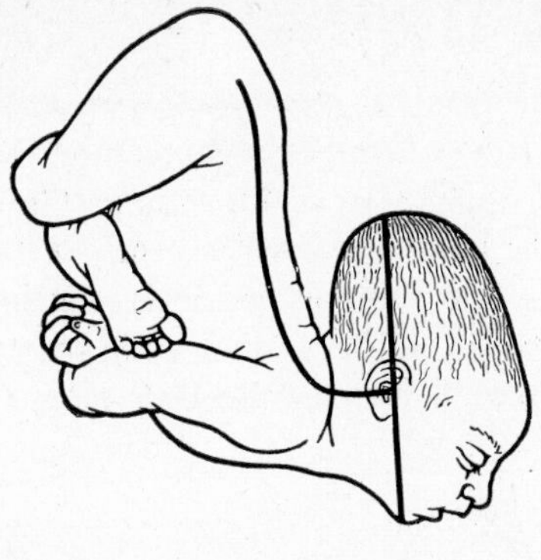

Fig. 409.

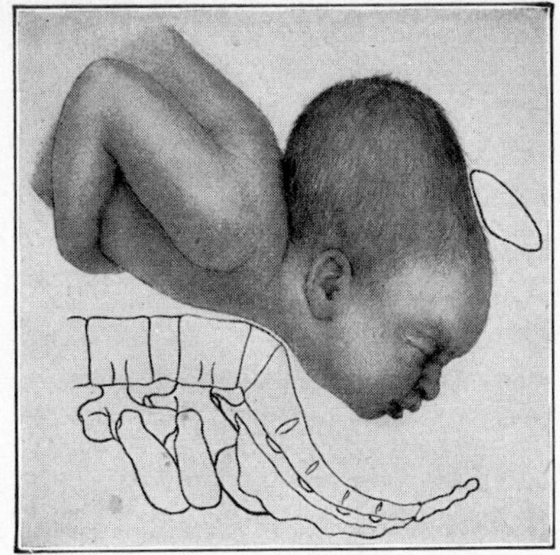

Fig. 410.

Fig. 409.—Face Presentation. Occiput on the Long End of Head Lever.

Fig. 410.—Face Presentation, Chin Directly Posterior, Showing Impossibility of Spontaneous Delivery, Unless Rotation Occurs.

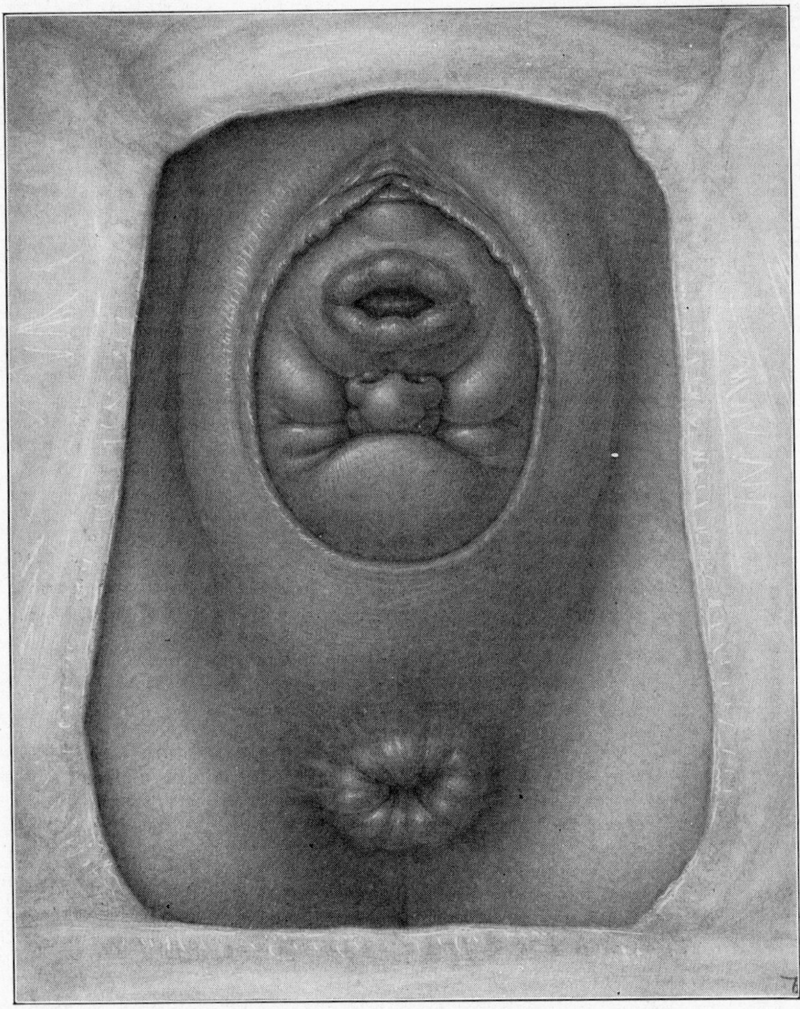

Fig. 411.—Distention of Vulva in Face Presentation.

The mechanism in these cases consists of the *cardinal movements*—descent, internal rotation and flexion—and the *accessory movements*—extension and external rotation. Descent is brought about by the same factors as in vertex presentations, while extension results from the relation which the body of the child bears to its deflected head, the latter being converted as it were into a two-armed lever, the longer arm of which extends from the occipital condyles to the occiput so that when resistance is encountered the occiput must be pushed upward, while the chin descends (Fig. 409).

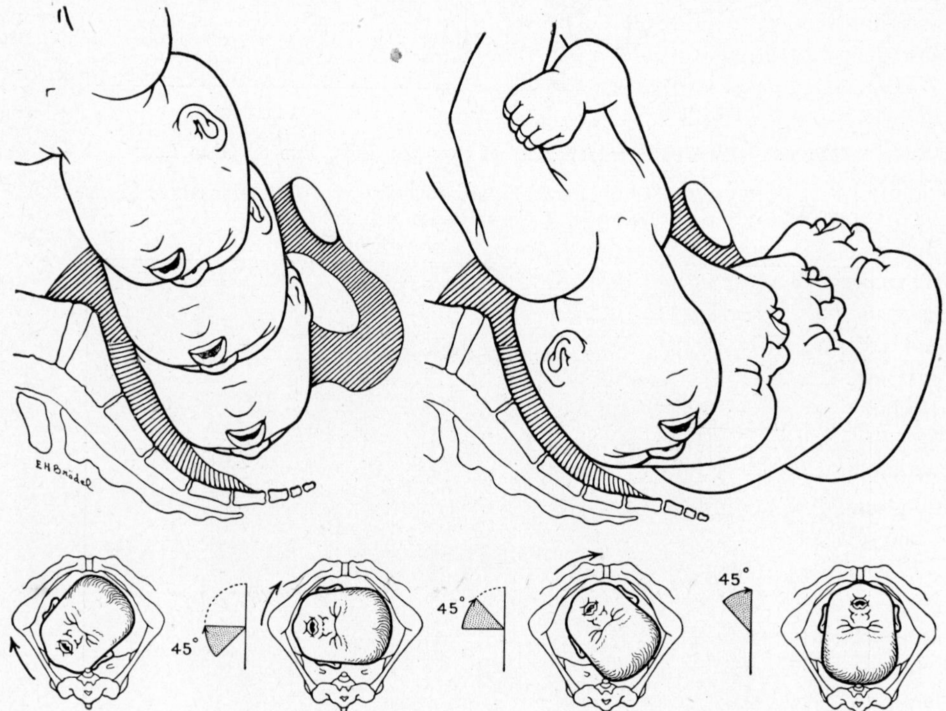

Fig. 412.—Mechanism of Labor for Right Mentoposterior Position.

Internal rotation has for its object the rotation of the face in such a manner as to bring the chin under the symphysis pubis, since otherwise, natural delivery cannot be accomplished. Only in this way can the neck subtend the posterior surface of the symphysis pubis. If the chin rotates directly posteriorly, the relatively short neck cannot span the anterior surface of the sacrum which measures 12 cm. in length; hence, the birth of the head is manifestly impossible unless the shoulders can enter the pelvis at the same time, which is out of the question except when the child is premature or macerated (Fig. 410). Internal rotation in a face presentation is due to the same factors that bring this about in vertex presentations, and Sellheim holds that, as bending in face presentations occurs most readily between the base of the neck and the chin, that portion of the child must inevitably rotate to the front in order to accommodate itself to the "knee" of the birth canal.

After anterior rotation and descent the chin and mouth appear at the vulva, the under surface of the chin becomes stemmed against the symphysis, and the head is delivered by a movement of flexion, the nose, eyes, brows, bregma, and occiput appearing in succession over the anterior margin of the perineum (Fig. 411). After the birth of the head the occiput sags backward toward the anus, and in a few moments the chin, by a movement of external rotation, turns to the side toward which it was originally directed, after which the shoulders are born as in vertex presentations.

In mental positions the face becomes distorted owing to the effusion of serum beneath the skin, which when marked completely obliterates the features and may readily cause confusion with a breech presentation. At the same time, the skull undergoes considerable molding which is manifested by an increase in length of the mento-occipital diameter and a diminution in the vertical diameters of the head.

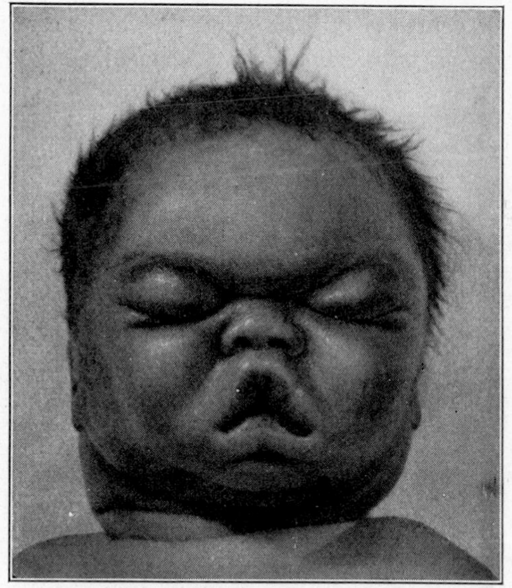

FIG. 413.—FACIAL EDEMA AND DISCOLORATION IN FACE PRESENTATION. AFTER DELIVERY.

Prognosis. Until the latter part of the eighteenth century, face presentations were considered extremely unfavorable, and most authorities advised their conversion into some other variety. But about that time a number of obstetricians in France and in Austria, pointed out that most of them would end spontaneously if left alone. This doctrine was definitely established by Johann Lucas Boer who reported that he had observed spontaneous labor in 79 out of a series of 80 face presentations and had applied forceps in only a single instance.

Deep tears in the perineum are of frequent occurrence, and are often erroneously attributed to excessive distention of the vulvar outlet by the largest circumference of the head—the mento-occipital. In reality, however, the trachelobregmatic is the circumference concerned, and, as it is but little larger than the suboccipitofrontal which is concerned in vertex presentations, some other factor must be invoked to explain the greater incidence of perineal tears. The explanation is probably to be found in the greater downward protrusion of the pelvic floor, as in face presentations the presenting part must descend very deeply before flexion of the neck under the symphysis can occur. (See Figs. 411 and 412.)

Owing to the prolongation of labor the fetal mortality is markedly increased, being usually estimated at about 14 per cent.

In dealing with face presentations it should always be borne in mind that internal rotation does not occur until the pelvic floor is well distended by the advancing face; frequently, when the chin is obliquely posterior, it may not take place until the obstetrician has almost abandoned hope of its occurrence. Nor should it be forgotten that the face must occupy a lower level than the vertex before one can feel assured that the greatest circumference of the head has passed through the superior strait. This can be readily appreciated from a study of Figs. 414 and 415 in which it is seen that the distance from the parietal boss to the vertex is only 3 cm., whereas a line drawn from the same point to the face will measure 7 cm.

Treatment. In the anterior varieties, spontaneous delivery is the rule, and, even when the chin is obliquely posterior, anterior rotation usually occurs, although often not until a very late period. In view of the serious prognosis attending failure of the chin to rotate anteriorly, and particularly when the face rotates into the hollow of the sacrum, an attempt may be made to substitute a vertex presentation. When the face is not deeply engaged, provided there exists no disproportion between its size and that of the pelvis, and the amniotic fluid has not long since drained away, this can sometimes be readily accomplished, either by pushing up the chin or by making traction upon the occiput and so bringing about flexion of the fetal head.

On the other hand, when the chin is directed anteriorly, attempts at conversion are not advisable, as they would merely substitute an occipitoposterior position which is but slightly more favorable than the original face presentation, not to speak of the increased danger of infection attending the manipulation. In obliquely posterior face positions, on the contrary, conversion is usually indicated and should be attempted as soon as it becomes clear that rotation has not occurred despite a reasonable period of labor.

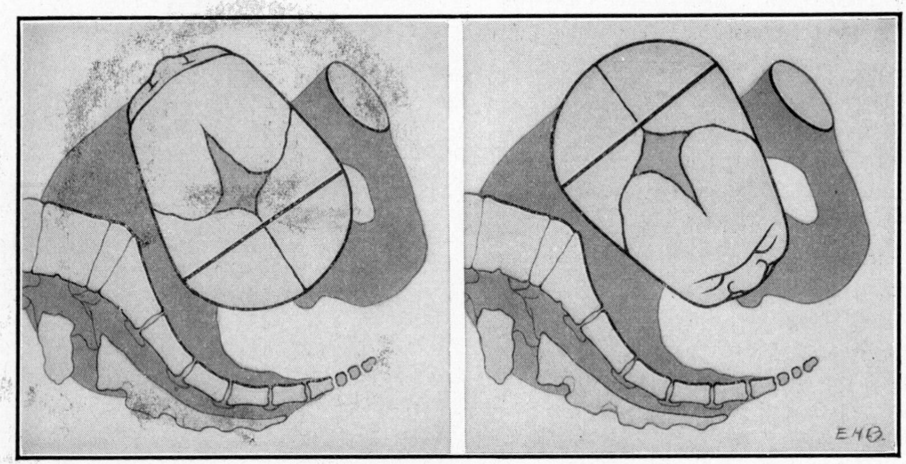

Fig. 414.—Diagram Showing That When the Vertex Is on the Line Joining the Ischial Spines, the Greatest Diameter of the Head Has Passed the Superior Strait.

Fig. 415.—Diagram Showing That When the Face Is on the Level of the Ischial Spines, the Greatest Diameter of the Head Is Still Above the Superior Strait.

From time to time numerous methods of conversion have been suggested, the oldest and most effectual, advocated by Baudelocque and revived by Thorn, Weiss, and others, being the following: Attempts are made to push up the chin by two fingers introduced into the vagina; if this does not succeed the patient is anesthetized, the whole hand introduced, and the head dislodged, after which the vertex is grasped and drawn down. At the same time, the external hand of the operator or the assistant carries the back in the opposite direction, so as to facilitate flexion. Satisfactory results have been reported from this maneuver, and its adoption in suitable cases can be recommended, especially in multiparae (Fig. 416). In our experience, however, it has proved efficacious in only about half the cases.

If the face is too deeply engaged in the pelvis to admit of the Baudelocque maneuver, the patient should be let alone and descent allowed to take place, in the hope that anterior rotation will occur when the face reaches the pelvic floor. If, however, this does not take place after a reasonable delay, manual rotation may be attempted followed by forceps, or cesarean section may be performed, depending on the circumstances of the case. In most persistent mentum posterior cases in primigravidae, cesarean section is the procedure of choice, provided the child is alive and no evidence of infection is present. Employed judiciously, it is preferable to local manipulations as well as to version. If the child is dead, craniotomy is indicated.

As stated above, in most persistent mentum posterior cases in primigravidae, cesarean section is the operation of choice. Moreover, in multiparae also, if there is any pelvic contraction or a large baby, abdominal delivery is advisable. In former times, when cesarean section was a more dangerous operation than it is today, version and extraction was often employed, both as a primary procedure and following unsuccessful attempts at conversion. When, in a multiparous woman with a normal pelvis and a baby which is not excessive in size, a posterior face presentation does not rotate after a reasonable period of labor, this operation still has a place, but the place is a small one because under the circumstances cited spontaneous rotation is the rule. In Reddock's large series of face presentations, the fetal mortality associated with version and extraction was extremely high, but in the series reported by Hellman, Epperson, and Connally the results were good, provided the pelvis was normal.

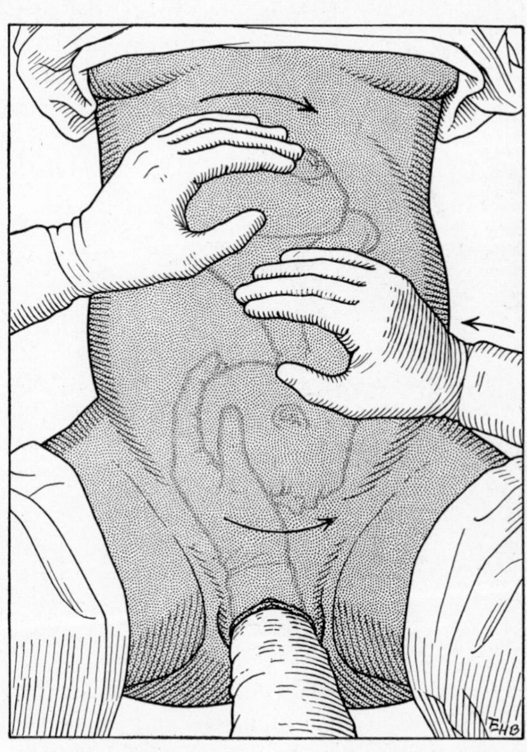

Fig. 416.—Thorn's Maneuver Showing Direction of Pressure in Conversion of a Face into a vertex Presentation.

To recapitulate, the management of face presentations comprises the following steps: (1) x-ray pelvimetry to establish or rule out pelvic contraction; (2) if any significant degree of pelvic contraction with disproportion is present, cesarean section; (3) if the pelvis is normal and the chin anterior, spontaneous delivery or an easy low forceps should be anticipated, no treatment being necessary; (4) if the pelvis is normal and the chin posterior, spontaneous rotation and an easy vaginal delivery should again be anticipated because this will occur in two thirds of these posterior cases (Since only about one third of all face presentations have the chin posterior, and since two thirds of this one third undergo spontaneous rotation, a case of persistent mentum posterior is encountered only once in about 10 face presentations); (5) if the chin persists as a posterior in a primigravida, cesarean section is usually the best procedure; (6) if the chin persists as a posterior in a multipara with a normal pelvis, conversion to a vertex, rotation with forceps, or version and extraction may be employed if the baby is not excessive in size, but in the event that it is, cesarean section is the method of choice in many cases; and (7) if the chin persists as a posterior and the child is dead, perforation of the fetal skull should be effected and extraction carried out by means of the cranioclast (see Chapter 43).

Brow Presentations. In brow presentations the head occupies a position midway between flexion and extension; hence, the portion situated between the orbital ridge and large fontanel presents at the superior strait. As nearly every child which is born by the face has gone through a preliminary stage of brow presentation, the latter must occur more frequently, later undergoing spontaneous conversion into either a face or

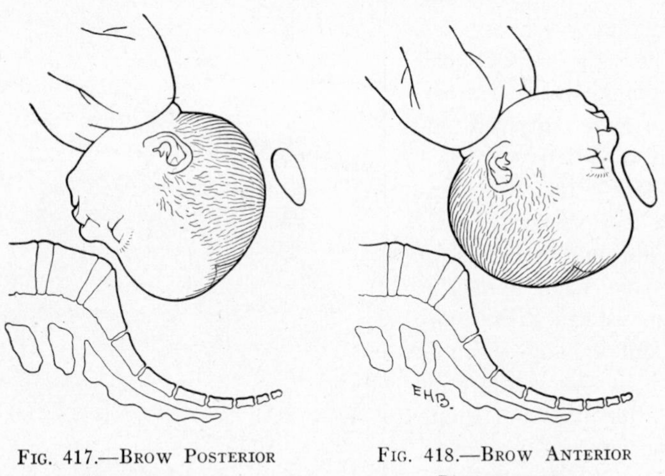

FIG. 417.—BROW POSTERIOR PRESENTATION.

FIG. 418.—BROW ANTERIOR PRESENTATION.

a vertex presentation. On the other hand, persistent brow presentations are rare, their incidence being approximately once in every 1,000 labors. The incidence of brow presentation in Stander's series was 0.1 per cent, or 1 in 968 cases of labor.

The causes of this presentation, which have been carefully studied by Ahlfeld and Neumann, are practically identical with those giving rise to face presentations, and depend upon any factor which interferes with flexion or promotes extension of the head. Neumann, in 1929, pointed out that heads of a certain shape predispose to the occurrence of brow presentations—notably hypsicephalus and oxycephalus, in which the head is tower-shaped or conical. In twin pregnancies not infrequently one or both children may present in this manner, and Ahlfeld maintains that the anterior surfaces of the two fetuses coming in contact mutually disturb the normal flexed attitude, so that extension is facilitated. Usually the brow is directed toward one or the other extremity of the transverse diameter of the superior strait.

Diagnosis. The presentation can occasionally be recognized by palpation, but vaginal examination is usually necessary, as the data obtainable from palpation are less characteristic than in the more common presentations. The palpatory findings are similar to those observed in face presentations, except that the cephalic prominence is less marked on the side of the back, while the resistance offered by the chin can be felt on the same side as the small parts. On vaginal or rectal touch the frontal suture and the anterior portion of the sagittal suture are encountered in the transverse diameter, at one end of which the large fontanel or the portion of the skull just posterior to it may be felt, while at the other the orbital ridges, the root of the nose, and the eyes may be distinguished. It is not possible to palpate the mouth or chin, for when these are within reach we have to deal with a face presentation.

Mechanism. The mechanism of labor in brow presentations differs materially with the size of the fetus, which Ahlfeld and most observers have stated is usually below the normal. Weiss and Neumann, on the other hand, maintain that large children are the rule. The average baby weight in Stander's cases of brow presentation was 3,410 gm., as compared with an average weight of 3,456 gm. for all full-term babies delivered in his service during a 12-year period. In the case of small children the course of labor, as a rule, is easy, while in larger babies it is usually very difficult. The cause of the difficulty is apparent when we consider that the circumference of the head which engages at the superior strait is the mento-occipital, whose greatest diameter averages 13.5 cm. in length, and that, consequently, engagement is impossible until after marked molding has taken place, by which the mento-occipital diameter has become diminished and the fronto-occipital increased in length.

After molding and descent have occurred the brow sometimes rotates anteriorly, and the forehead, orbital ridges, and root of the nose appear at the vulva. One of the superior maxillary bones then becomes stemmed against the inferior margin of the symphysis, and the rest of the head is born by a movement of extreme flexion, the brow, bregma, and occiput appearing in succession over the anterior margin of the perineum. After the birth of the occiput, the mouth and chin descend from behind the pubic arch by a movement of extension. In other words, we have a mechanism somewhat similar to that observed in the less frequent mode of delivery in the case of posterior occiput positions which had rotated into the hollow of the sacrum. Sometimes, however, as reported by Neumann and others, the brow descends to the outlet with the frontal suture directly transverse and is born in that position, or partial anterior rotation occurs, bringing the root of the nose to about the middle of the ischiopubic ramus, when the occiput is delivered posteriorly by a movement of extreme flexion, after which the face escapes following extreme extension. In either event, the second stage tends to be unduly prolonged.

As has already been pointed out, a large child cannot enter the birth canal without considerable molding of the head. This adds materially to the length of labor and results in the birth of children with characteristically deformed heads. The caput succedaneum is found over the forehead and extends from the orbital ridges to the large fontanel, and in many cases is so marked as to render diagnosis by vaginal touch almost impossible. In these cases, the forehead is very prominent and square, the mento-occipital diameter being diminished and the fronto-occipital diameter increased in length.

Prognosis. In the transient varieties of brow presentation, the outlook depends upon the presentation which ultimately results, and on whether the face or vertex enters the birth canal; in the persistent forms the outlook is generally considered to be bad, unless the fetus is small. It should always be remembered that disproportion between the size of the head and the pelvis is an important factor in the production of such presentations; under identical mechanical conditions the possibility of a spontaneous outcome is always much less in a brow than in a vertex presentation. Fink reports that in a series of 130 brow presentations, spontaneous delivery occurred in only 43 per cent of the patients.

Rational methods of treatment, similar to those indicated in face presentations, and, more particularly, stricter attention to aseptic technic have led to a marked improvement in the prognosis of the persistent varieties. Weiss has reported 29 cases, without a death of fetus or mother.

Treatment. If the brow is recognized at the superior strait, the treatment will vary according as the presentation promises to be transient or persistent. The former should be left alone, as the child will probably be born spontaneously by the vertex or face. On the other hand, in persistent cases, particularly if the brow is obliquely posterior, attempts at conversion may be made or cesarean section performed on a basis similar to that described in the treatment of persistent mentum posterior cases.

Transverse Presentation. In this condition the long axis of the fetus crosses that of the mother at about a right angle. When it forms an acute angle we speak of an *oblique* presentation. However, this is usually only transitory, becoming converted into a longitudinal or transverse presentation when labor supervenes.

In transverse presentations the shoulder usually occupies the superior strait, the head lying in one and the breech in the other iliac fossa. Accordingly, such a condition is commonly spoken of as a *shoulder,* less frequently as a *lateral plane,* and technically as an *acromion* presentation. The latter designation is chosen for the reason that the acromion process is one of the most characteristic features of the shoulder, the position being right or left according to the side of the mother toward which the acromion is directed. Moreover, as, in either position, the back may be directed anteriorly or posteriorly, it is customary to distinguish between the *dorso-anterior* and *dorsoposterior* varieties. The recognition of the position of the back is of great importance in connection with the proper performance of version, a procedure often used in this condition. According to Schroeder, the shoulder is directed toward the left side of the mother 2.6 times more frequently than toward the right, while the back looks anteriorly 2.5 times more frequently than posteriorly.

Etiology. The common causes of transverse presentation are three in number: abnormal relaxation of the abdominal walls due to great multiparity, pelvic contraction, and placenta previa. The incidence of transverse presentation augments greatly with parity, the condition being 10 times more frequent in patients with a parity of four or more than it is in primigravidae. Relaxation of the abdominal walls with a pendulous abdomen allows the uterus to fall forward so that the long axis of the fetus is deflected, away from the axis of the birth canal, into an oblique or transverse position. Placenta previa and pelvic contraction act in a similar manner by preventing engagement. It occasionally happens that a transverse or oblique presentation develops in labor following an initial longitudinal presentation, the head or breech migrating to one or another iliac fossa. This almost always indicates pelvic contraction.

Diagnosis. The diagnosis of a transverse presentation is usually readily made, inspection alone frequently causing one to suspect its existence. The abdomen is seen to be unusually wide from side to side, while the fundus of the uterus scarcely extends above the umbilicus.

On palpation, the first maneuver reveals the absence of a fetal pole in the fundus. On the second maneuver a ballottable head will be found in one and the breech in the other iliac fossa, while the third and fourth maneuvers are negative, unless labor

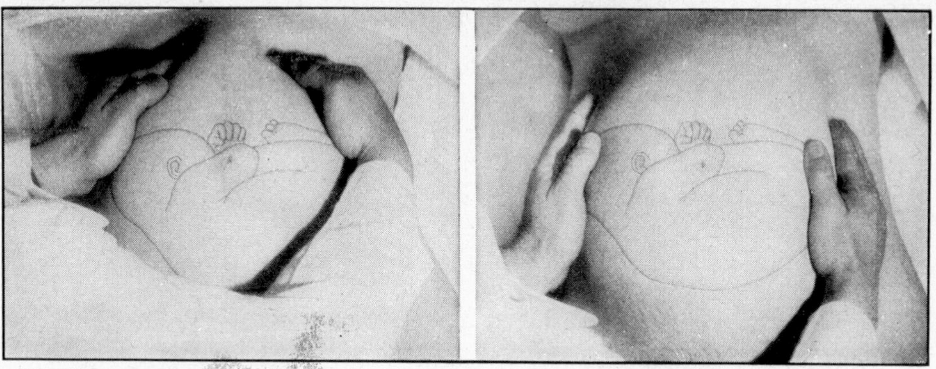

First Maneuver Second Maneuver

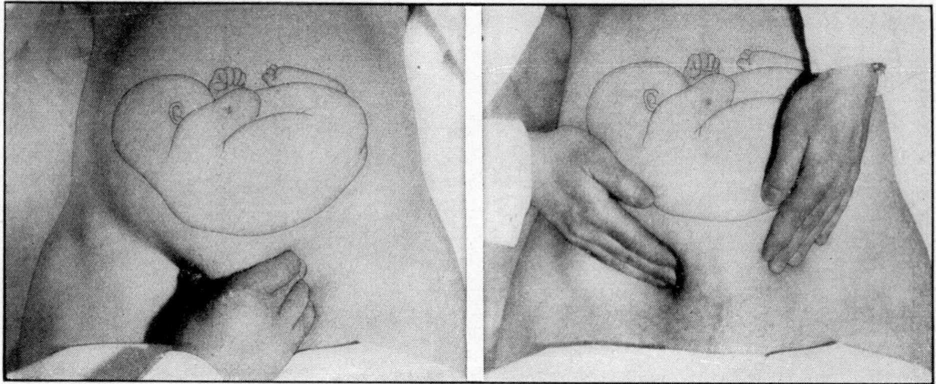

Third Maneuver Fourth Maneuver

Palpation in Right Acromiodorso-Anterior Position.

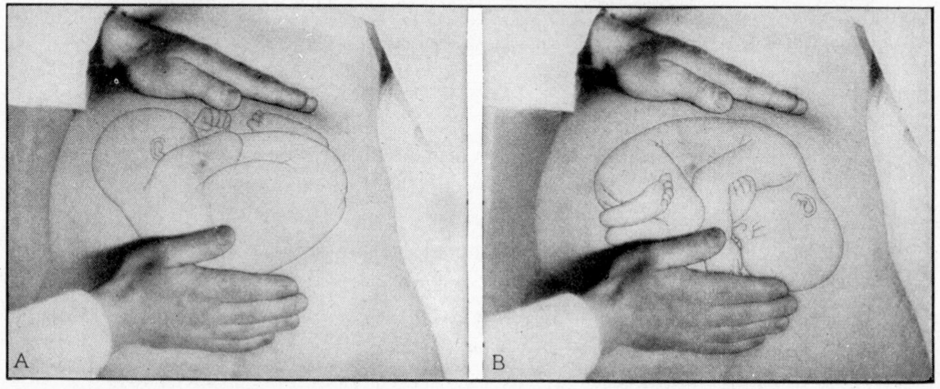

Palpation of Back in Dorso-Anterior (A) and in Dorsoposterior (B) Positions.

Fig. 419.—Palpation Maneuvers and Palpation of Back in Transverse Position.

has been in progress for some time and the shoulder has become impacted in the pelvis. At the same time the position of the back is readily determined. When it is situated anteriorly a hard resistant plane will be felt extending across the front of the abdomen; when it lies posteriorly irregular nodulations, representing the small parts, will be felt in the same location (Fig. 419).

On vaginal touch in the early stages of labor, the side of the thorax, readily recognizable by the "gridiron" sensation afforded by the ribs, can be made out at the

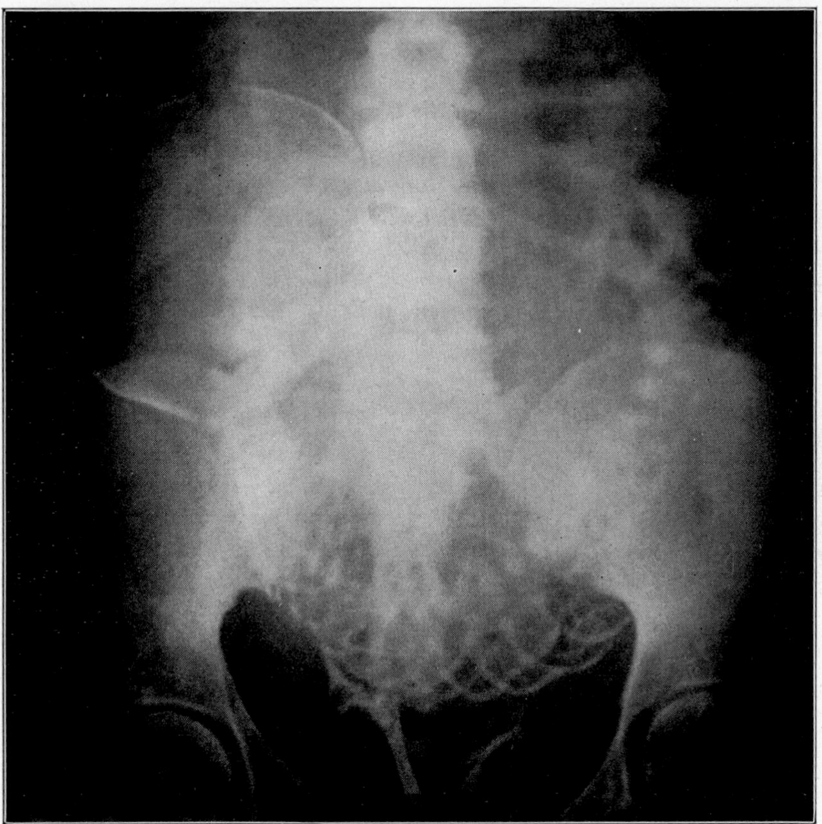

Fig. 420.—Roentgenogram of Transverse Presentation Showing Posterior Elbow in the Cervix.

superior strait. When dilatation is further advanced the scapula can be distinguished on one and the clavicle on the other side of the thorax, while the position of the axilla will indicate toward which side of the mother the shoulder is directed. Later in labor the shoulder becomes tightly wedged in the pelvic canal, and a hand and arm frequently prolapse into the vagina and through the vulva; whether it is the right or left can be readily determined by ascertaining to which one of the obstetrician's it corresponds, just as in shaking hands.

Course of Labor. With very rare exceptions, the spontaneous birth of a fully developed child is impossible in persistent transverse presentations, since expulsion cannot be effected unless both the head and trunk of the child enter the pelvis at the same time, which is manifestly impossible. Accordingly, both the fetus and mother must almost inevitably perish if appropriate measures are not instituted. On the other hand, small, premature, and, particularly, macerated children are frequently born spontaneously.

Throughout the first stage, but particularly during the early period of the second stage of labor, preliminary, but futile, preparations are made for spontaneous delivery. These consist in a molding of the fetus in anticipation of the engagement of the presenting shoulder, which results in the approximation of the head to the ventral surface of the child, by which the transverse diameter of the fetal ovoid becomes diminished and the vertical diameter increased in length. After rupture of the membranes, if the patient is left to herself, the shoulder is forced down into the pelvic cavity, and

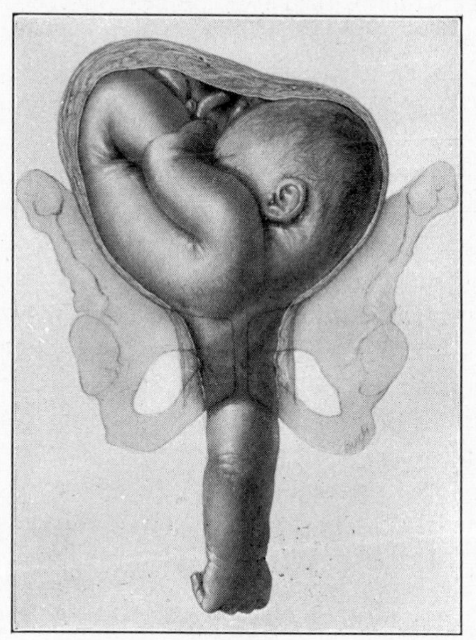

Fig. 421.—Prolapse of an Arm in Transverse Presentation.

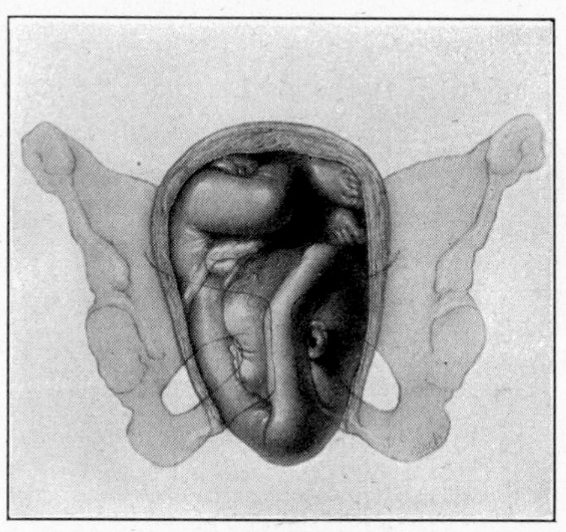

Fig. 422.—Conduplicato Corpore.

the corresponding arm frequently prolapses (Fig. 421). After a certain amount of descent, the shoulder becomes arrested by the margins of the superior strait, with the head in one iliac fossa and the breech in the other, and, with the continuance of labor, becomes firmly impacted in the upper part of the pelvic cavity. The uterus then contracts vigorously in the attempt to overcome the obstacle, but in vain. After a certain time the physiological retraction ring rises higher and higher and becomes more marked (pathological retraction ring), the lower uterine segment becomes more and more stretched and eventually gives way, when a part or the whole of the product of conception escapes into the abdominal cavity. In such circumstances the patient usually succumbs within a short time to intraperitoneal hemorrhage, while in other instances death from infection occurs after a longer period. (See Fig. 397.)

Possibly once in many thousand cases, the uterus may cease to contract before the membranes rupture, and the child, being retained within the uterus, may eventually become mummified. Such a missed labor is very rare in human beings, though it is well known to the veterinarians. On the other hand, such an occurrence would be out of the question had the amniotic sac been opened, as in such circumstances bacteria would gain access to the uterus and give rise to infection, which, if not terminating in the death of the patient, would lead to the gradual casting off of the product of conception by suppurative processes, supposing that the woman could be so long neglected.

It has long been realized that in very rare instances, if the child is very small and the pelvis large, spontaneous delivery may occasionally be accomplished in spite of the persistence of the abnormal presentation. In such cases the child becomes compressed upon itself with the head tightly pressed against the abdomen so that a portion of the thoracic wall below the shoulder becomes the most dependent part and appears at the vulva. The head and thorax then pass through the pelvic cavity at the same time, and the child, which is doubled upon itself, is expelled—*conduplicato corpore* (Fig. 422). Manifestly, such a mechanism is possible only in the case of very small children, and is occasionally observed when the second child in a twin pregnancy is prematurely born.

Also, on rare occasions, a dead child of moderate or average size may be expelled spontaneously by another mechanism, which is designated as *spontaneous evolution*. This, however, is met with so rarely, demands such peculiar conditions, and is attended by such risks to the mother that its occurrence should never be counted upon in actual practice, although very occasionally in neglected cases it may occur unexpectedly and even rapidly. Several cases have been observed in Williams' service, two of which are described in Stephenson's article; in one of them a 2,700 gm. child was born eight hours after the onset of labor. Eastman described three additional cases, and reported an incidence of spontaneous evolution, in the Johns Hopkins Hospital, of 5 in 147 consecutive cases of transverse presentation, or 3.4 per cent.

Spontaneous evolution was first mentioned by Denman in 1772; its mechanism was accurately described by Douglas, in 1811. It is generally stated that spontaneous evolution may be effected by either of two mechanisms—that of Denman or that of Douglas. The difference between the two processes seems to be that in the one the breech appears immediately after the prolapsed shoulder (the mechanism of Denman) while in the other the lateral aspect of the thorax follows the prolapsed shoulder, the breech being born after the thorax and abdomen have been delivered (the mechanism of Douglas). The two mechanisms are illustrated in Figs. 423 and 424.

In both mechanisms, the first stage consists in the molding of the fetus and impaction of the shoulder with prolapse of the arm, as described in a preceding paragraph. Then, under the influence of strong uterine contractions, the child rotates about its vertical axis, so that one side of the head comes to lie over the horizontal ramus of the pubis with the breech in the region of the opposite sacro-iliac joint, while the neck subtends the inner surface of the symphysis pubis (Fig. 423). Coincident with excessive stretching of the neck, the prolapsed arm continues to descend until eventually the corresponding shoulder emerges under the pubic arch. The escape of the arm and shoulder affords room for the entrance of the rest of the body of the child into the pelvic cavity. At this juncture in the mechanism, the crucial process takes place, namely, an extreme lateral flexion of the spinal column. This lateral flexion may occur in two directions, the breech being forced either toward or away from the prolapsed arm. If the breech is forced in the direction of the prolapsed shoulder, it is born before the lateral aspect of the thorax; while if lateral flexion takes place in the opposite direction, the breech cannot be delivered until the lateral aspect of the thorax is born (the mechanism of Douglas). Most students of the subject point out that the former mechanism, by which the breech is born before the lateral aspect of the thorax, should not be designated by the name of Denman, as that author reported only that the "breech and inferior extremities are expelled before the head." They also lean to the view that these two methods are variations of but one mechanism, an extreme lateral flexion of the spinal column, and that various gradations may exist, depending

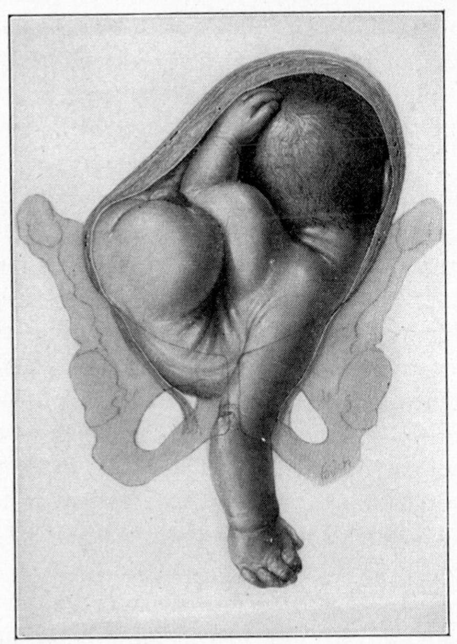

FIG. 423.—DOUGLAS' METHOD OF SPONTANEOUS EVOLUTION IN TRANSVERSE PRESENTATION.

Extreme lateral flexion of vertebral column with birth of lateral aspect of thorax before buttocks.

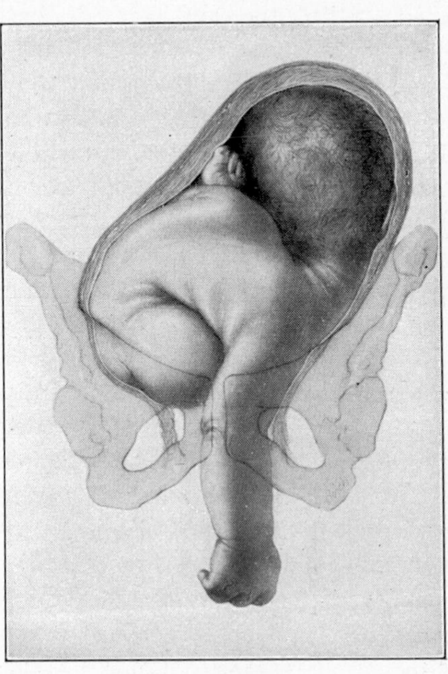

FIG. 424.—DENMAN'S METHOD OF SPONTANEOUS EVOLUTION IN TRANSVERSE PRESENTATION.

Same extreme lateral flexion of vertebral column as in Fig. 423, but in opposite direction so that buttocks are born before thorax.

upon the degree of lateral flexion. Following the breech or the side of the thorax the remaining arm is delivered, and finally the head is born spontaneously or is extracted manually, according to the exigencies of the case (Fig. 424).

In such cases the prolapsed arm is immensely swollen and a *caput succedaneum* develops over the presenting shoulder. From our studies it would appear that spontaneous evolution is possible only when the child is not unduly large and in the presence of strong uterine contractions and an unusually elastic neck. Herrgott has reported an instance in which the child weighed 3,300 gm.

Prognosis. Transverse presentations, even in competent hands, increase somewhat the maternal risk and aggravate tremendously the fetal hazard. Most maternal deaths from this complication occur in neglected cases, from spontaneous rupture of the uterus or from traumatic rupture consequent upon late and ill-advised version and extraction. Even with the best care, however, the maternal mortality will be increased to a slight but appreciable degree because of the frequent association of transverse presentation with placenta previa, because of its greater incidence in older women in whom other complications, such as hypertension and myomata, may aggravate the outlook, and because of the almost routine necessity of major operative interference.

With vaginal delivery the fetal mortality is extremely high and approximates 30 per cent. The main causes responsible for these infant deaths are prolapse of the umbilical cord, trauma in association with version and extraction, and anoxia consequent upon the tetanic state which the uterus often assumes in this presentation. The hazard for the baby increases directly with the duration of time between rupture of the membranes and delivery. If the membranes remain intact until complete dilatation and if delivery by version and extraction can be effected shortly thereafter, the prognosis for a full-term infant is relatively good for this condition, that is, less than 10 per cent mortality. Contrariwise, if the membranes rupture before the onset of labor or even at its onset, the fetal mortality soars to above 60 per cent. Since the shoulder of a baby in transverse presentation occludes the inlet very imperfectly, premature rupture of the membranes is very common, a fact which lends especial pertinence to this relationship between premature rupture of the membranes and fetal prognosis.

Treatment. Transverse presentation in a primigravida should always excite the suspicion of pelvic contraction and dictate x-ray pelvimetry. Any significant degree of pelvic contraction in a primigravida with a persistent transverse presentation constitutes an indication for elective cesarean section several days before term. Moreover, any primigravida with a normal pelvis whose baby at the onset of labor is in transverse presentation should also be delivered abdominally. This attitude toward transverse presentation in a primigravida is understandable on several grounds. The shoulder is a poor dilating wedge and, especially in a primigravida, the first stage is likely to be prolonged as well as incomplete. During this prolonged interval rupture of the membranes is very prone to occur with its threat to the baby. Moreover, version and extraction may be dangerous both to mother and infant because of incomplete cervical dilatation. In primigravidae attempts to convert the presentation to a longitudinal one by abdominal manipulation or postural therapy are rarely successful.

The management of transverse presentation of multiparae may be more elastic. Thus, attempts at external version both late in pregnancy and early in labor are occasionally rewarded by success and are worthy of trial. If, early in labor, the head can be brought into the pelvic brim by abdominal manipulation, it should be held there by a competent person for the next half dozen pains—a measure which will tend to prevent a return to the previous presentation. If this measure fails, as it often does, the management of the case will depend chiefly on the state of the membranes. Because of the extremely high fetal mortality associated with premature rupture of the membranes in this presentation, it is my feeling that any multipara with a persistent transverse presentation whose membranes rupture before the cervix is 4 cm. dilated is best delivered by cesarean section. If the membranes rupture after the cervix is 4 cm. dilated, labor should usually be allowed to continue until full dilatation, at which time version and extraction is performed. Because of the transcendent importance of intact membranes, various procedures have been recommended to maintain their integrity—especially a vaginal bag to exert counterpressure against any bulging bag of forewaters. I have tried this but have found it too painful to be practical. In cases in which the membranes rupture before complete dilatation, it has also been recommended that an intra-uterine bag be inserted to expedite cervical dilatation and prevent prolapse of the cord. This may occasionally prove desirable, especially if dilatation is slow, but it carries with it the drawback that the necessary manipulations may actually cause prolapse of the cord. The management of prolapse of the cord will be discussed in a subsequent section of this chapter.

In the hours succeeding rupture of the membranes in transverse presentations, the uterus retracts down more and more on the fetus; the shoulder becomes more and more impacted in the pelvis; and the lower uterine segment becomes thinner and thinner. Sooner or later an arm usually prolapses into the vagina, and meanwhile, intra-uterine infection develops. This state of affairs is referred to as a *neglected transverse presentation*. The first step in the management of such cases is the administration of a massive dose of penicillin or aureomycin followed by intravenous glucose. Since operative procedures in these depleted patients often provoke shock, blood for transfusion should be made available. In advanced degrees of neglected transverse presentations, the baby is usually dead, and decapitation by means of the sharp hook or sickle knife comprises the operative management (Fig. 659). Because of the thinned-out lower uterine segment and the consequent danger of uterine rupture imposed by the operation such cases should never be treated by version and extraction. If the baby is alive, the problem is indeed a grave one. As a rule, the best treatment is either extraperitoneal cesarean section or cesarean hysterectomy preceded and followed by chemotherapy. If the patient has three or more children, the latter is probably the preferable operation in most hands.

Compound Presentations. By this term is understood the prolapse of an extremity alongside of the presenting part, both entering the pelvic canal simultaneously. In a study of compound presentation carried out by Goplerud in our clinic, it was found that in the course of 42,410 viable deliveries 55 cases occurred in which a hand or arm had prolapsed alongside the vertex, an incidence of once in every 744 deliveries. Much less common is prolapse of one or more lower extremities alongside a vertex presentation, only 6 cases having been observed in the above series, or one in 7,068 deliveries. In addition to these 61 cases, there were 4 cases in which a hand prolapsed alongside a breech presentation. Compound presentations are frequently accompanied by prolapse of the umbilical cord, and whether or not this accident occurs is the determining factor in fetal outlook. The cord prolapsed in 15 of the 65 cases just enumerated, or in almost one quarter.

As might be expected, the predisposing causes of compound presentation are those conditions which prevent complete filling and occlusion of the pelvic inlet by the presenting part, to wit, multiparity (through lax abdominal walls and a high head), pelvic contraction, and small infants. In the series cited above, premature infants were encountered twice as frequently as would ordinarily be expected. In many cases, however, no cause is demonstrable.

In most cases the prolapsed part should be left alone since it will rarely interfere with labor. Thus, in Goplerud's series of 50 cases not associated with prolapse of the cord, 24, or approximately one half, had no treatment; normal delivery ensued in all with the loss of but one infant. If the entire arm is prolapsed alongside the head, replacement may become necessary. Under such circumstances, the condition should be observed closely to ascertain whether the arm rises out of the way with descent of the presenting part, as will sometimes occur. If it does not, and if it appears to be preventing descent of the head, the prolapsed arm should be pushed upward and simultaneously the head should be pushed downward by fundal pressure. In the absence of prolapse of the cord, the fetal mortality is not elevated in compound presentation, being 3.2 per cent in Goplerud's cases in which the infant was mature. With prolapse of the cord, the fetal mortality rate as well as the treatment is the same as in that accident.

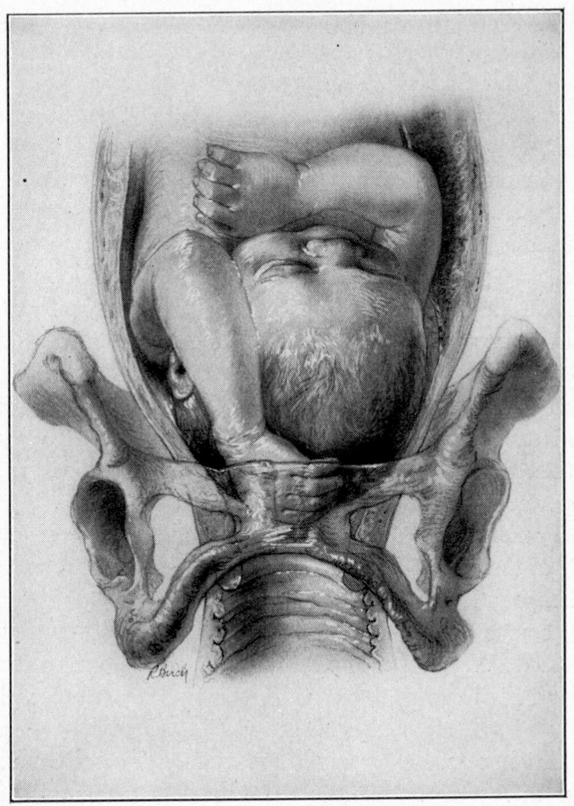

Fig. 425.—Compound Presentation.

ABNORMALITIES OF DEVELOPMENT

Excessive Development. As stated previously, the child at birth rarely exceeds 11 pounds (5,000 gm.) in weight, although authentic accounts of much larger infants are to be found in the literature.

Provided the pelvis is not contracted, it is very exceptional for a normally formed child weighing less than 10 pounds (4,500 gm.) to give rise to dystocia by its mere size. In overdeveloped children the difficulty is generally due to the fact that the head tends to become not only larger but harder and, consequently, less malleable with increasing weight. However, it sometimes happens that, after the head has passed through the pelvic canal without difficulty, the dystocia may be due to the arrest of the unusually large shoulders either at the pelvic brim or outlet.

Excessive development of the fetus can usually be traced to one of three causes: large size of one or both parents, multiparity, or diabetes in the mother.

Koff and Potter, in a study of 20,219 births, found that 0.94 per cent of the infants weighed more than 4,500 gm. and that in the mothers of these excessive-sized children the duration of pregnancy, calculated from the first day of the last menstrual period, averaged 288 days, or only eight days more than the average. This, as well as other studies, indicates that so-called "post-maturity" is not an important cause of excessive size in the infant, and per se calls for no treatment. It is our practice to designate all newborn infants weighing 4,000 gm. or more as "excessive-sized" and the incidence of these in 31,932 deliveries was 11.9 per cent, while the incidence of children weighing 4,500 gm. or more was 1.6 per cent.

The question sometimes arises as to whether excessive size of the child may be due to overeating on the part of the mother. Slemons and Fagin, in a study of the infant's birth weight and the mother's gain during gestation, concluded that, although diet control does not serve to determine precisely the size of the fetus, it does help to prevent its overgrowth. What apparently cannot be influenced by the mother's diet is the size of the fetal head, as expressed by the biparietal diameter. Although we are unable to control head size, and can, perhaps, only partly influence the body weight of the offspring, diet control during pregnancy is one of the most important factors in adequate antenatal care.

Although, in the case of a normal pelvis, a moderate increase in the size of the child is usually without practical significance, when any degree of contraction exists such a condition may make all the difference between an easy and a very difficult labor. At the same time, in multiparous women the dystocia is often due, in great part, to the loss of tone of the uterine musculature incident to repeated childbearing. On the other hand, it should always be remembered that quite as serious dystocia may arise when an excessively large head attempts to pass through a normal pelvis, as when a head of average size is arrested by a definitely contracted superior strait.

Inasmuch as our means of determining the size of the child, and particularly of its head, are at times still inaccurate, the diagnosis of excessive development is often not established until after fruitless attempts at delivery have been made. Nevertheless, thorough examination in which careful palpation, Müller's method of impression, and roentgenologic cephalometry, if available, are employed, should ordinarily enable the trained obstetrician to arrive at fairly accurate conclusions and prepare him to meet this complication.

Treatment. In multiparous women with normal pelves whose history shows that excessive fetal development was the cause of the previous difficult labors, the size of the child may very occasionally be regulated by restricting the diet during the last two months of pregnancy, although, in general, it has been our experience that regulation of the mother's diet produces little or no effect upon the size of her offspring. If the fetus of a diabetic mother is obviously large in the last three weeks of pregnancy, cesarean section is usually indicated.

Malformations of the Fetus. *Double Monsters.* For practical purposes three groups of double monsters may be distinguished: (1) Incomplete double formations at the upper or lower half of the body (*diprosopus, dipagus*); (2) twins which are united together at the upper or lower end of the body (*craniopagus, ischiopagus,* or *pygopagus*); and (3) double monsters which are united by the trunk (*thoracopagus* and *dicephalus*).

Although the existence of a multiple pregnancy may have been suspected, the diagnosis of any one of these conditions is rarely made until difficulty experienced in attempting delivery has led to careful exploration, under anesthesia, with the entire hand in utero. As such monstrosities frequently present minor deformities as well, the detection of a clubfoot, harelip, etc. should direct one's attention to the possible existence of some still more serious abnormality.

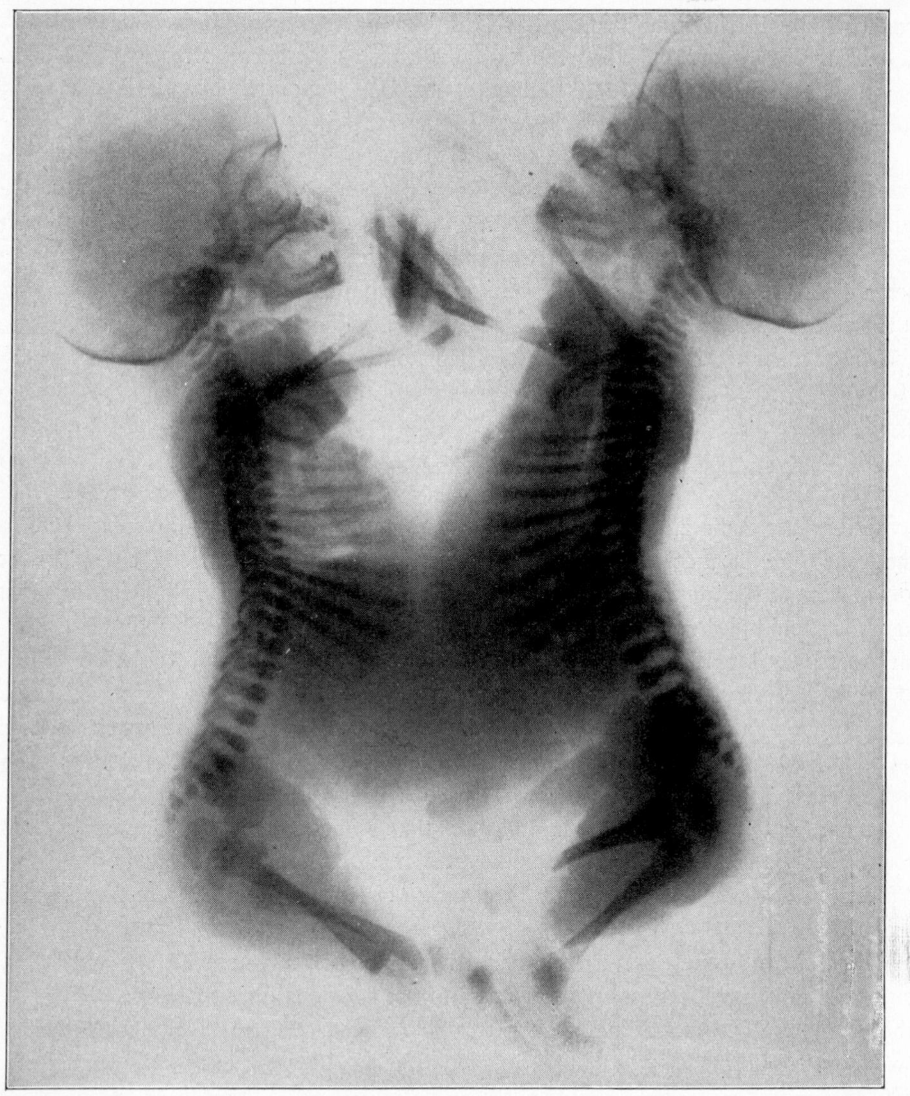

Fig. 426.—Roentgenogram of Thoracopagus Monster.

(From Shaw, Brumbaugh and Novey, *American Journal of Obstetrics and Gynecology.*)

Fortunately, the delivery of many monstrosities is sometimes much more readily accomplished than would appear possible at first sight. In the first place, such pregnancies rarely go on to full term, so that the monstrosity may not exceed a normal child in size. In the second place, the connection between the two halves is often of such a character as to permit of sufficient motility between the component parts as will make their successive delivery possible.

On the other hand, in the first group the large size of the doubled portion of the monster may lead to serious mechanical obstacles. The fused head in a *diprosopus* is, as a rule, much more readily delivered when it forms the aftercoming part than when it presents primarily. In the second group a *craniopagus* presenting by the head usually causes only a moderate amount of difficulty; whereas *ischiopagi* and *pygopagi,* as a rule, call for complicated and difficult maneuvers before delivery can be effected.

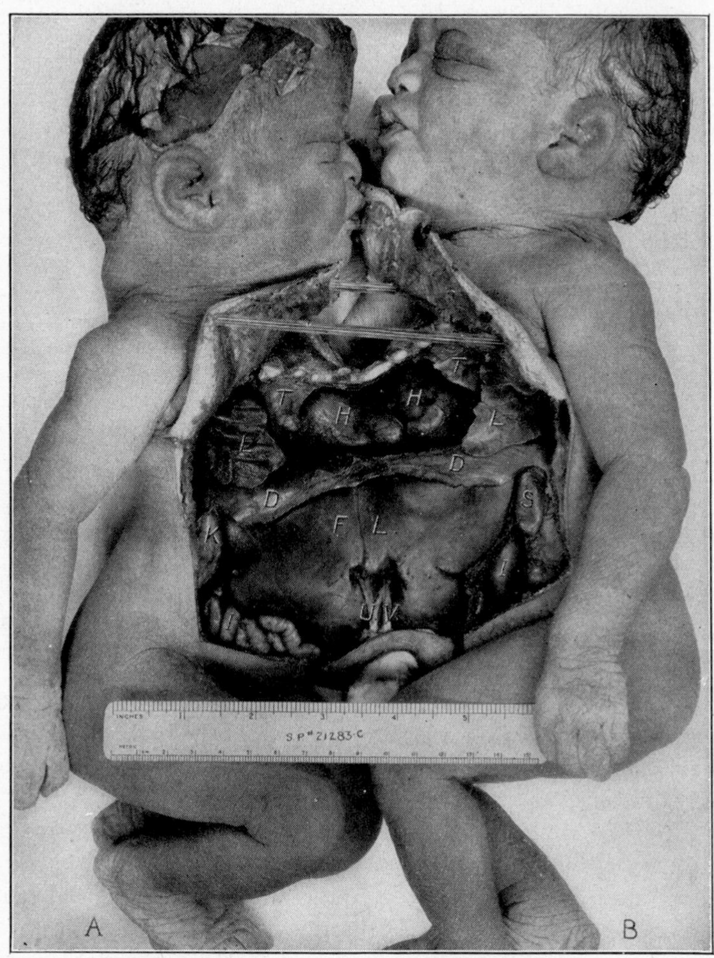

FIG. 427.—DISSECTION IN SITU OF MONSTER SHOWN IN FIG. 426.

The conjoined heart (*H*), lungs (*L*), and the thymus glands (*T*) lie above the common diaphragm (*D*). The fused liver (*F.L.*), a portion of intestine (*I*), the right kidney (*K*) of Twin A and the spleen (*S*) of Twin B are seen lying in the peritoneal cavity. The umbilical veins (*U.V.*) enter the anterior surface of the liver. (From Shaw, Brumbaugh and Novey, *American Journal of Obstetrics and Gynecology.*)

In the third group, the delivery of *dicephalic* monsters is facilitated when they present by the breech, as in many cases first one, and then the other head can be extracted. On the other hand, in cephalic presentations the two heads may mutually interfere with each other and thus prevent engagement until one has been diminished in size by craniotomy. When engagement of one head occurs, delivery can be partially effected by forceps, but as a rule the head cannot be delivered beyond the pubic arch for the reason that further descent is prevented by the arrest of the second head at the superior strait. Under such circumstances, it is advisable to amputate the first head, after which delivery of the rest of the monster is, as a rule, best accomplished by version, unless the uterus is too firmly contracted and there exists danger of rupture of the organ.

Thoracopagi usually offer a less serious obstacle to delivery, for the reason that they are frequently so loosely connected with one another that considerable motility is possible. Indeed, it is not unusual for the two children to present in a different manner. When possible, it is advisable to bring down all four feet at the same time and to effect extraction in such a way that the posterior head is first delivered. In cephalic presentations the head and the body of the first child are expelled, and the second child is then born very much as in an ordinary twin pregnancy. If, however, the latter presents transversely, its delivery can be effected only by version and extraction.

Other Deformities of the Fetus. In this place attention will be directed only to those abnormalities in fetal development which may give rise to difficult labor; other deformities that do not produce dystocia have been discussed in a later section. An *acardiacus* is a monster which is sometimes developed in single-ovum twin pregnancies as the result of inequalities in the communicating placental circulation. One twin is well developed and normal, while the other is imperfectly formed and possesses either a rudimentary heart or no heart at all, being designated as hemiacardius or holoacardius, respectively.

The holoacardiac monsters may occur as acephali, amorphi, or acormi. Of these the most common variety is the *acephalicus* or headless fetus. Less common is the *amorphus* monster, which possesses neither a head nor extremities but is round in shape and presents upon its surface a number of small nodules, which represent the rudimentary extremities. The umbilical cord may be attached to any portion of its surface. The interior of the monstrosity contains a rudimentary intestinal tract, cystic cavities, vertebrae, etc., but no trace of a heart. The rarest variety of acardiacus is the *acormus* or trunkless monster which consists of an imperfectly developed head and a rudimentary body, the umbilical cord being attached to the cervical region.

As a rule, such monsters do not attain any notable size, although exceptionally, as the result of obstruction in the umbilical vein, they may become edematous and give rise to dystocia.

The *anencephalus* or *hemicephalus* is a monster possessing a trunk, but only an imperfectly developed head, from which a large part of the brain and skull is lacking. Ordinarily such beings are of moderate size, but occasionally the shoulders may be so excessively developed as to give rise to serious dystocia.

Since the time of Morgagni it has been known that more than three quarters of such monsters are females. It is generally stated that the adrenals are lacking. Kratsch, however, found them in all of the 17 specimens which he studied, but much smaller than usual, particularly in the cortical portion.

Owing to the absence of the cranial vault the face is very prominent and somewhat extended; the eyes often protrude markedly from their sockets, and the tongue hangs from the mouth. The brain is in a rudimentary condition, and the base of the skull is accessible to the examining finger, so that the sella turcica can be distinguished. Owing to the exposed condition of the base of the brain and the upper part of the medulla, there is frequently a marked increase in the amount of amniotic fluid, its production being analogous to that noted in the piqûre experiments of the physiologists.

In view of the abnormal shape of the head, face presentations are frequently observed, while those of the vertex are less common than with a normal fetus. Other abnormal presentations, particularly transverse and foot, are likewise not unusual.

When the monstrosity presents by the face or head a correct diagnosis is frequently made by vaginal touch, the characteristic bulging of the eyes being noted in the face, and the absence of the cranial vault and the presence of the sella turcica in the head presentation. As the deformity is frequently accompanied by hydramnios, the occurrence of that condition should arouse suspicion as to the possibility of fetal abnormalities. In such cases, x-ray examination frequently leads to the recognition of anencephalic, hydrocephalic, or dicephalic children. (See Figs. 428, 535 and 536.)

Delivery, as a rule, occurs much more readily when the monster presents by the breech, for the reason that the imperfectly developed head is not an efficient dilating agent, though in many cases rapid and spontaneous delivery is observed. Even when the enlarged shoulders give rise to dystocia, delivery can usually be accomplished by means of version without any great difficulty.

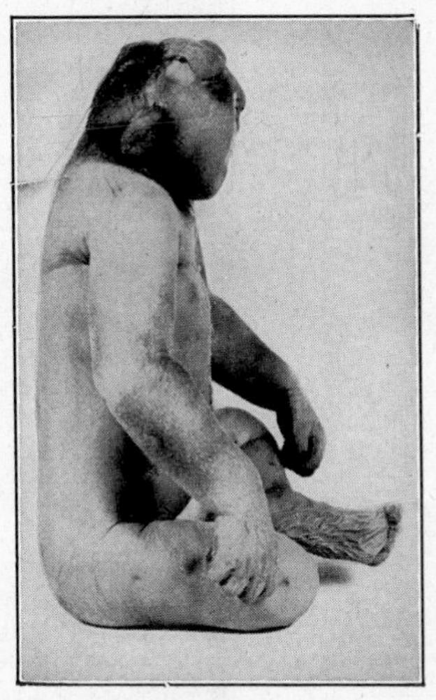

Fig. 428.—Anencephalic Monster. × ¼.

Note protruding eyes and relatively long arms which usually accompany this deformity.

Hydrocephalus. *Hydrocephalus internus*, or an excessive accumulation of cerebrospinal fluid in the ventricles of the brain, with consequent enlargement of the cranium, is encountered in one fetus in 2,000, approximately, and accounts for some 12 per cent of all malformations met at birth. Associated defects are common, spina bifida being present in about one third of the cases. Varying degrees of cranial enlargement are produced and not infrequently the circumference of the head exceeds 50 cm., sometimes reaching 80 cm. The amount of fluid present is usually between 500 and 1,500 cc., but as much as 5 liters has been reported. Since the distended cranium is too large to fit into the pelvic brim, breech presentations are exceedingly common, being observed in about one third of such cases. Whatever the presentation, gross disproportion between the size of the head and that of the pelvis is the rule and serious dystocia the usual consequence.

Diagnosis. Since the treatment of this complication of labor, once recognized, is clear-cut and simple, early diagnosis is all-important and upon it may rest the life of the mother. In this condition more than any other, possibly, an empty bladder facilitates both abdominal and vaginal examination; catheterization, therefore, is a desirable preliminary to examination in any suspected case. In vertex presentations, abdominal palpation reveals a broad, hard tumor high about the symphysis; the thickness of the abdominal walls usually prevents detection of the thin, elastic, parchment-like consistency of the hydrocephalic cranium. The high-riding head forces the body of the infant upward, so that the fetal heart is often heard loudest above the umbilicus, a circumstance which not infrequently leads to the suspicion of a breech. As labor advances the lower uterine segment becomes rigid and tender. Rectal examination reveals an empty pelvic cavity. Vaginally, the broad dome of the head conveys the impression of tenseness to the examining fingers, but more careful palpation will reveal the wide fontanels, the stretched suture lines, and the indentable, egg-shell craniotabes of hydrocephalus. It is occasionally necessary to introduce the entire hand into the uterus to make sure of the diagnosis, but if this is done, the utmost care must be exercised not to overstretch the already distended, lower uterine segment. In vertex presentations (but not in breech), the x-ray provides invaluable confirmatory evidence, showing a large, globular head with a cranial outline so thin that it is sometimes scarcely visible.

In breech presentations, the diagnosis is usually overlooked until it is found that the head cannot be extracted. X-ray outlines of the head when the baby lies in breech position are misleading unless steps are taken to correct distortion; indeed, in ordinary flat plates, the normal head in the upper pole of the uterus may appear huge and, as shown by Dippel, grave errors have resulted. The mistake may be avoided by using

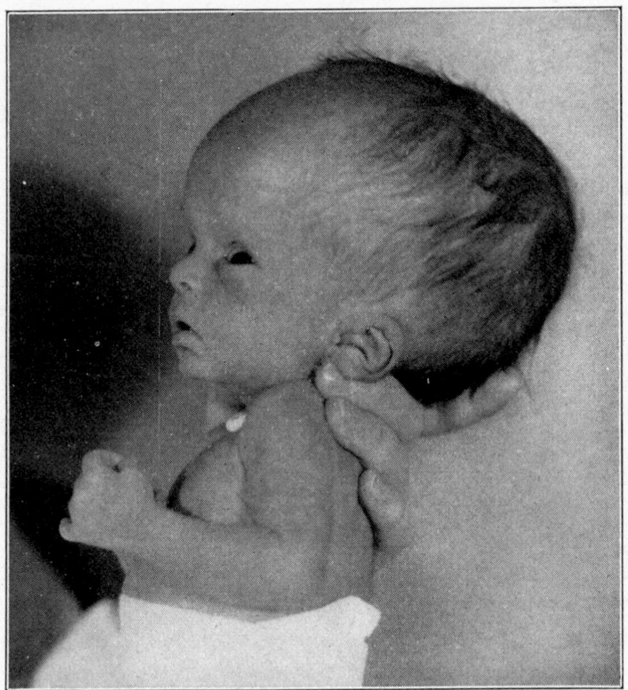

FIG. 429.—HYDROCEPHALUS OF NEWBORN CHILD.

"precision" methods of encephalometry, or by neglecting altogether the size of the cranial shadow and paying attention to the following criteria: (1) the face of the hydrocephalic infant is very small in relation to the large head. (2) the hydrocephalic cranium tends to be globular in shape, whereas the normal head is ovoid. (3) the shadow of the hydrocephalic cranium is often so thin that it may scarcely be visible.

Failure to recognize dystocia from fetal hydrocephalus is more often the result of negligence than of ignorance. It will rarely be missed if the obstetrician *will but think of the possibility whenever*: (1) the head remains high, despite a normal pelvis and good pains; (2) a floating head feels unusually broad; and (3) spina bifida is encountered as the trunk of a breech is being extracted.

Prognosis. Rupture of the uterus is the great danger and is the outcome of almost all untreated cases. Among 73 examples of the condition collected by Schuchard, there were 14 ruptures, an incidence of 19 per cent; eight were spontaneous and six were caused by attempted forceps operations; 12 of the mothers died. The hydrocephalic head predisposes to rupture, not only because of the disproportion produced, but also because the great transverse diameter of the cranium overdistends the lower uterine segment. Rupture not infrequently occurs before complete dilatation of the cervix is reached, and in one of the author's cases it was clearly imminent when the cervix was only 7 cm. in diameter. Because fetal hydrocephalus is frequently overlooked, with consequent rupture of the uterus, the mortality has been lamentably high. Kleinhaus' collected statistics on 254 cases show 46 maternal deaths, a mortality rate of 18 per cent.

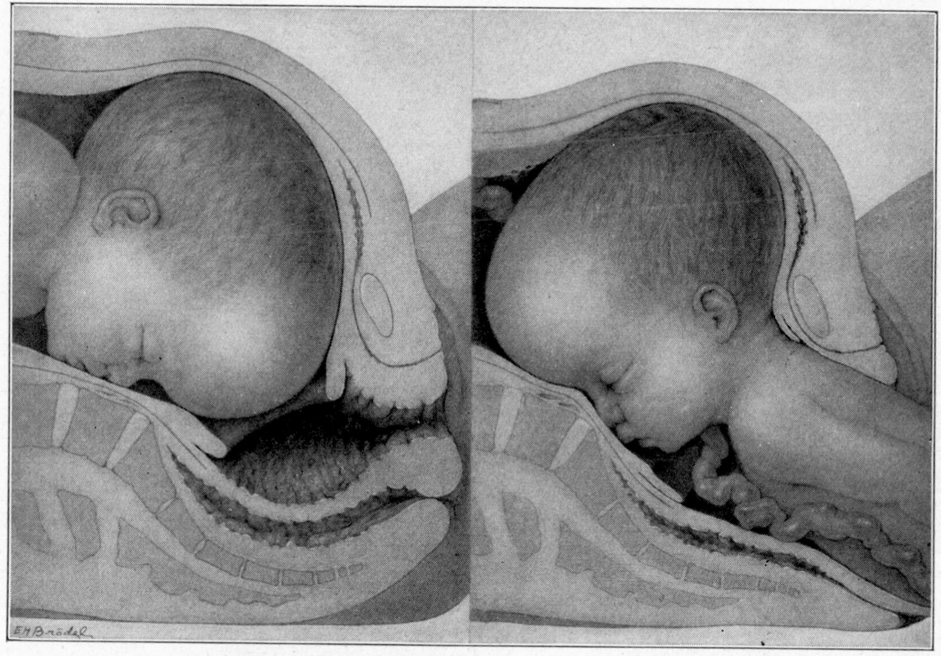

FIG. 430A. FIG. 430B.

FIG. 430A.—HYDROCEPHALUS CAUSING DYSTOCIA IN VERTEX PRESENTATION.

FIG. 430B.—HYDROCEPHALUS CAUSING DYSTOCIA IN AFTERCOMING HEAD OF BREECH PRESENTATION.

Rare cases are on record in which the force of the uterine contractions caused the hydrocephalic head to burst, with the result that spontaneous delivery ensued. Almost always, however, it is the uterus rather than the cranial sac, which ruptures. Minor degrees of hydrocephalus may cause no dystocia, but these are mostly incipient cases in which the diagnosis is not completely established until some days after birth.

Treatment. The progress of labor should be followed with utmost care, having in mind the possibility of rupture of the uterus. In clear-cut examples of this disorder, perforation should always be performed as soon as the cervix is completely dilated, but occasionally signs of threatened rupture may appear at 6 or 8 cm. dilatation and necessitate carrying out the procedure at this time or puncturing the head with a spinal-puncture needle. In such event no attempt should be made to deliver the baby immediately after the perforation, but labor should be allowed to proceed as usual; if actual perforation of the head has been performed with Smellie scissors the subsequent course may often be expedited if the collapsed cranial walls be grasped by a

Jacobs' clamp or two and gentle traction exerted by means of a one-pound weight attached by a tape to the forceps and hung over the foot of the bed. The cranioclast should not be used because of the danger of injuring the thin lower segment with such a heavy instrument. For the same reason, version is contraindicated.

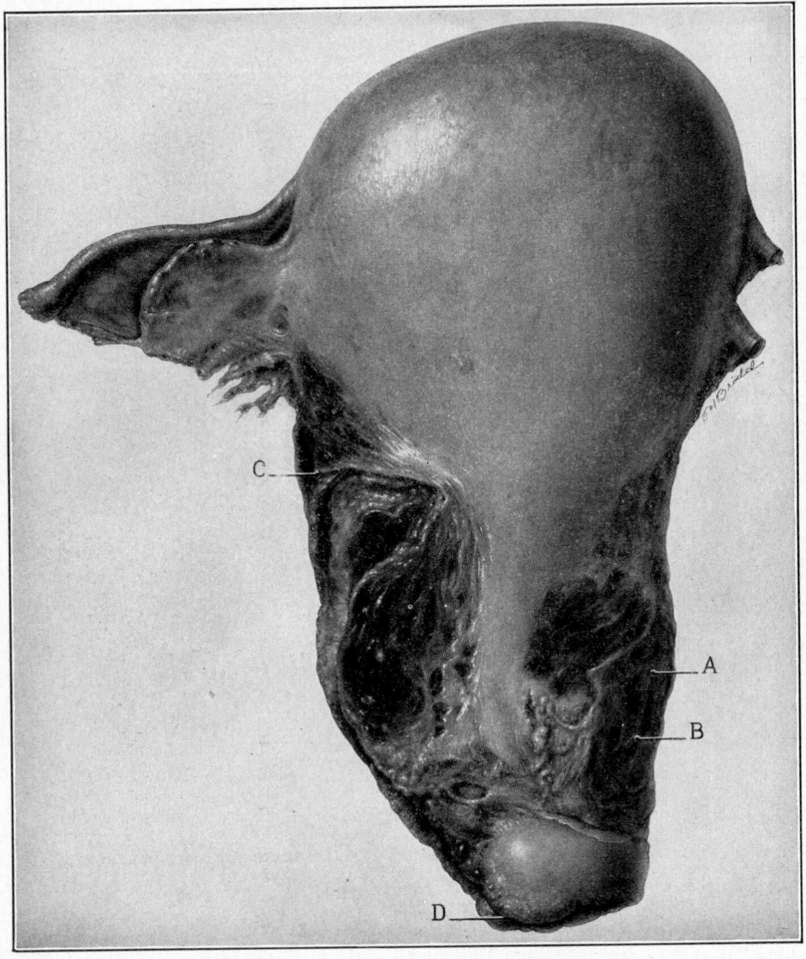

FIG. 431.—RUPTURE OF UTERUS CAUSED BY HYDROCEPHALIC HEAD.
Right tear *A-B* is 3 cm. long; left tear *C-D* extends through cervix into vagina.

Although the older writers recommended puncturing the hydrocephalic head with a trocar, the Smellie scissors would seem to be preferable, because they are better adapted to destroying the medulla, a procedure which should always follow the perforation. In vertex presentations perforation should be done through a fontanel or suture line; and on the aftercoming head, through a point behind the ear. (For technic of craniotomy, see page 1126.)

Enlargement of the Body of the Fetus. Enlargement of the abdomen sufficient to cause grave dystocia is usually the result of ascites, a very much distended bladder, or of tumors of the kidneys or liver.

Whenever the abdominal distention is excessive, spontaneous labor is out of the question, but, unfortunately, the condition usually escapes detection until fruitless attempts at delivery have demonstrated the existence of some obstruction and have led the obstetrician to introduce his entire hand into the uterus in the hope of discovering its nature.

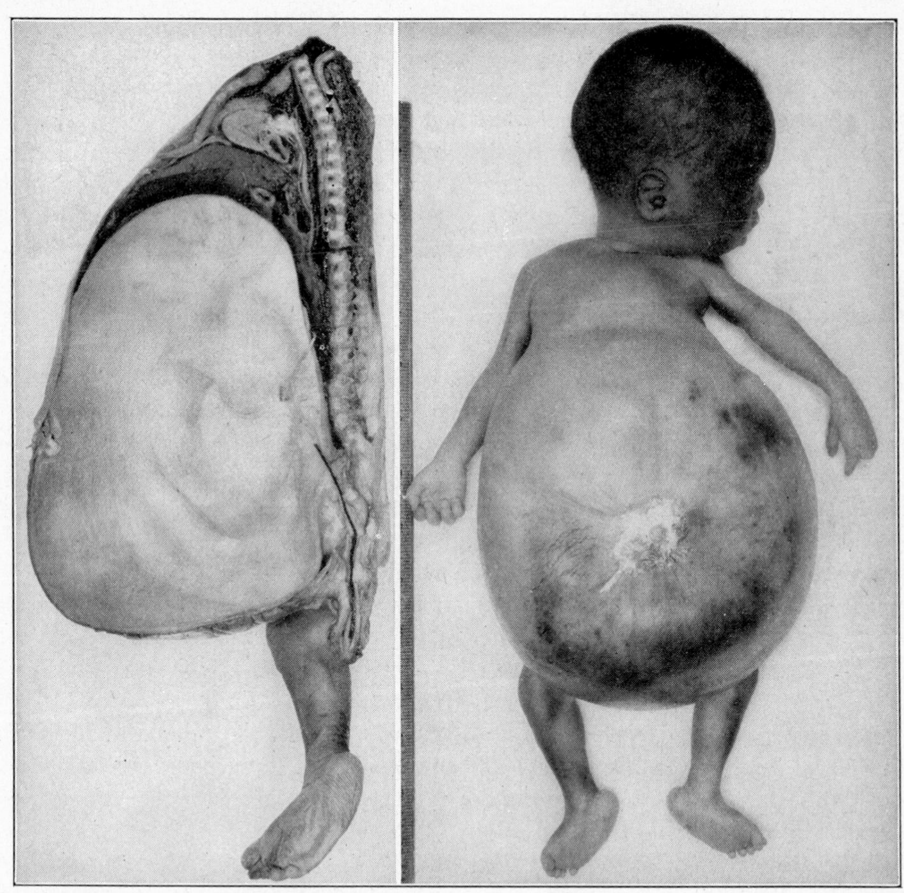

FIG. 432.—TWENTY-EIGHT WEEKS' FETUS WITH IMMENSELY DISTENDED BLADDER.

Delivery made possible by expression of fluid from bladder through perforation at umbilicus. Median sagittal section shows interior of bladder and compression of organs of abdominal and thoracic cavities. A black thread has been laid in the urethra. (From Savage, *American Journal of Obstetrics and Gynecology.*)

Occasionally a fetus affected with *general dropsy* may attain such immense proportions that spontaneous delivery is impossible. A number of such cases are recorded in the monographs of Ballantyne, Schumann, and Dorland. In very rare instances a child suffering from *chondrodystrophia foetalis* may become so edematous as to give rise to dystocia.

As the result of the dilatation of the superficial lymphatics associated with edema of the subcutaneous tissues, the fetus may assume immense proportions and take on a bizarre shape. This condition, which is designated as *elephantiasis congenita cystica,* has been studied in detail by Ballantyne and is a very rare cause of difficult labor.

Defective development of the lower portion of the urinary tract may lead to the *retention of urine* accompanied by distention of the abdomen sufficient to render normal delivery impossible (Fig. 432).

A more frequent cause of abdominal enlargement is the presence of *congenital cystic kidneys*. The growth, which is histologically an adenocystoma, may involve one or both organs and give rise to tumors of immense size. The condition is frequently associated with dilatation of the ureters and with dropsical effusions into the various body cavities. Congenital cystic kidneys may cause great abdominal enlargement as in a child which Williams delivered and which was described by Lynch, in 1906, together with an analysis of 50 other cases reported in the literature.

In rare cases the abdominal enlargement may be due to *tumors of the liver,* Porak and Couvelaire having reported a case of congenital cystic liver associated with a similar condition of the kidneys. Moreover, large tumors, arising from any of the abdominal organs, may give rise to dystocia. Occasionally, the invasion by *Bacillus aerogenes capsulatus* may be followed by such an extensive production of gas that the size of the fetus becomes more than doubled and spontaneous delivery is impossible.

In all of these conditions, if the dystocia is marked, delivery can be accomplished only after opening the body of the fetus and allowing the fluid to escape, or removing a portion, at least, of the offending tumor formation. The latter operation is not always easy, for, owing to the constrained position of the hand in utero and the dense consistency of the growth in many cases, great difficulty may be experienced.

In rare instances abnormal growths arising from various portions of the body of the fetus may interfere with delivery. Cases are on record in which lipomata, carcinomata, angiomata, and various other tumors have given rise to such an enlargement.

PROLAPSE OF THE UMBILICAL CORD

It is customary to distinguish between *presentation* of and *prolapse* of the funis or umbilical cord. In the former the cord can be palpated through the cervical canal, while in the latter a loop of it protrudes through the cervix into the vagina, and exceptionally emerges from the vulva.

In general it may be said that any factor which interferes with the accurate adaptation of the presenting part to the superior strait predisposes to prolapse of the cord. Accordingly, the accident occurs most commonly in transverse and foot, and less often in frank breech presentations. On the other hand, it is rarely observed when the child presents by the head, unless accommodation is interfered with as a result of contracted pelvis, excessive development of the fetus, hydramnios, or abnormal flaccidity of the lower uterine segment. For this reason, it is much more common in multiparous than in primigravidous women. Mengert and Longwell found the incidence of prolapse of the cord to be 0.37 per cent in cephalic, 4.54 per cent in breech and 14.27 per cent in transverse presentations.

Prolapse of the cord is without appreciable effect upon the course of labor so far as the mother is concerned. On the other hand, it is one of the frequent causes of fetal death, compression between the presenting part and the pelvic wall interfering with the circulation to such an extent that asphyxia and inevitable death often follow unless prompt delivery is effected. The danger is greater in vertex than in other presentations, for the reason that there is more likelihood that the cord will be compressed when the pelvic canal is filled out by the hard, rounded head than by the softer and more irregularly shaped part in breech and other presentations.

Presentation of the funis is diagnosed whenever on palpation a soft, pulsating, cord-like body can be felt through the cervix. In many instances, however, its recognition is only possible when the cord is in direct contact with the presenting part.

Prolapse of the cord, on the other hand, is readily recognizable, since on vaginal or rectal examination the fingers come directly in contact with a loop, while exceptionally it may be seen protruding from the vulva. In the latter event, the condition is self-evident, while in the former, mistakes are hardly possible, provided the fetus

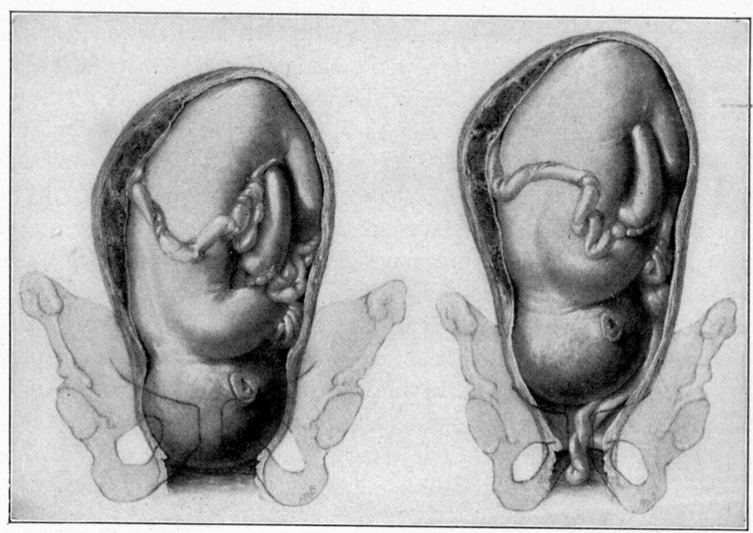

FIG. 433.—AN ENGAGED HEAD (LEFT), BY FILLING PELVIC CAVITY, PREVENTS PROLAPSE OF CORD. AN UNENGAGED HEAD (RIGHT), AS IN CASE OF CONTRACTED PELVIS, SHOWN HERE, TENDS TO FAVOR PROLAPSE OF CORD AFTER RUPTURE OF MEMBRANES.

is alive, as distinct pulsations are felt, although in their absence the condition is sometimes overlooked on superficial examination.

The possibility of prolapse of the cord should be particularly borne in mind in otherwise normal, multiparous women in whom the membranes rupture while the head is still freely movable above the superior strait. In such cases, the sudden cessation of the fetal heart beat renders the diagnosis almost certain, even without vaginal examination.

Treatment. The treatment to be pursued in any given case depends mainly upon the degree to which the cervix is dilated, and to a lesser extent upon the presentation of the child. In all instances, the head of the table should be lowered in order to relieve or minimize the pressure of the presenting part upon the cord and thus prevent, insofar as possible, the danger from impaired circulation to the child. In cases of presentation of the funis there is no immediate danger of compression so long as the membranes remain intact, and every precaution should be taken to avoid their premature rupture, vaginal examinations being made with the utmost gentleness. Furthermore, the obstetrician should hold himself in readiness to effect delivery as soon as the cervix is sufficiently dilated.

In the absence of serious disproportion, if the cord prolapses under the observation of the obstetrician after the cervix has become fully dilated, the life of the child can usually be saved. No attempt at reposition should be made, but delivery should be effected at once. In cephalic and transverse presentations, version is usually the operation of choice, but forceps are indicated when the head is already deep down in the pelvic canal. In frank breech presentations, a foot, or preferably both feet, should be brought down and extraction promptly completed. Undue haste in delivery must be avoided, as it is often attended by irreparable harm to the child.

On the other hand, when the cervix is only partially dilated, the chances of a favorable outcome for the child are greatly diminished. Should the cervix be soft and sufficiently dilated to admit the operator's hand, manual dilatation may sometimes be readily effected without undue injury. In instances where this cannot be accomplished, due to the condition of the cervix, Dührssen's incisions may at times be indicated. In either case, prompt delivery of the child, by the methods described in the preceding paragraph, must be effected. On the other hand, if the condition of the cervix precludes manual dilatation, the chances for the child are poor unless cesarean section is promptly done. In a few of these patients, particularly elderly primigravidae and those in whom a subsequent pregnancy appears undesirable, cesarean section is indicated when the cord has prolapsed early in labor and no contraindication to the operation exists. When the cord is still within the vagina, a vaginal instillation of an antiseptic solution, such as 1 per cent acriflavine in glycerine, should precede the section. In addition, should the cord be outside the vulva, its prolapsed portion should be cleansed with a mild antiseptic solution and placed within the vagina which in turn contains, as indicated, acriflavine. The danger of pulling such a cord through the uterus has been greatly exaggerated. While preparations are being made for cesarean section, the finger of an attendant should be kept in the vagina to support the head and keep it from pressing against the cord. When cesarean section is deemed inadvisable in these cases, the only hope lies in replacing the cord, and retaining it in place until the cervix dilates. If the cord has prolapsed to the extent of being outside the vulva it must be cleansed before reposition is attempted. If the presenting part is not deeply engaged, the head of the table is lowered, the entire hand introduced into the vagina, and an attempt made to push the cord up into the uterus and, if possible, to carry it over some projecting portion of the child's body. If the cord remains in place the patient should be made to lie upon the side toward which the child's back is directed in the hope of avoiding compression, and all danger is past if the head engages.

In the majority of cases, however, the prolapse recurs as soon as the hand is removed. In such circumstances an improvised repositor will sometimes serve in good stead, although the results attending its use are usually unsatisfactory. A piece of ribbon or tape is firmly attached to the free end of a sterile bougie in such a manner as to leave a loop several inches long. This is then passed around the prolapsed cord and slipped over the tip of the bougie. By this means the cord can be carried up into the uterus, after which it may be freed from the repositor by bringing the loop in contact with a portion of the child and making traction so as to cause the loop to slip off from the tip of the bougie. Unfortunately, the condition usually recurs as soon as the repositor is removed; to insure against such an accident the bougie may be left in the uterus, but even this is only a forlorn hope. Various cord repositors have been devised from time to time, such as Schoeller's, Poullet's, and Braun's, to mention only a few. With the majority of these we have had no experience, although most of them utilize the principle of reposition described above. The determining factor in the outcome is not the type of repositor, but rather the condition and dilatation of the cervix, the presenting part and the extent of its descent into the pelvis and the judgment and skill of the obstetrician.

If the pulsations in the cord are weak or have ceased altogether, no attempt at reposition should be made, inasmuch as the child has either already perished or will die before delivery can be effected. If, however, the cervix is fully dilated, such limitations do not hold good, as occasionally a child that is apparently hopelessly lost may be rescued by immediate delivery. On the other hand, if cesarean section is considered, no time should be lost in attempting such maneuvers, but immediate preparations for operation should be made. After their completion, the child's heart should be listened to, and the operation proceeded with only when its sounds are strong and regular, as it is unjustifiable to subject the mother to an added risk and then to deliver a dead child. Furthermore, it should always be remembered that such interference is justifiable only in hospital practice, and then only when clearly indicated.

BIBLIOGRAPHY

Ahlfeld, F. Die Entstehung von Stirnund Gesichtslagen. Leipzig, 1873.

Ballantyne, J. W. General Foetal Elephantiasis. The Diseases of the Foetus. Edinburgh, 1892, Vol. I, pp. 182-219.

Boer, J. L. Sieben Bücher über natürliche Geburtshülfe. Vienna, 1834.

Brakeman, O. Haltung und Konfiguration des Kindliche Kopfes bei der Beckenendlage. Ztschr. f. Geburtsh. u. Gynäk., 1936, 112:154.

Caldwell, W. E., and Studdiford, W. E. A Review of Breech Deliveries during a Five Year Period at the Sloane Hospital for Women. Am. J. Obst. & Gynec., 1929, 18:623.

Calkins, L. A. Occiput Posterior. Am. J. Obst. & Gynec., 1939, 38:993.

——— Occiput Posterior—A Normal Presentation. Am. J. Obst. & Gynec., 1942, 43:277.

Capon, N. B. Intracranial Traumata in the Newborn. J. Obst. & Gynaec. Brit. Emp., 1922, 29:572.

Crothers, B., and Putnam, M. C. Obstetrical Injuries of the Spinal Cord. Medicine, 1927, 6:41.

Denman, T. Observations to Prove that in Cases Where the Upper Extremities Present, at the Time of Birth, the Delivery May Be Effected by the Spontaneous Evolution of the Child. London M. J., 1785, 5:64 and 301.

Dippel, A. L. Errors in Diagnosis of Hydrocephalus in the Breech Presentation. Am. J. Obst. & Gynec., 1939, 38:1047.

Dorland, W. A. Watery Accumulations in the Fetal Abdomen Obstructing Labor. Am. J. Obst., 1919, 79:474.

Douglas, J. C. An Explanation of the Real Process of the "Spontaneous Evolution of the Foetus." 2nd Ed. Dublin, 1819.

Duncan, M. On the Production of Presentation of the Face. Mechanism of Natural and Morbid Parturition. Edinburgh, 1875, pp. 218-231.

Eastman, N. J. Transverse Presentation. Am. J. Obst. & Gynec., 1932, 24:40.

——— Spontaneous Evolution of the Fetus in Transverse Presentation. Am. J. Obst. & Gynec., 1933, 25:382.

Goethals, T. R. The Risk of the Infant in Breech Delivery. Surg., Gynec. & Obst., 1936, 62:525.

Goplerud, J., and Eastman, N. J. Compound Presentation. In preparation.

Gordon, C. A., Galick, R., and Oginz, P. An Analysis of 3,301 Breech Deliveries in the Hospitals of Brooklyn. Am. J. Obst. & Gynec., 1934, 28:140.

Hanson, S. The Transversely Contracted Midpelvis with Particular Reference to Forceps Delivery. Am. J. Obst. & Gynec., 1936, 32:385.

Hellman, L. M., Epperson, J. W., and Connally, F. Face and Brow Presentation. Am. J. Obst. & Gynec. In press.

Herrgott, A. Un Cas d'Evolution Spontanée. Ann. de gynéc. et d'obst., 1918, 13:193.

Holland, E. Cranial Stress in the Foetus During Labor, etc. J. Obst. & Gynaec. Brit. Emp., 1922, 29:551.

Irving, F. C., and Goethals, T. R. Elimination of the Second Stage of Labor in Breech Presentations. Am. J. Obst. & Gynec., 1926, 10:80.

Kerr, J. M. M. and Moir, J. C. Operative Obstetrics. 5th Ed. Bailliere, Tindall and Cox, London, 1949; Williams and Wilkins, Baltimore, 1950.

Kleinhaus, F. Winckel's Handbuch. Bd. 2, Teil 3, p. 1631.

Koff, A. K., and Potter, E. L. The Complications Associated with Excessive Development of the Fetus. Am. J. Obst. & Gynec., 1939, 38:412.

Kratsch, A. Nebennierenbefunde bei Anenzephalie. Ztschr. f. Geburtsh. u. Gynäk., 1928, 92:579.

Le Lorier. Presentation du Siège. Brindeau, La Pratique de l'Arts des Accouchements, 1927, T. I., pp. 413-440.

Lynch, F. W. Dystocia from Congenital Cystic Kidney of the Foetus. Surg., Gynec. & Obst., 1906, 3:628.

Macafee, C. H. G., and McClure, H. I. A Critical Survey of 349 Cases of Breech Delivery. Brit. M. J., 1937, 2:1112.

Mengert, W. F., and Longwell, F. H. Prolapse of the Umbilical Cord. Am. J. Obst. & Gynec., 1940, 40:79.

Moore, W. T., and Steptoe, P. O. The Experience of the Johns Hopkins Hospital with Breech Presentation. South M. J., 1943, 36:295.

Nandi, G. Habitual Breech Presentation. Calcutta M. J., 1936, 31:289.

Neumann, H. O. Die Stirnlagen Geburt. Arch. f. Gynäk., 1929, 135:334.

——— Die Stirnlagengeburt. Arch. f. Gynäk., 1929, 135:334.

Petitjean. Étude Statistique concernant le Case de Presentation de la Face ayant lieu à la clinique Baudelocque. Thèse de Paris, 1904.

Piper, E. B., and Bachman, C. Prevention of Fetal Injury in Breech Delivery. J.A.M.A., 1929, 92:217.

Posner, A. C., and Buch, I. M. Face and Persistent Brow Presentations. Surg., Gynec. & Obst., 1943, 77:618.

Reddock, J. W. Face Presentation. Am. J. Obst. & Gynec., 1948, 56:86.

Rudolf, S. J., Jr. Face Presentation. Am. J. Obst. & Gynec., 1947, 54:987.

Ryder, G. H. Breech Presentations Treated by Cephalic Versions in the Consecutive Deliveries of 1700 Women. Am. J. Obst. & Gynec., 1943, 45:1004.

Schuchard. Schwierigkeit der Diagnose und die Haufigkeit der Uterruptur bei fötaler Hydrocephalie. Diss. Berlin, 1884.

Siegel, I. A., and McNally, H. B. Breech Presentation and Prophylactic External Cephalic Version. Am. J. Obst. & Gynec., 1939, 37:86.

Slemons, J. M., and Fagin, R. H. A Study of the Infant's Birth Weight and the Mother's Gain during Pregnancy. Am. J. Obst. & Gynec., 1927, 14:159.

Stephenson, H. A. The Mechanism of Labor in Spontaneous Evolution. Bull. Johns Hopkins Hosp., 1915, 26:331.

Thorn, W. Zur manuellen Umwandlung der Gesichtslagen in Hinterhaupslagen. Ztschr. f. Geburtsh. u. Gynäk., 1886, 13:186.

Tompkins, P. The Intrinsic Risk of Breech Delivery. Am. J. Obst. & Gynec., 1943, 46:695.

Urnes, M. P., and Timerman, H. J. Breech Delivery. A Comparative Study of Local and General Anesthesia. J.A.M.A., 1937, 109:1616.

Walsh, J. W., and Kuder, K. Breech Presentation in the Elderly Primipara. Am. J. Obst. & Gynec., 1944, 47:541.

Way, S. Influence of Minor Degrees of Failure of Fusion of the Müllerian Ducts on Pregnancy and Labor. J. Obst. & Gynaec. Brit. Emp., 1945, 52:325.

31

DYSTOCIA DUE TO PELVIC CONTRACTION

Since the process of labor resolves itself into the passage of the infant through a bony birth canal, it would appear obvious that any substantial diminution in the size of that canal may constitute an impediment to the egress of the infant. For practical purposes, the common types of pelvic contraction may be classified in four main groups:

1. **Contraction of the inlet.**
2. **Contraction of the midpelvis.**
3. **Contraction of the outlet.**
4. **Combinations of inlet, midpelvic and outlet contraction.**

INLET CONTRACTION

Definition. Inlet contraction is defined as a diminution of the obstetrical conjugate measurement to 10.0 cm. or less. Since the anteroposterior diameter of the pelvis is frequently measured by the diagonal conjugate (roughly 1.5 cm. greater than the obstetrical conjugate), inlet contraction is also defined as diminution of the diagonal conjugate measurement to 11.5 cm. or less. These are not arbitrary figures, but are based on the fact that the biparietal diameter of an infant's head is occasionally as large as 10.0 cm. (average 9.25 cm.) and hence it might prove difficult, or even impossible, for such an infant to pass through the inlet unless the anteroposterior diameter of the latter exceeds 10.0 cm. Except in rare instances, inlet contraction is most marked in the anteroposterior diameter; hence the above definition covers almost all cases. Moderate degrees of transverse contraction of the inlet, however, are often seen in association with anteroposterior contraction, and naturally have an important bearing on the space available for the passage of the infant.

Etiology. The most common cause of inlet contraction is rickets. About 2 per cent of white women and about 15 per cent of colored women have pelvic contraction as the result of this disease suffered in infancy or early childhood.

Due to the mechanical action of various forces upon the softened bones and the traction or compression exerted by various muscles and ligaments, the rachitic pelvis shows characteristic changes.

The most important changes are to be noted in the sacrum which differs from the normal in that it is broader and less concave from side to side, thinner from behind forward, and shorter from above downward. The longitudinal axis of the bone is so altered as to form a greater angle with the obstetrical conjugate; consequently, the promontory lies at a level lower than usual, approaches the symphysis pubis, and encroaches markedly upon the area of the superior strait. Usually the entire sacrum is sharply bent upon itself in the neighborhood of its third vertebra so that its vertical concavity becomes markedly accentuated. At the same time, the bodies of the individual vertebrae extend out beyond the level of their alae, thereby diminishing the lateral concavity of the sacrum, and generally converting it into a pronounced convexity. In the latter event the spinous processes project less far than usual beyond the posterior surface, which tends to become concave. Occasionally, however, the increase in vertical concavity does not occur and in such cases the sacrum may be quite straight from base to tip.

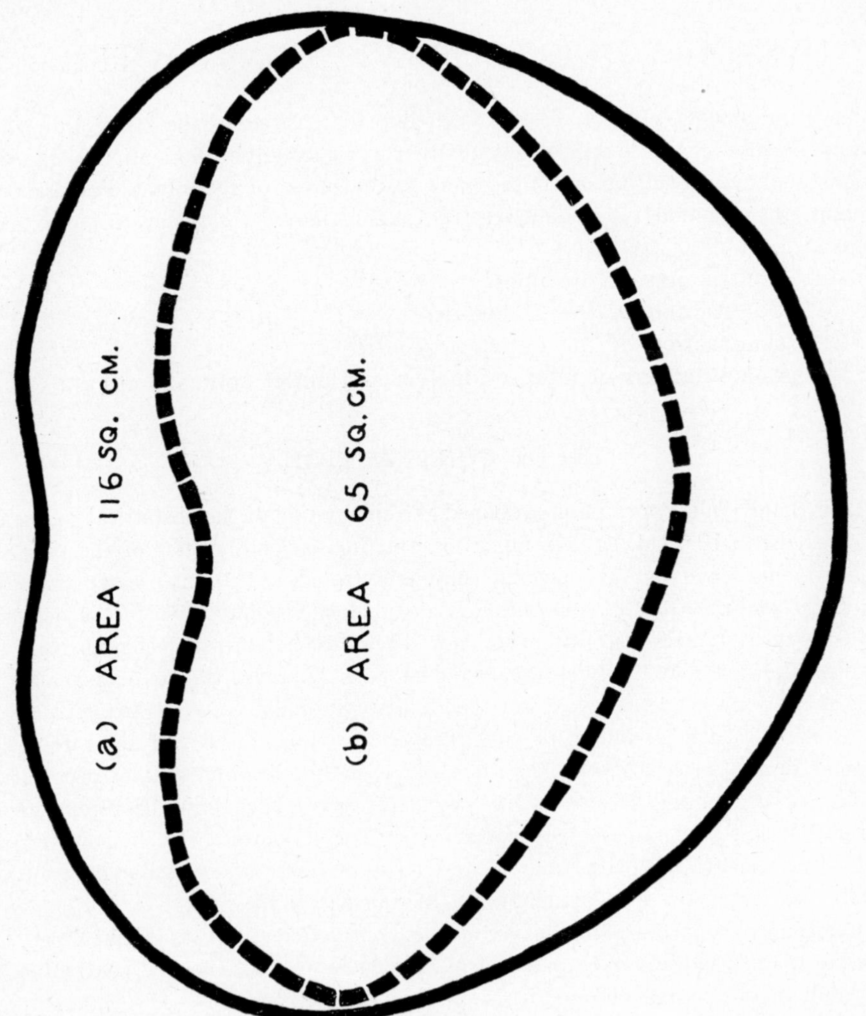

FIG. 434.—AREAS (ACTUAL SIZE) OF NORMAL PELVIC INLET (a) AND CONTRACTED INLET (b).

The extreme degree of inlet contraction in (b) occurred in a 26-year-old colored woman who had severe rickets in childhood (J.H.H. 283193).

Occasionally the body of the first sacral vertebra is displaced further forward than those below it, so that its lower margin projects beyond the general surface, and can be felt as a *false,* or *double promontory.* In such circumstances the distance between this false promontory and the symphysis pubis may be shorter than the obstetrical conjugate, in which case the distance to the false promontory is taken as the measurement of clinical importance since interest always centers on the smallest diameter through which the infant must pass. The presence of a false promontory is usually indicative of the assimilation of an extra vertebra of the sacrum.

The iliac bones are smaller and frequently more delicately shaped than normal, the vertical heights of the pelvis as well as the length of the iliac crest being diminished. The iliac fossae are more concave and frequently present a pronounced sharp depression just in front of the sacro-iliac joint. At the same time, the anterior portion of the ilium flares out at the expense of the crest, so that the distance between the anterior superior spines approaches and occasionally even exceeds that between the crests.

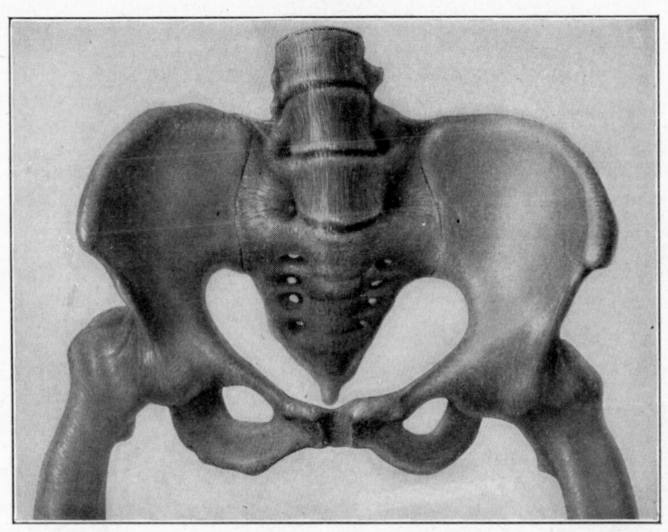

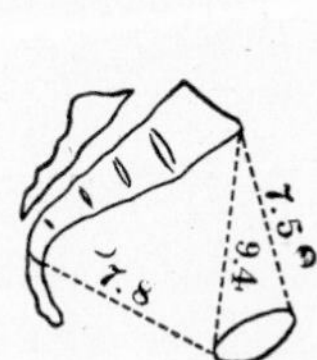

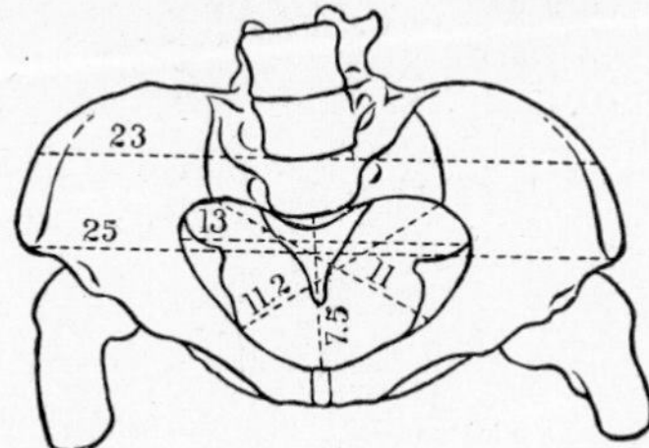

FIGS. 435, 436, AND 437.—FLAT RACHITIC PELVIS.

The diminution in the size of each iliac bone is best appreciated by studying its "terminal length" (page 265). Normally, the three components of this terminal length are practically of the same length, but in rickets the pubic portion retains its normal dimensions, the sacral portion is slightly shorter than usual, while the iliac portion is greatly shortened and occasionally presents only a fraction of its normal length. In many cases the iliac bones bend just in front of the sacroiliac synchondrosis so that the iliopectineal line, instead of following a gentle curve, forms a sharp angle at that point, thus adding materially to the flattening of the superior strait. At the same time, the acetabula are displaced forward and come to lie upon the anterior instead of upon the lateral portion of the pelvic ring.

According to the degree of the displacement of the promontory of the sacrum a decided influence is exerted upon the shape of the pelvic cavity, the effect being most marked in the superior strait, which may become oval, reniform, or even heart-shaped in outline. The obstetrical conjugate is always shortened while the transverse diameter seems to be enlarged, although this is usually only relative. Owing to the approach of the anterior and posterior walls of the pelvis, the oblique diameters of the inlet are also shortened.

In extreme cases the pubic arch may be relatively, and sometimes actually, wider than normal, and the tubera ischii may be so everted that the transverse diameter of the outlet appears to be exaggerated. In view of the upward and backward dislocation of the tip of the sacrum, the anteroposterior diameter of the outlet is also either relatively or absolutely increased in length. Consequently, in contrast with the flattened superior strait, the pelvic outlet may appear wide and gaping, but this is variable and occasionally a rachitic inlet may be seen in association with a contracted outlet.

Contraction of the pelvic inlet may be due also to generally poor development. In this case all of the pelvic measurements are more or less proportionately shortened so that a miniature pelvis results. It is usually met with in small women, although one is occasionally surprised to find it in those of large stature. Such a pelvis is often referred to as a "generally contracted pelvis."

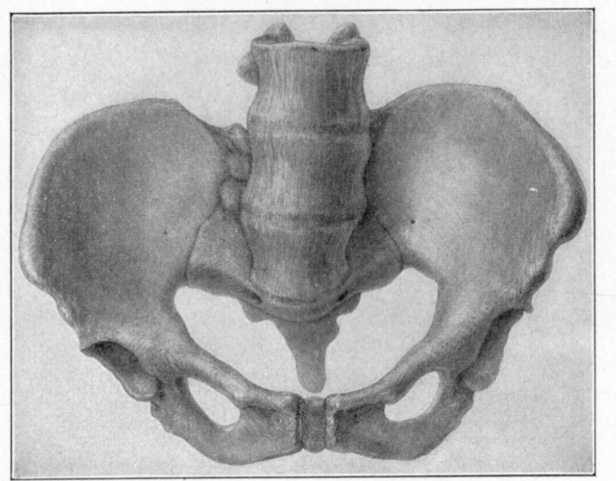

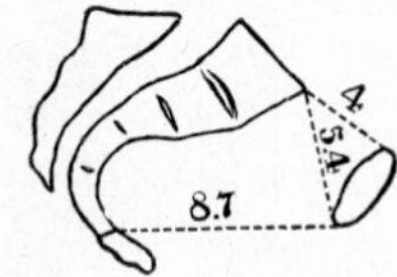

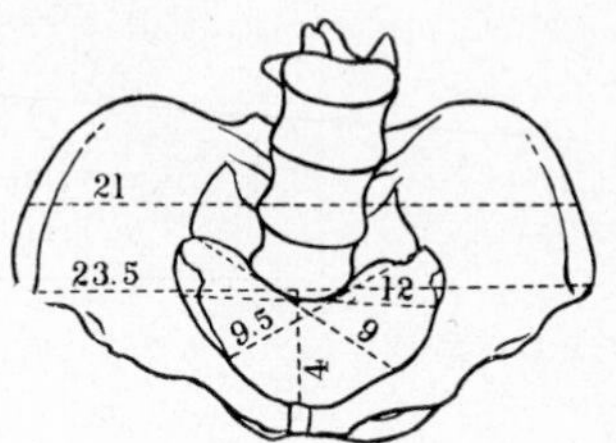

Figs. 438, 439 and 440.—Generally Contracted, Flat Rachitic Pelvis.

Not infrequently, especially in colored women, rachitic changes are superimposed on such a miniature or generally contracted pelvis. In that event, extreme degrees of contraction are sometimes encountered, the obstetrical conjugate occasionally being reduced to 5 cm. or less.

In occasional instances of inlet contraction, simple flattening may occur without evidence of rickets—a "simple flat pelvis." Although the etiology of this variety of inlet contraction is not known, it has been thought that it may be of congenital origin.

Effect on the Course of Pregnancy. Marked degrees of pelvic deformity exert a pronounced influence upon the course of pregnancy as well as upon the mechanism of labor. Indeed, to be unaccompanied by more or less definite effects the contraction must be minimal.

Position of the Uterus. Rarely in the early months of pregnancy a pronounced degree of pelvic malformation may interfere with the normal rising up of the uterus, particularly if the promontory of the sacrum projects so far into the superior strait as to overhang markedly the pelvic cavity. In these rare cases, as the uterus increases in size it may assume a position of pronounced retroflexion which later may give rise to characteristic symptoms of incarceration.

Later in pregnancy, when the deformity is sufficient to interfere materially with the descent of the presenting part into the pelvis, marked abnormalities in the position of the uterus are observed. Particularly in primigravidae, the fundus occupies a higher position than usual, and serious respiratory and circulatory disturbances often result. At the same time, owing to the fact that the lower portion of the uterus is not fixed by the engaged head, it is frequently found that the entire organ is more freely movable than usual.

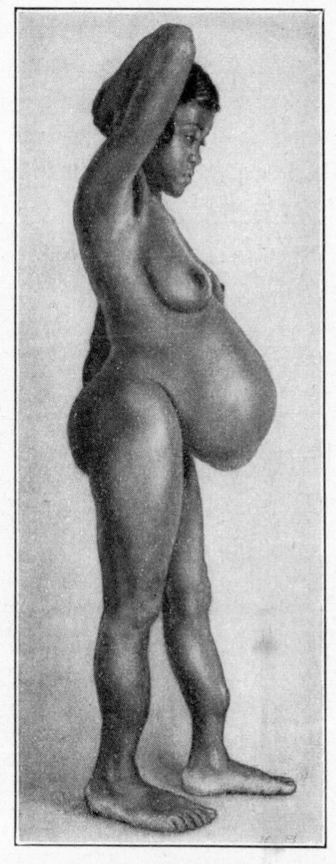

FIG. 441.—PENDULOUS ABDOMEN IN A PRIMIPARA WITH A GENERALLY CONTRACTED RACHITIC PELVIS.

More important, however, is the sharply anteflexed position which the uterus may assume. This is particularly the case in small women presenting marked lumbar lordosis, whereby the capacity of the abdomen is so diminished that the growing uterus seeks to gain room by pushing forward the anterior abdominal wall. Consequently, the presence of a pendulous abdomen is a sign of considerable importance in primigravidous women, and should always cause one to suspect the existence of marked pelvic deformity. The converse, however, does not necessarily indicate that no disproportion exists. On the other hand, the same condition may have no great significance in multiparous women, being generally due to a loss of tonicity of the uterine and abdominal walls as a result of previous pregnancies.

Position and Presentation of the Fetus. A contracted pelvis plays an important part in the production of abnormal presentations. In normal primigravidous women, the presenting part, as a rule, descends into the pelvic cavity during the last six weeks of pregnancy; but when the superior strait is considerably contracted this does not occur at all, or not until after the onset of labor. Vertex presentations still predominate, but since the head floats freely above the superior strait, or rests upon one of the iliac fossae, very slight influences may cause the fetus to assume other positions. According to Michaelis, vertex presentations are rarer by 10 per cent in contracted than in normal pelves, while face, breech, and transverse presentations occur two or three times, and prolapse of the cord and the extremities four to six times more frequently in the former than in the latter.

In 2,735 labors complicated by contracted pelvis in the New York Lying-In Hospital between 1932 and 1943, the following incidence for the various presentations was noted:

Vertex:	92.8%	instead of	94.6%
Breech:	4.4%	instead of	4.5%
Face, Brow, Parietal:	0.7%	instead of	0.4%
Tranverse:	0.6%	instead of	0.2%
Compound and Other:	0.2%	instead of	0.1%
No Record:	1.3%	instead of	0.2%
	100.0		100.0

In other words, face, brow, and parietal presentations were noted twice and transverse presentations three times as frequently as under normal conditions.

Since abnormal presentations occur more frequently in multiparous than in primigravidous women even under favorable conditions, they become still more common when the pelvis is contracted. Schauta estimated that they are three times more frequent in the fifth than in the first pregnancy.

In primigravidous women face and transverse presentations possess a peculiar significance, as their occurrence is often associated with serious disproportion between the size of the head and the pelvis, so that whenever either variety is encountered one can suspect that the head is unusually large or the pelvis abnormally small.

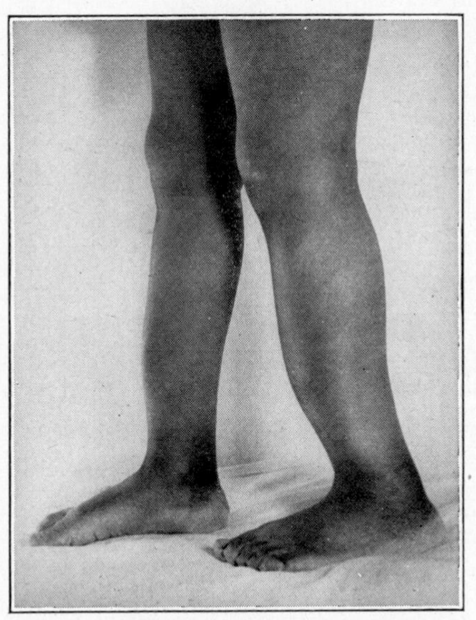

Fig. 442.—Saber Shins, a Frequent Accompaniment of Rachitic Pelvic Contraction. Shown Also in Fig. 441.

Size of the Fetus. Women with inlet contraction tend to have smaller children than do those without inlet contraction. This is probably due to the fact that the contracted pelvis represents only one of the many stigmata of degeneration which characterize the patient. Thoms, in a study of 362 white primigravidae, found the average weight of the offspring to be 278 gm. less in women with small pelves than in those with medium or large pelves. Furthermore, he observed that the relationship between maternal height and the weight of the newborn parallels that between the size of the pelvic inlet and the weight of the newborn. In this connection it is interesting to note that in veterinary obstetrics it has been frequently observed that the maternal size determines the fetal size.

Mechanism of Labor. Inasmuch as in a simple flat pelvis the contraction is practically limited to the anteroposterior diameter of the superior strait, it is evident that the obstacle to the passage of the child's head must be offered by the shortened conjugata vera. When this measures less than 9 cm. it becomes out of the question for the biparietal diameter of the normal head to pass through it unless it undergoes some diminution in size. Accordingly, when engagement is occurring, the head may gradually move to one side so as to bring the shorter bitemporal diameter into relation with the conjugata vera. As a result, the long arm of the head lever becomes displaced to the side of the occiput so that, under the influence of the uterine contractions, the anterior portion of the head descends while the occipital portion rises up. This means that more or less extension of the head takes place. This, indeed, is the mechanism responsible for the increased frequency of face presentation in inlet contraction. The large fontanel becomes more readily accessible to the examining finger on one side of the pelvis, and the small fontanel less so on the other. At the same time, the head tends to accommodate itself to the transverse diameter of the superior strait, so that its long axis, as indicated by the sagittal suture, comes to lie transversely.

More characteristic still is the abnormal attitude which the head assumes when the disproportion is at all marked in a flattened pelvis, when we may have what is known as an *anterior parietal presentation.* In this the sagittal suture comes to lie just in front of the promontory of the sacrum, with the result that the head assumes an eccentric position with the anterior parietal bone occupying the greater part of the superior strait. In such circumstances the anterior shoulder is readily distinguished upon external palpation. According to the explanation generally accepted, this condition is brought about by the abnormal relation borne by the axis of the anteflexed uterus to the plane of the superior strait, as the result of which the posterior portion of the head is arrested against the promontory of the sacrum, while its anterior portion is forced into the pelvis.

This presentation is simply an exaggeration of the so-called *Naegele's obliquity,* and the mechanism of descent is readily understood when we compare the passage of the head through the abnormal superior strait to the maneuver necessary to pass a stick of a certain length through a ring of a somewhat shorter diameter. To do so, one must depress one end so as to allow the stick to enter the ring obliquely, and after it has partially passed its other end will descend without difficulty. In other words, lateral flexion of the head is essential to its descent into the pelvis.

In order for descent to occur, the posterior parietal bone is firmly pressed against the promontory of the sacrum, while under the influence of the uterine contractions the anterior portion of the head is slowly forced down into the pelvis along the internal surface of the symphysis pubis (lateral flexion backwards). After this is accomplished the posterior portion passes over the promontory and enters the pelvis, the sagittal suture at the same time moving forward. Accordingly, when the contraction is marked, the posterior portion of the head must be subjected to considerable pressure, as is shown by the presence after birth of a more or less well-defined curved depression just beyond the coronal suture, upon the side of the head which was in contact with the promontory. After the posterior parietal bone has passed the superior strait, all resistance has been overcome, and owing to the fact that the lower portion of the pelvis is usually relatively large, the rest of the labor is promptly accomplished.

In about one fourth of the labors occurring in flat pelves, according to Litzmann, the reverse condition—the *posterior parietal presentation*—is observed. The sagittal suture now lies almost in contact with the symphysis pubis while the posterior parietal bone occupies the superior strait, and in pronounced cases the posterior ear of the child can be felt just above the promontory, causing the condition to be spoken of sometimes as an *ear presentation.* The long axis of the child's body forms an obtuse angle with its head, and upon palpation the anterior portion of the latter can be felt as a prominent tumor lying above the symphysis. In this event, the head cannot enter the pelvis until its posterior portion is pushed down past the promontory of the sacrum, after which its anterior portion descends along the symphysis pubis, while at the same time the sagittal suture approaches the midline of the pelvis. After this has occurred labor takes place in the usual manner.

The mode of production of this abnormality is not definitely understood, although it is observed most frequently when the grade of contraction is marked, the pelvic inclination considerably increased, and the abdomen not pendulous. It is generally considered as very unfavorable by the Germans, since the line along which the uterine contractions are transmitted is given another direction at the neck, which is much less advantageous than when the spinal column and head form a continuous axis. Tarnier and Varnier, on the other hand, held that the posterior parietal presentation occurs more frequently than the anterior and is without ominous prognostic significance. In an extensive roentgenologic study of the mechanism of labor, Caldwell, Moloy and Swenson found that both extreme positions, anterior (Naegele's obliquity) and posterior (Litzmann's or Varnier's obliquity) parietal presentations, are rare but that modern degrees of asynclitism occur in the majority of normal labors.

These recent roentgenological observations indicate that in the majority of patients with a flat pelvis, slighter degrees of asynclitism than those described above occur, and that the mechanism of labor depends upon lateral flexion of the fetal head as one of

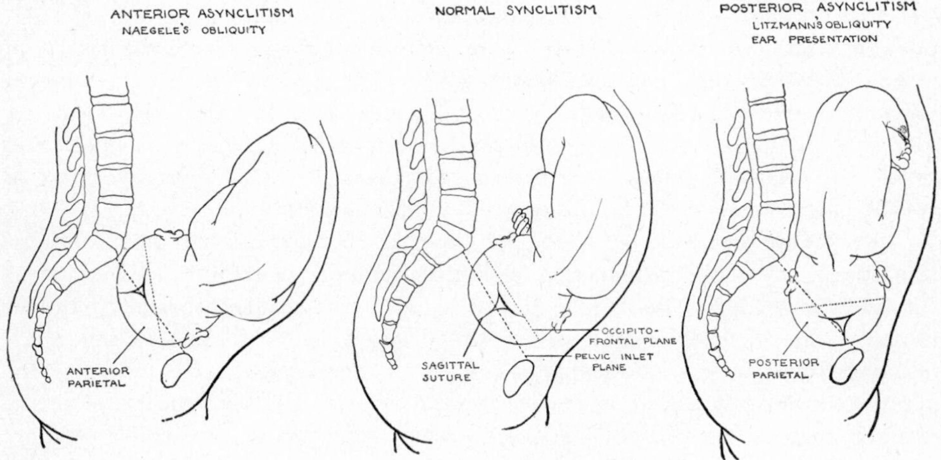

FIG. 443.—ASYNCLITISM.

the accessory movements. In this type of pelvic contraction, the head, as stated above, presents over the inlet of the pelvis in L. O. T. position before engagement, with its sagittal suture lying transversely toward the symphysis and with the posterior parietal bone presenting (posterior asynclitism). The force of the uterine contractions is along a line in the direction of the symphysis, with the resultant force backward. Engagement of the head, therefore, is effected by lateral flexion backward accompanied by ordinary flexion. The sagittal suture is now in synclitism, and descent occurs to the sacrococcygeal platform (below the spines) so that the anterior parietal bone presents (anterior asynclitism). Again the uterine drive meets resistance at the sacrococcygeal platform and the resultant force is directed forward; the head, therefore, flexes laterally again, this time forward. The posterior parietal bone now impinges on the left ischial spine. This forms a new point of resistance, with another resultant force toward the symphysis which initiates the movement of internal rotation through an arc of 90 degrees, bringing the occiput under the symphysis along the gentle curvature of the ischiopubic ramus, as originally pointed out by Smellie. Disengagement, or extension, and expulsion occur in the anteroposterior diameter of the outlet. This concept of the normal mechanism of labor for a transverse position of the vertex, based upon the x-ray findings obtained during parturition, coincides closely with the earlier views of Pinard and Varnier regarding abnormal labor.

When the promontory of the sacrum protrudes into the superior strait in such a way as to render it reniform in outline, it is impossible for the head to assume its usual transverse position, and the sagittal suture must occupy an oblique diameter. In rare instances the deformity is so great that the superior strait resembles the figure 8. In such circumstances only one side of it is available for the passage of the head, and Breisky has designated the condition as *extramedian engagement*. It naturally serves to exaggerate the degree of disproportion.

Breech presentations likewise complicate matters to some extent, since the imperfect adaptation of the breech to the superior strait facilitates prolapse of the cord or of one or more of the extremities. In such circumstances, although the prognosis for the mother remains favorable, the child's life is seriously endangered. In breech presentations, unfortunately, we cannot utilize Müller's method of impression of the head to estimate the presence and extent of any marked *cephalopelvic disproportion*. When the pelvic contraction is marked, great difficulty may be experienced in extracting the aftercoming head which, in passing through the contracted superior strait, may follow a mechanism analogous to that observed in anterior parietal presentations. In other words, its posterior portion is arrested at the promontory, while its anterior portion passes down behind the symphysis, after which its posterior portion descends (Fig. 444).

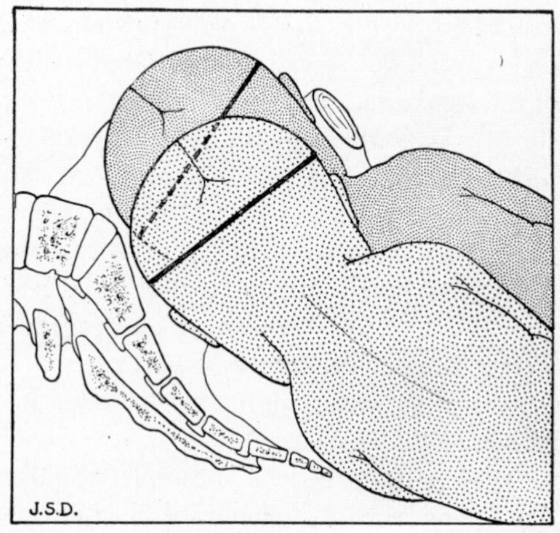

Fig. 444.—Passage of Biparietal Diameter of Aftercoming Head through Pelvic Inlet.

The effect of the generally contracted, or justominor, pelvis upon the course of labor is very characteristic. Owing to the fact that all of the diameters of the superior strait are shortened, the head encounters more or less equal resistance from all sides of the pelvic inlet. Consequently it enters it in an oblique diameter and in a sharply flexed position, so that on vaginal examination the small fontanel is readily felt while the large fontanel is almost or quite out of reach. Moreover, as the contraction involves all portions of the pelvic canal, labor is not rapidly completed after the head has passed the superior strait. The prolongation is due not only to the resistance offered by the pelvis but also in many instances to the faulty character of the uterine contractions incident to the imperfect development of the uterus, which frequently characterizes such patients.

Course of Labor. When the pelvic deformity is not absolute, but is sufficiently pronounced to prevent the head from entering the superior strait during the last few weeks of pregnancy, or at the onset of uterine contractions, the course of labor is usually unduly prolonged. In the first stage this is due to uterine inertia and to imperfect dilatation of the cervix, and in the second to the time required to so mold and configure the head as to render possible its passage through the pelvic cavity.

Abnormalities in Dilatation of Cervix. Normally, dilatation of the cervix is brought about by the unruptured membranes acting as a hydrostatic wedge, and after their rupture, by the direct action of the presenting part. In contracted pelves, on the other hand, when the head is arrested at the superior strait, the entire force exerted by the uterus acts directly upon the portion of membranes in contact with the internal os and, consequently, as the force is not broken by the intervening head as in normal labor, *premature rupture* frequently results, occurring in 23.7 per cent of Stander's cases, and is frequently followed by *intrapartum infection,* to which reference will be made later.

After rupture of the membranes, further dilatation cannot take place until the presenting part is able to exert a direct pressure upon the cervix, and this is out of the question until a succession of strong pains has molded the head sufficiently to permit its descent, or has led to the formation of a *caput succedaneum* upon its most dependent portion. Conversely, this absence of pressure by the fetal head against the cervix and lower uterine segment predisposes to poor pains and hence further dilatation of the cervix may proceed very slowly or never take place. By way of supporting this statement, 49 labors at the Johns Hopkins Hospital have been studied in women with contracted pelves in which cesarean section was finally performed after 30 or more hours of labor. It was found that the cervix had reached full dilatation in only 8 of these cases, or in one sixth; in 29 cases or over one half, the dilatation was less than 5 cm.; in 13, or over one fourth, it was less than 3 cm. even after 30 hours of labor. Stated briefly, **in degrees of contracted pelvis incompatible with vaginal delivery, the cervix rarely dilates satisfactorily.** By the same token, the behavior of the cervix has a certain prognostic value in regard to the outcome of labor in women with inlet contraction.

Even after the cervix is completely dilated further delay may occur, and it sometimes requires hours to mold the head to the pelvis. In flat pelves the labor is promptly terminated as soon as the contracted superior strait is passed, whereas in the generally contracted varieties the hindrance persists throughout the entire pelvic canal.

Abnormalities in Uterine Contraction. In many instances the course of labor is still further prolonged owing to faulty uterine contractions. In prolonged labors the contractions occasionally become abnormally frequent and severe, so that in extreme cases the uterus becomes *tetanically contracted.* This is an extremely serious condition since it cannot lead to the termination of labor and, at the same time, greatly increases the danger of uterine rupture. If this complication does not yield promptly to the administration of sedatives, it affords an imperative indication for the termination of labor.

Danger of Uterine Rupture. Abdominal thinning of the lower uterine segment frequently constitutes a very serious danger during a prolonged second stage. When the disproportion between the head and the pelvis is so pronounced that engagement and descent do not occur, the lower uterine segment becomes more and more stretched, and the danger of rupture becomes imminent. In such cases the contraction or *pathologic retraction ring* can be felt as a transverse or oblique ridge extending across the uterus somewhere between the symphysis and the umbilicus, while sometimes its position is clearly visible. Thinning of the lower uterine segment is particularly liable to occur in the generally contracted variety of rachitic pelves, since the lower end of the cervix may be caught between the child's head and the pelvic brim, and thus be prevented from retracting. Whenever this condition is noted, prompt delivery is urgently indicated; and if this is not effected by some type of cesarean section, great caution is necessary on the part of the physician lest his intra-uterine maneuvers give rise to traumatic rupture.

Production of Fistulas. When the presenting part is firmly wedged into the superior strait, but makes no advance for a long time, portions of the birth canal lying between it and the pelvic wall may be subjected to undue pressure. As a result, the circulation is so interfered with that necrosis follows, which may manifest itself a few days after labor by the appearance of *vesicovaginal, vesicocervical,* or *rectovaginal fistulas,* depending upon the part involved. In former times, when operative delivery was deferred as long as possible, such complications were of frequent occurrence, but at present they are rarely seen except in neglected cases. In general, injurious pressure is unlikely to occur so long as the membranes remain intact, but is liable to follow a very prolonged second stage.

Intrapartum Infection. Infection is another serious danger to which the patient is exposed in prolonged labors complicated by premature rupture of the membranes, particularly when examined repeatedly by those who do not observe stringent aseptic technic. If the amniotic fluid becomes infected, febrile symptoms appear during labor, while in other cases the micro-organisms pass through the fetal membranes and invade the uterine walls, giving rise later to the characteristic manifestations of puerperal infection. Intrapartum infection is serious not only for the mother but is also an important factor in causing intra-uterine death of the child since, as stated previously, bacteria can make their way through the amnion and invade the walls of the vessels in the chorionic membrane, and thus give rise to fetal bacteriemia.

In other instances, gas producing bacteria may gain access to the uterine cavity, which soon becomes distended with gas, and presents a peculiar "gurgling" feel to the examining fingers, as well as a tympanitic note upon percussion—*tympanitis uteri* or *physometra.* It usually follows infection with the colon bacillus or with the *Streptococcus putridus,* although the *Bacillus aerogenes capsulatus* may sometimes be concerned, particularly when the child is dead. It is always a serious condition and demands intensive treatment with penicillin and one of the sulfonamides. It should not be taken necessarily as indication to terminate labor, since the trauma of major operative procedures may prove fatal in the presence of a virulent uterine infection. Time, fluids, and the drugs mentioned constitute the best immediate treatment in the hope that easy vaginal delivery may ensue. If it does not, after a reasonable period, extraperitoneal section may become necessary, depending on a number of factors.

Rupture of the Pelvic Joints. In rare instances, particularly when the pelvis is contracted in its lower portion, spontaneous rupture of the symphysis pubis or of one or both sacro-iliac joints has been observed. However, in the great majority of cases the injury is produced by injudicious methods of delivery. Kehrer in 1915 collected from the literature 100 cases of rupture of the symphysis pubis, 17 of which occurred during the course of spontaneous labor. He considers that the predisposing cause for the accident consists in unusual softening or in the development of cavities in the pubic cartilage.

Effect of Labor upon the Child. So long as the membranes remain intact the child suffers but little from the prolonged labor, but after their rupture, continued uterine contractions may exert a deleterious influence upon it. This is due in great part to interference with the placental circulation, which sooner or later leads to manifestations of asphyxiation. Now and again premature separation of the placenta occurs, causing certain death to the child. Particularly during the second stage of labor, prolonged pressure exerted upon the head is not without influence upon the child, in some cases leading to vagus stimulation with its resulting slow pulse and consequent gradual asphyxiation, while in others death results from intracranial hemorrhage.

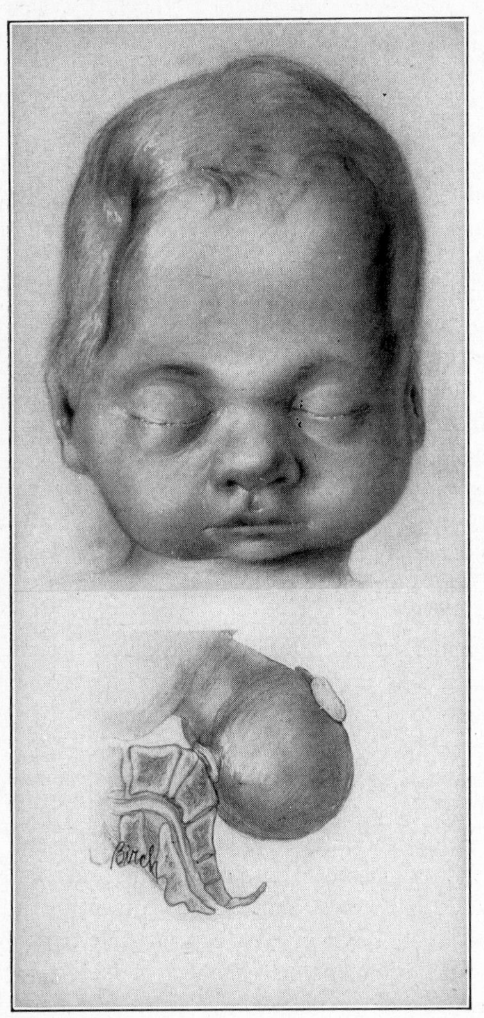

Fig. 445.—Depression of Skull Caused by Labor in a Contracted Pelvis.

Prolapse of the Cord. A much more serious complication for the child is prolapse of the cord, the occurrence of which is facilitated by imperfect adaptation between the presenting part and the pelvic inlet. The condition exerts no influence upon the course of labor, but unless prompt delivery can be accomplished, death of the child results from compression of the cord between the presenting part and the margin of the pelvic inlet. This must be regarded as a frequent cause of fetal death in spontaneous labor in contracted pelves.

Changes in Scalp and Skull. As has already been stated, a large caput is frequently developed upon the most dependent part of the head, and allusion has been made to the part which it sometimes plays in the dilatation of the cervix. In many instances it may assume very considerable proportions and lead to serious diagnostic errors. For example, *it may reach almost to the pelvic floor while the head is still only partially engaged, so that an inexperienced physician may mistake it for the head itself and be tempted to resort to ill-timed operative measures.* After delivery such a caput has no effect upon the child's well-being, since it disappears within a few days after birth.

When the disproportion between the size of the head and the pelvis is considerable, it is apparent that the head can only pass through after a process of *molding* and accommodation, which is usually spoken of as *configuration.* In exceptional cases the head may descend into the pelvic cavity comparatively early in pregnancy and, since it cannot readily escape, it undergoes further development in that position, and in consequence presents characteristic deformities at birth, the part within the pelvis being markedly flattened while that above is unusually large, as shown in Fig. 445.

Under the influence of the strong uterine contractions the various bones comprising the skull come to overlap one another at the various sutures. As a rule, the median margin of the parietal bone, which is in contact with the promontory, becomes overlapped by that of its fellow, and the same occurs with the frontal bones. The occipital bone, on the other hand, becomes shoved under the parietal bones, so that the posterior margins of the latter frequently overlap it. These changes are frequently accomplished without detriment to the child, though when the distortion is marked, they may lead to tentorial tears and, when vessels are involved, to fatal intracranial hemorrhage. Experience shows that this process of molding of the fetal head may yield a diminution in the biparietal diameter of 0.5 cm. without detriment to the brain, but when greater degrees of compression are demanded, the likelihood of cerebral injury is substantial.

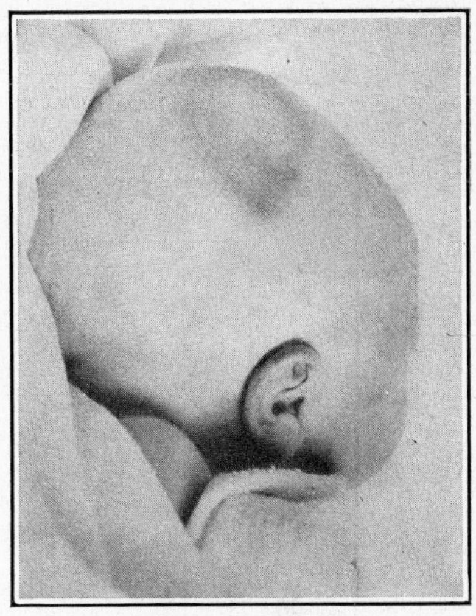

FIG. 446.—DEPRESSED FRACTURE OF SKULL CAUSED BY LABOR IN A CONTRACTED PELVIS.

The infant did well after immediate elevation of the depressed bone by neurosurgeon (J.H.H. 23443).

Coincident with the molding of the head, the parietal bone, which was in contact with the promontory, may show signs of having been subjected to marked pressure, sometimes becoming very much flattened. Configuration is more readily accomplished when the bones of the head are imperfectly ossified, in rare instances the skull being so soft that it yields to pressure far more readily than does the normal fetal head. This process is of great importance, and serves to explain the difference in the course of labor in two apparently similar cases in which the pelvis and the head present identical measurements. In the one the head is soft and readily molded, so that spontaneous labor can result; in the other the more resistant head retains its original shape, and radical operative interference becomes necessary for its delivery.

Reference has already been made to the pressure marks upon the scalp covering the portion of the head which passes over the promontory of the sacrum. These are very characteristic in appearance, and from their location frequently enable one to determine the movements which the head has undergone in passing through the superior strait. Much more rarely, similar marks appear on the portion of the head which has been in contact with the symphysis pubis. Such marks have no influence upon the well-being of the child, and usually disappear a few days after birth, although in exceptional instances the pressure may have been so severe as to lead to necrosis and sloughing of the scalp.

Fractures of the skull are occasionally met with and usually follow forcible attempts at delivery, though sometimes they may occur spontaneously. The fractures are of two varieties, appearing either as a shallow gutter-like groove or as a spoon-shaped depression just posterior to the coronal suture. The former is relatively common and, since it involves only the external plate of the bone, is not very dangerous; whereas the latter, if not operated upon, leads to the death of the child in over one half of the cases, since it extends through the entire thickness of the skull and gives rise to projections upon its inner surface, which exert injurious pressure upon the brain. Accordingly, it is often advisable as soon as convenient after labor, to elevate or remove the depressed portion of the skull as may be indicated, in the hope of preventing pressure symptoms as well as relieving the effects of hemorrhage.

Prognosis. The term "prognosis of labor" in inlet contraction connotes, in the main, whether or not vaginal delivery can be effected safely for mother and child, and with relative ease. In any given case, the outlook will depend on many factors in addition to the absolute size of the pelvis. Among these are the size and position of the infant, the outcome of past labors if any, the quality of the uterine contractions, the condition of the cervix, the extent to which the head descends over various time limits, the mobility of the head and whether or not it can be pushed manually through the inlet. Although pelvic size is but one of many factors which determine prognosis

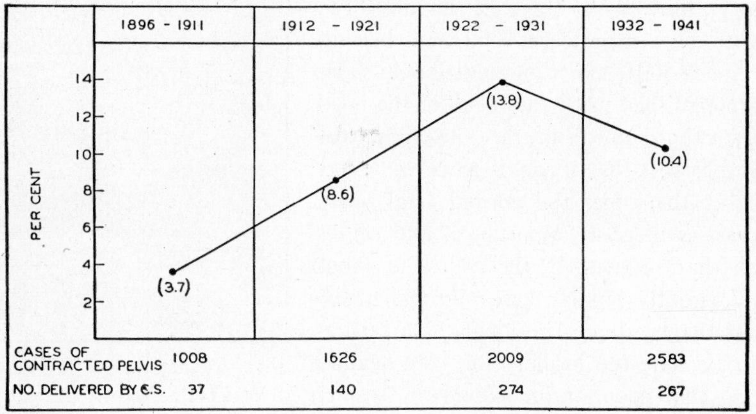

Fig. 447.—Incidence of Cesarean Section in Inlet Contraction at the Johns Hopkins Hospital in Four Periods.

Diagonal conjugate of 11.5 cm. or less. (Manahan, Connally and Eastman.)

in any given case, it is the only factor which can be determined with precision in advance of labor and, other circumstances being equivocal, it is the determining factor in the outcome.

In general, about 90 per cent of patients who fall under the definition of inlet contraction may be expected to deliver vaginally without great increase in risk to mother and child. In 2,583 cases of inlet contraction managed at the Johns Hopkins Hospital between 1932 and 1941, which were studied by Manahan, Connally and Eastman, 90.1 per cent were delivered vaginally with a total infant loss of 5.0 per cent (Fig. 447). This loss represents an increase of only 20 per cent over the total fetal mortality rate which was obtained in the clinic over the period mentioned. There was, however, one maternal death in this series which was the direct result of pelvic contraction. In the early years of the century cesarean section carried a much higher mortality than it does today; hence, it was justifiable to take greater risk with the baby. The results of such a policy are shown in the left hand columns of Figs. 447 and 448, where it may be seen that a cesarean section rate of 3.7 per cent was associated with a fetal mortality in excess of 12 per cent. On the other hand, the extension of cesarean section in borderline cases will not necessarily improve the fetal outlook,

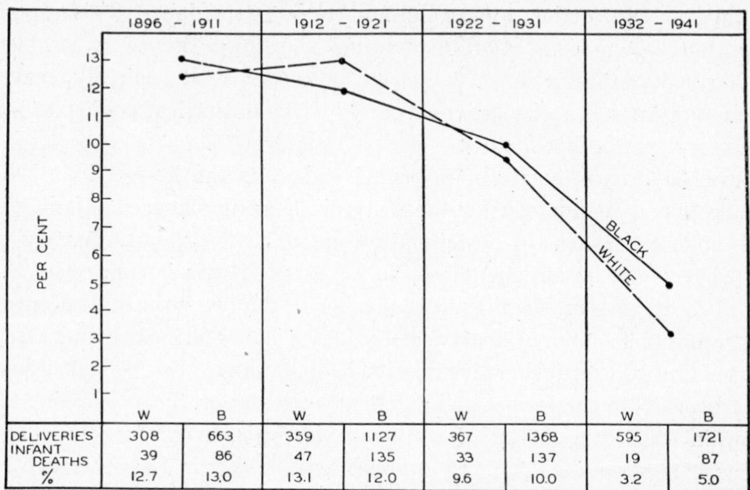

Fig. 448.—Stillbirth and Neonatal Mortality in 6,508 Cases of Inlet Contraction Delivered Vaginally at the Johns Hopkins Hospital.
(Manahan, Connally and Eastman.)

as evidenced by the fact that in the third period illustrated, with a cesarean section rate of 13.8 per cent, the fetal mortality was higher than in the fourth period when a section rate of 10.4 per cent was obtained. Among other factors, the advent of x-ray pelvimetry made possible a more intelligent selection of cases for abdominal delivery, and is largely responsible for this apparent paradox, namely, a decrease in cesarean section for inlet contraction in association with a greatly decreased fetal mortality.

As shown in Fig. 449, in the 2,583 cases of inlet contraction managed between 1932 and 1941, there were no vaginal deliveries in patients with diagonal conjugate measurements under 10.0 cm., or, generally speaking, with an obstetrical conjugate of less than 8.5 cm. In many of these cases of advanced inlet contraction, the decision

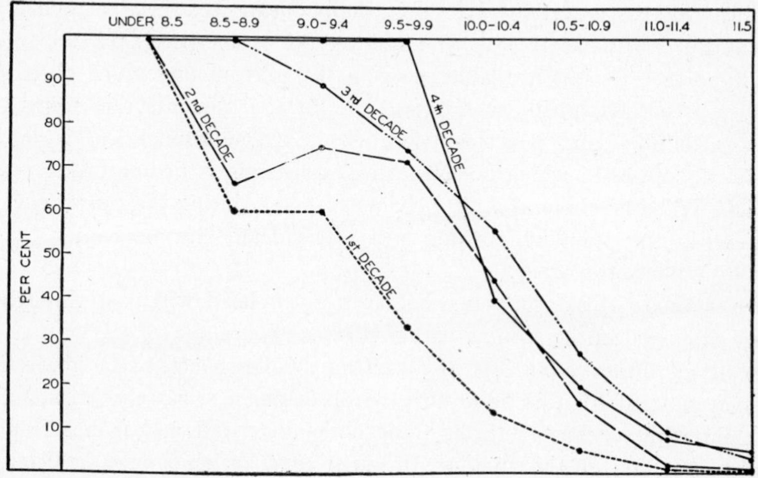

Fig. 449.—Incidence of Cesarean Section in Cases of Inlet Contraction at the Johns Hopkins Hospital According to Period and Diagonal Conjugate Measurement.

to perform cesarean section was made only after a trial labor. This experience, together with the high fetal mortality during the third decade, when many cases with a diagonal conjugate down to 9.0 cm. were delivered vaginally, makes us feel that no mature infant can be delivered safely if the obstetrical conjugate is less than 8.5 cm., regardless of other factors.

If an obstetrical conjugate of 8.5 cm. is taken as the lowest limit below which cesarean section is mandatory for the delivery of an undamaged infant, the reverse prognosis holds true when the obstetrical conjugate is 9.5 or above, namely, successful vaginal delivery can be anticipated, in so far as the pelvis is concerned, in some 95 per cent of cases. In sum, the prognosis of labor in the two groups mentioned, namely, cases of severe contraction (obstetrical conjugate under 8.5 cm.) and cases of very mild contraction (obstetrical conjugate of 9.5 cm. or above) can be stated dogmatically as almost hopeless in the former and excellent in the latter. There remains the borderline group in which the obstetrical conjugate lies between 8.5 and 9.5 cm., and here the prognosis is often as difficult to establish as it is easy in the other two categories. At the midpoint in this group, that is, in patients with an obstetrical conjugate of 9.0 cm., about one half require abdominal delivery. In this borderline category the prognosis of labor must be established on the basis of a number of associated circumstances, some of which have already been mentioned. They are: (1) If the patient has had a previous full-term labor (a small minority of cases), the outcome of that previous labor is of substantial significance. On the other hand, it may be misleading since, if it was easy, the happy outcome may have been attributable to a much smaller baby than the present one; or if it was difficult, the dystocia may have been due to poor management of labor rather than to small pelvic size. (2) The size of the infant is naturally of extreme importance. (3) Premature rupture of the membranes in inlet contraction (but not otherwise) is an unfavorable prognostic sign since it suggests considerable overriding of the head. (4) The quality of the labor pains may be a determining factor and, as mentioned, uterine inertia is common. (5) Again as stated, the behavior of the cervix in labor has great prognostic significance; satisfactory progress in dilatation usually indicates that vaginal delivery will be feasible, whereas a stationary cervix usually means that vaginal delivery cannot be accomplished with safety. (6) The architecture of the pelvis plays a role; in the android type there is less available space in the inlet at any given obstetrical conjugate measurement than in other types. (7) Intrapartum infection seems to inhibit uterine contractility and is a bad sign. (8) Extreme asynclitism is unfavorable. (9) Naturally, cases in which the obstetrical conjugate is nearer to 8.5 than to 9.5 will do less well. (10) Lateral x-ray pelvimetry taken during the course of labor with the patient in the standing position will often demonstrate whether the head is engaged or is likely to engage.

Other methods of ascertaining whether a given head will pass through a given pelvis are discussed in the ensuing paragraphs.

Methods of Determining Size of the Head. Müller's method of impression often affords material aid. In this procedure the obstetrician seizes the brow and occiput of the child with his fingers through the abdominal wall and makes firm pressure downward in the axis of the superior strait, the effect of which may be determined by a finger in the rectum. If there is no disproportion, the head will readily enter the pelvis and spontaneous labor may be predicted. On the other hand, the fact that the head cannot be forced into the superior strait does not necessarily indicate that spontaneous labor is out of the question. Demonstration of overriding of the fetal head, as shown in Fig. 450, is of value if the findings are positive, but absence of overriding is of little significance since it may be due to anterior asynclitism. Pressure at the same time upon the fundus by an assistant is often of great additional help.

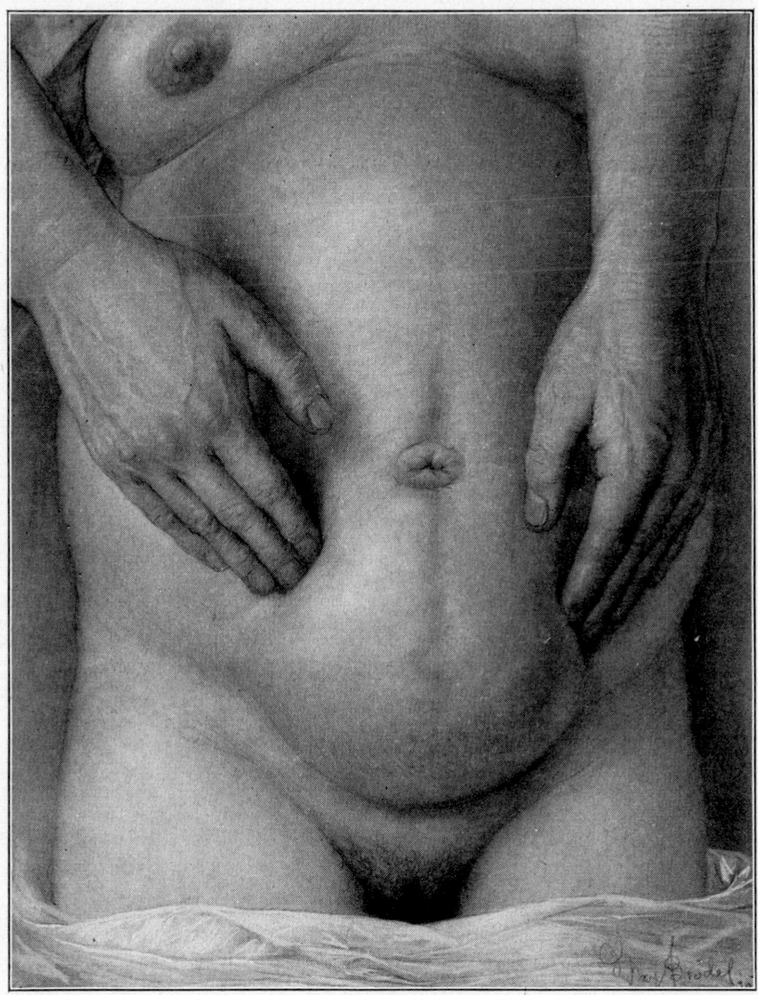

FIG. 450.—METHOD OF DETERMINING DEGREE OF DISPROPORTION BY ASCERTAINING THE EXTENT TO WHICH THE HEAD OVERRIDES THE SYMPHYSIS.

In general, x-ray measurements of the absolute diameters of the fetal head have proved disappointing, although several authors believe that this technic is helpful. The precision of roentgencephalometry is decidedly less than that of x-ray pelvimetry, showing an error of plus or minus 0.5 cm. in most hands. On the other hand, as stated, a lateral film of the pelvis with the patient in standing position will often afford valuable information in regard to the size of the head in relation to the size of the particular inlet concerned.

In many cases of borderline inlet contraction, it is desirable to allow a "trial labor." By this is meant a period of labor long enough to afford evidence, on the basis of the prognostic criteria enumerated, as to whether or not vaginal delivery may be anticipated with safety to mother and child. The period of time required for such evidence to accrue will vary between 6 and 18 hours. In former years, a so-called "test of labor" was often used which entailed allowing labor to continue until complete dilatation and two hours thereafter. This has no place in the modern management of pelvic contraction for two reasons. In the first place, as already explained, many labors with advanced inlet contraction do not reach complete dilatation even after 30 hours. Second, the fetal mortality resulting from this program is appalling, exceeding 30 per cent in our clinic in the days when it was employed.

Breech and Face Presentations in Contracted Pelves. The existence of a breech presentation in moderate degrees of pelvic deformity should be regarded as a complication especially unfavorable for the child, inasmuch as in the early stages of labor prolapse of the cord is facilitated, and in the later stages serious delay may be encountered in the extraction of the aftercoming head, which is often followed by the loss of the child. Moreover, since the head is not in contact with the superior strait, it is difficult to determine the degree of disproportion. For these reasons, one is justified in being much more liberal in the indications for elective cesarean section. Face and brow presentations should be regarded as much more serious complications, as their existence usually indicates a considerable degree of disproportion, and unless the baby is very small or dead, cesarean section is indicated.

Treatment. The management of cases of inlet contraction resolves itself almost entirely into establishing the prognosis for safe vaginal delivery and acting thereupon. If, on the basis of the criteria which have been reviewed, a delivery which will be safe for both mother and child cannot be anticipated, cesarean section should be done or, if the baby is dead, craniotomy. In present-day obstetrics, the latter operation is rarely necessary. In many instances, the prognosis in a given case can be reached before the onset of labor, and section can be done electively at an appointed time; on the other hand, a test of labor is desirable in many borderline cases. No analgesic drugs should be given to any parturient with any form of pelvic contraction because of the likelihood of inertia resulting. It will be recalled that patients with inlet contraction are especially prone to suffer from weak uterine action even in the absence of such medication and these patients often need all the uterine forces they can muster. The course of labor should be followed carefully from hour to hour and the prognosis established as soon as reasonably possible. Almost always this can be done within 18 hours and sometimes after 6 hours. Although signs of impending uterine rupture should always be looked for if the pains are strong, the danger of this accident is very remote in primigravidae. Indeed, in the many thousand labors associated with inlet contraction managed in our clinic, many of which received prolonged tests of labor, there has not been a single instance of spontaneous rupture of the uterus in a primigravida. With greater parity, however, the likelihood of the accident increases. Finally, it is scarcely necessary to add that the administration of pituitary extract in the presence of any form of pelvic contraction will prove tantamount in many cases to the murder of both mother and infant.

Definitions. From the obstetrical standpoint, the plane of the midpelvis extends from the inferior margin of the symphysis pubis, passes through the ischial spines, and touches the sacrum in the neighborhood of the junction of the fourth and fifth vertebrae, according to individual sacral conformation (Mengert). This is at slight variance with the anatomic description which places the posterior limits at the tip of the sacrum. The interspinous line divides the midplane into a fore and hind portion. The former is bounded anteriorly by the lower border of the symphysis pubis and laterally by the ischiopubic rami. The hind portion is bounded posteriorly by the sacrum, as noted above, and laterally by the sacrospinous ligament, forming the lower limits of the sacrosciatic notch. Average midpelvic measurements are: transverse (interspinous) 10.5 cm.; anteroposterior (from the lower border of the symphysis pubis to the junction of the fourth and fifth sacral vertebrae) 11.5 cm.; and posterior sagittal (from the midpoint of the interspinous line to the same point on the sacrum) 5.0 cm. Although the definition of midpelvic contraction has not been established with the precision which is possible in inlet contraction, it may be considered to be present when the sum of the interischial spinous diameter and the posterior sagittal diameter of the midpelvis (normally, 10.5 cm. plus 5.0 cm. equals 15.5 cm.) falls to 13.5 cm. or below (Guerriero). There is reason to suspect midpelvic contraction whenever the interischial spinous diameter falls below 10.0 cm. and when it is lower than 9.5 cm., it is very probably present.

It should be emphasized that the above definition of midpelvic contraction does not mean that dystocia will necessarily occur in such a pelvis, but simply that it may develop depending upon the size of the forepelvis, the degree of the midpelvic contraction, the size of the baby and other factors.

There is no satisfactory manual method of measuring midpelvic contraction, thus making x-ray pelvimetry necessary. It is true that DeLee once devised a pelvimeter to measure midpelvic contraction, which he regarded as one of the essential internal dimensions. In 1930 Hanson recommended a pelvimeter for the same purpose, and in 1936 reported that interspinous diameters of 9.5 cm. or less were present in 16.1 per cent of 1,120 consecutive patients measured by this instrument. Nevertheless, for adequate recognition of the clinical import of midpelvic contraction, especially the posterior sagittal diameter of the midpelvis, x-ray mensuration is essential. A suggestion of midpelvic contraction, however, can sometimes be obtained by ascertaining on vaginal palpation that the spines are prominent, that the side walls converge or that the sacrosciatic notch is narrow. Moreover, Eller and Mengert point out that the relationship between the intertuberous and interspinous diameters of the ischium is sufficiently constant so that contractions of the latter dimension will seldom be missed if x-ray pelvimetry is limited to patients whose intertuberous diameter is 8.5 cm. or less.

Prognosis. Midpelvic contraction in white women is more common than inlet contraction and is frequently a cause of transverse arrest of the head, and of difficult midforceps operations. In a notable case reported by Eller and Mengert, in which the sum of the interischial spinous diameter and the posterior sagittal diameter of the midpelvis was 12.3, grave dystocia necessitated craniotomy of a 3,130 gm. infant. Although such extreme degrees of dystocia in midpelvic contraction are rare, we have performed three cesarean sections because of the condition in which the interischial spinous diameter was 9.0 cm. or less.

Treatment. In the management of labor complicated by midpelvic contraction, the main injunction is to allow the natural forces to push the biparietal diameter through the interspinous obstruction. Forceps operations may be very difficult when applied to a head whose greatest diameter has not yet passed a contracted midpelvis. Hanson has observed the same difficulty with forceps and has explained it on two grounds: (1) forceps pull destroys flexion whereas pressure from above increases it; (2) the few millimeters occupied by the thickness of the forceps blades diminish still further the available space for the passage of the baby's head. In this connection it should be recalled that only when the head has been allowed to descend until the perineum is bulging and the vertex is actually visible, can one be certain that the head has passed the obstruction; only then is it safe to apply forceps. If necessary, suprafundic pressure can be used with pains to help attain this end. It is often more efficacious and always safer than forceps in such pelves.

OUTLET CONTRACTION

Definitions. Contraction of the pelvic outlet is defined as diminution of the interischial tuberous diameter to 8.0 cm. or less. By consulting Figs. 452 and 454, it will be seen that the area of the outlet (not actually a plane) may be likened to two triangles. The interischial tuberous diameter constitutes the base of both. The sides of the anterior triangle are the pubic rami, and its apex, the under surface of the symphysis pubis. The posterior triangle has no bony sides but is limited at its apex by the tip of the last sacral vertebra (not the tip of the coccyx). With this concept in mind, it is apparent that diminution in the intertuberous diameter with consequent narrowing of the anterior triangle must inevitably force the infant's head posteriorly; and whether delivery can take place or not depends partly on the size of the latter triangle. Moreover, since the posterior triangle has no bony sides, the above statement is tantamount to saying that the possibility of delivery will depend, in good part, on the size of the altitude of the posterior triangle. In other words, as was true of midpelvic contraction, the degree to which outlet contraction may cause dystocia will depend, not on one measurement alone, but on two, the interischial tuberous diameter and the posterior sagittal diameter of the outlet.

This concept in regard to outlet contraction has been stated by Thoms as follows: Whenever the sum of the interischial tuberous diameter and the posterior sagittal diameter of the outlet is less than 15.0 cm., dystocia may result. It does not necessarily develop, of course, for it is quite possible for a mature infant to be delivered easily through an outlet in which the sum of these two diameters is only 13.0 cm. However, with a large baby and other unfavorable pelvic factors present, dystocia may very likely develop if the sum of these two diameters falls appreciably below 15 cm. As already stated, a loose relationship exists between the size of the outlet and that of the midpelvis; and there is increasing evidence that a contracted outlet may cause dystocia not so much on its own account as through the midpelvic contraction, which is very often an accompaniment.

Contractions of the pelvic outlet are seen with equal frequency in both white and colored women, the general incidence being between 3 and 5 per cent. Even when the disproportion is not sufficiently great to give rise to serious dystocia, it may play an important part in the production of perineal tears. In such cases, with the increasing narrowing of the pubic arch, the occiput cannot emerge directly beneath the symphysis pubis, and accordingly must stem itself further and further down upon the ischiopubic rami, and in extreme cases must rotate around a line joining the ischial tuberosities. Consequently, the perineum must become more and more dis-

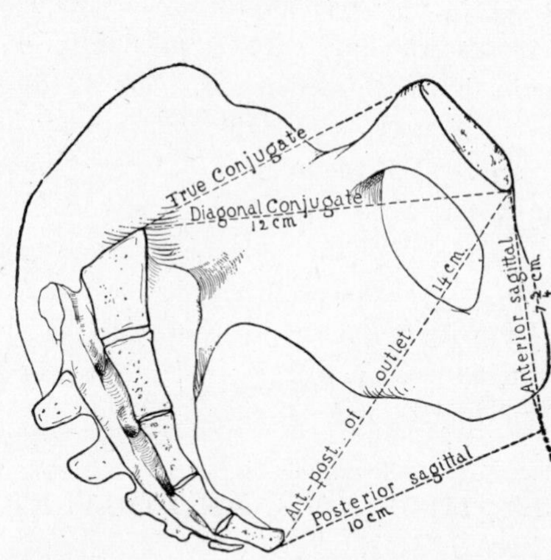

Fig. 451.—Diagram Showing the Significance of Anterior and Posterior Sagittal Diameters. × ⅓.

Spontaneous labor through a transverse diameter of 5.5 cm.

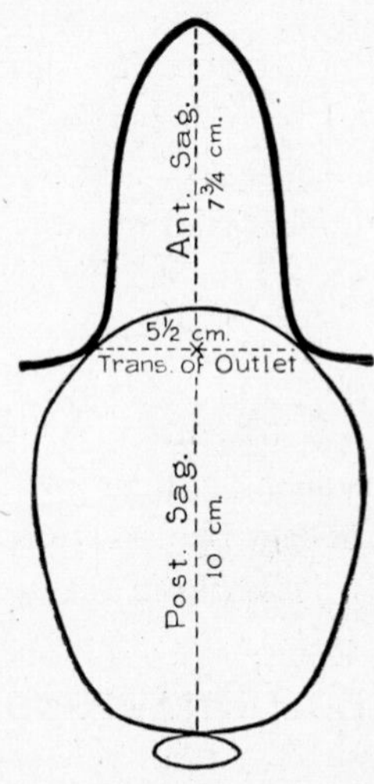

Fig. 452.—Diagram of Pelvic Outlet of Same Case, Illustrating Possibility of Spontaneous Labor Owing to Long Posterior Sagittal Diameter. × ⅓.

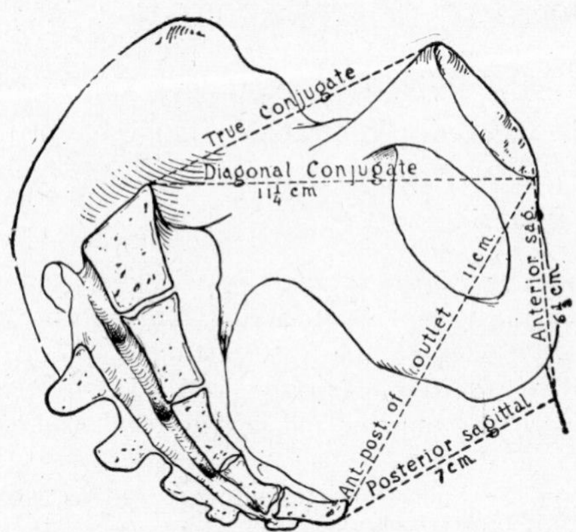

Fig. 453.—Diagram Showing the Significance of Anterior and Posterior Sagittal Diameters. × ⅓.

Cesarean section in spite of a transverse diameter of 6.5 cm.

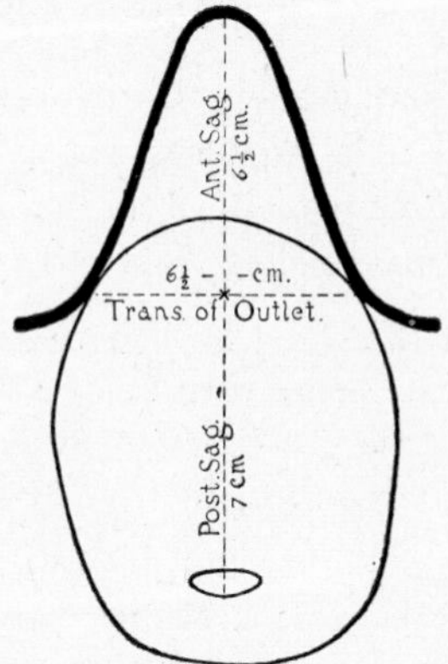

Fig. 454.—Diagram of Pelvic Outlet of Same Case, Illustrating Necessity for Cesarean Section. × ⅓.

tended, and thus be exposed to great danger of extensive rupture. Schumacher believes that this type of pelvis has a serious effect upon the mechanism of labor by hindering the anterior rotation of obliquely posterior occipital presentations, and states that it was present in one third of his cases of persistent deep transverse presentations.

In view of the frequency and practical significance of outlet contractions, palpation of the pubic arch, as described previously, should form an integral part of the preliminary examination of every pregnant woman. If any abnormality is detected the various diameters of the pelvic outlet should be carefully measured (see Fig. 196).

In general, it may be said that in multiparous women with a history of previous severe outlet dystocia, clear-cut outlet contraction may afford an indication in rare instances for cesarean section; while in women who have not been previously subjected to the final test of delivery through the birth canal, intelligent conduct of the second stage of labor is of the utmost importance. The necessity for the application of forceps increases. As the head is brought under the rami of the pubis, a deep episiotomy, frequently going below the level of the anus, lateral to the sphincter muscle, facilitates delivery and prevents the third degree lacerations of the perineum that so frequently develop in patients with funnel pelves. In rare instances an elective cesarean section may be definitely indicated; however, the rarity of such a procedure may be gathered from the fact that cesarean section on this indication was resorted to twice in 21,436 (ward) deliveries in the New York Lying-In Hospital.

COMBINATIONS OF INLET, MIDPELVIC AND OUTLET CONTRACTION

Combinations of inlet, midpelvic and outlet contraction are frequently seen and tend to aggravate the prognosis of labor in proportion to the additive effects which the several types of malformation may be expected to produce.

RARE TYPES OF PELVIC CONTRACTION

Transversely Contracted or Robert Pelvis. Imperfect development of both sacral alae produces a pelvis which is markedly contracted transversely; this is sometimes described as the *double Naegele pelvis,* but is more commonly known as the Robert pelvis. This variety is extremely rare.

In the pelvis described by Robert, both alae of the sacrum were lacking, and the innominate bones were firmly synostosed with the rudimentary sacrum. The anterior surface of the latter was convex in both directions. Owing to the imperfect development of the sacrum, the pelvis was markedly contracted transversely, and only slightly anteroposteriorly, the transverse and anteroposterior diameters of the superior and inferior straits measuring 7 and 9.7, and 5.1 and 10.6 cm., respectively.

Just as in the Naegele pelvis, two views are held as to its etiology; some consider it the result of a primary defect in the development of the sacral alae, while others, particularly Breus and Kolisko, hold that it is always the result of inflammatory processes. Indeed, bony union between the sacrum and innominate bones is not an essential characteristic, and is occasionally lacking, sometimes on one, much more rarely on both sides. Where there is a difference in the development of the alae on the two sides, it can readily be understood how an asymmetrically transverse contracted pelvis may result.

The diagnosis is readily made, all of the transverse external measurements being markedly shortened, while the external conjugate remains practically normal. Internal examination shows the conjugata vera to be only slightly changed, while it is hardly possible for the close approach of the ischial spines and tuberosities to one another to escape recognition. In all cases thus far reported the transverse narrowing of the pelvis was so great as to preclude the possibility of the birth of a living child per vaginam.

Split Pelvis. In rare instances union between the pubic bones at the symphysis does not occur, and the anterior portions of the pelvis gape widely (Fig. 457). This condition is usually associated with ectopia of the bladder and imperfect development

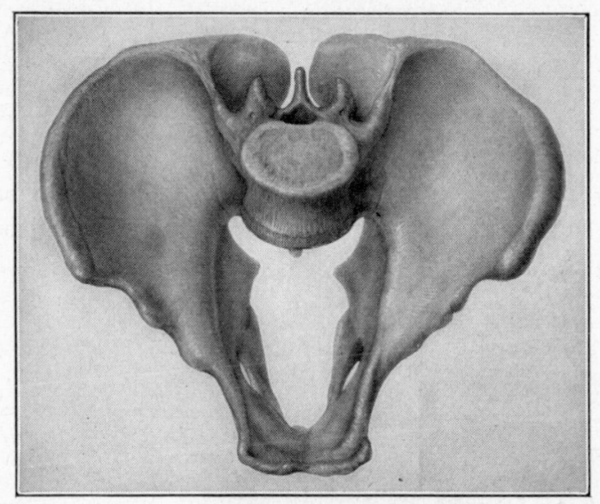

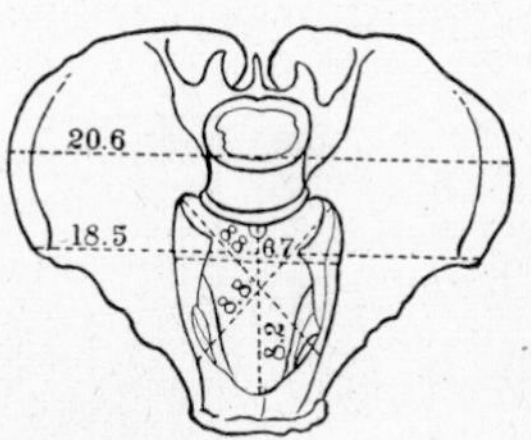

FIGS. 455, 456.—TRANSVERSELY CONTRACTED PELVIS (Robert).

of the lower portion of the anterior abdominal wall. As such abnormalities greatly diminish the probability of prolonged life, the condition is more common in young children than in adults. We are indebted to Litzmann for the first accurate description of a pelvis of this character from an obstetrical point of view.

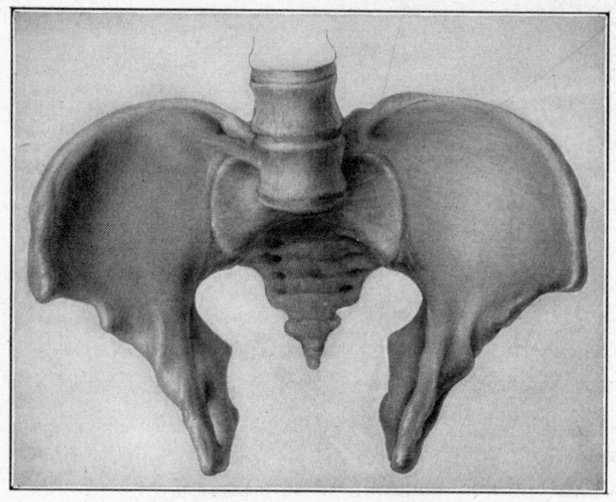

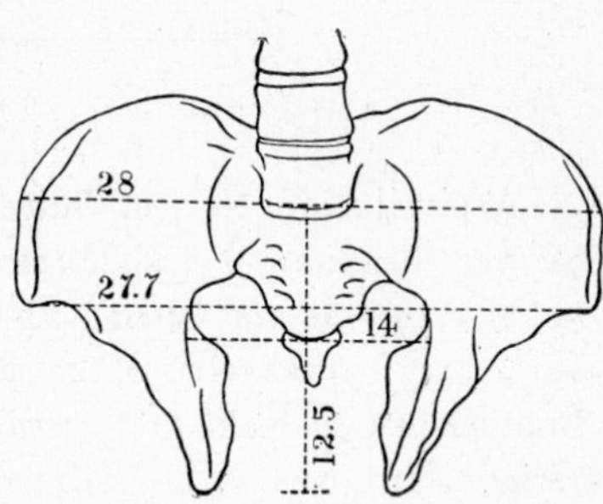

FIGS. 457, 458.—SPLIT PELVIS (Breus and Kolisko).

In the split pelvis, owing to the descent of the promontory of the sacrum and the absence of union at the symphysis, there is marked transverse widening of the posterior portion of the pelvis, while its anterior portions extend more or less parallel. External pelvimetry in such cases shows a pronounced flaring of the anterior superior spines of the ilium, and were the defective condition of the symphysis pubis not clearly evident a rachitic pelvis might be suspected.

The distance between the extremities of the pubic bones varies considerably, and occasionally is as great as 14 cm. This space is usually filled by a fibrinous band. For practical purposes the pelvis may be considered as generally enlarged, the dystocia being due to abnormalities of mechanism resulting from the absence of a resistant anterior pelvic wall. Gemmel and Paterson in 1913 described a remarkable case in which the entire generative tract as well as the bladder was doubled. In this patient successive pregnancies occurred in either uterus and all eventuated in spontaneous labor.

Imperfect Development of Vertebral Bodies of the Sacrum. Litzmann has described a remarkable pelvis in which almost the entire sacrum was lacking. This defect was associated with considerable transverse contraction, which increased as the inferior strait was being approached, the transverse diameter of the superior strait measuring 10.5 cm., while the distance between the ischial spines and ischial tuberosities was 6.5 and 8.5 cm., respectively (Fig. 459).

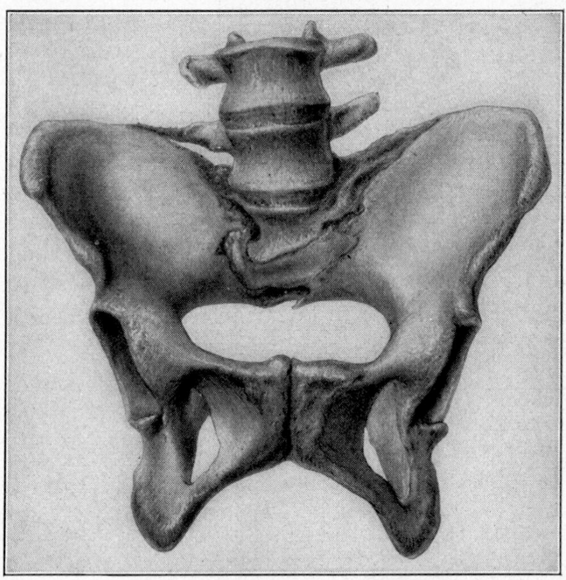

FIG. 459.—CONTRACTED PELVIS DUE TO ABSENCE OF BODIES OF SACRAL VERTEBRAE (Litzmann).

Assimilation Pelvis. Quite frequently the transverse processes of the last lumbar vertebra may be transformed into structures similar to the lateral masses of the sacral vertebrae and fused with them. In this event the former assumes the functions of the first sacral vertebra, the sacrum being now composed of six instead of five pieces. In other instances the first sacral vertebra may take on the characteristics of a lumbar vertebra and become assimilated to the lumbar column, so that there are six lumbar and only four sacral vertebrae. Occasionally the first coccygeal vertebra may become assimilated with the sacrum, but this has no effect upon the character of the pelvis. The assimilation pelvis is rarely a cause of dystocia.

Unless the entire vertebral column is available for study, it is frequently difficult to determine with which variety of assimilation one has to deal, as it is impossible to ascertain whether what corresponds to the first sacral vertebra is the twenty-fifth vertebra, as normal, or is the twenty-fourth or twenty-sixth vertebra, as the case may be.

Assimilation is the most common of all pelvic abnormalities, and is noted in at least every fifth or sixth pelvis; indeed, Paterson noted it in 38 per cent of all dried pelves which he studied. In a series of 217 Indian squaw pelves, Emmons found that its incidence was 21.7 per cent; while in the New York Lying-In Hospital McLane observed, by means of the x-ray, six sacral vertebrae in 24.4 per cent of a series of 164 cases studied.

When the last lumbar is assimilated with the first sacral vertebra—*high assimilation*—so that the sacrum consists of six pieces, important changes in the shape of the pelvis result, which depend in great part upon the manner in which the sacrum and innominate bones articulate, as well as upon the width of the former. In some cases the condition gives rise to a pelvis which is very high in its posterior portion, and whose superior strait is almost round, the walls of its inferior portion converging, thus producing a funnel-shaped pelvis. In other cases the condition gives rise to a pelvis

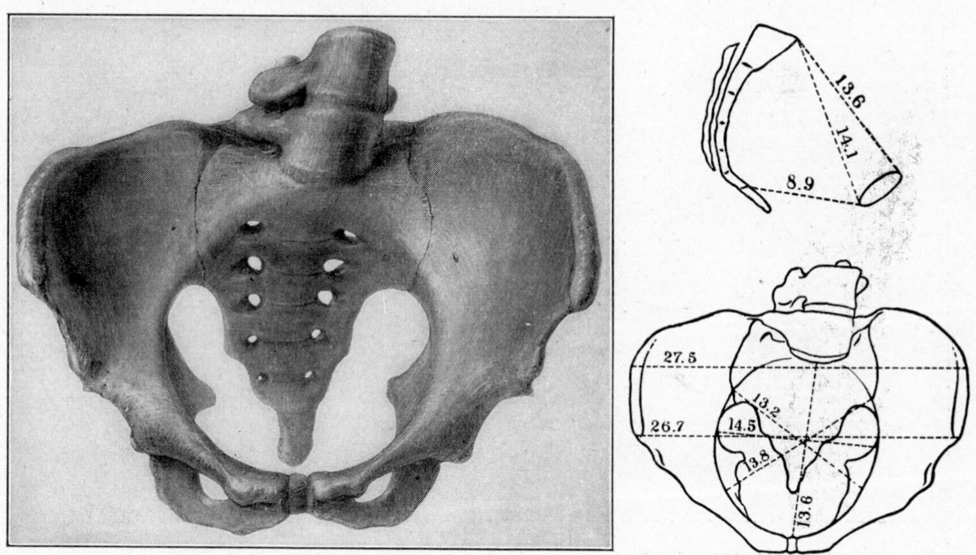

FIGS. 460, 461 AND 462.—HIGH ASSIMILATION PELVIS.

with a somewhat transversely contracted superior strait, in which the conjugata vera is either relatively or absolutely longer than the transverse diameter. Fabre and Bourret have carefully studied this type of pelvis from a clinical point of view, and state that it favors engagement of the head with the sagittal suture directed anteroposteriorly, instead of transversely or obliquely as usual; so that it should be regarded as an essential factor in the production of primary anterior or posterior occipital positions.

On the other hand, when the first sacral vertebra is assimilated with the lumbar column—*low assimilation*—a pelvis results which is very shallow in its posterior portion, but which offers no particular obstacle to labor.

Occasionally the assimilated vertebra may undergo only a partial change, one side of it retaining the characteristics of a lumbar or sacral vertebra, as the case may be, while the other side undergoes considerable modification. Under such circumstances asymmetric pelves result, which are frequently obliquely contracted and sometimes associated with scoliosis.

Obliquely Contracted or Naegele Pelvis. Naegele in 1803 was the first to recognize the significance of this variety of pelvis, and in 1839 published a monograph upon the subject based upon the study of 35 specimens, one of which had been obtained from an Egyptian mummy. Thomas in 1861 was able to collect from the literature a description of 50 such pelves. Since then, additional specimens have been described, Thoms having observed four during a relatively short period.

The Naegele pelvis presents the following characteristics: the sacral ala on one side is normal, while the other is either lacking or imperfectly developed, and the corresponding sacral foramina are smaller. In the great majority of cases the sacrum and the innominate bone are firmly synostosed on the affected side. At the same time, the latter is pushed upward and backward as well as inward from the region of the

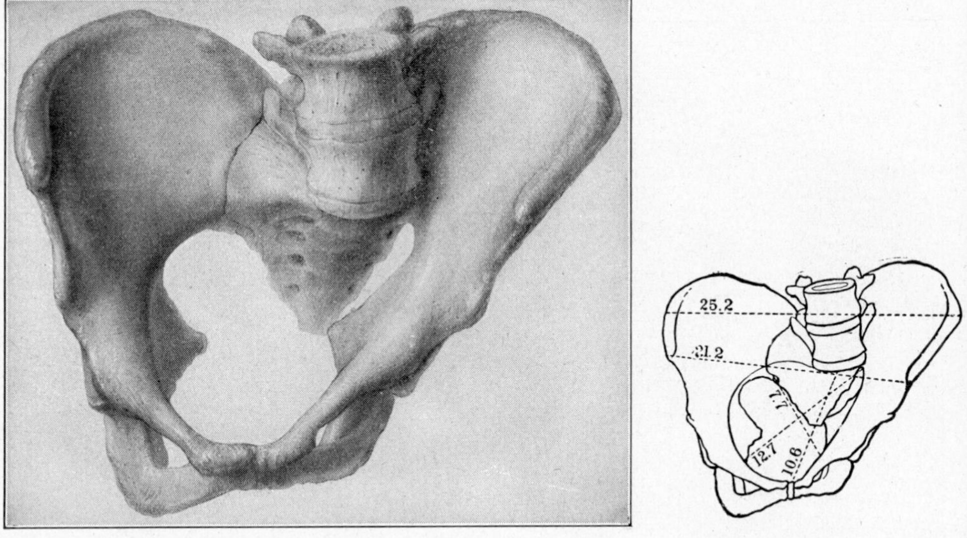

Figs. 463, 464.—Anterior View of Obliquely Contracted Pelvis (Naegele).

acetabulum, so that its crest is at a higher level than that of its fellow. The iliopectineal line is almost straight when the deformity is marked, while on the opposite side the curvature is accentuated, particularly in the anterior portion. Corresponding with the change in position of the innominate bone on the affected side, the ischial tuberosity and spine are displaced inward, upward, and backward, thereby approaching the outer margin of the sacrum and narrowing the sacrosciatic notch. The symphysis pubis is displaced toward the well side, while the pubic arch instead of facing directly forward is directed toward the abnormal side of the sacrum. The sacrum itself is displaced toward the ankylosed side, while its anterior surface is directed more or less obliquely toward it.

As a result of these changes the pelvis becomes obliquely contracted, the superior strait being ovate in shape, with its small pole directed toward the abnormal sacro-iliac joint and its large end toward the horizontal ramus of the pubis on the well side. Consequently, its oblique diameters are of unequal length, the shorter extending from the sacro-iliac synchondrosis of the well side to the iliopectineal eminence on the diseased side, while the conjugata vera is usually somewhat lengthened and is directed obliquely.

The walls of the pelvis converge below, so that the contraction involves the entire pelvic cavity, but is relatively greater in the plane of least pelvic dimensions, and in the inferior strait than at the superior strait. The acetabulum on the diseased side is directed more anteriorly, while that on the well side looks almost directly outward.

The distances from the promontory of the sacrum to the acetabulum and from the tip of the sacrum to the ischial spine are markedly diminished on the diseased side. At the same time, the distance between the tubera ischii of the diseased side and the opposite posterior superior spine is less than that between the tubera ischii of the well and the corresponding spine of the diseased side. Moreover, the tip of the spinous process of the last lumbar vertebra is nearer the anterior superior spine of the ilium on the diseased than on the well side, while the distance from the lower margin of the symphysis to the posterior superior spine is less upon the well side.

Mode of Production. The genesis of this variety of pelvic deformity has given rise to a great deal of discussion, some writers claiming that the defect in the sacrum is primary and the synostosis secondary; others, that the synostosis results primarily from inflammatory changes which bring about more or less destruction of the sacral ala. The present tendency is to regard the abnormality as the result of inflammatory processes about the sacro-iliac joint, and to consider the synostosis as entirely secondary. On the other hand, Williams and Thoms described cases supporting the idea of congenital origin. Furthermore, evidences of malformation in other parts of the body, as noted by Reinberger and others, suggest an embryonic origin. In general, it may be said that the congenital origin of the condition is tenable only when all signs of a previous osteitic process are lacking.

The mechanism by which the deformity is produced is as follows: owing to the asymmetry of the sacrum, there is a compensatory scoliosis of the lumbar portion of the vertebral column with its convexity on the diseased side. This causes the pelvis to assume an angle with the horizon, thereby bringing about a lowering of the acetabulum on the diseased side. As a consequence, greater pressure is exerted by the femur on that side, which gradually brings about an upward, backward, and inward displacement of the corresponding innominate bone. Owing to the increased pressure, the synovial membrane at the sacro-iliac synchondrosis gradually undergoes pressure necrosis, and synostosis eventually results.

Diagnosis. Generally speaking, the condition is readily recognizable, provided one's attention is directed to its possible existence. Unfortunately, such patients rarely limp, show no great external deformity and, as a rule, give no history suggestive of trouble at the sacro-iliac joint. Consequently, since the customary external measurements give no clue to its presence, the diagnosis of a justominor pelvis is usually made, unless the asymmetry of the outlet or the actual occurrence of dystocia leads one to make a more complete examination. On the other hand, the existence of scoliosis, a variation in the height of the hips, or a difference in the distance between the spine of the last lumbar vertebra and the posterior superior spine on either side, should cause one to suspect its possibility, when a radiogram will settle the question.

Naegele suggested five measurements which should be made in such cases: (1) from the tubera ischii of one side to the opposite posterior superior spine; (2) from the anterior superior spine of one side to the opposite posterior superior spine; (3) from the spine of the last lumbar vertebra to the anterior superior spine on either side; (4) from the trochanter to the opposite posterior superior spine; (5) from the lower margin of the symphysis pubis to the posterior superior spines on either side. Normally these various measurements should be the same on both sides, but they differ considerably in obliquely contracted pelves.

Owing to the difficulty of definitely locating their end points, the first, fourth, and fifth measurements are rarely employed; but the information obtained from the second and third is of very considerable value. A difference of more than 1 cm. between these measurements on the two sides indicates an obliquely contracted pelvis, but is not sufficient to enable one to differentiate between the Naegele and the other varieties. On internal examination the conjugata vera is not shortened, but on measuring the diagonal conjugate it is found that the symphysis pubis, instead of being situated directly in front of the promontory, lies considerably to one side of it. On palpation it is found that the sacrum is asymmetric, and that the lateral wall of the pelvis, as well as the ischial spine and tuberosity, approaches it much more closely on the diseased than on the opposite side, while the iliopectineal line is markedly flattened. At the same time, the distance between the tubera ischii is greatly diminished.

Effect upon Labor. When the deformity is pronounced, the side of the pelvis corresponding to the small end of the oval is so contracted as to be useless for the passage of the child, so that engagement, if it is to occur at all, must take place on the opposite side. In effect, the pelvic inlet becomes converted into one of the generally contracted type, and an idea of its available space is gained by measuring, not the conjugata vera, but the distance between the symphysis pubis and the sacro-iliac synchondrosis on the normal side. Owing to the contraction in the lower portion of the pelvis, still further difficulty is experienced when the head attempts to pass between the ischial spines and tuberosities and the possibility of delivery also depends upon the distance between these points.

Prognosis. If the deformity is pronounced the prognosis is bad, unless cesarean section is performed. The fact that the patient has previously had spontaneous labor does not necessarily imply that she will do likewise in the future. Williams' patient had given birth to six small children spontaneously, only to perish from rupture of the uterus at a seventh labor, when the child was 500 gm. heavier than any of her previous children.

Generally speaking, spontaneous labor is out of the question unless the short oblique diameter measures at least 8.5 cm., and even here the prognosis will depend upon the size of the child. Below this limit cesarean section is the only rational method of treatment provided the child is alive and the patient in good condition.

Osteomalacic Pelves. Inasmuch as osteomalacia gives rise to the most marked pelvic deformities with which we are familiar, it was only natural that the attention of obstetricians should have been directed to it at an early date. Cooper performed cesarean section for this condition in 1768, but for the main pioneer work we are indebted to Stein, Kilian, Litzmann and Maxwell and Miles.

Nature and Clinical History of Osteomalacia. Osteomalacia is a disease due to calcium deficiency, which manifests itself by neuritic changes, muscular atrophies, and particularly by characteristic changes in the bones, which become soft, yielding, and occasionally brittle, and consequently undergo marked changes in shape as the result of the action of the various mechanical forces to which they are subjected.

The disease is one of adult life, and is very rarely met with in children. It occurs far more frequently in women than in men, especially during pregnancy or the puerperium. It may occur in any part of the world, but is especially frequent, and may even be said to be endemic, in certain localities, notably in the Rhine Valley, the Ergolz Valley in Switzerland, the Olona Valley and Calabria in Italy, and in North China. It is very rarely observed in this country, England, or France.

No satisfactory explanation for its endemic occurrence has been adduced, although it seems to be intimately connected with unsanitary surroundings and dietary deficiency. Maxwell and Miles noted it in 1 to 3 per cent of the women in North China and consider it a diet deficiency disease probably due to a lack of fat-soluble vitamins and possibly of calcium itself. In 1934 Hannon and his co-workers studied the calcium, phosphorus and nitrogen metabolism in a case of early osteomalacia. They observed lack of absorption of calcium through the intestinal tract, with no increase in endogenous calcium excretion. They regard the absence of calcium excretion in the urine with a normal serum calcium as an attempt to conserve endogenous calcium elimination. Their patient received beneficial effect upon vitamin D, resulting in increased absorption of calcium with consequent calcium and phosphorus retention and deposition in the bone. Since 1934 additional studies have been reported by this group of investigators and in the last two of these, by Liu and associates, the observations have been extended to the period of lactation. This recent work has amply corroborated their original contention that the disease is associated with vitamin D deficiency and disturbed calcium and phosphorus metabolism. The causal relationship between osteomalacia in the mother and fetal rickets, first shown by Maxwell and his co-workers, has likewise been substantiated, as well as the fact that such fetal rickets can be influenced beneficially by vitamin D therapy administered to the mother.

Osteomalacia may affect any portion of the skeleton, but seems to select more particularly the pelvis, vertebrae, and ribs. The fresh bones are yellowish or yellowish-brown in appearance, and very soft and brittle. In advanced cases their consistence is that of leather or wax, so that they can readily be cut with a knife. In the later stages of the disease the

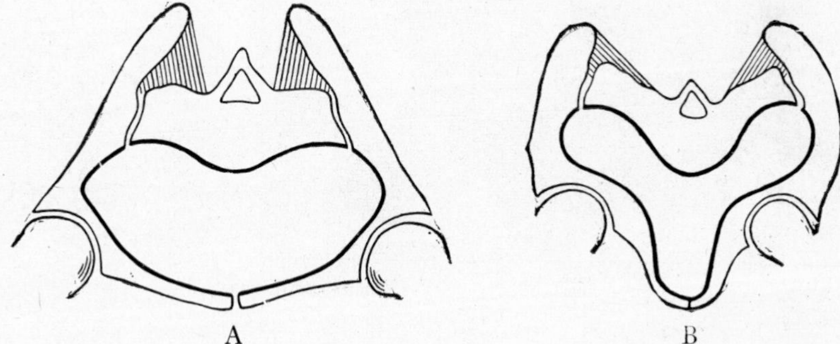

Fig. 465.—Diagrams Showing Changes in Shape in (A) Rachitic and (B) Osteomalacic Pelves (Schroeder).

spongy bones present a markedly areolated appearance on section, and in some instances are so rarefied that only the outer layers remain intact. At the same time they become much lighter, the specific gravity being frequently reduced by one half.

Under the microscope the marrow spaces are found to be greatly enlarged, and there is a marked increase in vascularity. The most important change, however, consists in the substitution of osteoid tissue in place of the true bone surrounding the haversian canals.

In its earliest stages it is characterized by peculiar muscular palsies, which more especially affect the iliopsoas, and which are often accompanied by contractions of the abductor muscles of the thigh and by increased patellar reflexes. A little later rheumatoid pains make their appearance in various portions of the body, and at the same time the pelvis, ribs, and vertebral column become very sensitive upon pressure. As the disease advances still further and the bones become softer, various deformities appear, which are particularly marked in the vertebral column and pelvis.

A history of rheumatoid pains and difficult locomotion requiring rest in bed during pregnancy, associated with a decrease in height, is almost pathognomonic of osteomalacia.

Changes in the Shape of the Pelvis. The extent of the deformity resulting from osteomalacia depends entirely upon the degree of softening which the various pelvic bones have undergone. According to Kehrer, in the early stages of the disease the pelvis is simply flattened as the result of the forcing downward and forward of the promontory of the sacrum.

In the later stages of the disease, when the bones have become very soft, the pelvis takes on a characteristic compressed appearance. The body weight presses the promontory still further downward and forward, while the upward and inward force exerted by the femora pushes the lateral walls of the pelvis inward, so that the superior strait assumes a trefoil appearance, and in extreme cases becomes almost

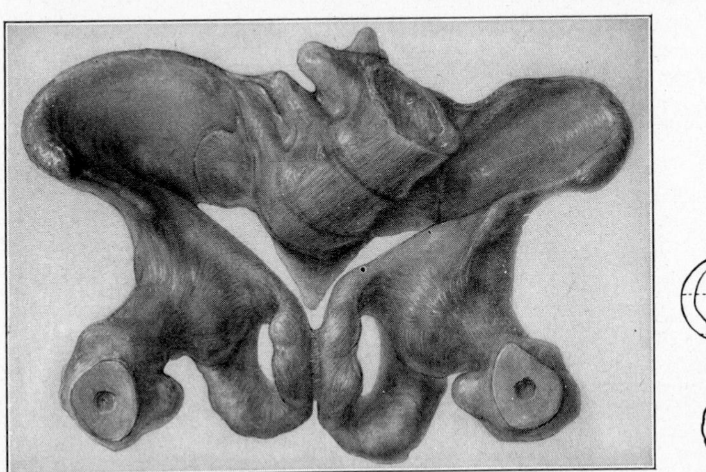

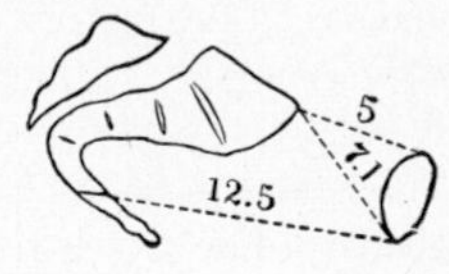

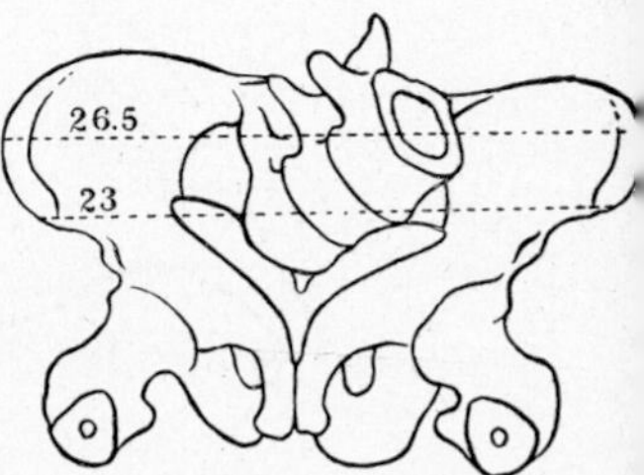

Figs. 466, 467 and 468.—Osteomalacic Pelvis.

entirely obliterated. At the same time the ischiopubic rami are approximated, and the pubic arch is converted into a narrow slit into which it is sometimes impossible to insinuate the fingers. The pubic rami are pushed markedly forward, giving rise to a beak-like protuberance upon the anterior wall of the pelvis. Coincident with these

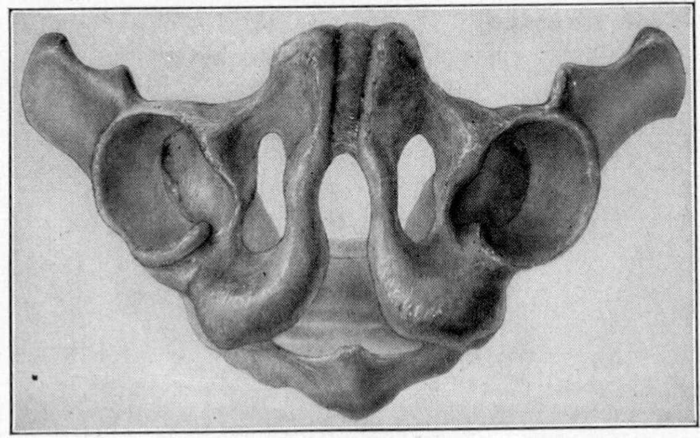

Fig. 469.—Osteomalacic Pelvis, Inferior Strait. × 0.28.

changes, there is a marked diminution in the size of the pelvic cavity and of the inferior strait, though in not a few cases, owing to constant sitting upon the softened bones, the tubera ischii are relatively flared out. In advanced cases the very deformed pelvis may present any one of an almost infinite variety of bizarre shapes.

Diagnosis. The diagnosis is readily made, as careful inquiry will usually elicit the characteristic clinical history of the disease; while examination of the pelvis will show that it is markedly compressed in all directions, and the pathognomonic changes in the pubic arch can hardly escape detection. Indeed, the only form of pelvis with which it might be confounded is the very rare transversely contracted Robert pelvis, but the clinical history and the lack of anteroposterior shortening in the latter will usually enable one to differentiate between them.

Pelvic Anomalies Secondary to Abnormalities of the Vertebral Column

Kyphosis or humpback, the result of spinal caries, plays an important part in the production of pelvic abnormalities for, when situated in the lower portion of the vertebral column, it is usually associated with a characteristically funnel-shaped distortion.

Kyphotic Pelvis. The effect exerted upon the pelvis by kyphosis differs according to its location. When the gibbus or hump is situated in the thoracic region, it is usually compensated for by pronounced lordosis beneath it, so that the pelvis itself is but little changed. On the other hand, when situated at the junction of the thoracic and lumbar portions of the vertebral column its effect upon the pelvis becomes manifest, and is still further accentuated when the kyphosis is lower down, being most marked when it is at the lumbosacral junction. If the vertebral caries is in the latter region the upper arm of the gibbus may overlie the inlet and give rise to *pelvis obtecta,* as shown in Fig. 472.

Characteristics. The characteristic feature of the kyphotic pelvis is a retropulsion and rotation of the sacrum, by which the promontory becomes displaced backward and the tip forward. At the same time, the entire bone becomes elongated vertically, and narrowed from side to side. These changes are associated with a rotation of each innominate bone about an axis, which extends through the symphysis pubis and either sacro-iliac articulation, so that the iliac fossae become flared outward while the lower portions of the ischial bones are turned in toward the middle line.

When the kyphosis is in the dorsolumbar region, marked lordosis below it indicates an attempt at compensation, but as this is imperfect, the body weight is transmitted to the sacrum in such a manner that the latter becomes retroposed and lengthened, its promontory being farther backward and at a higher level than usual. At the same time, its anterior surface loses its normal vertical concavity and becomes straight or even convex, while its lateral concavity is obliterated by the projection of the vertical bodies beyond the alae. The bodies themselves are considerably narrower than usual, and the alae of the first sacral vertebra appear to be drawn out and to extend obliquely upward to the promontory.

Owing to its backward displacement the posterior surface of the sacrum approaches the superior posterior spines of the ilium, thereby relaxing the iliosacral ligaments. As a result, the posterior extremities of the innominate bones are pushed apart, and their upper portions rotate outward and the lower portions inward, so that the crests are flared out and occupy a lower level than usual, while the ischial spines and tuberosities approach the middle line. This tendency is still further accentuated by the increased tension exerted by the iliofemoral ligaments resulting from a diminution of the pelvic inclination. The acetabula also are shifted slightly and look more to the front than usual. Coincident with the displacement of the sacrum, the iliopectineal line becomes longer, particularly in its iliac portion.

These changes give rise to a funnel-shaped pelvis, in which, as the result of the increased length of the conjugata vera, the superior strait becomes round or oval in shape, with the long diameter running anteroposteriorly, while the transverse diameter remains unchanged or may even be shorter than usual. There is also a gradual diminution of all the anteroposterior diameters of the pelvis below the superior strait, but the most characteristic change is the shortening of the distance between the ischial spines, and to a somewhat less extent of that between the ischial tuberosities.

Mode of Production. A kyphosis in the dorsal region is usually compensated for by a marked lordosis below it, so that the body weight is transmitted to the sacrum in the usual manner. On the other hand, when the hump is situated lower down, the body weight is transmitted through its upper limb, and on reaching the gibbus becomes re-

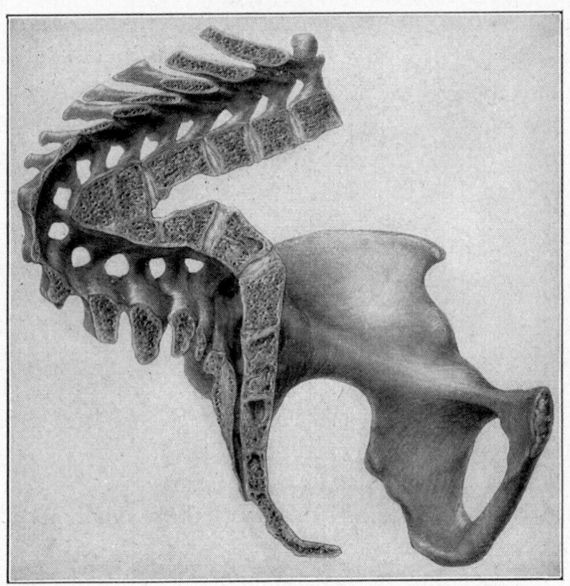

Fig. 470.—Longitudinal Section through Pelvis and Spinal Column in Dorsolumbar Kyphosis (Breus and Kolisko).

solved into two components, one of which is directed downward and the other backward. This latter force draws the promontory of the sacrum backward and upward, thus leading to rotation and elongation of the entire bone.

Diagnosis. The diagnosis is usually easy, for the external deformity is readily visible and should at once suggest the possible existence of a funnel pelvis.

External pelvimetry is of great value, for in pronounced cases it shows that the distance between the iliac crests is equal to or exceeds that between the trochanters, whereas normally the reverse is true. Consequently, in a patient suffering from this deformity, lines drawn through the iliac crests and trochanters will meet somewhere in the neighborhood of the feet, instead of near the head as is the case in normal women.

On palpation of the pubic arch the transverse narrowing of the pelvic outlet will be noted, while internal examination will reveal the lengthening of the conjugata vera. In lumbosacral kyphosis the promontory no longer exists, and the bodies of the lower lumbar vertebrae overhang the superior strait. Accordingly, in this type of deformity particular attention should be devoted to the length of the "pseudoconjugate"—the distance from the upper margin of the symphysis pubis to the nearest portion of the vertical column. Occasionally the condition may be confounded with spondylolisthesis, and the differential diagnosis will be considered under the latter heading.

Effect upon Labor. The mechanical conditions favor abnormal positions of the fetus, and Klien, in 100 longitudinal presentations, found 90 vertex, 4 face, and 6 breech presentations.

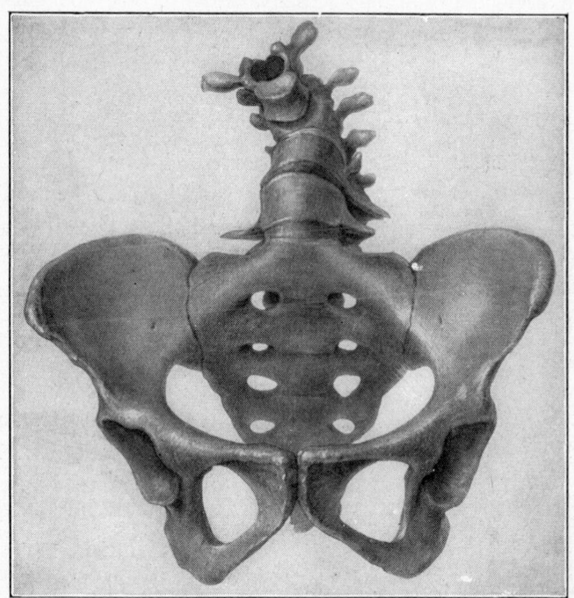

Fig. 471.—Kyphotic Pelvis Showing Elongation of Conjugata Vera.

It is interesting to note that left occipito-anterior presentations occur in only one third of the cases, while in the other two thirds right anterior and posterior presentations are encountered with equal frequency. It is difficult to give a satisfactory explanation for the unusual frequency of the right anterior position, but the production of posterior positions is attributed to the pendulous abdomen, for in such circumstances

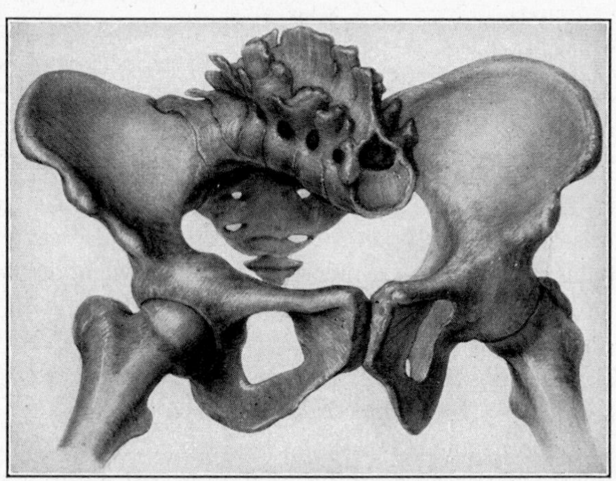

Fig. 472.—Pelvis Obtecta (Fehling).

the concave ventral surface of the child tends to apply itself to the convex inner surface of the anterior wall of the uterus.

Except in pelvis obtecta, or in patients presenting a very pendulous abdomen, the presenting part experiences no difficulty in entering the superior strait at the time of labor, and no obstacle is met with until it reaches the neighborhood of the ischial spines. If the transverse contraction in that locality is not too marked to prevent descent, further difficulty is encountered when the head reaches the pelvic outlet, for owing to the approach of the tubera ischii, the pubic arch has become more angular than usual, so that the head is prevented from filling it out and must descend lower than usual in order to be born. This fact readily explains the deep perineal tears so frequently observed.

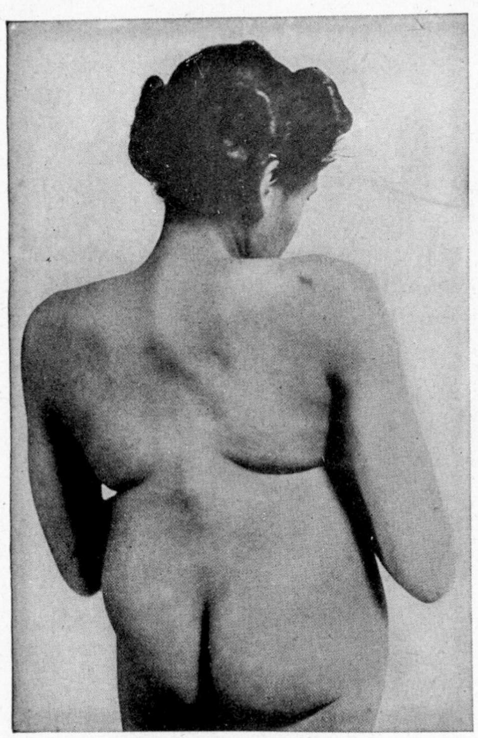

Fig. 473.—Patient with Obliquely Contracted Kyphotic, Funnel Pelvis.

Note presence of double gibbus. The lumbosacral one is concerned in producing the funnel pelvis.

Generally speaking, it may be said that when the distance between the tubera ischii is less than 8 cm. labor becomes difficult or impossible, according to the degree of transverse contraction of the outlet. In such cases the dystocia is more pronounced than in typical funnel pelves presenting identical measurements, for the reason that the anterior displacement of the tip of the sacrum is inevitably associated with shortening of the posterior sagittal diameter. Owing to the narrowing of the pubic arch, occipito-anterior are less favorable than occipito-posterior presentations, since in the latter, the smaller brow, instead of the wider biparietal, accommodates itself to the pubic arch. According to Klien face presentations are still more favorable for the same reason, a belief shared by others.

Effect upon Heart. Because of the dramatic pelvic changes which may accrue when the gibbus of kyphoscoliosis is located in the lumbar region, the error may be made of neglecting the grave effects which kyphoscoliosis often exerts upon the heart. In 50 fatal cases of kyphoscoliosis associated with pregnancy, collected by Jensen, at least 31 were due to heart failure—far more than were caused by pelvic dystocia.

Owing to the collapse of the vertebral column, the volume of the thoracic cage in thoracic kyphoscoliosis is diminished, with consequent pressure exerted on the lungs and heart. As a result, the vital capacity is decreased to one-half the normal value, as shown by the studies of Chapman, Dill, and Graybiel. This reduction applies to both the absolute and relative vital capacity. Thus, in 5 patients with thoracic kyphoscoliosis studied by them, it was found that the vital capacity constituted from 35 to 53 per cent of the total lung volume in these patients, whereas in the normals studied the amount was 57 to 69 per cent of the total. The ratio of residual air to vital capacity was 1.3 in kyphoscoliotic patients and 0.6 in the normal subjects. In other words, in these deformed women the usual mechanism of respiration is altered by the great limitation of costal movement. The ribs move only ineffectively, and breathing is accomplished largely by movements of the diaphragm. Partial collapse and infection are but natural results of these poorly aerated lungs.

Chapman, Dill, and Graybiel believe that the hypertrophy and ultimate failure of the right ventricle which are observed in these patients result from the increased work and pressure which have to be maintained by the right ventricle in order to support the arterial oxygenation through the cramped and undeveloped lungs. The important injunction here is simply to be aware of the cardiac hazard which these patients face in pregnancy. Hence special cardiac evaluation is indicated in this group of women.

Prognosis. All in all, the kyphoscoliotic patient is a poor subject for childbearing. If the condition is entirely thoracic, cardiac complications are a threat; if entirely lumbar, midpelvic contraction is common and, if low down, may be extreme; while in the cases in which the gibbus is thoracolumbar, both heart and pelvis may be sources of trouble; and in any type of the disease, faulty alignment of the uterus with the birth canal may cause uterine inertia.

Treatment. When the distance between the spines and tuberosities of the ischium does not fall below 8 cm., spontaneous labor, or at least a probable delivery with low or midforceps, can be looked for, provided the posterior sagittal diameter is not too shortened; but when the measurements are below this limit operative interference becomes necessary. Unless the child is very small, elective cesarean section is the operation of choice. If, however, the patient is not seen until late in labor, and the child is already dead, craniotomy is indicated.

Kyphorachitic Pelvis. Kyphosis is nearly always of carious origin, but when due to rachitis it is usually associated with a greater or lesser degree of scoliosis. In the rare cases of pure rachitic kyphosis, however, the pelvic changes are slight, as the effect of the kyphosis is counterbalanced to a great extent by that of the rachitis, the former leading to an elongation and the latter to a shortening of the conjugata vera, while tending, respectively, to narrow and to widen the inferior strait. Thus it may happen that a woman presenting a markedly deformed vertebral column of this character may have a practically normal pelvis. The two processes, however, do not always counteract each other and, as a rule, when the kyphosis is high up the pelvic changes are predominantly rachitic.

Scoliotic Pelvis. Pronounced scoliosis, or lateral curvature of the spine, is usually of rachitic origin; but minor degrees of the deformity are often observed which have no connection with rickets. When the scoliosis involves the upper portion of the vertebral column, it is usually compensated for by a corresponding curvature in the opposite direction lower down, thus giving rise to a double or S-shaped curve. In such cases the body weight is transmitted to the sacrum in the usual manner, so that the pelvis is not implicated. But when the scoliosis is lower down and involves the lumbar regions, the sacrum takes part in the compensatory process and accordingly assumes an abnormal position which leads to slight asymmetry of the pelvis.

Kyphoscoliotic Pelvis. In this type, the distortion of the pelvis will vary according to whether the kyphosis or the scoliosis is the predominant factor in the deformity of the spinal column. When the former is more pronounced the pelvis will partake of the kyphotic character, and vice versa. When the two deformities are approximately equal, however, the kyphotic changes in the pelvis predominate, although the influence of the scoliosis tends to counteract, to a certain extent, the transverse narrowing of the inferior strait.

Kyphoscoliorachitic Pelvis. This variety of pelvic deformity has been studied more particularly by Leopold and Barbour. As has already been pointed out, a kyphosis due to rachitis is nearly always complicated by a scoliosis and the latter usually predominates in the production of the pelvic deformity, for the reason that the kyphosis and the rachitis tend mutually to counteract each other in their effect upon the pelvis. Accordingly, the resulting pelvis does not differ materially from

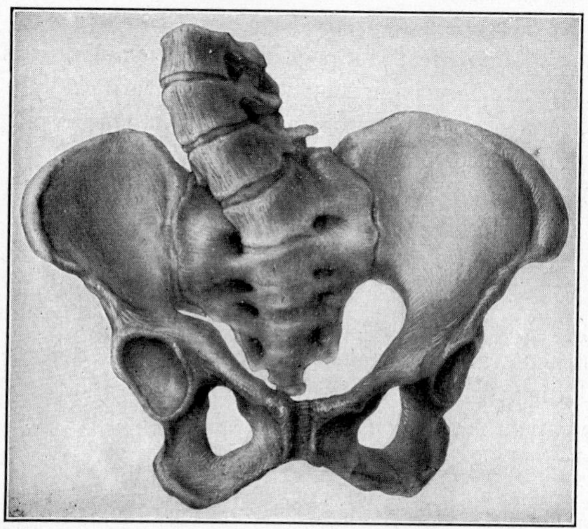

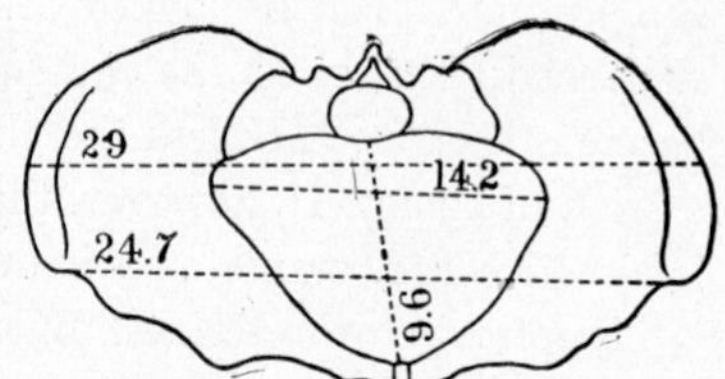

FIGS. 474, 475.—KYPHOSCOLIORACHITIC PELVIS (Leopold).

that observed in scoliorachitis, except that the tendency to anteroposterior flattening is partially counteracted by the action of the kyphotic vertebral column. Nevertheless, owing to the presence of the scoliosis, the oblique deformity of the superior strait is usually quite marked. Generally speaking, this type of pelvis is more favorable from an obstetrical standpoint than that due to scoliorachitis alone.

Spondylolisthetic Pelvis. The term spondylolisthesis (from σπόνδυλος, vertebra, and ὀλισθησις, slipping or sliding) was introduced by Kilian in 1853, in describing a pelvis in which the last lumbar vertebra had become displaced downward over the anterior surface of the sacrum.

Characteristics. The degree of displacement may vary greatly. When the deformity is slight the anterior inferior margin of the last lumbar vertebra merely projects a short distance beyond the anterior margin of the promontory of the sacrum; in pronounced cases the entire body of the vertebra is displaced downward and forward into the pelvic cavity, so that its inferior surface comes in contact with, and more or less completely covers, the body of the first, and occasionally that of the second, sacral vertebra. As a consequence, a greater or lesser portion of the lumbar column comes to occupy the upper portion of the pelvic cavity, the superior strait becoming markedly obstructed and assuming a reniform shape.

The lower lumbar vertebrae may overhang the pelvic inlet to such an extent that the obstetrical or pseudoconjugate will be represented by a line drawn from the upper margin of the symphysis to the lower margin of the fourth, third, or even of the second lumbar vertebra, as the case may be. The displacement of the last lumbar vertebra is due not to luxation, but to the lengthening and bending of its interarticular portions. Its inferior articular processes still retain their normal relation to the superior articular processes of the first sacral vertebra, whereas its body and its superior articular processes, together with the rest of the vertebral column, become displaced forward and eventually downward. As a result of the new position assumed by the body of the last lumbar vertebra, the superior and anterior surfaces of the promontory become worn away by friction, the defect being frequently followed by ankylosis which definitely checks further displacement. In advanced cases the inferior articular processes of the last lumbar and the superior articular processes of the first sacral vertebra are usually firmly synostosed together, as are also the inferior articular processes of the fourth and the superior articular processes of the fifth lumbar vertebra.

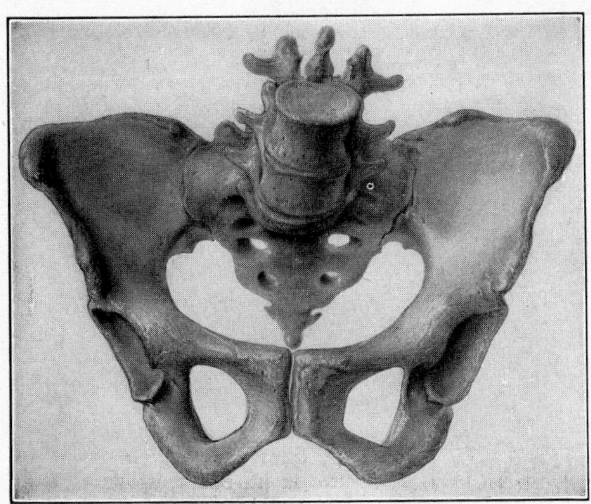

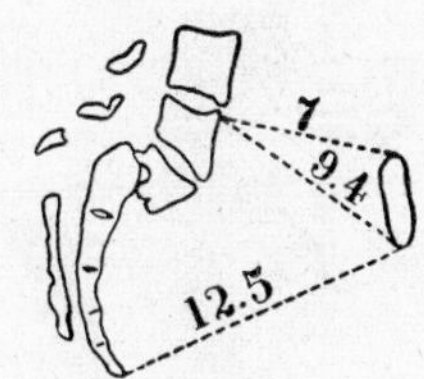

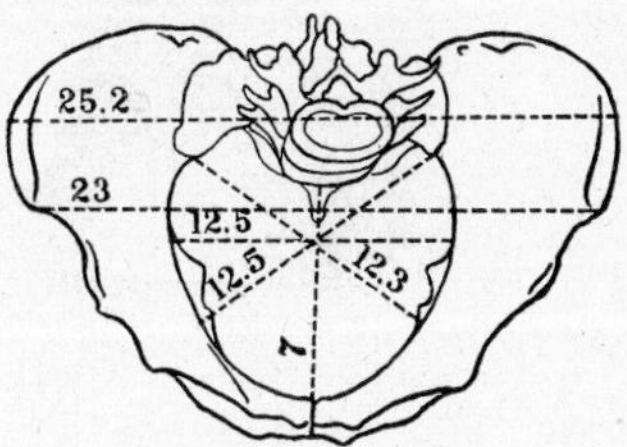

FIGS. 476, 477 AND 478.—WILLIAMS' SPONDYLOLISTHETIC PELVIS. (See Figs. 479, 480.)

Owing to the collapse of the vertebral column into the pelvic cavity, the center of gravity falls in front of instead of just behind the acetabula, and consequently the pelvis must be tilted backward in order that the individual may retain an upright position. In other words, the pelvic inclination must be diminished, and when the deformity is marked, the plane of the superior strait becomes parallel to, or even forms an obtuse angle with, the horizon. This is rendered possible by changes in the iliofemoral ligaments, which are manifested on the one hand by a marked roughening of the portions of the pelvis to which they are attached, and on the other by characteristic changes in the gait of the patient.

Since the inferior surface of the last lumbar vertebra is in contact with the anterior instead of the superior surface of the first sacral vertebra, the action of the body weight tends to force the promontory of the sacrum backward, thereby causing it to rotate about its transverse axis, so that its tip approaches the lower margin of the symphysis pubis. This rotation, together with the increased traction exerted by the iliofemoral ligaments, causes each innominate bone to rotate about an axis extending from the symphysis to the sacro-iliac joint, and tends to give the pelvis a funnel shape, just as in kyphosis, the inferior strait becoming contracted both transversely and anteroposteriorly.

Etiology. Neugebauer showed conclusively that in the vast majority of cases the deformity was rendered possible by a lengthening and thinning out of the interarticular portions of the last lumbar vertebra, by which its superior and inferior articular processes become separated by a long, thin lamina of bone instead of being almost in the same vertical line

(Fig. 480). This condition he attributed to imperfect development of the interarticular portion (spondylolysis) or to its fracture, with subsequent stretching of the callus. He considered that the former was the more frequent cause, as he was able to demonstrate it in many vertebrae which presented no signs of spondylolisthesis. Chiari has shown that it can occasionally follow fracture of the articular processes without the characteristic changes in the vertebra. At the same time, he considered that spondylolysis is the usual cause.

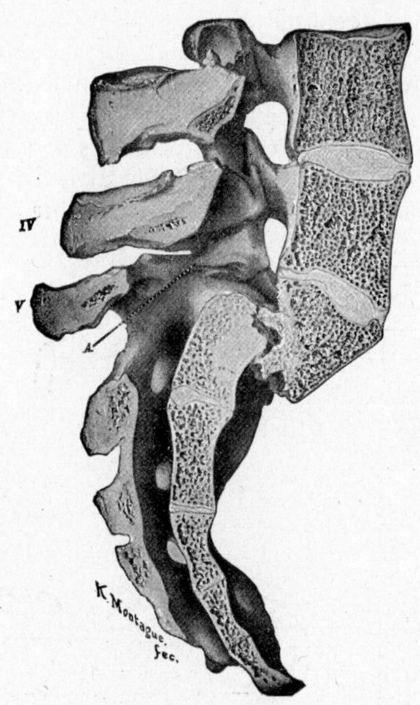

FIG. 479.—SPONDYLOLISTHESIS; VERTICAL SECTION THROUGH LAST THREE LUMBAR VERTEBRAE AND SACRUM. × ½. (Williams' Case.)

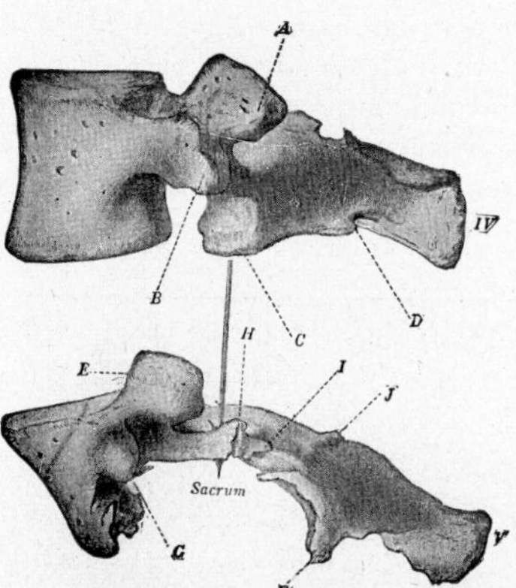

FIG. 480.—FOURTH AND FIFTH LUMBAR VERTEBRAE FROM WILLIAMS' CASE OF SPONDYLOLISTHESIS. × ½.

A, superior articular process; *B*, transverse process; *C*, inferior articular process; *D*, lamina of fourth lumbar vertebra; *E*, superior articular process; *F*, inferior articular process; *G*, transverse process; *H*, *I*, *J*, fissures in inter-articular portion of last lumbar vertebra. (See Fig. 479.)

Frequency. Neugebauer in 1893 was able to collect 115 cases of spondylolisthesis, most of which were clinical observations. In 1899 Williams collected 123 cases, which Chiari in 1912 increased to 150, including 17 cases occurring in males—11.3 per cent. According to Breus and Kolisko, only 20 indisputable anatomic specimens of this condition were in existence in 1900, including 2 which they described for the first time. In about 20,000 consecutive deliveries Stander had one spondylolisthetic pelvis, proven by x-ray as well as by clinical manifestations (Figs. 481, 482).

Effect upon Labor. When the condition is but slightly marked, its effect upon labor is similar to that of a flat pelvis, for the greatest contraction is in the conjugata vera, although it should be remembered that it is likewise associated with considerable contraction of the inferior strait. When the deformity is pronounced and the lower lumbar vertebrae overhang the superior strait, the degree of contraction, from an obstetrical point of view, is to be reckoned not by the distance between the symphysis pubis and the anterior portion of the last lumbar vertebra, but by the length of the pseudoconjugate, whose posterior extremity may be the fourth, third, or even second lumbar vertebra, and in many cases is so short as absolutely to preclude the possibility of the head entering the pelvis.

Diagnosis. In typical cases mere inspection of the patient should lead one to suspect the existence of this deformity, inasmuch as there is always marked lumbar lordosis and the entire trunk seems to have caved in, so that the ribs may come almost in contact with the iliac crests. When viewed from the front the abdominal walls usually appear redundant. Such patients have a peculiar ducklike or waddling gait, to which Neugebauer first directed attention. Since the posterior portion of the last lumbar vertebra retains its normal position while the rest of the vertebral column sinks forward, its spinous process will sometimes form a marked prominence just above the sacrum. The condition, however, may be confounded with a deep-seated kyphosis.

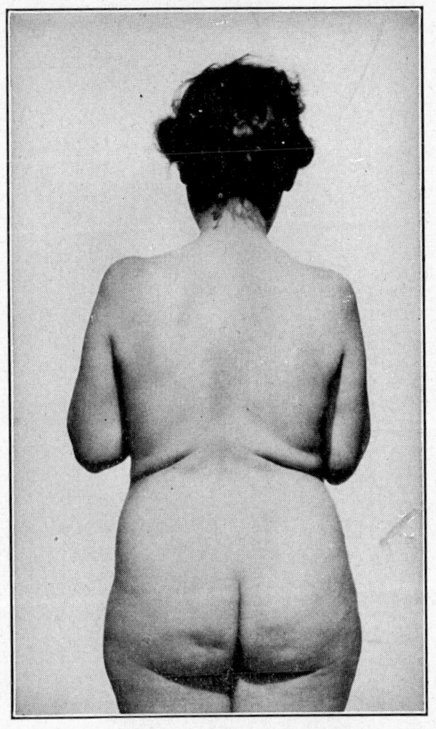

FIG. 481.—BACK VIEW OF WOMAN WITH SPONDYLOLISTHESIS.

Note depression in lumbar area. (Courtesy of Dr. H. C. Williamson.)

On internal examination the diagnosis, as a rule, is readily made. On attempting to measure the diagonal conjugate, the body of the last lumbar vertebra will be found lying in front of the anterior and upper portion of the sacrum. At the same time the iliopectineal line ends abruptly at the margins of the overhanging vertebral body, instead of continuing uninterruptedly to the promontory of the sacrum.

Owing to the marked lordosis, which frequently accompanies the condition, the bodies of the lower lumbar vertebrae can readily be palpated and counted, and the bifurcation of the aorta, or at least the common iliac arteries, are frequently readily accessible to the examining finger.

Occasionally, pronounced rachitic changes in the sacrum may simulate spondylolisthesis, but a correct diagnosis can usually be arrived at. In such cases, careful palpation, under anesthesia if necessary, will show that the ileopectineal lines terminate at the promontory of the sacrum instead of at the sides of the prolapsed body of the last lumbar vertebra.

A somewhat similar condition is presented in certain cases of lumbosacral kyphosis, particularly in the pelvis obtecta. Under such circumstances the promontory of the sacrum is destroyed, but a correct diagnosis can usually be made by carefully palpating the anterior surface of the sacrum and tracing the alae to the body of the first vertebra, which, of course, is impossible in spondylolisthesis. The x-ray is a valuable aid in diagnosis.

Prognosis. Generally speaking, spontaneous labor can occur only when the deformity is minimal, and accordingly, in pronounced cases the outlook is uniformly bad for both mother and child unless radical operative measures are undertaken. Other things being equal, a spondylolisthetic pelvis offers a worse prognosis than a rachitic one with the same anteroposterior measurements, for the reason that in the former the inferior strait is also contracted, while in the latter it is usually enlarged.

In considering the probable outcome of labor, one should measure the pseudoconjugate with particular care, inasmuch as it usually offers the greatest obstacle to labor. The fact that a patient with spondylolisthesis has had one or more spontaneous labors does not necessarily imply that the labor in question will be uneventful, for the

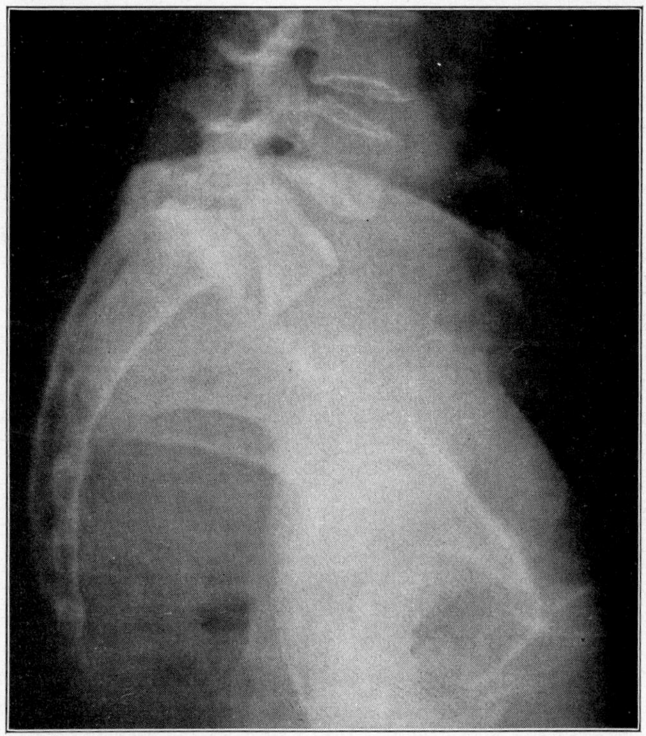

Fig. 482.—Roentgenogram of Spondylolisthesis, Lateral View, Showing Forward Displacement of Lower Lumbar Vertebrae. (Same case as Fig. 481.)

reason that the degree of deformity frequently increases with age, as happened in a patient of Williams.

Treatment. With a pseudoconjugate of more than 8 cm., the possibility of spontaneous labor should be borne in mind; but when it falls below that limit, cesarean section should be done at an appointed time.

Pelvic Anomalies Due to Abnormal Forces Exerted by Femurs

Normally, in the case of an individual standing erect, the upward and inward force exerted by the femurs is of equal intensity on either side, and is transmitted to the pelvis through the acetabula. In walking or running, the entire body weight is transmitted alternately first to one and then to the other leg. On the other hand, in a person suffering from disease affecting one leg, the sound one has to bear more than its share of the body weight, and consequently the upward and inward force exerted by the femur is, as a rule, greater upon that side of the pelvis. To these mechanical factors are due the changes in shape which accompany certain forms of lameness, provided the lesion, which gives rise to the latter, appears at an early period of life while the pelvic bones are still in a formative state.

The defect may be either unilateral or bilateral; in the former case it is usually due to coxitis, luxation of the femur, infantile paralysis, or shortening of one leg from various causes, while in the latter case common causes are luxation of both femurs and double clubfoot.

Pelvic Deformities Due to Unilateral Lameness. *Coxalgic Pelvis.* Coxitis occurring in early life nearly always gives rise to an obliquely contracted pelvis. If the disease makes its appearance before the patient learns to walk, or if the child is obliged to keep to its bed for a prolonged period, the entire organism may suffer

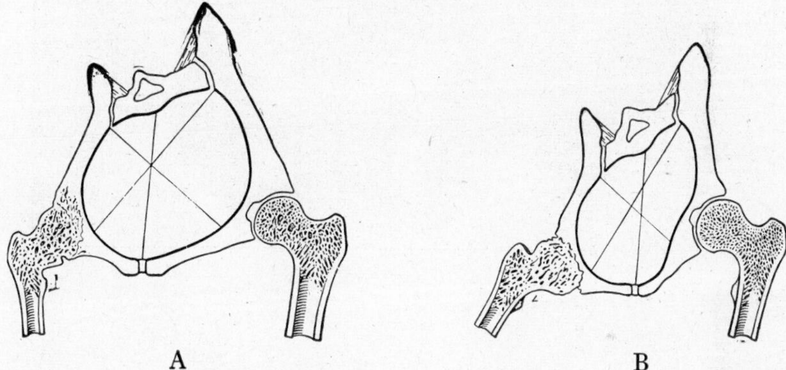

FIG. 483.—DIAGRAM SHOWING COXALGIC PELVIS, A, BEFORE AND B, AFTER THE INDIVIDUAL HAS WALKED.

from imperfect development, which also manifests itself in the pelvis and leads to the production of the generally contracted, or justo-minor type, to which are added the mechanical effects and atrophic changes resulting from the unilateral disease. These are manifested by imperfect development of the diseased side of the pelvis, the innominate bone being smaller than its fellow and the iliopectineal line forming the arc of a circle having a smaller radius than upon the well side. At the same time, the sacral alae are less developed upon the affected side, and the entire bone is somewhat rotated about its vertical axis, so that its anterior surface looks toward the well side.

When the individual begins to stand, the body weight is transmitted in great part to the well leg, owing to the actual shortening of the diseased leg or to fear of placing it firmly upon the ground. As a result, the pelvis becomes obliquely tilted, being higher on the well side, and a compensatory scoliosis appears. At the same time, the upward and inward force exerted by the normal femur tends to push that side of the pelvis upward, inward, and backward, whereby the iliopectineal line is markedly flattened and the asymmetry of the sacrum still further increased, thus giving rise to an obliquely contracted pelvis. The contraction is not limited to the superior strait, but involves also the lower portion of the pelvis, the spine and tuberosity of the ischium being displaced toward the midline, resulting in an oblique contraction of the pelvic outlet.

Not uncommonly these changes are accompanied by irritative processes at the sacro-iliac articulations, which may eventually lead to ankylosis. As a general rule, the oblique contraction is to be found on the well side of the pelvis but, according to Tarnier and Briggs, the reverse is the case when the affected leg is ankylosed in a position of adduction and internal rotation (Fig. 484).

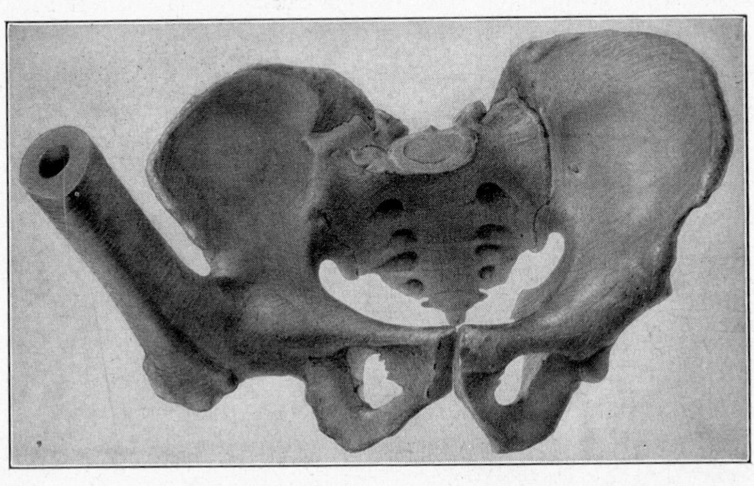

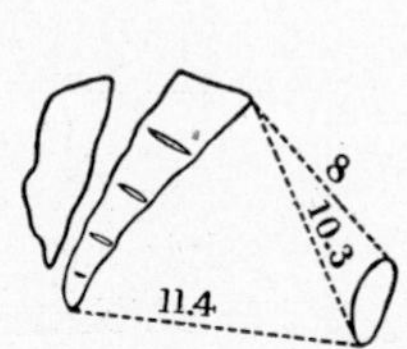

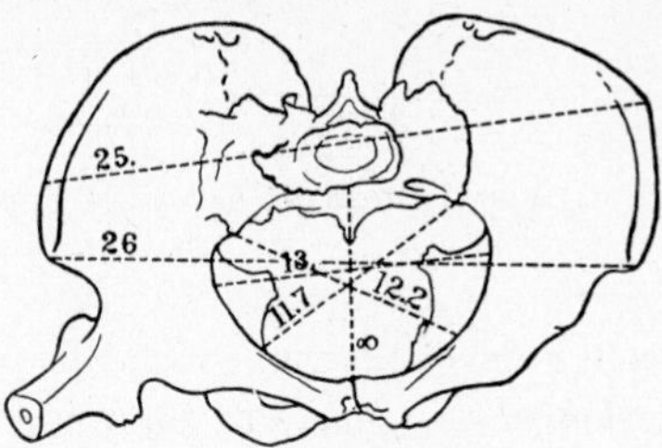

Figs. 484, 485 and 486.—Coxalgic Pelvis with Ankylosed Femur.

Oblique contraction of the pelvis may also develop when *unilateral luxation* of the femur occurs in early life, although it is usually less pronounced than that following coxitis. Under such circumstances the head of the bone is displaced backward and upward upon the outer surface of the ilium, where a new joint surface may occasionally be formed. The affected leg becomes considerably shortened, and accordingly an undue share of the body weight is transmitted through the well leg, which forces the corresponding side of the pelvis upward, inward, and backward, and leads to an oblique contraction, as in coxalgia.

Unless the patient has had the benefit of proper orthopedic treatment in unilateral *infantile paralysis,* as well as in those cases in which disease at the knee or ankle joint or amputation early in life has caused shortening of one leg, similar changes occur in the pelvis, though they rarely assume the extreme degree of obliquity which characterizes the coxalgic variety.

Diagnosis. A limping gait at once suggests an obliquely contracted pelvis, and when, upon questioning the patient, it is found that the condition has been present since early childhood, the existence of pelvic deformity upon the side corresponding to the sound leg becomes highly probable.

More accurate information can be obtained by careful examination of the patient, naked, when the posture of the involved leg can be noted, as well as the relative position of the posterior or superior spines and the crests of the ilia. At the same time, the presence or absence of compensatory scoliosis can be noted and, finally, the extent of the oblique contraction can be determined by the employment of the measurements suggested by Naegele for the detection of the obliquely ovate pelvis per se.

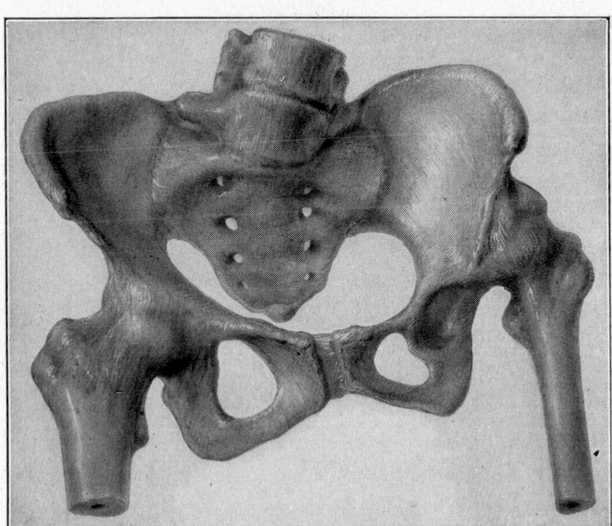

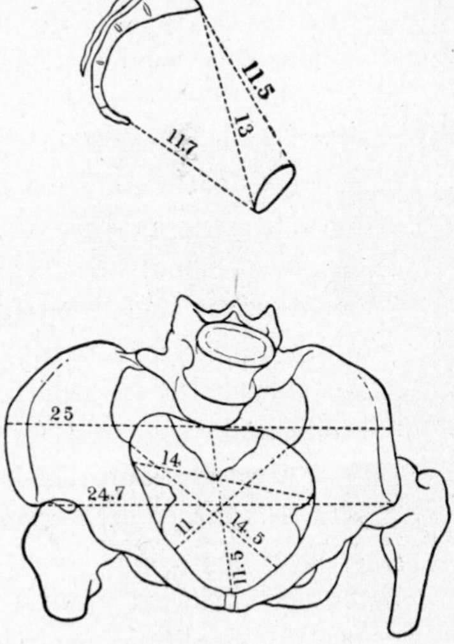

Figs. 487, 488 and 489.—Obliquely Contracted Pelvis, Due to Unilateral Luxation of Femur.

An accurate conception concerning the degree of contraction, however, can be obtained only by careful exploration of the interior of the pelvis, preferably with the patient under the influence of an anesthetic, although in many coxalgic patients this may be extremely difficult on account of the ankylosis of one leg. X-ray pelvimetry is, of course, of particular value in such cases.

Effect upon Labor. The effect of this type of pelvis upon labor varies with the extent and position of the deformity. If the affected side is so contracted as to prevent its being occupied by a portion of the presenting part, we have for all practical purposes a generally contracted pelvis, and engagement, if it can occur at all, will take place more readily when the biparietal diameter of the head is in relation with the long oblique diameter of the superior strait. But even after descent has occurred, all obstacles to labor have by no means been overcome, since in many cases the inward projection of the ischium may lead to abnormalities in rotation. Generally speaking, these pelves are not excessively contracted, Prouvost reporting that 40 out of 50 cases of labor complicated by them ended spontaneously.

Treatment. Although the pelvic contraction is usually not very pronounced, serious dystocia may occur. For this reason, if engagement has not occurred during the last weeks of pregnancy, the patient should be examined and, if possible, the entire interior of the pelvis carefully palpated. If facilities are available, careful roentgenologic examination of the pelvis should, of course, be carried out in all cases. If it appears probable that the engagement will not occur, cesarean section should be performed before the onset of labor. Fortunately, this is rarely indicated, unless the fetus is unduly large, or the history of previous labors has shown that the birth of a living child is out of the question. When the obstacle to the engagement of the head is not serious, version gives better results than forceps. This is especially true in coxalgic pelves when the awkward position of the ankylosed leg, as well as the asymmetry of the pubic arch, may make the application of forceps extraordinarily difficult.

Coxarthrolisthetic Pelvis. Very exceptionally, as the result of localized softening near the acetabulum, the base of one or both acetabula yields to the pressure exerted by the head of the femur and projects into the pelvic cavity, thus leading to a unilateral or bilateral transverse contraction, which when pronounced may give rise to serious dystocia. Eppinger, who studied the condition exhaustively in 1903, designated such pelves as coxarthrolisthetic, and attributed their production to delayed and deficient ossification of the base of the acetabulum. The deformity was known to A. W. Otto as early as 1824, and Breus and Kolisko have shown that it is usually dependent upon gonorrheal coxitis, instead of upon arthritis deformans or tuberculous processes, as was formerly believed. Chiari, however, in 1912 described a specimen which he held had resulted from tabetic arthritis. The condition is rare, and Benda has collected cases reported up to 1926 and has critically considered their mode of production.

Pelvic Deformities Due to Bilateral Lameness. Occasionally children are born with *luxation of both femurs,* the heads of the bones lying, as a rule, upon the outer surfaces of the iliac bones, above and posterior to their usual situation. In some cases the acetabula are entirely absent but more frequently they are present in a rudimentary condition, new but imperfect substitutes being formed higher up. Strange to say, the condition does not usually seriously interfere with the individual in the matter of learning to walk at the usual age, though the gait is more or less wobbly.

Owing to the fact that the upward and inward force exerted by the femurs is not applied in its usual direction through the acetabula, the pelvis becomes unduly wide, and more or less flattened anteroposteriorly. The transverse widening is particularly marked at the inferior strait, while the flattening, as a rule, is not very pronounced. Hence, this pelvis rarely offers any serious obstacle to labor.

Verning in 1928 directed attention to the fact that when the patient is placed in the obstetrical position, the heads of the femurs may slip through the sacrosciatic notches and so encroach upon the pelvic cavity as to cause dystocia. Fortunately, this accident should not lead to serious trouble, as experience teaches that a change in the position of the legs effects reduction of the luxation.

The patient presents a characteristic appearance which is suggestive of that observed in spondylolisthesis. Owing to the displacement of the femurs, the trochanters are more prominent than usual, and the width of the buttocks is increased. At the same time, owing to the increase in the pelvic inclination, there is marked lordosis, the back of the patient appearing considerably shortened and presenting a marked saddle-shaped depression just above the sacrum.

Atypical Deformities of the Pelvis

In rare instances the pelvis may be more or less deformed by the presence of bony outgrowths at various points, and less frequently by tumor formations. *Exostoses* are most frequently observed upon the posterior surface of the symphysis, in front of the sacro-iliac joints, or upon the anterior surface of the sacrum, though in occasional cases they may be formed along the course of the iliopectineal line.

Kilian in 1854 directed attention to the fact that such structures may form sharp, more or less knifelike projections. He designated the condition as *acanthopelys* or *pelvis spinosa.* Such formations are rarely sufficiently large to offer any obstacle to labor, but owing to their peculiar structure may do considerable injury to the maternal soft parts. In fact, in several of the cases reported, they have cut through the lower portion of the uterus.

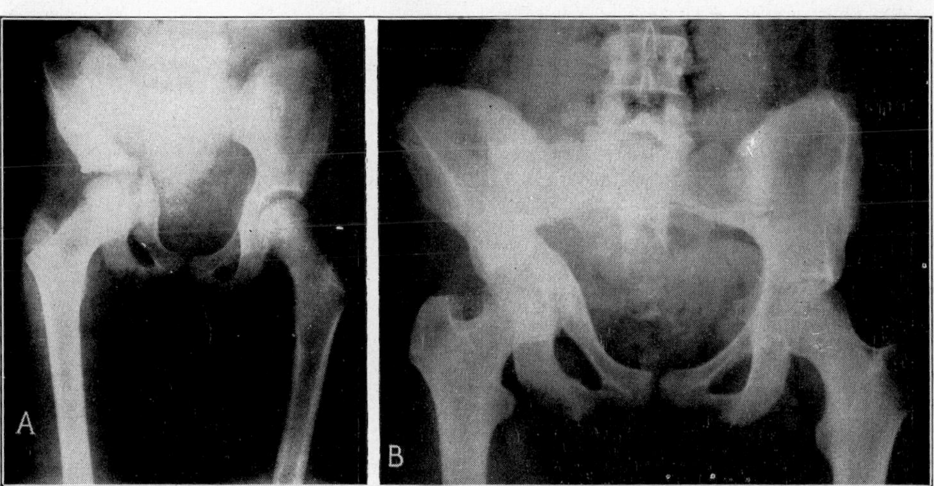

FIG. 490.—FRACTURE OF RIGHT ILIUM, PUBIC RAMUS, AND ACETABULUM.

A, Age 8 years; B, Age 22 years, showing residual asymmetry of pelvis. (Courtesy of Dr. L. A. Wing.)

Rarely, *callus* formation, resulting from inflammatory process within the pelvis, may attain such proportions as to lead to serious pelvic obstruction, as in a case reported by Ahlfeld.

Tumor formations of various kinds may spring from the walls of the false or true pelvis, and so obstruct its cavity as to render labor impossible. Fibromata, osteomata, enchondromata, carcinomata, and osteosarcomata of the pelvis have been described, and sometimes assume very considerable proportions, and occasionally become cystic. Enchondromata occur more frequently than other varieties of tumor formation.

Unless cesarean section is performed, the prognosis is very grave when the pelvis is obstructed by tumors from its walls, 50 per cent of the mothers and 89 per cent of the children having perished in the cases collected by Stadfeld, while in only 11 cases labor terminated by spontaneous delivery, forceps, or version.

Occasionally, healed *fractures* of the pelvis may offer an insuperable obstacle to the birth of the child, owing either to an excessive formation of callus or to the projection of the broken ends of the bones into the pelvic cavity. Recently Voegelin and McCall directed attention to the increasing incidence of fracture of the female pelvis as a result of several factors, such as automobile accidents, and the decreased mortality in such cases. According to Speed, they comprise 3 per cent of all fractures. The effect upon labor depends upon the location of the fracture and its manner of healing. Figure 490 shows the pelvis of an 8-year-old child with a fracture of the right acetabulum, ilium and pubic ramus, and gives an idea of the extent of the changes which sometimes result, and the residual deformity 14 years later. Each case of fracture of the pelvis must be evaluated clinically as well as by means of the x-rays before the onset of labor and a decision reached as to the type of delivery best indicated. As Voegelin and McCall point out, operative delivery is the exception rather than the rule in such acquired anomalies of the pelvis.

Dwarf Pelvis. According to Breus and Kolisko, several varieties of dwarfs must be distinguished, *i.e.*, the "true," the hypoplastic, the chondrodystrophic, the cretin, and the rachitic dwarf.

In the "true" dwarf there is a proportionate lack of general development, which is particularly characterized by the fact that the various epiphyses do not undergo ossification, but remain cartilaginous, until an advanced age.

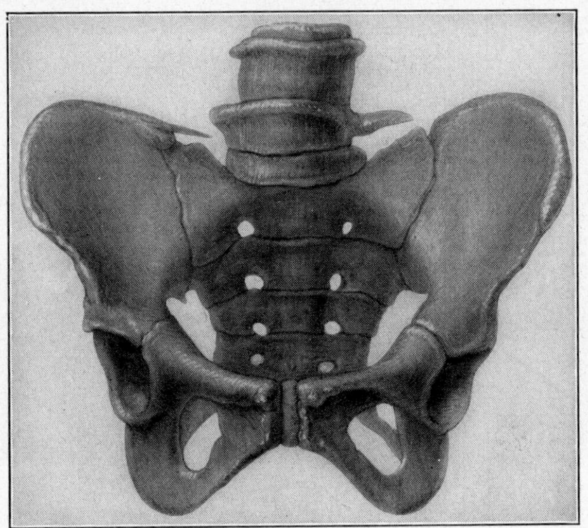

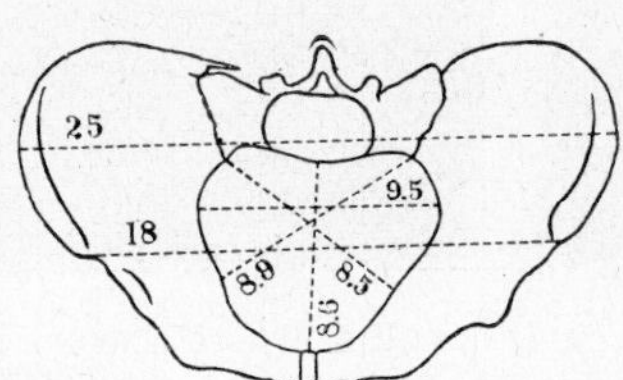

FIGS. 491, 492.—TRUE DWARF PELVIS (Boeckh).

In the *hypoplastic* dwarf the changes are quantitative instead of qualitative, so that the individual differs from the normal only in her miniature appearance.

In the chondrodystrophic dwarf the deformity results from chondrodystrophia foetalis, achondroplasia, or fetal rachitis, as the disease has been variously designated. The affection is not allied to rachitis, but is an entirely independent disease which begins in utero, and whose etiology is as yet unknown, although many recent writers are inclined to attribute it to abnormalities in the function of the endocrine glands. It is characterized by changes in the epiphyseal cartilages, which interfere with the normal apposition of bone, with the result that the shafts of the long bones are imperfectly developed so that the individual presents a normally formed body, while the extremities are short and stumpy. In many instances the head is brachycephalic, with a prominent forehead and saddle nose. The musculature is often excessively developed, so that chondrodystrophic dwarfs may be unusually strong. It is sometimes hereditary, and in such cases the tendency is usually transmitted through the father. Persons presenting the abnormality are frequently exceptionally fertile, and thus contrast markedly with cretin dwarfs, in whom sterility is the rule.

In the *cretin dwarf* the lack of development is general. The bony changes are allied to those observed in the true dwarf, but are less marked.

The term *rachitic dwarf* should not be applied to individuals whose short stature is due to skeletal deformities, but should be restricted to those who would fall far below the normal height even if one imagined the deformities straightened out.

Each of these varieties of dwarfs has a characteristically shaped pelvis, which is more or less generally contracted.

True Dwarf Pelvis (Pelvis Nana). This variety of pelvis is extremely rare, only four well-marked specimens being in existence. The pelvis is generally contracted and tends toward the infantile type, but its most characteristic feature is the persistence of cartilage at all the epiphyses.

Hypoplastic Dwarf Pelvis. According to Breus and Kolisko this variety of pelvis is observed in very small individuals, and is simply a normal pelvis in miniature. It differs materially from that of the true dwarf in that it is completely ossified.

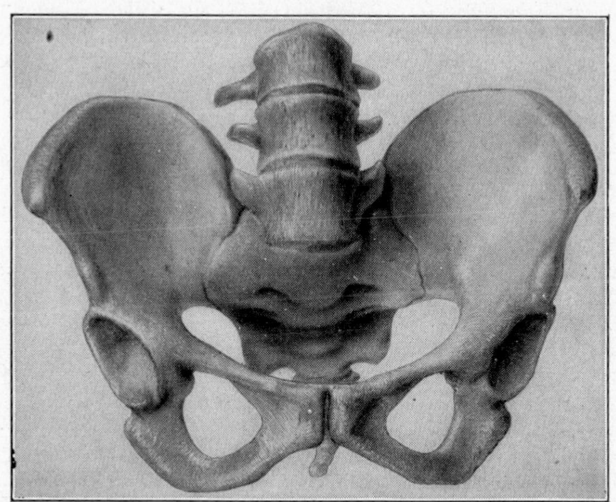

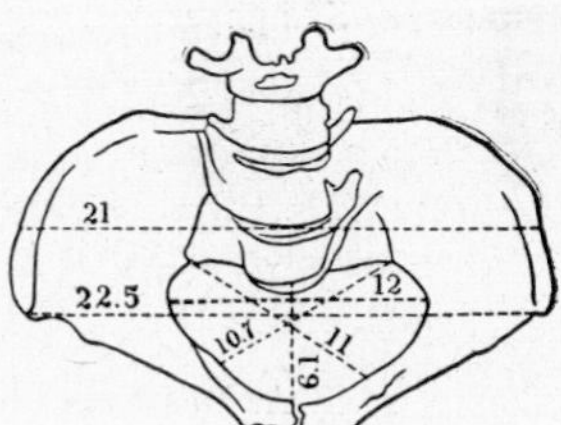

FIGS. 493, 494.—CHONDRODYSTROPHIC PELVIS (Breus and Kolisko).

Chondrodystrophic Dwarf Pelvis. This variety of pelvis is characterized by an extreme anteroposterior flattening, so that on first glance one might believe that one had to deal with a rachitic pelvis. On closer examination, however, it is seen that the flattening is due to the imperfect development of the portion of the iliac bone entering into the formation of the iliopectineal line, owing to which the sacral articulation is brought much nearer the pubic bone than usual. In six pelves of this character described by Breus and Kolisko the conjugata vera varied from 4 to 7 cm., while the transverse diameter of the superior strait was but slightly shortened, varying from 11 to 12 cm.

Cretin Dwarf Pelvis. This is a generally contracted pelvis with poorly developed and imperfectly formed bones. Unlike that of the true dwarf, it does not present infantile characteristics, but shows signs of a steady though imperfect growth throughout early life. Unossified cartilage may be present here and there in young subjects, but it disappears with advancing age and is never found in all the epiphyses as in the true dwarf pelvis.

Rachitic Dwarf Pelvis. True rachitic dwarfs are rare, and possess generally contracted rachitic pelves, which do not differ, except by their small size, from those described previously.

BIBLIOGRAPHY

General Literature

CALDWELL, W. E., and MOLOY, H. C. Anatomical Variations in the Female Pelvis and Their Effect in Labor with a Suggested Classification. Am. J. Obst. & Gynec., 1933, 26:479.

CALDWELL, W. E., and MOLOY, H. C. Classification of the Pelvis, the Mechanism of Labor and the Influence of Pelvic Abnormalities on Pelvic Arrest. In Gynecology and Obstetrics, C. H. Davis, Editor. W. C. Prior Co., Inc., Hagerstown, Md., 1946, Vol. 1, p. 61.

CALDWELL, W. E., MOLOY, H. C., and D'ESOPO, D. A. Studies on Pelvic Arrests. Am. J. Obst. & Gynec., 1938, 36:928.

——— MOLOY, H. C., and SWENSON, P. C. The Use of the Roentgen Ray in Obstetrics. Am. J Roentgenol., 1939, 41:305, 505, 719.

DANFORTH, D. N. The Practical Application of X-ray Pelviography to Clinical Obstetrics. Quart. Bull. Northwestern Univ. Med. School, Chicago, 1948, 22:223.

EASTMAN, N. J. Pelvic Mensuration: A Study in the Perpetuation of Error. Obst. & Gynec. Surv., 1948, 3:301.

ELLER, W. C., and MENGERT, W. F. Recognition of Midpelvic Contraction. Am. J. Obst. & Gynec., 1947, 53:252.

——— MENGERT, W. F., ANDREW, W. H., and JENNETT, R. J. Experience with Midpelvic Dystocia. Am. J. Obst. & Gynec., 1947, 53:823.

EMMONS, A. B. A Study in the Variations in the Female Pelvis, etc. Biometrika, 1913, 9:34.

FABRE et BOURRET. Bassin à diamètre antéropostérieuré prédominant. Bull. Soc. d'obst. et de gynec. de Paris, 1913, 16:108.

GUERRIERO, W. F., ARNELL, R. E., and IRWIN, J. B. Pelvicephalography; Analysis of 503 Selected Cases. South. M. J., 1940, 33:840.

HANSON, S. An Internal Outlet Pelvimeter. Am. J. Obst. & Gynec., 1933, 26:736.

——— A Combined Inlet and Outlet Pelvimeter. Am. J. Obst. & Gynec., 1934, 28:608.

——— Internal Pelvimetry as a Basis for the Morphologic Classification of Pelves. Am. J. Obst. & Gynec., 1938, 35:228.

HART, D. B. On Inversion of the Ilium and Sacrum and Ischium and Pubis as Causes of Deformities of the Female Pelvis. Edinburgh M. J., 1916, 16:9.

KEHRER. E. Symphysenlockerung und Symphysenruptur. Monatschr. f. Geburtsh. u. Gynäk., 1915, 42:321.

MANAHAN, C. P., CONNALLY, H. F., and EASTMAN, N. J. The Experience of the Johns Hopkins Hospital with Cesarean Section. Am. J. Obst. & Gynec., 1942, 44:999.

MENGERT, W. F. Pelvic Measurements of 4144 Iowa Women. Am. J. Obst. & Gynec., 1938, 36:260.

——— Estimation of Pelvic Capacity. J.A.M.A., 1948, 138:169.

——— and ELLER, W. C. Graphic Portrayal of Relative Pelvic Size. Am. J. Obst. & Gynec., 1946, 52:1032.

MICHAELIS, G. A. Das Enge Becken, Leipzig, 1865.

MOIR, J. C. The Use of Radiology in Predicting Difficult Labour. J. Obst. & Gynaec. Brit. Emp., 1946, 53:487; and idem, 1947, 54:20.

——— A Comment on a Recent Criticism of Brim Pelvimetry. J. Obst. & Gynaec. Brit. Emp., 1946, 53:496.

RIGGS, T. A Comparative Study of White and Negro Pelves, etc. Johns Hopkins Hosp. Rep., 1904, 12:421.

STEELE, K. B., and JAVERT, C. T. Roentgenography of the Obstetric Pelvis—A Combined Isometric and Stereoscopic Technique. Am. J. Obst. & Gynec., 1942, 43:600.

THOMS, H. A Statistical Study of the Frequency of Funnel Pelves and the Description of a New Outlet Pelvimeter. Am. J. Obst., 1915, 72:121.

——— The Obstetrical Significance of Pelvic Variations. A Study of 450 Primiparous Women. Brit. M. J., 1937, 2:210.

——— Outlet Pelvimetry: A Commentary, and the Presentation of a Pelvimeter for Measuring the "Symphysis and Sacral Biparietal Distance." Surg., Gynec. & Obst., 1946, 83:399.

——— and SCHUMACHER, P. C. The Clinical Significance of Midplane Pelvic Contraction. Am. J. Obst. & Gynec., 1944, 48:52.

WEINBERG, A., and SCADRON, S. J. The Value and Limitations of Pelvioradiography in the Management of Dystocia, with Special Reference to Midpelvic Capacity. Am. J. Obst. & Gynec., 1946, 52:255.

WILLIAMS, E. R., and PHILLIPS, L. G. The Value of Antenatal Radiological Pelvimetry: A Comparative Survey of the Prediction and Event in 300 Successive Pelvimetric Studies at Queen Charlotte's Maternity Hospital. J. Obst. & Gynaec. Brit. Emp., 1946, 53:125.

WILLIAMS, J. W. Frequency of Contracted Pelves in the First One Thousand Women Delivered in the Obstetrical Department of the Johns Hopkins Hospital. Obstetrics, 1899, I, Nos. 5, 6.

——— Frequency, Aetiology and Practical Significance of Contractions of the Pelvic Outlet. Surg., Gynec. & Obst., 1909, 8:619.

——— The Funnel Pelvis. Am. J. Obst., 1911, 64:106.

——— and SUN, K. A Statistical Study of the Incidence and Treatment of Labor Complicated by Contracted Pelvis in the Obstetric Service of the Johns Hopkins Hospital from 1896 to 1924. Am. J. Obst. & Gynec., 1926, 11:735.

Anomalies of Development

BREUS, C., u. KOLISKO, A. Die pathologischen Beckenformen, 1900, Bd. I: Spaltbecken, ff. 107-139; Assimilationsbecken, ff. 169-256; Zwergbecken, ff. 259-366.

——— Das ostitisch-synstotische Becken. *Ibid.*, 1904, Bd. II, Heft 1, ff. 135-290.

LITZMANN, C. C. T. Das schrägovale Becken. Kiel, 1853.

——— Das gaspaltene Becken. Arch. f. Gynäk., 1872, 4:266.

——— Ein durch mangelhafte Entwickelung des Kreuzbeines querverengtes Becken. Arch. f. Gynäk., 1885, 25:31.

NAEGELE, F. C. Das schrägverengte Becken. Mainz, 1839.

RISCHBEITH and BARRINGTON. Dwarfism. Eugenic Laboratory Memoirs, London, 1912, Vol. 15.

ROBERT, F. Beschreibung eines im höchsten Grade querverengten Beckens, etc. Karlsruhe u. Freiburg, 1842.

THOMS, H. The Naegele Pelvis. A Summary and a Description of a Case. Yale J. Biol. & Med., 1938, 10:513.

——— The Obliquely Ovate or Naegele Pelvis. A Commentary and a Report of Four Cases. J.A.M.A., 1944, 124:294.

WAGNER, G. A. Ueber familiäre Chondrodystrophie. Arch. f. Gynäk., 1913, 100:70.

WILLIAMS, J. W. A Clinical and Anatomic Description of a Naegele Pelvis. Am. J. Obst. & Gynec., 1929, 18:504.

Rachitic and Osteomalacic Pelves

BREUS, C., u. KOLISKO, A. Rachitis-becken. Die pathologischen Beckenformen. Leipzig u. Wien, 1904, Bd. 1, Teil 2, ff. 435-636.

CHU, H. I., LIU, S. H., YU, T. F., HSU, H. C., CHENG, T. Y., and CHAO, H. C. Calcium and Phosphorus Metabolism in Osteomalacia. X. Further Studies on Vitamin D Action: Early Signs of Depletion and Effect of Minimal Doses. J. Clin. Invest., 1940, 19:349.

FEHLING, H. Die Entstehung der rachitischen Beckenform. Arch. f. Gynäk., 1877, 11:173.

FRASER, J. R. The Ovary in Osteomalacia. Am. J. Obst. & Gynec., 1927, 14:697.

HANNON, R. R., LIU, S. H., CHU, H. I., WANG, S. H., CHEN, K. C., and CHOU, S. K. Calcium and Phosphorus Metabolism in Osteomalacia. I. Effect of Vitamin D and Its Apparent Duration. Chinese M. J., Peiping, 1934, 48:623.

HOLT, L. M., Jr., and MCINTOSH, R. Holt's Diseases of Infancy and Childhood. 10th Ed., Appleton-Century, New York, 1933.

KAUFMANN, E. Untersuchungen über die sogenannte fötale Rhachitis. Berlin, 1892.

KEHRER, F. A. Zur Entwickelungsgeschichte des rhachitischen Beckens. Arch. f. Gynäk., 1873, 5:55.

LITZMANN, C. C. T. Die Formen des Beckens, nebst einem Anhange über Osteomalacie. Berlin, 1861.

——— Die Geburt bei engem Becken. Leipzig, 1884, f. 36.

LIU, S. H., CHU, H. I., SU, C. C., YU, T. F., and CHENG, T. Y. Calcium and Phosphorus Metabolism in Osteomalacia. IX. Metabolic Behavior of Infants Fed on Breast Milk from Mothers Showing Various States of Vitamin D Nutrition. J. Clin. Invest., 1940, 19:327.

MAXWELL, J. P., and MILES, L. M. Osteomalacia in China. J. Obst. & Gynaec. Brit. Emp., 1925, 32:433.

MICHAELIS, G. A. Das enge Becken. Leipzig, 1865.

OGATA, M. Ueber das Wesen der Rachitis und Osteomalacie. Beitr. zur. Geburtsh. u. Gynäk., 1912, 17:23.

PARK, E. A., and HOWLAND, J. Radiographic Evidence of Influence of Cod Liver Oil. Bull. Johns Hopkins Hosp., 1921, 32:341.

PARK, E. A. Some Aspects of Rickets. Canad. M. A. J., 1932, 26:3.

PORAK. De l'achondroplaisie. Nouv. arch. d'obst. et gynéc., 1889, 4:551.

RECKLINGHAUSEN. Rachitis und Osteomalacie. Jena, 1910.

SCHMORL, G. Die path. Anatomie der rachitischen Knochenerkrankung. Ergebn. d. inn. Med., 1909, Bd. 4.

Pelvic Anomalies Secondary to Abnormalities of the Vertebral Column

BOWMAN, W. B. Spondylolisthesis—a Common Lumbro-sacral Lesion. Am. J. Roentgenol., 1924, 11:223.

BREISKY, A. Ueber den Einfluss der Kyphose auf die Beckengestalt. Ztschr. d. Gesellsch. d. Aertze in Wien, 1865, Bd. I.

BREUS, C., u. KOLISKO, A. Die pathologische Beckenformen. 1900. Bd. III, I. Teil, Spondylolisthesis, ff. 17-159; Kyphosen-Becken, ff. 163-307; Skoliosen-Becken, ff. 311-352; Kyphoskoliosen-Becken, ff. 355-359.

CHAPMAN, E. M., DILL, D. B., and GRAYBIEL, A. Decrease in Functional Capacity of Lungs and Heart Resulting from Deformities of Chest: Pulmonocardiac Failure. Medicine, 1939, 18:167.

CHIARI, H. Die Aetiologie und Genese der sogenannten Spondylolisthesis lumbosacralis. Ztschr. f. Heilk., 1892, 13:199.

——— Spondylolisthesis. Bull. Johns Hopkins Hosp., 1911, 22:41.

Fehling, H. Pelvis obtecta. Arch. f. Gynäk., 1872, 4:1.
Goldthwait, J. E. The Lumbo-sacral Articulation, etc. Boston M. & S. J., 1911, 164:365.
Hayek, H. Ueber Spondylolysis Zentralbl. f. Gynäk., 1928, 52:2511.
Hergott, A. Du spondylizème. Arch. de tocol. et de gynéc., Par., Fév.-Mars, 1877.
Jensen, J. The Heart in Pregnancy. C. V. Mosby Co., St. Louis, 1938, pp. 333-341.
Klein, P. Ueber das Cor Kyphoscolioticum in der Gestation. Arch. f. Gynäk., 1927, 130:653.
Klien, R. Die Geburt beim Kyphotischen Becken. Arch. f. Gynäk., 1896, 50:1.
Leopold, C. G. Das skoliotisch und kypho-skol. rachitische Becken. Leipzig, 1879.
——— Weitere Untersuchungen über das skoliotische und kypho-skol. rachitische Becken. Arch. f. Gynäk., 1880, 16:1.
Neugebauer, F. L. Zur Entwickelungsgeschichte des spondylolisthetischen Beckens und seiner Diagnose. Halle u. Dorpat, 1882.
——— Spondylolisthesis et spondylizème. Paris, 1892.
——— Die heutige Statistik der Geburten bei Beckenverengerung infolge von Rückgratskyphose. Monatschr. f. Geburtsh. u. Gynaek., 1895, 1:317.
Rokitansky, C. Anomalien der Gestalt des Rückgrats und seiner Theile. Lehrbuch der path. Anat., III. Aufl., 1856, Bd. II, ff. 162-172.
Williams, J. W. A Case of Spondylolisthesis, with Description of the Pelvis. Am. J. Obst., 1899, 40:145.
——— Spontaneous Labor Occurring through an Obliquely Contracted, Kyphotic, Funnel Pelvis. Bull. Johns Hopkins Hosp., 1922, 33:190.

Pelvic Anomalies Due to Abnormal Forces Exerted by Femora. Atypical Deformities.

Ahlfeld, F. Das durch Knochenauswüchse verengte Becken. Lehrbuch der Geburtshülfe, II. Aufl., 1898, f. 336.
Benda, R. Beitrag zur Kasuistik und Pathogenese der coxitischen Pfannenprotrusion. Arch f. Gynäk., 1927, 129:186.
Breus, C., u. Kolisko, A. Coxitis-Becken. Die pathologische Beckenformen. Leipzig u. Wien, 1912, Bd. III, ff. 474-593.
Briggs, H. The Coxalgic Pelvis. J. Obst. & Gynaec. Brit. Emp., 1914, 26:212.
Chiari, H. Pelikologische Mittheilungen. Verhandl. d. deutsch. path. Gesellsch., 1912, 9:318.
Delmas, J. Sur l'anatomie obst. du bassin à luxation coxo-fémorale congénitale double. Obstétrique, Par., 1911, n. s. 4:729.
Goder. Von dem Becken ausgehende Tumoren als Geburtshinderness. D. I., Halle, 1896.
Kleinwächter. Das Luxationsbecken, etc. Prager Vierteljahrsschr. f. Heilkunde, Bd. 118, 119.
Meurers, Carl. Beitrag zur geb. Bedeutung der Frakturbecken. D. I., Heidelberg, 1904.
Peabody, C. W. Bilateral Defect of Femoral Heads. J. Bone & Joint Surg., 1927, 9:288.
Sassmann, E. Das Becken bei angeborener doppelseitiger Hüftgelenksluxation. Arch. f. Gynäk., 1873, 5:241.
Schoppig, S. Das Becken-enchondrom, besonders als Geburtshindernis. Monatschr. f. Geburtsh. u. Gynaek., 1907, 25:845.
Stadfeld, A. Die Geburt bei Geschwülsten des Beckens. Zentralbl. f. Gynäk., 1880, 4:417.
Verning, P. Recherches sur la luxation coxo-fémorale congénitale bilatérale. Gynéc. et obst., 1928, 17:292.
Voegelin, A. W., and McCall, M. L. Some Acquired Bony Abnormalities Influencing the Conduct of Labor. Am. J. Obst. & Gynec., 1944, 48:361.
Wahrsinger, P. B. Naegele Pelvis Associated with Rudimentary Femur. Am. J. Obst. & Gynec., 1944, 47:427.

32

DYSTOCIA DUE TO ABNORMALITIES OF THE GENERATIVE TRACT

Vulva. Complete atresia of the vulva or the lower portion of the vagina is usually congenital, and unless corrected by operative measures would constitute an insuperable obstacle to conception. More frequently vulvar atresia is incomplete and is due to adhesions and cicatricial changes resulting from injury or inflammatory processes. The defect may offer a considerable obstacle to labor, but the resistance is usually overcome by the continued pressure exerted by the head, though frequently only at the expense of deep perineal tears.

Especially in elderly primiparae, the vulvar outlet may be very small, rigid, and altogether lacking in elasticity. This may cause dystocia and predispose to extensive laceration unless it is avoided by deep episiotomy. As the result of various factors, the vulva may become extremely edematous, but as discussed on page 729, this rarely causes difficulty. The formation of thrombi or hematomata about the vulva, although more common during the puerperium, occasionally occurs during the latter part of pregnancy or at the time of labor, and may give rise to some difficulty (page 590). Inflammatory lesions about the vulva as well as malignant new growths may have a similar effect.

Vagina. Complete vaginal atresia is nearly always congenital in origin and is an effectual bar to pregnancy. Incomplete forms, on the other hand, are sometimes manifestations of faulty development, but more frequently result from accidental complications (see Figs. 362, 363).

Occasionally the vagina is divided into two halves by a longitudinal septum extending from the vulva to the cervix; more often the structure is incomplete, being limited to either the upper or lower portion of the canal. Such conditions are frequently associated with other abnormalities in the development of the generative tract, and their presence should always lead to careful examination with a view to determining whether partial or complete duplicity of the uterus exists.

A complete longitudinal septum rarely gives rise to dystocia, as the half of the vagina through which the child descends gradually undergoes satisfactory dilatation. On the other hand, an incomplete septum occasionally interferes with the descent of the head, becoming stretched over it as a fleshy band of varying thickness. Such structures are usually torn through spontaneously, but occasionally are so resistant that they must be ligated and severed by the obstetrician.

Occasionally the vagina may be obstructed by ringlike strictures or bands of congenital origin. These, however, rarely offer a serious obstacle to labor, since they usually yield before the oncoming head, though in extreme cases incision may be necessary.

Sometimes the upper portion of the vagina is separated from the remainder of the canal by a diaphragmlike structure with a small central opening. Such a condition is occasionally mistaken by inexperienced observers for the vaginal fornix, and at the time of labor for the undilated external os. On careful examination, however, one should be able to pass a finger through the opening and to distinguish the cervix. After the external os has become completely dilated, the head impinges upon the abnormal structure and causes it to bulge downward. If it does not yield, slight pressure upon its opening will usually lead to further dilatation, but if this is not effectual, crucial incisions may be necessary in order to allow delivery.

Accidental atresia is always secondary in origin and results from the formation of cicatrices following injuries or inflammatory processes. It sometimes follows severe puerperal infections during the course of which a great part of the lining of the vagina may have sloughed off, so that as healing occurs its lumen becomes almost entirely obliterated. A similar result is sometimes noted after diphtheria, smallpox, cholera, and syphilis, while in rare instances, as in a case reported by Schenck, it may be due to the action of corrosive fluids injected into the vagina in the hope of inducing abortion. That the most frequent cause of atresia is injury or inflammatory conditions following labor is shown by the fact that 209 of the 1,000 cases collected by Neugebauer presented such a history.

The effects of such atresia vary greatly. In the majority of cases, owing to the softening of the tissues incident to pregnancy, the obstruction is gradually overcome by the pressure exerted by the presenting part; less often, manual or hydrostatic dilatation or incisions may become necessary. If, however, the structure is so resistant that spontaneous dilatation appears improbable, cesarean section should be performed at the onset of labor.

Among the rare causes of serious dystocia vaginal neoplasms are worthy of mention. The obstruction may be due to the presence of cystic structures, fibromata, carcinomata, sarcomata, or hematomata, arising from the vaginal walls or the surrounding tissues. When the tumor is accessible, it is best treated by excision, no matter what its origin. If this is not practicable and the growth is cystic, tapping becomes the operation of choice. The presence of a solid tumor may occasionally afford an indication for cesarean section. Sasonoff observed a case in which a vaginal hematoma developed so rapidly after the birth of one twin as to interfere seriously with the delivery of the second child.

Exceptionally, tetanic contraction of the levator ani muscle may seriously interfere with the descent of the head. In this condition, which is analogous to the vaginismus of nonpregnant women, a thick, ring-like structure completely encircles and markedly constricts the vagina several centimeters above the vulva. Hué in 1906 collected a number of such cases. Ordinarily the condition yields under the influence of anesthesia, although in one of Stander's patients the obstruction persisted in spite of profound anesthesia, and it was only after steady pressure had been exerted upon it for some minutes that it relaxed sufficiently to permit the passage of the hand folded in the shape of a cone.

Although not one of the generative organs, a distended bladder is a common cause of arrested labor, as shown in Fig. 495.

Cervix. Inasmuch as complete atresia of the cervix is incompatible with conception, it must be assumed, whenever such a condition is met with in a pregnant woman, that conception had occurred before its formation, or that the atresia is only relative. Davis and Haszard reported a case which they described as one of congenital absence of the cervix with a very small external os. After 10 hours of strong labor pains without any dilatation of the external os, cesarean section was performed.

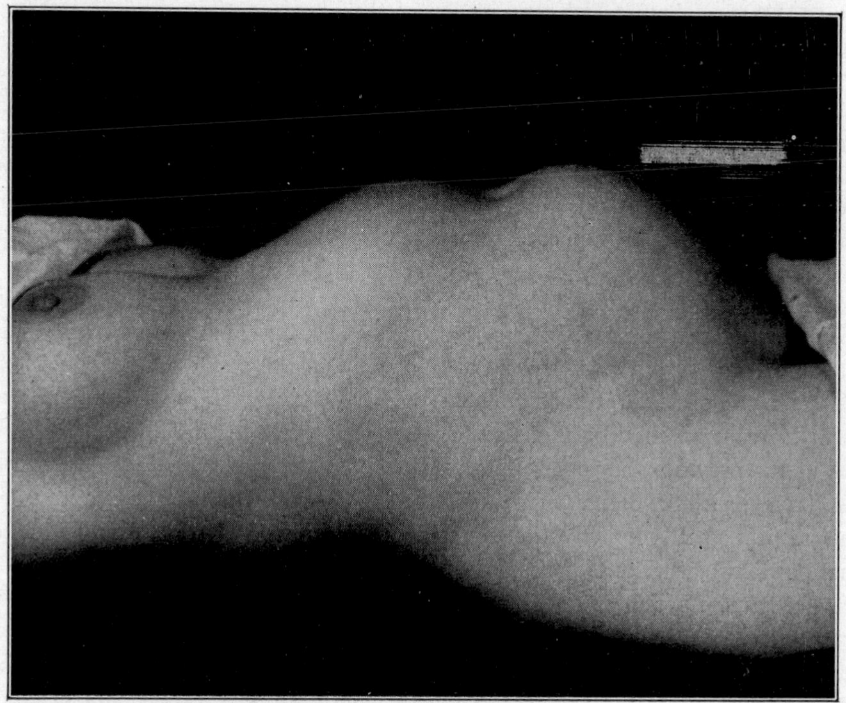

Fig. 495.—Dystocia Due to Bladder Distention.

This patient was sent to the hospital after three days of ineffectual labor at home. The cervix had been dilated, it is believed, for 24 hours, yet no progress had been made. Catheterization of the greatly distended bladder yielded 1,000 cc. of urine. Following this, the baby's head descended at once and delivery was easy. (J.H.H. 217811.)

A good illustration of relative atresia is afforded by the so-called *conglutinatio orificii externi*. In this condition the cervical canal undergoes complete obliteration at the time of labor while the os remains extremely small with very thin margins, the presenting part being separated from the vagina only by a thin layer of cervical tissue. Formerly, this appearance was attributed to the existence of adhesions between the lips of the external os, but Schroeder was probably right in stating that it is simply due to a very small and resistant opening. Ordinarily, complete dilatation promptly follows pressure with a finger tip, although in rare instances manual dilatation or crucial incisions may become necessary.

Cicatricial stenosis of the cervix frequently follows difficult labor associated with infection and considerable destruction of tissue. Less frequently it is due to syphilitic ulceration and induration. Now and again it results from the employment of corrosive substances for the purpose of producing abortion, while occasionally it is a sequel to gynecologic operations.

Ordinarily, owing to the softening and succulence of the tissues incident to pregnancy, the stenosis, whatever its cause, gradually yields to the natural forces. In rare instances, however, the stenosis may be so pronounced that it appears improbable that it can be overcome, and in such cases elective cesarean section is the procedure of choice. Such advanced degrees of atresia are likely to be observed in cases in which the atresia followed high amputation of the cervix or other cervical surgery.

Rigidity of Cervix. Reference has already been made to the unyielding cervix resulting in *cervical dystocia,* as well as to the cervical rigidity often seen in elderly primiparae. Occasionally, still greater rigidity is encountered in patients who have suffered from inflammatory lesions, though such conditions rarely give rise to serious dystocia. On the other hand, in certain cases of hypertrophic elongation of the cervix spontaneous dilatation does not occur although, as a rule, one is surprised to see how completely the abnormally elongated cervix may be effaced during the course of pregnancy.

Uterine Displacements. *Anteflexion.* Marked anteflexion of the uterus is usually associated with a pendulous abdomen. In primigravidae the condition is usually indicative of disproportion between the size of the head and the pelvis, whereas in multiparae it is more often an accompaniment of the flaccidity of the abdominal walls incident to repeated childbearing. In the latter class of cases, the abnormal position of the uterus prevents the force of its contractions from being properly transmitted to the cervix, hence the dilatation of the latter is interfered with. Marked improvement in this respect usually follows the maintenance of the uterus in an approximately normal position by means of a properly fitting abdominal bandage.

Retroflexion. As was stated in an earlier section, persistent retroflexion of the pregnant uterus is usually incompatible with advanced pregnancy since, if spontaneous or artificial reposition does not occur, the patient either aborts or presents symptoms of incarceration before the end of the fourth month. In very exceptional instances, however, pregnancy may go on to term, in which event the adherent fundus remains attached to the floor of the pelvis, while the anterior wall hypertrophies to such an extent as to afford room for the product of conception. In this condition, which is known as *sacculation,* the head of the child may occupy the displaced fundus, while the cervix is so drawn up that the external os lies above the upper margin of the symphysis pubis. Consequently, at the time of labor the contractions tend to force the child through the most dependent portion of the uterus, while the cervix dilates only partially, so that spontaneous birth is out of the question, and rupture of the uterus may occur, as in a case reported by Campbell. For these reasons cesarean section will afford the most conservative method of delivery, and at the same time make possible the reposition of the organ.

Dystocia Due to Operations for the Relief of Retroflexion of the Uterus. Unfortunately, several of the operations which have been suggested for the relief of retroflexion of the nonpregnant uterus, while rectifying the condition, occasionally give rise to serious dystocia. This is particularly true of those operations in which there is fixation of the round ligaments close to the uterus or the uterus itself to the anterior abdominal wall. While the Watkins-Wertheim interposition operation, in which the vesicovaginal fold is opened, the uterus drawn forward into the space thus formed and firmly sutured to the anterior vaginal wall, is seldom performed to rectify retroflexion, it is a common procedure for the cure of cystocele and prolapsus. It should never be performed before the menopause as it always gives rise to serious dystocia if the woman so treated subsequently becomes pregnant. Due to the many instances of dystocia following the ventrofixation procedures it is safe to say that these should seldom be performed during the childbearing period without sterilizing the patient. With any form of suspension, or indeed with any operation in which a lower abdominal incision is made at or near the midline, it may happen in very rare instances that, as a result of infection or some other unknown factor, firm adhesions form in consequence of which the uterus becomes firmly attached to the anterior wall. In this event, serious difficulty may arise at the time of labor in one of three ways. Most frequently, the anterior wall of the uterus below the area of fixation is unable to expand, so that the enlargement of the organ is effected solely at the expense of its posterior wall. At the same time, the anterior wall undergoes hypertrophy, and eventually forms a thick pad of muscle extending from the point of fixation to the cervix, and obstructs the superior strait. Furthermore, as the uterus expands, traction is made upon the cervix, which is gradually drawn upward from its normal position until the external os is on a level with, or even above, the promontory of the sacrum, so that in extreme cases its posterior lip may be opposite the second or third lumbar vertebra. When labor sets in, dilatation of the cervix is effected very imperfectly since the bag of waters and the presenting part, instead of impinging upon it, are forced down upon the thickened anterior uterine wall. Accordingly, the uterine contractions, no matter how strong they may be, are unable to effect the completion of labor, and unless suitable operative aid is forthcoming, rupture of the uterus will occur, as in the cases reported by Dickinson and others. Less frequently, as in the case reported by Lynch, the anterior wall of the uterus does not hypertrophy, and in such cases the dystocia will be due entirely to the upward dislocation of the cervix.

In other instances, as in the case which Williams reported in 1906, both walls hypertrophy, and because of the limited space available between the area of fixation and the cervix, the anterior wall buckles and becomes folded upon itself instead of forming a thick muscular pad in front of the cervix. In such circumstances, the lower part of the uterine cavity is divided by a crescentic fold, with a sacculation in front of it in which portions of the fetus may lie, and thus is inaccessible to the operating hand. Moreover, the dystocia is exaggerated by the upward displacement of the cervix, as well as by the fold itself interfering with the engagement of the presenting part, as indicated in Fig. 496.

Andrews in 1905 collected the histories of 395 cases of pregnancy following ventral fixation or suspension. In the 359 patients who went to full term, delivery was effected by cesarean section in 20, by forceps in 21 instances, and once by craniotomy. This, however, does not exhaust the untoward effects of the operation, as the uterus ruptured in three other cases, and transverse presentations were noted in 10 instances. In 1906 Williams was able to increase still further the list of complications, and collected from the literature 36 cases of cesarean section, as well as two additional cases of craniotomy. Since that time, many more cases have been reported, and the condition is now recognized as a definite factor in the production of dystocia (Fig. 496).

In view of such experiences, the question arises whether the performance of suspensory operations of any kind is justifiable in women during the childbearing period.

Pregnancy may and frequently does occur in a uterus which has been previously suspended by the Olshausen or Gilliam technics, or some modification of them. In prin-

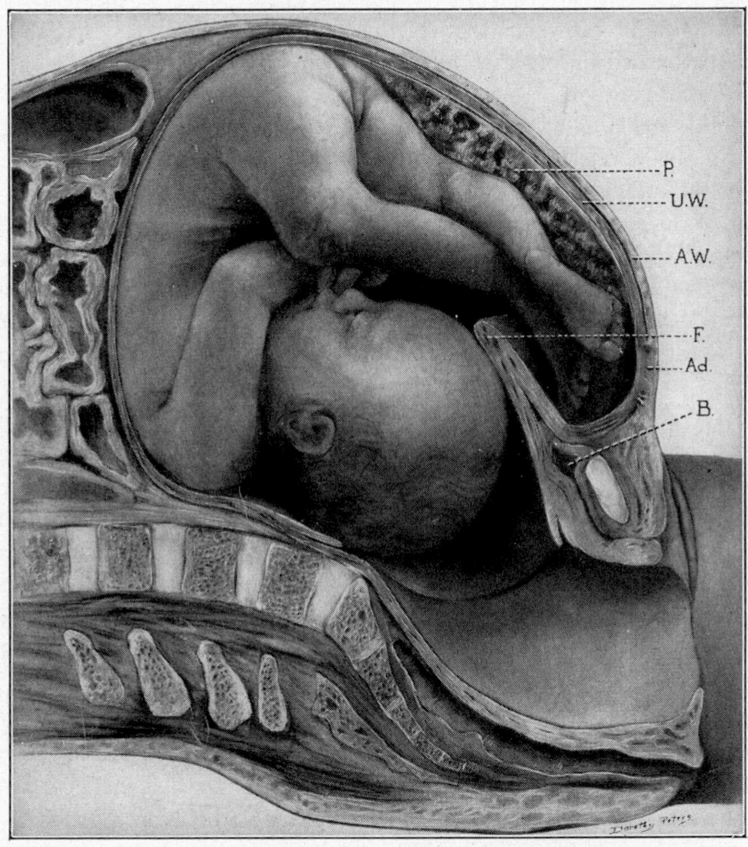

FIG. 496.—DYSTOCIA FOLLOWING VENTROSUSPENSION. SACCULATION OF ANTERIOR UTERINE WALL. × 1/3.
Ad., adhesion between uterus and anterior abdominal wall; *A.W.*, abdominal wall; *U.W.*, uterine wall; *B.*, bladder; *F.*, folded anterior uterine wall; *P.*, placenta.

ciple, these operations depend upon the fixation of the round ligaments at some distance from the uterus to the anterior sheath of the rectus muscle, after drawing them through a small incision made at the lateral edge of the rectus muscle. Again, quite as commonly, the Simpson operation has been done in which the slack round ligament is drawn snug through the internal inguinal ring and fixed to the inner surface of the anterior rectus sheath. Any of these operations should and usually do provide sufficient length of round ligament so that hypertrophy may take place and allow the normal elevation of the fundus into the upper abdomen. However, there are a number of writers who have felt that these operations, as well as those of the ventrofixation type, were frequent sources of dystocia and have created the impression that any form of suspension operation was contraindicated before the menopause. This is not true. If the large number of patients who have had uterine suspension operations without sterilization performed during the childbearing period is considered in connection with the incidence of serious dystocia ascribable to the operation, one must come to the conclusion that the latter group is very small. When the suspension operation is definitely indicated, there should be no hesitation because of possible future gestation, provided the Olshausen or Gilliam operations or some modification of these procedures can be carried out.

Prolapse. Pregnancy cannot go on to full term when the uterus is completely prolapsed, but it may do so in cases of incomplete prolapse. In the latter event the fundus occupies its usual level while the protrusion from the vulva is made possible by elongation of the hypertrophied cervix. As a rule, the latter becomes retracted as pregnancy advances, though in rare cases it may continue to protrude from the vulva and become so edematous and swollen as to give rise to dystocia. Under such circumstances multiple incisions may be necessary in order to effect delivery but this is rare. Even though dystocia may not result, the condition greatly increases the danger of labor. One of Stander's patients, who was delivered spontaneously at term, was suffering from intrapartum infection when admitted to the service and died a few days later from a streptococcus infection. Although she had not been examined vaginally, the fact that the external os protruded from the vulva afforded a rational explanation for the occurrence of the intrapartum infection.

Dystocia Due to Tumors of the Generative Tract and Pelvis. *Carcinoma of the Cervix.* The effect of this condition upon pregnancy and labor and its appropriate treatment has been considered in an earlier section.

Fibromyomata of the Uterus. Myomata were observed by Schauta and Pinard in 0.1 and 0.6 per cent of 55,311 and 13,915 consecutive labors, respectively. Pierson in 1927 reported an incidence of 0.68 per cent in 50,000 labors occurring at the Sloane Hospital for Women, while Kuder and Duckering noted an incidence of 1.4 per cent at the New York Lying-In Hospital. It is a matter of general observation that women suffering from this condition are relatively sterile. Seventy-five per cent of Schauta's patients were over 30 years of age when the first pregnancy occurred.

In many instances the association of myomata and pregnancy is without significance, while in others they are of considerable obstetrical importance for the following reasons: (1) they diminish the chances of conception; (2) they increase the probability of abortion; (3) under the influence of pregnancy, they may increase so rapidly in size as to produce serious pressure symptoms; (4) if situated in the lower segment or cervix, they may give rise to serious dystocia; (5) they favor the occurrence of abnormal presentations; (6) no matter where situated, they may so interfere with the efficiency of the uterine contractions as to give rise to inertia; (7) if submucous or interstitial in location, they may so interfere with the separation of the placenta as to render radical operative interference necessary; and finally, (8) they may undergo degenerative changes during pregnancy and particularly during the puerperium.

The obstacle to conception is most marked when the tumor is of the submucous or interstitial variety, and is in part due to changes in the endometrium which interfere with the implantation of the ovum. The correctness of such a view is demonstrated by the fact that the removal of such tumors is frequently followed by conception. Moreover, when pregnancy occurs the incidence of abortion is considerably increased, which is attributable to hemorrhagic and other pathologic changes in the decidua, which may be associated with imperfect nidation. Furthermore, when the tumor projects markedly into the uterine cavity and the placenta is implanted above it, spontaneous separation may become impossible, and manual removal may be so difficult that the exigencies of the condition are best met by supravaginal amputation of the uterus.

On the other hand, pregnancy is not without influence upon the tumors themselves, which frequently increase rapidly in size and give rise to serious pressure symptoms.

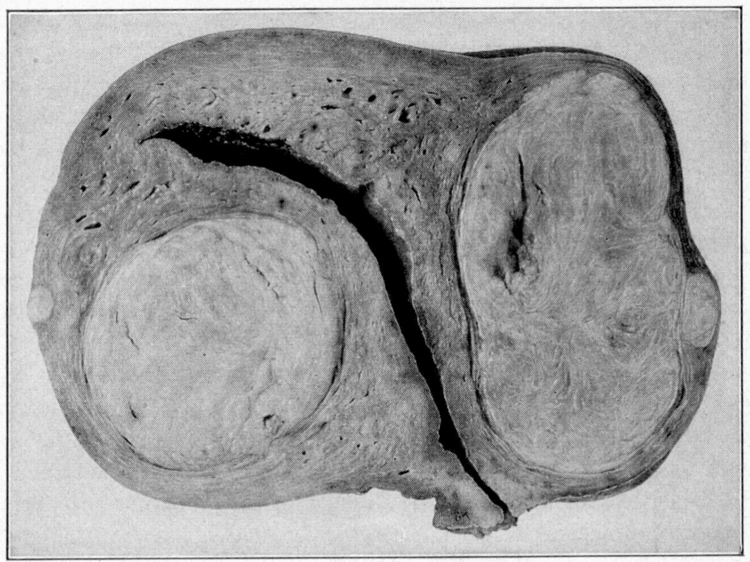

FIG. 497.—INTRAMURAL MYOMATA.

Puerperal uterus containing large myomata removed on third postpartum day, following spontaneous delivery at term, because of uterine infection. (From Traut and Kuder, *New International Clinics,* J. B. Lippincott Co., Philadelphia.)

This is in part due to actual hypertrophy which is sometimes accentuated by the occurrence of edema. Furthermore, owing to the pressure to which they are subjected by the growing ovum, the softened tumors may undergo considerable changes in shape, some showing so-called hemorrhagic or *carneous degeneration.* This form of degeneration, when it is the source of pain, low grade fever, leukocytosis and greatly increased sedimentation time, may occasionally necessitate operative removal but, as a rule, the signs and symptoms subside after two or three days of mild sedation and rest in bed. Occasionally the pedicle of a subserous myoma may become twisted, and gangrene and peritonitis may ensue.

At the time of labor the effect exerted by myomata depends entirely upon their size and situation. Generally speaking, subserous tumors are without great significance, except when their large size leads to pressure symptoms, or when a pedunculated tumor prolapses into the pelvic cavity. On the other hand, interstitial myomata situated in the cervix or lower uterine segment, may so obstruct the pelvic cavity that normal delivery will be impossible. As a result of the uterine contractions, a submucous myoma may become partially separated from its bed and protrude from the cervix as a polypoid mass. In such circumstances, since it effectively prevents the descent of the head, it must be removed by cutting through the pedicle.

Even when the tumor, by its size and situation, does not interfere with the course of labor, it predisposes to the occurrence of abnormal presentations. Olshausen, in tabulating the cases reported in the literature, found only 53 per cent of vertex presentations as compared with 24 and 19 per cent of breech and transverse presentations, respectively. Schauta, however, noted abnormal presentations in only 8 per cent of his personal cases. In Stander's 180 cases, which were of clinical importance, 26 abnormal presentations occurred, namely, 2 face, 8 transverse, and 16 breech presentations. The mere presence of the tumor may so interfere with the character of the uterine contractions as to cause inertia, as well as to favor the occurrence of postpartum hemorrhage. The latter is due partly to the fact that the myomatous nodules interfere with the normal contraction and retraction of the uterus, and partly because they may offer a mechanical obstacle to the separation and expulsion of the placenta. In addition, bleeding can occur from the myomatous nodule itself.

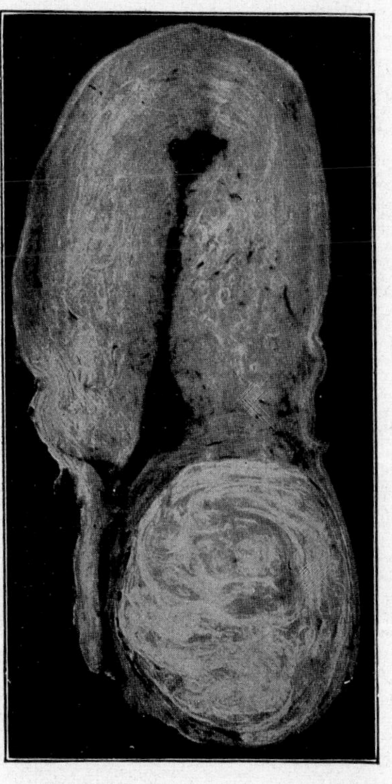

Fig. 498.—Uterus Removed by Supravaginal Amputation Following Cesarean Section Necessitated by Myoma in Posterior Wall of Cervix. × ½.

In the puerperium, myomata frequently undergo degenerative changes, and if they have been subjected to prolonged pressure, may become gangrenous. On the other hand, in certain cases the effect of pregnancy is beneficent, as the tumors may undergo puerperal involution, and thus become smaller or occasionally disappear.

The diagnosis of the association of pregnancy and myomata is not always easy. Hemorrhage may occur at intervals as the result of changes in the endometrium, and be mistaken by the patient for the menstrual flow, so that the idea of pregnancy may not suggest itself for months or until an abortion occurs. On the other hand, a sudden increase in the rapidity of the growth of the uterine tumor should direct attention to the possibility of pregnancy, and the diagnosis becomes assured when careful palpation shows the presence of soft areas interspersed between the firmer myomatous nodules. Subperitoneal myomata occasionally escape observation, being mistaken for the small parts, or sometimes for the head of the fetus, so that a diagnosis of multiple pregnancy may be made.

Myomectomy and enucleation are frequently followed by abortion or miscarriage, but do not necessarily destroy all chance of saving the life of the child. The duration of pregnancy, the size, number and location of the myomata, the age and obstetrical past history of the patient, and the type and severity of symptoms are among the factors which determine the procedure of choice in any given case. Child and Douglas reported that among 40,000 pregnant women admitted to the New York Lying-In Hospital over an 11-year period, there were 20, or 0.3 per cent, who required surgical or gynecological operative treatment during the course of their gestation. Among the cases in whom the complicating factor was myoma and operation was indicated, there were 9 patients in whom myomectomy was performed during the antenatal period, 7 who had a cesarean section and hysterectomy, and 7 a cesarean section and myomectomy at term. Of the 9 patients who were subjected to a myomectomy during pregnancy, 4 aborted following the operation. In addition to these 23 patients in whom the myomata were removed either before or at the time of delivery, there were 8 in whom a cesarean section was performed and the tumor not removed and of these one died of peritonitis, the only maternal death in the entire group of operative cases.

If serious symptoms do not supervene during pregnancy, operative interference should be deferred until shortly before the expected onset of labor, since the tumor may so change its shape or position as to render an operation unnecessary from an obstetrical point of view. In one of our patients, a tumor the size of a fist was found in the upper part of the cervix at the fifth month, and gave every promise of offering a serious obstacle to delivery. However, when she returned at the end of pregnancy for a cesarean section, the tumor had risen out of the pelvis, so that operation was not thought necessary, and a few days later an easy spontaneous delivery occurred.

So fortunate an outcome cannot always be expected. In any event, the patient should be examined thoroughly, and under anesthesia if necessary, shortly before the expected date of confinement. If the tumor is found to be firmly impacted in the pelvis, cesarean section should be performed before labor sets in, followed by supravaginal amputation, if indicated. Large myomata, which are liable to become degenerated and lead to severe infection of the uterus, usually necessitate hysterectomy. On the other hand, we do not favor extensive myomectomy or enucleation at the time of cesarean section because this leads to an increased incidence of puerperal infection. A pedunculated myoma may, of course, be removed with impunity, but any dissection in the uterine wall should be avoided.

On the other hand, if there is apparently no danger of impaction and spontaneous delivery seems probable, the patient should be allowed to go into labor spontaneously. If a mistake in prognosis has been made and symptoms of obstruction occur, cesarean section should be promptly performed in preference to attempts at delivery by the more usual obstetrical procedures.

It should be remembered that the completion of labor does not necessarily indicate that all danger is passed since, as has previously been indicated, the tumor may undergo gangrenous changes during the puerperium. Consequently, the occurrence of fever and abdominal pain should direct one's attention to such a possibility and make one consider the advisability of laparotomy.

Ovarian Tumors. The presence of an ovarian tumor is a serious complication of pregnancy since it increases the probability of abortion, frequently undergoes torsion and may offer an insuperable obstacle to delivery at the time of labor. Moreover, even after a spontaneous labor, its presence may give rise to disturbances during the puerperium.

While any variety of ovarian tumor may complicate pregnancy and labor, dermoid cysts have been described comparatively frequently in this connection. In 107 cases collected by McKerron in which the nature of the tumor was stated, there were 47 cystomata, 46 dermoid cysts, 9 malignant tumors, 5 fibromata, and 2 colloid cysts; while Spencer observed dermoid cysts in 12 of his 41 patients and Child and Douglas in 7 of their series of 23 patients.

Of the 321 pregnancies complicated by ovarian tumors which were collected by Remy, spontaneous abortion or premature labor occurred in 17 per cent of the cases. As has been indicated, tumors may also give rise to serious dystocia at the time of

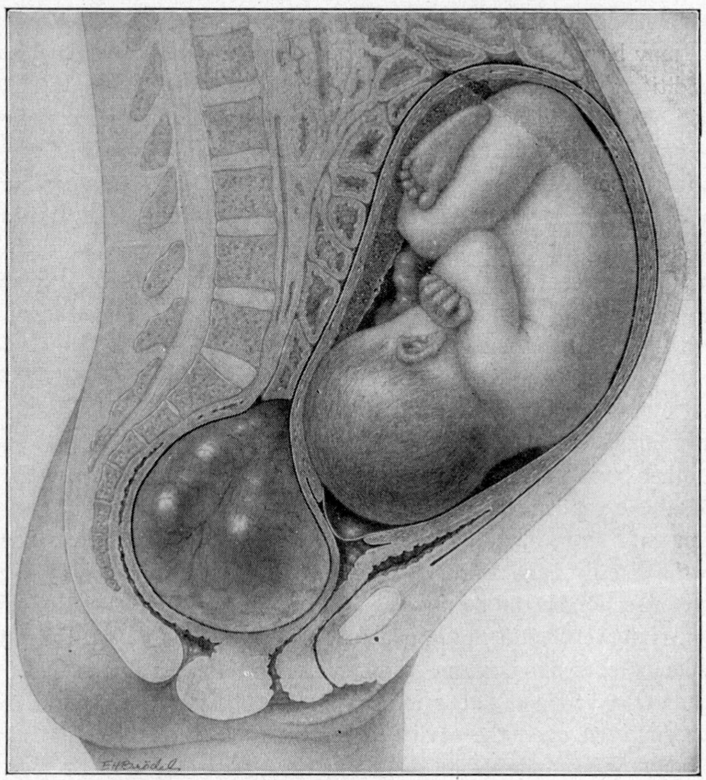

Fig. 499.—Ovarian Cyst Producing Dystocia.

labor. Moreover, the danger to the patient does not end with the birth of the child, for in not a few cases peritonitis follows gangrene of the tumor resulting from excessive pressure, while in other cases torsion of the pedicle may lead to a fatal termination.

Again, the cyst may rupture and extrude its contents into the peritoneal cavity during a spontaneous labor or as the result of operative interference. This event is a matter of indifference with the ordinary cystomata, but in the case of a dermoid it is frequently followed by fatal peritonitis. When the tumor occupies the pelvic cavity it may lead to rupture of the uterus or, if that does not occur, the tumor may be forced into the vagina and occasionally even into the rectum. While spontaneous rupture may occur it is surprising that it is not more frequent. In one of Stander's patients a thin-walled unilocular cyst, which was impacted in the pelvic cavity, led to rupture of the uterus instead of its own walls, although the latter did not exceed 1 mm. in thickness.

Unfortunately, the presence of an ovarian tumor complicating pregnancy often remains entirely unsuspected. Nevertheless, careful examination of all pregnant women, particularly when they are first registered, and again four or six weeks before the calculated date of confinement, should certainly eliminate a large proportion of these errors. Moreover, failure of the presenting part to engage, when the pelvis is known to be normal, suggests an obstructing mass. On the other hand, if the tumor does not occupy the pelvic cavity, the diagnosis may be extremely difficult, as the abdominal enlargement may be attributed to the presence of twin pregnancy or hydramnios, and the true condition is not recognized until after labor.

Inasmuch as the incidence of abortion following oophorocystectomy is relatively high, Child and Douglas concluded from their study and a review of the literature that the safest time to perform this operation is during or after the fourth month of gestation, provided operation can be postponed until that time. It has been objected that such a procedure increases the chances of premature delivery which occurred in 19.47 per cent of Heil's cases, but in only half as many of Syzmanowicz's personal cases. It should, however, be remembered that a similar accident may take place even if the patient is not interfered with, having been noted in 17 per cent of Remy's cases. This difference is so slight that the chances for the child are little, if at all, impaired by operation performed at the optimum time, while those of the mother are markedly improved.

On the other hand, when the diagnosis is not made until late in pregnancy, it is usually advisable except in the case of the malignant tumors of the ovary to postpone the operation until term, for the reason that the fresh abdominal cicatrix is not well-adapted to the strain of parturition. Consequently, if the tumor is impacted in the pelvis, cesarean section should be done at an appointed time, followed by the removal of the tumor. If, however, it is not impacted, it is preferable to allow the patient to go into spontaneous labor and to remove the tumor late in the puerperium.

Tumors of Other Origin. Labor is occasionally obstructed by tumors of various origin which encroach upon the cavity of the pelvis to such an extent as to render delivery difficult or even impossible. Among these, *pelvic ectopic kidney* is a rare complication of pregnancy, Anderson, Rice, and Harris having been able to collect only 98 cases from the literature to which they added 14 which have occurred in our clinic. Since such a kidney may occasionally block the birth canal and also be injured by the passage of the child, the condition has important obstetric aspects. In the 209 full-term deliveries recorded in the above series, spontaneous vaginal delivery occurred in 153, or in about three quarters, cesarean section was employed in 32 cases, the remainder having terminated in vaginal operative procedures. The maternal mortality was 8.9 per cent and the total fetal loss, 14.3 per cent. Both these figures are high, but it should be noted that no maternal death attributable to this condition has been recorded since 1927. In the 14 deliveries in seven mothers in our clinic, no maternal or fetal deaths occurred. In the opinion of Anderson, Rice, and Harris, the majority of these patients will deliver vaginally without hazard, but if all the kidney tissue the patient has is in the pelvis, abdominal delivery is probably the wiser course.

In rare instances a normal-sized or enlarged spleen may prolapse into the pelvic cavity and offer an obstacle to labor. Bland-Sutton has reported the removal of a prolapsed spleen in the second month of pregnancy, which might have given rise to serious dystocia at the time of labor had it remained *in situ.*

Echinococcus cysts are occasionally implanted in the pelvic cavity. Franta in 1902 collected 22 cases noted during pregnancy and discussed their effect upon the course of labor.

Reference has been made to those cases in which an old extra-uterine gestation sac so obstructed the pelvic canal as to interfere with the delivery of a subsequent intra-uterine pregnancy.

Enterocele, or hernia through the vaginal walls, occasionally give rise to dystocia, though in the majority of cases the prolapsed intestine can be replaced and the obstacle temporarily overcome. Where this is not possible, cesarean section is indicated as a more conservative procedure than forcibly dragging the child over a large irreducible hernia.

In occasional instances tumors of the bladder may offer an impediment to the passage of the child, though it is rarely serious enough to demand operative interference. On the other hand, it has sometimes been necessary to remove a large calculus from the bladder before delivery could be effected. In Neer's case the stone was almost spherical in shape and measured 2.75 inches at its greatest diameter.

A large rectocele or cystocele, though occasionally offering slight obstacle to labor, can generally be replaced while delivery is being effected.

Tumors arising from the lower part of the rectum or pelvic connective tissue may likewise give rise to serious dystocia, as reported by Pederson in 1922 after having collected a series of cases in which carcinoma of the rectum rendered cesarean section necessary.

BIBLIOGRAPHY

Anderson, G. W., Rice, G., and Harris, B. Pregnancy and Labor Complicated by Pelvic Kidney. A Review of the Literature. Obst. & Gynec. Surv., 1949, 4:737.

Andrews, H. R. The Effect of Ventral Fixation of the Uterus on Subsequent Pregnancy and Labour. J. Obst. & Gynaec., Brit. Emp., 1905, 8:97-125.

Bland-Sutton, J. The Surgery of Pregnancy and Labour Complicated with Tumours. Lancet, 1901, 1:382-386, 452-456, 529-532.

Brindeau, A. De l'atrésie acquise du vagin au point de vue obstétrical. Obstétrique, 1901, 6:97-122.

Campbell, J. Rupture of an Incarcerated Retroverted Gravid Uterus. J. Obst. & Gynaec. Brit. Emp., 1908, 14:403.

Carter, P. J. Conglutinatio Orificii Externi as a Factor in Delayed Labor. Am. J. Obst. & Gynec., 1941, 41:606.

Child, C. G., and Douglas, R. G. Surgical Problems Arising During Pregnancy. Am. J. Obst. & Gynec., 1944, 47:213.

Cragin, E. B. Congenital Pelvic Kidney Obstructing the Parturient Canal. Am. J. Obst., 1898, 38:36-41.

Davis, D. W., and Haszard, J. F. Congenital Absence of the Cervix Uteri Complicating Pregnancy. Canad. M. A. J., 1936, 35:425.

Dickinson, R. L. Pregnancy Following Ventrofixation. Am. J. Obst., 1901, 44:34.

Heil. Beitrag zur Ovariotomie in der Schwangerschaft. München med. Wchnschr., 1904, 51: No. 3.

Hué. Quelques recherches sur l'ampliation du diaphragme pelvien, etc. Paris, 1906.

Lynch, F. W. Kaiserschnitt und schwere Geburtsstörung infolge Ventro-fixation und Suspension. Monatschr. f. Geburtsh. u. Gynäk., 1904, 19:521.

McKerron, R. G. Pregnancy, Labour and Childbed with Ovarian Tumour. London, Rebman, 1903.

Neer, C. S. Dystocia from Large Bladder Stone Impacted in the Pelvis. J.A.M.A., 1919, 77:479-480.

Neugebauer, F. L. Zur Lehre von dem angeborenen und erworbenen Verwachsungen und Verengerungen der Scheide. Berlin, 1895.

Oldham. Sacculation of the Uterus. A Case of Retroflexion of the Gravid Uterus. Tr. Obst. Soc. Lond., 1860, 1:317-322.

Pederson. Dystocia Caused by Diseases of the Rectum. Acta Gyn. Scandinav., 1922, 1:445-458.

Pierson, R. N. Fibromyoma and Pregnancy; a Study of 250 Cases. Am. J. Obst. & Gynec., 1927, 14:333.

Remy. De la Grossesse Compliquée de Kyste Ovarique. Paris, 1886.

Sasonoff. Étude du thrombus de la vulve et du vagin. Ann. de gynéc. et d'obst., Par., 1884, 22:447-467.

Schroeder, K. Conglutinatio Orificii Externi. Lehrbuch der Geburtshülfe, 13. Aufl., 1899, pp. 590-592.

Spencer, H. R. Ovarian Tumors Complicating Pregnancy, Labor and the Puerperium. Surg., Gynec. & Obst., 1909, 8:461-466.

Szymanowicz, J. Kystes de l'ovaire et gestation. Gynéc. et obst., 1922, 6:405-419.

Ward. Atresia Vaginae Complicating Labour. Obstetrics, N. Y., 1899, 1:623-625.

Weibel, W. Ueber Schwangerschaft und Geburt nach Interpositio uteri vesicovaginalis. Arch. f. Gynaek., 1916, 105:65-73.

Williams. Dystocia Following Ventral Suspension and Fixation of the Uterus. Tr. South Surg. & Gynec. Ass., 1906, 19.

33

INJURIES TO THE BIRTH CANAL

With the exception of the most superficial varieties, which are limited to the mucous membrane of the fourchet, all perineal lacerations are accompanied by varying degrees of injury to the lower portion of the vagina. Such tears rarely occur in the median line but extend a variable distance up one or both vaginal sulci, being sufficiently deep to involve some fibers of the levator ani muscle. Bilateral lacerations of this variety are usually unequal in length and are separated from one another by a tongue-shaped portion of mucosa which represents the lower end of the posterior column of the vagina (Fig. 294).

These injuries should always be looked for, and their repair should form a part of every operation for the restoration of a lacerated perineum. If this precaution is neglected and the external wound alone is sutured the patient will eventually present symptoms due to *relaxation of the vaginal outlet,* even though the perineum proper may be in perfect condition.

Isolated tears involving the middle or upper third of the vagina, and unassociated with lacerations of the perineum or cervix, are very rarely observed. They are usually longitudinal and result from injuries sustained during a forceps operation though now and again they follow spontaneous delivery. They frequently extend deeply into the underlying tissues and may give rise to a copious hemorrhage which, however, is readily controlled by a few sutures. Their presence is readily overlooked, inasmuch as they can be recognized only after the vaginal walls have been spread apart by means of a speculum.

More important are the *injuries to the levator ani muscles,* which are not associated with tears through the vaginal mucosa, and which consequently usually escape immediate detection. As a result of overdistention of the birth canal there may occur a submucous separation of certain fibers of the muscle, or at least so great a diminution in its tonicity that it can no longer properly fulfil its function as the pelvic diaphragm. In such cases the patient sooner or later suffers just as severely from symptoms of relaxation as if a deeply lacerated perineum had been left unrepaired. Although the accident can sometimes be avoided by an intelligent use of forceps when the second stage of labor is unduly prolonged, it frequently follows spontaneous and rapid delivery.

Lesions of the upper third of the vagina are extremely uncommon unless they represent the extension of deep cervical tears into the fornix. In very rare instances, however, the cervix may be entirely or partially torn loose from its vaginal attachment, rupture in other cases occurring in either the anterior, posterior, or lateral fornix. Hugenberger in 1875 collected 40 cases of this accident and designated it as *colporrhexis,* while Gamble has made an extensive survey of the literature up to 1927.

The accident is somewhat analogous to rupture of the lower uterine segment and follows energetic efforts on the part of the uterus to overcome some obstacle to the passage of the child. In Gamble's patient it was due to overstretching of the posterior fornix incident to an unusually pendulous abdomen. As a result of the retraction of Bandl's ring, so great a strain may be exerted upon the cervix that it is torn loose from its vaginal attachment. It is commonly taught that colporrhexis is possible only in those cases in which the lips of the cervix are not compressed between the presenting part and the pelvic wall, but are free to follow the retracting uterus. While colporrhexis sometimes occurs spontaneously, it more frequently follows brutal and unskillful use of forceps.

The symptoms are identical with those following rupture of the uterus and will be considered under that heading. Immediately following the rupture the child may escape into the peritoneal cavity, after which the intestines may protrude into the vaginal canal as in a case reported by Ross.

The diagnosis is made solely by the sense of touch as the clinical symptoms do not differ from those following rupture of the uterus. The prognosis is extremely unfavorable, a large proportion of the cases reported in the literature having ended fatally.

Most authorities recommend treating the condition by means of a vaginal pack, a procedure which probably explains in part the high mortality. We, however, agree with Schick that laparotomy offers the best chance for successfully coping with this emergency since in that way one can obtain an accurate idea of the extent of the injury, when the torn surfaces may be united by sutures, or failing that, the uterus may be removed.

LESIONS OF THE CERVIX

Slight degrees of cervical laceration must be regarded as an inevitable accompaniment of childbirth. Such tears, however, heal rapidly and rarely give rise to symptoms. In healing they cause a material change in the shape of the external os and thereby afford a means of determining whether a woman has borne children or not.

In other cases the tears are deeper, implicating one or both sides of the cervix and may extend up to or beyond the vaginal junction. In rarer instances the laceration may extend across the vaginal fornix or into the lower uterine segment, and occasionally open up the base of the broad ligament. Such extensive lesions frequently involve vessels of considerable size, and are then associated with profuse hemorrhage.

Deep cervical tears occasionally occur during the course of spontaneous labor and under such circumstances their genesis is not always clear. More usually, however, they follow rapid manual or instrumental dilatation. Moreover, they are apt to result from attempts at delivery through an imperfectly dilated cervix, no matter whether forceps or version be employed.

Occasionally, even in spontaneous labors, the edematous anterior lip of the cervix may be caught between the head and the symphysis pubis and be compressed until it undergoes necrotic changes and separation occurs. In still rarer instances the entire vaginal portion may be torn loose from the rest of the cervix, and be cast off. According to Boudreau, this so-called annular or *circular detachment of the cervix* usually occurs in elderly primiparae when the pains are strong and a serious obstacle to delivery is offered by an imperfectly dilated os externum.

Symptoms. In all lesions involving the cervix there is usually no escape of blood until after the birth of the child, when the hemorrhage may be profuse. In many cases, however, the bleeding is so slight that the condition would pass unrecognized were it not detected upon vaginal examination. When one lip of the vaginal portion of the cervix is torn off, there is usually very little hemorrhage for the reason that the tissues have been so compressed before the occurrence of the accident that the vessels have undergone thrombosis. Likewise, in our case of circular detachment of the cervix

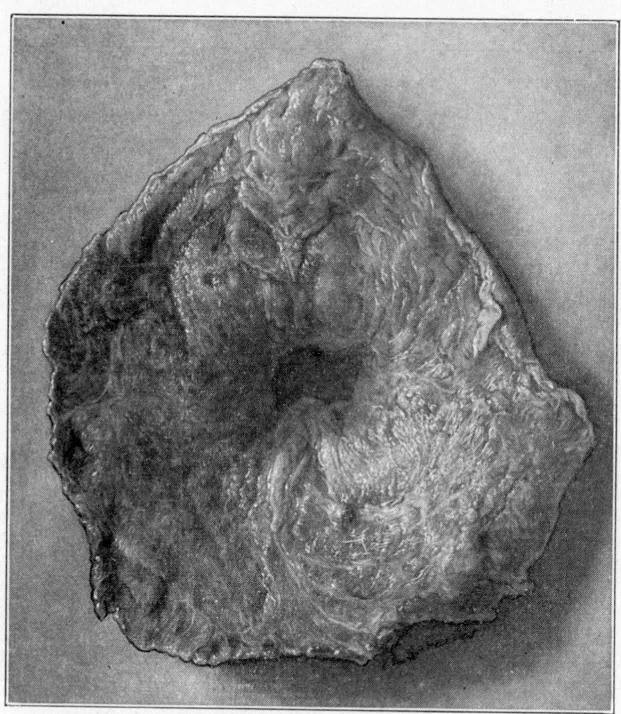

Fig. 500.—Annular Detachment of Cervix.

Specimen cast off before the birth of child, showing undilated and rigid external os and obliterated cervical canal seen from within. × 1.

figured in this section, there was no bleeding and the nature of the cast-off tissue was not recognized until after examination in the laboratory.

Slight cervical tears heal spontaneously and extensive lacerations have a similar tendency but perfect union rarely results. They afford to any pathogenic micro-organisms which may be present a ready portal of entry into the lymphatics at the base of the broad ligament.

The development of erosions at the site of the old tears is frequently the cause of persistent leukorrhea. Consequently at the end of the puerperium it is advisable as a matter of routine to examine the cervix by means of a speculum, and if such areas are found to cauterize them as a prophylactic precaution.

Diagnosis. A deep cervical tear should always be suspected in cases of profuse hemorrhage coming on during the third stage of labor if the hand applied over the lower abdomen feels that the uterus is firmly contracted. For a positive diagnosis, however, a thorough examination is necessary. Owing to the flabby condition of the cervix immediately after delivery mere digital examination is often unsatisfactory and the extent of the injury can be fully appreciated only after drawing the cervix down to the vulva and carefully subjecting it to direct inspection.

In view of the frequency with which deep tears follow all but the more simple operative procedures, the cervix in all such cases should be inspected as a matter of routine at the conclusion of the third stage, even if there be no bleeding; and if a tear is discovered it should be united by sutures as a prophylactic measure. Annular de-

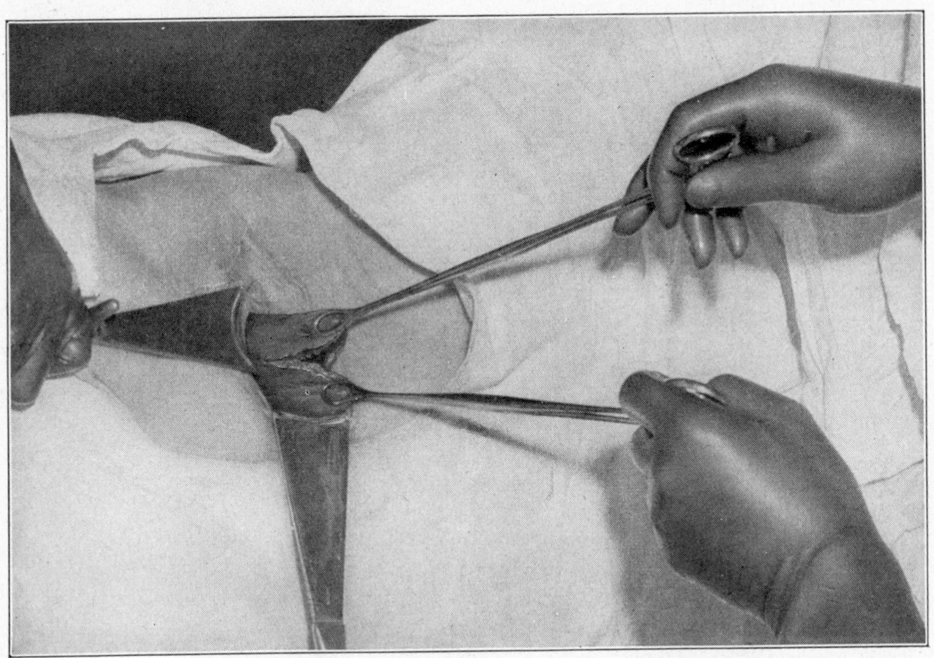

Fig. 501.—Cervical Laceration Exposed for Repair.

tachment of the vaginal portion of the cervix should be diagnosticated whenever an irregular mass of tissue having a circular opening in its center is cast off before or after the birth of the child.

Treatment. Deep cervical tears accompanied by hemorrhage should be immediately repaired, the introduction of a few sutures readily checking the flow of blood. On the other hand, if there be no hemorrhage, the condition usually escapes detection unless specifically looked for. We have already indicated the advisability of inspecting the cervix after all operative procedures; but we consider its routine employment unnecessary after normal labor, because we believe that the benefits following the repair of all tears will be more than counterbalanced by the increased incidence of infection resulting from the necessary manipulations. Moreover, the majority of such tears heal spontaneously and in the exceptional cases in which this does not occur better results are obtained by a secondary operation performed at a later date.

The treatment of cervical tears associated with hemorrhage varies with the extent of the lesion. When the laceration is limited to the cervix, or even when it extends well into the vaginal fornix, satisfactory results are obtained by the introduction of sutures after bringing the cervix into view at the vulva. This is effected by having an assistant make firm downward pressure upon the uterus, while at the same time the operator exerts strong traction by means of a fenestrated ovum or sponge forceps applied to either lip of the cervix, the vaginal walls being held apart by means of suitable retractors (Fig 501). As the hemorrhage usually comes from the upper angle of the wound it is advisable to apply the first suture in that situation since, if the suturing is begun at the free end of the tear, a dead space is often left toward its upper extremity from which subsequent hemorrhage may occur. Interrupted chromicized catgut sutures should be employed as they do not have to be removed. The beginner is cautioned against too great a regard for appearances in attempting to give the cervix a normal look, inasmuch as the involution and retraction occurring within the next few days may lead to such constriction of its lumen as to cause retention of the lochial discharge.

Many authorities recommend a tight vaginal pack in these cases. No doubt it will usually check the hemorrhage and may be employed in an emergency, but it does not compare in efficiency with repair by suture. In the rare cases in which the wound extends through the broad ligament into the peritoneal cavity a tight pack may be introduced provided there is no serious hemorrhage; but in all other cases the only satisfactory method of dealing with the condition is by laparotomy.

The treatment of tears of the upper part of the cervix which involve the lower uterine segment will be considered in the following section.

RUPTURE OF THE UTERUS

The term *rupture of the uterus* is usually employed to denote rupture after the period of viability of the fetus. This definition eliminates from consideration such conditions as rupture of interstitial pregnancies, traumatic perforations in the course of abortion, etc. which may occur in the early months of pregnancy.

This accident is one of the most serious the obstetrician meets. Its actual incidence among pregnant and parturient women is difficult to assess, as published hospital statistics vary greatly and are modified by the type of patients and number of referred cases received. The combined figures of four published series (Acken, Bill, Barney and Melody, Delfs and Eastman, and Sheldon) from different areas give a total of 117 ruptures of the uterus in 190,454 deliveries, that is, once in 1,627 deliveries. The last two of these papers also give figures for registered cases under observation before rupture occurred, and their combined data show an incidence of once in 2,198 deliveries. This latter figure is probably more nearly the actual incidence throughout the population than is the figure which precedes it. In spite of its infrequent occurrence, rupture of the uterus looms as a major cause of death in present-day obstetrics; it is responsible for at least five per cent of all maternal deaths.

Various classifications of rupture of the uterus have been made, but one of the most useful from a clinical standpoint is based upon the time of rupture as follows:

A. Rupture during pregnancy

1. Spontaneous rupture of
    a. Previous cesarean section scar
    b. The intact uterus

2. Traumatic rupture

B. **Rupture during labor**

1. Spontaneous rupture of
    a. Previous cesarean section scar
    b. The intact uterus
2. Traumatic rupture

Rupture of the scar from previous cesarean section, either in pregnancy or in labor, is a special situation with some differences in etiology, symptoms, and prognosis from other types of rupture. It is discussed under cesarean section (page 1120).

Spontaneous rupture of the intact uterus during pregnancy is exceedingly rare. Pregnancy in a poorly developed horn of a bicornuate uterus has been reported as causative, as has adenomyosis of the fundus. Some cases have presented no discernible cause. In rupture during pregnancy the lesion is almost always in the body of the uterus, either fundal or on the anterior or posterior wall. This is in contrast to ruptures during labor which are characteristically in the lower uterine segment.

The symptoms and signs of rupture during pregnancy are the same as those occurring with ruptures during labor (see below). A few cases have been reported, however, in which intraperitoneal hemorrhage was slight and symptoms minimal so that hours or even days elapsed before the patient presented herself. In very rare cases the fetus may be extruded into the abdomen while the placenta remains in the uterus, and the gestation continues as a utero-abdominal pregnancy (Leopold, Gepfert). Escape into the abdomen is almost always accompanied by death of the fetus because the retraction of the uterus critically reduces the maternal circulation to the placental area.

Traumatic rupture of the uterus during pregnancy is quite uncommon but may occur at any stage beyond the early months. A blow or fall on the abdomen or an automobile accident may cause rupture. The tear may occur at the site of the blow or elsewhere in the body of the uterus by contrecoup. It is surprising how resistant the uterus is to external trauma, yet, occasionally, apparently slight force causes rupture. One patient seen in our clinic fell on a curb but was unaware of injury at the time. She came to the hospital eight hours later because of faintness. She was in shock and at laparotomy had in the fundus a ragged laceration through which a fetal arm and shoulder protruded. Any pregnant woman who is involved in an automobile accident should be watched carefully for signs of ruptured uterus.

In the past spontaneous rupture during labor has been somewhat less common than traumatic rupture but this may no longer be true with the modern trend away from difficult vaginal operating. Delfs and Eastman found 40 per cent of ruptures during labor to be spontaneous (17 of 43 cases). Most of these patients were in the older age group and of great parity (average 6.4). None were primigravidae. Some contraction of the pelvis was a contributory factor in 41 per cent. Though all had had previous vaginal deliveries, in most cases the present infants were somewhat larger than these women had previously delivered. Even slight mechanical difficulties may not be surmounted safely in the uterus which has been weakened by repeated childbearing. This point is emphasized because it has been customary teaching to stress as causes of spontaneous rupture only the more obvious dystocia factors, such as transverse presentation, hydrocephalus, impacted tumors, brow or face presentation, etc.

Pathologic Anatomy. The important predisposing role played, in uterine rupture, by excessive stretching of the lower uterine segment with the development of a

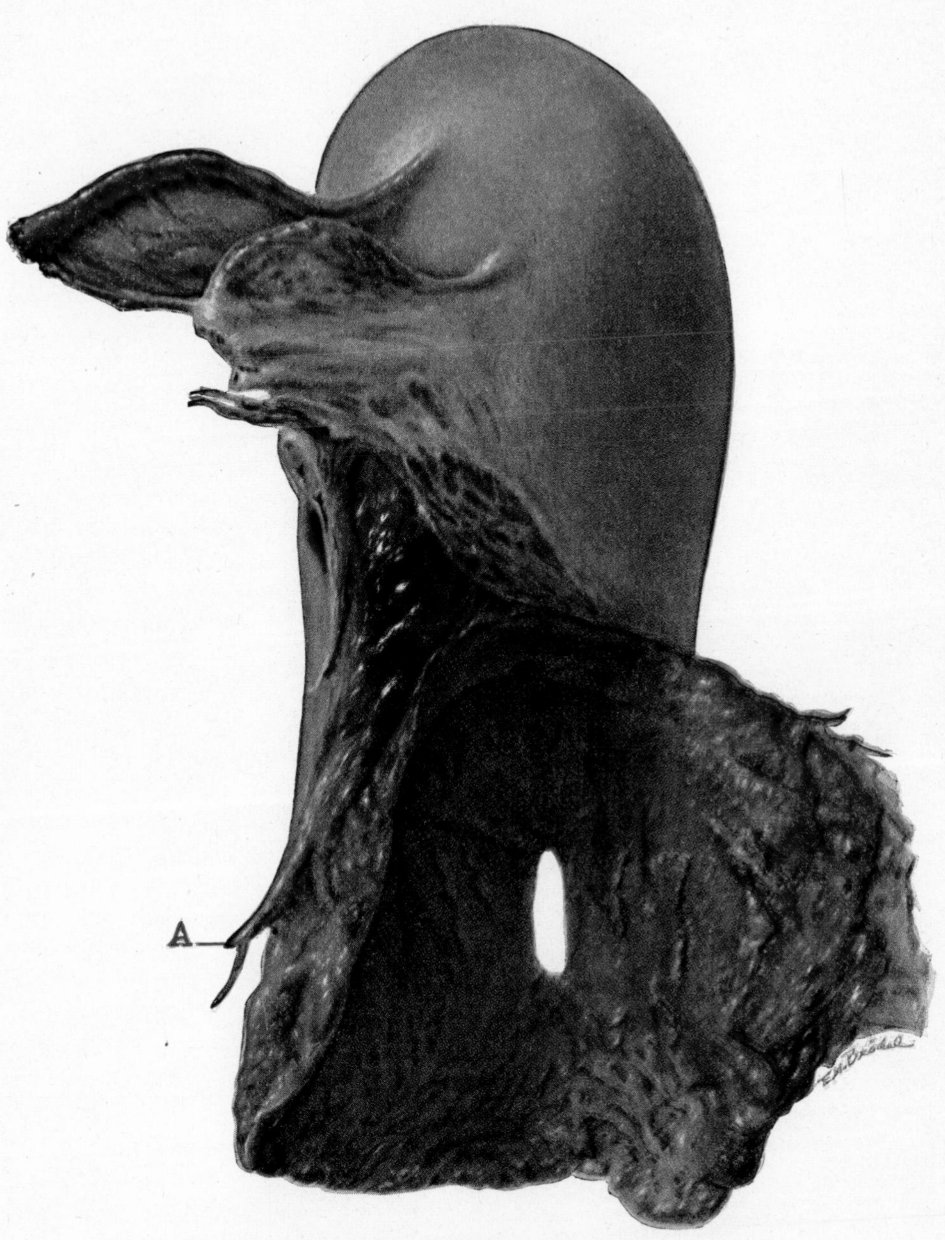

FIG. 502.—RUPTURE OF UTERUS, BILATERAL.
A. Laceration extends through left uterine artery. (Same case as Fig. 431.)

pathologic retraction ring has already been stressed in Chapter 29. Rupture of the uterus occurring at the time of labor is limited almost entirely to the lower uterine segment, the rent usually pursuing an oblique direction, although when it is in the immediate vicinity of the cervix, it frequently extends transversely. On the other hand, it is usually longitudinal when it occurs in the portion of the uterus adjacent to the broad ligament. Although occurring primarily in the lower uterine segment, it is not unusual for the laceration to extend further upward into the body of the uterus or downward through the cervix into the vagina. The tear itself usually presents jagged, irregular margins which are stained with blood (Fig. 502).

It is customary to distinguish between *complete* and *incomplete rupture,* according as the laceration communicates directly with the abdominal cavity or is separated from it by the peritoneal covering of the uterus or broad ligament. Of 106 ruptures occurring at the New York Lying-In Hospital, Davis found that 88 were complete and 18 incomplete and that 24 of the complete ruptures had occurred through former cesarean section scars.

Incomplete ruptures frequently extend into the broad ligament; in such circumstances the hemorrhage often occurs less rapidly than in the complete variety, the blood slowly accumulating between the leaflets and leading to the separation of the peritoneum from the surrounding viscera, with the consequent formation of a large *subperitoneal hematoma.* Occasionally an effusion of blood sufficiently copious to cause the death of the patient may be enclosed in such a structure. More frequently, however, the fatal issue does not occur until secondary rupture of the hematoma relieves the pressure, which had previously, to some extent, restrained the bleeding, and permits the blood to escape into the peritoneal cavity.

Following complete rupture, the uterine contents may escape into the peritoneal cavity but, when the presenting part is firmly engaged, only a portion of the fetus may escape, the rest remaining in the uterine cavity. On the other hand, in the incomplete variety, the product of conception may remain within the uterus or come to lie beneath the serous covering of the uterus or between the leaflets of the broad ligament.

Clinical Picture. If the accident occurs at the time of labor the patient, after presenting for some time the premonitory signs of the accident, suddenly, at the height of an intense uterine contraction, complains of a sharp, shooting pain in the lower abdomen, and frequently cries out that something has given way inside her. At the same time the lower uterine segment becomes much more sensitive to pressure. Immediately following these symptoms there is cessation of the uterine contractions and the patient, who had previously been in intense agony, suddenly experiences great relief. At the same time there is usually some external hemorrhage, although in many cases it is very slight in amount.

Palpation or vaginal examination shows that the presenting part has slipped away from the superior strait and has become movable while a hard, round body, which represents the firmly contracted uterus, may be felt alongside the fetus which is often more easily palpated than usual. Naturally, if the uterine contents have escaped into the abdominal cavity, the presenting part cannot be felt on vaginal examination. Vaginal examination sometimes reveals the existence of a tear in the uterine wall through which the fingers can be passed into the abdominal cavity where they come in contact with the intestines, although failure to detect the tear by no means indicates its absence.

As a rule, shortly after the occurrence of complete rupture the patient presents symptoms of collapse: the pulse increases in rapidity, loses tone, and takes on a filiform character; the face becomes pallid, assumes a drawn appearance, and is often covered with beads of sweat. If the hemorrhage has been copious she may complain of chilliness, disturbance of vision, and air hunger and eventually pass into an unconscious state. Symptoms of collapse, however, do not always appear immediately but are sometimes deferred for several hours after rupture, being less marked when the child remains partially within the uterus. After incomplete rupture, moreover, the immediate symptoms are sometimes very slight but increase in severity as the subperitoneal hematoma becomes larger. This fact—that many uterine ruptures remain silent for many hours—demands especial emphasis because failure to make the diagnosis in these cases is responsible for many fatalities. In general, the most constant clinical symptom is pain coupled with abdominal tenderness rather than shock. In cases in which there is any possibility of uterine rupture it is desirable to secure a catheterized urine specimen. If this is grossly bloody it lends strong support to the diagnosis of rupture, but a clear specimen, of course, by no means rules rupture out. When rupture has occurred in labor and is overlooked, the first sign of the condition may be abdominal distention in the puerperium consequent upon the irritation produced by retroperitoneal blood.

Traumatic Rupture. Traumatic rupture during labor is most commonly produced by version and extraction. In our clinic 11 of 26 (42 per cent) traumatic ruptures occurred with version and extraction. Although the accident is most likely to occur in cases attempted after rupture of the membranes or with impaction of a transverse presentation, it may also happen in more favorable cases when the operator has taken pains to proceed with great gentleness. Other causes of traumatic rupture are Braxton Hicks version, breech extraction, and difficult or unsuccessful forceps. Unfortunately, administration of pituitrin in the first or second stage of labor continues to be a cause of traumatic rupture. Use of the bag or bougie has occasionally produced rupture.

Since patients who suffer traumatic rupture in labor are usually under anesthesia, pain and tenderness are not immediately exhibited, and the condition makes itself manifest by bleeding and evidence of shock. In this condition also, blood in the urine is an important positive finding.

Prognosis. The chances for the child are almost uniformly bad. On the other hand, if it has survived up to the time of the accident, its only chance of living is afforded by immediate laparotomy; otherwise, anoxia, the result of the separation of the placenta, is inevitable. If left to themselves, the vast majority of the mothers die from hemorrhage or infection; however, spontaneous recovery has been noted in exceptional cases. In 23 maternal fatalities due to uterine rupture studied in our clinic by Delfs and Eastman, death was due to shock and hemorrhage in 57 per cent and to infection in 43 per cent. In Delfs and Eastman's 43 cases of ruptured uterus (excluding rupture of section scars), the maternal and fetal mortality rates were 53 per cent and 83 per cent, respectively. In 26 cases of rupture of the uterus recorded by Sheldon, the maternal mortality was 42.3 per cent and the fetal death rate, 82 per cent. Bill and his associates reported 23 cases of rupture of the uterus with a maternal mortality of 21.7 per cent and a fetal mortality of 62 per cent. Gordon and Rosenthal believe that rupture of the uterus is a more common cause of death than is ectopic gestation. Earlier diagnosis, immediate operation, the availability of large amounts of blood from blood banks, and chemotherapy should greatly improve maternal prognosis in rupture of the uterus.

Treatment. *Prophylactic.* Intelligent care during labor should largely do away with this accident. Whenever there is a possibility of the existence of an obstacle to the birth of the child the obstetrician should always be on the alert for symptoms indicative of impending rupture. He should be especially wary about the possibility of this accident in labors in which the fetus presents transversely or is hydrocephalic; and in vertex presentations, failure of engagement after one hour of strong second-stage pains should call for careful watching of the lower uterine segment. If it balloons out or if the pathologic retraction ring rises up, labor should be promptly terminated by the most conservative procedure. In very neglected cases, decapitation in transverse and craniotomy in head presentations often promise the best results, as the infants are usually already dead.

Curative. Whether the child is alive or dead and whether it is still within the ruptured uterus or has already escaped into the abdominal cavity, no attempt should be made to extract it per vaginam, but laparotomy should be performed immediately. After removal of the child, whatever operative procedures may be deemed necessary are carried out. The procedure will usually consist of hysterectomy, but in selected cases suture of the lacerated wound may be performed. After the latter procedure, however, the value of the uterus for future childbearing is questionable; repeated ruptures of such repaired tears are on record.

Blood transfusion is of lifesaving importance in the treatment of a ruptured uterus. It should be started at once if shock is present, and in any case, *blood should be running in throughout the operation.* Many cases may require three to six or more pints to give adequate support. In this connection it should be stressed that many patients who appear to be relatively free of shock, collapse completely when the abdomen is opened. Ample chemotherapy and antibiotics should be given before and after operation, since infection is present in many cases and traumatized tissues and vessels in the pelvic floor are fertile sites for infection.

INSTRUMENTAL PERFORATION OF THE UTERUS

Reference has already been made to perforation of the uterus following attempts at criminal abortion or in the effort to remove placental tissue by means of curet or polypus forceps after an incomplete abortion. Similar accidents occasionally are the result of want of skill on the part of the obstetrician in full-term labor when either the uterus or the vaginal vault may be perforated. As has been pointed out, in cases of this character, loops of intestine frequently prolapse through the rupture. In such circumstances laparotomy is the ideal treatment though, in the absence of prolapse of the intestines, cases are recorded in which recovery occurred spontaneously under what were apparently most unfavorable circumstances.

A graphic idea of the variety and extent of such injuries is afforded by the illustrations in Liepmann's book on criminal abortion, while the literature up to 1936 is critically considered in Taussig's book on abortion.

PERFORATION OF THE GENITAL TRACT FOLLOWING NECROSIS

In the obstructed labor the tissues in various portions of the genital tract may be forcibly compressed between the head and the bony canal. If the pressure is transitory it is without significance; but if it is long-continued, necrosis results and after a few days the area implicated sloughs away so that perforation follows.

In most cases of this character the perforation occurs between the vagina and the bladder, giving rise to a *vesicovaginal fistula.* Less frequently the anterior lip of the cervix is compressed against the symphysis pubis, and an abnormal communication is eventually established between the cervical canal and the bladder—*cervicovesical fistula.*

If the patient is not infected the fistulous tract frequently heals without further treatment. In other cases, however, it may persist, and a subsequent plastic operation becomes necessary for its cure.

Occasionally the posterior wall of the uterus may be subjected to so much pressure against the promontory of the sacrum that necrosis results and a connection is established with Douglas' cul-de-sac. If infection occurs the accident is usually followed by septic peritonitis. Fortunately recovery usually follows without further complications, inasmuch as a localized peritonitis leads to the formation of adhesions between the posterior wall of the uterus and the pelvic peritoneum, thereby doing away with the possibility of a general peritoneal infection. It should be remembered that similar lesions may occur in the rare cases in which exostoses or bony spicules protrude from the walls of the birth canal, as in *pelvis spinosa.*

BIBLIOGRAPHY

ACKEN, H. S. Rupture of the Pregnant Uterus. Am. J. Surg., 1940, 49:423.

BANDL. Ueber Ruptur des Uterus und ihre Mechanik. Wien, 1875.

BILL, A. H., BARNEY, W. R., and MELODY, G. F. Rupture of the Uterus. Am. J. Obst. & Gynec., 1944, 47:712.

BOUDREAU, Louis. L'Arrachement Circulaire du Col Utérin pendant l'Accouchement. Thèse de Toulouse, 1902.

DAVIS, A. B. The Ruptured Uterus. Am. J. Obst. & Gynec., 1927, 13:522-528.

DELFS, E., and EASTMAN, N. J. Rupture of the Uterus (An Analysis of 53 Cases). Canad. M. A. J., 1945, 52:376.

GAMBLE, T. O. Colporrhexis, or Rupture of the Vault of the Vagina. Am. J. Obst. & Gynec., 1927, 14:766-773.

GEPFERT, J. R. Antepartum Rupture of the Uterine Scar Following Low Flap Cesarean Section. With a Report of a Case Giving Rise to a Secondary Abdominal Pregnancy. Am. J. Obst. & Gynec., 1939, 37:466.

GORDON, C. A., and ROSENTHAL, A. H. Rupture of the Uterus. An Analysis of 30 Maternal Deaths. Surg., Gynec. & Obst., 1943, 77:26.

LEOPOLD, G. Ausgetragene secundäre Abdominalschwangerschaft nach Ruptura uteri traumatica, etc. Arch. f. Gynäk., 1896, 52:376-388.

LIEPMANN, W. Die Abtreibung. Berlin u. Wien, 1927.

MAHON, R. Complex Birth Injuries of the Vagina. Bull. de la Soc. d'Obst. et de Gynéc., 1939, 28:224.

MCNEILE, L. G., and MCBURNEY, R. D. Statistical Study of Uterine Ruptures. California & West. Med., 1935, 42:73.

PEHAM, H., und KATZ, H. Die instrumentelle Perforation des graviden Uterus und ihre Verhütung. Wien, 1926.

PETTIT, R. D. Repeated Secondary Rupture of the Pregnant Uterus. Am. J. Obst. & Gynec., 1943, 45:334.

Riddel, J. Rupture of the Uterus during Pregnancy. J. Obst. & Gynaec., Brit. Emp., 1926, 33:1.

Schäfer, P. Zur Aetiologie der Schwangerschaftsrupturen. Arch. f. Gynäk., 1918, 109:284-301.

Sheldon, C. P. A Record of 26 Cases of Rupture of the Uterus. Am. J. Obst. & Gynec., 1936, 31:455.

Taussig, F. J. Abortion. Spontaneous and Induced. St. Louis, 1936.

Whitacre, F. E., and Fang, L. Y. Management of Rupture of the Uterus. Report of 44 Cases. Arch. Surg., 1942, 45:213.

Woodhull, R. B. Traumatic Rupture of the Pregnant Uterus Resulting from an Automobile Accident. Surgery, 1942, 12:615.

34

ABNORMALITIES OF THE THIRD STAGE OF LABOR

POSTPARTUM HEMORRHAGE

Postpartum hemorrhage is defined as bleeding from the birth canal in excess of 500 cc. during the first 24 hours after birth. Hemorrhages subsequent to the first 24 hours are called *late hemorrhages* and are discussed under disorders of the puerperium on page 974.

Postpartum hemorrhage is the most common cause of blood loss in obstetrics. As a direct factor in maternal mortality it looms large, being responsible through exsanguination for about one quarter of the deaths in the obstetric hemorrhage group (postpartum hemorrhage, placenta previa, abruptio placentae, ectopic pregnancy, abortion hemorrhage, and rupture of the uterus). In addition, as stressed in Chapter 1, it is probably an even more important indirect cause of death since, by weakening the patient's resistance to infection and necessitating operative manipulations in the birth canal, it predisposes to puerperal infection. In Douglas and Davis' analysis of 183 cases of puerperal infection, postpartum hemorrhage was the most important underlying cause; indeed, it may be said categorically that losses of 1,000 cc. or more, unless replaced by transfusions, are almost invariably followed by puerperal infection, while even after losses of the magnitude of 600 cc. the postpartum morbidity rate rises sharply. For example, Stander found an incidence of puerperal infection of 27.2 per cent following hemorrhages of 600 cc. and more, in contrast with a figure of only 8.3 per cent for all hospital deliveries during the same period. These facts make manifest the transcendent importance of the old dictum: *Save blood.*

Incidence. Postpartum hemorrhage, as defined, is of frequent occurrence and is observed in about 10 per cent of all deliveries. Larger hemorrhages are less common, the average figures from a number of reports ranging as follows: 600 cc. or more in 5 to 6 per cent; 1,000 cc. or more in 1.5 per cent; 1,500 cc. or more in 0.3 per cent or once in about 335 deliveries; and 2,000 cc. or more in 0.07 per cent or once in about 1,400 deliveries.

Immediate Causes. The immediate causes of postpartum hemorrhage are three in number:

1. Uterine atony.
2. Vaginal and cervical lacerations.
3. Retention of placental fragments.

The most common of these causes is the first, which is responsible for over 90 per cent of the cases. Vaginal and cervical lacerations constitute the main source of postpartum bleeding in about 6 per cent. Retention of a placental fragment is an uncommon cause of postpartum hemorrhage as defined but is frequently responsible for late bleeding.

Somewhat akin to vaginal lacerations as a source of bleeding at delivery is episiotomy blood loss. Although a large part of the bleeding from the episiotomy incision occurs before the birth of the child, it is not generally feasible to measure this blood separately and it is usually regarded as making up a portion of the total postpartum blood lost. While it is uncommon for an episiotomy to produce alone sufficient bleeding to be called postpartum hemorrhage, blood so lost averages about 200 cc. and, when added to uterine blood flow, often puts the aggregate in the category of postpartum hemorrhage. Odell and Seski find the average blood loss from episiotomy to be 253 cc. and believe that it probably constitutes the chief source of bleeding in most primiparous patients. This is doubtless true in blood losses under 500 cc.

Predisposing Causes. The predisposing causes of postpartum hemorrhage fall into two main groups: (1) those which are predetermined and beyond the control of the obstetrician, and (2) those which are directly under his surveillance.

In the former category the most important predisposing cause of postpartum hemorrhage is the size of the baby. This general relationship was noted by Ahlfeld as early as 1904 and has since been substantiated by the statistical study of Calkins, Litzenberg and Plass, and Reich. The latter author found that the likelihood of postpartum hemorrhage with a baby of five pounds or less was one in 21, whereas with a baby of nine pounds or more the chances of excessive bleeding were one in four. Multiple pregnancy is likewise associated with an increased frequency of postpartum bleeding. Guttmacher, in a study of 234 twin pregnancies at the Johns Hopkins Hospital, found that the incidence of postpartum hemorrhage in excess of 600 cc. was 14.5 per cent, whereas in the clinic population at large it was 6.3 per cent. He made the observation, however, that in the last 40 cases of multiple pregnancy, there was not a single case of excessive bleeding. Since the only alteration in procedure during the period covered by the 40 cases lay in the administration of pitocin immediately after the birth of the baby, he was inclined to attribute the improved results to this medication. This observation suggests that the increased frequency of postpartum hemorrhage following multiple birth (and probably also after the delivery of large babies) is not caused by the increased size of the placental site but by atony of the uterus consequent upon overdistention of the organ. In this connection, it is well known, of course, that hydramnios is frequently followed by postpartum hemorrhage. Other conditions in which it is extremely frequent are abruptio placentae (about once in four cases) and placenta previa (possibly as often as once in two cases).

Among the controllable causes of postpartum hemorrhage the most important are: operative delivery, deep ether anesthesia, prolonged labor with maternal exhaustion, and mismanagement of the third stage of labor. The statistics of Pastore, Reich, and others indicate that excessive bleeding is about three times more common after operative delivery than after spontaneous termination of labor. While anesthesia and lacerations both contribute to this end, there is general agreement that the former is a most important factor, particularly ether anesthesia. Internal podalic version is followed by serious postpartum hemorrhage in such a high percentage of cases that any patient in whom such an operation is contemplated should have blood ready for transfusion and every preparation made to combat bleeding. With the possible exception of rectal ether, which Irving, Berman, and Nelson have shown causes an increased incidence of postpartum atony, modern analgesia per se cannot be incriminated in this respect. However, insofar as it increases the incidence of operative delivery, it may well be a factor. Colvin and Bartholomew, on the other hand, report a very low incidence of hemorrhage in their series of paraldehyde cases and are inclined to attribute the gratifying results to the greater amount of rest obtained during labor and the smaller quantity of ether used.

In prolonged labor with maternal exhaustion the uterus often takes part in the general fatigue and does not contract satisfactorily. In this type of case the triad of exhaustion, infection, and hemorrhage often spells the death of the mother. The most common way of mismanaging the third stage of labor is to try to hasten it. Constant kneading and squeezing of a uterus that is already contracted are likely to bring about incomplete degrees of placental separation and in general interfere with the physiologic mechanism of placental detachment.

Clinical Picture. Postpartum hemorrhage may occur prior to the birth of the placenta and is then called *third stage bleeding,* or it may take place after delivery of the placenta, or at both times. Whether it occurs before or following delivery of the placenta, it is most important to note that the usual picture, contrary to general opinion, is not one of sudden massive hemorrhage but of slow, steady, moderate bleeding. This is especially true of hemorrhage after the birth of the placenta in which the constant seepage of blood, the continuous drop, drop, drop, may amount, over a period of an hour or two, to unbelievable quantities. This fact has been emphasized particularly by Beecham in his survey of the 52 deaths occurring in his Philadelphia study of postpartum hemorrhage. The average interval between delivery and death in this series was 5 hours and 20 minutes. Only six patients, 11.5 per cent, died within two hours of delivery and none in less than one and one-half hours. In other words, there would have been ample time for intensive treatment in any of these cases, had the attendant realized how much blood was being lost.

The effect of hemorrhage will depend upon the condition of the patient, the status of her blood as revealed by the erythrocyte count, cell volume, or hemoglobin content at the time of admission to the labor room, as well as upon the actual quantity of blood lost. Thus, a woman who is already exhausted by a prolonged labor or weakened by antecedent anemia or chronic disease may succumb after a loss of less than 1,000 cc. which others would bear with impunity. As a rule, the loss of a moderate amount of blood is not attended by serious symptoms, but when the hemorrhage is profuse the pulse becomes rapid and compressible, the face becomes pallid and assumes a drawn appearance while, at the same time, the woman may complain of chilliness, shortness of breath, and disturbed vision. As the situation becomes more dire, air hunger develops and not infrequently a frantic restlessness, and then the patient passes into unconsciousness, as a rule, just before the fatal termination.

A treacherous feature of postpartum hemorrhage is that the pulse and blood pressure may show only moderate alterations until large amounts of blood have been lost. Then, as the compensatory vascular mechanisms are no longer able to accommodate themselves to further decline in blood volume, the pulse suddenly soars and shortly becomes impalpable, while the blood pressure falls precipitously.

In rare instances in which the fundus has not been palpated at all after delivery, or it has been left to an inexperienced attendant, the blood may not escape vaginally but collects within the uterus. In such a case the uterine cavity may be ballooned out by 1,000 cc. or more of blood, while an incompetent attendant is massaging a roll of abdominal fat. This is an error which must be checked if the postpartum uterus has to be left to an inexperienced person.

Diagnosis. Except in cases in which a uterus ballooned out with blood is not recognized, the diagnosis of postpartum hemorrhage offers few problems. The differentiation between bleeding from uterine atony and from uterine lacerations is made tentatively on the condition of the fundus; if bleeding persists, despite a firm, well-retracted uterine body, the source of the hemorrhage is probably lacerations. Bright red blood suggests lacerations, while venous blood points to the uterine cavity as its source. To establish or rule out lacerations as a cause of bleeding, careful inspection of the cervix and vaginal walls is essential. Sometimes both types of bleeding may occur at once, especially following major operative delivery. Routine inspection of the cervix should be done after midforceps, version and extraction, or other difficult vaginal operation, as well as in cases in which arterial bleeding occurs during the second stage or is present immediately after the birth of the child. Many authorities believe that routine inspection of the cervix should be done after every delivery, not only as a preventive against hemorrhage from cervical lacerations but also to ensure complete restoration of the integrity of the cervix.

Prognosis. The older estimates of prognosis in postpartum hemorrhage, based on the amount of blood a woman can lose without dying and on maternal mortality figures at various blood losses, are meaningless today with the ready availability of blood transfusion. In modern obstetrics no woman should die from postpartum hemorrhage. It is true that in every several thousand deliveries, a hemorrhage of 2,000 or even 2,500 cc. may be encountered, but before half this blood is lost a transfusion should actually be running into the patient's vein (or veins), and at no time should the blood deficit be more than 1,000 cc. With large quantities of blood readily available, it should be possible to save every woman with postpartum hemorrhage even though in some instances hysterectomy may be necessary. To obtain this objective, however, requires assiduous watching of all puerperae postpartum, a good institutional or municipal blood bank, and alert action by an experienced team of attendants.

Management of Third Stage Bleeding. A certain amount of bleeding occurs during the third stage of every labor, as the result of transient partial separation of the placenta which is an inevitable stage, if momentary, of the physiologic process of detachment. In cases in which the placenta is extruded by the Schultze mechanism this blood follows the delivery of the placenta, but in the Duncan mechanism it flows out immediately. Accordingly, blood losses of 50 to 200 cc. during the third stage of labor cannot be regarded as necessarily pathologic. In our opinion, as previously stated, the routine administration of 1 cc. of pitocin (10 units) intramuscularly as soon as the baby is born, aids materially in keeping this blood loss to a minimum and in expediting placental separation.

In the presence of any external hemorrhage during the third stage the uterus should be massaged if it is not firmly retracted, and, if the signs of placental separation are present, expression of the placenta should be attempted by pressure with the palm of the hand downward against the fundus of the uterus; however, the organ should not be squeezed as in the classical Credé procedure. If, with the placenta undelivered, bleeding continues, the blood should be measured (Fig. 291), or at least carefully estimated, and if the amount reaches the neighborhood of 400 cc., manual removal of the placenta is indicated. Let it be emphasized again that attempts to deliver the placenta by squeezing and kneading the uterus through the abdomen, as entailed in the original Credé procedure, are not only futile as a rule but traumatize the myometrium and often aggravate the difficulties.

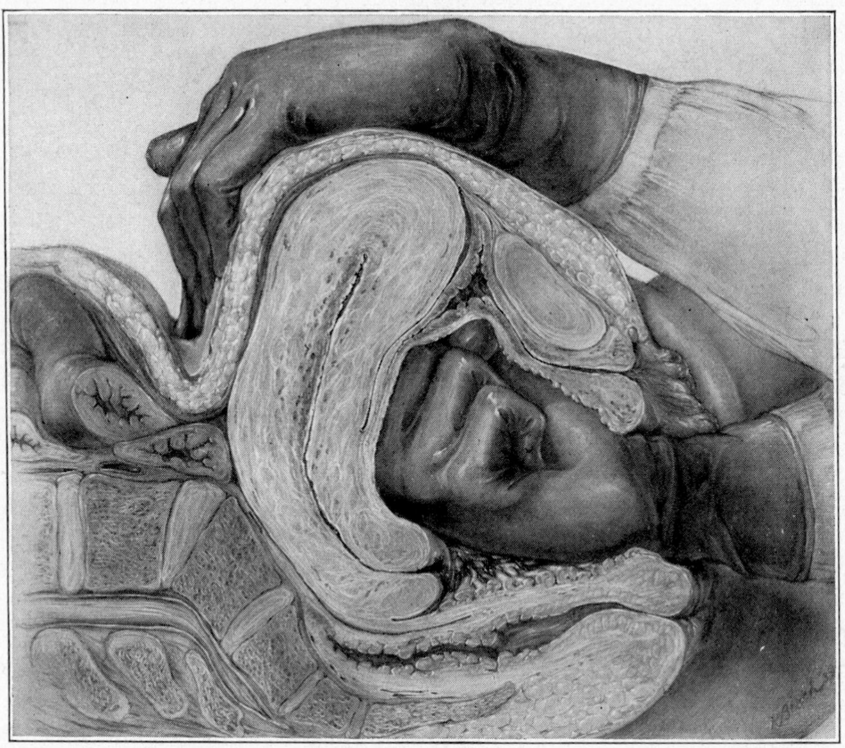

Fig. 503.—Bimanual Compression of Uterus.

Management after Placental Delivery. In every labor, following the delivery of the placenta, the fundus is palpated to make certain that it is well retracted; if it is not firm, massage with the fingertips is carried out. In addition 0.2 mg. of ergonovine is administered routinely, either by the intramuscular or intravenous route, as a further preventive against postpartum hemorrhage. If bleeding persists, the ergotrate may be repeated; if it is, regardless of the manner of its previous administration, it should be given, this time, intravenously. In addition, 3 minims (no more) of pitocin (not whole pituitary extract) in 10 cc. of normal saline may be injected intravenously. Larger doses of pitocin, or even a 3-minim dose of whole pituitary extract, when given intravenously may cause "pituitrin shock." Meanwhile, massage of the uterus is continued. These simple measures will control postpartum hemorrhage in the great majority of cases.

In the event that bleeding persists despite the above procedure, no time should be lost and bimanual compression of the uterus should be employed immediately. The technic of this procedure is shown in Fig. 503. It consists simply of massage of the posterior aspect of the uterus with the abdominal hand and massage of the anterior uterine aspect with the other fist, the latter being rotated in such a manner that the knuckles rub against the uterine wall; this provides not only twice the amount of uterine stimulation that can be accomplished with abdominal massage alone but, by compression of the venous sinuses of the uterus, allows the organ to contract on these vessels more effectively than would otherwise be possible. Although this procedure was described by Hamilton in 1861 and has enjoyed wide usage in England and Europe, it has received scant attention in this country where packing of the uterus has been the orthodox procedure whenever the simpler measures mentioned in the foregoing paragraphs have not proved effectual. As an example of the British point of view, Berkeley, Bonney, and MacLeod, in their book *The Abnormal in Obstetrics,* evaluate the two procedures as follows:

> "The uterus should never be packed for postpartum haemorrhage. Bimanual compression if properly applied and for sufficient time will suffice. Moreover, the uterus immediately after delivery cannot be packed adequately since it dilates under the packing and however carefully it is done it is almost certain to lead to infection."

Similarly, in *Midwifery by Ten Teachers* the following recommendations are made:

> "In the rare cases in which the uterus is distended with blood, the hand may be introduced into the uterus, if perfect asepsis is assured, to clear out clot, otherwise the clot should be squeezed out by bimanual compression, which is carried out as follows. Insert one hand into the vagina, close it, making a fist with the back of the hand directed posteriorly and the knuckles in the anterior fornix; put the other hand on the abdomen resting on the posterior surface of the uterus and press the anteverted uterus down on to the fist by the external hand. In this way the posterior wall is pressed against the anterior, and haemorrhage checked. *In cases of severe flooding it should be performed as soon as the placenta is removed, without wasting time on less effective methods of treatment.* Compression properly carried out is absolutely efficient, and has great advantages over plugging the uterine cavity, in that the danger of sepsis is almost completely avoided and a foreign body is not left in the uterus. It should be kept up until the uterus contracts; this, however, is tiring to perform, and after a quarter to half an hour, an assistant may be required to press on the obstetrician's arms in order to maintain continued firm pressure."

After an extended experience with bimanual compression of the uterus, as well as with packing the uterus, I am convinced that the claims of the British school of obstetrics in behalf of the former procedure are fully justified and that it constitutes, aside from hysterectomy, the most efficacious method at our disposal to combat postpartum hemorrhage. Despite the time-honored place which packing the uterus has held in American obstetrics, its efficacy is questionable and its disadvantages many. The drawbacks to packing the uterus have been set forth so lucidly by Cosgrove that his attitude toward this question is quoted (with permission) verbatim as follows:

> "At about this juncture most authorities advise packing the uterus. This, I do not approve. It seems to me entirely unphysiological. Up to this time all

effort has been made completely to empty the uterus in order to permit it to contract down, and by its contraction to squeeze shut the bleeding sinuses and permit their occlusion by clots formed in the mouths thereof. Now, to reverse this physiological effort to empty the uterus, and proceed to introduce a large mass of foreign material with the avowed purpose of stimulating the uterus to contract and of controlling bleeding by direct pressure of the foreign mass against the sinuses, necessarily mechanically held wide open by the pressure of that mass, does not seem to me good sense.

"If the uterus is so truly atonic as not to be capable of response to the mechanical stimulation of manual control already described and powerfully acting oxytoxcis, one can hardly expect that it will be capable of responding to the less efficient irritation of a wad of gauze pushed into it. If it does not so contract, it will merely balloon more and more as blood accumulates above the pack, and the supposed function of direct pressure of the packing against the whole surface of the uterus will be nullified. In this way the packing may do little more than stop the obvious flow of blood escaping from the uterus and lull the operator into a false sense of security.

"The best descriptions I have been able to find of the technique of packing insist on the necessity of the attendant's staying with the patient and exerting manual pressure of the fundus against the packing from above and the provision of counter-pressure against it from below by tight vaginal packing or manual manipulation.

"Thus, the packing cannot be depended upon to function without the constant presence of the attendant, and the use by him of manual manipulation applied directly to the uterus. It would therefore seem to me self-evident that his continued presence for the same length of time, and his manual manipulation applied to the uterus without the intervention of the packing, would be definitely more effective and physiological than with the use of the packing. Besides all this, packing of the uterus is one of the gravest invitations to infection."

Likewise, Leff believes that it is unphysiologic to pack the uterus. He recalls that the natural mechanism by which postpartum hemorrhage is controlled consists in a contraction and retraction of the uterine muscle fibers with the result that the blood sinuses of the uterus are eliminated; packing, he points out, has the opposite effect, that is, distention of these sinuses. Behler and Reiles, although granting the advisability of uterovaginal tamponade in selected cases, emphasize its disadvantages. They believe that the hemostatic effect is due to reinstatement of good contractions rather than to direct action of the tampon. If the uterus after being packed with gauze does not respond actively, it is technically impossible to fill it to the limits of elasticity, and in any case this help would come too late. Indeed, the authors find that the most important disadvantage of tamponade is the slowness with which the hemostatic effect is obtained; they attribute the loss of five patients to this fact. They feel, furthermore, that it is a traumatizing procedure which may lead to serious lesions of the genital organs.

In any case of postpartum hemorrhage in which abdominal massage of the uterus and oxytocic agents do not control the bleeding, arrangements for blood transfusion should be initiated immediately and the blood started if 800 cc. or more appears to have been lost. With blood running into the patient's vein at the same time that manual compression of the uterus is being carried out, the situation is under control and it is rarely that other measures have to be considered. If the operator's hand becomes tired, as often happens, an assistant can take over the procedure and alternate with the operator over a period of 10 to 15 minutes if necessary.

In rare instances, all the measures described above to combat postpartum hemorrhage may fail and the question arises as to the justification of hysterectomy. In the past this operation has been used for the most part as a last resort in exsanguinated women who have not been supported with adequate amounts of blood and many of whom have died on the operating table. However, with the help of massive, continuing transfusions, it is a life-saving procedure in occasional instances of this complication. If performed on a woman without pulse or blood pressure who is about to die from postpartum hemorrhage, it will of course only hasten the end and in a few such cases may even bring about the death of patients who would otherwise have survived with more conservative treatment. However, in cases in which the patient has been protected with adequate blood, has a palpable pulse and a readable blood pressure, and in which all other measures have failed to meet the intractable hemorrhage, rapid supravaginal hysterectomy will prevent many deaths.

Bleeding from Cervical Lacerations. In any case in which bleeding persists in the presence of a tightly retracted uterus and/or in which the blood is arterial in color, inspection of the cervix should be made and any cervical lacerations greater than 1 cm. in extent repaired. Moreover, in any case of protracted hemorrhage, even though the obstetrician may feel certain that it is due entirely to uterine atony, inspection of the cervix is a wise precaution to make sure that a laceration has not been overlooked. Proper exposure of the cervix and the repair of such lacerations calls for the help of an assistant. Two retractors are inserted into the vagina and its walls separated widely. A sponge forceps is then placed on the anterior aspect of the cervix and another on its posterior lip. Any cervical laceration which is obviously bleeding or which is longer than 1 cm. should be repaired. Interrupted sutures are employed, it being very important to place the highest one slightly above the apex of the tear because bleeding from cervical lacerations usually has its source in a vessel at this point. The importance of cervical lacerations as a cause of postpartum hemorrhage should not be minimized since they sometimes cause profuse bleeding and, if extensive and multiple, the blood loss may be enough to prove fatal.

Postpartum Hemorrhage from Retained Placental Fragments. Immediate postpartum hemorrhage is rarely due to retained placental fragments but, as indicated, a remaining piece of placenta is the most common cause of late bleeding in the puerperium. If, upon routine inspection of the placenta after delivery, a piece of placenta is plainly missing, the uterus should be explored and the placental fragment removed. This is all the more necessary in the presence of persisting postpartum bleeding, but in my experience this cause of bleeding is not sufficiently common to warrant routine exploration of the uterus to rule it out. On the other hand, several authorities believe that the retention of a succenturiate lobe may occasionally be responsible for postpartum hemorrhage and feel that this possibility should be ruled out in the management of all cases of persisting postpartum hemorrhage. In years gone by when packing of the uterus was a routine in our clinic, the uterus was always explored for this possibility and with rare exceptions no placental fragments were demonstrable.

RETENTION OF THE PLACENTA

By retention of the placenta is meant failure of the placenta to be expelled within one hour after delivery of the child. This condition is sometimes called "adherent placenta," but, since most of these cases are believed to be due to faulty uterine behavior rather than to any actual adhesions between the placenta and uterine wall, the more general terminology "retention of placenta," or "retained placenta," seems preferable. The cause of the great majority of these cases is obscure, but it is assumed that uterine retraction is not sufficiently intense to bring about placental detachment. A certain percentage of these cases (just what proportion has not been established) may be the result of partial placenta accreta. This condition, as described in the following section, is characterized by the fact that the decidua is absent, scanty, or defective, so that the chorionic villi attach themselves directly to the uterine muscle. Under these circumstances the physiologic line of cleavage, the spongy layer of the decidua, is lacking and as a consequence a dense union results between the villi and the muscle. It seems conceivable that various minute areas of placenta accreta may occur more frequently than is realized and result in multiple fibrous bands between the placenta and uterus. In separating a retained placenta manually it is not uncommon to feel such bands.

Placental retention is not uncommon, being seen in about 1 per cent of all deliveries. If, after waiting one hour, during which time repeated massage of the uterus has been carried out, it is impossible to express the placenta by downward pressure on the fundus, manual separation of the organ is indicated. Vigorous attempts to separate the placenta by the original Credé maneuver are usually of little avail and may be harmful as already emphasized.

Manual Removal of the Placenta. Widely divergent views have been advanced concerning the risks incurred in manual removal of the placenta. Until very recent years, many authors maintained that this is the most dangerous of obstetric procedures and substantiated their statements by such mortality figures as these: Hegar, 11 per cent; Vogel, 13.5 per cent; Rosenthal, 13.0 per cent; Peckham, 10.76 per cent; and Jaschke, about 10 per cent (in general practice). In 1919 Liepmann claimed that the intervention is so hazardous that a retained placenta without hemorrhage is by no means an indication for removal. He stated that 12 hours is too short a time to wait before attempting manual extraction and recorded two cases in which expression of the placenta was successfully carried out after 10 hours. Other authors, rather than employ manual removal, have let the placenta remain in utero for such periods as 5 days (Polak), 7 days (Fromont), and 10 days (Hegar), without untoward results. In sharp contrast to this viewpoint is the opinion of Gheorghiu, who considers it so harmless to insert a hand into the uterus that, in 1932 at the Société de Gynécologie et d'Obstétrique de Bruxelles, he claimed that after every delivery one should systematically examine the uterine cavity by inserting a hand into the uterus. An identical practice has recently been recommended by Leff, of New York, on the basis of an exceedingly large personal experience.

Several recent reports from the Scandinavian countries indicate that manual removal of the placenta, although a formidable procedure, carries a much lower mortality than formerly supposed, at least in uncomplicated cases. For instance, at the University Hospital in Oslo, during the decade 1927-1936, there were a total of 17,133 deliveries in which manual removal of the whole placenta was performed in 189 cases, that is, in 1.1 per cent. In his study of these cases, Schie found that only three patients, or 1.58 per cent, died after the intervention, all three deaths being due to puerperal infection. Similarly, Block has reviewed 386 cases of manual removal of the placenta (whole or part) occurring in 50,545 deliveries, the incidence being 0.76 per cent. There were 14 deaths, a mortality of 3.6 per cent. In six of the fatal cases the intervention was

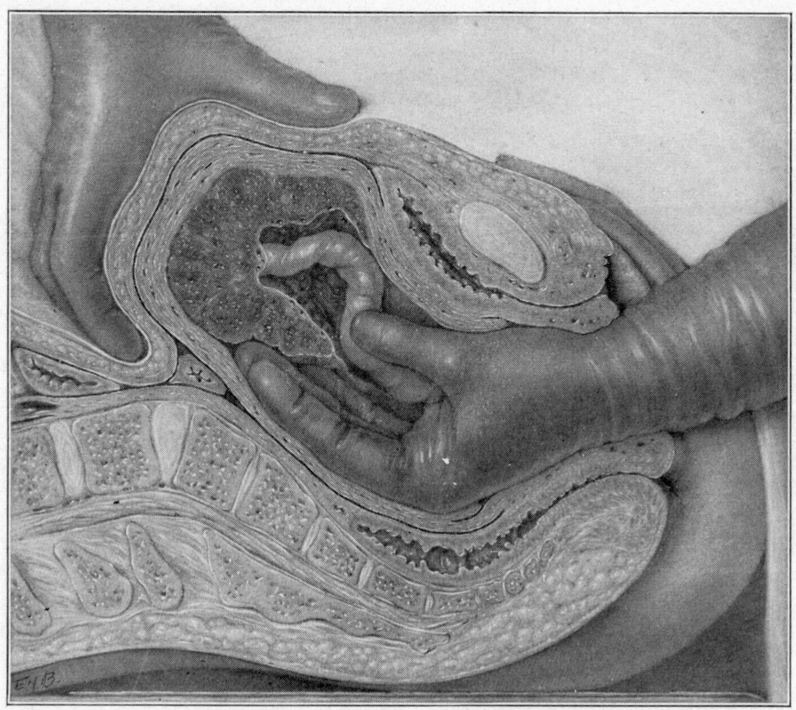

Fig. 504.—Manual Removal of Placenta.

prompted by hemorrhage and this, rather than the operation, was the cause of death. The remaining eight women died of infection. When Block divided the cases according to whether the whole placenta or placental fragments were removed, he reached the conclusion that the latter procedure is not nearly so dangerous as believed. Of his 386 cases, 267 involved removal of the complete placenta and 119 of placental remnants; the mortality of the former group was 4.9 per cent and of the latter 0.8 per cent. Dreyfus, Kristensen, and others also report that exploration of the uterine cavity after delivery, when done under good conditions and on uncomplicated cases, carries slight risk.

On the basis of experience such as the above, the opinion is growing that the danger of manual removal of the placenta depends largely on the degree of antecedent hemorrhage and infection. Accordingly, in the presence of marked bleeding before separation has occurred, the present tendency is to carry out manual removal at once, certainly before the blood loss has attained 500 cc. Although there are cases in the older literature, as noted above, in which prolonged retention of the placenta (without bleeding) appeared to be innocuous, there are an equal number in which retention of the organ for periods as short as 12 hours was followed by fatal sepsis. Today, as stated, manual removal is ordinarily resorted to whenever the third stage lasts longer than one hour.

Technic of Manual Removal. When this operation becomes necessary, the strictest attention should be given to every aseptic detail. The external genitalia should be rigorously cleansed, the hands and forearms of the operator redisinfected and encased in freshly boiled rubber gloves. After grasping the uterus through the abdominal

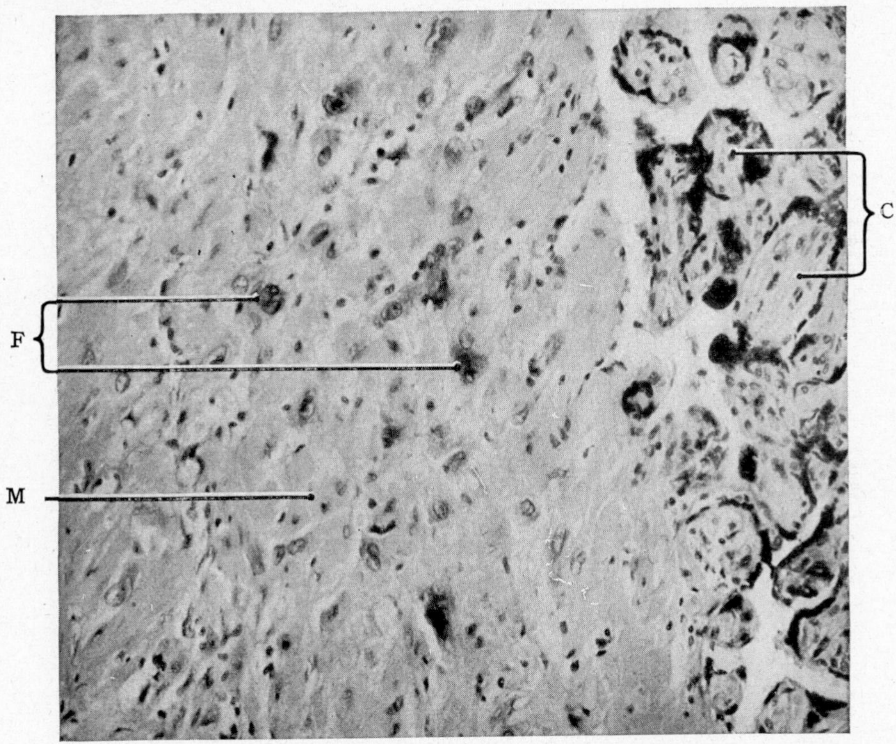

FIG. 505.—PHOTOMICROGRAPH OF UTERINE WALL IN CASE OF PLACENTA ACCRETA SHOWING CHORIONIC ELEMENTS IN DIRECT CONTACT WITH AND INVADING MUSCULATURE.

F, fetal giant cells; *C,* chorionic villi; *M,* uterine muscle.

wall with one hand, the other, suitably lubricated, is introduced into the vagina and passed into the uterus, following the umbilical cord. As soon as the placenta is reached, its margin should be sought for, and the ulnar margin of the hand insinuated between its margin and the uterine wall. Then, with the back of the hand in contact with the latter, the placenta should be peeled off from its attachment by a motion similar to that employed in cutting the leaves of a book. After its complete separation, the placenta should be grasped in the entire hand, but not extracted immediately, the operator waiting until the uterus contracts down firmly over the hand which should then gradually be withdrawn.

Placenta Accreta. Placenta accreta is defined as an abnormal adherence of the placenta to the uterine wall due to absent, scanty, or faulty decidua as the result of which the chorionic villi become attached directly to the uterine muscle. By *placenta* *increta* is meant a condition in which the chorionic villi have not only made contact with, but have actually penetrated the uterine muscle. By *placenta percreta* is meant a condition in which the chorionic villi have penetrated the whole thickness of the uterine wall and reached its serosal covering, sometimes rupturing into the peritoneal cavity. Placenta accreta may be complete or partial. The partial variety of the disorder has been described in the foregoing section. Total placenta accreta is an extremely rare complication of the third stage; Kaltreider found only 177 cases in the literature up to 1945. In the course of over 70,000 deliveries at the Johns Hopkins Hospital not a single case of complete placenta accreta has been observed. Placenta increta and percreta are still more rare.

The clinical picture of placenta accreta is failure of the placenta to separate, with no hemorrhage whatsoever. Attempts to separate the placenta manually are futile and, if persistent, lead only to digging into the uterine muscle with the obvious hazard of perforation. The usual treatment is immediate hysterectomy. The suggestion has recently been made that no therapy be instituted in cases of placenta accreta and that the organ be allowed to slough out. The results which accrued from this practice several decades ago were very unfavorable but with the use of modern chemotherapy this program may well have a place in the management of this complication, especially in primigravidae.

INVERSION OF THE UTERUS

This condition is a very rare, but important, cause of postpartum shock. McCullagh estimates that it occurs about once in 30,000 labors and in patients delivered on our service it has occurred once in the last 20,000 cases. Many obstetricians with large practices have never seen a case. On the other hand, it is much more frequently noted in the practice of ignorant midwives.

Now and again the fundus of the uterus becomes inverted and comes into close contact with or may protrude through the external os; in rare instances the entire organ appears outside of the vulva, the condition being respectively designated as *incomplete* and *complete inversion,* and *prolapse of the inverted uterus* (Figs. 506, 507, and 508). In not a few cases the placenta remains attached to the inverted organ.

Etiology. For the production of the accident three factors are necessary: marked laxity or thinness of the uterine walls, particularly at the placental site; pressure from above or traction on the cord or placenta; and a patulous cervical canal. Its occurrence is also favored by a fundal insertion of the placenta. Inversion may occur spontaneously as the result of the intra-abdominal pressure or from the mere weight of the intestines, but in most cases it is attributable to violence resulting from the too vigorous employment of Credé's maneuver or to traction upon the cord. Occasionally, inversion may recur in the same patient.

Beckmann believes that in the majority of instances the accident occurs spontaneously, while Vogel, in a similar review, holds that most cases are due to violence. His contention appears to be confirmed by Beckmann's statistics, as only 3 of the 100 cases which he analyzed occurred in hospital practice. Indeed, the accident is excessively rare when labor is properly conducted. As stated in the discussion on the treatment of this stage of labor, it is imperative that the fundus of the uterus be held or kept above the pelvis and not be violently pushed downward in attempts to expel the placenta. Harer and Sharkey, in a study of 21 cases, found that 76 per cent were due to faulty technic and, therefore, avoidable.

The complication usually follows a full-term labor, although a number of cases are recorded in which it was noted after abortion. It is interesting that more than 50 per cent of the cases recorded by both Beckmann and Vogel were in primiparous women.

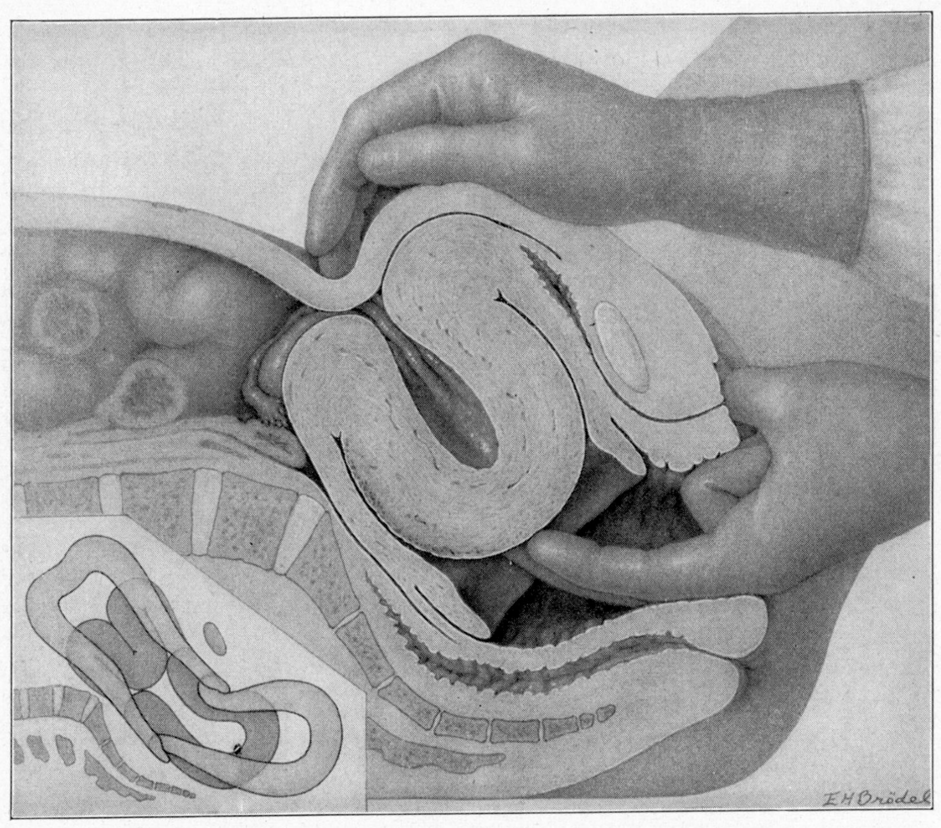

Fig. 506.—Incomplete Inversion of the Uterus.

Diagnosis by abdominal palpation of crater-like depression and vaginal palpation of tumor in the cervix. Insert shows progressive degrees of inversion.

Symptoms. As a rule, inversion of the uterus is promptly followed by alarming symptoms, the patient presenting evidences of shock out of proportion to the amount of blood lost, with a rapid pulse and a tendency to syncope. In many cases severe uterine pain occurs and profuse hemorrhage is frequently noted. On the other hand, the symptoms are sometimes slight, and in rare instances the condition may continue for several days without causing any serious annoyance to the patient.

Occasionally the cervix may so retract about the completely inverted uterus that strangulation occurs, followed by gangrene. In other cases this does not take place but the condition becomes chronic, necessitating operative procedures later.

Diagnosis. The diagnosis of complete inversion of the uterus is usually simple, as the organ is frequently extended through the vaginal orifice. On the other hand, incomplete inversion may remain unrecognized, unless careful abdominal palpation reveals the absence of the fundus or shows a crater-like depression above or behind the symphysis. Unexplained shock, following delivery, should suggest the possibility of inversion of the uterus and make imperative an immediate vaginal examination by which means the diagnosis is readily established.

Prognosis. If the condition is detected promptly, and the uterus replaced immediately, the prognosis is good. Cosgrove reported complete recovery in eight cases in which the condition was promptly recognized and the uterus immediately replaced, and the death of only one case, in which he ascribes the outcome to delayed diagnosis and treatment. In the eight cases which occurred in 31,932 consecutive deliveries at the New York Lying-In Hospital, prompt recognition and immediate reposition of the uterus led to their complete recovery. On the other hand, if strangulation or gangrene occurs the outlook is ominous.

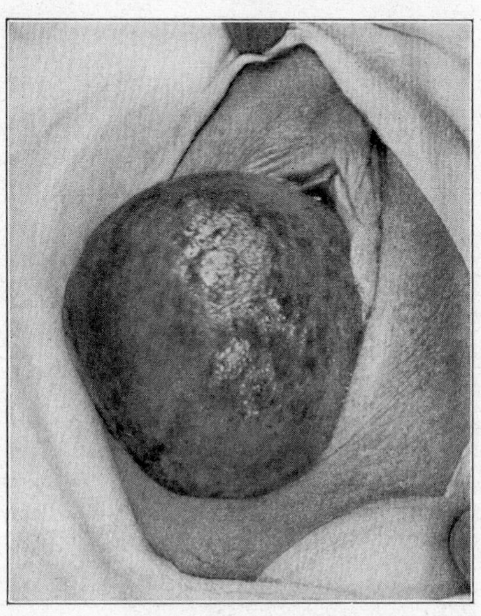

Fig. 507.—Complete Inversion of the Uterus.

Treatment. Immediately following inversion, reposition can frequently be effected without difficulty by pressure exerted by several fingers in the vagina; it is important to remember that the force should be directed upward in the axis of the superior strait. Neglect of this precaution undoubtedly accounts for a certain number of failures. As the procedure is generally painful, anesthesia should be employed. On the other hand, if several hours have elapsed, reposition may be difficult or impossible. In this event, the patient is usually profoundly shocked, so that morphine and transfusion should be given before beginning the anesthesia; if much blood has been lost, it is advisable to postpone manipulative procedures until after transfusion and recovery from the marked shock, provided that such recovery occurs promptly. If the patient is still in shock after 30 minutes of liberal administration of blood, either manual reposition or the Huntington operation as described below should be done.

If the placenta is still attached to the uterus, it is generally advisable to defer its separation until reposition has been effected, because the contractile function of the inverted uterus being in abeyance, there is always the risk of profuse hemorrhage. That the shock is not necessarily the result of hemorrhage, is proven by the fact that it may develop in the absence of any excessive bleeding, and may disappear promptly following reposition.

If, however, the patient is not seen until several days after the accident, the cervix may have so contracted about the neck of the organ that reposition by manual manipulation is impossible, and radical interference becomes necessary.

In cases of acute inversion of the uterus where vaginal reposition is unsuccessful, the operative technic devised by Huntington may be used to advantage or it may well be employed electively. In this operation the abdomen is opened and the crater formed by the inversion of the uterus exposed. The operator and his assistant, by means of Allis clamps, grasp the surface of the uterus inside the crater at a depth of 2 cm. Then, by simultaneous upward traction, a portion is drawn out of the ring. The pro-

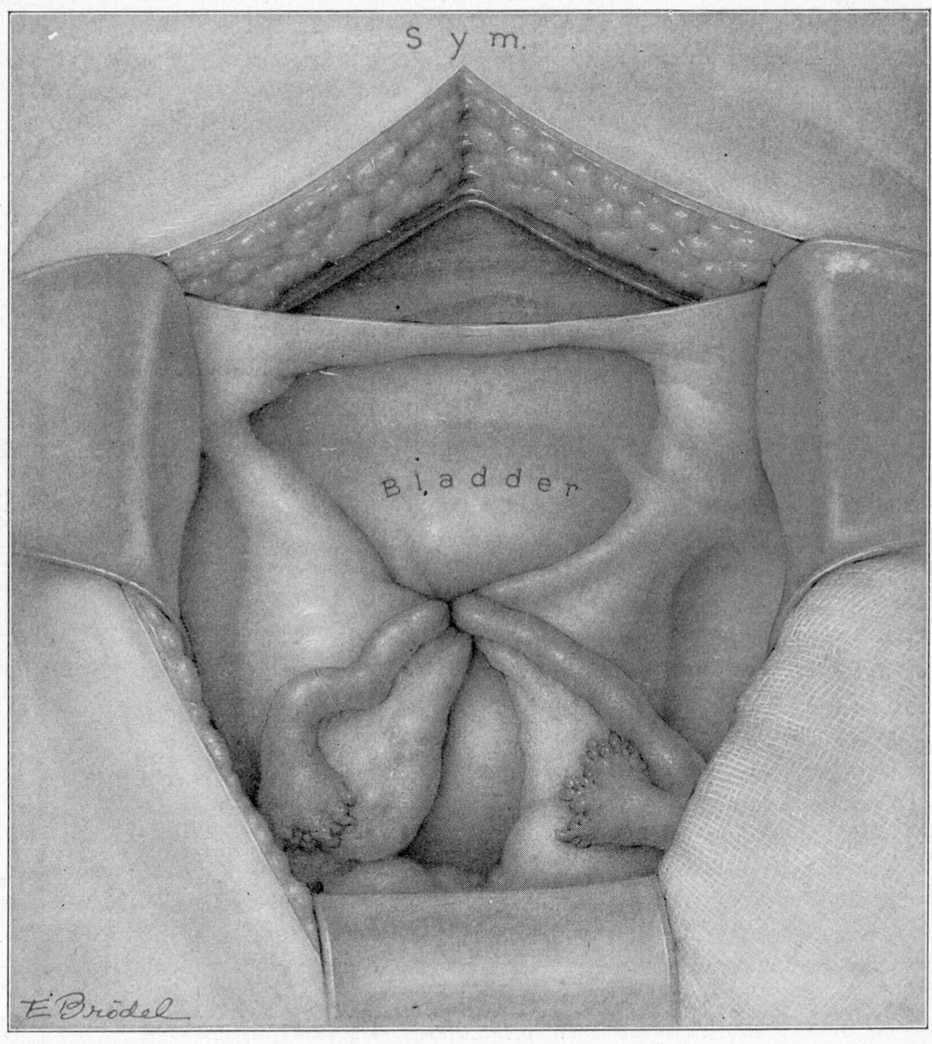

Fig. 508.—Complete Inversion of the Uterus.

Operative findings in same case as Fig. 507.

cedure is repeated by the successive application of clamps until the whole organ is restored to the peritoneal cavity.

In chronic or long standing inversion, as well as in some cases of shorter duration, it frequently becomes necessary to utilize the technic of Haultain by which, after the abdomen is opened, the cervical ring is incised posteriorly and the uterus elevated to its normal position either by pressure from below, through the vagina, or by inserting the finger through the cervical incision at a point below the fundus and exerting upward pressure. This procedure is followed by closure of the cervix in layers. Phaneuf reports good results, in chronic inversion of the uterus, by means of the vaginal operative approach utilizing the Spinelli anterior colpohysterotomy.

AMNIOTIC FLUID OR MECONIUM EMBOLISM

At any time after the membranes have ruptured, and more especially after the infant and placenta have been delivered, there is the possibility that amniotic fluid may enter the gaping venous sinuses of the placental site, be drawn into the general circulation, and in this way reach the pulmonary capillaries. Since the amniotic fluid invariably contains particulate matter, such as lanugo hair and particles of vernix caseosa and meconium, multiple miliary emboli may conceivably reach the lungs in this manner.

In 1941 Lushbaugh and Steiner introduced the concept that this accident was an occasional cause of sudden death during and shortly after labor and documented their claims with a mass of convincing evidence. The clinical characteristics of the condition are sudden dyspnea, cyanosis, pulmonary edema, shock, and uterine relaxation with postpartum hemorrhage. Some subsequent authors find that these cases are frequently associated with failure of the blood to coagulate in addition to the other signs and symptoms mentioned. Lushbaugh and Steiner advanced the belief that the phenomena which follow in the train of amniotic fluid emboli are due to anaphylactoid shock from the sudden deposition of the amniotic material in the pulmonary arterioles. This anaphylactoid reaction in turn causes the vascular collapse and this in turn the postpartum atony and hemorrhage. Experimental studies by Hanzlik and Karsner indicate that the injection of finely divided particulate matter, such as suspensions of charcoal particles or India ink, produces, because of the large surface area of the particles, various blood chemical changes, such as lessened coagulability of the blood, and also dramatic systemic phenomena such as restlessness, tremors, marked dyspnea, convulsions, and often death.

There is evidence, therefore, both clinical and experimental, that sudden pulmonary blockage by extremely small particles may cause a wide variety of grave signs and symptoms. Just how frequently, however, cases of amniotic fluid embolism actually occur is not established and there has been a regrettable tendency to put in this category many unexplained sudden deaths in association with childbirth. Although amniotic fluid embolism still remains something of a moot question, the evidence suggests that sudden death in association with labor is occasionally due to this accident. The only treatment is oxygen and supportive measures and, as a rule, these are of no avail.

BIBLIOGRAPHY

Beecham, C. T. Postpartum Hemorrhage As a Cause of Death. Am. J. Obst. & Gynec., 1939, 37:258.

Block, E. Ueber Manuelle Losung der Placenta und Intrauterine Revision Postpartum. Acta obst. et. gynec. Scandinav., 1937, 17: Suppl. 342.

Bohler, E., and Reiles, M. Suppression du Tamponnement Utero-vaginal au Profit de la Revision Uterine Combinée a l'Injection Intraveineusse d'Hypophysine. Gynéc. et obst., 1934, 29:393.

Calkins, L. A., Litzenberg, J. C., and Plass, E. D. Management of the Third Stage of Labor with Special Reference to Blood Loss. Am. J. Obst. & Gynec., 1931, 21:175.

Colvin, E. D., and Bartholomew, R. A. Improvements in the Paraldehyde Method of Relief of Pain in Labor. Am. J. Obst. & Gynec., 1938, 35:589.

COSGROVE, S. A. Obstetric Hemorrhage and Its Management. South. M. J., 1936, 29:1219.
——— Management of Acute Puerperal Inversion of the Uterus. Am. J. Obst. & Gynec., 1939, 38:912.
DOUGLAS, R. G., and DAVIS, I. F. Puerperal Infection. Etiologic, Prophylactic and Therapeutic Considerations. Am. J. Obst. & Gynec., 1946, 51:352.
EASTMAN, N. J. Obstetric Hemorrhage. New Internat. Clin., 1939, 3:265.
HAMILTON, G. Postpartum Haemorrhage. Edinburgh M. J., 1861-62, 7:313.
HANZLIK, P. J., and KARSNER, H. T. Anaphylactoid Phenomena from the Intravenous Administration of Various Colloids, Arsenicals and Other Agents. J. Pharmacol. & Exper. Therap., 1920, 14:379, 425, 449, 463 and 479: *Ibid.,* 1924, 23:173.
HARER, W. B., and SHARKEY, J. A. Acute Inversion of the Puerperal Uterus. A Record of Twenty-one Cases. J.A.M.A., 1940, 114:2289.
HUNTINGTON, J. L. Acute Inversion of the Uterus. Boston M. & S. J., 1921, 184:376.
——— IRVING, F. C., and KELLOGG, F. S. Abdominal Reposition in Acute Inversion of the Puerperal Uterus. Am. J. Obst. & Gynec., 1928, 15:34.
IRVING, F. C., BERMAN, S., and NELSON, H. B. The Barbiturates and Other Hypmotics in Labor. Surg., Gynec. & Obst., 1934, 58:1.
IRVING, F. C., and HERTIG, A. T. Study of Placenta Accreta. Surg., Gynec. & Obst., 1937, 64:178.
KALTREIDER, D. F. Placenta Accreta. Bull. School Med. Univ. Maryland, 1945, 30:1.
KRISTENSEN, B. Regarding Manual Detachment of the Placenta and Intrauterine Palpation. Acta obst. et gynec. Scandinav., 1935, 15:165.
LEFF, M. Management of the Third and Fourth Stages of Labor. Surg., Gynec. & Obst., 1939, 68:224.
LIEPMANN, W. Zur Indicationsstellung für die Manuelle Placentarlösung bei Placenta Adhaesiva. Berl. Klin. Wchnschr., 1919, 56:300.
LUSHBAUGH, C. C., and STEINER, P. E. Additional Observations on Maternal Pulmonary Embolism by Amniotic Fliud. Am. J. Obst. & Gynec., 1942, 43:833.
McCULLAGH, W. McK. H. Inversion of the Uterus: A Report of Three Cases and an Analysis of 233 Recently Recorded. J. Obst. & Gynaec. Brit. Emp., 1925, 32:280.
McLENNAN, C. E., and McKELVEY, J. L. Conservative Treatment of Inversion of the Uterus. J.A.M.A., 1942, 120:679.
ODELL, L. D., and SESKI, I. Episiotomy Blood Loss. Am. J. Obst. & Gynec., 1947, 54:51.
PASTORE, J. B. A Study of the Blood Loss in the Third Stage of Labor and the Factors Involved. Am. J. Obst. & Gynec., 1936, 31:78.
——— The Cell Volume Following Delivery and Its Relation to Blood Loss and Postpartum Infection. Am. J. Obst. & Gynec., 1936, 32:859.
PECKHAM, C. H. Statistical Survey of 186 Cases of Manual Removal of the Placenta. Bull. Johns Hopkins Hosp., 1935, 56:224.
——— and KUDER, K. Some Statistics of Postpartum Hemorrhage. Am. J. Obst. & Gynec., 1933, 26:361.
PHANEUF, L. E. Inversion of the Uterus: A Report of Five Personal Cases. Surg., Gynec. & Obst., 1940, 71:106.
REICH, A. M. A Critical Analysis of Blood Loss Following Delivery. Am. J. Obst. & Gynec., 1939, 37:224.
SCHIE, E. On the Prognosis of Manual Removal of the Placenta and Possible Predisposing Factors of Retained Placenta. Acta obst. et gynec. Scandinav., 1939, 19:28.
(For further—especially, older—literature, see Eastman and Schie references.)

Section Eight: ABNORMALITIES OF THE PUERPERIUM

35

PUERPERAL INFECTION

Definition. Puerperal infection, one of the commonest causes of death in childbearing, is a postpartum wound infection of the parturient canal (usually of the endometrium) which may remain localized but often extends along various avenues to produce diverse clinical and pathological pictures. Febrile reactions of greater or less severity are the rule, and the outcome varies according to the portal of entry, the type, virulence, and number of the invading organisms, the reaction of the tissues, and the general resistance of the patient. Commonly used, but less satisfactory synonyms are: puerperal fever, puerperal sepsis, puerperal septicemia, and childbed fever.

Since the great majority of temperature elevations in the puerperium are due to puerperal infection, the incidence of fever after childbirth is a reliable index of the incidence of the disease. For this reason it has become customary to group all puerperal fevers under the general term, *puerperal morbidity,* and to evaluate the frequency of puerperal infection on this basis. Several definitions of puerperal morbidity have been established on the basis of the degree of pyrexia reached. The Joint Committee on Maternal Welfare, United States, has defined morbidity as a "temperature of 100.4° F. (38.0° C.), the temperature to occur on any two of the first 10 days postpartum, exclusive of the first 24 hours, and to be taken by mouth by a standard technic at least four times daily." This is probably the most commonly employed standard in the United States. The British Medical Association recommends the following definition of morbidity: "The puerperal morbidity should include all fetal cases and also all cases in which temperature exceeds 100° F. on any two of the bidaily readings from the end of the first to the eighth day after delivery."

These definitions may suggest that all fever in the puerperium is due to puerperal infection. Strictly speaking, this is not true since elevations in temperature are occasionally the result, beyond all question, of extraneous causes, such as pyelitis and upper respiratory infections; and it is for this reason that "corrected morbidity statistics" are sometimes reported. However, the practical difficulties of differentiating extraneous causes of fever from puerperal infection are often great and depend upon a variable subjective factor. For this reason, total morbidity figures are unquestionably the most reliable index of the incidence of the disease. It should be the rule, moreover, to regard every fever in the puerperium as due to puerperal infection unless proof positive can be advanced that it is the result of some extraneous cause.

History. It is probable that puerperal infection has occurred almost as long as children have been born, and passages in the works of Hippocrates, Galen, Avicenna, and many of the old writers clearly have reference to it. As early as 1676, Willis wrote on the subject of *febris puerperarum,* although the English term "puerperal fever" was probably first employed by Strother in 1716.

The ancients regarded the affection as the result of retention of the lochia, and for centuries this explanation was universally accepted. In the early part of the seventeenth century Plater taught that it was essentially a metritis, and was followed in the next century by Puzos with his milk metastasis theory. From the time of Plater, until Semmelweis had proved its identity with wound infection, Pasteur had cultivated the streptococcus, and Lister had demonstrated the value of antiseptic methods, all sorts of theories were suggested concerning its origin and nature, which are comprehensively dealt with in the monographs of Eisenmann, Silberschmidt, Burtenshaw, and Peckham.

Although John Leake (1772) first made the suggestion of the contagiousness of puerperal infection, it remained for Alexander Hamilton to make the earliest positive statement on this subject in 1781. Alexander Gordon of Aberdeen clearly stated in a treatise on epidemic puerperal fever in 1795 the idea of the infectious and contagious nature of the disease, which preceded the papers of Holmes and Semmelweis by a half century. Charles White (1773) of Manchester believed puerperal fever to be an absorption fever dependent on stagnation of the lochia. He advised the semirecumbent posture to facilitate drainage, insisted on rigorous cleanliness and ventilation of the lying-in room and complete isolation of infected patients. Although many other British observers also had vague ideas upon the subject, it was not until the middle of the nineteenth century that such views were strongly urged. In 1843, Oliver Wendell Holmes read a paper before the Boston Society for Medical Improvement, entitled "The Contagiousness of Puerperal Fever," in which he clearly showed that at least the epidemic forms of the affection could always be traced to the lack of proper precautions on the part of the physician or nurse. Four years later Semmelweis, then an assistant in the Vienna Lying-In Hospital, began a careful inquiry into the causes of the frightful mortality attending labor in that institution, as compared with the comparatively small number of women succumbing to puerperal infection when delivered in their own homes. As a result of his investigations he concluded that the morbid process was essentially a wound infection, and was due to the introduction of septic material by the examining finger. Acting upon this idea he issued stringent orders that the physicians, students, and midwives should disinfect their hands with chlorine water—the forerunner of Dakin's solution—before examining parturient women. In spite of immediate surprising results—the mortality falling from over 10 to 1 per cent—his work, as well as that of Holmes, was scoffed at by many of the most prominent men of the time, and his discovery remained unappreciated until the influence of Lister's teachings and the development of bacteriology had brought about a revolution in the treatment of wounds.

BACTERIOLOGY

The vast majority of puerperal infections are caused by the streptococcus. The term *Streptococcus,* however, is merely a morphological designation and includes a wide variety of micro-organisms. Some of these are pathogenic, others are not; some possess hemolytic properties, others do not; some are vulnerable to chemotherapeutic agents, while others are resistant. Moreover, some types of pathogenic streptococci are normal inhabitants of the vagina in a large proportion of women, while other forms are never normally present in the birth canal but must be brought there from without; in view of this fact, precise knowledge of the type of the streptococcus concerned in a given case of puerperal infection is often of extreme importance in determining the source of the infection and in establishing responsibility for the case. Since the clinical course, prognosis, and treatment of puerperal infections are also closely related to the type of the streptococcus involved, it becomes apparent that an acquaintance with the several varieties of these bacteria and their characteristics is prerequisite to an understanding of the disease.

Classification of Streptococci. It is customary to divide streptococci into two main groups according to whether oxygen is helpful or injurious to their growth, that is, into aerobic and anaerobic groups. Further subdivision is based on the ability of the organism to produce hemolysis in blood agar plates; two types of hemolysis are recognized and have been called by *alpha* and *beta;* streptococci which produce no change whatsoever in the surrounding blood agar are called *gamma*. By *alpha* type of hemolysis is meant a somewhat greenish discoloration and *partial* hemolysis of the blood corpuscles immediately surrounding the colony, forming a rather definitely bounded zone 1 to 2 mm. in diameter outside of which is a second, narrow, clearer, not discolored zone. The *beta* type of hemolysis is characterized by the fact that the colonies are surrounded by a zone of hemolysis which is sharply defined, clear, colorless, and 2 to 4 mm. in diameter. Under the microscope no intact red cells can be seen in this zone. *Beta* hemolysis develops more rapidly than the *alpha* type and is often well established after 18 hours of incubation. Ever since this form of hemolysis was first described by Schottmüller in 1903, the streptococci which are capable of producing it have been known as *hemolytic streptococci,* whereas streptococci which produce the *alpha* type of hemolysis, or none at all, are called *non-hemolytic*. The hemolytic streptococci, of course, occupy a pre-eminent place among harmful bacteria because they are responsible for some of the gravest human infections, such as erysipelas, scarlet fever, and "streptococcal sore throat"; they may also cause some of the most fulminating forms of puerperal infection. On the other hand, not all types of hemolytic streptococci are pathogenic for man. In a series of meticulous bacteriological studies, Lancefield and Hare have shown, by means of precipitin and biochemical reactions, that there are some nine different groups of hemolytic streptococci of which only one group, Group A, is definitely pathogenic in the human; the other groups, designated by succeeding letters of the alphabet, may be present as saprophytes in the human but are rarely the cause of serious infections; they play, however, an important role in certain diseases of lower animals. The aerobic, nonhemolytic streptococci (that is, the alpha and gamma types) are not infrequently isolated from mild cases of puerperal infection, as shown in Table 21, but are seldom responsible for severe examples of the disease.

Anaerobic streptococci have been recognized as entities since they were first described by Kronig in 1895. One of the earliest investigators to demonstrate the presence of these organisms in the normal vagina of gravidae was J. Whitridge Williams who, in 1898, showed that three of his patients harbored in the vagina streptococci which would grow in anaerobic media but not under aerobic conditions. Like other observers of this period, however, he regarded these bacteria as harmless saprophytes and it was not until the classic article of Schottmüller appeared in 1910 that the important role played by the anaerobic streptococcus in human infections was stressed. Schottmüller's paper reported 25 cases of anaerobic streptococcal infections of which 16 followed abortion; seven of these latter cases died, a mortality rate of 44 per cent. In six of the fatal cases and in one of the patients who survived, he was able to obtain the organism from the blood, as well as from the cervix, and in five instances the blood showed pure cultures of anaerobic streptococci. In view of these facts, Schottmüller reached the conclusion that anaerobic streptococci are not harmless saprophytes but virulent pathogenic organisms capable of producing fatal infections.

Organism	Count	Percent
Anaerobic streptococcus *	386 or	68.0%
Aerobic nonhemolytic streptococcus	136 or	24.0%
Anaerobic staphylococcus	97 or	17.0%
Staphylococcus albus	91 or	16.0%
Anaerobic diphtheroid	84 or	14.8%
Colon bacillus	78 or	13.8½
Streptococcus viridans	77 or	13.4%
Aerobic diphtheroid	42 or	7.4%
Lactobacillus	26 or	4.5%
Anaerobic gram negative rod	24 or	4.1%
Alpha prime streptococcus	23 or	4.0%
Staphylococcus aureus	12 or	2.1%
B. Welchii	9 or	1.5%
Beta-hemolytic streptococcus	6 or	1.0%
Enterococcus	4 or	0.7%
B. aerogenes	4 or	0.7%
B. proteus	4 or	0.7%
Gonococcus	3 or	0.5%
Monilia albicans	3 or	0.5%
B. Friedlander	1 or	0.2%
Pneumococcus Group IV	1 or	0.2%
No growth	23 or	4.0%

TABLE 21. INCIDENCE OF ORGANISMS IN THE UTERINE LOCHIA OF 565 PATIENTS WITH PUERPERAL INFECTION WHO WERE DELIVERED SPONTANEOUSLY OR BY OPERATIVE MEANS. (21 different organisms.) (Courtesy of Dr. R. Gordon Douglas.)

* Includes both facultative and obligatory anaerobes. Where two strains were isolated from one patient they are counted as one. A few strains were hemolytic, some produced pigment but for the most part they represent nonhemolytic strains.

Despite the convincing character of Schottmüller's work, his views received little acceptance at the time. During recent years, however, the studies of Schwarz and Dieckmann, of Harris and J. H. Brown, of Colebrook, of T. K. Brown, and of Douglas and Rhees, all appearing between 1926 and 1939, leave little doubt that Schottmüller was correct; indeed, the opinion is established that the anaerobic streptococcus is the most common cause of puerperal infection.

The anaerobic streptococci doubtless embrace as many subgroups as the aerobic variety, but they have been little studied by bacteriologists and the available data are insufficient to permit of any systematic classification or nomenclature. It is characteristic of most strains that they produce abundant gas in fluid culture, differing sharply in this way from the aerobic species. It is for this reason that such names as *Streptococcus putridus* and *Streptococcus foetidus* have been assigned to some of them. They are usually non-hemolytic, Colebrook and Hare having found that only two of 60 strains studied by them produced hemolysis. The pathogenicity of different strains of anaerobic streptococci for laboratory animals seems to differ widely and in all probability many forms are not pathogens. In 1909 Wegelin injected anaerobic streptococci into the peritoneal cavities of mice and produced small abscesses. One strain examined by Marwedel and Wehrsig caused an acutely fatal infection in a guinea pig. Prevot finds pathogenic lesions of a suppurative, gangrenous, or edematous type, sometimes fatal, with most of his strains. Harris and J. H. Brown found that three of 57 strains obtained from cases of puerperal infections killed mice within 24 hours. Colebrook and Hare tested seven puerperal strains by subcutaneous injections into mice. Two of them produced small caseous foci at the site of the injection, but none of the mice died.

From what has been said it is apparent that there are only two types of streptococcus which commonly cause severe puerperal infection, namely the Group A hemolytic streptococci and the anaerobic streptococci. Although these are occasionally obtained in pure culture from the uterus in cases of puerperal infection, it is much more common to meet them in association with other invaders such as the colon bacillus, non-hemolytic aerobic streptococci, and diphtheroids.

Hemolytic Streptococci. The hemolytic streptococcus is the most common cause of fulminating puerperal infection as well as of epidemics of the disease. **Virulent forms of this organism are never normal inhabitants of the birth canal, their presence there invariably meaning that they have been introduced from without.** It is true that investigators have occasionally found hemolytic streptococci in the vagina of normal women during pregnancy and immediately postpartum, but evidence has never been advanced that these bacteria were pathogenic and today it seems certain that they did not belong to Group A of Lancefield and Hare, but to other non-pathogenic groups. In other words, puerperal infection due to the hemolytic streptococcus is always exogenous in etiology.

The validity of this statement has been demonstrated by Lancefield and Hare in an extensive series of cases at the Isolation Block of the Queen Charlotte's Hospital, London. In an examination of 855 normal pregnant women, 13 had hemolytic streptococci in the upper part of the vagina. Twelve of these women with positive cultures subsequently had an afebrile puerperium, although hemolytic streptococci were still present after delivery in the majority of them. The other carrier had some fever during the puerperium, but it was slight and there were no other signs of puerperal infection. None of the strains in this series fell into Group A. On the other hand, among 46 strains obtained from typical cases of puerperal infection (many of which were fatal), all except one strain were classified as Group A. In the one exception, the patient was suffering from an overwhelming infection with the *Staphylococcus aureus,* while the hemolytic streptococcus, a Group C, was present merely as a secondary invader. In addition, vaginal swabs were made from a series of 837 puerperal women who were afebrile or who had only a slight increase in temperature; streptococci giving areas of hemolysis on blood agar plates were isolated from 85 of them. Only one of these 85 was definitely infected and she later died of peritonitis. Now, this fatal case was the only one in the 85 which showed a Group A streptococcus. The remaining 65 totally afebrile cases and the 18 barely febrile cases harbored hemolytic streptococci, but these belonged to other groups (B, C, D, F, or G).

It is, therefore, evident that hemolytic streptococci may be harbored in the birth canal either before or after delivery without causing disease *provided* they belong to serological groups other than Group A. Group A hemolytic streptococci, on the contrary, are rarely if ever found in the vagina antepartum, but, if present in the birth canal postpartum, almost always give rise to serious puerperal infection. (Since the name *hemolytic streptococcus* has obtained wide currency in clinical medicine, the term *hemolytic streptococcus, Group A* is preferred by many writers in designating the particular organism which alone among the hemolytic streptococci can cause definite puerperal infection in the human species. On the other hand, not a few bacteriologists would rather use the term *Streptococcus pyogenes* for this group, the name which Rosenbach originally gave to streptococci isolated from suppurative lesions. Since hemolytic streptococci, Group A, possess all the characters of *Streptococcus pyogenes,* the two terms are synonymous and may be used interchangeably.)

If Group A hemolytic streptococci are not normal inhabitants of the vagina, from what source are they carried to the birth canal? The most common source in modern practice is the human nasopahrynx. Colebrook, Maxted, and Johns find that 3 to 5 per cent of normal persons are carriers of Group A hemolytic streptococci in the nose, while 5 to 10 per cent harbor the organism on their tonsils and posterior nasopharynx. The incidence in persons with recent upper respiratory infections is naturally much higher. As the result of droplet dispersion of the organism from the nose and throat, it is not infrequently met on the hands, the same authors finding that 3.8 per cent of 181 persons had Group A hemolytic streptococci on the skin of their hands. It is not present, however, on the perianal or perineal skin, nor in the feces of healthy persons.

Since approximately one individual in 10 harbors Group A hemolytic streptococci in his nasopharynx, and since women during labor and the puerperium usually come in contact with 10 or more persons, the likelihood of obstetrical patients' being exposed to carriers of this organism is excellent. To assume, however, that a given puerperal infection is the result of some specific contact of this character is unjustifiable because there can be no assurance that actual transfer took place. If there were some way of identifying the particular organism in the patient and in the carrier, such a causal relationship might be established with more certainty. Griffith, by means of agglutination tests, has shown that there are 27 different antigenic types of the Group A hemolytic streptococcus (*Streptococcus pyogenes*) and each of these can be readily identified by these tests. To be sure, the prevalence of each of these 27 types of streptococci is probably not the same, but, nevertheless, since any one of them may be met in both patient and carrier, it is very unlikely that the type isolated from both would be the same unless actual transfer had taken place. (The likelihood would be one in 729 if the types were equally prevalent.) Using this method of identifying the streptococcus, Smith has shown that in 39 of 49 cases of puerperal infection due to the *Streptococcus pyogenes*, a strain antigenically identical with that obtained from the patient could be demonstrated in the nasopharynx of the doctor, nurse, midwife, or other attendant, or, more rarely, in the nose or throat of the patient herself. In a similar study of 63 cases of puerperal infection, Dora Colebrook has shown that in 57.1 per cent, a strain antigenically identical to that causing the infection of the patient could be isolated from some attendant.

Accordingly, it seems certain that the most common source of puerperal infection with the hemolytic streptococcus is the nose or throat of some person in attendance. The second most common source of Group A hemolytic streptococci is found in actual infections due to the organism, such as other cases of puerperal infection, infected wounds, autopsy material, and the like. According to Colebrook, the dust and even the air of a room which has housed a case of infection with this organism may harbor it for weeks.

Anaerobic Streptococcus. While the hemolytic streptococcus is the most common cause of fulminating and epidemic puerperal infection, **the most common cause of puerperal infection, in general, is the anaerobic streptococcus.** In a series of 165 uterine cultures from cases of puerperal infection, Schwarz and Dieckmann were able to demonstrate this organism in approximately 40 per cent; in severe infections, moreover, they were often able to regain it from the blood stream in pure culture. Subsequent studies by T. K. Brown, working in Schwarz's clinic, indicate that the St. Louis workers continue to find the anaerobic streptococcus the most common offender in puerperal infection. The same is true in England, according to Leonard Colebrook. Summarizing the combined aerobic and anaerobic blood cultures made on 76 cases of puerperal infection, he states that he was able to recover anaerobic streptococci from the blood in no fewer than 17 cases, either in pure or mixed culture, whereas the *Streptococcus pyogenes* (hemolytic streptococcus, Group A) was obtained only 12 times. Among 3,764 women delivered between 1928 and 1930, he obtained a pure culture of aerobic streptococci from the blood during life in six cases, with three deaths, while the anaerobic streptococcus was obtained in pure culture from the blood in 13 cases with five deaths. In this period, therefore, two thirds of Colebrook's puerperal infections (blood stream) were due to anaerobic streptococci and but one third to the hemolytic streptococcus. Douglas and Rhees have reached similar conclusions on the basis of the routine bacteriological work that has been carried out at the Woman's Clinic of the New York Lying-In Hospital from September 1, 1932 to April 1, 1933. An analysis of the uterine cultures from febrile puerperae showed that 65.5 per cent of the organisms recovered were anaerobic streptococci. An additional 8.1 per cent were classed as anaerobic streptococci, but were facultative aerobes, so that the combined incidence of anaerobic streptococci, including the facultative group, was 73.6 per cent. In addition, uterine cultures were taken 20 times at cesarean section and here also the anaerobic streptococcus was found more often than any other organism. As shown in Table 21, more recent observations by Douglas on 565 patients with puerperal infection confirm the earlier statistics by showing that 68.0 per cent of these puerperae had anaerobic streptococci in their uterine cultures.

Not only is the anaerobic streptococcus the most common organism met in puerperal infection, but it is frequently found in the vagina of normal pregnant women and in uterine cultures taken from normal, afebrile puerpera. T. K. Brown, in the course of examining 103 normal gravida, found obligatory anaerobic streptococci in the vagina of 39.5 per cent, a figure in close agreement with that of Armstrong and Burt-White (35.9 per cent) and with the earlier figure of Rosowsky (40 per cent). Weinstein, using special culture media (cystine-glucose agar), found anaerobic streptococci in the vagina of 93 per cent of normal gravida. Likewise, it is encountered very frequently in uterine cultures from normal, afebrile puerperae, Guilbeau and Schaub having demonstrated it in 81.3 per cent of our patients during the first three days of the puerperium. The fact that the anaerobic streptococcus is an inhabitant of the birth canal in a large proportion of normal gravidae and puerperae points a most important clinical lesson. These organisms are ordinarily nonpathogenic and give no clinical evidence of their presence. The determining factor in their becoming pathogenic and invading the maternal tissues appears to be the presence of traumatized, devitalized tissues. This circumstance should logically lead to greater restraint and greater gentleness in operative interference.

Staphylococcus. The older writers believed that the staphylococcus was a rather common cause of puerperal infection, Zangemeister estimating that 15 per cent of cases were caused by it in comparison to 70 per cent due to the streptococcus, and in 1928 Sommer went so far as to state that the hemolytic *Staphylococcus aureus* was a more frequent cause of fatal puerperal infection than the *Streptococcus hemolyticus*. It is true, furthermore, that these ubiquitous organisms, both the *Staphylococcus albus* and *aureus*, are often present in the vaginas of normal gravidae. Thus, in the course of 375 vaginal examinations, Weinstein isolated staphylococci 254 times. Of the total number of strains isolated, 208 were found to resemble non-hemolytic *Staphylococcus albus* strains, while 12 strains were identified as hemolytic *Staphylococcus aureus*. It is informative to note that none of the women who harbored the *Staphylococcus aureus* (hemolytic) exhibited puerperal fever or any other complication.

It is present-day experience that staphylococci are rather uncommon causes of puerperal infection except for stitch abscesses in perineal and vaginal wounds. In Douglas and Rhees' bacteriological study of 171 postpartum cases, mostly instances of infection, the *Staphylococcus aureus* was recovered in only one uterine culture and the *Staphylococcus albus* but eight times. As shown in Table 21, a later study by Douglas revealed the former organism in but 2.1 per cent of 565 patients with puerperal infection.

Bacterium coli and Related Organisms. Contrary to what one might expect because of the proximity of the rectum, the *Bacterium coli,* or colon bacillus, is not a common inhabitant of the female generative tract. Thus, in Weinstein's study of the bacterial flora of the human vagina, among 375 women, he found *Bacterium coli* in only 27 cases and *Bacterium aerogenes* in only 14 cases. He was unable, moreover, to correlate the presence of these bacteria in pregnancy with any subsequent puerperal fever. In Douglas and Rhees' study mentioned above, among 171 postpartum cases, mostly febrile, uterine cultures showed the colon bacillus in 8.7 per cent, but following operative delivery it was met three times as often. Tables 21, 22, and 23 show similar findings. It is rather common experience that the colon bacillus is a more frequent cause of intrapartum than of postpartum infection; and, when found in the latter condition, it is usually, but not always, associated with the anaerobic streptococcus as a secondary invader.

Bacillus welchii. Synonyms: *Bacillus aerogenes capsulatus* (the name originally given the organism in 1892 by Welch and Nuttal and still used extensively in English-speaking countries); *Clostridium welchii* (bacteriologic species name); Fränkel's bacillus (German name); *Bacillus perfringens* (French name).

The Welch bacillus is an uncommon cause of puerperal infection, but the dramatic course and the high mortality which usually attend such infections in the puerperium make this organism of signal interest to the obstetrician. It is a normal inhabitant of the intestinal tract of humans as well as of the lower animals. It can be isolated consistently from soil and has been found repeatedly in the dust swept from floors of hospital wards and laboratories. Although some difference of opinion has been expressed concerning the presence of the Welch bacillus in the birth canal of healthy pregnant women, recent research shows clearly that about 1 gravida in 20 harbors the organism in the vagina. Among 253 prenatal patients Falls found the organism in the vagina of 15, an incidence of 5.9 per cent; among 78 gynecologic patients he demonstrated it 13 times, or in 16.6 per cent; while in 17 incomplete abortions he recovered it in 5 cases, or in 29.4 per cent. Similarly, Bysshe found *B. welchii* in the genital tract of 25 patients (mostly prenatal) among 547 examined, an incidence of 4.5 per cent. In our own clinic Sadusk and Manahan have not only studied the incidence of *B. welchii* in the vagina of normal gravidae but have attempted to evaluate the virulence of the organism found. Among 132 colored patients examined, the organism was isolated in 12, or in 9.1 per cent; in 6 of these 12 cases the organism was lethal for a guinea pig in less than 48 hours, with characteristic findings at autopsy. Of 87 white patients, 7, or 8.1 per cent, showed *B. welchii,* 3 of the strains being lethal to guinea pigs.

In view of the widespread distribution of the Welch bacillus, particularly its prevalence in the genital tract of normal women, one would expect that puerperal infections from this source would be much more frequent than they are. Their comparative rarity is due to the fact that the organism exhibits the most extraordinary variation in pathogenicity. On the one hand, it may produce the most cataclysmic of clinical pictures: rapid hemolysis, profound vasomotor collapse, metastatic gas gangrene, and

Organism	Number		Percent
Anaerobic streptococcus *	242	or	77.0%
Aerobic nonhemolytic streptococcus	78	or	25.0%
Anaerobic staphylococcus	68	or	21.0%
Anaerobic diphtheroid	60	or	19.0%
Streptococcus viridans	48	or	15.0%
Staphylococcus albus	48	or	15.0%
Colon bacillus	23	or	7.0%
Aerobic diphtheroid	23	or	7.0%
Lactobacillus	20	or	6.0%
Anaerobic gram negative rod	17	or	5.0%
Alpha prime streptococcus	9	or	2.5%
Staphylococcus aureus	4	or	1.2%
B. Welchii	3	or	0.9%
Enterococcus	2	or	0.6%
Gonococcus	2	or	0.6%
Beta-hemolytic streptococcus	2	or	0.6%
Monilia albicans	1	or	0.3%
No growth	9	or	2.5%

TABLE 22. INCIDENCE OF ORGANISMS IN THE UTERINE LOCHIA OF 314 PATIENTS WITH PUERPERAL INFECTION WHO WERE DELIVERED SPONTANEOUSLY. (17 different organisms.)
(Courtesy of Dr. R. Gordon Douglas.)

* See footnote to Table 21.

Organism	Number		Percent
Anaerobic streptococcus *	144	or	60.0%
Aerobic nonhemolytic streptococcus	58	or	24.0%
Colon bacillus	55	or	27.0%
Staphylococcus albus	43	or	18.0%
Anaerobic staphylococcus	29	or	12.0%
Streptococcus viridans	29	or	12.0%
Anaerobic diphtheroid	24	or	9.9%
Aerobic diphtheroid	19	or	7.8%
Alpha prime streptococcus	14	or	5.8%
Staphylococcus aureus	8	or	3.3%
Anaerobic gram negative rod	7	or	2.9%
B. Welchii	6	or	2.4%
Lactobacillus	6	or	2.4%
B. aerogenes	4	or	1.6%
B. proteus	4	or	1.6%
Beta-hemolytic streptococcus	4	or	1.6%
Enterococcus	2	or	0.8%
Monilia albicans	2	or	0.8%
Gonococcus	1	or	0.4%
B. Friedlander	1	or	0.4%
Pneumococcus Group IV	1	or	0.4%
No growth	14	or	5.8%

TABLE 23. INCIDENCE OF ORGANISMS IN THE UTERINE LOCHIA OF 241 PATIENTS WITH PUERPERAL INFECTION WHO WERE DELIVERED BY OPERATIVE MEANS. (21 different organisms.)
(Courtesy of Dr. R. Gordon Douglas.)

* See footnote to Table 21.

sometimes death within 24 hours. On the other hand, it sometimes behaves as a harmless parasite. Even in cases in which the organism is cultivated from the blood, the patient may show no serious symptoms. In one case reported by Falls, a woman in the hospital four weeks under observation for cardiac disease aborted spontaneously. The fetus was emphysematous and smears and cultures showed Welch bacillus, yet there was no fever previous to or following the abortion. Although it is doubtless true that the virulence of different strains of *B. welchii* varies greatly, the most important determining factor in the production of an actual infection would seem to be the presence of traumatized or dead muscle tissue, which augments enormously the pathogenicity of the organism. In keeping with this fact, the vast majority of serious puerperal infections caused by it follow criminal abortion or traumatic operative delivery. In most such cases, moreover, the bacteriologic findings show a mixed infection with some other organism, usually a streptococcus, and it seems probable that the association of the two enhances the virulence of both.

The Welch bacillus is a more common cause of postabortal than of puerperal infection, approximately two thirds of the cases occurring in association with abortion. The organism liberates two toxins, one a myotoxin which liquefies protein with the production of gas, and the other a hemotoxin which destroys red blood cells. It is these toxins which account in large measure for the characteristic clinical picture produced.

Gonococcus. It has been estimated that the gonococcus is the cause of 5 to 10 per cent of all fevers occurring in the puerperium. Around the turn of the century, moreover, most writers on the subject were of the opinion that about one half of women who go into labor with cervical gonorrhea suffer an extension upward of the infection during the second week of the puerperium, the extension manifesting itself in the form of a salpingitis in about one case in three. It is doubtless true that the gonococcus exhibits a predilection for the fallopian tube in the puerpera just as it does in the nonpregnant, but a study of Overstreet in our clinic would suggest that the above figures are much higher than obtain today. In analyzing various aspects of 114 cases of gonorrheal ophthalmia neonatorum, in all of which the causative agent was definitely identified by bacteriological study, he found that 40 of the mothers had febrile puerperia, an incidence of 33.4 per cent. With very few exceptions, the endometritis produced was mild, the temperature elevation moderate (under 102° F.) and of one or two days' duration only; the peak of temperature was usually reached around the fifth day. It should be noted, moreover, that the majority of these patients were colored women (73.6 per cent) and, in our hands, they ordinarily exhibited, at the time this study was made, a morbidity incidence of about 20 per cent; it seems likely, therefore, that many of these cases of endometritis were due to the ordinary invaders rather than to the gonococcus. More remarkable was the fact that the classical picture of second week fever due to gonococcal salpingitis, was a rarity among these patients. In the entire series there was only one case of clear-cut salpingitis and but five others in which the findings were in any way suggestive of tubal disease. Likewise, Tucker, Trussell, and Plass observed 20 patients, from whom they had cultured the gonococcus before labor and during the puerperium and found the postpartum course was not different from that of a control group. Douglas also has observed afebrile puerperia in cases where the gonococcus was cultured from the lochial discharge. It is quite possible and even probable that an endosalpingitis with subsequent tubal occlusion may occur during the puerperium in the absence of any febrile reaction or disturbing subjective symptoms. Williams demonstrated the gonococcus in the tissues of cases of decidual endometritis, and others have made similar observations. As a rule, gonorrheal infection in the puerperium pursues a favorable course, but occasionally fatal septicemia may result, as in two cases reported by Harris and Dabney, and J. T. Smith. In our experience, puerperal salpingitis of gonococcal origin is more likely to follow abortion than full-term delivery.

Pneumococcus. In a study of 20,364 deliveries occurring at the Boston Lying-In Hospital, Nuckols and Hertig encountered three cases of pneumococcal puerperal infection, an incidence of one case to 6,788 deliveries. These authors suspect that such infections are more common than these figures would indicate, owing to failure to identify correctly organisms loosely classed as "non-hemolytic" or "green streptococci." The majority of cases of pneumococcal puerperal infection are secondary to pneumococcal infections elsewhere in the body, such as lobar pneumonia, otitis media, or nasopharyngeal conditions. Puerperal infections caused by this organism carried a grave prognosis prior to the present era, Nuckols and Hertig finding a mortality of 67.6 per cent among cases reported in the literature; in postabortal pneumococcal infections, the death rate was 82.3 per cent. Localization of the infection into an abscess improves the outlook, mortality in this group being 26.0 per cent.

Bacillus typhosus. Although the typhoid bacillus is occasionally found in uterine cultures, it is almost always associated with some other organism, often an anaerobic streptococcus. In so far as its role in puerperal infection is concerned, it behaves much more benignly in the birth canal than in the intestinal tract and resembles the colon bacillus in its pathogenicity.

Bacillus diphtheriae. Current prophylaxis against diphtheria has made the Klebs-Loeffler bacillus an exceedingly rare cause of puerperal infection in modern practice. In the early years of this century, however, it was encountered from time to time, Gude being able to collect 42 cases in 1911. The disease is characterized by the formation of a membrane on the vagina and endometrium and responds readily to antidiphtheric serum.

Bacillus tetani. Thanks to modern asepsis, puerperal infection due to the tetanus bacillus is so rare that it requires mention from an historical viewpoint only. In 1894 Vinay reported 106 cases with a mortality of 88.7 per cent; in 20 patients the placenta had been removed manually and in another 17 an intra-uterine tampon had been inserted. In 1898 an epidemic occurred in Prague and 28 women died forthwith. During a stay in China I saw one case, delivered by a Chinese midwife, and heard of a few others.

Diphtheroids. Very frequently organisms are found in the lochia which resemble the Klebs-Loeffler bacillus in appearance and have hence been called *diphtheroids;* in mixed cultures they are very common. They appear to be normal inhabitants of the birth canal and are not pathogenic.

MODES OF INFECTION

It is the physician himself who is most likely to carry infection to the parturient uterus. He may do so in two ways. In the first place, gloved and sterile though his hands may be, he may carry the already present anaerobic streptococcus from the vagina to the uterus through vaginal examinations or operative manipulations. Secondly, his hands and the instruments he uses may become contaminated by virulent streptococci as the result of droplet infection, dispersed by himself or some of the attendants, and in this manner he may be responsible for introducing bacteria to the birth canal. Unless the utmost vigilance is used in masking all attendants in the delivery room (both nose and mouth) and in excluding therefrom all persons suffering or recovering from an upper respiratory infection, the latter mode of infection is a constant source of danger. Although a less common means of transfer today than a few decades ago, careless physicians and nurses have been known to carry bacteria to the parturient from countless extraneous contacts: from other cases of puerperal infection, from suppurative postoperative wounds, from cases of sloughing carcinoma, from patients with scarlet fever, from infants with impetigo neonatorum, from umbilical infections of the newborn, and finally, from the autopsy table. The physician himself may have the infection on his own person, such as an infected hangnail or felon.

Among certain classes, coitus late in pregnancy is more common than is ordinarily believed and may introduce extraneous organisms to the birth canal or carry upward bacteria already present on the vulva or in the lower vagina. The observations of Carl Ruge II on this practice in Germany are almost unbelievable: among 410 married women, more than one half admitted coitus in the last month of pregnancy; 31.5 per cent in the last week, 20 per cent in the last three days and 9.5 per cent on the day before delivery. Of the women who had had intercourse in the three days prior to delivery, more than 20 per cent suffered a severe puerperal infection. Many fatal cases of puerperal infection are on record in which infection was introduced in this manner, and in some the penis even ruptured the membranes. It is well known that the penis is never sterile, pathogenic streptococci having repeatedly been cultured from the prepuce.

Tub baths, particularly in multiparae with gaping vulvae, may permit the wash water to gain access to the vagina and thus introduce surface bacteria from the whole body. Another way in which the patient may infect herself is through the introduction of one or more of her own fingers into the vagina during labor. During the second stage of labor the chances of fecal matter being transferred to the vagina are, of course, excellent. The evidence would indicate, however, that this is a source of milder infections only. In the course of examining the feces of 100 women in labor, Hare and Maxted found hemolytic streptococci in 29 cases, but in no instance was a Group A organism isolated. The latter type of streptococcus, however, is found occasionally in the feces of individuals suffering from, or recovering from, scarlet fever or upper respiratory infections. On the other hand, transfer of fecal matter from rectum to vagina is the most common cause of colon bacillus infections. Proof that such *B. coli* infections are usually autogenous has been supplied by G. Smith, who, in 13 out of 14 cases investigated, showed serological identity between the *B. coli* in the genital infection and a strain in the urine or feces. As has been indicated, such transfer is much more likely to occur in operative deliveries.

PREDISPOSING CAUSES

The most important predisposing causes of puerperal infection are hemorrhage and trauma at the time of labor. Spontaneous delivery followed by minimal blood loss is rarely followed by fever, but women who have suffered a hemorrhage of 1,000 cc. or more almost always become infected. Thus, Reich found that the puerperal morbidity among 1,154 patients without postpartum hemorrhage was 15.1 per cent, but among 135 patients with hemorrhage it reached 41.9 per cent. In this connection it should be recalled that most methods of treating obstetric hemorrhage (for instance, uterine tamponade) entail intra-uterine manipulations which often inflict shock and introduce infection. Working hand in hand with hemorrhage is the other great predisposing factor, trauma. Trauma not only creates more portals of entry for bacteria but means dead tissue and dead tissue means that harmless organisms become pathogenic and pathogenic bacteria more virulent. The associated shock, moreover, together with the absorption of toxins from dead tissues, serves further to weaken the resistance of the host and pave the way for invasion.

Labors which last more than 24 hours, particularly if the membranes have been ruptured throughout most of the period, provide vaginal bacteria with readier and more prolonged access to the uterus, promote exhaustion, and are followed by an increased incidence of puerperal infection. Unfortunately, moreover, such cases are often terminated by difficult operative means, so that the triad of exhaustion, trauma, and hemorrhage combine to form the soil par excellence for bacterial growth.

Retention of the placenta, in whole or in part, predisposes to infection in a number of ways. In the first place, vigorous and repeated efforts to express the placenta traumatize the uterus. Secondly, if manual removal becomes necessary, the insertion of the hand between the naked placental site and the placenta is the surest means of conveying bacteria to the most vulnerable site in the uterus. And finally, if small fragments of placenta or membrane are retained, these undergo necrosis and readily become infected. Superimposed on these accidents of the third stage, moreover, there is usually hemorrhage.

Pre-existing anemia, undernutrition, and other debilitated states also make puerperal infection more likely. In our own clinic, Bickerstaff has shown that the incidence of puerperal morbidity, other things being equal, is in direct proportion to the degree of anemia existing in the last month of pregnancy.

PATHOLOGY

Following completion of the third stage of labor, the area of placental attachment is represented by a raw, elevated area, deep red in color, and about 4 cm. in diameter. Its surface is nodular, owing to the presence of numerous gaping veins, many of which are occluded by thrombi. These form admirable culture media for bacteria and constitute the most common portal of entry for pathogenic organisms. At this time, furthermore, the condition of the entire endometrium is peculiarly favorable to bacterial invasion since it is less than 2 mm. in thickness, is infiltrated with blood, and presents numerous small wounds. Since the cervix rarely escapes some degree of laceration in labor, it is another ready site for bacterial invasion. Vulvar, vaginal, and perineal wounds offer still other portals of entry.

The pathology of puerperal infection is that of any wound infection. Accordingly, the inflammatory process may remain localized in the wounds mentioned above, or may extend through the blood stream or lymphatics to tissues far beyond the original lesion. **Whether or not such extension occurs is of decisive importance; indeed, it is the determining factor not only in the pathological changes wrought, but in the whole clinical course, prognosis and treatment of the**

disease. So important is this matter of extension that it is desirable to regard puerperal infection as falling into two main categories:

1. Local processes (inflammatory lesions of the perineum, vulva, vagina, cervix, and endometrium).
2. Extensions of the original process (along the veins to produce **thrombophlebitis** and **pyemia**, through the lymph vessels to produce **peritonitis** and **parametritis**, and along the surface of the endometrium and endosalpinx to produce **salpingitis**).

Lesions of the Perineum, Vulva, Vagina, and Cervix. The most common puerperal lesion of the external genitalia is a localized infection of a repaired laceration or episiotomy wound. The apposing wound edges become red, brawny and swollen; the sutures cut through the edematous, expanding tissues, allowing the necrotic edges of the wound to gape so that greenish-yellow pus can be seen exuding from the crevice of the wound. In this manner, complete breakdown of the wound may occur, with profuse serous and purulent discharge. Following traumatic operative delivery, wounds and contusions of the vulva are common; the entire vulva may become edematous, ulcerated, and covered with a grayish exudate. Lacerations of the vagina are very frequent after operative delivery and may become infected directly or by continuity from the perineum. The mucous membrane becomes swollen and intensely red; sloughs and necrotic debris are present and purulent secretions are discharged in large amounts from ulcerated areas. A pseudodiphtheritic membrane is occasionally present, as in vulvar lesions. Extension may occur by infiltration, lymphangitis resulting, but as a rule the infection remains local. However, it is occasionally followed by the formation of large cicatrices with irregular contractions and atresia of the vagina.

Cervical infection is probably more common than is realized. Moreover, since deep lacerations of the cervix often extend directly into the cellular tissue at the base of the broad ligament, infection of such wounds may form the starting point for lymphatic infection, parametritis, and bacteremia.

Endometritis. The most common manifestation of puerperal infection is endometritis. After an incubation period which may vary from a few hours to several days, the bacteria invade the tissues of an endometrial wound (usually the placental site) and a typical wound reaction ensues. The blood vessels and lymphatics in the vicinity of the infected area become engorged and an effusion of serum is poured into the tissues and on to the surface of the wound. Whether the process begins at the placental site or elsewhere, it spreads rapidly to involve the entire endometrium. Meanwhile, leukocytes migrate through the capillary walls into the underlying tissues and form a dense protective barrier. In addition to this leukocytic wall and the effusion of antibody-containing serum, a third important protection is found in the tight contraction of the interlacing muscle bundles of the uterus which tend to close the lymphatics and blood vessels. These three mechanisms represent nature's effort to restrict the infection to the more superficial layers of the endometrium; if the process is limited to the endometrium, the superficial necrotic tissues are cast off within a week or so and the episode is closed.

The appearance of the endometrium varies widely. In some cases the mucosa is sloughing and necrotic, the debris abundant, the discharge foul, profuse, bloody, sometimes frothy; the color of the necrotic material covering the endometrium is yellowish green, as a rule, but may be black from decomposed blood. The cervix is usually involved in the process and if lacerations have occurred they are ulcerated and sloughing. As a rule, involution is greatly retarded but, occasionally, may be little affected. Microscopic sections show first a thick layer of necrotic material containing bacteria, then a thick zone of leukocytic infiltration—nature's wall of defense, so to speak—beneath which is normal tissue. At the other extreme are cases in which the endometrium is smooth and clean, the necrotic layer thin or absent, and the discharge scant and odorless. Microscopic examination shows a very thin layer of necrotic material containing bacteria, with a zone of leukocytic infiltration which is either poorly developed or entirely lacking.

The older writers regarded these two extremes of endometrial change as representing two different types of infection and designated the former as *putrid endometritis* and the latter *septic endometritis*. They differentiated between the two in the belief that in the putrid type saprophytic organisms multiplied in the superficial debris of the uterine cavity but did not invade the living tissues of the endometrium. On the other hand, they considered that septic endometritis was the result of invasion of the endometrium by highly pathogenic organisms capable of penetrating living tissues. This differentiation is gradually being abandoned since true infection, even of the slightest degree, must entail invasion of living tissue. It seems probable that in so-called "putrid endometritis" bacteria of low virulence invade tissues with high powers of resistance so that the process is limited to the surface; anaerobic streptococci, colon bacilli, and other gas-producing organisms are the usual offenders and account for the profuse and fetid discharge. On the other hand, in "septic endometritis" highly virulent organisms penetrate tissues of weakened resistance so rapidly that minimal pathologic changes are produced in the endometrium; overwhelming infection with the beta hemolytic streptococcus is the classical example of this type of endometritis. In other words, these two pathologic pictures represent merely extremes in the balance between virulence of the invader and resistance of the host; between the two, all gradations exist.

It must be recalled, furthermore, that in cases of puerperal infection of long duration, metastatic processes in the lungs and elsewhere may effect a fatal outcome while the original endometrial lesion becomes healed. The endometrium in such cases will appear quite normal at autopsy, a frequent finding in thrombophlebitis. Among 163 cases of puerperal infection studied at autopsy by Halban and Köhler, the endometrium was entirely normal in 20.2 per cent.

Thrombophlebitis and Pyemia. In modern obstetrics the most common mode of extension of puerperal infection is along the veins, with resultant thrombophlebitis. It would appear, indeed, that from 30 to 50 per cent of all deaths from puerperal infection are attributable to this type of extension. Thus, at the Johns Hopkins Hospital, 41 per cent of our fatal cases of puerperal infection have been associated with thrombophlebitis. Halban and Köhler, in autopsies on 163 women who had died from puerperal infection, found 82 instances of thrombophlebitis, an incidence of approximately 50 per cent; in 36 of these cases thrombophlebitis represented the only mode of extension, while in 46 there was a coexisting lymphatic involvement. The frequency of the condition is attributable to two facts: (1) the most vulnerable wound of the endometrium after delivery—the placental site—is a mass of thrombosed veins; and (2) the anaerobic streptococcus, which, as we have seen, is frequently a normal inhabitant of the vagina, seems to have an especial predilection for veins. In keeping with the latter statement, the vast majority of cases of puerperal thrombophlebitis are due to the anaerobic streptococcus.

Two groups of veins are principally involved: (1) the veins of the uterine wall and broad ligament (the ovarian, uterine, and hypogastric veins); and (2) the veins of the leg (femoral, popliteal, and saphenous veins). It is customary to differentiate between involvement of these two groups of veins by calling the former *pelvic thrombophlebitis* and the latter *femoral thrombophlebitis* ("phlegmasia alba dolens"). This differentiation is highly important since the pathology, clinical course, prognosis, and treatment of the two sets of conditions differ widely.

The vein most commonly involved in pelvic thrombophlebitis is the ovarian since it drains the upper part of the uterus and sinuses of the placental site. The process is usually unilateral, one side being affected as often as the other. Extension of the process in the left ovarian vein may reach its junction with the renal vein with involvement of that vessel and consequent renal complications; or, if the right ovarian vein is affected, the thrombosis may extend well into the inferior vena cava. Not infrequently, thrombosis of the uterine and lymphatic vessels extends far into the common iliac. In most cases several veins are involved in various combinations.

The pathology of pelvic thrombophlebitis is the same as that of thrombophlebitis elsewhere in the body. As the inflammatory process progresses, the thrombosis extends higher and higher, a mechanism designed to prevent wide dissemination of the infecting organisms. Where resistance is high, the thrombosis of the infected vein may limit the advance of the infection so that the thrombus undergoes organization. In other cases, extension of the inflammation converts the thrombus into a mass of pus while the surrounding vein wall becomes edematous and necrotic. As the process continues small emboli sooner or later break off into the blood stream and are disseminated to various parts of the body. This discharge of emboli into the blood stream is such a constant accompaniment of pelvic thrombophlebitis that the whole process is often spoken of as *pyemia*. The most common sites of metastases from pelvic thrombophlebitis are the lungs, kidneys, and the heart valves. Although large emboli may occasionally reach the pulmonary artery and cause sudden death, this is uncommon in pyemia. More often, small emboli reach the terminal branches of the pulmonary vessels and produce hemorrhagic infarcts. Lung abscesses are extremely frequent sequelae and are found at autopsy in more than one half of such cases; pleurisy and pneumonia are also common.

Femoral thrombophlebitis may arise in one of three ways: (1) as a simple thrombophlebitis of the great saphenous or femoral vein secondary to a bacteriemia of low virulence; (2) as an extension of a thrombophlebitis of the uterine vein, the process extending thence to the hypogastric, external iliac, and femoral veins; and (3) as a periphlebitis of the femoral vein consequent upon the extension of parametritic infection to the connective tissue surrounding the femoral vein. The first two mechanisms are more common than the third, but as to which of the former two is the more frequent, there is wide difference of opinion. Indeed, since few patients die of femoral thrombophlebitis, per se; the underlying pathological anatomy of the condition has been inadequately studied and is poorly understood. Agreement is general, however, that it is always the manifestation of an infection and is caused by organisms of low virulence, usually by the anaerobic streptococcus. The condition

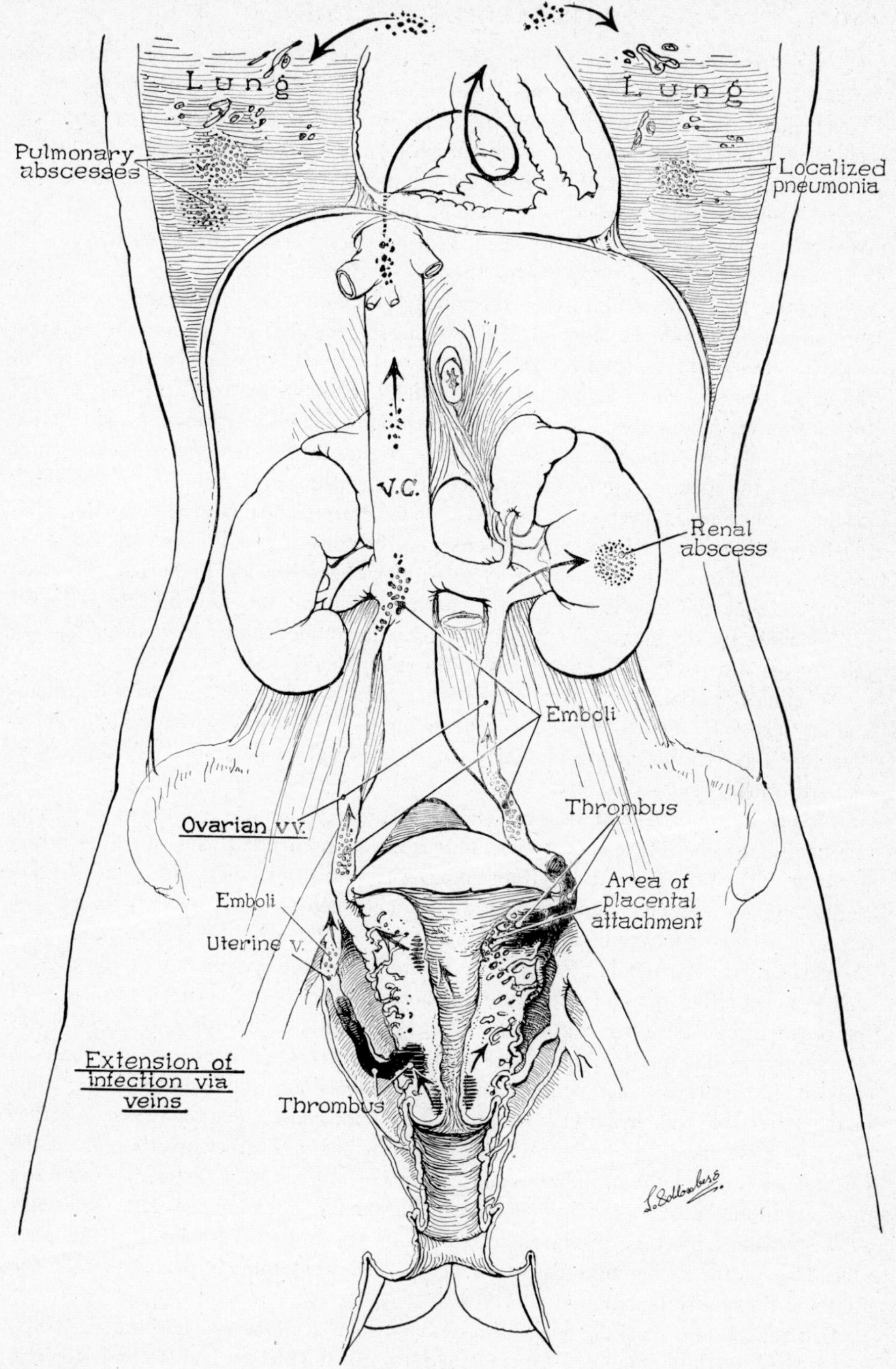

FIG. 509.—DIAGRAMMATIC ILLUSTRATION OF EXTENSION OF PUERPERAL INFECTION IN UTERINE THROMBOPHLEBITIS.

is always preceded by a low-grade infection of the birth canal, commonly of the endometrium; in the course of this, bacteria are apparently emitted into the blood stream and may, accordingly, reach the thigh by way of the general circulation, as well as through extension of a pelvic thrombosis. By way of explaining the occurrence of a primary thrombophlebitis of the leg veins, Widal has shown that organisms are particularly prone to attack the wall of the femoral vein near the inguinal ligament since the blood flow is very sluggish at this point, especially when the patient first stands on her feet after delivery; the high fibrinogen content of the blood in the puerperium facilitates still further thrombus formation. The obstructed venous return invariably produces more or less swelling of the leg, but this varies in type with the underlying mechanism and the vessel involved. In primary thrombosis of the femoral or saphenous vein, the edema usually begins in the toes and then spreads to the foot, calf, and thigh. If the femoral thrombophlebitis represents a direct extension of a pelvic thrombosis, the swelling begins in the femoral area and later extends to the calf. As might be expected, the extension of a cellulitis to the thigh produces a localized phlegmon in that area. In general, the edema of femoral thrombophlebitis is brawny and pits with difficulty. Although the condition at the outset is usually unilateral, it is exceedingly common for the other leg to become involved about the time the first is returning to normal. Femoral thrombophlebitis is rarely accompanied by discharge of emboli and consequent metastatic phenomena and in this respect differs decidedly from pelvic thrombophlebitis.

In clinical parlance the term *phlegmasia alba dolens* ("white, painful inflammation") is often used in a loose way to designate any variety of femoral thrombophlebitis; the term *milk-leg* is similarly employed by physicians and laity alike, particularly when edema is marked.

Closely allied to femoral thrombophlebitis is the very rare and grave condition, puerperal gangrene of the extremities. This is due to a carrying over of the infection to the arteries of the leg with resultant endarteritis and thrombosis. Although infection is the common etiologic factor, the indiscriminate use of ergot in the presence of infection seems to have played an important role in the causation of certain cases.

Peritonitis. Puerperal infection may extend along the lymphatics of the uterine wall to reach either the peritoneum or the loose cellular tissues between the leaves of the broad ligaments, in the former instance producing a peritonitis and in the latter a parametritis. The peritonitis may be localized to the pelvic region or may be generalized. In the former case, organisms of low virulence are usually responsible, while in the latter the beta hemolytic streptococcus is the most common cause. Whether pelvic or generalized, the peritonitis may be due either to a direct involvement of the peritoneum through the lymphatics of the uterine wall or to a secondary extension to the peritoneum of a thrombophlebitic or parametric infection. On rare occasions, pelvic peritonitis may be produced by escape of pus from the lumen of a fallopian tube. One of the commonest causes of generalized peritonitis is perforation of the uterus in the course of criminal abortion.

Generalized peritonitis is one of the gravest complications of childbearing, being the cause of death in about one third of the fatal cases. Thus, in Halban and Köhler's series of 163 autopsies previously mentioned, it was present in 60 cases. The pathology of puerperal peritonitis is essentially the same as that of surgical peritonitis in general. The intestines are distended with gas and their peritoneal coat reddened. The usual luster of the peritoneum is dulled by the exudation of a layer of fibrin, while the intestinal loops are matted together by fibrinous or purulent lymph. In some cases, encysted collections of pus may form, either in the pelvis or between the coils of bowel. The pouch of Douglas, the subdiaphragmatic space and the fold between the infundibulopelvic and broad ligaments are common sites for such accumulations. By and large, the more virulent the causative organism, the less is the peritoneal reaction; thus, in peritonitis due to the beta hemolytic streptococcus, the peritoneum

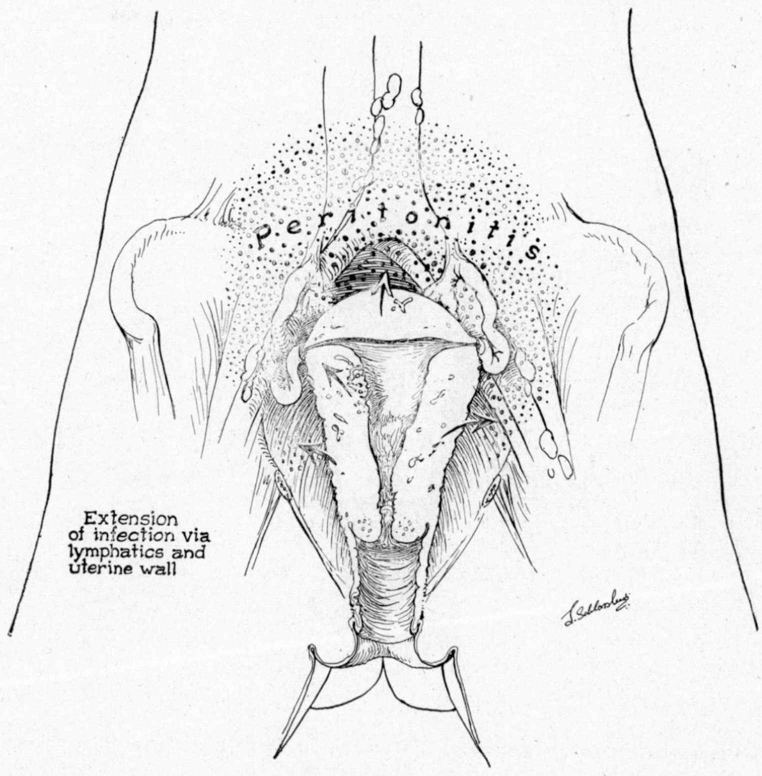

FIG. 510.—DIAGRAMMATIC ILLUSTRATION OF EXTENSION OF PUERPERAL INFECTION IN PERITONITIS.

may be only reddened with little exudate, while with organisms of less virulence the peritoneal cavity may become actually filled with pus. Recalling the huge absorptive area represented by the peritoneal surface, it is readily understood that the blood stream in such cases is inundated not only by overwhelming amounts of bacterial toxins but also by large numbers of bacteria themselves, with the result that a bacteremia is an invariable accompaniment.

Pelvic Cellulitis (Parametritis). It will be recalled that the pelvic connective tissue is a loose fibro-areolar network forming a complete subserous investment of the pelvic organs and providing sheaths for the blood vessels, nerves, and lymphatics. It is most abundant at the sides of the pelvis and in the lower part of the broad ligaments surrounding the cervix and upper portion of the vagina. Infection of this pelvic connective tissue may be brought about in three main ways: (1) It is most commonly caused by the lymphatic transmission of organisms from an infected cervical laceration. Similar lymphatic extension from an endometritis may also be responsible but is probably less frequent. Although lacerations of the perineum or vagina may be a cause of localized cellulitis, the process is usually limited to the paravaginal cellular tissue and rarely extends deeply into the pelvis. (2) Since cervical lacerations not infrequently extend well into the connective tissue at the base of the broad ligaments, this tissue may be laid bare to direct invasion by whatever pathogenic organisms are in the vagina. Quite analogous results are frequently seen in cases of criminal abor-

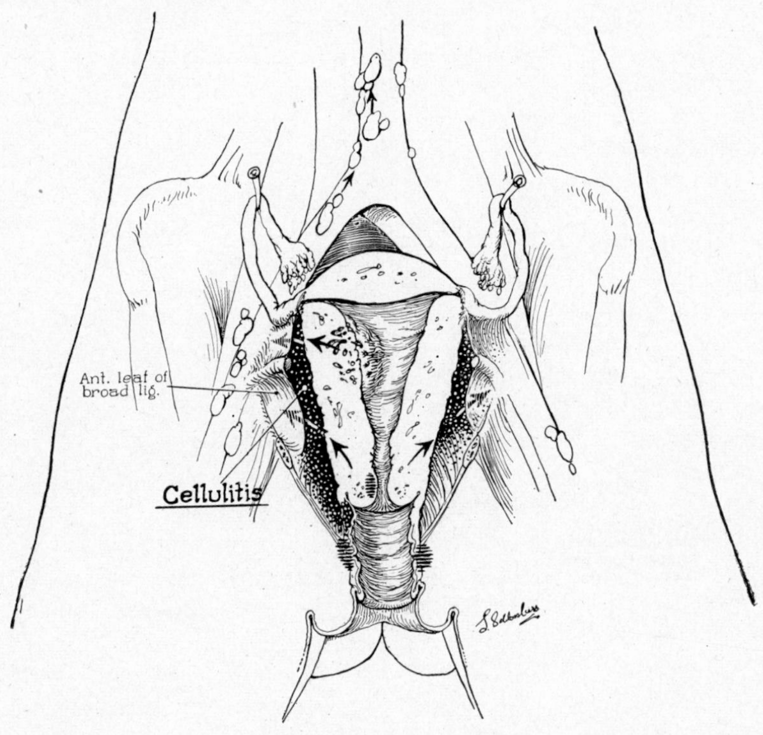

Fig. 511.—Diagrammatic Illustration of Extension of Puerperal Infection in Pelvic Cellulitis (Parametritis).

tion in which a sharp instrument has followed a false passage and penetrated the connective tissue at one or another side of the cervix. (3) Pelvic cellulitis may be secondary to a pelvic thrombophlebitis. Indeed, the latter condition is rarely seen without some degree of cellulitis and if the thrombi become purulent, the vein wall may undergo such necrosis as to permit massive egress of organisms into the surrounding connective tissue. As a rule, the organisms involved are either the beta hemolytic streptococcus or the anaerobic streptococcus. The former is the common offender in cases of lymphatic extension, the latter in cases in which the cellulitis is secondary to a thrombophlebitis.

Hyperemia, edema, and the effusion of serum are the natural reaction of the connective tissue to the infection. The swelling thus produced is at first soft but within a few days becomes firm from the deposition of fibrin. The process may remain limited to the base of the broad ligament, but, if the inflammatory reaction is at all substantial, the very bulk of the exudate forces extension along natural lines of cleavage. The most common form of extension is directly lateral along the base of the broad ligament, with a tendency to extend to the lateral pelvic wall; as the mass increases in size it distends the leaves of the broad ligament and, raising the anterior leaf upward, dissects its way forward to reach the abdominal wall just above Poupart's ligament. The uterus is, naturally, pushed to the opposite side and fixed. In other cases, high intraligamentary exudates spread from the region of the uterine cornua to the iliac fossae. Retrocervical exudates tend to invade the rectovaginal septum with the development of a firm mass posterior to the cervix. Occasionally, involvement of the precervical connective tissue results in a cellulitis of the space of Retzius with extension upward, beneath the anterior abdominal wall, as high as the umbilicus. Or, again, the process may extend out through the sciatic foramen into the thigh.

Inflammatory exudates in the pelvic connective tissue, such as we have described, follow a slow, indolent course but ultimately undergo either resolution or suppuration; resolution is the more common. If suppuration occurs, the most frequent outcome is "pointing" just above Poupart's ligament; the skin over the inguinal region becomes edematous, red, and tender, while fluctuation sooner or later indicates that the abscess is ready for opening—or rupture. A somewhat less common outcome is "pointing" in the posterior cul-de-sac. In one of our cases a high intraligamentary abcess ruptured directly into the peritoneal cavity, with fatal outcome.

Pelvic cellulitis is ordinarily unilateral but involves both sides in about one case in four. One side is as likely to be affected as the other. Minor degrees of the condition are very frequent and represent the most common cause of prolonged, unexplained fever in the puerperium. It is encountered at autopsy in about one third of all fatal cases of puerperal infection, sometimes alone but rather more often in association with thrombophlebitis or peritonitis. Since most cases of pelvic cellulitis are secondary to cervical lacerations, the condition is encountered more frequently in primiparae than in multiparae.

Salpingitis. Surface extension of bacteria from the puerperal endometrium or cervix to the fallopian tube with resultant endosalpingitis is a rare phenomenon, even in the case of the gonococcus. Although contrary to the viewpoint held some years ago, this statement is in accord with most modern evidence, particularly with the rarity of adnexal signs and symptoms in puerperae whose infants develop gonorrheal opthalmia (page 938). It is likewise in keeping with the observation of Tucker, Trussell, and Plass on the postpartum course of 20 patients from whom the gonococcus had been cultured before labor; the puerperia of these women differed in no way from a control group. To be sure, pre-existing salpingitis may manifest exacerbations in the puerperium, especially postabortal, but it would appear that initial attacks of endosalpingitis are a less common puerperal phenomenon than previously believed. On the other hand, the tube often becomes inflamed as the result of peritonitis or pelvic cellulitis with the development of a perisalpingitis. Loose, filmy adhesions are thus produced between the tube and surrounding structures, but, since the endosalpinx is usually unscathed, closure of the tubal lumen is uncommon. In exceptional instances, however, the fimbriated extremity may become sealed as the result of a contiguous peritonitis.

Other Modes of Extension. Bacteremia is a frequent accompaniment of pelvic thrombophlebitis, peritonitis, and, to a lesser extent, of pelvic cellulitis, and, whenever blood stream infection is encountered in the course of puerperal infection, it may almost invariably be charged to one of these three processes. However, in rare instances, when the invading bacteria are exceedingly virulent and the resistance of the host very weak, such a rapid transit of organisms into the blood may occur as to leave no time for the development of these processes; the patient is simply overwhelmed by bacterial toxins and death follows quickly—this is the so-called *sepsis foudroyante* of the French. Occasionally small abscesses in the myometrium develop, due either to the breaking down of a thrombophlebitic process or to lymphatic infection. Extension to the peritoneal surface often occurs with the formation of adhesions to surrounding structures; less commonly, direct perforation into the peritoneal cavity ensues with resultant peritonitis. In Halban and Köhler's series of 163 fatal cases of puerperal infection, endometrial abscesses were present in seven. *Metritis dissecans,* or *gangrene of the uterus,* is a rare and grave form of puerperal infection in which not only the endometrium but also part of the myometrium undergoes necrosis; in some cases the entire endometrium becomes detached and is expelled as a complete cast of the uterine cavity. Clinically, the condition is characterized by the expulsion of large pieces of necrotic tissue, usually during the second or third week of the puerperium.

CLINICAL COURSE

Sapremia (Toxinemia, Retention Fever). There are occasional instances in which a patient manifests evidence of uterine infection but with the expulsion of a blood clot, a piece of membrane, or an abortus, shows an immediate drop in temperature with no further signs or symptoms. In incomplete abortions this is an exceedingly common phenomenon. The very rapid and permanent subsidence of fever in such cases would indicate that we are not dealing with infection of living tissues, but with absorption of toxins from necrotic material lying free in the uterine cavity. These toxins are ordinarily produced by putrefactive processes in the dead tissue due to the action of saprophytic organisms but may result from the invasion of this tissue by anaerobic streptococci and other bacteria. The symptoms are almost identical with those of endometritis and it is usually impossible to differentiate the two conditions until the passage of a piece of membrane or other necrotic material makes plain the situation. However, the persistence of after-pains in the presence of a low grade fever may suggest retention of membranes, while profuse, bloody lochia, plus fever, may hint that a piece of placenta has been left behind.

Lesions of the Perineum, Vulva, Vagina and Cervix. Pain, burning on urination and a sensation of local heat are the common symptoms. Provided drainage is good, the reaction in these local conditions is seldom severe, the temperature remaining below 101° F. and the pulse under 100. If, however, purulent material is dammed back by perineal or vaginal suture, the complication may be signalized by a chill and a sharp rise of fever to 105° F. or 104° F., simulating the onset of a grave infection.

Endometritis. The clinical picture of puerperal endometritis depends chiefly on the type and virulence of the offending organism. It may vary from mild cases in which temperature elevations between 100.4° F. and 101° F. persist from the third to fifth day with no other signs or symptoms, to cases which are ushered in by a chill, fever between 104° F. and 105° F., and other evidence of a fulminating infection. In the average case, the temperature begins to rise about 48 hours postpartum and mounts with morning remissions, "saw-tooth" fashion, to reach levels between 101° F. and 103° F. on the fourth or fifth day. The pulse rate tends to follow the temperature curve, but in grave infections it is usually rapid from the first. The uterus is almost always large but, contrary to orthodox teaching, may occasionally be involuted satisfactorily despite outright endometritis. There is more or less tenderness over the uterus and very frequently after-pains are severe and prolonged. Changes in the lochia are observed even in the early stages and may afford valuable information as to the nature of the infecting bacteria. As a rule, the discharge is increased in amount and is hemorrhagic or dark brown in color. The presence of an offensive smell has long been regarded as an important sign of endometrial infection and is due, of course, to the invasion of the uterine cavity by putrefactive bacteria, particularly certain strains of anaerobic streptococci and the colon bacillus. However, some of the severest infections, notably cases of beta hemolytic streptoccal endometritis, are frequently associated with scanty, odorless lochia. Indeed, the gravity of a case of endometritis is in almost *inverse* proportion to the amount and putridity of the lochia. Leukocytosis may range from 15,000 to 30,000 cells per cubic millimeter, but in view of the physiologic leukocytosis of the puerperium these figures are difficult to interpret. In simple endometritis, blood cultures are almost invariably negative; as already indicated, a positive culture points to lymphatic or thrombophlebitic extension.

The general symptoms of endometritis are variable and depend on the nature and amount of the bacterial toxins absorbed. Many patients feel well and have no complaints whatsoever. The common symptoms are: headache, varying degrees of insomnia, and more or less anorexia. Except in very mild cases, milk secretion is suppressed. Chilly sensations and, more rarely, actual chills may be seen at the onset of endometritis, but after the first day or two, chills invariably mean extension, usually thrombophlebitis. If the process remains localized in the endometrium, the temperature falls by lysis, the uterine discharge diminishes, and, by the end of a week, or at the most 10 days, the episode is over.

Pelvic Thrombophlebitis. The clinical picture of pelvic thrombophlebitis is characterized by repeated, severe chills, hectic temperature swings, a tendency toward metastatic pus formation, particularly in the lungs, and a prolonged course. Chills are a constant feature of the disease and may total as many as 100; the initial chill is likely to be very severe, lasting 30 or 40 minutes; the interval between chills may be only a few hours but is sometimes as long as three days, the patient being almost afebrile in the interim. The temperature swings are often tremendous with steep climbs from 96.0° F. to 105.0° F., followed by a precipitous fall within an hour. Although the onset is ordinarily in the second week, a survey of the temperature chart will almost always show that the condition has been preceded by a low-grade fever of endometritis type. Between the episodes of chills and high fever, the patient may look and feel quite well. Pelvic examination profits little, as a rule, since the vein most commonly affected, the ovarian, is too high to reach. (Our records show many instances in which experienced examiners *thought* they felt the thrombosed vein, only to find at autopsy that the thrombosed vessel was on the opposite side or in some entirely different location). Although leukocytosis is sometimes present, it is our experience that the majority of these patients show white counts under 10,000 cells per cubic millimeter. Bacteria are unquestionably present in the blood stream during the chills, but positive blood cultures are notoriously difficult to obtain; the optimum time to take the blood is early in the chill or, better yet if one is lucky, just before the chill begins. The offending organism is usually the anaerobic streptococcus.

Metastatic pulmonary complications are exceedingly common, particularly lung abscesses, pleurisy, and pneumonia. The next most common site for metastasis is the left kidney—heralded, as a rule, by sudden renal pain followed by albuminuria and hematuria. The joints, eyes, and subcutaneous tissues may also be affected by mycotic emboli. As these metastatic infections become established, the temperature curve assumes a more steady character.

The typical case of pelvic thrombophlebitis lasts between one and three months, the outcome being fatal in about half the cases (but see section on prognosis). The common cause of death is some metastatic pulmonary condition, usually pneumonia. Some patients, however, succumb to the inanition and exhaustion consequent upon the prolonged course of chills and fever.

Femoral Thrombophlebitis. About the tenth day, but sometimes as late as the twentieth, the puerpera shows a rather abrupt rise of temperature to 102° F. or 103° F. and complains of pain in one of her legs, usually the left. The leg is kept slightly flexed and rotated outwards and can be moved only with difficulty. Even in the early stages, the affected leg is hotter than the other, differences of 1° F. to 3° F. having been reported. This persists throughout and may be a valuable diagnostic sign. Palpation reveals tenderness along the course of one of the leg veins, and the vein itself may be traced as a firm, tender cord in the upper part of the thigh. Edema is variable; it sometimes precedes the pain, sometimes follows; it may be almost imperceptible, or may be so great as to produce a huge swelling of the leg. Edema may be first recognized, as a rule, in the upper part of the thigh but more commonly commences in the toe and ankle and extends from below upward.

The general condition of the patient remains good. An initial chill may or may not occur, but subsequent rigors are rare. The temperature is moderately elevated for seven to 10 days, gradually returning to normal. The edema is slow to disappear and may persist for many weeks, or even months. Indeed, long after the attack the leg may show a tendency to swell prior to menstruation and after exposure to cold. Bilateral thrombophlebitis occurs in about one fifth of the cases, but the two legs are rarely involved simultaneously; generally the process starts in the second leg about the time it is subsiding in the first.

Peritonitis. Puerperal peritonitis resembles surgical peritonitis in general, except for the fact that abdominal rigidity is slight or absent altogether—presumably as the result of the flaccid state of the abdominal musculature postpartum. In peritonitis of the general variety the symptoms seldom appear later than the third day. There is a definite chill, a temperature from 103° F. to 105° F. or over without marked remissions, and a pulse of 140 or more which soon becomes weak and compressible. Not only does pressure on the abdomen cause exquisite pain, but sudden release of the pressure produces even severer pain—so called *rebound tenderness*. Pain is quite constant and often of an excruciating character; tympanites is uniformly present and frequently associated with a paralytic ileus, although intractable and exhausting diarrhea may occur. Vomiting is frequent, eventually stercoraceous in character, and often projectile in type. The other classical symptoms of general peritonitis are also present, such as hiccough, sleeplessness, restlessness, the pinched Hippocratic facies, glassy eyes, and a furred tongue. Bacteremia is invariable and consequent lung involvement frequent. Delirium and coma usually precede death. Sometimes, shortly before exitus, the temperature drops from 105° F. or over to below normal, crossing on the chart the rapidly mounting pulse line and thereby forming the so-called "cross of death." Now and then grave symptoms may be entirely absent; the patient seems in a state of euphoria and only from the expression of the facies and the rapid and thready pulse may the true gravity of the situation be deduced. On rare occasions in the course of a pelvic cellulitis, an abscess may rupture into the peritoneal cavity and produce general peritonitis with a cataclysmic picture.

Pelvic Cellulitis. As has been said, minor degrees of pelvic cellulitis (parametritis) are the most common cause of prolonged, sustained fever in the puerperium, and whenever steady temperature elevations persist for longer than a week the condition should be suspected. In mild cases the findings are limited to moderate but persistent, temperature elevations in association with more or less local tenderness. The invasion of the parametrial tissue may be marked with a chill, but more often it is difficult to determine precisely when the extension occurred, the course seeming to represent merely the continuation of the original endometrial infection. The height of the temperature varies with the degree of cellulitic involvement, but in the average case runs in the neighborhood of 102° F. with moderate morning remissions. There is pain or tenderness in one or both sides of the abdomen and marked tenderness on vaginal examination. As the process advances, other findings on vaginal examination become more characteristic: fixation of the uterus by the parametrial exudate, thickening in one or the other fornix, and the development of a hard, unyielding mass in the broad ligament. The exudate may extend upward and an area of resistance may be felt along the upper border of Poupart's ligament. Not infrequently it extends backwards into the lower part of the broad ligament along the sacro-uterine folds and into the cellular tissue surrounding the uterus. In these cases a rectal examination is very helpful.

Absorption of the exudate occurs in about two thirds of the cases but may require months; in this process the swelling often becomes of stone hardness, gradually diminishing in size from week to week. Not infrequently the end result is dense scar tissue in the parametrium which pulls the uterus to one or the other side and causes other gynecologic difficulties. Suppuration of the parametrial mass occurs in the remaining third of the cases and is also a slow process. Indeed, pointing of the abscess may not occur until six or eight weeks after the commencement of the illness. Suppuration may be suspected under the following circumstances: a change in the temperature curve to the constant type, often in association with chills; spontaneous, intense pain; leukocytosis in excess of 20,000 cells per cubic millimeter; and general deterioration of the patient with rapid loss of weight and a characteristic sallow complexion. As the abscess points above Poupart's ligament, the skin becomes red and edematous. After the abscess has been opened recovery is usually prompt.

Salpingitis. Initial attacks of gonorrheal salpingitis during the puerperium are probably less common than was formerly believed (page 938), but they are seen from time to time, particularly after abortion. Most instances of puerperal salpingitis represent exacerbations of old processes which have been lighted up by changes incident to labor and the puerperium. The onset occurs late, ordinarily between the ninth and fifteenth days and is characterized by pain and tenderness in the lower abdomen, usually bilateral, together with fever in the neighborhood of 103.0° F. or 104.0° F. Rebound tenderness is likely to be present as the result of some degree of pelvic peritonitis. Chills are uncommon. Joint involvement—a knee or a wrist—clinches the diagnosis, but this is seen only in a minority of the cases.

The life of the patient is rarely jeopardized, the acute symptoms subsiding within a week or two as a rule. Residual changes in the tubes frequently leave the patient a gynecologic invalid and, depending on the intensity of the inflammation, sterility may ensue as the result of tubal closure—the so-called "one-child sterility." But, as pointed out by Curtis, one-child sterility is much more frequently the result of gonorrhea contracted subsequent to the obstetrical episode than to gonorrheal salpingitis developing in the puerperium.

Welch Bacillus Infections. The classical picture of puerperal infection due to the Welch bacillus is catastrophic and resembles somewhat that of acute yellow atrophy of the liver. Within two or three days after delivery, most frequently postabortal, the patient develops jaundice which becomes most marked on the face and body, least marked on the legs. This develops rapidly and is soon accompanied by slightly dusky cyanosis of the fingers and toes. Within a few hours the skin may become darkened to a bronze or mahogany and the conjunctiva be of the shade of chocolate. The temperature is not exceedingly high, averaging between 101.0° F. and 102.0° F., and it may be normal or even subnormal. The pulse, however, is rapid, 140 or above. The patient sinks into a state of extreme prostration and within a day or two, the cyanosis deepens, circulatory collapse ensues, and the respirations become rapid and shallow; consciousness, however, is usually clear to the last. Catheterization yields but an ounce or two of strongly acid, port wine colored urine containing hemoglobin and fragments of destroyed red cells. Anemia often progresses with unbelievable rapidity, Frankel and Lehman having noted a red-cell fall of over two million within six hours. Leukocytosis is regularly present and is often extreme. Renal failure is a well-nigh constant finding with a rise of the nonprotein nitrogen of the blood to high levels. Although the presence of gas bubbles in the tissues or uterus, as shown by crepitus or tympani uteri, has long been regarded as an important diagnostic sign, this is demonstrable ante mortem in one fourth or one fifth of the cases only. Not infrequently the gas manifests itself by excruciating skeletal-muscle pain before crepitus can be elicited; when this is widespread ("metastatic gas gangrene") the course is extremely rapid and death may ensue within 10 hours after the onset of the muscle pain. Before modern chemotherapeutic agents were available, the severer forms of puerperal Welch bacillus infection were almost uniformly fatal within five or six days; even the "milder" types used to carry a mortality of some 20 per cent.

DIAGNOSIS

The vast majority of fevers occurring after childbirth are due to puerperal infection, and this diagnosis should be assigned to all puerperal elevations of temperature unless incontrovertible proof can be adduced that the fever is due to an extragenital focus. The diagnosis of puerperal infection can often be made without difficulty. This is especially true if the signs and symptoms cited are present and if the preceding labor has been attended by extensive vaginal or uterine manipulation; in mild cases, however, fever may be the only sign. In any event, every puerpera whose temperature rises to 100.4° F. should be given a complete physical examination in order to rule out extrapelvic causes of fever and to establish the diagnosis definitely by the process of exclusion.

The most common extragenital causes of fever in the puerperium are: respiratory infections (la grippe, tonsillitis, pneumonia), pyelitis, mastitis, and pulmonary tuberculosis. In modern practice, typhoid fever and malaria are less common offenders. Among this list, pyelitis offers the most difficult problem in differential diagnosis and occasionally it may be almost impossible to rule it out. In the typical case, of course, the cloudy urine loaded with clumped pus cells, the colon bacilluria, the costovertebral-angle tenderness, and the spiking temperature point clearly to pyelitis. However, varying degrees of this clinical picture are seen; a moderate number of clumped pus cells may be found in the catheterized urine of even normal puerpera, while the same is true of colon bacilluria; moreover, chills and fever are common to puerperal infection and pyelitis alike. Because of these facts, we believe that the diagnosis of pyelitis in the puerperium should be made with great caution and should be limited to cases in which there are 50 clumped pus cells per high-power field in addition to the usual clinical syndrome, that is, spiking fever and costovertebral-angle tenderness. Despite authoritative opinion to the contrary, it is our belief that mammary engorgement may occasionally give rise, in association with breast symptoms, to a single, brief, temperature spike at any time during the first 10 days; the picture is characteristic in that it never lasts longer than 24 hours, the temperature readings on the days preceding and following being absolutely normal. The temperature curve of true mastitis is usually sustained and associated with mammary signs and symptoms which become clear-cut within 24 hours.

During the first 10 days of puerperal infection, digital examination of the vagina yields little information of value and may do harm by breaking up healed abrasions and opening up new avenues of infection. However, it is our firm conviction, based on many years of experience, that the gentle introduction of a small tube into the uterine cavity for the purpose of bacteriological diagnosis is of great value. This procedure is even more important today than it was some years ago because the intelligent and effective use of modern therapeutic agents demands accurate knowledge of the offending bacteria. It should be carried out in every case in which, between the second and sixth days inclusive, a temperature of 100.4° or above is maintained for 24 hours. Such cultures are of little value following the sixth day because after that period a variety of organisms, of vaginal origin, are normally present in the uterus.

Equipment. The instrument used in obtaining material from the uterine cavity consists of: (1) a stainless-steel or chrome-plated tube 12 inches in length with a ¼-inch bore, curved on one end; (2) a sharp steel stylet which projects very slightly beyond the end of the metal tube when inserted; (3) a steel wire with a small loop on one end which will project ¼ inch beyond the end of the tubing and through the loop of which a small piece of cloth (*i.e.,* cord tie) may be tied. These are sterilized by autoclaving along with a gauze sponge on a clamp and several 6-inch pieces of braided silk cord.

As will be described, rubber finger cots are used to protect the tip of the metal tube from cervical contamination while being inserted into the uterus. These finger cots are unrolled

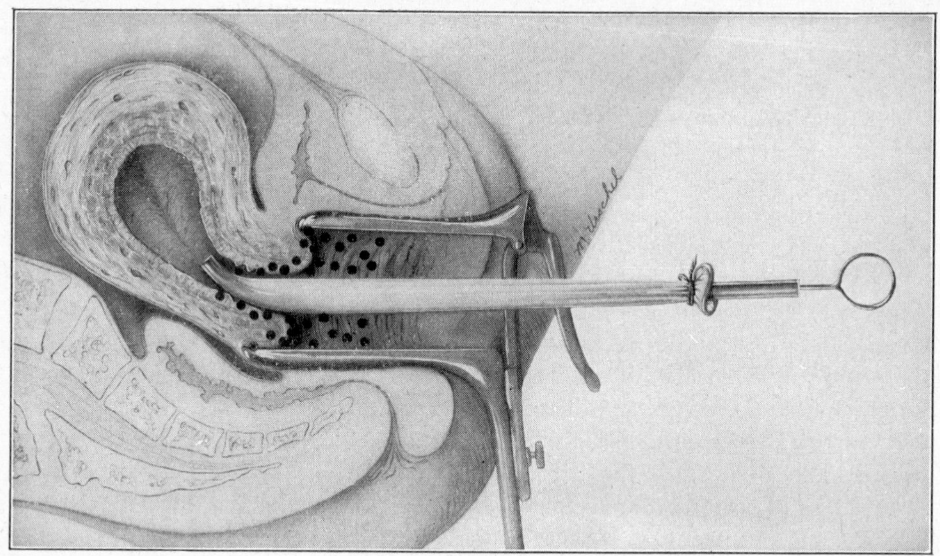

FIG. 512.—TECHNIC OF UTERINE CULTURE.

Diagrammatic cross section showing culture tube through cervix beyond the internal os. Finger cot has been drawn taut and the stylet partially inserted preparatory to perforating the stretched rubber protecting the end of the metal tube. Vaginal and cervical flora indicated by dots (Guilbeau and Schaub).

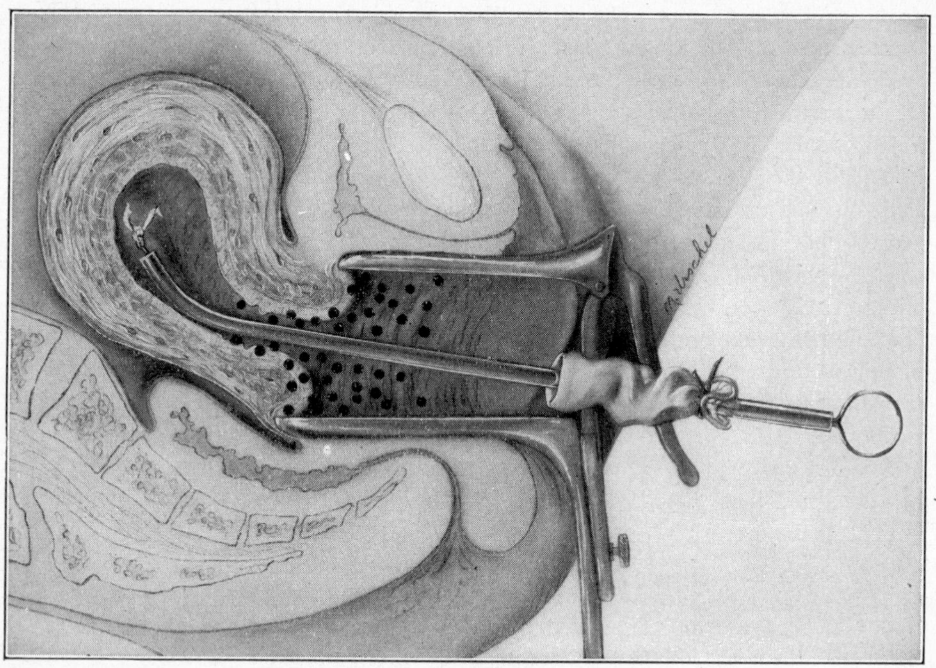

FIG. 513.—TECHNIC OF UTERINE CULTURE.

Diagrammatic cross section revealing stiff wire loop in place following perforation and retraction of the finger cot which is shown retracted into the vagina. Contamination with vaginal and cervical flora is thus avoided and a culture representing true uterine flora is obtained. Vaginal and cervical flora indicated by dots (Guilbeau and Schaub).

and sterilized by soaking in an aqueous 1:1,000 zephiran chloride solution for 48 hours. They are dried immediately before using. Repeated tests have shown finger cots treated in this manner to be sterile, and it has been demonstrated that no disinfectant is carried over into the culture medium to inhibit the growth of any organisms which may be present. Heat sterilization and other chemical methods were found to give incomplete sterilization, or to affect the elasticity of the rubber.

Other equipment used in taking the uterine cultures includes sterile gloves, a sterile bivalve speculum, and tubes of thioglycollate medium for inoculation.

Procedure. The patient is placed in dorsal lithotomy position and draped in the conventional manner. A sterile bivalve speculum is introduced into the vagina and the cervix is visualized. Blood clots and/or products of conception are gently removed from the cervix with a sterile sponge. Sterile gloves are then donned and a sterile, dry, finger cot is drawn taut over the tubing and tied in place. The tube is then inserted through the cervical canal and past the internal os for a centimeter or so in order to be past the bacterial flora of the vaginal and cervical canals (Fig. 512). The sharp stylet is then introduced into the tube and the rubber closing the tip of the tube is pierced. The taut rubber retracts instantaneously on the tubing, leaving a sterile end, uncontaminated by vaginal or cervical flora. The stylet is removed and the wire loop containing the wick is introduced through the tube. The tube is then advanced several centimeters more into the uterus and the wire loop is twisted from side to side in the uterine cavity in order to collect sufficient material on the wick (Fig. 513). The wire loop is then withdrawn, leaving the tubing still in place, and the material collected on the wick is implanted in thioglycollate medium. Finally the tube is removed. Definite evidence that sufficient material for culture is obtained is revealed by a serosanguineous, soaked wick which frequently has blood clots adhering to it.

Using this procedure, we have caused no apparent morbidity from carrying bacteria into the uterine cavity, and have seen no endometritis or injury resulting from the technic.

Blood cultures should be taken in all cases in which the temperature reaches 103° F. In pelvic thrombophlebitis and, indeed, in all anaerobic streptococcal infections, positive blood cultures are notoriously difficult to obtain and repeated attempts are usually necessary. In thrombophlebitis, the optimum time to take the blood is at the very beginning of the chill, or, if one could have clairvoyant foresight, 15 minutes or so beforehand.

PROGNOSIS

The most dependable prognostic guide in puerperal infection is the pulse rate. As long as it remains under 100, the outlook is excellent, whereas rates of 130 and more—especially those which do not fall as the temperature recedes—carry an ominous prognosis. Almost as important is the time and fulminance of the onset. Cases characterized by a sharp rise of temperature to 103.0° F. or more during the first 48 hours after delivery are usually grave infections, while a later, more gradual onset suggests a more benign process. Sustained high fever carries a worse prognosis than does the remitting type. By and large, chills are a bad sign, particularly if repeated, since they invariably mean extension of the infection; insomnia is likewise unfavorable. Icterus is invariably a grave omen.

The laboratory may afford prognostic help in three ways: the hemoglobin level, the blood culture, and the leukocyte count. Since the more virulent bacteria are usually hemolytic, the graver infections are often associated with low hemoglobin concentrations, sometimes in spite of blood transfusions; low hemoglobin levels, moreover, mean lessened resistance and often reflect the blood loss and trauma sustained at delivery. If positive, the blood culture is of serious import, but if negative, little conclusion can be drawn since the organism may have been missed. Repeatedly negative blood cultures in the presence of an infection which is obviously severe usually mean that the anaerobic streptococcus is the offender. Very low leukcocyte counts (under 8,000 per cubic millimeter) and extremely high ones (over 30,000 per cubic millimeter) are unfavorable signs; the former suggests low resistance and the latter a virulent infection; counts between these figures are of little significance since they may or may not be due to the normal leukocytosis of the puerperium. Differential study of the leukocytes, such as the Arneth count, has proved disappointing.

Of the several clinical types of puerperal infection, general peritonitis is the most grave and prior to the days of modern chemotherapy was almost uniformly fatal. Pelvic thrombophlebitis with pyemia also carries a serious prognosis. The final outcome is determined in large measure by the nature and extent of the metastases; as long as they are absent the outlook is moderately good, but with the development of lung abscesses and pneumonia it becomes correspondingly bad. The outcome of femoral thrombophlebitis is almost always favorable, but pulmonary emboli have been known to cause sudden death when the patient first gets up. Although pelvic cellulitis often entails a prolonged febrile course of several months, the great majority of the patients survive. Occasionally, however, the development of multiple abscess pockets at inaccessible sites causes death as the result of the prolonged febrile course, constant pain, inanition, and exhaustion. We have seen two cases in which such abscesses ruptured into the peritoneal cavity with rapid exitus, but we have reason to believe that this accident is rather rare. Gonococcal salpingitis in the puerperium almost invariably runs a benign course, insofar as life is concerned. The local infections, such as endometritis and lesions of the cervix, vagina, vulva and perineum, are serious only because they are potential foci from which extension may occur; per se they never cause death.

PREVENTION

During Pregnancy. Since anemia predisposes to puerperal infection, blood studies should be carried out on every pregnant woman and low hemoglobin levels combatted by the administration of iron. Although the evidence that specific vitamin deficiencies predispose to puerperal infection may not be altogether convincing, the general nutritional status of the patient is unquestionably an important factor and the necessity of a well-balanced, vitamin-rich diet should be emphasized to every expectant mother. Sexual intercourse shortly before the onset of labor has precipitated some of the most fulminating infections on record, and, since one can never be sure precisely when labor will begin, coitus should be strictly forbidden during the last two months of pregnancy. Vaginal douches at this time are likewise dangerous. In regard to tub baths, it is best to omit them during this same period for two reasons: in the first place, especially in multiparae with relaxed pelvic floors, the contaminated bath water may ascend the vagina and thus introduce extraneous bacteria to the birth canal; the second objection (which has nothing to do with puerperal infection) is that the patient may slip and be injured, her equilibrium being naturally impaired at this period. In most clinics it is customary to give ward patients a bath at the onset of labor. This is best done by placing her on a slab or very shallow bath tub;

the nurse then washes her with a gentle, warm spray in such a manner that the external genitals are never submerged in water.

During Labor. The three main principles to follow are: first, limit to a minimum the number of bacteria introduced into the birth canal; second, limit to a minimum the wounds inflicted; and third, save blood.

The first of these principles demands, of course, rigid aseptic technic, but it demands, in addition, that the birth canal be regarded as forbidden territory whose invasion by finger or instrument should be undertaken only on strict indication. Every introduction of the finger into the vagina during labor is attended by some risk of conveying infection, for, as we have seen, even though the gloved hand be bacteriologically sterile, it may readily carry pathogenic bacteria from the lower to the upper reaches of the vagina. Insofar as is possible, therefore, labor should be conducted by abdominal and rectal examinations only, and in 19 cases out of 20 these methods will yield all the information necessary. (This teaching should not be pushed too far, however; if there is reason to believe that labor is not proceeding normally and that rectal examinations are not revealing the true state of affairs, a careful, sterile vaginal examination may be essential.) For half a century and more, efforts have been made to reduce the bacterial content of the vagina by means of vaginal instillations and douches. The most noteworthy among recent advocates of this practice are Mayes, who employs prophylactic instillations of 4 per cent mercurochrome during labor, and T. K. Brown who uses a 1 per cent solution of acriflavine in glycerine. Although the results reported by these authors would seem gratifying, the same procedures in other hands have not yielded the results which were hoped for. Opponents of vaginal instillations believe that such instillations not only fail to reach bacteria buried between vaginal rugae but may be actually dangerous, through irritating the vaginal mucosa and through diluting and removing the natural protective properties of the vaginal secretions. In our own clinic, a three-year trial of Dettol, a British antiseptic recommended by Colebrook as a vaginal instillation in labor, has had no effect on puerperal morbidity. In summation, it is our opinion that vaginal instillations are not essential to the routine conduct of labor and had best be avoided, at least until more convincing evidence of their value becomes available. Perineal pads should not be worn during labor since they slip around so much that they serve only to carry bacteria from the thighs, buttocks, and rectum to the vaginal orifice.

Since the nasopharynx of attendants is the most common source from which extraneous bacteria are brought to the birth canal, the wearing of masks by obstetrician and nurses is imperative; this rule should apply not only to the period of actual delivery but to any other occasion when the external genitalia are exposed (as when rectal or vaginal examinations are done). The mask must cover the nose as well as the mouth. If an attendant has an actual upper respiratory infection, masking is of little avail and such persons should be watched for vigilantly and excluded from the delivery suite.

Every wound of the birth canal represents a portal of entry for infection, means additional blood loss, and predisposes to shock. This triad of trauma, hemorrhage, and shock provides the setting par excellence for puerperal infection, and it goes without saying that the wounds inflicted must be kept at a minimum if infection is to be avoided. This means the avoidance of unnecessary operations, the utmost gentleness in indicated procedures, the immediate repair of all wounds, and the conduct of the third stage in such a manner as to conserve blood. If, despite these precautions, hemorrhage is excessive, the blood should be replaced within 24 hours after delivery. In our own clinic the following general rule is followed: every postpartum hemorrhage of 1,000 cc. or more demands blood transfusion, the amount given to be never less than one half the estimated blood loss (it is usually more); in small women weighing under 130 pounds an 800 cc. loss is usually an indication for transfusion, while if pre-existing anemia is present even smaller hemorrhages may call for replacement of blood.

During the Puerperium. The birth canal remains a wounded surface for many days after delivery, but this is well protected against extraneous bacterial invasion by the closed vulva, *provided* meddling fingers do not open this barrier. The fingers may be those of the patient herself and she should be warned accordingly. They are more often those of a nurse who, over-zealous in the toilet of the perineum, separates the vulva and permits contaminated wash water to enter the vagina. It must be emphasized that the aim of routine perineal care in the puerperium is not antisepsis but comfort and cleanliness. Accordingly, elaborate and "thorough" methods are unnecessary and may even do harm. As a rule the simplest procedure is the best, with the reservation that the nurse who carries out the perineal toilet follows an aseptic technic and wears a mask at the time. The perineal pads must be sterile and should be changed frequently—at least every four hours during the first week and thereafter every eight hours. Preferably, bed pans should be cleansed and sterilized after each use. If this is not feasible, each patient should have a labelled, individual bed pan throughout, this bed pan to be sterilized once a day and cleansed and scalded after each use. Douches should never be given in the first 10 days, but thereafter low-pressure douches are usually permissible for purposes of cleanliness; it is important that the douche bag be hung at a low level, not more than 18 inches above the introitus.

Every infected patient should be isolated and all precautions taken (in the way of gowns and hand disinfection) to make sure that organisms are not carried to other patients. This requires careful study and everlasting vigilance.

TREATMENT

The advent of the sulfonamides and penicillin has so revolutionized the treatment as well as the prognosis of puerperal infection that the attitude is likely to develop that these drugs constitute the sum total of therapy in these conditions. Actually, these agents, while effective in most cases of puerperal infection, are not invariably so, and it is prudent in every case to supplement these drugs with all those measures which proved efficacious prior to the present era. In other words, cases of puerperal infection are best treated by a number of well-established supportive measures to which one of the sulfonamides and penicillin may well be added.

Except for the colon bacillus, penicillin is effective against most organisms responsible for puerperal infection. Its efficacy against the hemolytic streptococcus, the Welch bacillus, and staphylococci are well known. Most strains of the anaerobic streptococcus are also vulnerable to penicillin, as has been shown convincingly in a recent study carried out in our clinic by Guilbeau, Schaub, and Andrews. Uterine cultures were taken from 86 postpartum patients, 54 of whom received varying amounts of penicillin, and 32 of whom received no antibiotic therapy. From 30 of the 32 cultures in the control series from untreated patients, various bacteria were isolated; most were anaerobic streptococci and bacteroides. Of the uteri of 54 patients who had received varying amounts of penicillin during and after labor, 32 were sterile, aerobically and anaerobically, and eight showed only pleuropneumonia-like organisms which are not pathogenic. Only 14 cultures in the penicillin series showed significant bacteria, four of which were penicillin resistant coliform organisms. All but one of the penicillin-sensitive organisms occurred in cultures taken more than 48 hours after delivery, from patients receiving small amounts of penicillin. In actual cases of puerperal infection, including endometritis, pelvic cellulitis, and perineal infections, Harris and Shook, as well as many other authors, have found penicillin highly effective, if begun early in the disease process. By the prophylactic administration of penicillin Keetel, Scott, and Plass have been able to reduce greatly their puerperal morbidity, and their results suggest that penicillin may be given profitably to any woman with intrapartum fever, prolonged labor, postpartum hemorrhage, or difficult operative delivery. Patients with desperate postabortal infections who have been admitted to our clinic in a condition which, a decade ago, would certainly have eventuated fatally, have in most instances responded dramatically to penicillin and sulfadiazine.

Since penicillin is not efficacious against the colon bacillus, and since it is less effectual against other commonly encountered organisms than are the sulfonamides, penicillin is always combined with one of the sulfonamides—preferably sulfadiazine at the present writing—in order to afford full coverage for all organisms which may be present. The dosage of penicillin employed will depend upon the severity of the case. In obviously severe infections, the dosage should not be less than one million units a day, while in milder infections an initial dose of 200,000 units followed by 50,000 units every four hours is usually adequate. The dosage of sulfadiazine is 3 to 4 gm. daily in divided doses combined with an equal amount of sodium bicarbonate. In the rare instances in which the combination of these two drugs does not prove efficacious, streptomycin will often prove helpful. At the present writing it would appear that aureomycin may also have an important place in the treatment of puerperal infection.

Lesions of the Perineum, Vulva, and Vagina. These infected, external wounds should be treated in the same manner as any infected surgical wound, that is, by establishing drainage. All stitches must be removed and the wound surface laid open. Reluctance to do this may lead not only to infection of the cellular tissue about the cervix and vagina but to a worse anatomical result than removal of the stitches would have caused. Daubing the wound surfaces with 3 per cent hydrogen peroxide, followed by gentle external flushings with a mild antiseptic solution, will aid in keeping the wound clean, but vaginal douches are obviously contraindicated. Relief of pain can be afforded either by warm compresses of 20 per cent magnesium sulfate, or by exposure of the perineum to a sun lamp for periods of half an hour two or three times a day.

Endometritis. Cases which are obviously mild (temperature under 101.0° F., pulse under 100, no chills) are best handled by simple measures. In this group it is unnecessary to take the baby off the breast. Isolation, however, is desirable in order to protect other patients and give the mother more opportunity for rest. She is placed in the Fowler position to facilitate lochial drainage; given Ergonovine, 0.2 mg. four times daily for two days to promote uterine tone; and fluids forced to 4,000 cc. or more daily. It is customary to place an ice bag over the lower abdomen, but this measure is of questionable value. As stated previously, we feel that, even in these mild cases, an intra-uterine culture should be taken, for one can never forecast with absolute certainty what the next day or two may bring, and, if the patient should become worse, knowledge of the organism involved is of the utmost help in directing therapy. Following this procedure, moreover, the temperature occasionally returns to normal, suggesting that, in certain of these cases, drainage is at fault. Penicillin and one of the sulfonamides should be given if the temperature exceeds 101.0° F.

In severer cases, isolation is imperative. Breast feeding is discontinued, not only because it exhausts the mother but also because it is usually futile in the presence of high fever. In addition to carrying out the measures described in the preceding paragraph, penicillin and one of the sulfonamides should be given and the desirability of blood transfusions considered. If the hemoglobin concentration is below 75 per cent a transfusion is indicated, preferably two small ones of 300 cc. each, on successive days.

Pelvic Thrombophlebitis. Since thrombophlebitis is usually due to the anaerobic streptococcus, it is rarely affected by the sulfonamides but may be by penicillin. A most salutory remedy in this condition is repeated small blood transfusions, 250 cc. every other day, as long as chills and fever persist. In some cases as many as 20 or 30 transfusions may be necessary. Nursing care is highly important since the prolonged course predisposes to bed sores.

Femoral Thrombophlebitis. In addition to the usual routine, the leg is elevated on a pillow, or better, on a cushioned, inclined trough and pressure of the bed clothing relieved by a cradle over the leg. Massage is contraindicated because of the danger of a pulmonary embolism. The patient must be kept in bed until she has been afebrile for a week. Again, nursing care is of prime importance. In severe cases in which there is substantial pain, continuous caudal anesthesia will relieve vasospasm, and thereby stop the pain. In many cases, moreover, it exerts a beneficial effect on the progress of the condition.

Ochsner and his associates have emphasized the two main forms of intravascular thrombosis, one due to bacterial, chemical, or traumatic injury to the vascular endothelium (thrombophlebitis) and the other brought about by venous stasis or alterations in the blood constituents leading to an increase of the clotting tendency (phlebothrombosis). In thrombophlebitis the clot is more firmly attached to the vessel wall than in phlebothrombosis, while the latter is more insidious in its development. Thrombophlebitis is invariably accompanied by fever, pain, and swelling of the involved part, while phlebothrombosis elicits minimal symptoms and signs, these usually being anxiety, restlessness, increased pulse rate, and, sometimes, slight tenderness over the involved vein. This latter condition, because of its insidious onset, too often is not recognized until the development of a pulmonary infarction. Phlebography, the visualization of the veins, may prove to be of great value in the early diagnosis of phlebothrombosis. While the treatment of the thrombophlebitis, as stated above, generally consists of conservative measures, that of phlebothrombosis, according to most authorities, should be more radical, such as proximal ligation of the involved vein or thrombectomy. Anticoagulants, such as heparin and dicumarol, may be of use in the prevention of further thrombi, although having no effect upon the already-formed thrombus in both forms. Sympathetic block, either by paravertebral injections as advocated by Ochsner or by the introduction of anesthetic agents into the epidural space in the sacral canal as used by Hingson, may be of great value in the alleviation of the symptoms and signs of thrombophlebitis.

General Peritonitis. Since the common cause of general peritonitis in the puerperium is the beta hemolytic streptococcus, massive doses of penicillin together with sulfadiazine should be started at the first sign of this complication. Time is all important and every effort should be made to attain a therapeutic tissue-concentration as soon as possible; since withdrawal of food and fluids by mouth is part of the treatment, the therapeutic agents must be given subcutaneously or intravenously. Fluids to the extent of 4 to 5 liters daily are introduced in the same manner. As a rule, half of this amount can be given intravenously in the form of 5 per cent glucose in normal saline, employing three intravenous infusions of 750 cc. each; the remainder can be administered as subcutaneous infusions of normal saline or 2.5 per cent glucose in normal saline. Instillation of fluid per rectum is not advisable because of the likelihood of stimulating peristalsis. The stomach should be kept empty by lavage, the small nasal tube of Levin being very useful for this purpose. An additional procedure of great value is the Wangensteen constant-suction apparatus, which can be attached to the nasal tube. With this in operation, the patient can drink water as desired and quench her thirst, which is often intolerable; the water, of course, is removed at once by the tube. The Miller-Abbott tube is also an effectual means of combating distention. Efforts to combat distention by the use of drugs (pituitrin, prostigmine, and physostigmine) are dangerous as well as futile, and steps in this direction should be limited to small saline enemas. Morphine is given liberally, not only to control pain and restlessness but to diminish peristalsis. Nourishment by mouth should be withheld until flatus is being passed spontaneously by rectum.

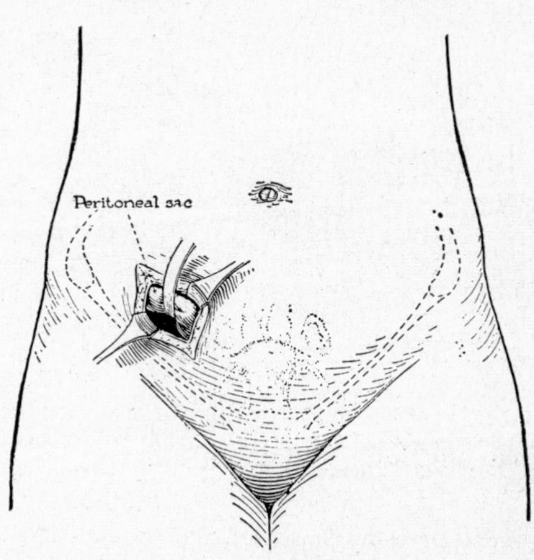

Fig. 514.—Technic for Opening Localized Collections of Pus Pointing above the Inguinal Ligament.

(After Cullen, *Surg., Gynec. & Obst.*, 1917, 35:134.)

Pelvic Cellulitis. In addition to the usual supportive measures, including blood transfusions for anemia, penicillin and one of the sulfonamides should be used. The physician should follow a program of patient, watchful expectancy, being on the alert for signs of beginning suppuration. This is suggested by spontaneous, severe pain, continuous temperature, and high leukocytosis, but the actual diagnosis of an abscess must rest upon the presence of fluctuation. Very often the mass is so tender that brief anesthesia (nitrous oxide or sodium pentothal) is necessary to elicit this sign.

In the majority of cases, abscesses of this type are best opened by an incision just above and parallel to Poupart's ligament, but occasionally a bulging, fluctuant mass in the posterior cul-de-sac will indicate the desirability of that approach. In the latter instance the incision should be made in the midline, to avoid possible injury to a ureter or large blood vessel. After the pus collection has been reached by cautious, blunt-scissor dissection, drainage is established by cigarette drains. If pus is not reached, a drain should, nevertheless, be left in contact with the mass and, as a rule, the resultant pressure necrosis results in spontaneous rupture of the abscess at this point.

Procedures to Avoid. Although countless local therapeutic measures have been recommended—such as intra-uterine douches, swabbing of the endometrium with antiseptic solutions, continuous irrigation of the uterine cavity, instillations of glycerin, drainage with rubber tubes, and curettage—these have all been abandoned since experience has shown them to be dangerous as well as futile. In the main, they tend to disseminate rather than halt the infectious process. Nor does surgery merit a place in the treatment of puerperal infection, save for the opening and drainage of abscesses. Hysterectomy serves only to spread infection and promote shock; it has killed many women who would otherwise have survived and has saved scarcely any. Almost the same statement is applicable to incision and drainage of the abdomen in cases of general peritonitis; such rapid encapsulation of the drainage tube occurs that the real purpose of the operation is defeated. Attempts to ligate the involved veins in thrombophlebitis have likewise met with failure, the mortality in the operated cases being higher than in those left alone.

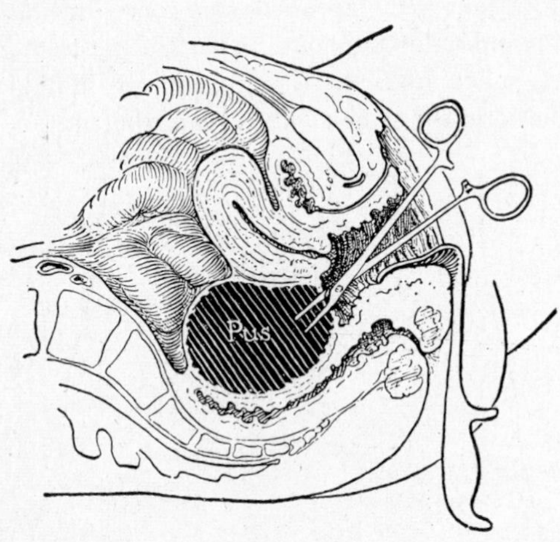

Fig. 515.—Technic for Opening Collection of Localized Pus in the Cul-de-sac of Douglas (Posterior Colpotomy).

BIBLIOGRAPHY

Armstrong, R. R., and Burt-White, H. The Problem of Puerperal Sepsis; The Bacteriology of the Puerperium, Brit. M. J., 1929, 1:592.

Bickerstaff, H. J. The Relationship between Late Prenatal Hemoglobin Levels and Febrile Puerperal Morbidity. Am. J. Obst. & Gynec., 1942, 43:997.

Bigger, J. W., and Fitzgibbons, G. An Investigation into the Aetiology of Puerperal Sepsis. J. Obst. & Gynaec. Brit. Emp., 1925, 32:318.

Bingold. Die Bedeutung anaërober Bakterien als Infektions-erreger septischer internen Erkrankungen. Virchow's Arch. f. path. Anat., 1921, 234:332.

Blumer, G. A Case of Mixed Puerperal and Typhoid Infection, in Which the Streptococcus and Typhoid Bacillus Were Isolated Both from the Blood and Uterine Cavity. Am. J. Obst., 1899, 39:42.

Bondy, O. Ueber puerperale Infektion durch anaerobe Streptokokken. Monatschr. f. Geburtsh. u. Gynaek., 1911, 34:536.

——— Die Bedeutung der Pneumokokken für die puerperale Infektion. Ztschr. f. Geburtsh. u. Gynäk., 1912, 72:631-644.

Brown, T. K. The Incidence of Puerperal Infection Due to Anaerobic Streptococci. Am. J. Obst. & Gynec., 1930, 20:300.

——— Bacteriology of the Uterus at Cesarean Section. Am. J. Obst. & Gynec., 1939, 38:969.

Butler, H. M. The Bacteriological Diagnosis of Severe Clostridium Welchii Infection following Abortion. Med. J. Australia, 1941, 1:33.

——— Further Bacteriologic Studies of Severe Clostridium Welchii Infections following Abortion. J. Obst. & Gynaec. Brit. Emp., 1943, 50:105.

BYSSHE, S. M. The Significance of Clostridium Welchii in the Genital Tract of Pregnant and Puerperal Women. Am. J. Obst. & Gynec., 1938, 35:995.

COLEBROOK, L. Prevention of Puerperal Sepsis. J. Obst. & Gynaec. Brit. Emp., 1936, 43:691.

——— and HARE, Ronald. The Anaerobic Streptococci Associated with Puerperal Fever. J. Obst. & Gynaec. Brit. Empire, 1933, 40:609.

COLEBROOK, L., and PURDIE, A. W. Treatment of 106 Cases of Puerperal Fever by Sulphanilamide (Streptocide). Lancet, 1937, 2:1237, 1291.

COLEBROOK, L., MAXTED, W. R., and JOHNS, A. M. The Presence of Hemolytic and Other Streptococci on the Human Skin. J. Path. & Bact., 1935, 41:521.

DOUGLAS, R. G. Bacteriologic Findings in the Uterus during Labor and the Early Puerperium. Am. J. Obst. & Gynec., 1934, 27:203.

——— and RHEES, H. S. Experimental Evaluation of the Use of Some Vaginal Antiseptics during Labor. A Preliminary Report. N. Y. State J. Med., 1934, 34: No. 23.

ELLIS, G. J., and SHEFFERY, J. B. Acute Pelvic Thrombophlebitis Treated with Continuous Caudal Anesthesia. Am. J. Obst. & Gynec., 1944, 48:241.

FALLS, F. H. Endometritis and Physometra Due to Welch Bacillus. Am. J. Obst. & Gynec., 1933, 25:280.

FRY, R. M. Fatal Infections by Hemolytic Streptococcus Group B. Lancet, 1938, 1:199.

GOLDSBOROUGH, F. C. Thrombosis of the Internal Iliac Vein during Pregnancy. Bull. Johns Hopkins Hosp., 1904, 15:193.

GUILBEAU, J. A., and SCHAUB, I. Uterine Culture Technic: Simple Method for Avoiding Contamination by Cervical and Vaginal Flora. Am. J. Obst. & Gynec., 1949, 58:407.

——— and ANDREWS, M. C. Penicillin Treatment in the Obstetrical Patient. A Study of Its Effect on the Bacterial Flora of the Postpartum Uterus. Am. J. Obst. & Gynec., 1949, 58:101.

HAGEMAN, P. O., MARTIN, S. P., and WOOD, W. B., Jr. Penicillin: Clinical Study of Its Therapeutic Effectiveness. J.A.M.A., 1944, 124:798.

HALBAN, J., and KOHLER, R. Die Pathologische Anatomie des Puerperalprozesses. Vienna and Leipzig, 1919.

HARE, Ronald. The Haemolytic Streptococci from the Vagina of Febrile and Afebrile Parturient Women. The Ability of Haemolytic Streptococci Found in Infected Throats to Resist the Bactericidal Power of Normal Human Blood. J. Path. and Bacteriol., 1934, 38:129, 143.

——— Alterations in the Bactericidal Power of the Blood Which Occurs during Haemolytic Streptococcal Infections in the Puerperium. J. Path. and Bacteriol., 1935, 41:61.

——— and COLEBROOK, Leonard. The Biochemical Reactions of Haemolytic Streptococci from the Vagina of Febrile and Afebrile Parturient Women. J. Path. and Bacteriol., 1934, 39:429.

HARRIS, J. W., and BROWN, J. H. The Bacterial Contents of the Vagina and Uterus on the Fifth Day of the Normal Puerperium. Bull. Johns Hopkins Hosp., 1928, 43:190-200.

——— A Clinical and Bacteriological Study of 113 Cases of Streptococci Puerperal Infection. Bull. Johns Hopkins Hosp., 1929, 44:1-31.

——— Description of a New Organism That May Be a Factor in the Causation of Puerperal Infection. Bull., Johns Hopkins Hosp., 1927, 40:203-215.

HARRIS, L. M., and SHOOK, D. M. Role of Penicillin in Obstetrics. Am. J. Obst. & Gynec., 1949, 57:1186.

HARRIS, N. MACL., and DABNEY, W. M. Report of a Case of Gonorrheal Endocarditis in a Patient Dying in the Puerperium. Bull. Johns Hopkins Hosp., 1901, 12:68.

HILL, A. M. Post-abortal and Puerperal Gangrene. J. Obst. & Gynaec. Brit. Emp., 1936, 43:201.

HOFBAUER, J. The Defensive Mechanism of the Parametrium during Pregnancy and Labor. Bull. Johns Hopkins Hosp., 1926, 38:255-272.

HOLMES, O. W. Puerperal Fever as a Private Pestilence. Boston, 1855.

HUGGINS, R. R. Ligation of Pelvic Veins in Thrombophlebitis. Am. J. Obst. & Gynec., 1926, 12:562-570.

JOHNSTON, E. K. W. Prevention and Control of Puerperal Sepsis, Including its Medico-legal Aspects. Brit. M. J., 1938, 2:331.

JOHNSTON, R. A., and MORGAN, H. J. Acute Lobar Pneumonia and Hematogenous Puerperal Infection. Bull. Johns Hopkins Hosp., 1922, 33:106-109.

KEETEL, W. C., SCOTT, J. W., and PLASS, E. D. Evaluation of Prophylactic Penicillin Administration to Parturient Women. Am. J. Obst. & Gynec., 1949, 58:335.

LANCEFIELD, Rebecca, and HARE, Ronald. The Serological Differentiation of Pathogenic and Non-pathogenic Strains of Hemolytic Streptococci from Parturient Women. J. Exper. M., 1935, 61:335-349.

LEFEVRE, Louis. Diphtheritic Endometritis. Review of the Recent Literature and Report of a New Case. J.A.M.A., 1928, 90:1015.

MAYES, H. W. Prevention of Obstetric Infection by the Use of Vaginal Antisepsis. West. J. Surg., 1942, 50:568.

MELENY, F. L., and STEVENS, F. A. Postoperative Hemolytic Streptococcus Wound Infections and Their Relation to Streptococcus Carriers Among Operating Personnel. Surg., Gynec. & Obst., 1926, 43:338-342.

NUCKOLS, H. H., and HERTIG, A. T. Pneumococcus Infection of the Genital Tract in Women Especially during Pregnancy and the Puerperium. Am. J. of Obst. & Gynec., 1938, 35:782.

PASTEUR, L. Septicémie puerpérale. Bull. Acad. de méd., Par., 1879, pp. 260-271.

PASTORE, J. B. The Cell Volume Following Delivery and Its Relation to Blood Loss and Postpartum Infection. Am. J. Obst. & Gynec., 1936, 32:859.

PECKHAM, C. H. A Brief History of Puerperal Infection. Buli. Inst. Hist. Med., 1935, 3:187.

RIVETT, L. C., WILLIAMS, L., COLEBROOK, L., and FRY, R. M. Puerperal Fever,—A Report upon 533 Cases Received at the Isolation Block of Queen Charlotte's Hospital. Proc. Roy. Soc. Med., 1933, 26:1161.

ROSENTHAL, A. H., and STONE, F. M. Puerperal Infection with Vegetative Endocarditis. Report of Sulfanilamide Therapy in Two Fatal Cases Due to Streptococcus Haemolyticus Groups B and C. J.A.M.A., 1940, 114:840.

SADUSK, J. F., Jr., and MANAHAN, C. P. Sulfanilamide for Puerperal Infections Due to Clostridium Welchii. J.A.M.A., 1939, 113:14.

——— Observations on the Occurrence of Clostridium Welchii in the Vagina of Pregnant Women. Am. J. Obst. & Gynec., 1941, 41:856.

SCHOTTMÜLLER, H. Zur Bedeutung einiger Anaeroben in der Pathologie, insbesondere bei puerperalen Erkrankungen. Mitt. a. d. Grenzgeb. d. Med. u. Chir., Jena., 1910, 21:450-490.

SCHWARZ, O. H., and DIECKMANN, W. J. Puerperal Infection Due to Anaerobic Streptococci. Am. J. Obst. & Gynec., 1927, 13:467-485.

SEMMELWEIS, I. P. Die Aetiologie, der Begriff u. die Prophylaxis des Kindbettfiebers. Pest, Wien u. Leipzig, 1861.

STIEVE, H. Das Mesenchym in der Wand der menschlichen Gebärmutter. Zentralbl. f. Gynäk., 1929, 53:2706.

TUCKER, W. W., TRUSSELL, R. E., and PLASS, E. D. Latent Gonorrhea in Obstetric Patients. Am. J. of Obst. & Gynec., 1939, 38:1055.

WATSON, B. P. An Outbreak of Puerperal Sepsis in New York City. Am. J. Obst. & Gynec., 1928, 16:157.

WEINSTEIN, L. The Bacterial Flora of the Human Vagina. Yale J. Biol. & Med., 1938, 10:247.

WELCH, W. H. Morbid Conditions caused by Bacillus Aerogenes Capsulatus. Boston M. & S. J., 1900, 143:73-87.

WILLIAMS, J. W. Puerperal Infection considered from a Bacteriological Point of View, with Special Reference to the Question of Auto-infection. Am. J. M. Sc., 1893, 106:45.

——— The Cause of the Conflicting Statements concerning the Bacterial Contents of the Vaginal Secretion of the Pregnant Woman. Am. J. Obst., 1898, 38:807.

——— The Bacteria of the Vagina and Their Practical Significance, Based upon the Bacteriological Examination of the Vaginal Secretion in Ninety-two Pregnant Women. Am. J. Obst., 1898, 38:449.

——— Diphtheria of the Vulva. Am. J. Obst., 1898, 38:180-185.

——— Ein Fall von puerperaler Infektion, bei dem sich Typhusbacillen in den Lochien fanden. Zentralbl. f. Gynäk., 1898, Bd. 22, Nr. 34.

——— Ligation or Excision of Thrombosed Veins in the Treatment of Puerperal Pyemia. Am. J. Obst., 1909, 59:758-789.

WRIGLEY, A. J. Puerperal Infection by Pathogenic Anaerobic Bacteria. Proc. Roy. Soc. Med., 1930, 23:61.

36

DISORDERS OF THE PUERPERIUM OTHER THAN PUERPERAL INFECTION

DISORDERS OF THE BREASTS

Engorgement of the Breasts. For the first 24 or 48 hours following the development of the lacteal secretion it is not unusual for the breasts to become immensely distended, and to offer on palpation a firm, nodular resistance. This condition, which is commonly known as "*caked breast,*" often gives rise to a considerable degree of pain, but is usually unaccompanied by any elevation of temperature. The disorder represents an exaggeration of the normal venous and lymphatic stasis of the breasts which is a regular precursor of lactation. It is not due to any overdistention of the lacteal system with milk.

Treatment consists of supporting and compressing the breasts by means of a binder or brassière, applying an ice bag and, if necessary, the oral administration of 60 mg. (1 grain) of codeine sulfate. In addition 5 mg. of stilbestrol may be given twice a day for 48 hours. It is unwise to continue it for a longer period for several reasons: (1) the span of time cited is adequate to relieve the discomfort; (2) stilbestrol depresses lactation and in borderline cases this may militate against breast feeding; and (3) when given for a long time in the puerperium, as shown by Rutherford, estrogens interfere with regeneration of the uterine mucosa and may cause irregular bleeding. Even without treatment the condition usually subsides within a day or two.

Drying Up the Breasts. After the death of the child, or in cases in which for one reason or another the continuance of lactation is thought inadvisable, steps must be taken for checking the lacteal secretion, or "drying up the milk," as it is usually designated.

When it is desired to "dry up" the breasts, it is best simply to leave them absolutely alone and ask the patient to restrict all fluids to a bare minimum. In the course of 24 hours they become more or less engorged, and sometimes very painful. If the pain is severe, 1 grain (0.060 gm.) of codeine is administered and repeated if necessary, but the breast pump or massage is not employed unless the pain is unbearable. Within a few hours the engorgement so compresses the vessels within the breasts that the secretory activity is checked after which the engorgement subsides and the pain diminishes, and within 24 or 36 hours the breasts become soft and painless. With each succeeding day the secretion becomes less and less abundant and practically disappears in the course of a week. After considerable experience with stilbesterol for this purpose,

I gave it up because (1) its withdrawal is often followed by a return of milk secretion, and (2) irregular uterine bleeding is a common sequel.

Occasionally the use of an ice bag is indicated, and when the breasts are large and pendulous they are supported by means of a binder, which does not exert pressure upon them.

Inflammation of the Breasts. *Mastitis.* Parenchymatous inflammation of the mammary glands is a rare complication of pregnancy, but is frequently observed during the puerperium and lactational period. In 20,258 patients delivered at the Johns Hopkins Hospital prior to the introduction of the sulfonamides and penicillin, 113, or 1 in 179 developed suppurative mastitis (Dippel and Johnston). Seven of the 113 breast abscesses developed in pregnancy. Seventy-nine, or 70 per cent of the cases occurred in association with the first pregnancy confirming the older observation of Winckel that two thirds of the cases occur in primiparae.

The symptoms of mastitis rarely appear before the end of the first week of the puerperium, and as a rule not until the third or fourth week. Marked engorgement usually precedes the inflammatory trouble, the first sign of which is afforded by chilly sensations or an actual rigor which is soon followed by a considerable rise in temperature and an increase in the rate of the pulse. The breast becomes hard, its surface is reddened, and the patient complains of acute pain. In some cases the constitutional symptoms attending a mammary abscess are pronounced, and very exceptionally, if neglected, lead to a fatal termination. On the other hand, the local manifestations may be so slight as to escape observation; such cases are usually mistaken for puerperal infection. In still another group of patients the process pursues a subacute or almost chronic course, the breast being somewhat harder than usual and more or less painful, but constitutional symptoms are either lacking or very slight. Under such circumstances the first indication of the true state of affairs is often afforded by the detection of fluctuation.

Etiology. Mastitis is always the result of infection, pathogenic bacteria from outside gaining access to the breast through fissured nipples by way of the lymphatics; or else some of those already present in the lactiferous ducts meet with conditions which enable them to invade the tissues. By far the most common offender is the *Staphylococcus aureus* which is encountered in 66 per cent of Dippel and Johnston's series, and in 93.4 per cent of 40 cases of mastitis studied by Douglas at the New York Lying-In Hospital. The hemolytic streptococcus is occasionally encountered and it is these cases which are likely to prove especially grave if neglected.

Mastitis can conveniently be classified as interstitial and parenchymatous. Both types are usually preceded by cracking or fissure of the nipple or areola. This admits micro-organisms to the subcutaneous lymphatics where they set up a marked reaction, characterized by high fever and occasionally a chill. Often this is the end of the process; on the other hand it may continue its course and set up an interstitial inflammatory reaction. This is usually a very edematous, tense process and in resolving sometimes suppurates to form abscesses in various parts of the breast. Parenchymatous mastitis, as its name suggests, refers to those infections which are located in the glandular and duct portions of the breast. Although having an origin similar to the interstitial type, the parenchymatous infections usually appear somewhat later in the puerperium. The explanation usually offered for this difference is that as long as the ducts of the breast afford drainage the process may be quite asymptomatic but once an infected duct is occluded the response is rapid. This sequence of events usually follows the institution of lactation and hence is seen from the fifth or sixth day onward. In marked contrast is the interstitial type which is common in the first days of the puerperium. Either variety may end in suppuration with the formation of abscesses in various parts of the breast, unless intensive treatment is started early in the disease.

TREATMENT. The occurrence of mastitis can be prevented in great part by suitable prophylactic measures which mainly consist in preventing the development of fissured nipples or treating them properly after they have appeared.

The routine care of the lactating breasts should include the use of 2 per cent boric acid solution or sterile water to cleanse the nipples before and after each nursing; the purpose of this is to remove encrusted flakes of inspissated milk which are irritating if attached to the nipple. If cracks or fissures develop, the affected nipple is covered with a paste of lanolin and tincture of benzozone, or one of bismuth subcarbonate and castor oil, or penicillin ointment, or one of the commercial preparations available for this purpose. The paste is removed before each nursing by washing with 70 per cent alcohol and boric acid solution. If the cracks bleed or the nipples become too tender to allow the infant to nurse directly, a nipple shield is used, or the breast pump employed. Fissured nipples usually respond to this treatment and only rarely is it necessary to discontinue breast feeding on this account.

The advent of penicillin has improved dramatically the prognosis in acute puerperal mastitis and, provided antibiotic therapy is started before suppuration begins, the infection can usually be aborted within 48 hours. Two hundred thousand units of aqueous penicillin should be administered intramuscularly as an initial dose and followed by 50,000 units every four hours. Often the signs and symptoms disappear entirely after the second or third injection of the antibiotic but it is wise to continue therapy for three days to make certain that all staphylococci responsible for the disease have been killed. Even if suppuration is present, as evidenced by a clear-cut fluctuation, it is still possible to avoid incision of the abscess by puncturing it, withdrawing the pus and replacing the pus is approximately two thirds of its quantity by an isotonic sodium chloride solution containing 100,000 units of crystalline sodium penicillin in 20 cc. Although the response to penicillin therapy in acute puerperal mastitis is usually prompt, Hesseltine has observed some failures and has demonstrated that certain strains of *Staphylococcus aureus* responsible for mastitis may be resistant to penicillin therapy. In the presence of an outright puerperal mastitis it is best to take the baby off the breast until the infection has been arrested.

In rare instances, as in Hesseltine's cases, it may still be necessary to incise a breast abscess despite penicillin therapy.

The incisions should be made radially, extending from near the areolar margin toward the periphery of the gland, in order to avoid injury to the lactiferous ducts. In early cases a single incision over the most dependent portion of the area of fluctuation is usually sufficient, but when multiple abscesses are present several incisions may be required. The operation should always be done under general anesthesia, and should not be considered as completed until the operator has introduced a finger through the incision and carefully explored the interior of the breast, breaking down the partition walls between the various pockets of pus, so that only a single abscess cavity is left to be dealt with. This should then be loosely packed with gauze and replaced at the end of 24 hours by a smaller pack. If the pus has been thoroughly evacuated, the abscess cavity becomes obliterated and a complete cure effected with a rapidity which is sometimes surprising.

Galactocele. Very exceptionally, as the result of the clogging of a milk duct by inspissated secretion, an accumulation of milk may take place in one or more lobes of the breast. Ordinarily this is limited in amount but may become excessive and form a fluctuant tumor which may give rise to pressure symptoms. In many instances the application of a tight binder will cause it to disappear, and we have never seen the structure attain such size that puncture was necessary.

Hypertrophy of the Breasts. This may be observed, but abnormal enlargement is nevertheless an infrequent occurrence. In a large proportion of the recorded cases the condition developed rapidly in young unmarried women, both breasts being implicated and occasionally attaining such immense proportions that amputation became necessary. Cases have been reported in which a single breast weighed more than 50 pounds. The hypertrophy sometimes recedes during lactation so that the abnormality does not always afford an absolute contraindication to suckling the child. Overdevelopment of the mammae is sometimes observed in men, a number of cases having been collected by Laurent.

Supernumerary Breasts. Probably one in every few hundred women has one or more accessory breasts, *polymastia*. Reference to 262 such cases is to be found in Goldberger's article.

The supernumerary breasts are sometimes so minute as to be mistaken for small pigmented moles and rarely attain any considerable size. They are often provided with distinct nipples, and are most commonly situated in pairs upon either side of the midline of the thoracic or abdominal walls, and usually below the main breasts; less frequently they are found in the axillae, and occasionally upon other portions of the body, on the shoulder, flank, or groin, and in rare instances the thigh. The number of supernumerary breasts varies greatly. When arranged symmetrically two or four are the commonest number, although Neugebauer has described a patient with 10.

The condition is usually regarded as an atavistic reversion though it is not associated with an increased tendency toward multiple pregnancy. In not a few instances an apparent hereditary influence can be traced. Not all observers, however, accept this view, Ahlfeld holding that the distribution of the mammary tissue is to be attributed to the transference at an early period of development by means of the amnion, of some of the cells which ordinarily go to form the breasts, to other portions of the body. The condition has no obstetrical significance though occasionally the enlargement of supernumerary breasts occupying the axillae may result in considerable discomfort. Quite frequently a tongue of mammary tissue may extend out into the axilla from the outer margin of a normal breast, while sometimes an isolated fragment will be found in the same location. Such structures undergo hypertrophy during pregnancy, and when lactation is being established become swollen and painful. Ordinarily, if let alone, they soon undergo regression and give no further trouble.

Abnormalities of the Nipples. The typical nipple is cylindrical in shape and projects well beyond the general surface of the breast, its exterior being slightly nodular but free from fissures. Variations from the normal, however, are not uncommon, some of them being so pronounced as to interfere seriously with the act of suckling.

In some women the lactiferous ducts open directly into an area which forms a depression at the center of the areola. In pronounced instances of this so-called *depressed nipple* nursing is out of the question, although when the depression is not very deep the breast may occasionally be made available by the employment of an electrically driven breast pump.

More frequently, although not depressed, the nipple is so *inverted* that it hardly projects above the surface of the breast, and in consequence can be seized by the child's mouth only with the greatest difficulty. In the presence of this anomaly daily attempts should be made during the last few months of pregnancy to draw the nipple out by traction with the fingers. This however is rarely successful so that, if the nipples cannot be made available by the temporary use of an electric pump, suckling will have to be discontinued.

Again it sometimes happens that nipples which are normal in shape and size may present so fissured or nodular a surface as to be especially susceptible to injury from the child's mouth during the act of suckling. In such cases small cracks or *fissures* almost inevitably appear, and render nursing so painful that the mother dreads the approach of the child, and the mental distress so induced often has a deleterious influence upon the secretory function. Moreover such lesions are still more serious in that they offer a convenient portal of entry for pyogenic bacteria which are liable to invade the breast and give rise to a mastitis. For these reasons every effort should be made to heal such fissures, and this is best effected by protecting them from further injury by the child by the use of a nipple shield, and soothing and antiseptic applications. If such measures are of no avail the child should not be permitted to nurse on the affected side; rather the breast should be emptied regularly by means of a suitable pump until the lesions are completely healed.

Abnormalities in the Mammary Secretion. Marked individual variations exist in the amount of milk secreted, many of which are dependent not upon the general health and appearance of the individual, but upon the degree of development of the glandular portions of the breasts. Thus we often find that a woman who possesses large, well-formed breasts and who apparently should be an excellent milk producer, secretes only a small quantity; while, on the other hand, one is often surprised at the abundant supply produced by another whose mammae are small and flat. It is a matter of common observation that stout women with redundant breasts usually have a deficient secretion, the bulk of the organ being made up of fatty tissue while the glandular elements are poorly developed. Deficient secretion is likewise frequently noted in very young women and in elderly primiparae. In the former the defect is to be attributed to imperfect development; in the latter to regressive and atrophic changes in the breasts.

In very rare instances there is an absolute lack of mammary secretion, *agalactia*. As a rule, however, the defect is not absolute, as it is nearly always possible to cause at least a small amount to exude from the nipple on the third or fourth day of the puerperium. On the other hand, relative deficiency is frequently observed, a large number of women secreting an amount of milk quite insufficient for the nutrition of the child. In an earlier section reference is made to the variations in the quantity of the milk as well as to the various factors which may be concerned in their production and to the endocrine control of mammary growth and lactation.

Occasionally the mammary secretion is excessive, *polygalactia,* and may even be so abundant that milk is constantly escaping from the nipples. This latter condition, which is known as *galactorrhea,* sometimes continues for years after the birth of the child and is extremely intractable to treatment. Very little is known as to its cause. Although in rare instances the health of the woman may remain unimpaired, as a rule she soon begins to show evidences of the continuous drain upon her system, becoming irritable, querulous, and eventually developing symptoms of cachexia.

Galactorrhea is best treated by not attempting to empty the breast completely, but by allowing it to become engorged, in the hope that the intramammary pressure will become so great as to compress the vessels and thus check secretion. At the same time the breasts should be supported by a bandage, and the total daily fluid intake limited to 1,000 to 1,500 cc., until the condition is corrected.

DISEASES AND ABNORMALITIES OF THE UTERUS

Subinvolution. This term is used to describe an arrest or retardation of the process of *involution,* by which the puerperal uterus is normally restored to its original proportions.

Involution is the result of an autolytic process, which leads to atrophy of the individual muscle cells, rather than to fatty degeneration, as was formerly supposed. Its possible cause is to be sought in the liberation of certain, as yet unknown, ferments associated with the sudden and marked diminution of the blood supply to the uterus. As this can be brought about only by satisfactory contraction and retraction of the organ, it is apparent that any interference with those functions may be followed by subinvolution of the uterus which is readily revealed on abdominal or vaginal examination.

Among the most frequent factors concerned in its production are imperfect exfoliation of the decidua, retention of portions of the after-birth, inflammatory lesions of the endometrium, the presence of myomatous nodules in the uterine wall, abnormalities of circulation which accompany displacements of the uterus, existence of pelvic inflammatory lesions, and insufficient rest during the puerperium. In other words, subinvolution is the result of local conditions and not of constitutional disorders. Accordingly, careful investigation will usually reveal the underlying cause, and appropriate treatment, if undertaken sufficiently early, will lead to its cure.

The existence of subinvolution is manifested by a prolongation of the lochial discharge beyond the usual period, and sometimes by profuse hemorrhage, its cessation being followed by persistent leukorrhea with pains in the back, a dragging down sensation, and a delayed return to perfect health. If the condition is not properly treated it may lead to permanent changes in the uterus and particularly in its vessels which are sometimes associated with such persistent hemorrhage as eventually to necessitate the removal of the organ. According to R. F. Smith, and Otto Schwarz, such uteri are abnormally large, contain much more fibrous and less muscular tissue than normally, while the arterial walls are so altered that the normal mechanism for the regulation of the circulation is in abeyance.

The diagnosis is established by bimanual examination, the uterus being found to be larger, softer, and more succulent than it should be at a given time following delivery. Inasmuch as subinvolution is dependent mainly upon local conditions very little can be expected from medicinal treatment, although the administration of ergonovine 0.2 mg. every three or four hours, together with copious hot vaginal douches for several days, is usually followed by improvement. Local measures afford much better results. If the uterus is displaced it should be put in proper position by bimanual manipulation and held in position by a suitably fitting pessary. When disease of the endometrium or retention of portions of the after-birth is responsible, prompt curettage offers the most efficient method of treatment. On the other hand, procrastination may lead to serious results, as the subinvolution may become permanent.

Lactation Atrophy of the Uterus. Ordinarily, in women who suckle their children, the uterus continues to involute after the completion of the puerperium, so that several months after delivery it may be smaller than in the virginal state. This condition is attributed to reflex irritation emanating from the breasts and incident to lactation and nursing. It usually disappears spontaneously after weaning although, when the child is nursed for a long period, the uterus may begin to increase in size after the fifth and sixth month even though lactation continues. It is probable that the cessation of menstruation, which is usually observed during the early months of lactation, should be partly attributed to this form of atrophy.

Lactation atrophy was first definitely described by Jacquet in 1871 and since the publication of his paper has been carefully studied by numerous investigators, particularly Thorn, Gottschalk, Döderlein, and Vineburg. In rare instances it may persist after weaning and become permanent, the uterine cavity sometimes measuring only a few centimeters in length. It is probable that it may occasionally be an important factor in the production of subsequent sterility, as well as in the unusually early appearance of the menopause. This condition is exceedingly rare.

Displacements of the Uterus. Immediately following the birth of the child, the lower uterine segment and cervix are represented by a flabby, collapsed structure which is freely movable upon the rest of the organ. In these circumstances a comparatively trivial cause, such as a slight increase in the intra-abdominal pressure or distention of the rectum, may lead to an excessive bending forward of the body of the uterus, *acute anteflexion*. The condition is usually without significance but occasionally the angle formed between the upper and lower portions of the organ may be so acute as to occlude the cervical canal and lead to the retention of the lochial discharge, *lochiometra*. As a rule the retention, when it occurs, is only transitory but if it be prolonged the lochia may undergo putrefactive changes, when the absorption of toxins may give rise to constitutional symptoms. The complication is readily overcome by allowing the retained discharge to drain away through a glass tube, inserted in the cervical canal.

So long as the body of the uterus lies above the superior strait, retrodisplacement cannot occur, as the falling backward of the enlarged fundus is prevented by the promontory of the sacrum. But as soon as the organ has become sufficiently involuted to descend into the pelvic cavity a *retroflexion* or *retroversion* becomes possible. The development of such displacements, which are rarely observed before the third week of the puerperium, is probably connected with excessive relaxation of some of the structures about the base of the broad ligaments incident to overdistention by the presenting part, and in all likelihood is favored by undue laxness of the walls of the uterine isthmus. Doubtless, prolonged distention of the bladder may act as an accessory cause. It is important to remember that it is not due to negligence on the part of the obstetrician at the time of delivery, nor is it by any means always due to trauma incident to operative procedures, as in our experience retroflexion quite as frequently follows normal spontaneous labor during which no apparent injury was sustained. In other cases the retroflexion merely represents a recurrence of a condition existing prior to pregnancy.

Backward displacement of the uterus occasionally gives rise to symptoms so long as the patient remains in bed. The earliest and the most characteristic manifestation is an increase in the amount of lochial discharge and its persistence for longer periods than usual. Sometimes the patient suffers from pain in the back and lower abdomen, although in other cases she may only be conscious that she is not regaining her strength as rapidly as she had expected. In many instances, however, the displacement does not give rise to symptoms, so that the patient may have no idea of its existence until it is detected during the course of a pelvic examination months or years later. In our experience such displacements occur in every fourth or fifth puerperal woman. A positive diagnosis can always be made upon vaginal examination, when the displaced uterus will be found to be larger and softer than normal, the condition which is usually associated with subinvolution.

In the absence of symptoms and of clear-cut evidence of subinvolution, no treatment is necessary. In the presence of symptoms (commonly, persistence of lochia) and/or subinvolution two weeks postpartum, the knee-chest position should be recommended for five minutes night and morning. If, four weeks postpartum, subinvolution is still evident, a properly fitting, hard rubber pessary should be inserted to hold the uterus in anterior position and allowed to remain in place two months. In a short time the subinvolution is usually corrected by this means, and with it any tendency to irregular bleeding. In some cases, at the end of two months the retroposition is also corrected, but, if not, it is usually symptomless and requires no treatment.

Relaxation of the Vaginal Outlet and Prolapse of the Uterus. Reference has already been made to the frequent occurrence of perineal lacerations at the time of labor and the consequent relaxation of the vaginal outlet which follows neglect to repair them. Furthermore, in the absence of any visible laceration it should always be remembered that pronounced relaxation sometimes follows overstretching or submucosal tearing of an inelastic or flabby pelvic floor. In such circumstances, as there was nothing to repair at the time of delivery, the condition will escape detection unless an examination is made at the end of the puerperium.

Moreover, the changes following childbearing predispose to the occurrence of *prolapse* of the uterus, and aggravation of the condition should be expected during the puerperium in women who have presented moderate degrees of descensus uteri before labor. In general, operative correction of the prolapse should be postponed till the end of the childbearing period, unless of course serious disability develops, necessitating intervention.

HEMORRHAGES DURING THE PUERPERIUM

Ordinarily, if there has been no serious loss of blood during the first hour or hour and a half following delivery, it may be assumed that the danger of postpartum hemorrhage has passed. Occasionally, however, in the latter part of the first week, and more often still later in the puerperium, more or less severe uterine hemorrhages are encountered. They are nearly always due to the retention of portions of a placental cotyledon or of a succenturiate lobule which may have been overlooked at the time of labor. If the retained tissue is not cast off spontaneously or removed manually, it undergoes gradual necrosis, while at the same time fibrin becomes deposited about its periphery giving rise to a polypoid growth of varying size, *placental polyp,* which so interferes with the involution of the adjacent portion of the uterus that bleeding continues so long as it remains in utero. This bleeding may be so profuse that immediate removal of the tissue and transfusion are necessary.

In a study of later postpartum hemorrhage by Wolfe and Pedowitz, the incidence of this complication was found to be once in about 1,000 cases. Most commonly, abnormal vaginal bleeding appeared in their cases between the sixth and tenth postpartum days. Shock (systolic blood pressure below 100, pulse above 100, pallor, cold skin) in varying degrees was present in 12 of 24 afebrile cases. All uteri were noted as subinvoluted.

The retention of large portions of the fetal membranes rarely gives rise to serious hemorrhage as the tissues gradually disintegrate and are cast off with the lochial discharge. On the other hand, a relatively small portion of the decidua may fail to undergo the usual regressive changes while the remainder of the mucosa regenerates normally. In such circumstances the condition is designated as endometritis postpartum or postabortum, according as it follows full-term labor or abortion. For reasons with which we are as yet unacquainted, it interferes with the involution of the uterus, and may give rise to severe hemorrhage. Frankl described such conditions in 1926, and we have been surprised to find that a portion of retained decidua only a few millimeters in diameter may lead to serious consequences.

The diagnosis of the retention of a placental remnant or the existence of a polyp can only be verified by the sense of touch. Therefore, whenever a patient suffers from an acute loss of blood during the puerperium, the interior of the uterus should be carefully palpated and/or curetted, and any abnormal tissue promptly removed.

The treatment of the slight hemorrhage following retroflexion and subinvolution of the uterus will be referred to under those headings. The excessive loss of blood associated with an endometritis postpartum demands curettage. If the patient bleeds excessively after the expulsion of an hydatidiform mole similar treatment is indicated. Furthermore, on account of the possibility of the development of a chorionepithelioma, the tissue removed should always be subjected to careful microscopic examination.

Puerperal Hematomas. A tumefaction resulting from the escape of blood into the connective tissue beneath the skin covering the external genitalia or beneath the vaginal mucosa is known as a *vulvar* or *vaginal hematoma.* This condition, first studied in detail by Deneux in 1830, is a rare complication of labor and the puerperium occurring about once in 1,500 or 2,000 cases. It occasionally originates during pregnancy and may attain such proportions as to interfere with the descent of the child. Very exceptionally, if medical aid is not available, fatal hemorrhage may follow its rupture at the time of labor, as in the cases reported by Künzig and others. The condition usually follows injury to a blood vessel during the act of labor without laceration of the superficial tissues and may follow spontaneous, as well as operative, delivery. Now and again it does not occur until later and is then attributable to the sloughing of a vessel which had become necrotic as the result of prolonged pressure.

Less frequently the torn vessel lies above the pelvic fascia. In this event the hematoma develops above it, and in its early stages gives rise to a rounded tumefaction which projects into the upper portion of the vaginal canal and may almost occlude its lumen. If the bleeding continues it spreads apart the broad ligament and separates the peritoneum from the adjacent tissues. In this way the effused blood may form a tumor palpable above Poupart's ligament, or it may make its way into the iliac fossae, gradually invade the renal region and eventually reach the lower margin of the diaphragm.

Vulvar hematomata of moderate size are usually absorbed spontaneously. Occasionally the tissues covering the tumor may undergo pressure necrosis and give way, profuse hemorrhage resulting, or the contents may be discharged in the form of large clots. In either event the interior of the hematoma is very prone to become infected, the condition sometimes ending fatally. If the tumor is large it not only causes discomfort by its mere size, but gives rise to great suffering which, as the result of the tearing and stretching of the tissues, becomes more intense the more rapidly the hematoma develops.

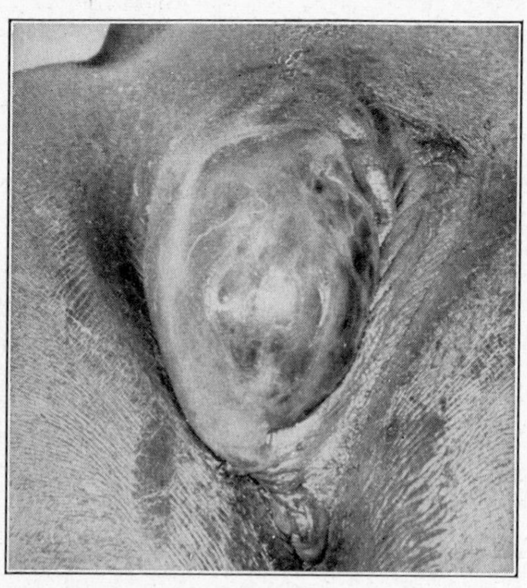

Fig. 516.—Vulvar Hematoma Bulging out the Right Vaginal Wall.

In the *subperitoneal* variety, such quantities of blood may be effused beneath the peritoneum that the patient rapidly succumbs to acute anemia. In other cases a fatal issue follows secondary rupture into the peritoneal cavity. Occasionally rupture occurs into the vagina, in which event the hematoma becomes infected, and the patient perishes if suitable treatment is not promptly instituted. In 33 cases of subperitoneal hematoma which Williams collected in 1904, the mortality was 56 per cent. It is interesting to note that more than 60 per cent of the cases occurred in primiparae, and 71 per cent after spontaneous labor. In Williams' patient the hemorrhage came from a vessel at the base of the bladder, which had become torn through during the course of a spontaneous labor.

A vulvar hematoma is readily diagnosticated by the sudden appearance of a tense, elastic, fluctuating, and sensitive tumor of varying size, covered by discolored skin. When the mass develops in the vagina it may escape detection for a time but the development of pressure symptoms soon leads to a vaginal examination when a round, fluctuant tumor is found, which encroaches upon the lumen. When the hematoma extends upward between the folds of the broad ligament it is liable to escape detection unless it gives rise to a tumor which can be felt upon abdominal palpation, or unless symptoms of anemia or infection appear. In Williams' case the uterus was displaced upward by the effused blood, and on bimanual examination a fluctuant tumor 15 cm. in diameter could be palpated beneath it.

The prognosis is usually favorable, though very large hematomata occasionally lead to death from hemorrhage, whereas in rare cases the fatal termination is the result of infection.

Treatment. Small hematomata should be left alone for spontaneous but slow resorption usually takes place, provided the parts be kept clean and infection avoided.

On the other hand, a steady increase in size indicates a continuance of hemorrhage, and in such cases the tumor should be laid widely open and packed with gauze as it is rarely possible to isolate and tie the bleeding vessel. The strictest antiseptic precautions are imperative inasmuch as infection is a frequent complication. In large subperitoneal hematomata, accompanied by acute anemia, laparotomy should be promptly performed, the blood clots removed, and the hemorrhage controlled by ligature or by packing the cavity with gauze.

DISEASES OF THE URINARY TRACT

The process of evacuation of the uterus is associated with stretching and trauma of the base of the bladder. Cystoscopic examination soon after delivery shows not only edema and hyperemia but frequently submucous extravasations of blood. At times the edema of the trigone is so marked as to be the cause of obstruction of the urethra and acute retention. In addition to these factors the puerperal bladder has an increased capacity and is not as sensitive to intravesical fluid tension as in the nonpregnant state, so that overdistention and incomplete emptying with the establishment of residual urine are common. The paralyzing effect of anesthesia and temporarily disturbed function of the nerve supply to the bladder are undoubtedly contributory factors.

Residual urine with the presence of bacteriuria in a traumatized bladder present the optimum conditions for the development of true bladder infection. Taussig found an incidence of cystitis of 3.8 per cent, while Prather reports 1.1 per cent.

The symptoms are often inability to urinate, frequent voiding in small amounts, dysuria, and a low-grade fever which rarely rises above 101°F. The treatment is usually confined to intermittent catheterization of the bladder every eight hours, followed by the instillation of 15 cc. of a 3 per cent solution of strong silver proteinate or some other mild antiseptic irritant. This is continued until the patient voids spontaneously in satisfactory amounts and catheterization once in 24 hours fails to show a residual urine of over 30 cc. In more severe cases it is occasionally necessary to place an indwelling catheter in the bladder so that constant drainage is established. When this is done, the bladder should be irrigated three or four times in each 24 hours with warm boric acid solution.

In view of the high incidence of bacteriuria, 11 per cent in the antepartum and 70 per cent in the postpartum woman, it is interesting to note the relatively small number of patients, approximately 3 per cent, who show an involvement of the bladder wall sufficiently severe to warrant the diagnosis of cystitis. Studies have shown the normal bladder to be very resistant to infection and that when inflammation of its tissues occurs it is due not only to the presence of infectious organisms, but also to stagnant urine or trauma. The diagnosis of cystitis, therefore, cannot be made upon the bacteriuria alone, but must involve the demonstration of pus cells associated with residual urine in the bladder. The treatment must therefore be concentrated upon the avoidance of accumulations of stagnant urine as well as trauma.

Incontinence of Urine. In multiparous women, during the early part of the puerperium, coughing, sneezing, or other factors leading to a sudden increase in the intra-abdominal pressure, often produce an involuntary discharge of a small quantity of urine. The condition usually passes off spontaneously but may sometimes necessitate operative intervention at a later date.

More marked incontinence at this time is usually the result of lesions about the neck of the bladder following operative delivery, though when the condition does not manifest itself until late in the first week it may be the first sign of the development of a *vesicovaginal fistula.* In this event scrupulous attention to cleanliness will frequently be followed by spontaneous recovery; but when the fistulous opening persists, a cure can be effected only by operative procedures at a later period.

DISORDERS OF THE NERVOUS SYSTEM

Obstetrical Paralyses. That branches of the sacral plexus sometimes suffer from pressure during labor is demonstrated by the fact that many patients complain of intense neuralgia or of cramplike pains extending down one or both legs as soon as the head begins to descend into the pelvic canal. As a rule the compression is rarely severe enough to give rise to grave lesions. In some instances, however, the pain continues after delivery and is accompanied by the development of paralysis in the muscles supplied by the external popliteal nerve—the flexors of the ankles and the extensors of the toes. Occasionally the gluteal muscles become affected to a lesser extent.

The subject has been carefully studied by Hünermann, H. M. Thomas, and Hösslin. Hünermann supplied a very satisfactory explanation of the common localization of the paralysis by showing that the external popliteal nerve receives fibers from the fourth and fifth lumbar roots, and that these on their way downward to join the sacral plexus pass over the brim of the pelvis, where they are exposed to danger from compression, whereas the lower roots which lie upon the pyriformis muscle are more protected.

Hünermann considers that the chances of injurious pressure are greatest where the pelvis is generally contracted, in which event the nerves are compressed between the head of the child and the pelvic brim. Moreover, as only one oblique diameter of the superior strait is occupied by the greatest diameter of the head, it is readily understood why the paralysis is usually limited to one leg, Thomas' case being the only instance in which both legs were affected which had been recorded up to 1900. The paralytic symptoms usually appear immediately after delivery and may become permanent unless suitable therapeutic measures, more particularly the use of electricity, are promptly instituted.

In other cases paralytic symptoms, accompanied by intense neuralgic pains along the course of the sciatic nerve, follow pelvic inflammatory troubles. The condition is sometimes due to the development of a neuritis affecting certain branches of the sacral plexus, while in other cases pressure exerted by an inflammatory exudate is responsible. We have seen a case of the latter character, which had persisted for years in spite of continuous treatment, disappear as if by magic after laparotomy and the separation of the adherent appendages from the posterior and lateral portions of the pelvic wall.

Winschied has directed attention to the rare cases of *neuritis* which follow delivery. The condition may be general or localized. In the latter only one or two nerves are affected, namely the median, ulnar, or crural; while in the former, since a number of nerves are implicated simultaneously, sometimes even those of the face not escaping, the symptoms may be manifold and the condition become most serious. In either event we are ignorant concerning the mode of production of the nerve lesions, although when generalized they may be due to toxemic influences being occasionally noted after toxemic vomiting and allied conditions. The prognosis is fair for the localized but often poor for the generalized variety, although even the latter occasionally undergo spontaneous cure. Vitamin deficiency, as previously noted, may be associated with nerve lesions, and in such event the treatment must of course include an adequate supply of the deficient vitamins, usually those of the B complex.

It is also important to bear in mind that separation of the symphysis pubis, or of one or the other sacro-iliac synchondrosis during labor may be followed by pain, and by so marked an interference with locomotion as at first sight to suggest the existence of paralysis. Moreover the disturbances in the function of the psoas muscles and the adductors of the thigh, which so frequently accompany the early stages of osteomalacia, might readily lead to a similar error.

In addition to these more localized processes the puerperal woman may occasionally suffer from paralysis of central origin. In most instances these result from various varieties of apoplexy, and occasionally from areas of cerebral degeneration incident to eclampsia and the other toxemias.

Puerperal Psychosis. According to statistics compiled by Berkley and Jones, this is noted once in every 616 and 1,100 labors, respectively. In the last 34,356 deliveries in the New York Lying-In Hospital, an incidence of puerperal psychosis of 0.12 per cent was found. Of these cases of puerperal psychosis, 34.8 per cent were idiopathic or of unexplained etiology, 25.6 per cent were in association with puerperal infection, while 39.6 per cent followed a toxemia of pregnancy. In former times it was a comparatively common complication, and it would seem that the introduction of aseptic methods into obstetrics is responsible for a reduction by one half in its incidence. The affection usually makes its appearance within the first two weeks following delivery.

Following Olshausen's contribution in 1891, it has been generally recognized that the causative factors concerned in production of puerperal psychoses fall into the three great groups of infectious, idiopathic, and toxemic. In the past the former was the most important, but with gradual improvement in aseptic technic it has lost a great part of its significance, although we have repeatedly seen puerperal insanity associated with infection due to a streptococcus alone or in combination with other organisms.

At present the idiopathic type is the most usual and it commonly occurs in women with hereditary tendencies or in those who are unable to accommodate themselves to the complications of married life. The toxemic type is best represented by the outbreaks of insanity which sometimes occur a day or so after the cessation of an eclamptic attack. Olshausen noted it in about 6 per cent of his eclamptic patients, while it occurred in 10 per cent of the eclamptic patients in the New York Lying-In Hospital.

The idiopathic psychoses do not differ from those occurring at other times and may occur in various forms and with varying degrees of intensity. The infectious types are usually characterized by great excitement during the first few days, associated with all sorts of hallucinations. Later the maniacal symptoms disappear, and the patient passes into a condition of depression, and frequently exhibits suicidal tendencies. The posteclamptics are sometimes very violent, and the delusions often have a religious tinge, while in others the color sense is affected.

The prognosis is most favorable in the cases following eclampsia, the majority of such patients recovering within a few weeks. The other cases, including those following infection, are very tedious and 20 to 40 per cent of the women fail to regain their mental equilibrium. It is not unusual for the disturbance to last for from three to six months, although the prospect for recovery is poor if the latter period is exceeded. In the idiopathic type the prognosis varies according to the underlying cause, and according to Saunders only about one half of the patients recover permanently. It was formerly stated that from 5 to 10 per cent of the patients suffering from the various types of puerperal insanity died, but with the present lessened mortality from puerperal infection and eclampsia such figures give an exaggerated idea of the danger.

In cases following infection the treatment should first be directed to the underlying condition, and the directions described in the previous section rigorously followed. The acute maniacal symptoms should be met by the administration of sedatives, and the patient should be watched most carefully throughout her entire illness, more particularly during the periods of depression, during which she should never be left alone for fear that she may do an injury to herself. If prompt improvement does not follow the disappearance of the symptoms ascribable to infection, the patient should be placed in charge of a competent psychiatrist.

MISCELLANEOUS CONDITIONS

Pulmonary Embolism. This accident, usually noted only later in the puerperium, but occasionally occurring shortly after labor, is due to the detachment of a small particle of thrombus situated in a uterine or pelvic vein or elsewhere, which is carried to the right side of the heart and leads to more or less complete occlusion of the pulmonary artery. It is usually associated with infective or thrombotic processes elsewhere in the body, though it may occur in women who were apparently perfectly well. Davis considers it the most frequent cause of sudden death in the absence of definite disease. Bunzel reported 32 cases in 31,716 pregnant patients, or an incidence of approximately 0.1 per cent, a figure in close agreement with the incidence of 0.12 per cent observed in 41,454 patients in the New York Lying-In service. He found pulmonary embolism to be three times more frequent in operative than in normal deliveries, an observation in agreement with the New York Lying-In experience.

With the occurrence of a pulmonary embolism the patient complains of intense and sudden dyspnea and eventually air hunger. Death may ensue within a short time, Nygarrd reporting that 70 per cent of his cases died within half an hour after the occurrence of the accident. A small embolus is not necessarily fatal although the patient may succumb to repeated attacks. An infected thrombus may lead to the development of a lung abscess.

Prophylaxis may play a role in the prevention of pulmonary embolism as circulatory stasis is undoubtedly a factor in its production. Toward this end some authorities advocate exercise early in the puerperium, Walthard and others advising it as early as within 24 hours after delivery. We, however, are of the opinion that such a regimen is unnecessary and inadvisable and believe that sitting up with a back-rest in bed as early as the second day of the puerperium, fairly unrestricted movements in bed on the sixth day and sitting out of bed on the tenth day is a schedule sufficiently satisfactory to overcome circulatory stasis due to enforced rest. Prophylaxis also consists in conservative obstetrics with a minimum of operative interference with its increased incidence of infection. Other prophylactic measures have been advocated from time to time, such as the Trendelenberg position, thyroid extract and sodium thiosulfate. In our opinion the maintenance of an adequate fluid balance after operative delivery is of definite value.

The treatment of pulmonary embolism consists in the immediate administration of high concentrations of oxygen by means of nasal catheter, followed by mask or tent. In addition, morphine may be given and general supportive measures instituted to combat shock. Dicumarol is usually indicated to prevent further embolism.

Gangrene of the Extremities. In very rare instances, as the result of extensive thrombosis of venous channels or of *embolism* of the arteries, the circulation in the extremities may become so impaired that gangrene results. This accident, first described by Churchill and studied more particularly by Wormser and Burckhard, is a most serious complication, and usually ends fatally. Wormser in 1904 collected 80 cases from the literature, 6 of which were apparently examples of Raynaud's disease, while of the remaining cases 66 occurred in puerperal, as compared with 6 in pregnant, women. The process usually involves one or both feet, although the hand or forearm may occasionally be implicated. Sixty-two per cent of the 34 patients mentioned in Lafond's thesis died, in spite of the fact that in several instances amputation was resorted to in order to check the further development of the process. In the preceding section reference was made to the production of the accident by excessive medication with ergot.

Scarlet Fever. Although scarlet fever is rarely encountered during the puerperium, its occurrence has given rise to a great deal of discussion and a very considerable literature. The interest manifested in the disease is largely to be accounted for by the fact that a scarlatiniform rash is occasionally observed during the course of a puerperal infection so that in many cases a differential diagnosis becomes very difficult.

The puerperal woman appears to be definitely more susceptible to scarlet fever than is the pregnant woman. Diddle, Trussell and Plass report an incidence of clinical scarlet fever of 1:140 in antepartum patients, 1:14 in puerperal patients and 1:83 among attendants in their hospital in a recent scarlet fever epidemic in Iowa.

It is generally stated that infection may occur in the usual manner, as well as by the entrance of the specific infecting agent through wounds about the genitalia. The belief in the possibility of the latter eventuality was based upon the supposition that the rash occasionally appears first in the neighborhood of the vulva, and thence spreads to other portions of the body. Moreover, the frequent association of pelvic inflammatory troubles, and the occasional localization of diphtheritic patches in the vulva or vagina, instead of in the throat, were advanced in support of this view. Modern bacteriologic investigation, however, has destroyed the force of this last argument, since it has shown that a specific hemolytic streptococcus is chiefly concerned in the causation of scarlet fever, and thereby makes it more difficult to distinguish symptoms due to frank puerperal infection and those due to scarlet fever.

In frank cases the diagnosis is readily made from the existence of a characteristic rash, which is later followed by desquamation. Moreover, the strawberry tongue, the development of pseudodiphtheritic patches in the pharynx, the appearance of albumin in the urine, together with a history of exposure to possible contagion, usually remove all doubt. On the other hand, in the absence of characteristic manifestations, a differential diagnosis cannot be made even when a distinct history of exposure to contagion can be elicited.

The advent of chemotherapy has revolutionized the prognosis of scarlet fever and with the prompt institution of modern methods of treatment the outlook is favorable.

Postpartum Pituitary Necrosis. In patients who have suffered profound shock at the time of delivery, the anterior lobe of the pituitary body may occasionally sustain such a degree of anoxia that necrosis ensues. Sheehan and Murdoch, in a follow-up of 128 patients who had experienced shock at delivery, found symptoms suggesting pituitary insufficiency in 41. The general picture is one of hypogonadism, hypothyroidism and anemia. The condition is rare in our experience, but is said to be resistant to treatment, death usually occurring from some intercurrent infection.

BIBLIOGRAPHY

Berkley. The Insanities of the Puerperal Period. A Treatise on Mental Diseases, 1900, pp. 307-328.

Bunzel, E. E. Pulmonary Embolism Complicating Pregnancy, Labor and the Puerperium. Am. J. Obst. & Gynec., 1927, 13:584.

Burckhard, G. Gangrän der unteren Extremitäten in Wochenbette. Zentralbl. f. Gynäk., 1900, 24:1381.

Diddle, A. W., Trussell, R. E., and Plass, E. D. Scarlet Fever in Obstetrics. Am. J. Obst. & Gynec., 1940, 39:608.

Dippel, A. L., and Johnston, R. A. Suppurative Mastitis as a Complication of Pregnancy and the Puerperium. Am. J. Obst. & Gynec., 1935, 29:258.

Döderlein. Die Atrophia uteri. Veit's Handbuch der Gynec., 1897, Bd. II, 391.

Frankl, O. Ueber Spät-blutungen postpartum et abortum. Arch. f. Gynäk., 1927, 129:87.

Goldberger, H. Ein Seltener Fall von Polymastic. Arch. f. Gynäk., 1895, 49:272.

Hesseltine, H. C., Freundlich, C. G., and Hite, K. E. Acute Puerperal Mastitis. Clinical and Bacteriologic Studies in Relation to Penicillin Therapy. Am. J. Obst. & Gynec., 1948, 55:778.

Hosslin, R. Ueber periphere Schwangerschaftslähmungen. München med. Wchnschr., 1905, Nr. 14.

Hünermann. Ueber Nervenlähmung im Gebiete des Nervus ischiadicus infolge von Entbindungen. Arch. f. Gynäk., 1900, 42:489.

Jones, R. Puerperal Insanity. J. Obst. & Gynaec. Brit. Emp., 1906, 3:109.

Nygarrd, K. K. Pulmonary Emboli. Proc. Staff Meet. Mayo Clin., 1938, 13:586.

Prather, G. E. Postpartum Bladder Complications. Am. J. Obst. & Gynec., 1929, 17:215.

Rutherford, R. N. Postpartum Breast Comfort Achieved by Sex Hormone Therapy. West. J. Surg., 1942, 50:282.

Saunders, E. B. Association of Psychoses with the Puerperium. Am. J. Psychiat., 1929, 8:669.

Schwarz, O. H. The Pathology of Chronic Metritis and Subinvolution. Am. J. Obst. & Gynec., 1919, 79:63.

Sheehan, H. L. Simmond's Disease due to Postpartum Necrosis of Anterior Pituitary. J. Obst. & Gynaec. Brit. Emp., 1943, 50:27.

——— and Murdoch, R. Postpartum Necrosis of Anterior Pituitary; Pathological and Clinical Aspects. J. Obst. & Gynaec. Brit. Emp., 1938, 45:456.

Smith, R. F. The Subinvoluted Uterus. Surg., Gynec. & Obst., 1910, 10:17.

Thomas, H. M. Obstetrical Paralysis, Infantile and Maternal. Bull. Johns Hopkins Hosp., 1900, 11:279.

Williams, J. W. Subperitoneal Hematoma Following Labor, Not Associated with Lesions of the Uterus. Tr. Am. Gynec., 1904, 29:186.

Wolfe, S. A., and Pedowitz, P. Late Postpartum Hemorrhage. Am. J. Obst. & Gynec., 1947, 53:84.

Wormser. Nochmals zur puerperalen Gangrän der unteren Extremitäten. Zentralbl. f. Gynäk., 1901, 25:110.

Section Nine: ABNORMALITIES OF THE NEWBORN

37

INJURIES SUSTAINED BY THE INFANT DURING LABOR

Various types of injury may be sustained by the infant in the course of labor and delivery. These may be grouped as follows:

1. Central nervous system injuries
    1. Narcosis
    2. Anoxia
    3. Cerebral hemorrhage
2. Peripheral injuries
    1. Cephalhematoma
    2. Trauma to peripheral nerves
    3. Skeletal fractures
    4. Trauma to soft parts

CENTRAL NERVOUS SYSTEM INJURIES

Apnea Neonatorum, the Sign Common to All Central Nervous System Injuries. With the exception of prematurity central nervous system injuries are by far the most common cause of stillbirth and neonatal death. The three causes of such injuries, narcosis, anoxia and brain hemorrhage, have in common the fact that the clinical picture they present in the newborn, at least during the first few minutes of life, is very similar and is characterized chiefly by apnea. Such babies, who do not breathe at birth, are usually referred to as being "asphyxiated" and the term "asphyxia neonatorum" is deeply rooted in the literature and in common parlance. Although questions of nomenclature are usually of academic interest only, occasionally a term is encountered which is so inept that it leads to incorrect thinking and an erroneous concept of the condition designated. Deeply entrenched as "asphyxia neonatorum" is in obstetric terminology, there is no reason to believe that it belongs in this unhappy category.

Few words have undergone such radical changes in meaning as *asphyxia*. The term comes from the Greek ἀσφυξία (ἀ, not + σφύζειν, to throb) and means literally absence of pulsation. It was used in this sense by Galen to describe the state of an artery distal to a tourniquet and, as late as the eighteenth century, seems to have carried no other meaning. Thus, in 1706 Phillips described asphyxia as "a cessation of the pulse throughout the whole body; which is the highest degree of Swooning and next to Death"; while Quincy in his *New Medical Dictionary*, published in 1730, defined the term as a "deficiency or privation of the pulse in some cases where it stops for a time." By 1778 the word was being used in a broader sense to convey the idea of apparent death, as from drowning, and in that year an essay by T. Brandt carried the title, "The Cure of Asphyxia, or Apparent Death by Drowning." In a later edition of Quincy's dictionary published in 1794, the earlier definition is entirely deleted and in its place we read that asphyxia "happens from a long failure of vital and animal power, as from drowning." With the beginning of the nineteenth century the import of the word centered more and more on the suffocation which results from drowning, and at the same time its connotation became extended to include suffocation from other causes, such as strangulation and noxious gases. This meaning, of course, has persisted to the present; but when it is recalled that the pulse in asphyxiated animals continues to beat long after all signs of respiratory action have ceased, it becomes apparent that our word *asphyxia* represents a most curious infelicity of etymology.

From a practical viewpoint a much more important objection to the term is the fact that obstetricians have taken further liberties with it and customarily refer to any baby who does not breathe at birth as "asphyxiated," whether the cause be lack of oxygen, cerebral hemorrhage, congenital defect or whatnot. This use of one etiologic condition to denote the whole syndrome of apnea at birth, from whatever cause, is not only illogical but disregards some of the most important etiologic factors. It ignores one of the gravest causes of apnea, birth trauma, as well as the commonest cause of *temporary* apnea in modern practice, namely, narcosis. Moreover, by focusing attention solely on the acute anoxic episode at birth, it tends to circumscribe unduly the scope of the problem.

In view of these facts, the simple term *apnea neonatorum,* which is merely descriptive and carries no implication in regard to etiology, seems preferable to the older designation. The use of the word *asphyxia* could then be restricted to those cases in which apnea was actually due to lack of oxygen as in, for instance, prolapse of the umbilical cord and premature separation of the placenta.

Narcosis. Although rarely the sole cause of death in full-term newborn infants, drugs given to the mother are frequently responsible for temporary apnea at birth and may occasionally account for the death of a premature child, as emphasized in the chapter on Analgesia and Anesthesia. In the well-known investigations by Irving and his associates, it was found that infants born of mothers who had received neither analgesic nor anesthetic drugs breathe immediately after birth in 98.1 per cent of the cases. On the other hand, in a series of 800 women who received barbiturate analgesia (sodium amytal or sodium pentobarbital) together with scopolamine, rectal ether or paraldehyde, it was discovered that only 50 to 65 per cent of the infants breathed immediately. It is well known that barbiturates pass within 15 minutes from mother to fetus and clinical experience shows that these drugs used as analgesics in labor retard the initiation of respiration at birth in about one half of the cases. This deleterious action on fetal respiration has been emphasized especially by Snyder who has shown that all sedative drugs inhibit intra-uterine respiration in experimental animals although the dosage may be so small as to have no effect whatsoever on the maternal respiration. As already indicated, the administration of such drugs to mothers in premature labor may prove the determining factor in the life or death of the infant. In a statistical study of the records of 304 premature infants, Clifford found that the intrapartum administration of morphine within one and one-half hours of delivery was found to be associated in every instance with the death of that infant. With the increasing use of terminal spinal anesthesia for delivery, it is becoming increasingly apparent that these sedative drugs are most likely to produce apnea neonatorum when a general anesthetic is superimposed upon them for delivery. Babies who are born of mothers under spinal anesthesia, although barbiturates may have been given previously for analgesia, usually breathe as well at birth as when no form of anesthesia or analgesia is administered.

Apnea neonatorum resulting from narcosis is usually transient, rarely lasting more than one minute. The babies are of good color and their muscle tone is normal. As will be described subsequently the treatment is the same as in apnea due to graver causes because it is never possible to be certain that narcosis is the only etiologic factor involved.

Anoxia. Lack of oxygen kills tissues as quickly as many active poisons and lack of oxygen during the birth process, sometimes acting alone and sometimes in conjunction with cerebral hemorrhage, is a common cause of fetal death and a much graver threat to the infant than is narcosis. The most obvious example of this condition is prolapse of the umbilical cord with impingement of the cord between the presenting part and pelvic brim; another is abruptio placentae; while still another is fluctuations in the maternal blood pressure; a more common cause of oxygen want during labor is abnormality of the uterine contractions, either in length or intensity, so that placental interchange is impaired.

If blood oxygen studies are made on umbilical vein blood taken immediately after birth, it will be found that the severer degrees of apnea (over two minutes) are usually consequent to profound depletion of oxygen at the moment of delivery. Whereas the normal oxygen saturation of the arterial blood of the fetus at birth is approximately 50 per cent, in the severer degrees of apnea neonatorum the blood oxygen is reduced to levels which represent only one fifth or even one tenth of this value. That such low concentrations of oxygen are insufficient for fetal needs is clearly shown by the fact that the blood of these infants taken at birth shows also high lactic acid, and a pH of such a low level as to be scarcely compatible with life. Partly because of an alkali deficit due to fixation of base by lactic acid and partly due to a primary carbon dioxide excess as the result of inadequate diffusion of this gas from fetus to mother, the tension or partial pressure of free carbon dioxide rises to levels far in excess of normal. While these changes in the lactic acid, pH and carbon dioxide tension of the blood are striking, it should be noted that they are purely secondary and that the primary blood chemical change in most cases of severe apnea neonatorum is an extreme reduction in the oxygen content of the infant's blood.

In addition to apnea, babies suffering from anoxia exhibit evidence of damage in the color of their skin, in their muscle tonus and in heart rate. In milder cases they are bluish in color; while in the graver examples of the condition, they are white, the "asphyxia livida" and the "asphyxia pallida" of the older writers. In the presence of any significant degree of anoxia the muscle tone is weak and in severe cases the infants are utterly limp. A very slow heart beat is a characteristic finding, the rate often being under 50 per minute. The bradycardia responds dramatically to oxygen insufflations even in cases in which the ultimate termination is unfavorable. Because anoxia causes the rectal sphincter to relax, these infants are often covered with meconium.

Since minor degrees of oxygen want increase the rate of respiration, it is often forgotten that profound levels of anoxemia (such as we have just described) invariably produce the opposite effect, namely, absence of respiration. And it is seldom recalled in viewing a grave case of asphyxia at birth, with the slow heart rate, the cold, white body covered with meconium, and the limp extremities, how precisely the clinical picture duplicates the reaction of any organism to anoxemia. In experimental animals, as well as in man, anoxemia has been the object of intensive study for over half a century. But, whether we consider the studies of Klug of Germany in 1883, or Lewis and Mathison of London in 1910, or of Greene and Gilbert of the United States in recent years, the results are the same; on few subjects has there been such complete agreement, for experimental anoxemia produces a constant, clear-cut train of phenomena which may be reduplicated in the laboratory at will.

The sequence of events in experimental anoxia may be described as follows. To mild degrees of anoxemia the body reacts by increased respiration and accelerated heart rate; these presumably are compensatory mechanisms, the first designed to bring more oxygen to the blood and the second to deliver more oxygen to the tissues. With increasing anoxemia a point is reached when these compensatory mechanisms fail to supply oxygen in amounts sufficient for cellular oxidation and then with dramatic suddenness, "the oxygen crisis" of

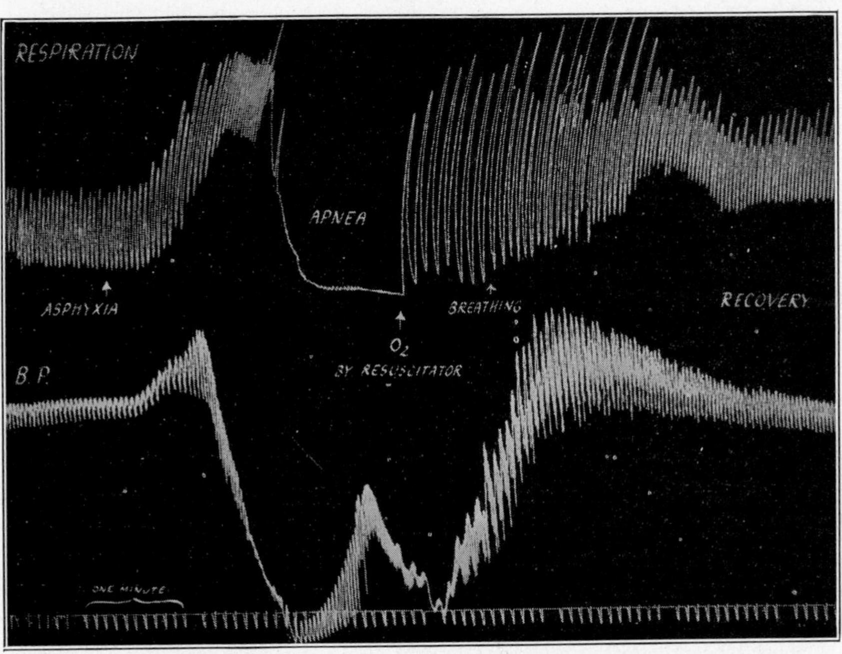

Fig. 517.—Experimental Apnea due to Anoxia Produced by Substituting 100 per cent Helium for Air. See text. (Eastman and Kreiselman.)

the physiologists, or what is termed the "reversal" by Schmidt, takes place and after this events occur rapidly. Consciousness is lost and respirations stop. Following respiratory failure there is an interval of from three to five minutes during which the heart continues to beat; but there is a marked slowing of the rate. In a typical case the slowing occurs by abrupt steps from 156 per minute before the crisis to 44 per minute in the post-crisis phase. Electrocardiographic studies of the heart at this stage show suppression of the pace-making function of the sino-auricular node and the assumption of that function by the auricular-ventricular node with its characteristic slow and regular rate. There is regularly partial or complete heart block with decrease in conduction in the internodal region to the point of suppression. Since this slowing of the heart in anoxemia does not occur in animals with the vagi cut, it is apparently due to vagospasm which suppresses the sino-auricular rhythm. After respirations cease, sometimes a little earlier, the blood pressure slowly declines through 40 to 60 seconds. It then may show a slight increase, but finally falls rapidly through two to three minutes, then more slowly for one or two minutes until a systolic pressure of 15 to 20 mm. Hg is reached. Concomitant with the drop in blood pressure the skin becomes blanched and cold, as in shock. Early in the post-crisis phase of experimental anoxemia another important change occurs: the nerve muscle endings of skeletal muscle cease to function with complete collapse of that muscular system. This results, of course, not only in flaccid extremities but in relaxation of the sphincter ani. Finally, it may be noted that a few whiffs of oxygen or air, administered by artificial respiration, restore the animal at once to normal provided this is done within three or four minutes following the oxygen crisis. To summarize the picture of experimental anoxemia in the post-crisis phase, there occur in rapid succession loss of consciousness, cessation of respiration, marked slowing of the heart, fall in blood pressure with the white, cold skin of shock, and skeletal muscle collapse causing general flaccidity of the extremities together with relaxation of the sphincter ani. Few clinical conditions can be simulated so completely as can asphyxia neonatorum by experimental anoxemia.

The experimental as well as the blood chemical evidence thus attests the fact that profound anoxemia regularly produces a condition very similar to that which obstetricians have long called "asphyxia pallida" in contradistinction to "asphyxia livida." These two terms occupy an old and honored place in the literature but underlying etiology is seldom discussed. Cruickshank, in his exhaustive survey, "The Cause of Neonatal Death," published in 1930, considers that "the essential difference between these two forms is that in the livid one the child may be regarded as having died of suffocation, while in the pallid form death is the result of shock. The distinction between the two forms," he continues, "is not an absolute one, however, and many cases of a combined or intermediate kind are found." This belief that "asphyxia pallida" is the result of shock is widespread and particularly the associated conception that it is due to brain hemorrhage. In the last analysis the latter view is doubtless correct since cases of cerebral hemorrhage show a similar, if not the same, syndrome. But so clear-cut is the role of anoxemia in producing the whole picture experimentally that it seems reasonable to believe that cerebral hemorrhage causes the condition through the intermediary action of anoxemia, or at least anoxia of the respiratory center. This may occur in two ways. In the first place, brain hemorrhage may produce such anoxia by arresting the cerebral circulation through generally increased intracranial pressure; in the second place, the direct pressure of free blood on the circulatory centers of the medulla oblongata may effect such a slowing of the umbilical circulation that marked anoxemia and consequent anoxia of all tissues is caused. Accordingly, it is suggested that "asphyxia pallida" is always an example of profound oxygen want, particularly of the respiratory center. To recapitulate, in some cases this is brought about by anoxemia alone as the result of some interference with the supply of oxygen from the placenta; in other instances it is caused by anoxemia due to sluggish flow of the fetal blood consequent to pressure of cerebral hemorrhage on the circulatory centers; and in still other cases the oxygen lack results from arrested cerebral blood flow secondary to generally increased intracranial pressure. What then is "asphyxia livida"? Blood oxygen studies carried out on actual cases of this disorder indicate that it is characterized by a considerable degree of anoxemia but one which is much less pronounced than that met in "asphyxia pallida." Accordingly, in my opinion, "asphyxia livida" represents a stage in the development of the pallid form. This would seem the more probable when it is recalled that in experimental anoxemia there occurs a brief moment after respiration ceases, but before the blood pressure falls, when the picture is that of "asphyxia livida." This explanation would explain the greater frequency of the livid form as well as its better prognosis.

The Vernix Membrane. It is believed that a significant number of anoxic neonatal deaths are caused by vernix caseosa plugging the bronchioles and lining the alveolar ducts and walls. The sequence of events which produce the phenomenon is described as follows: (1) intra-uterine anoxia stimulating deep respiratory movements on the part of the fetus, (2) aspiration of amniotic fluid containing dissolved vernix caseosa and epidermal cells, and (3) the subsequent deposition of a viscous layer of the aspirated material on the mucous membranes of the lower respiratory tract. When sections of the lungs are stained with hematoxylin and eosin, the membrane stains a clear pink and for this reason it is sometimes called also the "hyaline membrane." The membrane stains readily for fat.

In 119 consecutive autopsies on newborn infants, Dick and Pund encountered the condition in seven cases, or in 5.8 per cent. It seems to be somewhat more frequent following delivery by cesarean section. The vernix membrane is associated with a rather characteristic clinical picture. The babies may breathe normally or be slow to breathe at birth, but within the first day or two of life, there develops an increasing struggle for breath, presumably owing to the fact that the membrane is preventing adequate interchange of gases through the alveolar walls.

There are many questions about the vernix membrane which remain to be answered. Thus, the phenomenon is at variance with the concept of physiologic intra-uterine respiratory activity, unless the depth of the respiratory movements is the determining factor. It is not at variance with the trend of events in experimental anoxia, as described above; the apnea of experimental anoxia is immediately preceded by violent respiratory efforts. Some investigators even question the mechanism of formation of the vernix membrane, as just outlined. Hence, the condition is something of an enigma and constitutes a fertile field for research.

Cerebral Hemorrhage. The head of the fetus may sustain considerable molding (configuration) during its passage through the birth canal. Such molding is usually more marked in prolonged and difficult labors, especially when the pelvis is contracted. The shape of the head becomes altered with a considerable lengthening of the occipitofrontal and saggital diameters of the skull, so that stretching and even laceration of the tentorium cerebelli and less often of the falx cerebri may take place. Such injury is not uncommon following delivery by breech extraction, when the unmolded head is brought through the pelvis. Thus, no molding, as in breech, as well as marked molding in vertex presentations may be associated with intracranial injury. The skull bones, the dura mater and the brain itself permit considerable alteration in the dimensions of the fetal head without untoward results. This may be due in part to changes in the distribution of the cerebrospinal fluid. However, edema and hyperemia may occur in various parts of the brain with the development of fetal distress during labor, or asphyxia following delivery. Small petechial hemorrhages are not infrequently seen in the dura mater, especially along the skull sutures. Intracranial hemorrhages used to be encountered in 40 to 80 per cent of infants at autopsy but today is a less common cause of infant loss. The incidence of such hemorrhages is especially high in the premature child.

Injury to the tentorium and falx may be complicated by actual rupture of blood vessels, especially the great vein of Galen, which is most frequently involved, according to Ford, Crothers and Putnam, Potter, Monro and others; and infratentorial hemorrhage results in pressure on the vital centers of the medulla and pons. Subarachnoid hemorrhage may occur, while less frequently the cerebral veins, or the longitudinal, transverse or straight sinuses may be involved, should the skull be fractured.

Brain examination, by means of the window technic introduced by Benecke, has advanced materially our knowledge of the pathology of these lesions. According to Green, intracranial hemorrhage is sometimes the first indication of a hemorrhagic diathesis. This observation finds support in the high incidence of hemorrhagic disease in infants suffering from intracranial hemorrhage (19 to 44 per cent), as reported by Dembo, Warwick and Salomonsen.

The symptoms are variable and include drowsiness, apathy, feeble cry, pallor, failure to nurse, dyspnea, cyanosis, vomiting and convulsions. Atelectasis and asphyxia neonatorum and forceps abrasions on the face may be associated findings. In order to rule out diaphragmatic hernia, congenital heart disease, atelectasis and pneumonia, roentgenologic examination of the chest is desirable.

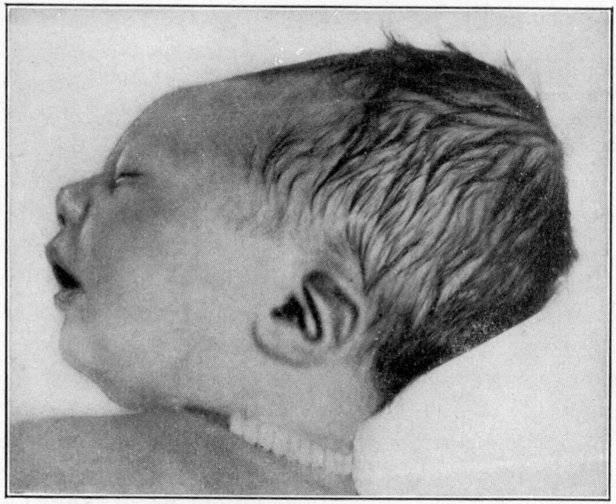

FIG. 518.—MOLDING OF HEAD, NEWBORN CHILD.

Treatment consists of sedation, supportive measures, and oxygen for the dyspnea and cyanosis. If the anterior fontanel is bulging, a lumbar puncture is indicated in order to relieve pressure. The intramuscular administration of vitamin K is always indicated, because in many of these cases slow oozing of blood from the ruptured vessel continues for several days and hence optimum coagulability of the blood is essential if the process is to be checked.

Prevention of this condition is of utmost importance since cerebral hemorrhage ranks with asphyxia neonatorum and prematurity as a cause of stillbirths and neonatal deaths, with a mortality rate of 50 per cent, according to most writers. The surviving infants may subsequently develop motor disturbances, while about 10 per cent of these infants have residual mental deficiency. It is also probable that certain cases of idiopathic epilepsy are due to intracranial injury sustained at birth. The proper indications for the forceps, as well as their correct application, the use of cesarean section when there is definite cephalo-pelvic disproportion, the correct management of breech delivery, and the limitation of internal version and extraction should contribute a great deal toward a reduction in the incidence of all birth injuries and especially intracranial hemorrhage.

Diagnosis. The importance of watching for manifestations pointing to threatened *intra-uterine anoxia* cannot be overestimated, inasmuch as *fetal distress* frequently affords the indication for operative delivery, without which the life of the child is inevitably lost.

The most characteristic sign is afforded by changes in the *fetal pulse rate.* At first, as a result of momentary compression of the brain or interference with the placental circulation, it becomes slower with each uterine contraction, but regains its normal frequency in the intervals between the pains. As the condition becomes more serious the remissions fail to occur and the pulse becomes slower and slower and eventually the heart ceases to beat. For practical purposes it is well to assume that a pulse rate of 100 or less for any great length of time is incompatible with life of the fetus, and under such circumstances delivery is indicated, provided it can be accomplished without risk to the mother. A rapid fetal heart rate, over 160, is not itself an indication of fetal distress; but when associated with alternate periods of bradycardia, anoxia is indicated according to the degree and duration of the slowing. Such rules, however, have only an approximate value and Baumm has pointed out their limitations stating that the fetal pulse may retain its normal rate notwithstanding the existence of severe intracranial hemorrhage, while in other cases, in which delivery has been effected on account of a very slow heart beat, the child may present no sign of asphyxia or of any other abnormality. Notwithstanding these generally recognized limitations the fetal heart rate constitutes the most available means of obtaining information concerning the condition of the child, and should be counted every hour or two during the first stage of labor, and at intervals of five to ten minutes during the second stage. To neglect of this latter precaution can be attributed the death of many children who otherwise could have been saved.

In vertex presentations another characteristic sign of impending asphyxia is the escape of *meconium.* This is due to relaxation of the sphincter ani muscle induced by faulty aeration of the blood. Accordingly, whenever the amniotic fluid presents a yellowish-green appearance and contains flakes of meconium, we may suspect that the child is in distress. In itself this sign is not an indication for delivery but demands very close watching of the fetal heart rate. In breech presentations, of course, this sign is without significance, as it is a purely mechanical result of pressure applied to the abdomen of the fetus.

Especially in difficult breech extractions, when delay is experienced in delivering the head, signs of anoxia may appear in a child which was apparently in excellent condition before the operation. In such circumstances the finger in the child's mouth can readily appreciate the fact that vigorous inspiratory movements are being made. A similar phenomenon may occasionally be observed in vertex presentations, when the head is arrested on the pelvic floor, the movements of the mouth being felt or seen through the thinned-out perineum.

Very exceptionally the child may not only make inspiratory efforts, but actually give utterance to sounds in utero, *vagitus uterinus.* For the production of this phenomenon it is essential that air gain access to the fetus, its entrance into the uterus sometimes resulting from the introduction of the hand or instruments. A very characteristic example of this phenomenon has been recorded by Ryder, who has summarized the reported cases, now totaling 123.

Apnea neonatorum due to anoxia and that due to cerebral hemorrhage present an identical clinical picture not only during the first few minutes of life but often for many hours and even days. This is attributable to the fact, as mentioned, that cerebral hemorrhage itself produces anoxia through interfering with the fetal circulation and thus preventing proper oxygenation of the blood in the placenta. Since, conversely, anoxia is a common cause of small cerebral hemorrhage, the situation is avowedly a complicated one and it is often difficult to determine positively the primary cause of the apnea in a given case unless it comes to autopsy. However this may be, from a practical viewpoint, the most important fact to bear in mind is that

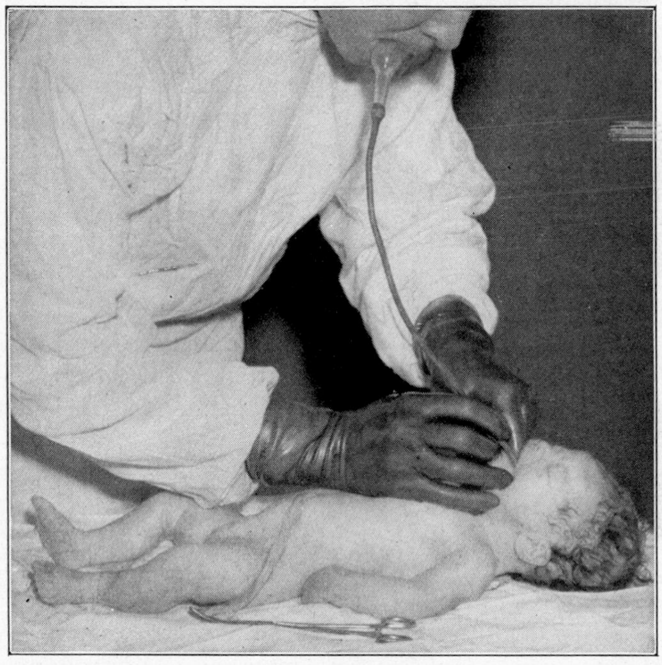

FIG. 519.—ASPIRATION OF PHARYNGEAL SECRETIONS PREPARATORY TO INSUFFLATION WITH OXYGEN IF NECESSARY.

most apneic babies are *anoxic*. As will be discussed presently, this is the dominant consideration in the treatment of the condition.

Treatment. In the presence of anoxia, apnea is resistant to all types of treatment other than correction of the anoxia itself. In a study of experimental anoxia by Kreiselman and myself, even convulsive doses of alpha-lobeline, metrazol and coramine, whether injected intravenously or directly into the carotid artery, were found to have no effect whatsoever on anoxic apnea; on the other hand, a few insufflations with oxygen produced immediate breathing. In other words, there is only one way in which respiration can be initiated when suppressed by anoxia and that is by the administration of oxygen or air. Insufflation with 100 per cent oxygen, therefore, transcends all else in the treatment of apnea at birth. Attempts to stimulate respiration by adding carbon dioxide to the oxygen are not only futile (because all forms of stimulation are futile in the presence of anoxia), but may even be dangerous since these babies are already overloaded with carbon dioxide; the first objection applies also to the drugs mentioned above.

The main desiderata in the treatment of apnea at birth would seem to be four in number: (1) *Warmth.* These babies are in a state of vascular collapse and should be treated as is any patient in shock. (2) *Posture.* The head should be declined about 30 degrees to favor gravity drainage of fluids in the trachea, but should not be placed so directly downward as to augment a preexisting cerebral hemorrhage. (3) *Aspiration of mucus.* Clear air passages are essential, and mucus must be removed by means of a catheter, employing either mouth suction or an electric aspirator. Intratracheal aspiration is rarely necessary and is not without hazard, moreover, since it predisposes to laryngeal edema. (4) *Delivery of 100 per cent oxygen to the pulmonary alveoli,* by an adequate apparatus is desirable, but mouth-to-mouth insufflation, provided it is done gently (never over 20 cm. of water pressure), is usually a satisfactory substitute. Other forms of artificial respiration such as jack-knifing the infant and manual compression of the thorax may be dangerous. Indeed, we have seen two fatal cases of rupture of the liver in newborn attributable to the jack-knifing procedure.

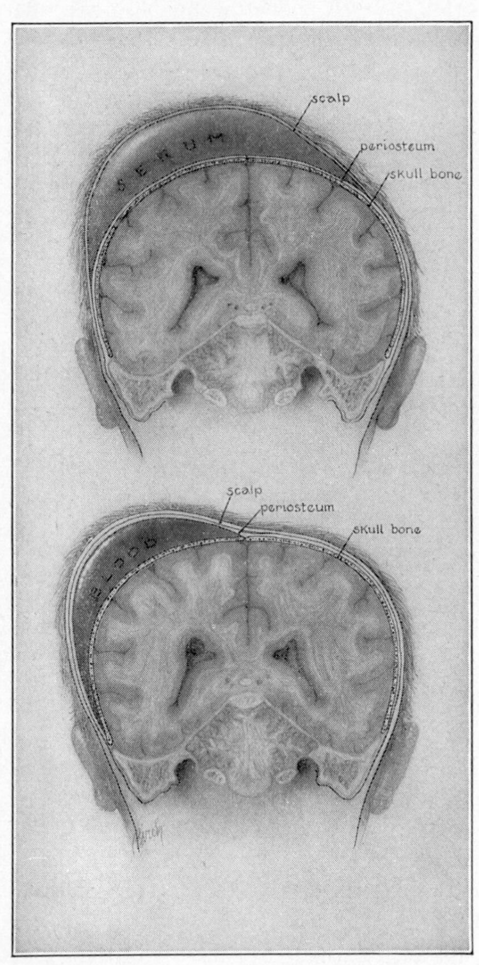

Fig. 520.—Diagrammatic Sketch to Illustrate Difference between Caput Succedaneum (above) and Cephalhematoma (below).

In a caput succedaneum the effusion overlies the periosteum and consists of serum; in a cephalhematoma it lies under the periosteum and consists of blood.

PERIPHERAL INJURIES

Cephalhematoma. Subperiosteal hemorrhages, when present, are usually found over one or both parietal bones with gradual increase in size during the first week of life. This lesion is differentiated from caput succedaneum by having periosteal limitations, with a definite palpable edge. Furthermore, it may not appear for hours or days after delivery, often grows larger and disappears after weeks or months while caput succedaneum is present at birth, grows smaller and disappears usually within a few hours. A cephalhematoma is due to injury to the periosteum of the skull during labor or delivery. No special treatment is required as this soft, nonpulsating, parchment-like tumor invariably disappears spontaneously, sometimes with antecedent calcification.

Spinal Column Injury. Overstretching of the spinal cord and associated hemorrhage may follow undue traction during a breech delivery, and actual fracture or dislocation of the vertebrae may occur. Complete data on such lesions are lacking, since even the most scrupulous autopsy does not always include examination of the spinal column. Pierson has reported spinal hemorrhages in nearly half of his autopsy material on infants delivered by breech extraction (Fig. 521). Injuries of the spinal cord are discussed in greater detail under "Obstetrical Paralyses."

Obstetrical Paralyses. As a result of a difficult labor, and exceptionally after an easy one, the child is sometimes born presenting an affection of the arm which is commonly known as *Duchenne's*, or *Erb's paralysis*. In this form, paralysis of the deltoid, infraspinatus, and the flexor muscles of the forearm causes the entire arm to fall close to the side of the body, and at the same time to rotate inward, while the forearm becomes extended upon the arm. The motility of the fingers is usually retained.

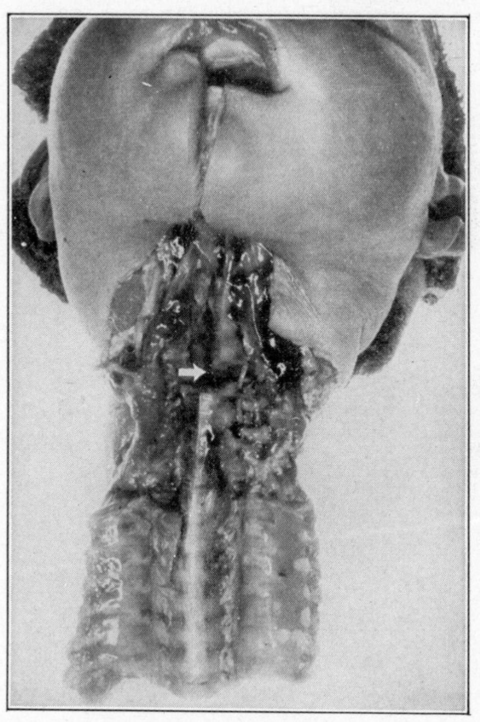

Fig. 521.—Fracture of Cervical Vertebra following Breech Extraction.

Erb pointed out that such a paralysis could be due only to a lesion involving the fifth and sixth roots of the brachial plexus, and showed that electrical stimulation at a point from 2 to 3 cm. above the clavicle and in front of the transverse process of the sixth cervical vertebra, now known as Erb's point, produces contractions of the muscles involved. He considered that the paralysis frequently followed compression of the plexus by the clavicle in the Prague method of extraction more particularly when the arms have become extended over the head, while in other cases it is due to traction with the fingers in the axilla of the child, and occasionally to the use of forceps. On the other hand, the experiments of Stolper show that the plexus cannot possibly be compressed by the tips of the forceps so long as the child presents by the vertex, although it may occur in face or brow presentations.

Carter in 1893 was the first to direct attention to the fact that the condition is due to stretching or tearing of the upper roots of the brachial plexus more frequently than to abnormal pressure. His results were confirmed by the experimental work of Fieux, Schumaker, and Stolper, all of whom demonstrated that the plexus was readily subjected to extreme tension as a result of pulling obliquely upon the head, thus sharply flexing it toward one or other shoulder. As traction in this direction is frequently employed in order to effect delivery of the shoulders in normal vertex presentations, it is readily seen that Duchenne's paralysis may follow spontaneous labor, and thus be in no way due to violence on the part of the obstetrician. In view of these considerations, therefore, in extracting the shoulders care should be taken not to bring about too great lateral flexion of the neck. Moreover, in breech extractions the

Prague maneuver should be employed only when absolutely necessary, and particular attention should be devoted to preventing the extension of the arms over the head, as it not only materially complicates delivery, but adds considerably to the danger of paralysis.

The prognosis is usually fair, many of the children recovering. Occasionally, however, a case may resist all treatment and the arm may remain permanently paralyzed. All of the instances which we have personally observed ended in recovery, but in some of them prolonged treatment was necessary. In this form of paralysis the child should be promptly put under the care of a competent orthopedic surgeon, as the intelligent use of postural treatment will insure a useful arm, even if degenerative changes occur in the nerves and muscles.

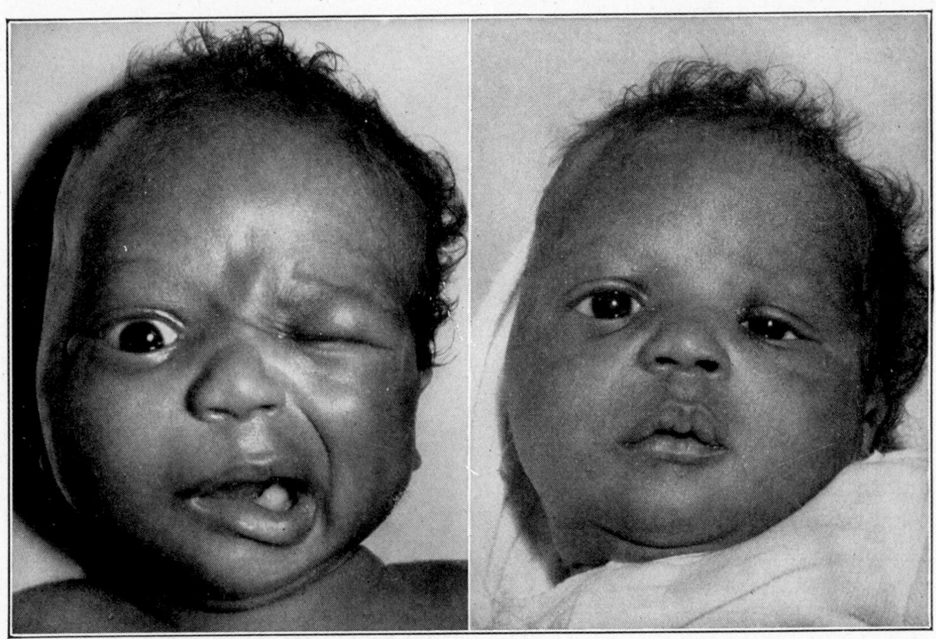

Fig. 522A. Fig. 522B.

Fig. 522A.—Paralysis of Right Side of Face 15 Minutes after Forceps Delivery.

Fig. 522B.—Same Infant 24 Hours Later; Recovery Was Complete in Another 24 Hours (J.H.H. 296226).

In 1925 Ford considered in detail the paralyses which may follow cerebral injury at the time of labor, and in the following year Crothers and Putnam studied those following injuries to the spinal cord. The former pointed out that there is no evidence that Little's palsy, or diplegia, follows birth injury, and that while cerebral damage is a frequent cause of fetal death within the first few days following delivery, it is only rarely concerned in such children as survive. Crothers and Putnam, on the other hand, showed very clearly that damage to the cord is a common cause of all sorts of infantile palsy, and is particularly prone to follow difficult breech extractions. In this country their publication has served a very useful purpose, and has impressed upon obstetricians the necessity for not employing undue force in the delivery of children presenting by the breech.

Occasionally the child may be born with *facial paralysis,* or the condition may develop shortly after birth. This is usually noted when the head has been seized obliquely, and is due to the pressure exerted by the posterior blade of the forceps upon the neighborhood of the stylomastoid foramen, through which the nerve leaves the skull. Not every facial paralysis, however, following delivery by forceps should be attributed to the operation as such a condition is occasionally encountered after a spontaneous labor, and may be due to intracranial causes quite independent of the use of instruments.

Skeletal Fractures. Fractures of the clavicle and those of the humerus are found with about the same frequency. Difficulty encountered in the delivery of the shoulders in vertex presentations and extended arms in breech are the main factors in the production of such fractures. These are often of the greenstick type, although complete fracture with overriding of the bones is occasionally seen. Routine palpation of the clavicles and long bones should be performed on all newborn infants, and any crepitation or undue irregularity should be investigated by means of the roentgenogram.

Treatment of the clavicular fracture is simple, consisting of abduction of the arm, with outward and backward rotation. This position can be maintained by fastening the garment of the forearm to the bassinette above the child's head. The fractured humerus is maintained in a hand on hip position by means of a triangular splint, which maintains the arm in adduction, and the application of a Velpeau bandage, for further immobilization.

The fractured femur is relatively uncommon and is usually associated with breech delivery. It may be treated satisfactorily by extension of the leg and flexion of the thigh on the abdomen, this position being maintained by traction in an upward direction, as provided in a Bradford frame. Adhesive tape is used to attach the pulley and weight mechanism to the skin of the legs and thighs. Unilateral fractures are treated as if they were bilateral, that is, traction is applied to both legs.

Muscular Injuries. Hemorrhage into the sternocleidomastoid muscle is the commonest variety, and consists of an extravasation into the muscle where it is limited by the fascial sheath. It is caused by excessive rotation of the head during delivery. A visible neck swelling develops and the child holds the head toward the affected side. Spontaneous regression occurs in a few weeks. Erroneously, this condition was once regarded as a frequent cause of "wry neck."

BIBLIOGRAPHY

Clifford, S. H. A Consideration of the Obstetrical Management of Premature Labor. New England J. Med., 1934, 210, 570.

Cruickshank, J. N. Child Life Investigations. The Causes of Neo-natal Death. Medical Research Council, London, 1930.

Dembo, L. H. An Analysis of 55 Cases of Hemorrhage in the Newborn. Am. J. Obst. & Gynec., 1933, 25:587.

Dick, F., Jr., and Pund, E. R. Asphyxia Neonatorum and the Vernix Membrane. Arch. Path., 1949, 47:307.

Eastman, N. J. Fetal Blood Studies. Bull. Johns Hopkins Hosp., 1930, 47:221; 1931, 48:261; 1932, 50:39.

——— Apnea Neonatorum. Am. J. Obst. & Gynec., 1940, 40:647.

Eastman, N. J., and Kreiselman, J. Treatment of Experimental Anoxia with Certain Respiratory and Cardiac Stimulants. Am. J. Obst. & Gynec., 1941, 41:260.

Erede, U. Treatment of Apparent Death in Newborn Infants. J.A.M.A., 1941, 117:814.

Flagg, P. J. Treatment of Asphyxia in the New Born. J.A.M.A., 1928, 91:788.

Flagg, P. J. Treatment of Asphyxia Neonatorum. J. Maine M. A., 1940, 31:1.

Ford, Crothers, and Putnam. Birth Injuries of the Central Nervous System. Medicine Monographs, Vol. 11. Williams and Wilkins Co., Baltimore, 1924.

Greene, C. W., and Gilbert, N. C. Studies on the Responses of the Circulation to Low Oxygen Tension. Arch. Int. Med., 1921, 27:517; Am. J. Physiol., 1921, 55:307; 1921, 56:475; 1922, 60:155.

Gumbiner, B., and Cutler, M. M. Spontaneous Pneumomediastinum in the Newborn. J.A.M.A., 1941, 117:2050.

Gustafson, G. W., and Garceau, G. J. Cerebral Spastic Paralysis. J.A.M.A., 1941, 116:374.

Henderson, J. L. Hepatic Haemorrhage in Stillborn and Newborn Infants. A Clinical and Pathological Study of Forty-seven Cases. J. Obst. & Gynaec. Brit. Emp., 1941, 48:377.

Henderson, Y. The Prevention and Treatment of Asphyxia in the Newborn. J.A.M.A., 1928, 90:583-586.

——— Inhalation Method of Resuscitation from Asphyxia. Am. J. Obst. & Gynec., 1931, 21:542.

Holland, E. Birth Injury in Relation to Labor. Am. J. Obst. & Gynec., 1937, 33:1.

Huber, C. P., and Shrader, J. C. Blood Prothrombin Levels in the Newborn. Am. J. Obst. & Gynec., 1941, 41:566.

Irving, F. C., Berman, S., and Nelson, H. B. The Barbiturates and Other Hypnotics in Labor. Surg., Gynec. & Obst., 1934, 58:1.

Lund, C. J. The Recognition and Treatment of Fetal Heart Arrhythmias Due to Anoxia. Am. J. Obst. & Gynec., 1940, 40:946.

——— Prevention of Asphyxia Neonatorum. A Study of the Etiologic Factors Observed in 2,000 Consecutive Deliveries. Am. J. Obst. & Gynec., 1941, 41:934.

——— Fetal Tachycardia During Labor. A Fallible Sign of Fetal Distress. Am. J. Obst. & Gynec., 1943, 45:636.

McPhail, F. L., and Hall, E. L. A Consideration of the Cause and Possible Late Effect of Anoxia in the Newborn Infant. Am. J. Obst. & Gynec., 1941, 42:686.

Macpherson, A. I. S. Observations on the Aetiology and Prophylaxis of Prothrombin Deficiency and Haemorrhagic Disease in the New-born. J. Obst. & Gynaec. Brit. Emp., 1942, 49:368.

Mengert, W. F., and Longwell, F. H. Prolapse of the Umbilical Cord. Am. J. Obst. & Gynec., 1940, 40:79.

Moloy, H. C. Studies on Head Molding During Labor. Am. J. Obst. & Gynec., 1942., 44:762.

Parks, J., and Sweet, L. K. Does the Antenatal Use of Vitamin K Prevent Hemorrhage in the Newborn Infant? Am. J. Obst. & Gynec., 1942, 44:432.

Potter, E. L. The Lessons to Be Learned from a Study of Infant Deaths. J.A.M.A., 1944, 124:336.

——— and Adair, F. L. Clinical-Pathological Study of Infant and Fetal Mortality for a Ten-year Period at the Chicago Lying-In Hospital. Am. J. Obst. & Gynec., 1943, 45:1054.

Potter, E. L., and Bohlender, G. P. Intrauterine Respiration in Relation to Development of the Fetal Lung. Am. J. Obst. & Gynec., 1941, 42:14.

Potter, E. L., Sage, E. C., Torpin, R., and Tyson, R. M. Abstract of Discussion of Papers. J.A.M.A., 1944, 124:356.

Pray, L. G., McKeown, H. S., and Pollard, W. E. Hemorrhagic Diathesis of the Newborn; Effect of Vitamin K Prophylaxis and Therapy. Am. J. Obst. & Gynec., 1941, 42:836.

Reifferscheid, W., and Schmiemann, R. Roentgenological Studies of So-called Intrauterine Respiration of the Fetus. Int. Abst. Surg. (Surg., Gynec. & Obst.), 1940, 71:278.

Ryder, G. H. Vagitus Uterinus. Am. J. Obst. & Gynec., 1943, 46:867.

Sage, Earl C. The Care of the Parturient Woman in Relation to Neonatal Mortality. J.A.M.A., 1944, 124:339.

Schmidt, C. F. The Influence of Cerebral Blood-Flow on Respiration. Am. J. Physiol., 1928, 84:202.

Shock, N. W. Fetal Aspiration of Amniotic Fluid. Am. J. Physiol., 1941, 134:769.

Smith, C. A., and Barker, R. H. Ether in the Blood of the Newborn Infant. Am. J. Obst. & Gynec., 1942, 43:763.

Snyder, F. F. The Rate of Entrance of Amniotic Fluid into the Pulmonary Alveoli During Fetal Respiration. Am. J. Obst. & Gynec., 1941, 41:224.

——— Obstetric Analgesia and Anesthesia. W. B. Saunders Company, Philadelphia, 1949.

Sontag, L. W. The Significance of Fetal Environmental Differences. Am. J. Obst. & Gynec., 1941, 42:996.

——— and Newbery, H. Normal Variations of Fetal Heart Rate during Pregnancy. Am. J. Obst. & Gynec., 1940, 40:449.

Speert, Harold. Swallowing and Gastrointestinal Activity in the Fetal Monkey. Am. J. Obst. & Gynec., 1943, 45:69.

SPEERT, Harold. Placental Transmission of Sulfathiazole and Sulfadiazine and Its Significance for Fetal Chemotherapy. Am. J. Obst. & Gynec., 1943, 45:200.

THOMPSON, L. R. Resuscitation of the Newborn. Case Report. Am. J. Surg., 1942, 58:140.

TYSON, Ralph M. Immediate Care of the Newborn in Relation to Neonatal Mortality. J.A.M.A., 1944, 124:351.

WINDLE, W. F., and BECKER, R. F. Rôle of Carbon Dioxide in Resuscitation at Birth after Asphyxia and after Nembutal Anesthesia. An Experimental Study in the Cat and Guinea Pig. Am. J. Obst. & Gynec., 1941, 42:852.

——— Asphyxia Neonatorum. An Experimental Study in the Guinea Pig. Am. J. Obst. & Gynec., 1943, 45:183.

38

DISEASES AND MALFORMATIONS OF THE NEWBORN

PREMATURITY

Definitions. A premature infant is one which has been born so early in the course of gestation that its organs have not reached full development so that its chances of survival, although not entirely hopeless as in an abortion, are less good than those of an infant which has enjoyed a full period of intra-uterine growth. Various criteria have been suggested for determining categorically whether an infant is premature or not, such as its gestational age as calculated from the mother's last menstrual period, its length, its weight, and various combinations of these factors. Since menstrual histories are often indefinite or unreliable, estimations of gestational age on this basis are sometimes highly erroneous. Likewise, measurements of the length of the infant are not regularly dependable because of inaccuracies in mensuration. Accordingly, the weight of a premature baby is usually taken as the main index of its gestational age, at least for purposes of classification. There is general agreement that 2,500 gm. (5 pounds, 8 ounces) should mark the upper boundary of prematurity, that is, the borderline between a premature and a mature infant. The rationale of this figure lies in the fact that infants weighing more than 2,500 gm., as shown by the statistical studies of Peckham and others, are about as able to cope with extra-uterine conditions as are larger infants and enjoy an outlook for survival which is about as good. On the other hand, infants weighing less than 2,500 gm. (in the white race at least) face a diminished likelihood of survival which becomes more and more evident as the birth weight falls further and further short of 2,500 gm.

The lower limits of prematurity, that is, the borderline between a premature infant and what is usually called an "abortus," is less definitely established. There are several ways of viewing this problem. Since an abortus is defined as a nonviable conceptus, the borderline between an abortus and a premature infant may be considered to be that weight level below which survival is utterly impossible. This figure may logically be set at 400 gm. because, on the one hand, no fetus weighing less than this amount has ever been known to survive and, on the other hand, one fetus weighing 397 gm. on the second day of life (and doubtless slightly more than 400 gm. at birth) has survived, as reported by Monro. As shown in Fig. 523, a fetus weighing 400 gm. has a gestational age of approximately 20 weeks. From the viewpoint of convenience this fact affords another reason for adopting this figure, since both national and state departments of vital statistics demand the reporting of all births in which the period of gestation is in excess of 20 weeks. Twenty weeks, of course, marks the midpoint of the normal duration of pregnancy in the human, counting from the last menstrual period. On the basis of the above reasoning, a premature infant would be defined as one which weighs between 400 and 2,500 gm. at birth.

Although it is true that infants weighing less than 800 gm. have been known to survive, such occurrences are extremely rare, and, even in the weight group between

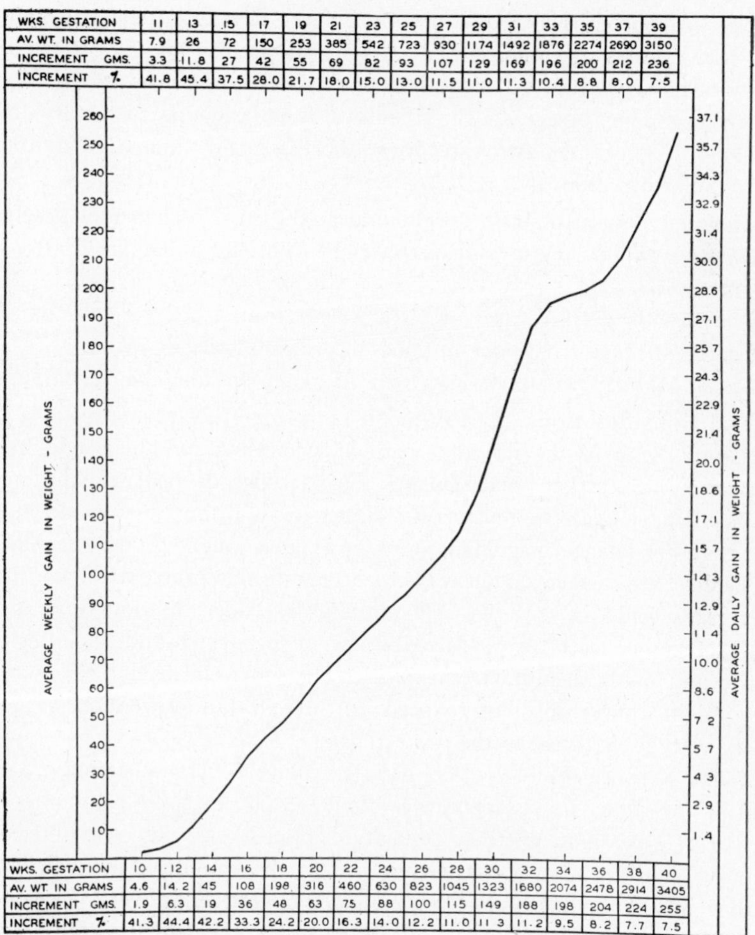

WKS. GESTATION	11	13	15	17	19	21	23	25	27	29	31	33	35	37	39
AV. WT. IN GRAMS	7.9	26	72	150	253	385	542	723	930	1174	1492	1876	2274	2690	3150
INCREMENT GMS.	3.3	11.8	27	42	55	69	82	93	107	129	169	196	200	212	236
INCREMENT %	41.8	45.4	37.5	28.0	21.7	18.0	15.0	13.0	11.5	11.0	11.3	10.4	8.8	8.0	7.5

WKS. GESTATION	10	12	14	16	18	20	22	24	26	28	30	32	34	36	38	40
AV. WT. IN GRAMS	4.6	14.2	45	108	198	316	460	630	823	1045	1323	1680	2074	2478	2914	3405
INCREMENT GMS.	1.9	6.3	19	36	48	63	75	88	100	115	149	188	198	204	224	255
INCREMENT %	41.3	44.4	42.2	33.3	24.2	20.0	16.3	14.0	12.2	11.0	11 3	11.2	9.5	8.2	7.7	7.5

FIG. 523.—AVERAGE DAILY AND WEEKLY FETAL GAIN IN WEIGHT, WITH AVERAGE WEIGHT OF FETUSES PLOTTED WITH MENSTRUAL AGE OF FETUSES.

(From figures in Table 1, Dr. George L. Streeter, Contrib. to Embryology, Vol. XI, Car. Inst. of Wash., Pub No. 274, 1920.)

800 and 1,000 gm., the probability of survival is only about one in 20. Accordingly, the attitude may be taken that there is such a small chance for the survival of an infant under 1,000 gm. that all fetuses in this category, generally speaking, should be classified as abortuses. Until very recently this view has been widely held and, on this basis, it has been customary to classify an infant as premature when it weighs between 1,000 and 2,500 gm. at birth; and to consider fetuses of less than 1,000 gm. as abortuses. As may be seen from Fig. 523, a fetus weighing 1,000 gm. has a ges-

tational age of approximately 28 weeks. Since 28 weeks has long been cited in statutes as the border line of viability, the figure of 1,000 gm. is in keeping with a time-honored concept. But when an abortus, as thus defined, occasionally survives, the inconsistency of this definition becomes apparent.

Although the problem of defining "prematurity" might seem to be of academic interest only, its ramifications are surprisingly wide since it enters into the definition of abruptio placentae, therapeutic abortion, fetal mortality, and other important obstetric terms. Much attention is being given this problem at the present time and uniformity of nomenclature will doubtless be evolved in the near future. Meanwhile, in order to meet some of the above difficulties, it is becoming customary to classify fetuses under 1,000 gm. in two categories, abortuses and "immature infants." This yields the following groups:

1. *Abortuses.* Fetuses of birth weight under 400 gm. No chance of survival.
2. *Immature Infants.* Fetuses of birth weight from 400 to 999 gm. Extremely poor chance of survival.
3. *Premature Infants.* Fetuses of birth weight from 1,000 to 2,499 gm. Chances of survival range from poor to good according to weight.
4. *Mature Infants.* Fetuses of 2,500 gm. or more. Optimal chances of survival.

General Considerations. It is common knowledge that prematurity is the principal cause of death in the neonatal period, accounting for about one half of all fatalities occurring at that time. During the past decade pediatricians and public health officials have made significant inroads on this toll, but they would be the first to affirm that the salvage, particularly in the smaller-weight groups, is still discouragingly small. There are two main ways of attacking this problem. In the first place, mortality rates could be lowered substantially by wider dissemination of existing knowledge, together with better distribution of personnel and facilities. This is a pediatric and public health responsibility. The other means by which premature mortality might conceivably be reduced is through the prevention of premature birth—obviously a challenge to the obstetrician.

Etiology. Between June 1, 1926 and December 31, 1945, among 28,493 total deliveries in our clinic, 3,331 premature infants (1,000 to 2,499 gm), were born, an incidence of 11.7 per cent. Of these premature infants, 11.9 per cent were associated with multiple gestations; in about 90 per cent of these multiple pregnancies the onset of labor was spontaneous, in the remainder operative. In 14.3 per cent of the total cases, premature delivery of single infants was effected artificially because of maternal disease, chiefly because of toxemia, placenta previa, and abruptio placentae. The remaining 73.8 per cent, or approximately three-quarters, were cases in which the premature labors were of spontaneous onset and the pregnancies single. What caused labor to start prematurely in these 2,457 gravidae? In evaluating this question it is important to recall that the simple association of premature labor and some complication of pregnancy does not necessarily mean that the complication was the cause of the premature parturition. Such a causal relationship can be postulated only if it can be shown that a given complication precedes premature labor much more frequently than would ordinarily be expected. This type of relationship could be established definitely in only 14 per cent of this last group. The diseases most frequently responsible for the onset of premature labor are chronic hypertension, syphilis, abruptio placentae, placenta previa, heart disease, and eclampsia.

By adding up the incidence of the causative factors of prematurity as listed in the foregoing paragraph, the resulting figures are as follows: multiple gestation, 11.9 per cent; maternal disease necessitating operative termination of pregnancy, 14.3 per cent; maternal disease, spontaneous onset of labor, 10.3 per cent of total; and congenital abnormalities, 1.6 per cent. In other words, in the whole series of 3,331 premature infants, a definite cause for the early termination of pregnancy was demonstrable in only 1,269 or in 38.1 per cent.

Other similar studies also indicate that a large proportion of premature births, perhaps 50 per cent or more, are without explanation. Although many investigations, including the above analysis, suggest that these labors are more common in the lower economic group and may possibly be associated with dietary deficiencies, proof of this contention is lacking.

Prognosis. The prognosis for a premature infant depends almost entirely on its gestational age and, by the same token, on its weight at birth. If the group of prematures between 1,000 and 2,499 gm. be considered, the over-all mortality is in the neighborhood of 20 per cent. Thus, in the preceding Johns Hopkins series it was 20.9 per cent during the last 10-year period investigated and 18.7 per cent in the most recent five-year interval.

Retrolental Fibroplasia. In 1942 Terry described a disease occurring in very premature infants in which an opaque tissue forms behind the lens of the eye during the first few months after birth. It is estimated that this condition, retrolental fibroplasia, develops in 10 to 15 per cent of infants weighing less than three pounds (1,360 gm.) at birth and in about one per cent of infants weighing from three to four and one-half pounds (1,360 to 2,000 gm.). The prognosis is grave; most of the infants affected become partially or totally blind. At the present writing the cause of retrolental fibroplasia is unknown and no method of prevention or therapy is available. However, the serious problem imposed by the disease is being vigorously attacked by many ophthalmologists. (See Owens and Owens.)

HEMOLYTIC DISEASE OF THE FETUS AND NEWBORN

Milton S. Sacks, M.D.*

Introduction. Approximately 0.5 per cent of all deliveries result in the birth of an infant affected, to a greater or lesser extent, by hemolytic disease of the fetus and newborn (erythroblastosis fetalis). Some infants affected by this disease are stillborn, while others who are born alive exhibit a clinical picture, during the first several days of neonatal existence, characterized by jaundice, anemia, and splenomegaly. The disease has an immunological basis dependent upon blood-group differences between the fetus and the mother. These differences, having once led to the birth of an affected infant, may result in the establishment of a pattern which will be repeated in subsequent pregnancies, thus effectively curtailing the normal childbearing career of the woman.

The physician must be equipped to deal not only with the problems of the disease

* Associate Professor of Medicine, University of Maryland School of Medicine; Director, Baltimore Rh Typing Laboratory.

Note: The use of "we" or "our" refers, in this section, to Dr. Sacks' experience in the Baltimore Rh Typing Laboratory.

in the infant, but also with the questions which necessarily arise concerning the outcome of future pregnancies of such a mother. Moreover, he must be aware of the particular hazards associated with the administration of a blood transfusion to this type of patient. The foundation for an understanding of the etiological basis of hemolytic disease was laid in 1940 with the discovery of one component member of the Rh-Hr antigen system of the human erythrocyte. Although much information has been gained since, the limits of the subject have not yet been reached and additions or modifications of current concepts can be expected in the future.

An adequate comprehension of this subject requires some knowledge of basic facts regarding blood groups. In 1900–1901 Landsteiner discovered the existence of the two antigens, known as A and B, in human red cells, and of the naturally occurring iso-agglutinins, anti-A and anti-B, in human sera. These findings permitted the division of all human blood into four groups: A, B, AB, and O. It will be observed that the groups are named on the basis of the antigen or antigens contained within the erythrocyte. In subsequent years slight differences were found in the antigenic structure of A and we now know that there are at least three such variants: A_1, A_2, and A_3. These variations are not of great clinical significance.

Studies were subsequently made of the mode of inheritance of these factors and it was established that their occurrence was governed by well-defined Mendelian principles. The genetic theory first proposed by Bernstein has since been supported by actual experimental observations. The basic tenets of this theory will be briefly cited since similar principles apply to the genetics of the Rh-Hr antigens. According to the Bernstein hypothesis, three genes, also named A, B, and O, determine the occurrence of the antigens, A, B, and O. These three genes can occur interchangeably in a particular chromosome and they are, hence, known as *allelic genes,* or *allelomorphs.* The definitive blood type of an individual, *i.e.,* his *phenotype,* represents a summation of two genes, one inherited from each parent. If, for example, an individual inherits gene A from both parents, his genotype is AA, his phenotype is A, and he is said to be *homozygous* for A. If he inherits gene A from one parent and gene O from the other, his genotype is AO, his phenotype is still A, and he is said to be *heterozygous* for A. In the case of the A-B-O genes, A and B are dominant over O so that the latter may exist in the genotype without being serologically detectable. We see, therefore, that phenotype A has two possible genotypes. It is impossible by serological means to distinguish heterozygous A from homozygous A. An important law derived from the Bernstein theory is that the erythrocytes of a child cannot contain an antigen which is not present in the red cells of one of the parents.

In 1927 two additional antigens were discovered by Landsteiner and Levine to be present in human erythrocytes. These were termed M and N, respectively. Only three groups are distinguishable, M, N, and MN, as there is no human blood which does not possess one or the other of these factors. There are no normally occurring iso-agglutinins for these antigens and they are, moreover, only weakly antigenic. Hence persons of differing M and N types can be interchangeably transfused without fear of reaction. At about the same time, another factor, P, was also found to be present in human erythrocytes. It is of interest to note that all of the antigens described thus far exist quite independently of each other in the erythrocyte and that the inheritance of each group or system (the A-B-O system, M-N system, etc.) likewise occurs independently. Space will, unfortunately, not permit further discussion of these problems. The interested reader will find a fuller exposition of the topic in the monograph of Wiener which is listed in the bibliography.

The search for new erythrocyte antigens continued and led, in 1940, to the discovery of the Rh antigen by Landsteiner and Wiener. This event had, to a certain extent, been foreshadowed by the report of Levine and Stetson in 1939. The latter described the presence of an atypical agglutinin in the blood of a woman who had just given birth to a stillborn, macerated fetus and who subsequently experienced a severe reaction when transfused with apparently compatible blood. This reaction was classified as an *intragroup hemolytic transfusion reaction* since both donor and recipient were of the same major (A-B-O) blood group. It was postulated by these observers that maternal immunization had resulted from the stimulation by some fetal antigen inherited from the father, but absent in the mother. This phenomenon is known as *iso-immunization* since the antigen originated from an individual of the same species as the patient. The antibody was found to react best at 37° C. (warm agglutinin) and produced agglutination of 80 per cent of a series of bloods with which it was tested. It appeared to be independent of the properties M, N and P. No name was given to the antigen or its antibody.

Since 1937 Landsteiner and Wiener had been studying a property of the red blood cell of the rhesus monkey which was apparently related to, but not identical with, human blood group antigen M. These investigators studied the reactions of a series of human bloods with a rabbit anti-rhesus immune serum. In 1940 they reported that the erythrocytes of 85 per cent of a group of Caucasoid individuals reacted positively with this anti-rhesus serum and therefore contained the antigen, while 15 per cent did not. The property of human erythrocytes thus discovered was termed Rh to indicate its relationship to a similar property of rhesus erythrocytes. Those who reacted were said to be Rh positive (Rh+) and those who did not were designated Rh negative (Rh—). It has since been determined that this antigen is only one member of an antigen system now known as the Rh-Hr system.

In 1940, Wiener and Peters reported that the Rh factor of human erythrocytes was antigenic, *i.e.*, repeated injection of Rh-positive cells into an Rh-negative person led to the production of an antibody capable of agglutinating and hemolyzing Rh-positive red blood cells. This discovery was of fundamental significance in explaining the etiology of the hitherto mysterious intragroup reactions referred to above. In their review of the pertinent literature these authors pointed out that one group of patients was prone to develop intragroup hemolytic reactions with the very first transfusion. These patients were invariably pregnant or parturient women, or women who had only recently been delivered. It was suggested that these women had previously been iso-immunized by an antigen which the fetus inherited from the father—an antigen which reached the maternal blood by the continual passage of small numbers of fetal red cells through microscopic breaks in the placental barrier.

During 1941, in a series of papers, Levine and his co-workers developed the concept of transplacental iso-immunization further and produced evidence of statistical significance which correlated the newly discovered Rh antigen with the pathogenesis of the disease, *erythroblastosis fetalis* (hemolytic disease of the fetus and newborn). Ninety-three per cent of a group of 153 mothers who had given birth to infants with erythroblastosis fetalis were found to be Rh negative. All husbands and infants tested in this group were Rh positive. Anti-Rh agglutinins were demonstrated in the blood of approximately 30 per cent of 141 patients tested. The theory was proposed that erythroblastosis fetalis, a hemolytic anemia of newborn infants, was due to the intra-uterine activity of anti-Rh agglutinins produced by the mother in response to antigenic stimulation by Rh-positive fetal erythrocytes. Subsequent studies have confirmed and extended this hypothesis.

It is of interest to note that as early as 1905 Dienst had called attention to the fact that a recently delivered mother of group O might show a rising titer of anti-A or anti-B if her infant belonged to group A or B respectively. The type of pregnancy, in which mother and fetus are of different blood groups, has been referred to for many years as a *heterospecific pregnancy*. The observations of Dienst have been confirmed in recent years by other investigators. In the decades preceding 1941 numerous studies were made of heterospecific pregnancies in an effort to discern a significant relationship to some of the toxemias of pregnancy, but the conclusions were, in the main, negative. The lack of apparent clinical effects of elevated anti-A and anti-B agglutinin titers upon the fetus has been explained in several ways. It is generally believed that a rise in titer of these normally occurring iso-agglutinins is not of the same significance as is the formation of new agglutinins due solely to an immune process. Furthermore the anti-A and anti-B agglutinins which enter the fetal circulation may find antigenic receptors in tissues and secretions other than the erythrocytes and hence their hemolytic potential is largely nullified. The recent increase in interest in the entire subject of hemolytic anemia of the fetus and newborn may, we suspect, alter certain previous ideas concerning the apparent benignity of these findings. Waterhouse and Hogben in a recent statistical study of the distribution of blood groups of the offspring of heterospecific pregnancies in which the mother was group O and the father group A, found a 25 per cent deficit of group A children when the theoretical and actual proportions were compared. The significance of this observation has yet to be determined. Finally, it is of interest to note briefly another type of heterospecificity which has not been exhaustively studied. Darrow, in 1938, published an extensive survey of theories concerning the pathogenesis of erythroblastosis fetalis and postulated that hemolytic anemia of the fetus and newborn might be due to differences in chemical structure between fetal and adult hemoglobin with resultant formation, in some cases, of maternal antibodies against fetal hemoglobin. Such differences do exist but their significance has not yet been established. This aspect of the problem was completely overshadowed, shortly after it was suggested, by the discovery of the Rh factor and its relationship to erythroblastosis fetalis.

Antigenic Components and Genetics of the Rh-Hr System. The use of immune rabbit sera as well as the early studies with the sera of sensitized Rh-negative women permitted the differentiation of only two Rh types (Table 24). Subsequent studies have shown that the sera used contained an antibody which was the result of immunization by only one of a group of closely related Rh antigens. The antigen first discovered has since come to be known as Rh_0 (D) and the antiserum, anti-Rh_0 (anti-D). **Of the entire constellation of Rh-Hr antigens, Rh_0 is the most important since it is the commonest cause of iso-immunization.** Studies of the sera of many more iso-immunized women soon led to the discovery of antibodies of differing specificities which were apparently due to antigenic stimulation by other Rh factors. In the period between 1941 and 1945 the discovery of new antigens occurred with such rapidity that constant revision of concepts regarding the antigenic components of the Rh-Hr system was the order of the day. It would serve no useful purpose to attempt to review these developments in detail. Suffice it to say that in a relatively brief time it was apparent that there were three basic Rh antigens which may occur either alone or in various combinations in Rh-positive erythrocytes. These basic antigens are now known as Rh_0(D), rh′(C), and rh″(E).

Genes	Genotypes	Phenotypes	Incidence
Rh	Rh Rh Rh rh	Rh positive (Rh +)	85%
rh	rh rh	Rh negative (Rh −)	15%

TABLE 24. ORIGINAL CONCEPT OF THE RH BLOOD TYPES (Landsteiner-Wiener, 1941) BASED ON STUDIES WITH A SINGLE ANTISERUM.

The use of three specific anti-Rh sera makes it possible to distinguish eight Rh blood types (Table 25). It will be observed that the first four of these types are represented in lower case letters, in accordance with the suggestions of Wiener, and are characterized, in common, by the absence of Rh_0, the most potent antigen of the group. The second group of four types contain this antigen either alone or in some combination. These are designated by capital letters. The purpose of this terminology, proposed by Wiener, is to indicate that all individuals in the first group can potentially be immunized by the Rh_0 antigen. Unfortunately, the apposition of lower case and capital letters in a presentation of blood-group phenotypes tends to carry with it a connotation of Mendelian dominance and recessiveness which is not borne out by the facts of the matter.

Rh types (Phenotypes)	Reactions with serums			Incidence NYC Whites
	anti-rh′ (C)	anti-rh″ (E)	anti-Rh_0 (D)	
rh (cde)	−	−	−	14.4%
rh′ (Cde)	+	−	−	1.1
rh″ (cdE)	−	+	−	0.4
rh′ rh″ (CdE)	+	+	−	0.02
Rh_0 (cDe)	−	−	+	2.5
Rh_1 (CDe)	+	−	+	51.2
Rh_2 (cDE)	−	+	+	16.5
Rh_1 Rh_2 (CDE)	+	+	+	14.9

TABLE 25. THE 8 RH TYPES AS DETERMINED BY REACTIONS WITH THREE ANTI-RH SERA.

The designations in parentheses are those of Fisher and Race, while the others are the names proposed by Wiener. See text for further discussion.

From a clinical standpoint the division of the Rh types into eight subtypes is, usually, entirely adequate. By using only a single antiserum, anti-Rh_0(D), it is possible to separate the eight types into two major groupings, *i.e.*, those which are Rh_0(D) negative and those which are Rh_0(D) positive. The significance of this division may be briefly stated in the following way: any individual who is Rh_0(D) negative, regardless of the presence or absence of the other antigens (rh′(C) and rh″(E)), can become iso-immunized by blood containing the Rh_0(D) antigen.

The discovery of new antisera led to further characterization of the Rh family of antigens. In 1941 Levine had studied the blood of an *Rh-positive* woman who had given birth to a typical erythroblastotic infant. Her serum contained an antibody which agglutinated the red blood cells of her husband who was Rh negative. The infant's erythrocytes were likewise agglutinated. Because this immunological situation was exactly the reverse of the usual pattern found in cases of Rh iso-immunization, Levine suggested the designation Hr for the antigen present in both the father's and the infant's blood cells but absent in the mother's blood. Subsequent studies by Race and Fisher demonstrated that the Hr antigen of Levine was actually an allelomorph of rh′ and should more properly be designated Hr′.

It is now believed that for each of the Rh antigens there is an allelomorphic Hr antigen. When these relationships were first proposed by Fisher the existence of Hr_0 and Hr″, the allelomorphs of the corresponding Rh antigens, could only be theoretically postulated. Since then sera of specificities anti-Hr_0 and anti-Hr″ have been discovered and the existence of the antigens thus verified. At the same time that the genetic relationships were proposed, Fisher and Race designated the Rh and Hr genes and antigens by new symbols. These symbols are as follows: Rh_0(D), rh′(C), rh″(E), Hr_0(d), Hr′(c), Hr″(e).

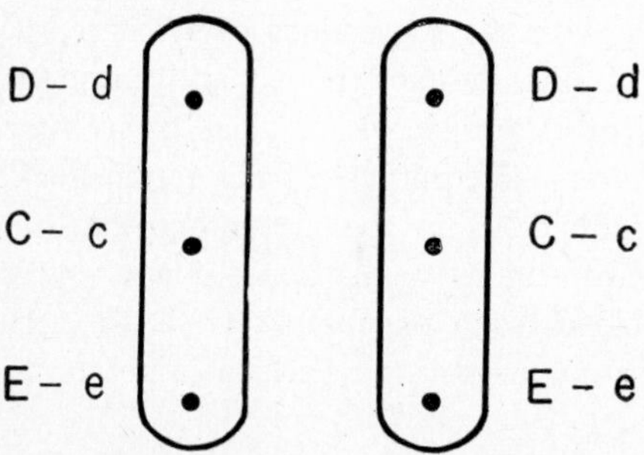

Fig. 524A.—Schematic Representation of the Fisher-Race Hypothesis of the Inheritance of the Rh-Hr Genes.

Two chromosomes are portrayed, each containing three loci for the Rh-Hr gene pairs. One or the other member of a pair can occur at a single locus.

Although the validity of the Fisher-Race genetic theory has yet to be definitively established, there is no doubt but that it has been of great value in clarifying the complexities of the Rh-Hr antigen system. According to this hypothesis three pairs of allelic genes occurring at closely linked loci determine the Rh-Hr type of an individual (Fig. 524A). Only one member of each pair can be present in a chromosome at a time. Since we inherit one such chromosome from each parent a variety of combinations of these three pairs of genes are possible. Each gene is responsible for the occurrence of a single antigen. It is, therefore, possible for some individuals to possess all six of the Rh-Hr antigens while others, because of duplications in the two chromosomes may possess only three to five. With the appropriate sera the presence of these antigens can be detected in the erythrocyte.

In Table 26 we have listed 27 Rh-Hr types which can be distinguished by the use of six specific antisera. Thus, by determining the presence or absence of the six antigens it is virtually possible to write a genotype symbol instead of a phenotype symbol. As yet, the anti-Hr sera are available only in small quantity so that definitive typing is not possible on a wide scale. This situation will undoubtedly improve in the near future, but it is certainly wise, at this stage, to emphasize that studies of this type should be done only by individuals with special training in the field. In the table we have listed the nomenclature of the 27 types in both the Fisher-Race and Wiener terminologies. Since both terminologies are in daily use a brief discussion of the basic differences is essential.

Rh Phenotypes		Expected Reactions with Antisera					
		Anti-rh′ (C)	Anti-rho (D)	Anti-rh″ (E)	Anti-hr′ (c)	Anti-Hro (d)	Anti-hr″ (e)
1. r r	$\left(\frac{cde}{cde}\right)$	−	−	−	+	+	+
2. r′ r′	$\left(\frac{Cde}{Cde}\right)$	+	−	−	−	+	+
3. r′ r	$\left(\frac{Cde}{cde}\right)$	+	−	−	+	+	+
4. r″ r″	$\left(\frac{cdE}{cdE}\right)$	−	−	+	+	+	−
5. r″ r	$\left(\frac{cdE}{cde}\right)$	−	−	+	+	+	+
6. r_y r	$\left(\frac{CdE}{cde}\right)$	+	−	+	+	+	+
7. r_y r′	$\left(\frac{CdE}{Cde}\right)$	+	−	+	−	+	+
8. r_y r″	$\left(\frac{CdE}{cdE}\right)$	+	−	+	+	+	−
9. r_y r_y	$\left(\frac{CdE}{CdE}\right)$	+	−	+	−	+	−
10. R_0 R_0	$\left(\frac{cDe}{cDe}\right)$	−	+	−	+	−	+
11. R_0 r	$\left(\frac{cDe}{cde}\right)$	−	+	−	+	+	+
12. R_1 R_1	$\left(\frac{CDe}{CDe}\right)$	+	+	−	−	−	+
13. R_1 r′	$\left(\frac{CDe}{Cde}\right)$	+	+	−	−	+	+
14. R_1 R_0	$\left(\frac{Cde}{cDe}\right)$	+	+	−	+	−	+
15. R_1 r	$\left(\frac{CDe}{cde}\right)$	+	+	−	+	+	+
16. R_2 R_2	$\left(\frac{cDE}{cDE}\right)$	−	+	+	+	−	−
17. R_2 r″	$\left(\frac{cDE}{cdE}\right)$	−	+	+	+	+	−
18. R_2 R_0	$\left(\frac{cDE}{cDe}\right)$	−	+	+	+	−	+
19. R_2 r	$\left(\frac{cDE}{cde}\right)$	−	+	+	+	+	+
20. R_z R_0	$\left(\frac{CDE}{cDe}\right)$	+	+	+	+	−	+
21. R_z r	$\left(\frac{CDE}{cde}\right)$	+	+	+	+	+	+
22. R_z R_1	$\left(\frac{CDE}{CDe}\right)$	+	+	+	−	−	+
23. R_z r′	$\left(\frac{CDE}{Cde}\right)$	+	+	+	−	+	+
24. R_z R_2	$\left(\frac{CDE}{cDE}\right)$	+	+	+	+	−	−
25. R_z r″	$\left(\frac{CDE}{cdE}\right)$	+	+	+	+	+	−
26. R_z R_z	$\left(\frac{CDE}{CDE}\right)$	+	+	+	−	−	−
27. R_z r_y	$\left(\frac{CDE}{CdE}\right)$	+	+	+	−	+	−

TABLE 26. THE EXPECTED REACTIONS OF THE 27 RH-HR PHENOTYPES WITH SIX SPECIFIC ANTISERA. ONLY THE FIRST FOUR SERA ARE AS YET GENERALLY AVAILABLE.

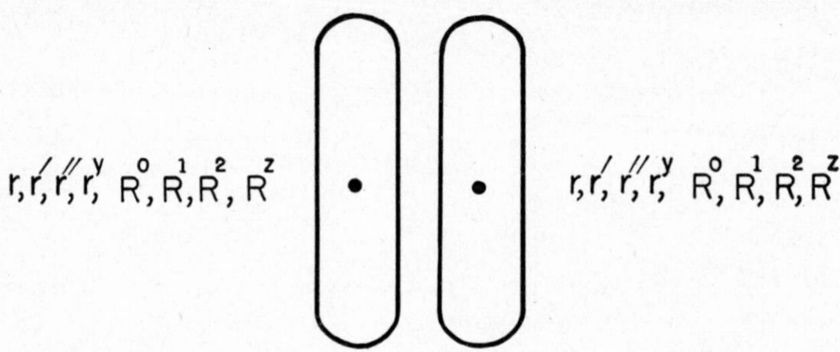

FIG. 524B.—SCHEMATIC REPRESENTATION OF THE WIENER THEORY OF THE INHERITANCE OF THE RH-HR GENES.

Two chromosomes are portrayed, each with a single locus. A series of eight allelic genes may interchangeably occupy this locus.

According to the Wiener theory, the Rh-Hr types are determined by a series of eight allelic genes occurring at a single locus in a chromosome (Fig. 524B). The relationship between these genes and the gene combinations of Fisher and Race are presented in Table 27. It will be observed that the Wiener gene symbol actually includes several genes believed to be present according to the Fisher-Race theory. The controversy over the mode of inheritance of the Rh-Hr antigens has not yet been resolved. No doubt the accumulation of further genetic data, based upon careful family studies, will permit settlement of these opposing views in the near future.

Wiener	r	r′	r″	r^y	R^o	R_1	R_2	R_z
Fisher-Race	cde	Cde	cdE	CdE	cDe	CDe	cDE	CDE
Strandskov	Rh^{cde}	Rh^{Cde}	Rh^{cdE}	Rh^{CdE}	Rh^{cDe}	Rh^{CDe}	Rh^{cDE}	Rh^{CDE}

TABLE 27. THE SERIES OF EIGHT RH-HR GENES POSTULATED BY THE WIENER MULTIPLE ALLELE THEORY OF RH BLOOD TYPE INHERITANCE.

For comparison, the corresponding Fisher-Race gene combinations are also listed. The nomenclature proposed by Strandskov is likewise shown.

The genetic controversy has unfortunately resulted in the establishment of two parallel systems of nomenclature, neither of which is entirely satisfactory. Aside from the necessity of awkwardly verbalizing the Fisher-Race nomenclature symbols as "big C, little c, etc.," a more valid objection to this terminology lies in the complete disregard of the symbol Rh which not only has historical significance, but has also become firmly related to the concept of the rhesus antigens. The Wiener nomenclature offers difficulty because of its somewhat confusing use of superscripts and subscripts, symbols which resemble each other so closely (Rh_z, Rh_2, etc.) as to be readily confused in printing, and, more importantly, because the gene symbols (Table 27) do not clearly indicate the antigenic activity of the alleles. Strandskov has recently proposed a nomenclature (Table 27) which retains the symbol Rh as the basic locus symbol and indicates the antigenic content by superscripts employing the CDE symbols of Fisher-Race—*e.g.*, R^1 (Wiener) = CDe (Fisher-Race) = Rh^{CDe}

(Strandskov), etc. This suggestion, which is of recent origin, appears to have considerable merit.

No mention has been made in this discussion of a number of "intermediate" or variant Rh antigens whose existence has recently become known. These variant genes, which have been detected at the C and D loci, seem, in the main, to be of genetic rather than clinical significance.

Biological and Anthropological Data. Efforts to extract the Rh antigen by chemical means from the erythrocyte indicate that its general structure is that of a lipoprotein. Additional studies of the chemical structure are currently in progress in connection with the extraction of Rh hapten from Rh-positive erythrocytes for therapeutic purposes. Further reference to this subject is made in another section. Data regarding the distribution of the antigen in the body leave this matter in an unsettled state. Wiener and Levine have both reported failure to demonstrate the antigen in saliva, spermatozoa, and seminal fluid and have concluded that it is confined to the erythrocyte. Boorman and Dodd, on the other hand, reported its presence in saliva, salivary glands, liver, and spleen. Further studies of this problem seem to be indicated. The antigen appears in the red cell quite early in fetal life. Stratton was able to detect its presence in a 48 mm. fetus. Bornstein and Israel reported the presence of the antigen in a 17 cm. fetus.

The Rh-Hr antigens exist and are inherited independently of all other blood-group antigens. There is apparently no difference in the distribution of the various Rh-Hr antigens with regard to sex. There are, however, important racial differences in the distribution of these antigens. Space limitations do not permit a complete presentation of these data, but a few examples will be cited. The Chinese and other Asiatic peoples thus far studied, are almost all Rh positive (99 per cent). Among American Negroes there is a lesser incidence of Rh negatives (7 to 8 per cent) than among American whites. Of all the racial groups studied thus far, the Basques show the highest incidence of Rh negative individuals (33.6 per cent). There is a direct correlation between the incidence of Rh negatives in a population and the occurrence of hemolytic disease.

No satisfactory explanation has yet been offered regarding the predominance of the Rh-Hr antigens over other blood-group antigens in the etiology of erythroblastosis fetalis. Nor is there any satisfactory biological explanation for the varying antigenic potency of the factors themselves. Wide experience has demonstrated that the various factors can be arranged as follows in order of diminishing antigenicity: Rh_0(D), rh′(C), rh″(E), hr′(c), hr″(e), hr_0(d).

Rh Antibodies. Immunization or sensitization by any of the Rh antigens, whether due to transfusions or pregnancy, is accompanied by the production of several varieties of antibodies. The earliest to be recognized, and yet the least in incidence, is the agglutinin which reacts with Rh-positive erythrocytes suspended in physiological saline solution. This antibody has acquired a number of descriptive names during the past few years. Some of these are based upon physical characteristics (heat-lability) while others describe theoretical concepts of their mode of action (bivalent antibodies). For purposes of clear differentiation, we have recently adopted the custom of characterizing the antibody by the medium in which its activity can be detected. We would therefore speak of the type of antibody mentioned above as a *saline agglutinin.* It was recognized quite early that the sera of many women whose infants displayed evidence of a hemolytic anemia did not contain saline agglutinins. In 1944 Race and Wiener independently described another variety of antibody to which they respectively applied the terms "incomplete" and "blocking." This antibody could only be detected by an indirect method. When a serum containing "blocking" antibodies is added to a saline suspension of Rh-positive red cells the blocking antibodies are adsorbed upon the erythrocytes and apparently saturate the antigenic receptors without producing visible agglutination. If, subsequently, a serum containing potent anti-Rh saline agglutinins is added to such a cell suspension, agglutination fails to occur. The activity of the saline agglutinin has been "blocked." Later studies have demonstrated that if pooled compatible human serum, human plasma, or bovine or human albumin solutions are substituted as a vehicle instead of normal saline solution, "blocking" antibodies will produce visible agglutination. The term "blocking antibody" has continued to be used even though it is now possible to demonstrate them by a direct method. Additional studies have demonstrated that there are least two varieties of "blocking antibodies." Some so-called "blocking antibodies" can only be demonstrated when the Rh-positive erythrocytes are suspended in a 20 to 30 per cent bovine albumin solution, and this type of antibody frequently fails to give a positive "blocking test" when the indirect technic outlined above is carried out. Antibodies which react only in an albumin medium and fail to give a positive blocking test can be referred to as *albumin agglutinins*. Antibodies which react in a human serum suspension vehicle and do give a positive "blocking test" may be referred to as *serum agglutinins*.

It has been demonstrated that at varying periods during and after antigenic stimulation the different varieties of antibodies mentioned above can be found alone or in combination in the serum of the immunized individual. Diamond regards the saline agglutinins as the early or "immune" response to antigenic stimulation; they frequently disappear and are replaced by either serum or albumin agglutinins which he looks upon as a "hyperimmune" response. We and others have studied patients who have apparently never developed saline agglutinins but have shown serum or albumin agglutinins from the very beginning of iso-immunization. Some iso-immunized patients show a mixture of saline agglutinins with the other types of antibodies throughout pregnancy. There is no doubt, however, that when the pregnancy and the period of antigenic stimulation is over, saline agglutinins, if present at all, tend to disappear, and subsequent studies, years later, demonstrate only serum or albumin agglutinins. The latter remain as more or less permanent evidences of Rh iso-immunization. Any subsequent pregnancy or transfusion involving the introduction of Rh-positive blood into the immunized person's circulation will result in a so-called "anamnestic" rise in titer of serum and albumin antibodies.

Evidence has now accumulated which indicates that antibodies of the types we have been discussing are not peculiar to Rh iso-immunization. Blocking antibodies have been detected, for example, in cases of brucellosis and acquired hemolytic anemia. The intensive study of Rh iso-immunization has undoubtedly stimulated, in recent years, the investigation of similar immune processes in other diseases.

Certain physicochemical characteristics of the Rh antibodies have been established. These antibodies, on the whole, react better at 37° C. and may therefore be classified as warm agglutinins. The saline agglutinins are thermolabile. Exposure to a temperature of 65° C. to 70° C. for 5 to 10 minutes will render them inactive. Blocking antibodies, on the other hand, are heat stable. These physical differences have only recently begun to be utilized in the clinical study of the sera of iso-immunized women. It has been reported that blocking antibodies are largely contained in the beta fraction of plasma globulin while the saline agglutinins are to be found almost exclusively in gamma globulin. Other biological properties and effects of the various types of antibodies are discussed in the following sections.

Rh Iso-immunization in Pregnancy. The incidence and consequences of Rh iso-immunization have been somewhat exaggerated among physicians as well as laymen, in recent years, as a result of unwise publicity in the lay press. In order to present this aspect of the problem in proper perspective we have analyzed data derived from studies made at the Baltimore Rh Laboratory during the four-year period, 1945 to 1949. During this time blood studies were made on 69,356 pregnant women. Of these, 13,167 were found to be Rh negative, an incidence of 18.9 per cent. This figure is somewhat higher than the usual incidence of approximately 15 per cent and is due to the fact that some women found to be Rh negative elsewhere were referred to this laboratory for routine study throughout pregnancy. The group is not selected in any other way. It represents a cross section of all economic strata in Baltimore and includes both white and Negro patients.

Six hundred and twenty-two iso-immunized Rh-negative women were discovered and studied during this period. In terms of the total Rh-negative group, this represents an incidence of iso-immunization of 4.72 per cent. Stated in a slightly different way, approximately one in 20 of all Rh-negative women studied in our laboratory displayed serological evidence of iso-immunization. This figure has been found to be virtually identical for both white and Negro patients. Among the 622 iso-immunized patients, 580 were multiparae and only 42 were primiparae. It will be observed that Rh iso-immunization is largely a phenomenon of multiparity. It has been suggested that iso-sensitization in primiparae is frequently due to the administration of Rh-positive blood at sometime earlier in life. A review of the histories of the 42 primiparae in our series disclosed a positive transfusion history only in 14, or 33 per cent. It has also been suggested, on theoretical grounds, that in the absence of a transfusion history, immunization may have been initiated by the intramuscular injection of blood in infancy. This theory does not readily lend itself to statistical verification. In this connection it should be pointed out that early abortion, whether spontaneous or induced, may be responsible for the initiation of immunization. This aspect of the history may be either unknown to or deliberately withheld by the patient. Among the 580 sensitized multiparae, 174, or 30 per cent, also had a positive transfusion history. In the latter group, of course, it is difficult to evaluate the relative importance of transfusion and pregnancy as a cause of iso-immunization.

We have analyzed the histories of a group of 557 sensitized multiparous women in an effort to determine when iso-immunization first occurred. The criteria used were: either an unmistakable history of the birth of an erythroblastotic infant in a previous pregnancy or the observation of the development of sensitization during the current pregnancy. The complete data are listed in Table 28. It will be observed that 74.8 per cent of the patients became sensitized by the third pregnancy. In the remainder, immunization occurred in a scattered fashion from the fourth to the twelfth pregnancy. In a group of 175 Rh-negative iso-immunized women, Potter found that the first erythroblastotic infant in 75 per cent of the cases had been born before the fourth

Pregnancy order	1st	2nd	3rd	4th	5th	6th	7th	8th	9th	10th	11th	12th	Total number of patients
Number of patients	57 (27 with history previous transfusion)	247	113	55	32	20	18	9	2	1	1	2	557
Per cent	10.2%	44.3%	20.3%	9.8%	5.9%	3.6%	3.2%	1.6%	0.3%	0.15%	0.15%	0.3%	100%

TABLE 28. THE PREGNANCY IN WHICH ISO-IMMUNIZATION FIRST OCCURRED IN 557 RH-NEGATIVE WOMEN WHO BECAME IMMUNIZED. IMMUNIZATION OCCURS IN ONLY ABOUT 5 PER CENT OF RH-NEGATIVE GRAVIDAE.

pregnancy. The significance of these data may be stated in the following way: although the over-all incidence of iso-immunization among all Rh-negative gravidae is approximately 5 per cent, the majority of those who do become sensitized do so by the fourth pregnancy.

Studies have been made by ourselves and others of the Rh genotypes of the husbands of immunized women. The data indicate that homozygous, positive males exceed heterozygous positives in this group by about three to one. Antibody specificity is routinely determined in all of our cases and the accumulated data demonstrate an overwhelming predominance of anti-Rh_0(D) antibodies. This variety of antibody usually occurs alone but may be occasionally accompanied by specific agglutinins for rh′(C) and rh″(E) antigens. On rare occasions the latter two varieties may occur alone. Immunization by Hr′(c) has been extremely rare in our experience, having been observed only twice in the four-year period. One such instance was associated with pregnancy and the other was due to transfusion. Analysis, as to the type of antibody formed, demonstrated, in a group of 271 women, that 190, or 70.9 per cent formed only serum or albumin agglutinins throughout pregnancy.

Early efforts to correlate the degree of iso-immunization, *i.e.*, the titer of antibodies during pregnancy, with the occurrence and degree of severity of hemolytic anemia in the newborn infant were not very successful. This was largely due to the fact that the only antibody which could be quantitated prior to 1944 was the saline agglutinin which, as we have already seen, is not present at all in a large proportion of iso-immunized women. Studies cited in another section of this chapter demonstrate, furthermore, that this type of antibody is rarely found in the newborn infant's blood. Obviously, therefore, no correlation between the potency of saline agglutinins in the maternal serum and hemolytic disease in the fetus or newborn is possible. This is not valid for serum or albumin agglutinins. There is a high degree of correlation between the maternal albumin agglutinin titer and the amount of this antibody which reaches the fetal circulation. Evidence for this statement is cited in a later section of the chapter.

Prenatal Antibody Titers		No. of Patients	Clinical Status of Infant	
			Erythroblastosis Fetalis	"Clinically Normal"
Serum Agglutinins and/or Albumin Agglutinins	< 10 units < 50 units	152	37 (24.3%)	115 * (75.7%)
Serum Agglutinins and/or Albumin Agglutinins	> 10 units > 50 units	298	254 (85.2%)	44 ** (14.8%)

TABLE 29. THE OUTCOME OF PREGNANCY IN 450 RH-NEGATIVE ISO-IMMUNIZED WOMEN WITH PARTICULAR REFERENCE TO PRENATAL ANTIBODY TITER.

* Includes 31 Rh-negative infants.
** Includes 23 Rh-negative infants.

We have assembled data regarding the outcome of pregnancy in 450 iso-immunized women (Table 29). It will be observed that there were 152 patients whose highest prenatal antibody titer was less than 10 units of serum agglutinins and/or 50 units of albumin agglutinins (the unit is equivalent to the reciprocal of the titer, *i.e.*, a titer of 1:10 is referred to as 10 units of antibody). One hundred and fifteen of the infants in this group, 75.7 per cent, were considered "clinically normal" by the attending pediatrician, *i.e.*, did not show sufficient evidence to warrant a clinical diagnosis of erythroblastosis fetalis or require specific treatment. Thirty-seven infants, 24.3 per cent, were said to have some degree of hemolytic anemia. On the other hand, 298 women demonstrated antibody titers in excess of 10 units of serum agglutinins and/or 50 units of albumin agglutinins. Two hundred and fifty-four, 85.2 per cent, gave birth to infants with hemolytic disease, while only 44, 14.8 per cent, had infants who were said to be "clinically normal."

Refinements in technics have given prenatal antibody studies increased validity. However, such studies must be done with considerable care and the utilization of multiple procedures in order to characterize completely the types of antibodies present. Only recently, procedures have been devised, based upon the differences in heat stability of the saline and albumin agglutinins, which permit more accurate analysis of the antibody content of a serum. This type of analysis has not yet had sufficient trial to permit the accumulation of analyzable data. Space limitations do not permit us to enter into the details of Rh-antibody testing. The interested reader is referred, for this purpose, to the several monographs listed in the bibliography.

Other factors in addition to antibody titer must be considered in attempts to evaluate the probable outcome of pregnancy. The previous obstetrical history, with particular reference to the birth of infants affected by hemolytic disease, is of great significance. It is the general experience that with the establishment of the iso-immunized state and/or the occurrence of some manifestations of hemolytic anemia in a previous infant virtually all succeeding Rh-positive infants will be more severely 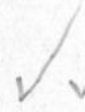 affected. Succeeding infants who may be Rh negative will be completely unaffected by the iso-immunized state of the mother. It is in this connection that the genotype of the Rh-positive husband becomes of great importance. The mating of a homozygous Rh-positive male and an Rh-negative female can result only in the birth of Rh-positive offspring. On the other hand, the mating of a heterozygous Rh-positive male and an Rh-negative female is potentially productive of infants, 50 per cent of whom may be Rh negative. We have noted above that analyses of the genotypes of husbands of iso-immunized women have demonstrated that homozygous positives predominate in a ratio of three to one.

Evaluation of the significance of prenatal antibody titers in a female married to a heterozygous, Rh-positive male presents particular interpretive hazards which should be appreciated by the physician attending the patient. The sera of such patients may contain elevated titers of albumin agglutinins which are simply residuals of a previous pregnancy which resulted in the birth of an infant affected by hemolytic disease. There is no absolutely certain way of determining whether such a patient is carrying an Rh-negative fetus in a subsequent pregnancy. A sharply rising titer in a succeeding pregnancy is suggestive, but not positive, evidence of the presence of an Rh-positive fetus in utero. These statements simply underscore the necessity for prompt serological study of the newborn infant of iso-immunized women.

Studies have been made in an effort to link Rh iso-immunization with other complications of the gravid state but have thus far failed to reveal any significant correlations.

Glass studied the incidence of abortion in a group of 209 Rh-negative immunized women seen in our laboratory and found no significant differences between this group and a comparable group of Rh-positive women. No definite relationship between Rh sensitization and any of the toxemias of pregnancy has been established.

Clinical Management of the Rh-Negative Pregnant Women. It has been estimated that approximately 13 per cent of all marriages in this country take place between an Rh-negative female and an Rh-positive male. The potentialities for isoimmunization, therefore, exist in a considerable proportion of pregnant women. In view of this fact the determination of the Rh type of every pregnant woman has become established as an imperative routine of prenatal care. Since a history of previous blood transfusion may be of significance with regard to the occurrence of immunization early in the obstetrical career of the patient, this fact should also be ascertained and noted in the patient's record. Routine Rh typing before transfusion has only become an established practice within the past several years. Hence a history of transfusion has, until recently, carried with it the strong possibility that an Rh-negative female may have received Rh-positive blood.

If typing has established the fact that a particular patient is Rh-negative it is then essential to type her husband. Should he also be found to be Rh-negative there will be no danger of hemolytic anemia in any infant since all offspring of such a union will be Rh negative. On the other hand, if he is found to be Rh positive an effort should be made to determine his genotype. This may be accomplished in several ways. If the husband's parents are living they should be typed since if one of them is found to be Rh negative, the male in question must be heterozygous positive. One may also approach the problem by Rh typing any living children of the couple. The detection of an Rh-negative child likewise implies that the husband is heterozygous positive. On the other hand, if all children are Rh positive no certain inferences can be drawn as to the husband's genotype. Serological methods are also applicable to this problem in some instances. If all six antisera listed in Table 27 were widely available the serological determination of genotypes would be possible with a relatively high degree of accuracy. The most important serum from this standpoint is anti-Hr_0(d) since with it one could distinguish the Rh_0 Rh_0(DD) genotype from the Rh_0 rh(Dd) genotype. Unfortunately, at present, only small quantities of this type of serum are available so that general use is not yet feasible. A somewhat indirect approach is possible through the use of the more readily available anti-hr′(c) serum. The use of this serum permits division of the relatively common phenotype, Rh_1(CDe), into two groups. Those who react negatively are probably homozygous positive, while those who react positively are probably heterozygous positive. There is, however, a certain margin of unavoidable error in the serological determination of genotypes. For example, no antiserum could distinguish between such genotypes as R^zr(CDE/cde) and $r^y R^o$(CdE/cDe).

How often should serological studies be done on the Rh-negative pregnant woman? The frequency of such examinations varies somewhat and is dependent upon a number of factors. Prominent among these factors are the question of the availability of special facilities for Rh studies and the cost entailed. The organization of a nonprofit central laboratory under the auspices of the Obstetrical and Gynecological Society, has made it possible, in Baltimore, to carry out complete studies on all patients at a nominal cost or at no cost whatsoever. The organization and method of operation of this laboratory have been published. In brief, after the initial typing and family studies as described above, tests on the pregnant women are done at monthly intervals during the first two trimesters of pregnancy and at biweekly intervals in the last trimester. It is thus possible for the attending physician to have a current picture of the immunologic status of his patient. Modifications of this routine are acceptable in certain circumstances. In view of the infrequency of sensitization of Rh-negative primiparae this routine may be curtailed, if desired, after the initial typing and serologic study. Serologic examinations may be limited to several tests made at intervals after the thirty-fourth week of pregnancy. In the case of an Rh-negative multipara, more frequent serological studies are desirable since they will furnish a sounder basis for the management of pregnancy and of the expected infant. However, if facilities are limited, the initial typing and examination for antibodies may be followed by more intensive studies only after the thirty-fourth week of pregnancy. This will allow an adequate interval for planning the management of the case.

Under some circumstances, delivery of the fetus before term may be desirable. Such a course of action should seldom be undertaken prior to the thirty-seventh or thirty-eighth week of pregnancy because of the serious hazards of prematurity superimposed upon hemolytic anemia. The indications for adoption of such a plan of action may be briefly listed: (1) a previous history of the birth of an infant with unmistakable evidences of erythroblastosis fetalis; (2) the existence during a considerable portion of the current pregnancy of a significant titer of antibodies (see previous section); (3) reasonably certain evidence of hemozygosity of the husband; and (4) progressive and even sharp rise in antibody titer during the last trimester of pregnancy. The choice of a method of delivery, *i.e.*, induction of labor or cesarean section, must depend upon the clinical judgment of the obstetrician but the latter operation is rarely indicated. Under any circumstances, if a decision to terminate pregnancy before term is reached, adequate facilities for the handling of premature infants should be available as well as the necessary equipment for carrying out an exchange transfusion should this prove essential.

On rare occasions, a question of induction of abortion on the basis of severe Rh iso-immunization may arise. This problem is apt to develop in the case of a patient who has already had one or more severely affected or even stillborn erythroblastotic infants; whose husband has unquestionably been shown to be homozygous positive; and who at the beginning of a new pregnancy shows serological evidence of strong immunization. Such a patient is virtually certain to have a badly affected, full-term infant or perhaps a premature, hydropic, stillborn infant. Under such circumstances, rather than permitting the mother to undergo another fruitless labor, the obstetrician may consider abortion within the first three months to be the best course of action. Such a decision can only be arrived at after complete and thorough evaluation of the individual situation.

We may consider here, briefly, some of the therapeutic efforts which have been made in the recent past to obviate the effects of Rh iso-immunization prior to delivery of the infant. It must be stated at once that as yet no satisfactory method exists for the in vivo neutralization or inhibition of Rh antibodies. Efforts to inhibit antibody formation and activity by the injection of such substances as typhoid vaccine, pertussis vaccine, and ethylene disulphonate have been uniformly unsuccessful. Recently, a somewhat more rational approach has been suggested, *i.e.*, the periodic injection of Rh hapten during pregnancy. This substance can be demonstrated to react with Rh antibodies in vitro, but is said to be non-antigenic. It is obtained by extraction from human Rh-positive erythrocytes. Clinical investigation of the usefulness of this material is in progress at present. Thus far, insufficient data have been accumulated for evaluation.

The obstetrician may be called upon, at times, for advice, by an apprehensive Rh-negative woman married to an Rh-positive male. As we have already noted, when no serological evidence of sensitization exists the prospects for a normal childbearing career are no different from those of the Rh-positive female. A recent study, by Glass in our laboratory, of the family size of Rh negative–Rh positive matings contrasted with Rh positive–Rh positive matings has demonstrated the interesting fact that family size in the former group was actually somewhat greater than in the latter group. When iso-immunization is found to exist, any advice must be based upon a thorough clinical and immunological study of the individual problem. It has been conclusively shown that the interval between pregnancies will not affect the outcome, hence there is no point in advising postponement of pregnancy. The patient who has already given birth to one or more severely affected infants and whose husband can be conclusively shown to be homozygous should, in the present state of our knowledge, be advised against future pregnancies. For such couples adoption or even artificial insemination, utilizing an Rh-negative donor, may be advised.

Hemolytic Disease of the Fetus and Newborn. Maternal iso-immunization results in the varied clinical and pathological manifestations of the syndrome collectively known as hemolytic disease of the fetus and newborn. Prior to the discovery of the paramount importance of Rh incompatibility in the etiology of this disease, it was recognized that at least three clinical varieties existed—*hydrops fetalis, icterus gravis neonatorum,* and *congenital anemia of the newborn.* One of the outstanding features of the disease, namely, the occurrence of increased numbers of nucleated erythrocytes in the peripheral blood, led to the use of the term *erythroblastosis fetalis* as a common name for the entire syndrome. Current thinking favors the name used as the heading of this section since it is more descriptive of the nature of the entity.

Maternal antibodies, particularly of the albumin agglutinin variety, gain ready access to the fetal circulation. In studies of the blood of newborn Rh-negative infants born to mothers who have been immunized by previous pregnancies or transfusions we have been able to demonstrate a high degree of correlation between the titer of antibodies in the maternal serum and in the newborn infant's serum. In the case of infants who are Rh positive, such antibodies can be shown, by appropriate technics, to be adsorbed upon the Rh-positive erythrocytes as well as to exist in a free form in the infant's serum. The latter fraction may be looked upon as representing a temporary surplus which is potentially able to become attached to antigenic receptors on the erythrocyte. The adsorbed antibodies act as hemolysins and lead to an accelerated rate of destruction of the red blood cells. The earlier this process begins in utero and the greater its intensity the more severe will be the effect upon the fetus, hence the variability of the syndrome. Earlier observers, lacking a knowledge of the common underlying mechanism, were led to describe as separate entities the clinical varieties of the disease mentioned above. Careful and widespread antenatal study of the maternal serum has led not only to the recognition of intermediate forms of the disease, but also to the detection of many cases which, because of their relatively mild nature, would probably have been overlooked in the past. Nevertheless, the clinical divisions mentioned above serve excellently for descriptive purposes. Before elaborating upon the clinical and laboratory aspects of the disease it may be well to discuss somewhat further at this point the behavior of Rh antibodies which enter the infant's circulation.

It has been demonstrated that maternal antibodies, detectable at birth, gradually disappear from the fetal circulation over a period of four to eight weeks. Their rate of disappearance is influenced considerably by the therapy employed in the management of the infant. Investigation has also demonstrated that saline agglutinins which may be present in the maternal serum are rarely found in the infant's serum. On the other hand, if free antibody is present at all, it is usually of the albumin agglutinin variety. Detection of adsorbed antibodies is best accomplished by the use of the Coombs' test. This technic employs, as the testing reagent, an immune rabbit serum prepared by the repeated injection of human serum. Maternal antibodies which are globulin in nature may be adsorbed or "coated" upon the infant's cells. Agglutination of such "coated" cells occurs upon addition of the anti-human serum. A word of caution is indicated here regarding the Rh typing of "coated" cells. Such cells, if tested with an anti-Rh saline agglutinin serum, may be reported, incorrectly, as Rh negative because of the "blocking" effect produced by the adsorbed antibody.

It is permissible to make the generalization that whenever albumin agglutinins are present in the maternal serum they will invariably cross over into the fetal circulation. If the fetus is Rh positive, maternal antibodies will be found adsorbed upon the erythrocytes, and, at times, in a free state in the serum. Thus, the detection of antibodies in both the maternal and fetal blood, provided the latter is Rh positive, is sufficient evidence for a presumptive diagnosis of hemolytic disease. The degree of severity of the process will be gauged by additional data of a clinical and hematological nature to be discussed in succeeding paragraphs.

The pathology of hemolytic disease of the fetus and newborn varies again with the severity of the process. A composite picture of the changes commonly observed may be given. The severely affected fetus or infant may show considerable subcutaneous edema as well as effusions into the serous cavities (hydrops fetalis). In these cases the placenta is likewise markedly edematous and boggy, and shows large, prominent cotyledons. If death has occurred sometime before delivery considerable maceration of the fetal tissues is observed. If, on the other hand, the infant has survived for several days after birth it will appear intensely jaundiced (icterus gravis neonatorum). There may be petechiae and purpuric lesions scattered over the skin. Excessive and prolonged hemolysis results in marked erythroid hyperplasia of the bone marrow as well as the appearance of large areas of extramedullary hematopoiesis which are particularly notable in the spleen and liver. In the latter organ, histological examination may show, in addition, fatty degenerative parenchymal changes as well as hemosiderin deposition and engorgement of the bile canaliculi with bile. Some cardiac enlargement may be present. Pulmonary hemorrhages are not uncommonly noted. Important lesions may occur in the brain. These are collectively known as kernicterus and consist of yellowish pigmentation of the basal nuclei as well as of other portions of the brain. A small proportion of infants who survive the neonatal period may later exhibit neurological abnormalities which have been shown to be due to neuronal degeneration in the areas mentioned with subsequent gliosis.

Many of the clinical aspects of the disease have been partially depicted in the preceding paragraphs. Severely affected infants (hydrops fetalis) may die in utero

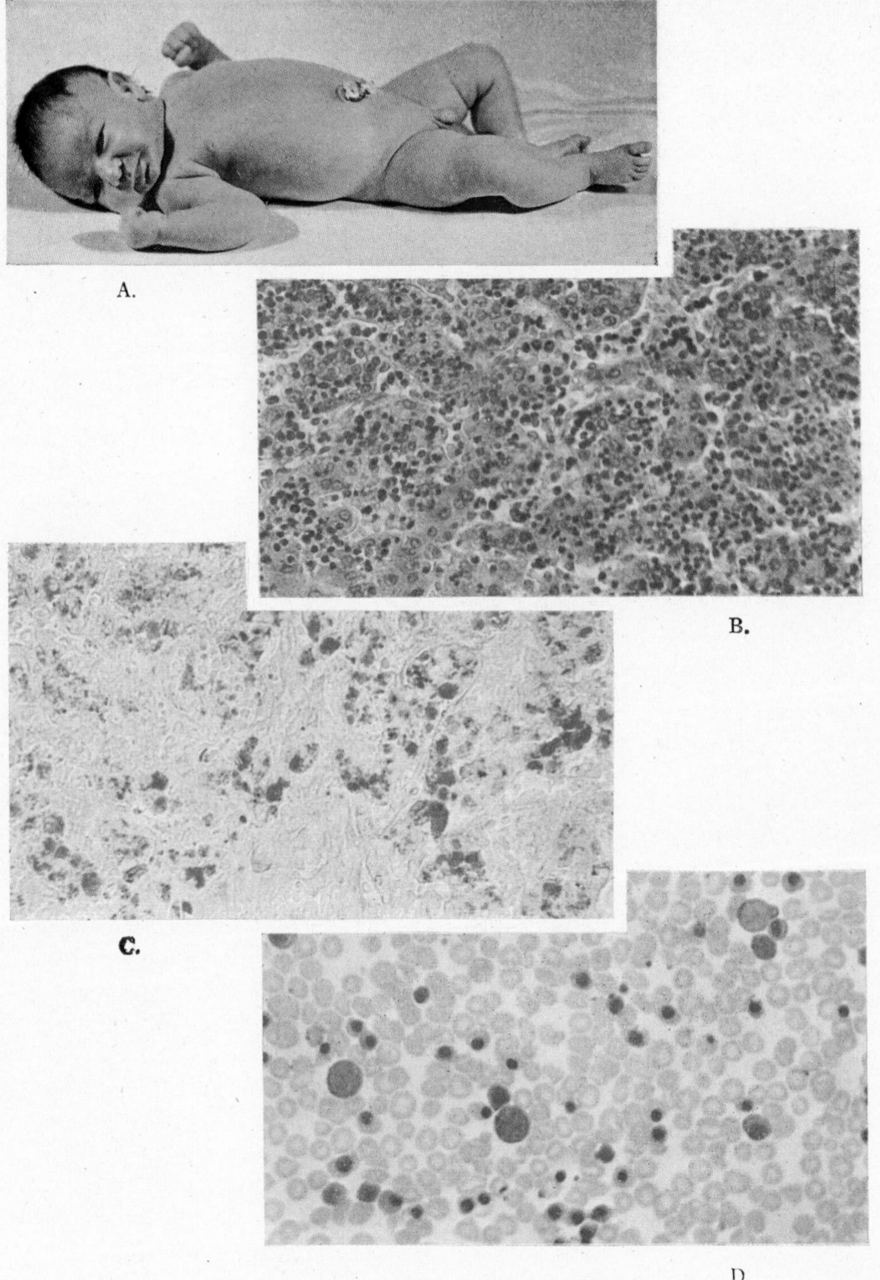

FIG. 525.—ERYTHROBLASTOSIS NEONATORUM.

A. Icterus of the skin on third day of life in an infant with erythroblastosis neonatorum.

B. Hematopoiesis in liver in hydrops type of erythroblastosis. × 190.

C. Intracellular pigment in liver. Some pigment remains unstained, the contrast suggests a difference in its nature. (Prussian blue stain. × 375.)

D. Photomicrograph of cord blood in erythroblastosis. Erythroblasts have large nuclei and a basophilic cytoplasm. Normoblasts are smaller and have pycnotic nuclei. (Wright's stain. × 315.)

(From Javert, *Surg. Gyn. Obst.*, 1942, 74:1-19. By permission of *Surgery, Gynecology and Obstetrics*. Copyright, 1942, by The Surgical Publishing Co. of Chicago.)

sometime between the twenty-sixth and thirty-fourth weeks of pregnancy. Those who are born alive usually survive only a few hours. The outstanding feature of such cases is the marked edema previously described. Other infants, not quite so severely affected, will be observed to become increasingly jaundiced within 12 to 36 hours after birth. Hepatomegaly and splenomegaly are regularly present. The characteristic hematological changes will be considered below. The course of the untreated disease may follow one of several pathways. It should be emphasized that the crucial period for these infants is during the first week of life. Most fatalities occur within the first three or four days. With each day of survival beyond this period the outlook for life becomes better. An unfavorable outcome is indicated by increasing lethargy, poor feeding, retraction of the head, spasticity of the extremities, and, at times, convulsions. These signs are usually indicative of central nervous system damage. Modification of the clinical picture by appropriate therapy is associated with the gradual disappearance of jaundice over a period of 10 to 14 days. Infants who are improving feed normally, show the usual weight gain, and fail to develop any signs of cerebral damage. In the great majority of infants who survive the neonatal period there will be no residual stigmata of the disease. The exact incidence of those demonstrating late residuals of cerebral injury cannot be stated with certainty. Most statistics in the literature are based upon series of cases accumulated prior to the widespread testing of women antenatally and hence probably included a disproportionate number of cases of moderate severity. Thus in the series of 29 cases reported by Stiller, four, or 14 per cent, were said to have demonstrated residual stigmata of kernicterus. It is quite likely that this figure is higher than the actual over-all incidence.

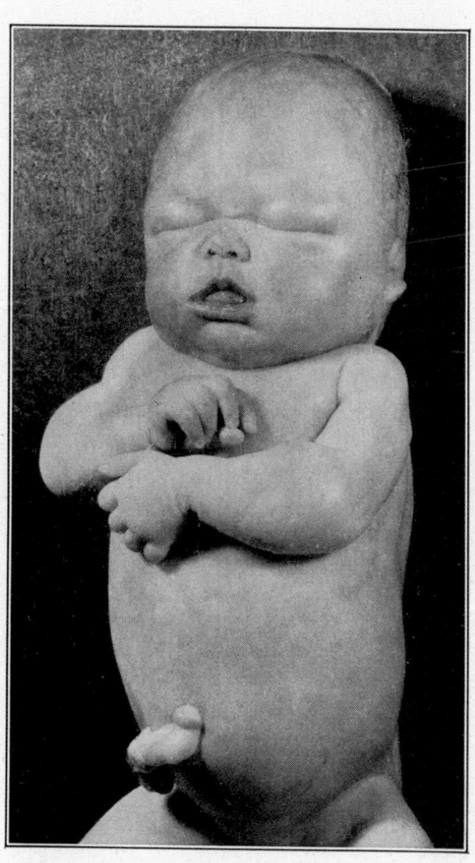

Fig. 526.—Fetus with Hydrops Type of Erythroblastosis.

Before describing the hematological changes seen in this disease, it may be well to note that hematological standards for the neonatal period differ from those of a later period of life. On the first day of life the average normal hemoglobin value is approximately 16.3 gm. per cent and the erythrocyte count 5.5 to 6.0 million per cubic millimeter. Infants with hydrops fetalis may show a red count as low as 1.0 million with a hemoglobin value as low as 4.0 gm. per cent. Infants less severely affected will show higher values on the initial examination immediately after birth. However, it is not uncommon for serial observations, made at 6 to 12 hour intervals during the first 48 hours of life, to show abrupt drops indicative of marked hemolysis. Examination of the blood smear in most cases reveals an increased number of normoblasts and erythroblasts. The normal newborn infant may, on the first day of life, show up to 10 nucleated erythrocytes per 100 leukocytes. Figures above this value are considered pathological. Other hematological changes likewise exist but are of

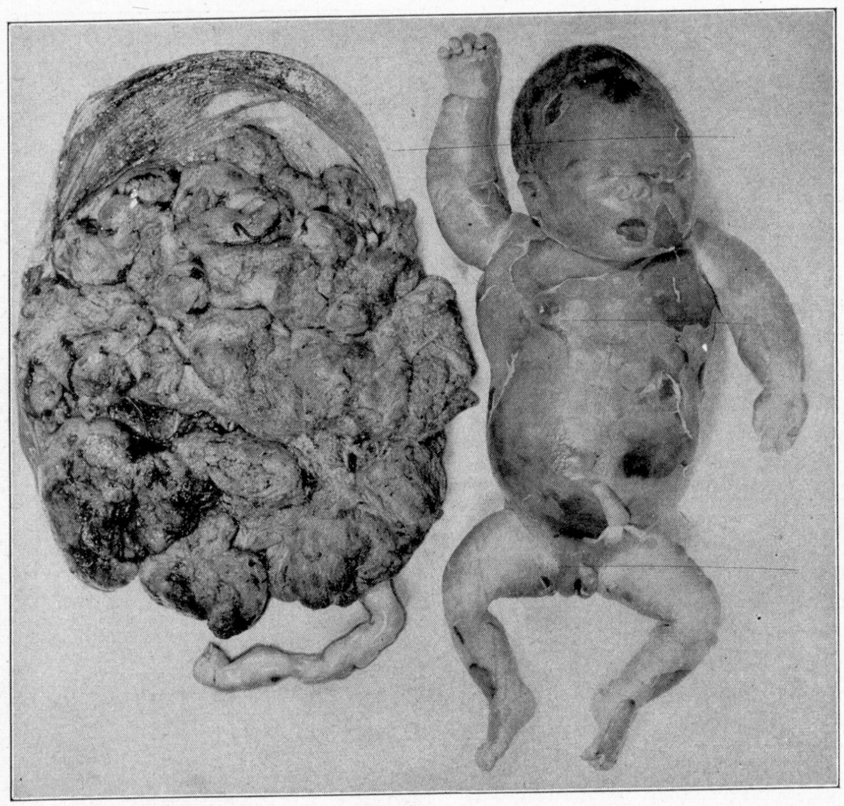

Fig. 527.—Macerated Fetus Weighing 2,750 Grams with Hydrops Type of Erythroblastosis. The placenta weighed 2,200 gms.

lesser significance. The most important biochemical abnormality is hyperbilirubinemia. The bilirubin is predominantly of the type which gives an indirect van den Bergh reaction, but there will also be a smaller increase in direct-reacting bilirubin.

No specific mention has as yet been made in this discussion of the mildest variety of hemolytic disease, namely, that type conveniently labelled congenital anemia of the newborn. If antenatal testing has not been done, these cases may be overlooked because of their mildness in the early neonatal period. It is not uncommon for such infants to be brought to the attention of the physician at the age of three or four weeks at which time they will be found to have a severe anemia with little or no associated jaundice. The spleen will be moderately enlarged. Nucleated erythrocytes may be present only in small numbers or not at all. The diagnosis in such cases is established by the demonstration of specific antibodies in the maternal serum as well as in the infant's blood.

Efforts have been made to relate hemolytic disease of the newborn with other clinical entities observed in later life. Of particular interest among these may be mentioned undifferentiated feeblemindedness. Several groups of investigators have reported a somewhat higher incidence than normal of Rh-negative mothers of Rh-positive, feebleminded individuals. The exact significance of these findings, however, remains to be determined.

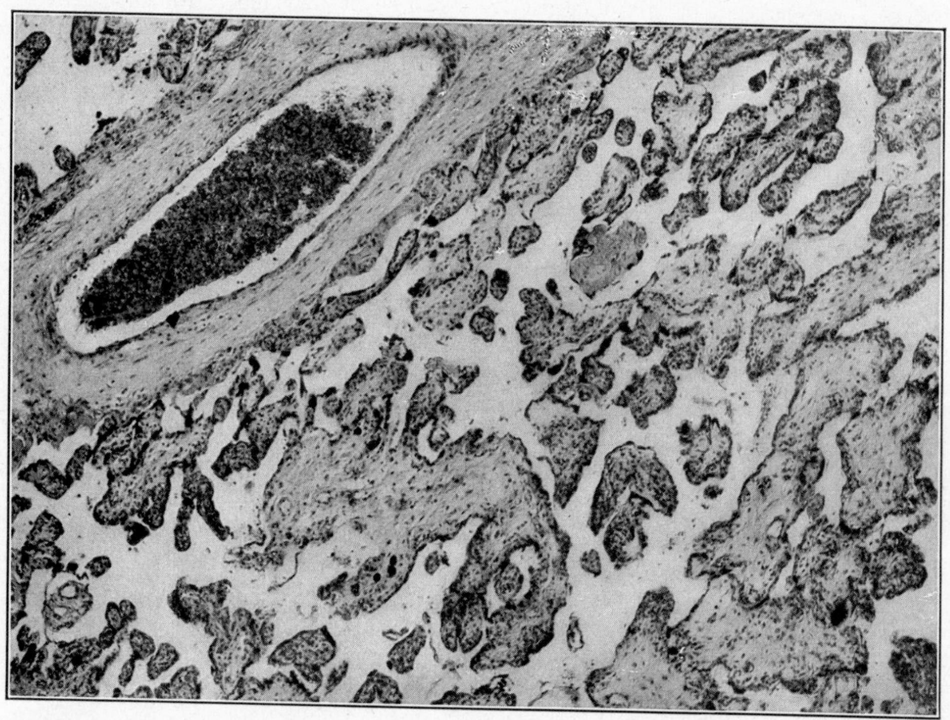

FIG. 528.—PHOTOMICROGRAPH OF A HYDROPIC PLACENTA.
Note the large edematous villi and fetal vessel filled with immature erythrocytes.

Any general consideration of the management of hemolytic disease should properly include some aspects of prevention. The increasing awareness of the role of transfusion in iso-immunization has already helped to diminish the frequency of this procedure as an etiological factor and should continue to do so in the future. Iso-immunization by heterospecific pregnancy cannot, of course, be prevented. Attempts at antenatal treatment have, thus far, been confined to efforts to either inhibit the formation of antibodies or to neutralize those already formed. This goal has not yet been achieved. Studies which are at present being carried on with a serologically specific, but non-antigenic substance derived from Rh-positive erythrocytes, Rh hapten, are at too early a stage for evaluation.

The practical management of hemolytic disease of the newborn, today, rests largely upon the transfusion of an adequate amount of Rh-negative blood when the proper indications exist. The decision to transfuse must be based upon a careful evaluation of a number of factors. As previously noted, the maternal past history, with particular reference to the birth of affected infants, is one such factor. Since it is generally true that following the birth of one erythroblastotic infant subsequent Rh-positive infants will be more seriously affected, this fact is, properly, a potent determinant in the decision to resort promptly to transfusions. Knowledge of the degree of elevation of maternal antibody titer during the present pregnancy will also be of value in planning the course of action. Hematological data obtained as promptly as possible after birth are invaluable as a guide to management. Hemoglobin values of 14.5 gm. per cent or less obtained on a sample of cord blood are indicative of an anemia which can be expected to become rapidly worse. Although the degree of erythroblastemia is generally considered unreliable, the presence of a very large number of nucleated erythrocytes accompanies other signs of severity. The prompt appearance of jaundice belongs in the same category. Serological studies of the infant's blood are very helpful in planning management. A strongly positive Coombs' test is indicative of the adsorption of considerable amounts of antibody. The amount of free antibody in the serum is too variable to be a reliable index of severity.

The evaluation of these data permits one to classify the case as mild or severe. If placed in the former category, the infant should be closely observed and transfused only if increasing evidence of anemia appears. The more severely affected infant should be treated, preferably by exchange transfusion. Exchange transfusion, as the name implies, is a procedure in which some other variety of blood is substituted for the infant's own. Since a major pathogenetic mechanism in this disease is the destruction of Rh-positive erythrocytes by specific antibodies, a rational plan of treatment is the removal of the infant's own blood and replacement, to as great an extent as possible, by Rh-negative blood which will remain relatively stable in content during the crucial neonatal period. It has been estimated that by the use of 500 cc. of Rh-negative blood, which represents approximately twice the total blood volume of the newborn infant, a 90 per cent substitution is accomplished, *i.e.*, 90 per cent of the blood remaining after completion of the procedure will be Rh-negative. By removing most of the Rh-positive erythrocytes, one obviates overloading of the infant's organs by breakdown products of red cell origin. Furthermore, the procedure results in the removal of a considerable proportion of free antibody. Following an exchange transfusion it may or may not be necessary to administer further small transfusions during the first several weeks of life. This can only be ascertained by serial blood counts during the neonatal period.

It is customary to employ fresh, type-specific, Rh-negative blood. If type-specific blood is not available, group O Rh-negative blood may be used. Although 500 cc. is usually given, amounts up to 1,000 cc. have been used for severely affected infants. Several technics have been proposed for exchange transfusion for this purpose. The technic recommended by Diamond utilizes a plastic catheter which is introduced into the inferior vena cava by way of the umbilical vein. Blood is introduced and withdrawn through this catheter. The umbilical vein may be used any time during the first 24 hours of life, but thereafter shrivelling of the tissues increases the likelihood of thrombosis of this vein. The technic recommended by Wiener utilizes the saphenous vein at the ankle for infusion and the radial artery for withdrawal of the blood. Other technics have also been described. The details of these procedures may be found in the original communications which are listed in the bibliography at the close of the chapter.

Other aspects of the therapeutic management may be briefly mentioned. In the course of an exchange transfusion, at times, signs of tetany may appear as a result of the injection of a large amount of sodium citrate. This may be remedied by the administration of small (5 to 10 cc.) amounts of a 10 per cent calcium gluconate solution. Penicillin or some other antibiotic should be administered as a prophylactic measure for 24 to 48 hours after an exchange transfusion. The administration of Vitamin K has been recommended by some authors to combat hypoprothrombinemia. Although it has been demonstrated that the breast milk of sensitized women contains antibodies, there is no conclusive evidence that these are absorbed through the infant's intestinal mucosa to any great extent. Until this has been conclusively determined, however, it would seem safer to recommend abstinence from breast feeding.

Maternal Iso-immunization by Other Blood Group Antigens. Although the vast majority of cases of hemolytic anemia of the newborn are due to Rh iso-immunization, some instances of iso-sensitization due to other blood group antigens have been reported. Iso-immunization by the antigens A and B occurs in heterospecific pregnancies occasionally and should be thought of when the more common type has been ruled out. Recently, Levine has described an instance of iso-immunization associated with another antigen system (Kell-Cellano) of the red cell. As a general rule, in atypical cases of hemolytic anemia of the newborn, the maternal serum should be studied for antibodies which will react with either the father's or infant's red blood cells since these are the probable source of the antigenic stimulus.

FETAL SYPHILIS

Syphilis is one of the frequent causes of fetal death in the later months of pregnancy and is probably always maternal in origin. The mother may be suffering from the disease at the time of conception or may contract it during the course of pregnancy; in either event transmission to the fetus occurs through the placenta. Colles' law, which postulates the possibility of paternal infection of the product of conception without infecting the mother, may be dismissed as unproven. The paternal transmission of syphilis to the fetus without the production or previous presence of the disease in the mother does not exist, according to the latest opinion of most authorities.

Another interesting possibility, which is well established, is that a woman who has had syphilis for many years may have a nonsyphilitic offspring. The probability that the child will be infected in utero diminishes as the years following the maternal infection pass. Thus it will be seen that the infection of the fetus is dependent to some extent upon the proximity of the infection of the mother. If the woman contracts syphilis shortly before, at the time of conception, or soon afterward, the fetus is almost sure to be infected during intra-uterine life. However, if the previously normal woman is infected after the sixth month of gestation, in the majority of instances the offspring will escape the disease. It is important to bear in mind in such cases that the infant may contract the disease during delivery, as a result of nursing, or in other ways.

It has long been known that a syphilitic infection exerts a most deleterious influence upon the product of conception. In 1915, Williams showed that it was the most important single factor concerned in the production of fetal death in hospital practice, and, in 1920, he demonstrated that it was responsible for 34 per cent of 302 consecutive fetal deaths in his service. Usually it leads to the untimely expulsion of a macerated premature fetus. Less commonly, the child is born alive, showing distinct manifestations of the disease, while in other cases they do not appear until a later period. Formerly, it was thought that syphilis played no role in the production of abortion. The recent reports of McCord tend to contradict this; he has demonstrated both long-bone changes and the organisms of syphilis in the bodies of 35 fetal abortions. In addition, he has found the treponemata abundant in the tissues of eight fetuses, each of which weighed less than 500 gm.

McCord states that he has not definitely demonstrated the organism of syphilis in fetuses under four months of age, while Dippel, in a study of 67 nonviable fetuses of luetic women, found no spirochetes in fetal tissues prior to the eighteenth week of gestation and noted that the incidence of infection of the fetus rose from 10 per cent in the first half to 50 per cent in the latter half of the miscarriage period. If we use the term abortion as referring to pregnancies terminating before or during the sixteenth week, and miscarriage between the sixteenth and the twenty-eighth weeks, one may say that syphilis definitely causes early as well as late miscarriage, but that the disease has not been proven to cause abortion. Dippel suggests that there may be some natural protection of the fetus against syphilis during the first seventeen weeks of pregnancy.

It is of the greatest importance that the practitioner should become thoroughly familiar with the characteristic lesions of fetal and placental syphilis; upon their recognition the future treatment of the patient often depends. This is a point especially worthy of emphasis, inasmuch as, in consequence of ignorance or design on the part of one or both parents, the first intimation that the physician may have of the existence of the disease is often afforded by the birth of a dead child, or the appearance of syphilitic stigmata in a living one, unless the Wassermann reaction is determined in all pregnant women. The laws of certain states now make it mandatory upon the physician that every pregnant woman under his care receive a serologic examination. The enactment of such legislation in other states and countries would be a great step toward the eradication of syphilis.

Syphilis not only gives rise to characteristic lesions of the fetus but also affects the placenta, so that frequently a diagnosis can be made from an examination of that organ. This fact is of special importance in those cases in which the fetus is born alive, or when an autopsy upon a dead child is not permitted. The appearance of the syphilitic fetus varies materially according as it is born alive or dead. In either instance it is markedly undersized, and the subcutaneous fat is poorly developed or entirely lacking. In the living child the skin usually presents a dry, drawn appearance and has a peculiar grayish hue. It is very brittle, especially at the flexor surfaces of the joints, where abrasions readily occur and expose the underlying corium. The skin covering the soles of the feet and palms of the hands is often thickened and glistening, and suggests the condition observed in the hands of washerwomen. In other cases, characteristic pemphigoid vesicles are noted in the same locations. If intra-uterine death has occurred, the fetus rapidly undergoes maceration, the skin peeling off upon the slightest touch and exposing the underlying discolored corium. It should be noted that maceration is by no means pathognomonic, since it occurs whenever a dead fetus is long retained in utero, no matter what the cause of death.

The lesions in the internal organs consist essentially in interstitial changes in the lungs, liver, spleen, and pancreas, and osteochondritis in the long bones. It is generally stated that the lungs frequently contain gummatous nodules. These, however, are usually lacking. Usually the lungs are enlarged, pale, and scarcely float when placed in water. On microscopic examination the alveoli are found filled with cast-off epithelial cells in all stages of fatty degeneration—catarrhal pneumonia, the *pneumonia alba* of Virchow. In other cases the lesion consists of an increase in the interstitial tissue associated with pronounced round-cell infiltration, by which the alveoli are

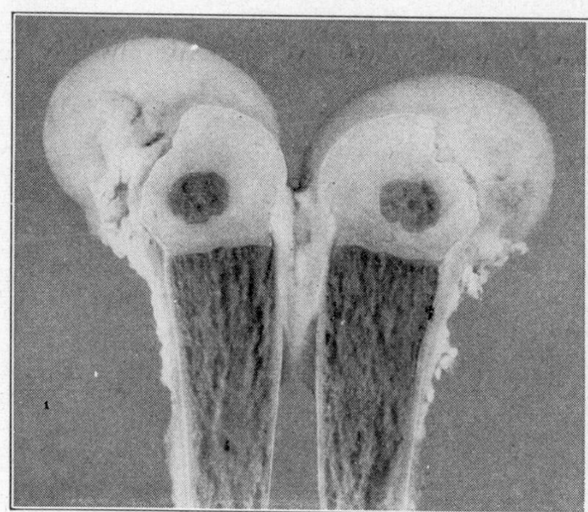

FIG. 529A.—NORMAL FETAL EPIPHYSIS. × 1.5.

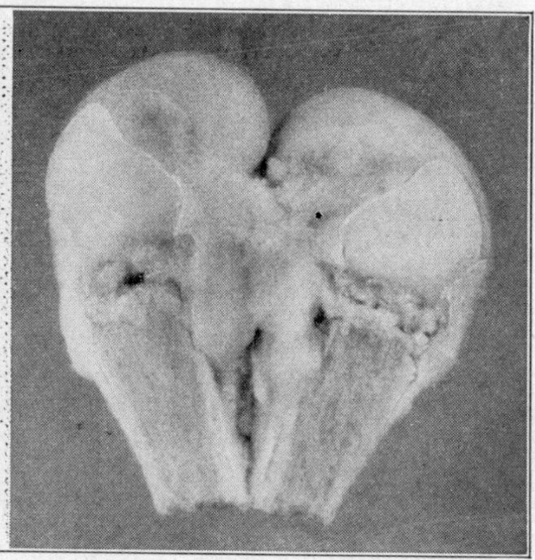

FIG. 529B.—SYPHILITIC FETAL EPIPHYSIS. × 1.5.

(Courtesy of Dr. Jacob Furth, Dept. of Pathology, Cornell University Medical College and The New York Hospital.)

compressed but do not quite become impervious to air. These changes have been exhaustively studied by Heller.

As the result of hypertrophic cirrhosis, the liver undergoes a marked increase in size, and, according to Ruge, its weight may equal one tenth or even one eighth of that of the whole body, instead of one thirtieth as is usual. Under the microscope there is a marked increase in the connective tissue surrounding the individual lobules and acini, with here and there small areas of round-cell infiltration. Many authorities lay great stress upon the presence of so-called blood islands—dilated capillaries containing red cells in all stages of development—but in our experience the condition is not pathognomonic.

The spleen likewise undergoes interstitial changes and increases markedly in size, so that it frequently weighs two or three times as much as usual, which, roughly speaking, is one three-hundreths of the body weight. The pancreas also presents interstitial changes, and is slightly larger than normal.

Tissier and Girauld state that prior to the middle of pregnancy, the *Spirochaeta pallida* is rarely found, but after that period the fetus may be said to suffer from a spirochetal septicemia and the parasites may be demonstrated in large numbers in the various organs and blood. They are most abundant in the adrenals, where they are noted in 97.5 per cent of all cases, according to Trinchese, and progressively less frequently in the lungs, pancreas, liver, and internal genitalia, respectively.

The recognition of the organic lesions requires some pathologic experience, though if the liver and spleen of a macerated fetus are markedly increased in size and weight the diagnosis is practically assured.

An equally characteristic sign, and one which is readily detected, is afforded by changes occurring at the junction of the epiphysis with the diaphysis in the long

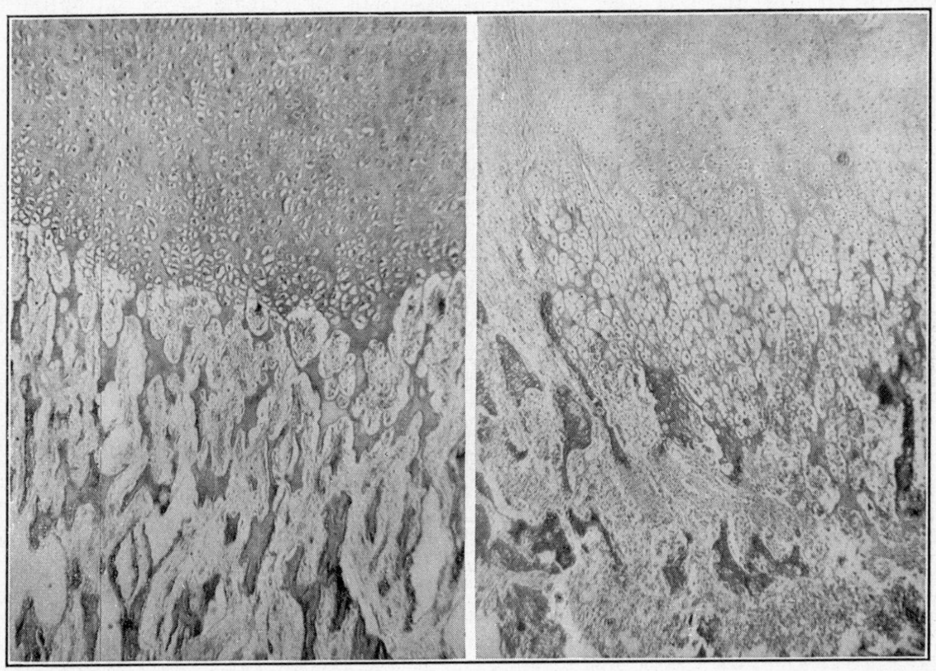

Fig. 530A.—Normal Fetal Epiphysis. × 45. Fig. 530B.—Syphilitic Fetal Epiphysis. × 45.

(Courtesy of Dr. Jacob Furth, Dept. of Pathology, Cornell University Medical College and The New York Hospital.)

bones—Wegner's bone disease. Normally the two are separated by a narrow, whitish, slightly curved line 0.5 to 1 mm. in diameter—Guérin's line—representing the zone of preliminary calcification, which constitutes the scaffolding upon which the new bone is developed. In syphilis, on the other hand, this becomes converted into an irregular, jagged, yellowish zone 2, 3, or more mm. in thickness. In advanced cases this alteration is associated with considerable softening and the formation of a soft pultaceous material, which sometimes leads to complete separation of the epiphysis (Fig. 529A and B).

Upon microscopic examination of the normal epiphysis, as shown in Fig. 530A, the cartilage cells are found to be arranged in parallel columns at right angles to Guérin's line, while below it is the typical bony structure of the diaphysis with its narrow cavities. The line itself is formed by a deposit of lime salts between the median ends of the rows of cartilage cells, and is gradually invaded by the newly formed bone.

In syphilis, as is illustrated in Fig. 530B, the changes are due to an osteochondritis, as the result of which there is no longer a sharply marked zone of preliminary calcification between the cartilage and the growing bone, but areas of bone formation, calcification, and leukocytic and small-cell infiltration are found scattered irregularly through the lower portion of the epiphysis, giving an irregular appearance to this region.

These changes, which have been carefully studied by Wegner and R. Müller, are most readily recognizable at the lower end of the femur, and at the lower ends of the tibia and radius. They are extremely characteristic, and their detection justifies one in making a positive diagnosis and placing the mother under specific treatment. Alexander has shown that the osseous lesions are widely diffused, occurring at the epiphyses of all the long bones, as well as in the phalanges of the hands and feet. Since the demonstration by Shipley and Pearson that the changes can readily be recognized by means of the x-ray, we have utilized the procedure as an accessory means of diagnosis. Accordingly, we take x-ray pictures of all dead children as a matter of routine—partly for diagnostic purposes but especially to permit comparison between the x-ray, placental, and autopsy findings. Furthermore, they are taken in the case of live children whenever anything in the history suggests the possibility of the existence of syphilis.

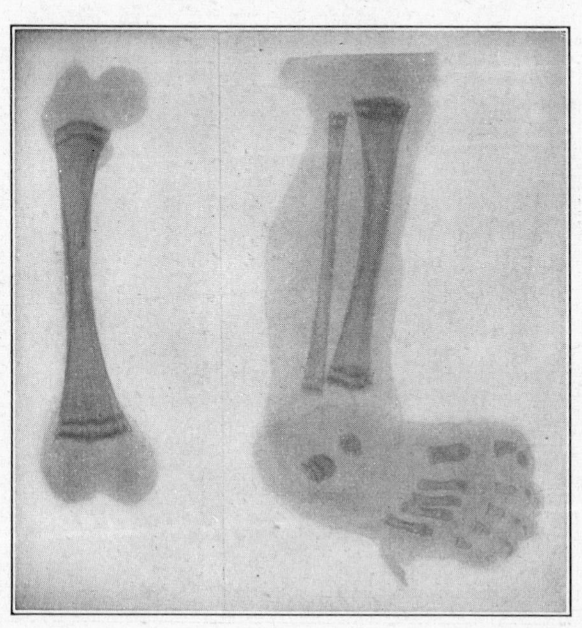

Fig. 531.—X-ray of Leg Bones of Syphilitic Fetus.

Many years' experience has convinced us that the procedure constitutes a most valuable addition to our diagnostic equipment, and, whenever lesions similar to those depicted in Fig. 531 are present, that the diagnosis of syphilis is assured.

Placental Syphilis. Under the influence of syphilitic infection the placenta undergoes characteristic changes. It becomes larger and paler in color, and often presents a dull, greasy appearance. It is always relatively, and frequently absolutely, increased in size, and, according to the researches of Schwab and Levy-Solal, which we confirm, instead of one sixth, it may represent as much as one fourth, one third or even one half, of the entire body weight of the fetus.

Still more characteristic, however, are the changes in the chorionic villi to which Fränkel called attention in 1873. During the last three or four months of pregnancy, when the syphilitic placentae are teased out in salt solution, the villi are seen to have lost their characteristic arborescent appearance and to have become thicker and more club-shaped. At the same time, there is a marked decrease in the number of blood vessels, which in advanced cases have almost entirely disappeared. This results partly from endarteritic changes, but principally from a proliferation of the stroma cells, which lose their normal stellate appearance, becoming round or oval in shape, and closely packed together.

The changes are still more characteristic when sections made from hardened specimens are studied. The individual villi are increased in size and almost devoid of blood vessels, while their stroma is made up of closely packed, round or oval cells. The appearance, while characteristic for the advanced cases of placental syphilis, par-

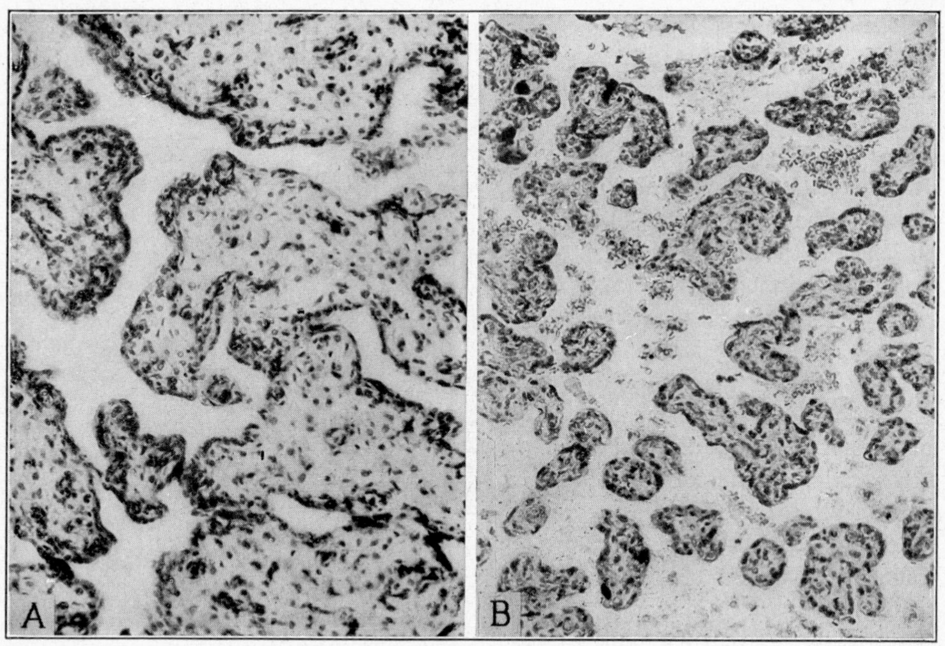

FIG. 532.—PHOTOMICROGRAPHS OF PLACENTAS AT TERM.

A, Syphilitic, showing large, club-shaped villi with increased amount of fibrous tissue in stroma. B, Normal placenta.

ticularly of the untreated types, is of only moderate value in early, mild, or treated cases of syphilis. McCord has demonstrated, most conclusively, the difficulties encountered in this connection. X-ray of the long bones is a far more definite criterion of fetal syphilis that are placental changes. On the other hand, it must be admitted that negative findings do not necessarily imply the absence of syphilis in the child. The lesions described afford a satisfactory explanation for the poor development of the fetus when born alive and, in association with the spirochetal septicemia and the organic involvement, readily explain the frequency of a fatal issue.

On the other hand, Mohn and others believe that the changes just described, while very suggestive, are not absolutely characteristic and hold that a positive diagnosis cannot be made unless the presence of the spirochetes can be demonstrated in the placenta. This has been attempted by many investigators, who have found that the spirochetes are so sparsely scattered through the organ that their recognition is most difficult, even when they are present in large numbers in the fetal organs. Trinchese states that they can always be found, if one is willing to study several hundred sections, but this has not been our experience. On the other hand, Philipp has shown that spirochetes in motion can be readily demonstrated by examining under the dark-field microscope scrapings from the intima of the vessels of the fresh cord.

HEMORRHAGIC DISEASE OF THE NEWBORN

There is a tendency toward spontaneous hemorrhages in a small group of newborn infants, which may be manifested clinically by bloody emesis, melena, skin petechiae, and less often by umbilical bleeding. Multiple ecchymoses and petechiae are found at autopsy in various organs, including the liver, spleen, adrenals, thymus, pleura, pericardium, and brain. These lesions are not regarded as pathognomonic, since they may also be found in infants dying of asphyxia neonatorum, and even following normal labor, according to Parmalee. The clinical and pathologic multiplicity of the hemorrhages suggests a generalized systemic process which may be associated with labor. The uterine contractions express blood from the placenta into the arterial and venous systems of the fetus, which intercommunicate by means of the ductus arteriosus, ductus venosus, and the foramen ovale; intravascular tension may be increased to the point of actual capillary endothelial separation, with escape of blood into organs and tissues. These hemorrhages may therefore be regarded as physiologic and an expression of the change from intra-uterine to extra-uterine existence, as has been discussed in the introduction to this section. The deranged bleeding and clotting mechanism characteristic of this period of life is probably responsible for these physiologic hemorrhages reaching, at times, pathologic proportions.

Bleeding in the newborn was discussed by Mauriceau as early as 1694, and omphalorrhagia, or umbilical bleeding, was first described by Watts in 1753. The latter condition is now quite rare, the lowered incidence being due to better technic in the care of the umbilical cord. Hemorrhagic disease of the newborn has been described in the literature under many headings, including: "hemophilia neonatorum," "idiopathic hemorrhage," "hemorrhagic diathesis," "melena neonatorum," "hemorrhagica neonatorum," "umbilical hemorrhage," and "morbus hemorrhagicus neonatorum." In 1894 Townsend reported 50 cases and called the condition "hemorrhagic disease of the newborn," a designation which is commonly used today.

Renewed interest in the disease followed Dam's discovery in 1934 that newborn chicks on fat-free diets developed hemorrhages from the mucous membranes and into soft tissues, with prolonged clotting time and a reduction of plasma prothrombin. These experimental hemorrhages were controlled by feeding alfalfa and spinach, and it was concluded that a "Koagulationsvitamine" was responsible, hence the name vitamin K. This work was confirmed by Almquist in 1935. Furthermore, investigations by Hawkins and Brinkhous on dogs with bile fistulae revealed a prothrombin deficiency, and these animals developed a bleeding tendency, which suggested to Quick that the absence of bile led to a faulty absorption of vitamin K. This situation also exists in patients with obstructive jaundice. The next development was the demonstration of the value of vitamin K in obstructive jaundice and bile fistula.

Earlier studies by Whipple in 1912 had shown a complete absence of prothrombin in a case of melena neonatorum and in the same year Richards stated that the prothrombin deficiency was probably due to thrombocytopenia. In 1921 Gelston was also impressed by the prolonged prothrombin time in a case of hemorrhagic disease. More recently Brinkhous, Smith, and Warner showed that the prothrombin concentration is normally low at birth, the values ranging between 14 and 39 per cent of the adult normal in cord blood. In our clinic, Javert and Moore obtained an average value of 23 per cent. A further decrease in the first days of life has been reported by Owen and co-workers, confirming the earlier report of Lucas (1921), who used the method of Howell. However, Quick, using his own method for determining coagulation time, has found prothrombin concentration to be nearly normal at birth.

Javert found the incidence of hemorrhagic disease in the New York Hospital to be 0.77 per cent, agreeing closely with Townsend's earlier figure of 0.67 per cent, and Salomonsen's incidence of 0.68 per cent. It is evidently more frequent in infants delivered in a hospital than in those born at home, probably because of a greater prevalence, in the former, of obstetrical abnormalities such as toxemia of pregnancy, prolonged labors, and forceps deliveries. The disease does not appear to be familial although Minot and Kugelmass have reported such occurrence.

Hemorrhagic disease of the newborn is thus a syndrome characterized by spontaneous internal or external bleeding accompanied by hypoprothrombinemia. It is generally believed that the onset takes place between the third and sixth days of life, although Javert found that fully one third of the infants began to bleed on the first day of life. This observation suggests an intra-uterine and parturitional course for the disease, such a view being supported by two cases recently observed in which bloody amniotic fluid was seen when the membranes ruptured. The relationship to labor is further established by a series of more than 700 infants delivered by cesarean section in this clinic, in which only one case of hemorrhagic disease occurred.

The infants are often full term and healthy in appearance, although a greater incidence of the disease has been noted in premature children. The bleeding and clotting times are usually within the elevated physiological range for newborn infants, although both occasionally may be markedly increased. The red cell count, hemoglobin, and white count are within the normal range for the newborn infant, unless continued hemorrhage has produced a secondary anemia. The platelets may be slightly decreased, and the prothrombin is probably markedly reduced, even below the very low values seen normally at birth. Icterus neonatorum is not more frequent. The placenta is usually of average weight, and shows no distinctive pathology. In the differential diagnosis, hemophilia, congenital syphilis, sepsis of the newborn, purpura, erythroblastosis, and traumatic intracranial hemorrhage must be considered.

In the treatment of hemorrhagic disease of the newborn, the intramuscular injection of synthetic vitamin K (2-methyl-1, 4-naphthoquinone) has proved the most efficacious therapy. Not only does Vitamin K, given orally or parenterally to the infant, raise the plasma prothrombin rapidly, but as shown in our clinic by Hellman, Moore and Shettles, the administration of vitamin K to the mother in pregnancy or labor also prevents hypoprothrombinemia.

Upon these facts, all observers agree. Whether, however, the prophylactic administration of vitamin K to mothers in pregnancy or labor will improve fetal mortality statistics, through reducing the incidence of certain types of cerebral hemorrhage, is a moot question. It is our opinion that it does practically eliminate the occurrence of hemorrhagic disease of the newborn and the extent to which this prophylactic practice will improve fetal mortality will naturally depend upon the frequency, in any given locality, of hemorrhagic disease in newborn infants. If the figures cited above by Javert and Townsend are valid indications of the frequency of this neonatal complication, the routine administration of vitamin K to mothers would seem well justified. On the other hand, other observers, notably Potter, regard hemorrhagic disease as a much rarer entity and question the justification of the routine use of vitamin K. We have employed vitamin K routinely in antenatal and parturient patients for a number of years, and when it is administered, we rarely encounter hemorrhagic disease of the newborn. On the other hand, in preceding years when it was not employed, hemorrhagic disease was not infrequent and was often fatal. Since vitamin K is cheap and does specifically prevent this serious, if uncommon, complication of neonatal life, we believe that its routine use is justifiable but are cognizant of the fact that many authorities take the opposite point of view.

EPIDEMIC DIARRHEA OF THE NEWBORN

Outbreaks of epidemic diarrhea of the newborn may occur at any time and several have been reported in this country during the past several years. Certain cities have recently enacted rigid sanitary codes for the conduct of maternity hospitals with the hope of preventing the occurrence of this disease. We regard the code of the Department of Health of the City of New York as adequate and commensurate with our present knowledge of the disease. This code, as well as the epidemiology and pathology of the condition, are fully described by Rice, Best, Frank, and Abramson. Full protection of the newborn demands that all maternity services adhere to a rigid regimen, such as that reported by these authors.

The etiology of the disease is as yet unknown. In 1935 Dulany and Michelson demonstrated *B. coli mutabile* in the stools of 67 per cent of the babies suffering from this condition. Baker, in 1939, studying three separate outbreaks of the disease, could find no definite pathogenic micro-organism in the stools of the full-term infants while in the stools of 70 per cent of the premature infants with the disease he noted *B. coli mutabile,* or hemolytic *B. coli,* or both. Recent work suggests that some cases of epidemic diarrhea are due to a filterable virus.

The clinical symptoms may be variable and usually appear from the second to the fourteenth day after birth, although it may occur later in premature babies. The stools, which are loose, and sometimes watery yellowish-green, with or without mucus, and occasionally blood-tinged, may vary in number from 7 to 11 or more per day. Vomiting is usually rare. Marked dehydration and acidosis may develop.

In the absence of proper treatment the prognosis is grave, mortalities as high as 50 per cent having been reported. In our experience, such treatment demands a personnel adequately trained to institute the necessary therapy. In the New York Hospital all babies suffering from this condition are immediately transferred to the Pediatric Department, necessary isolation precautions being taken to prevent the spread of the disease in the nurseries of the maternity service. The results obtained by Dr. S. Z. Levine in these babies have recently been reported by Baker. He records a mortality rate of zero for an outbreak, of apparently mild character, in 1935; a rate of 15.4 per cent for a more severe epidemic occurring in the premature nursery in 1937; and no deaths in an epidemic in 1938 in which all the infants involved were extremely ill.

As stated above, precautionary measures are essential in the prevention of this condition. Should a newborn child develop loose and frequent stools (seven or more a day) it must be immediately isolated and the necessary steps taken to prevent spread of the disease. The treatment of epidemic diarrhea, as employed by Levine, consists in complete starvation and no water by mouth until no stools have been passed for a period of 12 to 24 hours and the carbon dioxide content of the blood has returned to normal. During this interval of starvation the child is given hypodermoclysis of normal saline solution followed by intravenous injections of 10 per cent glucose solution in water. Molar sodium lactate solution is employed to combat acidosis, as shown by very low carbon dioxide content of the blood. In addition, transfusions of 20 cc. of citrated whole blood per kilogram of body weight are administered on the first and second days of the treatment, and thereafter if necessary. Following starvation regimen, the infant receives small quantities, starting with 5 cc. and increasing by 5 cc. at alternate feedings, of sterile distilled water every two hours until he receives his total fluid requirement by mouth. Then protein milk, skimmed milk, or preparations of hydrolyzed casein are gradually substituted for the water. Subsequently the two-hour feedings are slowly decreased until the infant is on six feedings a day.

SPONTANEOUS PNEUMOTHORAX

The possibility of spontaneous pneumothorax should always be borne in mind whenever a newborn infant shows persistence of dyspnea and cyanosis. The diagnosis will be made in most cases by the fluoroscope or roentgenogram since the physical findings are not always clear-cut and may be misleading. The etiology is often obscure since it may develop in infants who breathe spontaneously at birth and upon whom no artificial respiration has been used. It appears to be more common in males than in females. The prognosis of pneumothorax is believed to be somewhat better when it occurs in the neonatal period than when it develops later on, but it is always grave, the outcome being fatal in about half the cases. Although withdrawal of the air with a needle and syringe is often successful, the relief may be only temporary and the procedure may have to be repeated one or more times.

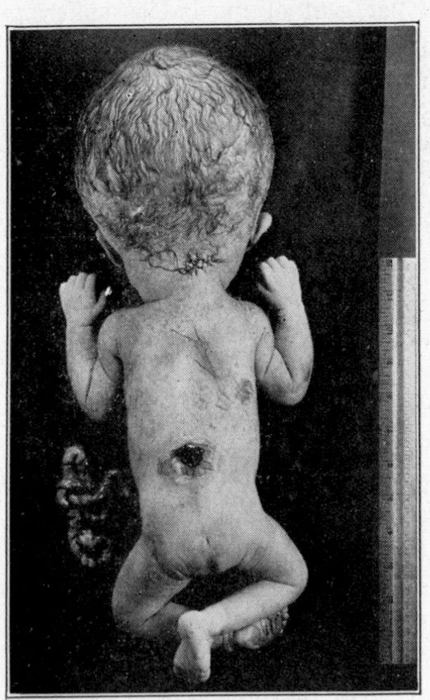

Fig. 533.—Hydrocephalus with Spina Bifida.

ABNORMALITIES OF DEVELOPMENT

In Chapter 30, "Dystocia Due to Abnormalities in Presentation or Development of the Fetus," fetal malformations, which may give rise to difficult labor, are discussed in some detail. Every newborn child must have a complete physical examination at the time of delivery, in order to insure it every opportunity for survival. In this initial examination any abnormalities are noted and recorded in the child's history. A report of the condition can likewise be given at once to the father of the child, which usually avoids mistrust should a serious lesion be discovered at a later time. For detailed description of the various anomalies, as well as the hereditary factors involved, the reader is referred to Murphy's excellent monograph on this subject (1940).

Hydrocephalus. This lesion is discussed in Chapter 30, "Dystocia Due to Abnormalities in Presentation or Development of the Fetus."

Meningocele. This is a herniation of the meninges in the suture lines, usually in the occipital region, less commonly at the root of the nose, or it may be associated with spina bifida. If brain substance is present in the sac, the condition is spoken of as an *encephalocele.* Any attempt at closure generally results in the development of hydrocephalus, and these infants usually die from meningitis.

Spina Bifida. This condition represents a hiatus, usually in the lumbosacral vertebrae, through which a meningeal sac protrudes (meningocele) and if the sac contains the spinal cord the condition is called a meningomyelocele. It is commonly associated with hydrocephalus and clubfeet. In other instances, the defect may be very slight and is then referred to as a *spina bifida occulta.* Treatment consists in prevention of trauma and infection by protecting the sac with cotton and alcohol, and having the infant lie, as much as possible, on its abdomen. If the infant survives, surgical closure is performed in the third month. A guarded prognosis is given to the parents, especially if a *myelocele* is also present; furthermore, a statement should be made regarding possible development of hydrocephalus following the operation.

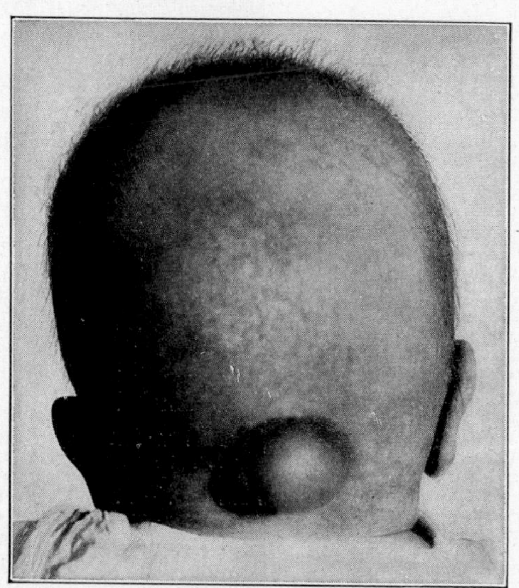

Fig. 534.—Meningocele. Infant Age Four Months.
(Courtesy of Dr. S. Z. Levine.)

Mongolian Idiot. This name has been given to infants who present a definite clinical picture, the configuration of their facies resembling that of a Mongol. Their eyes are set close together, with small slanting palpebral fissures. The hands are short and thick, especially the fingers. The tongue is large, fissured, and has a rough, beefy surface. The palatal arch is often high and there is generally an excess of adenoid tissue. These infants are defective in mentality as well as in other respects and, although they sometimes live past the age of puberty, the majority succumb earlier to some intercurrent infection. From an obstetrical point of view it is important to note that a clear-cut relationship exists between Mongolism and advanced maternal age, over a third of Mongolian idiots being born to mothers who are 40 years of age, whereas in the population at large the percentage of births to mothers of 40 or over lies somewhere between 2 and 4 per cent.

Harelip and Cleft Palate. A cleft in the lip, either unilateral or bilateral, may be associated with or without a cleft in the alveolar arch, and may or may not be associated with a cleft in the palate. It is a developmental defect. Closure of the lip is usually performed early for cosmetic reasons. The cleft palate may require the manufacture of a dental plate to facilitate nutrition prior to surgical closure at an opportune time in the first year of life.

Polydactylism. Supernumerary digits are occasionally seen and may consist of a small amount of skin and cartilage attached by a fine pedicle to the base of the fourth finger or toe. Simple ligation of the stalk with a silken thread will often suffice. If the base is broad and the digit well-developed, surgical removal is usually required.

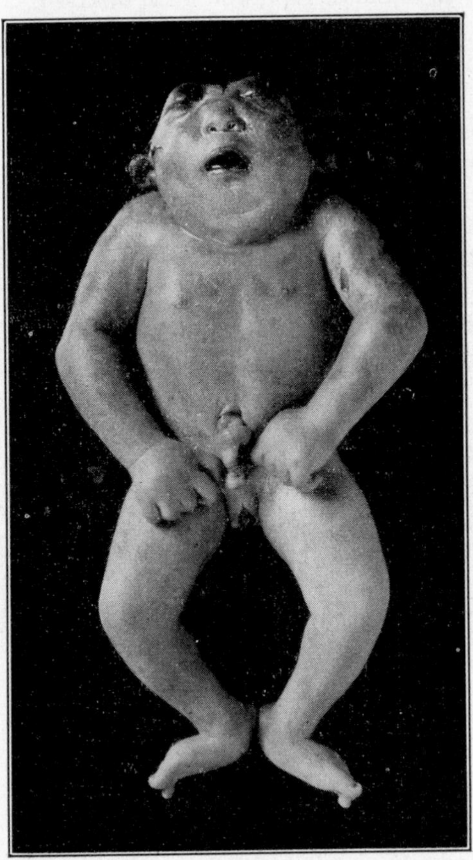

Fig. 535.—Anencephalus.

Clubfeet. Talipes equinovarus is the commonest type of clubfoot, although talipes equinovalgus, and talipes calcaneovarus and valgus deformities are sometimes seen. The cause is obscure, but congenital maldevelopment is thought to be responsible. On manipulating the feet, no muscle resistance is encountered, a finding which is important in differentiating actual deformity from an apparent one. Treatment consists of overcorrection by manipulation. This is repeated many times each day and may be performed by the mother if she is capable. The foot may also be maintained in a position of overcorrection by a cast. Operative correction is very rarely necessary.

Hernia: Umbilical and Inguinal. These herniae are usually discovered when the infant cries and are more frequent in the premature child. The umbilical hernia is

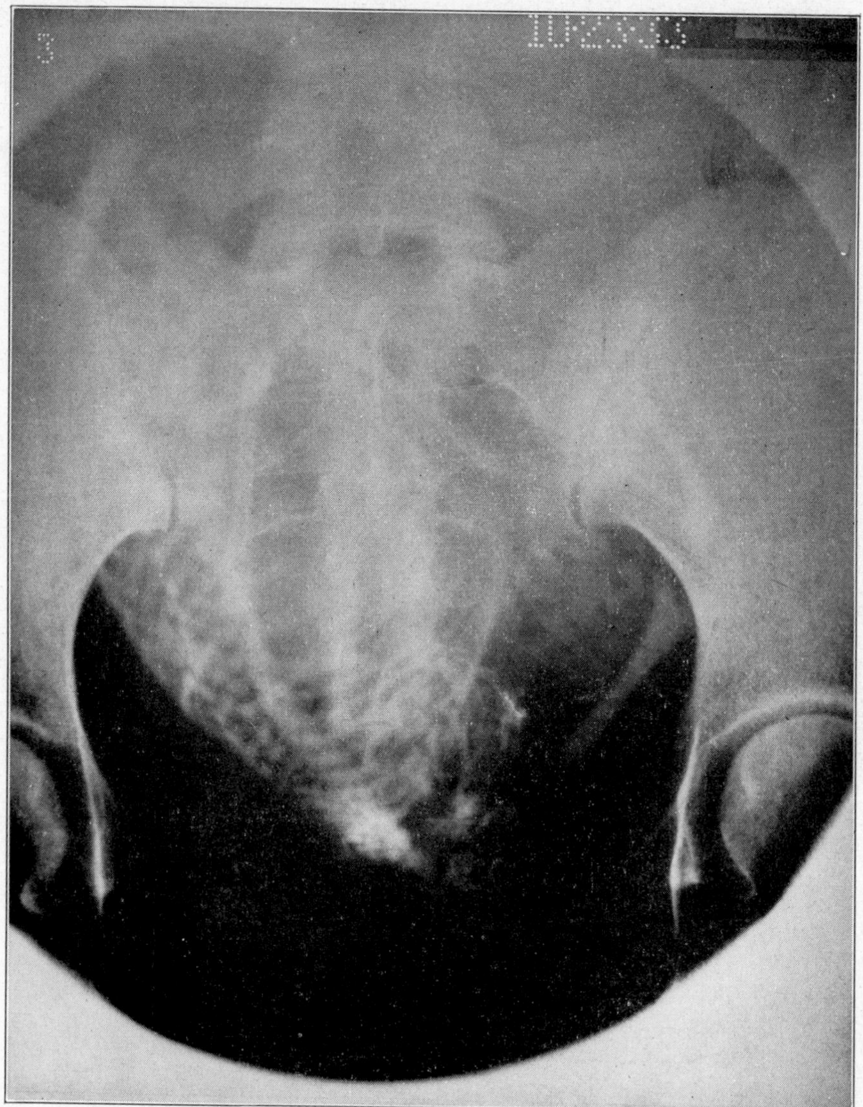

Fig. 536—X-ray Film of Pelvic Region of Antenatal Patient Showing Anencephalic Infant. The conspicuous nubbins of bone where the skull should be is diagnostic of this malformation.

treated by manipulating the recti muscles together and holding them in apposition with adhesive tape. It may be necessary to repeat this maneuver at intervals for six or eight weeks. The inguinal hernia frequently requires surgical reduction because of the danger of bowel strangulation, although a truss made of yarn is satisfactory in the less marked cases.

Undescended Testicles. Occasionally the testes do not descend in the first month of life, in which event expectant treatment should be continued until just before puberty when surgical replacement may be necessary. Endocrine treatment, in the form of chorionic gonadotrophin, with or without testosterone, has recently been considered to be of value in some cases. Inguinal hernia is often an associated condition.

Phimosis. A redundant foreskin may be so adherent as to interfere with micturition, while in other instances smegma collects, interfering with cleanliness. In such cases circumcision is usually indicated, although some prefer a more conservative

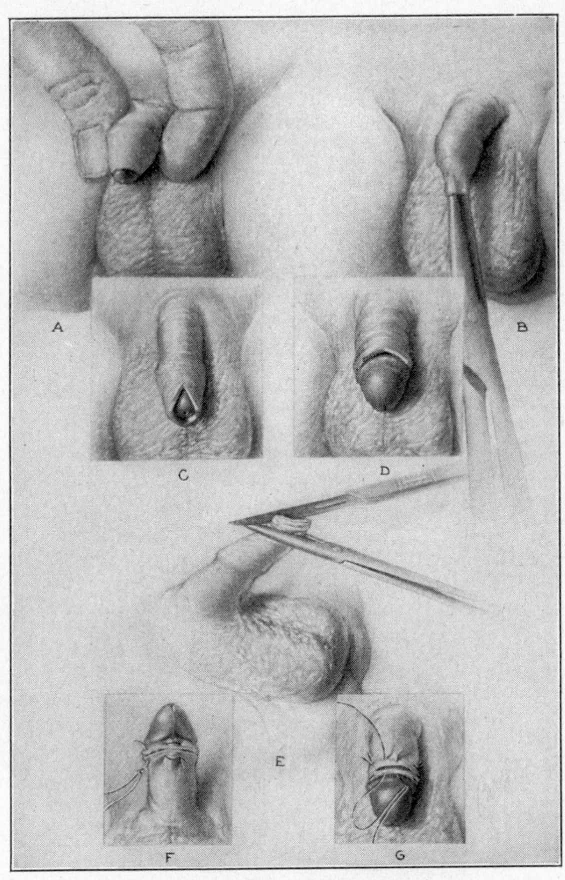

Fig. 537A.—Technic of Circumcision Using Hemostat, Scalpel and Sutures.

After cleansing penis and surrounding area, the prepuce is stripped back with the help of a partial dorsal slit (A to D). The prepuce is now clamped, and the excess prepuce cut off (E). The suture material generally used is plain 00 or 000 catgut in a very small needle (F and G), although some physicians prefer silk.

treatment consisting of breaking the preputial adhesions and stretching the foreskin with a mosquito clamp followed by retraction. If the latter procedure is carried out care should be exercised so that trauma to the urethra is avoided. Circumcision performed either for religious or other reasons or as a routine procedure is preferably carried out in the early part of the second week of life. We have had satisfactory results with the Yellon circumcision clamp.

Imperforate Anus. This abnormality consists of atresia of the anus, with the rectum ending in a blind pouch. Careful examination in the delivery room usually reveals the condition, or it is discovered at the time of the first rectal temperature. Surgical intervention is, of course, imperative.

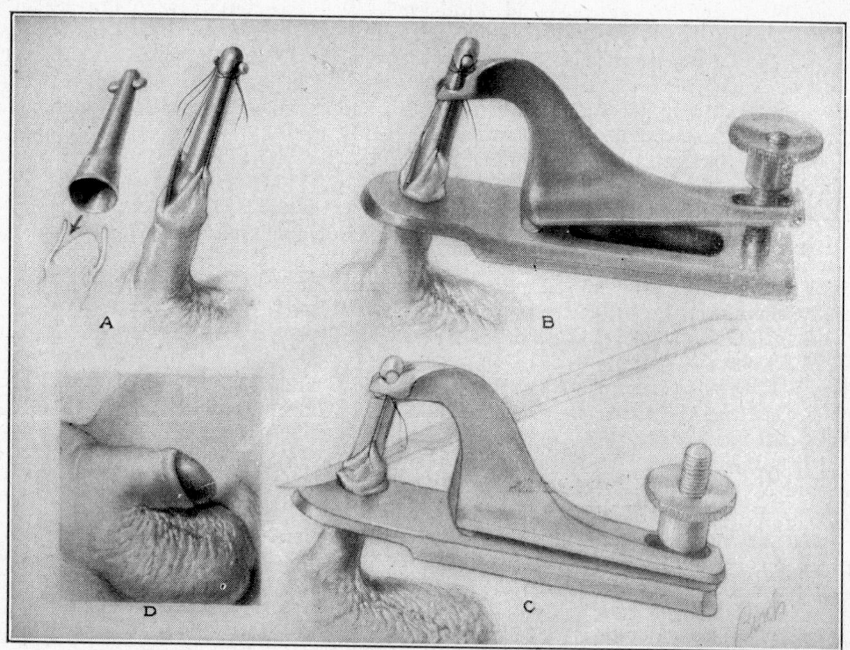

FIG. 537B.—TECHNIC OF CIRCUMCISION WITH YELLON CLAMP.

After cleansing area and stripping back prepuce as shown in Fig. 537A, the cone of the Yellon clamp is placed over the glans and the prepuce put on a stretch with sutures (A). The prepuce is now drawn through the bevelled hole of platform (B). Screwing down clamp crushes prepuce, producing hemostasis. Three to five minutes of such pressure are necessary to prevent subsequent bleeding. The excess of the prepuce is then cut away (C) and the clamp removed (D). (Yellon, H. S., *Am. J. Obst. & Gynec.,* 30:146.)

BIBLIOGRAPHY

Diseases and Malformations of the Newborn

BAKER, C. J. Epidemic Diarrhea of the Newborn. J. Pediat., 14:183.

BRINKHOUS, K. M., SMITH, H. P., and WARNER, E. D. Plasma Prothrombin Level in Normal Infancy and in Hemorrhagic Disease of the Newborn. Am. J. Med. Sc., 1937, 193:475.

CRUICKSHANK, J. N. The Hemorrhages of the Newborn. Lancet, 1923, 1:836.

DAM, H. Hemorrhages in Chicks Reared on Artificial Diets: New Deficiency Disease. Nature (London), 1934, 133:909.

——— The Antihemorrhagic Vitamin of the Chick. Biochem, J. 1935, 29:1273.

——— The Antihemorrhagic Vitamin of the Chick. Nature, 1935, 85:652.

D'ESOPO, D. A., and MARCHETTI, A. A. The Causes of Fetal and Neonatal Mortality. Am. J. Obst. & Gynec., 1942, 44:1.

DIPPEL, A. Louis. Relationship of Congenital Syphilis to Abortion and Miscarriage, and the Mechanism of Intrauterine Protection. Am. J. Obst. & Gynec., 1944, 47:369.

DULANEY, A., and MICHELSON, J. Study of *B. coli mutabile* from Outbreak of Diarrhea in Newborn. Am. J. Pub. Health, 1935, 25:1241.

DUNHAM, E. C. Premature Infants, A Manual for Physicians. Children's Bureau Publication No. 325, 1948. Federal Security Agency, Social Security Administration, Washington, D. C.

——— and MCALENNEY, P. F. A Study of 244 Prematurely Born Infants. J. Pediat., 1936, 9:717.

EASTMAN, N. J. Prematurity from the Viewpoint of the Obstetrician. Am. Practitioner, 1947, 1:343.

Gelston, C. F. On the Etiology of Hemorrhagic Disease of the Newborn. Am. J. Dis. Child., 1921, 22:351.

Green, R. M. Intracranial Hemorrhage in the Newborn. Boston M. & S. J., 1914, 170:682.

Hawkins, W. B., and Brinkhous, K. M. Prothrombin Deficiency the Cause of Bleeding in Bile Fistula Dogs. J. Exper. Med., 1936, 63:795.

Heller, A. Die Lungenerkrankungen bei angeborener Syphilis. Deutsch. Arch. f. klin. Med., 1888, 42:159.

Hellman, L. M., Moore, W. T., and Shettles, L. B. Factors Influencing Plasma Prothrombin in The Newborn Infant. Bull. Johns Hopkins Hosp., 1940, 66:379.

Hoffman, S. J., Greenhill, J. P., and Lundeen, E. C. A Premature Infant Weighing 735 Grams and Surviving. J.A.M.A., 1938, 110:283.

Javert, C. T. Hemorrhagic Disease of the Newborn. Am. J. Obst. & Gynec., 1938, 35:200.

Javert, C. T., and Moore, R. A. Prothrombin Concentration in Parturient Women and Their Newborn Infants. Am. J. Obst. & Gynec., 1940, 40:1022.

Kugelmass, I. N., and Tritsch, J. E. Prenatal Prevention of Potential Hemorrhagic Disease of the Newborn. Am. J. Obst. & Gynec., 1934, 28:259.

Levy-Solal, E. Contribution à l'Étude des Rapports de la Syphilis et de l'Hypertrophie Placentale. Gynéc. et obst., 1921, 4:94.

McCord, J. R. Syphilis of the Placenta. Am. J. Obst. and Gynec., 1934, 28:743.

Minot, F. On Hemorrhage from the Umbilicus in Newborn Infants, with an Analysis of 46 Cases. Am. J. M. Sc., 1852, 24:310.

Monro, J. S. Premature Infant Weighing Less than One Pound at Birth Who Survived and Developed Normally. Canad. M. A. J., 1939, 40:69.

Murphy, D. P. Congenital Malformations. Univ. of Pa. Press, Philadelphia, 1940.

——— Maternal Age at Conception of the Congenitally Malformed Child; Study Based on 607 Cases. Am. J. Dis. Child., 1936, 51:1007.

——— Intervals Between Pregnancies of Mothers Giving Birth to Congenitally Malformed Children. A Study of 531 Families. Surg., Gynec. & Obst., 1936, 63:593.

——— The Coincidence of Placenta Previa and Congenital Malformations. Am. J. Obst. & Gynec., 1938, 35:653.

Norris, R. F., and Rush, A. A Comparison of the Prothrombin Levels of Maternal and Cord Blood at Delivery. Surg., Gynec. & Obst., 1940, 70:1006.

Owen, C. A., Hoffman, G. R., Ziffren, S. E., and Smith, H. P. Blood Coagulation During Infancy. Proc. of the Soc. for Exper. Biol. and Med., 1939, 41:181.

Owens, W. C., and Owens, E. U. Retrolental Fibroplasia in Premature Infants. Trans. Am. Acad. of Ophthalmologists, Sept. & Oct., 1948.

Peckham, C. H. Statistical Studies on Prematurity. I. The Incidence of Prematurity and the Effect of Certain Obstetric Factors. II. The Mortality of Prematurity and the Effect of Certain Obstetric Factors. J. Pediat., 1938, 13:474.

Philipp, E. Die Diagnose der Lues bei Mutter und Kind. Zentralbl. f. Gynäk., 1928, 52:416.

Potter, E. Postmortem Examination of Stillborn and Newly born Infants. Arch. Path., 1938, 25:607.

——— The Effect on Infant Mortality of Vitamin K Administered during Labor. Am. J. Obst. & Gynec., 1945, 50:235.

Quick, A. J., Stanley-Brown, M., and Bancroft, F. W. A Study of the Coagulation Defect in Hemophilia and in Jaundice. Am. J. M. Sc., 1935, 190:501.

Rice, J. L., Best, W. H., Frant, S., and Abramson, H. Epidemic Diarrhea of the Newborn. J.A.M.A., 1937, 109:475.

Shipley, P. G., and Pearson, J. W. X-ray Pictures of the Bones in the Diagnosis of Syphilis in the Foetus and Young Infant. Bull. Johns Hopkins Hosp., 1921, 32:75-78.

Townsend, C. W. Hemorrhagic Disease of the Newborn. Arch. Ped., 1894, 11:559.

Turner, T. B., and McKelvey, J. L. Syphilis and Pregnancy: An Analysis of the Outcome of Pregnancy in Relation to Treatment in 943 Cases. J.A.M.A., 1934, 102:503.

Williams, J. W. The Significance of Syphilis in Prenatal Care and in the Causation of Foetal Death. Bull. Johns Hopkins Hosp., 1920, 31:141-145.

——— The Value of the Wassermann Reaction in Obstetrics, Based upon the Study of 4,547 Consecutive Cases. Bull. Johns Hopkins Hosp., 1920, 31:335-342.

——— The Influence of the Treatment of Syphilitic Pregnant Women upon the Incidence of Congenital Syphilis. Bull. Johns Hopkins Hosp., 1922, 33:383.

Yellon, H. S. Bloodless Circumcision of the Newborn. Am. J. Obst. & Gynec., 1935, 30:146.

Hemolytic Disease of the Fetus and Newborn

BERNSTEIN, F. Heredity of Blood Groups. Klin. Wschr., 1924, 3:1495.

BOORMAN, K. E., and DODD, B. E. The Group Specific Substances A, B, M, N, and Rh. Their Occurrence in Tissue and Body Fluids. J. Path. and Bact., 1943, 55:329.

BORNSTEIN, S., and ISRAEL, M. Agglutinogens in Fetal Erythrocytes. Proc. Soc. Exp. Biol. and Med., 1942, 49:718.

COOMBS, R. R. A., MOURANT, A. E., and RACE, R. R. A New Test for the Detection of Weak and "Incomplete" Rh Agglutinins. Brit. J. Exp. Path., 1945, 26:255.

DARROW, R. R. Icterus Gravis (erythroblastosis) Neonatorum. Arch. Path., 1938, 25:378.

DIENST, A. Eclampsia: Further Studies. Zentralbl. f. Gynäk., 1905, 29:353.

DIAMOND, L. K. Replacement Transfusion as a Treatment for Erythroblastosis Fetalis. Pediatrics, 1948, 2:520. (Technic of exchange transfusion via umbilical vein).

——— and DENTON, R. L. Rh Agglutination in Various Media with Particular Reference to the Value of Albumin. J. Lab. and Clin. Med., 1945, 30:821.

FISHER, R. A. The Rhesus Factor. Am. Scientist, 1947, 35:95.

GLASS, B. The Relation of Rh Incompatibility to Abortion. Am. J. Obst. & Gynec., 1949, 57:323.

LANDSTEINER, K. First Observations of Differences in Blood of Normal Human Beings. Zentralbl. f. Bakt., 1900, 28:357.

——— On the phenomenon of Agglutination in Normal Human Blood. Wien. klin. Wchnschr., 1901, 14:713.

LANDSTEINER, K., and LEVINE, P. On Individual Differences in Human Blood. J. Exp. Med., 1928, 47:757.

LANDSTEINER, K., and WIENER, A. S. An Agglutinable Factor in Human Blood Recognized by Immune Sera for Rhesus Blood. Proc. Soc. Exper. Biol. and Med., 1940, 43:223. (First publication on the Rh antigen as such.)

LANDSTEINER, K., and WIENER, A. S. Studies on an Agglutinogen (Rh) in Human Blood Reacting with Anti-Rhesus Sera and Human Iso-antibodies. J. Exp. Med., 1941, 74:309.

LEVINE, P. Iso-immunization in Pregnancy and the Pathogenesis of Erythroblastosis Fetalis, in H. T. Karsner and S. B. Hooker, 1941 Yearbook of Pathology and Immunology. Year Book Publishers, Inc., Chicago, 1941, p. 505. (First report in literature on Hr.)

——— A Survey of the Significance of the Rh Factor, in The Rh Factor in the Clinic and the Laboratory, Hill, J. M., and Dameshek, W. Grune & Stratton, New York, 1948, p. 3. (General review.)

——— BURNHAM, L., KATZIN, E. M., and VOGEL, P. The Role of Iso-immunization in the Pathogenesis of Erythroblastosis Fetalis. Am. J. Obst. & Gynec., 1941, 42:925.

LEVINE, P., and KATZIN, E. M. Iso-immunization in Pregnancy and the Varieties of Iso-agglutinins Observed. Proc. Soc. Exper. Biol. and Med., 1940, 45:343.

LEVINE, P., and STETSON, R. An Unusual Case of Intragroup Agglutination. J.A.M.A., 1939, 113:126.

LEVINE, P., and WALLER, R. K. Erythroblastosis Fetalis in the First Born. Blood, 1946, 1:143.

LEVINE, P., WIGOD, M., BOCKER, A. M., and PONDER, R. The Kell-Cellano (K-k) Genetic System of Human Blood Factors. Blood, 1949, 4:869.

LEVINE, P., and WONG, H. The Incidence of the Rh Factor and Erythroblastosis Fetalis in Chinese. Am. J. Obst. & Gynec., 1943, 45:832.

MOLLISON, P. L., MOURANT, A. E., and RACE, R. R. The Rh Blood Groups and Their Clinical Effects. Medical Research Council Memorandum No. 19. His Majesty's Stationery Office, London, 1948. (General review, technics of Rh typing and antibody study.)

POTTER, E. L. Rh—Its Relation to Congenital Hemolytic Disease and to Intra Group Transfusion Reactions. The Year Book Publishers, Inc., Chicago, 1947. (Monograph. See for details of Rh typing and antibody testing.)

——— Reproductive Histories of the Mothers of 322 Infants with Erythroblastosis. Pediatrics, 1948, 2:369.

RACE, R. R. An "Incomplete" Antibody in Human Serum. Nature, 1944, 153:771.

——— The Rh Genotypes and Fisher's Theory, in The Rh Factor in the Clinic and the Laboratory, Hill, J. M., and Dameshek, W. Grune and Stratton, New York, 1948, p. 27.

——— and TAYLOR, G. L. A Serum That Discloses the Genotype of Rh Positive People. Nature, 1943, 152:300.

SACKS, M. S., GUILBEAU, J. A., BRADFORD, G. T., and JAHN, E. F. Rh Iso-sensitization in the American Negro. Blood—in press.

SACKS, M. S., JAHN, E. F., and KUHNS, W. J. The Baltimore Rh Typing Laboratory—A New Community Public Health Service. J.A.M.A., 1946, 132:983.

Sacks, M. S., Kuhns, W. J., and Jahn, E. F. Studies in Rh Iso-immunization in Pregnancy. Am. J. Obst. & Gynec., 1947, 54:400.

Stiller, R. K. A Follow-up Study of 35 Erythroblastotic Infants. Amer. J. Dis. Child., 1947, 73:651.

Strandskov, H. H. Recent Views on the Genetics of the Rh-Hr Blood Factors. Bull. N. Y. Acad. Med., 1949, 25:249.

Waterhouse, J. A. H., and Hogben, L. Incompatibility of Mother and Fetus with Respect to the Iso-agglutinogen A and Its Antibody. Br. J. Sociol. Med., 1947, 1:1.

Wiener, A. S. A New Test (Blocking Test) for Rh Sensitization. Proc. Soc. Exp. Biol. and Med., 1944, 56:173.

——— Blood Groups and Transfusions, 3rd Ed. Charles C Thomas, Springfield, Ill., 1943.

——— Conglutination Test for Rh Sensitization. J. Lab. & Clin. Med., 1945, 30:662.

——— Heredity of the Rh Blood Types: VII—Additional Family Studies with Special Reference to the Genes R^z and r^y. Proc. of the Eighth International Congress of Genetics. Hereditas, Suppl. Vol., 1949, pp. 500-519. (Wiener genetic theory—present status.)

——— Recent Developments in the Knowledge of the Rh-Hr Blood Types: Tests for Rh Sensitization. Am. J. Clin. Path., 1946, 16:477. (General review.)

——— and Peters, H. R. Hemolytic Reactions following Transfusions of Blood of the Homologous Group, with Three Cases in which the Same Agglutinogen Was Responsible. Ann. Int. Med., 1940, 13:2306.

Wiener, A. S., and Wexler, I. B. Results of Therapy of Erythroblastosis with Exchange Transfusion. Blood, 1949, 4:1. (Technic of exchange transfusion.)

Section Ten: OPERATIVE OBSTETRICS

39

ARTIFICIAL TERMINATION OF PREGNANCY AND STERILIZATION

THERAPEUTIC ABORTION

Definitions. Therapeutic abortion is the termination of pregnancy prior to the period of viability for the purpose of saving the life of the mother or safeguarding her health, including her mental health or sanity. Since therapeutic abortion is homicide with respect to the fetus, it is a grave undertaking and must never be considered unless there is imminent danger of death of the mother as the result of pregnancy, or of great bodily or mental harm. The operation is governed by statute or common law in all states but the wording of the regulations varies widely. For this and other reasons, therapeutic abortion should never be performed without the written approval of two consultants. Neither the law nor medical ethics permits the procedure for sociological reasons such as illegitimacy, poverty, or rape. One English court, however, has acquitted a physician for performing therapeutic abortion in a particularly grievous case of rape.

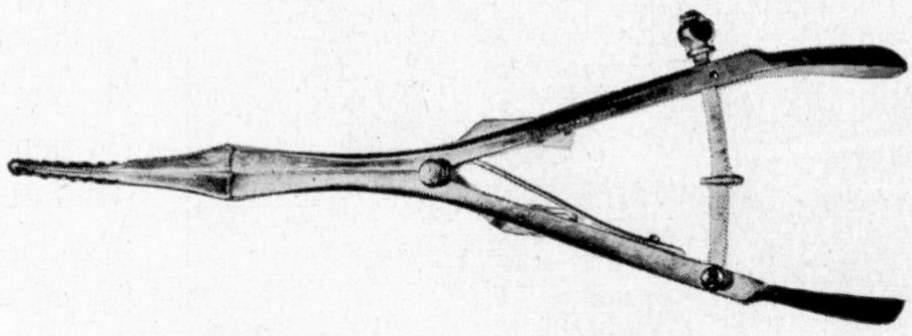

Fig. 538A.—Goodell's Dilator.

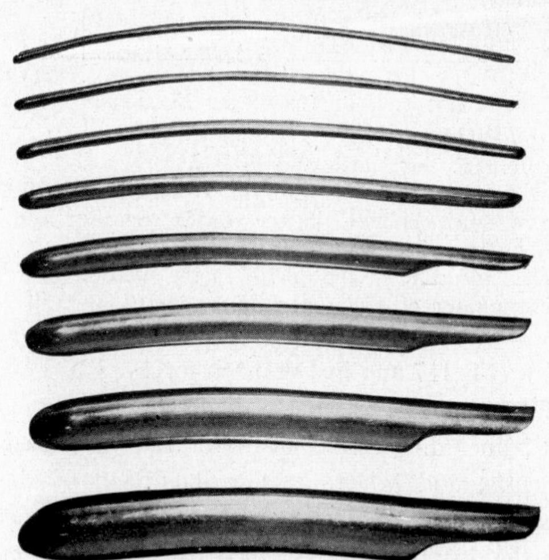

Fig. 538B.—Hegar's Graduated Dilators.

Indications. The indications for therapeutic abortion are discussed in connection with the diseases which most commonly prompt the operation. The best documented indication is perhaps rheumatic heart disease in the presence of a history of previous decompensation. Another commonly accepted indication is advanced hypertensive vascular disease, as discussed on page 698. Still another is carcinoma of the cervix. Other indications are more debatable.

Incidence. Therapeutic abortion is a greatly abused operation and the incidence of the procedure the country over is much higher than it should be. This fact has been emphasized especially by Cosgrove and Carter who cite an incidence of therapeutic abortion at the Margaret Hague Maternity Hospital of one to 16,750 deliveries. However, the frequency of the operation in most obstetrical clinics is much higher than this and probably averages one to every 150 or 200 deliveries. In the course of the last 10,000 deliveries in our own clinic, the incidence of therapeutic abortion was one to every 147 deliveries.

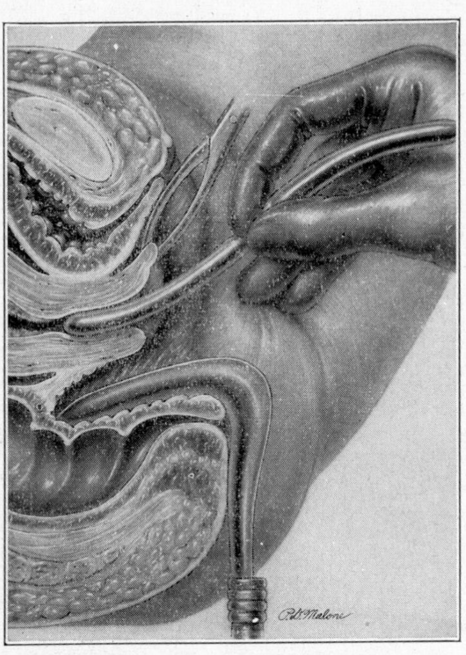

Fig. 539.—Dilatation of Cervix by Means of Hegar Dilator.

Note that the fourth and little fingers rest against the buttock. This is a most important safety measure because if the cervix relaxes abruptly, these fingers prevent sudden and uncontrolled thrusting of the dilator to the fundus, a common cause of perforation of the uterus.

In the country at large the incidence of therapeutic abortion probably approximates one to every 200 or so live births. In New York City every fetal death must be reported, regardless of the period of gestation, and the Bureau of Records and Statistics of the Department of Health possesses extensive data on all such cases. Dr. Christopher Tietze of our School of Public Health and Hygiene has recently compiled data from their reports of therapeutic abortion for the five-year period, 1943 through 1947. He finds that the ratio of therapeutic abortion to live births was 1:196 and to total known pregnancies was 1:213. Although observations such as this are susceptible to error of various sorts, especially incomplete registration, the figures cited are in keeping with those reported in Sweden and Denmark where reporting has long been mandatory and is believed to be reasonably accurate. The ratio of therapeutic abortions to live births in Sweden for 1939 to 1945 was 1:217 and in Denmark for 1932 to 1940 was 1:167.

Technic. The vaginal operation of therapeutic abortion is fraught with several hazards including danger of perforating the uterus, hemorrhage, retention of placental fragments, and infection. The likelihood of these complications augments sharply after the twelfth week and for this reason the procedure should never be done vaginally when the duration of pregnancy has exceeded that limit. If it has, and if interruption of pregnancy appears urgent, abdominal hysterotomy (miniature cesarean section) is the operation of choice.

If therapeutic abortion is performed in accordance with proper indications, the patients will, of necessity, be seriously sick women and hence the choice of the anesthetic is usually of great importance. Low spinal anesthesia, with minimal dosage, is often satisfactory, but the dosage should not exceed 50 mg. of procaine and, as a rule, 35 mg. is adequate. Fractional spinal anesthesia has great advantages in these cases because the initial dose can be as low as 10 mg. of procaine and the level built up gradually and cautiously from that amount.

In order to diminish the likelihood of uterine perforation, pituitary extract in the form of pitocin and in dosage of 0.5 cc. (5 units) is given 20 minutes before the start of the operation and repeated as the patient is being draped. After the usual preparations for a vaginal operation, the cervix is grasped with a tenaculum forceps and the depth of the uterine cavity measured by a sound. A mental image of this depth is retained and care taken that no instrument introduced into the uterus be advanced quite so far as that depth. The cervix is dilated with Hegar dilators, aided, if necessary, with a Goodell dilator. As shown in Fig. 539, the small fingers of the hand introducing the Hegar dilators should rest on the buttock as a further safeguard against uterine perforation. Although a dull curet is usually recommended, it is our feeling that a sharp curet is more efficacious and that its dangers are no greater than those of the dull type of instrument. Perforations of the uterus do not occur on the down-pull of the curet but may occur when any instrument is being introduced into the uterus; since the knife edge of a sharp curet is directed downward, it can have no bearing on this hazard. Any curet, however, is a dangerous instrument if injudicious force is applied to it and, as shown in Fig. 540, the necessary manipulations should be carried out with the strength in the thumb and forefingers only.

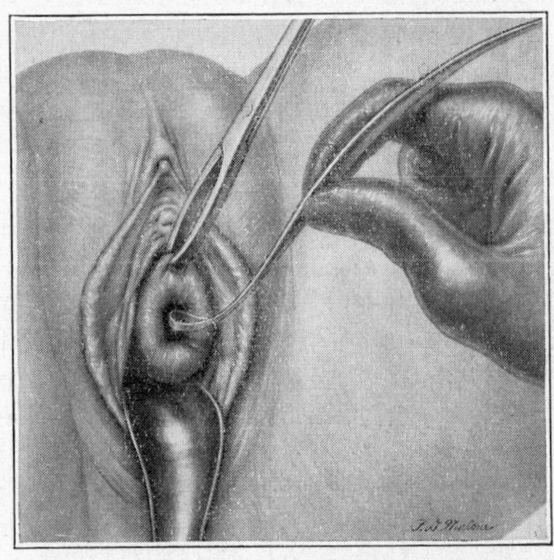

FIG. 540.—INTRODUCTION OF THE CURET.

Note that the instrument is held merely with the thumb and forefinger, and in the upward direction of the curet no more strength should be used than exists in these two fingers. Moreover, just as soon as the curet has actually entered the cervical canal, the fourth and last fingers will come to rest on the buttock as a further protective measure against uterine perforation. Still another safeguard is the administration of pituitary extract ½ cc. (7½ minims) 15 minutes before the operation and repeated as the patient is being draped.

In occasional cases, it may prove difficult to dilate the cervix to such an extent as to permit easy introduction of the curet and withdrawal of fetal parts. In that event, the uterus should be packed with ribbon gauze by means of fine forceps and a 24-hour period allowed to elapse. The presence of the packing will usually provoke contractions of sufficient intensity to soften and efface the cervix so that the operation can be performed without difficulty the next day.

INDUCTION OF LABOR

Provided that the cervix presents certain favorable conditions, it is often possible to induce labor in patients near term and sometimes in cases in which the infant is still in the range of prematurity. For a cervix to be favorable for induction, or "ripe," it is essential that it be soft, more than half effaced, and sufficiently dilated to admit one finger with ease. If all three of these conditions are not present, it is prudent to abandon any thought of trying to initiate labor because, in the absence of these conditions, any attempted induction may be unsuccessful and, if labor does ensue, it is likely to be desultory and prolonged.

The main indication for the induction of labor is preeclampsia, as discussed on page 660. Whether or not to induce labor in preeclampsia will depend again on the condition of the cervix and the general reaction of the patient to rest in bed, salt restriction, and medicinal therapy. If the patient is far from term, with a cervix which is long, firm, and closed, it is much wiser to persist with medicinal therapy than to risk dealing with the potentialities of such a cervix; if the preeclampsia is fulminating and resistant to other therapy, cesarean section may be indicated. There are a number of conditions in which induction of labor is thought to be indicated but which are actually contraindications. One of these is so-called "postmaturity" of the fetus, that is, the state in which the patient goes a week to a month beyond her expected date of confinement. The studies of Calkins and of others show that the infants in such cases are rarely larger than the normal range and that actually the "problem of postmaturity" is non-existent. And even in cases in which the infants prove to be excessive in size, labor of spontaneous onset is helpful because, in general, it is less likely to be associated with inertia in this type of case than is induced labor. Nor is rheumatic heart disease an indication for the induction of labor since the load on the heart tends to diminish, rather than increase, in the last weeks of gestation.

The procedure which is employed to induce labor is almost always artificial rupture of the membranes. This entails simply the introduction of a finger through the cervix, stripping the membranes from their uterine attachment for a distance of about two inches, and scratching them with a sharp hook until rupture occurs. The head should be held up slightly with the finger to allow as much fluid as possible to drain away. Provided the cervix is favorable, labor usually sets in within an hour or two after this procedure. If it has not begun within six hours, minute doses of pitocin (0.25 minim every 30 minutes) are advisable, or intravenous drip pitocin. Bags and bougies for the induction of labor are not recommended.

STERILIZATION

Most conditions which justify therapeutic abortion make permanent prevention of pregnancy also desirable. This is especially true of rheumatic heart disease and chronic hypertensive states. Other conditions which frequently warrant sterilization are a history of two or more previous cesarean sections, great multiparity (eight or more viable deliveries), and, less frequently, various mental states.

Great Multiparity. Justification of sterilization after the eighth viable delivery is based on the greatly increased maternal mortality rates which pregnancies beyond that number carry, as shown in Fig. 8. Pregnancies after the eighth are also associated with elevated stillbirth and neonatal death rates. The causes of death in these women of great parity follow a characteristic pattern and are due to three main conditions: chronic hypertensive vascular disease, rupture of the uterus, and placenta previa. Certain other complications, such as obesity, transverse presentations, and twins also augment with parity. The increasing frequency of chronic hypertensive vascular disease with age and parity, as well as the hazards which this disease introduces in childbearing, has already been discussed in Chapter 27. The higher frequency of rupture of the uterus in women of great parity is attested by all studies on the subject. For instance, in Davis' analysis of 57 cases of rupture of the uterus (postcesarean section cases excluded), approximately two thirds occurred in women whose parity was four or more. In our own clinic, in 17 spontaneous, noncesarean-scar ruptures, the average parity was 6.4 and the average age, 36.3. As pointed out by Kerr and Moir, an increase in fibrous tissue occurs normally after each pregnancy; hence, because of diminished elasticity of the uterine wall, after numerous pregnancies, there is a higher chance of rupture.

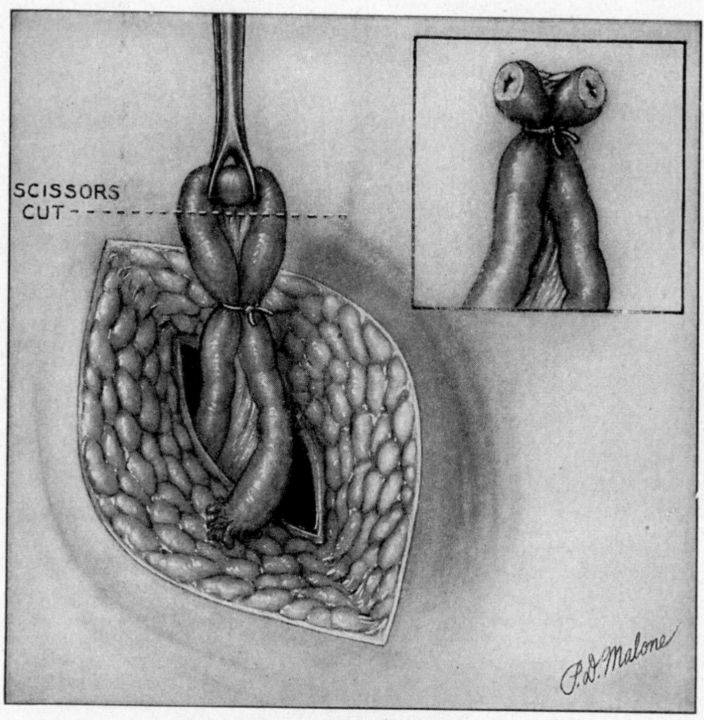

Fig. 541A.—Pomeroy Tubal Sterilization.

The tube has been withdrawn through a short midline incision and a knuckle ligated with catgut. Insert shows knuckle incised with divergent ends. (From Te Linde, R. W., *Operative Gynecology*, J. B. Lippincott Co., Philadelphia.)

Because of the high maternal and fetal mortality associated with bearing the ninth child and subsequent children, and in view of the transcendent value of such a mother to her family, it is my belief that mothers who have had eight or more viable deliveries should be offered tubal ligation; and, provided genuine permission can be obtained from the woman and her husband, that it should be performed early in the puerperium. On the other hand, the general recommendation that tubal sterilization be performed for great multiparity is avowedly subject to abuse. However, it is not likely to be abused, in my opinion, if "great multiparity" is rigidly defined as specified above. Although we have carried out this operation in more than 500 cases on the grounds of great multiparity, in no single instance have we performed it on this indication in women who had had less than eight viable infants.

Technic. Pregnancy has occurred after all types of sterilization, with the exception of bilateral oophorectomy. Failures have been reported after all varieties of tubal ligation, after wedge-shaped excision of the uterine cornua, burial of the uterine ends of the tubal stump, bisection of the tubes with the cautery, and bilateral salpingectomy. Even supravaginal hysterectomy has been followed by abdominal pregnancy.

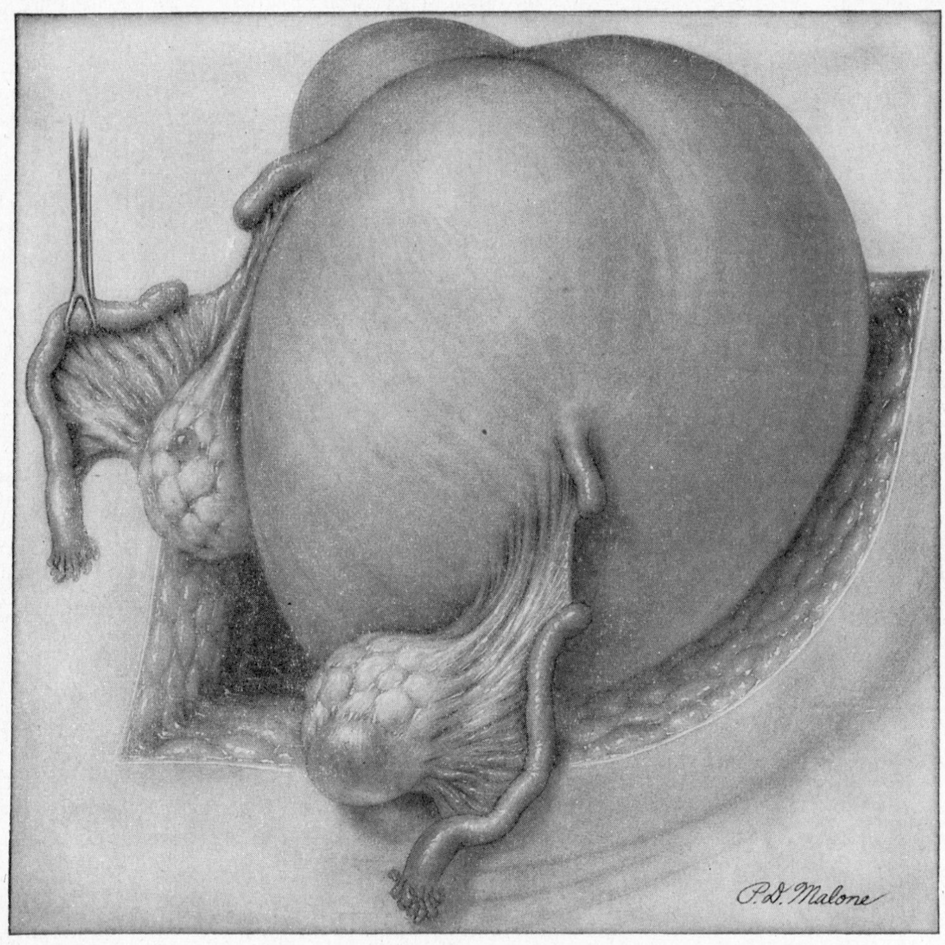

FIG. 541B.—END RESULT OF POMEROY STERILIZATION DONE THREE YEARS BEFORE.
This patient was observed at a hysterectomy for fibroids. (From Te Linde, R. W., *Operative Gynecology*, J. B. Lippincott Co., Philadelphia.)

The simplest and one of the most efficacious methods of performing tubal sterilization is the Pomeroy technic, as illustrated in Figs. 541A and 541B. It is important that catgut be used to ligate the knuckle of tube, the rationale of the procedure being based on absorption of the ligature and subsequent separation of the severed tubal ends which become sealed over by a fibrinous exudate. The Madlener operation for tubal sterilization is very similar to the Pomeroy in outward appearance but is quite different in principle and in efficiency. The technic of the Madlener procedure differs in three important respects from the Pomeroy: (1) In the Madlener operation, the tube is crushed with a Kelly clamp at the site of the intended ligation; in the Pomeroy technic, it is not crushed. (2) In the Madlener procedure, silk or other nonabsorbable suture is used; in the Pomeroy method, an absorbable suture is employed. (3) In the Madlener technic, the knuckle of tube is not cut; in the Pomeroy operation, the knuckle of tube is cut across in such a manner that the tubal stumps are completely severed. The objective of the Madlener operation is to produce occlusion of the tube by crushing and the use of a silk suture; the aim of the Pomeroy technic is separation of the tubal ends and their occlusion by exudate. In our hands the Pomeroy method has been much more dependable than the Madlener. Thus, a follow-up of more than 1,000 Pomeroy operations has revealed only four subsequent pregnancies, whereas 101 Madlener operations resulted in five failures, as reported by Dippel. Although many other technics have been recommended, the Pomeroy operation has proved so simple, bloodless, and efficient in our clinic that we see no reason to employ any other. The operation may be done at any time, but when performed following delivery, the optimum time seems to be during the first 48 hours. Most of our cases have been performed within that period.

BIBLIOGRAPHY

ALDRIDGE, Albert H. Temporary Surgical Sterilization with Subsequent Pregnancy. Am. J. Obst. & Gynec., 1934, 27:741.

CALKINS, L. A. Postmaturity. Am. J. Obst. & Gynec., 1948, 56:167.

COSGROVE, S. A., and CARTER, P. A. A Consideration of Therapeutic Abortion. Am. J. Obst. & Gynec., 1944, 48:299.

DAVIS, A. B. The Ruptured Uterus. Am. J. Obst. & Gynec., 1927, 13:522.

DIPPEL, A. L. Tubal Sterilization by the Madlener Method. Surg., Gynec. & Obst., 1940, 71:94.

EASTMAN, N. J. Hazards of Pregnancy and Labor in the "Grande Multipara." New York State J. Med., 1940, 40:1708.

GUTTMACHER, A. F., and DOUGLAS, R. G. Induction of Labor by Artificial Rupture of the Membranes. Am. J. Obst. & Gynec., 1931, 21:485.

KERR, J. M. M., and MOIR, J. C. Operative Obstetrics, Williams and Wilkins Co., Baltimore, 1950.

MORTON, D. G. A Comparison of the Results Obtained in the Induction of Labor by Means of Bougie or Bag. Am. J. Obst. & Gynec., 1929, 18:849-859.

——— Induction of Labor by Means of Artificial Rupture of the Membranes, Castor Oil, Quinine, and Nasal Pituitrin. Am. J. Obst. & Gynec., 1933, 26:323.

MURPHY, D. P. Ovarian Irradiation. Its Effect on Health of Subsequent Children. Surg., Gynec. & Obst., 1928, 47:201.

TIETZE, C. Unpublished data. Personal communication.

WILLIAMS, J. W. The Problem of Effecting Sterilization in Association with Various Obstetrical Procedures. Am. J. Obst. & Gynec., 1921, 1:783-793.

——— Indications for Therapeutic Sterilization in Obstetrics. J.A.M.A., 1928, 91:1237-1242.

40

FORCEPS

The obstetrical forceps is an instrument designed for the extraction, under certain conditions, of the child when it presents by the head. It consists of two branches which cross one another, and are designated right and left, respectively, according to the side of the pelvis to which each corresponds. They are introduced separately into the genital canal and are articulated after being placed in position. Each branch is made up of four portions—the *blade, handle, shank,* and *lock.*

The instruments vary considerably in size and shape, as will be seen when certain varieties of forceps are considered. The blades possess a double *curvature*—the *cephalic* and the *pelvic*—the former being adapted to the shape of the child's head, the latter to that of the birth canal. The blades are more or less elliptical in shape, tapering toward the shank, and are usually *fenestrated* so as to allow of a firm hold upon the head. Certain authorities, however, prefer *solid* blades in the belief that they can be made less bulky.

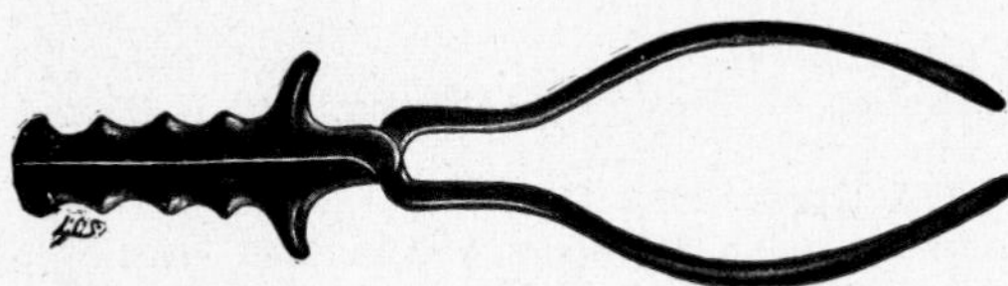

Fig. 542.—Simpson's Forceps, Cephalic Curve.

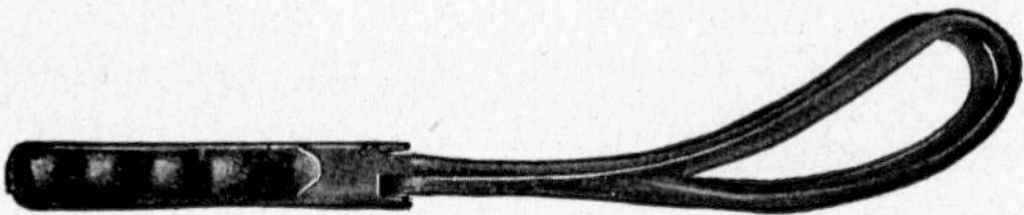

Fig. 543.—Simpson's Forceps, Pelvic Curve.

The cephalic curves should be such as to permit the head to be grasped firmly, but without serious compression. The greatest distance between the two blades should not exceed 7.5 cm. (3 inches), when they are articulated. The pelvic curve corresponds more or less to the axis of the birth canal, but varies considerably in different instruments. When the forceps is placed upon a plane surface, the tips of the blades should be about 8.8 cm. (3½ inches) higher than the handles. The latter are connected with the blades by the shanks, which give the requisite length to the instrument.

The two branches articulate at the lock, which varies widely in different instruments. The English type consists of a socket upon each branch, into which fits the shank of the other half of the instrument. This arrangement permits of ready articulation, but does not hold the blades firmly together. In the French lock a pivot is screwed into the shank of the left branch, while the right presents an opening which can be adjusted to it, the screw being tightened after articulation. The German lock is a combination of the two, the shank of the left branch bearing a pivot with a broad, flat head, while the right is provided with a notch which corresponds to the pivot.

When the instrument is properly articulated the handles should fall together in such a way as to be conveniently grasped by one hand of the operator.

History. Crude forceps were in use from an early period, several varieties having been described by Albucasis, who died in 1112; but, as their inner surfaces were provided with teeth intended to penetrate the head, it is evident that they were intended for use only upon dead children.

The true obstetrical forceps was devised in the latter part of the sixteenth or the beginning of the seventeenth century, by a member of the Chamberlen family. The invention, however, was not made public at the time, but was preserved as a family secret, through four generations, and did not become generally known until the early part of the eighteenth century. Prior to that time version had been the only method which permitted the artificial delivery of an unmutilated child, and accordingly when that operation was out of the question and delivery became imperative, it was accomplished by means of hooks and crotchets, which usually led to the destruction of the child. Thus, before the invention of forceps, the use of instruments was synonymous with the death of the child, and frequently of the mother as well, and tended to bring obstetrics into disrepute.

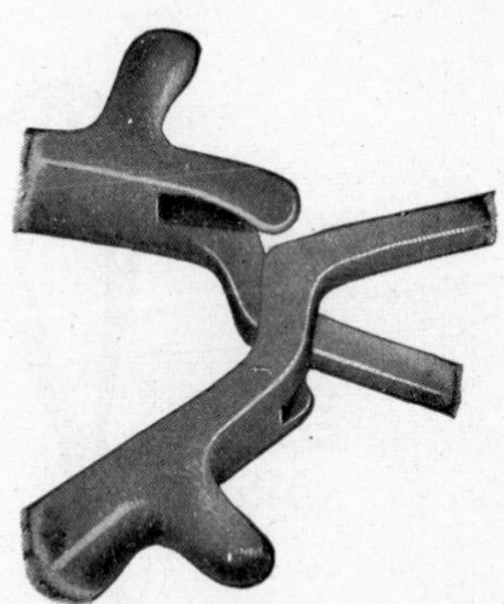

Fig. 544.—English Lock.

William Chamberlen, the founder of the family, was a French physician, who fled from France as a Huguenot refugee and landed at Southampton in 1569. He died in 1596, leaving a large family. Two of his sons, both of whom were named Peter, and designated as the elder and younger, respectively, studied medicine and settled in London. They soon became successful practitioners, and devoted a large part of their attention to midwifery, in which they became very proficient. They attempted to control the instruction of midwives, and in justification of their pretensions claimed that they could successfully deliver patients when all others failed.

The younger Peter died in 1626, and the elder in 1631. The latter left no male children, but the former was survived by several sons, one of whom, born in 1601, was likewise named Peter. To distinguish him from his father and uncle, he is usually spoken of as Dr. Peter, as the other two did not possess that title. He was well educated, having studied at Cambridge, Heidelberg and Padua, and on his return to London was elected a Fellow of the Royal College of Physicians. He was most successful in the practice of his profession, and counted among his clients many of the royal family and nobility. Like his father and uncle, he attempted to monopolize the control of the midwives, but his pretensions were set aside by the authorities. These attempts gave rise to a great deal of discussion, and many pamphlets were written as to the mortality of women in labor being attended by men, which he answered in a pamphlet entitled "A Voice in Ramah, or the Cry of Women and Children as Echoed Forth in the Compassions of Peter Chamberlen." He was a man of considerable ability, and united at the same time some of the virtues of a religious enthusiast with many of the devious qualities of a quack. He died at Woodham Mortimer Hall, Moldon, Essex, in 1683, the place remaining in the possession of his family until well into the succeeding century. Formerly he was considered the inventor of the forceps, but, as we now know, this view was incorrect.

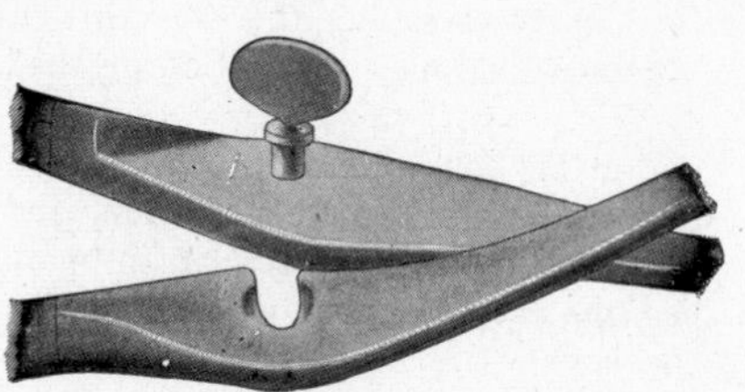

Fig. 545.—French Lock.

He left a very large family, and three of his sons—Hugh, Paul, and John—became physicians, and devoted special attention to the practice of midwifery. Of these Hugh (1630-?) was the most important and influential. Like his father, he possessed considerable ability, and at the same time took a practical interest in politics. Some of his views not being in favor, he was forced to leave England, and while in Paris, in 1673, attempted to sell the family secret to Mauriceau for 10,000 livres, claiming that by its means he could deliver in a very few minutes the most difficult cases. Mauriceau placed at his disposal a rachitic dwarf whom he had been unable to deliver, and Chamberlen, after several hours of strenuous effort, was likewise obliged to acknowledge his inability to do so. Notwithstanding his failure, however, he maintained friendly relations with Mauriceau, and on returning home translated the latter's book into English. In his preface he refers to the forceps in the following words: "My father, brothers, and myself (though none else in Europe as I know) have by God's blessings and our own industry attained to and long practiced a way to deliver women in this case without prejudice to them or their infants."

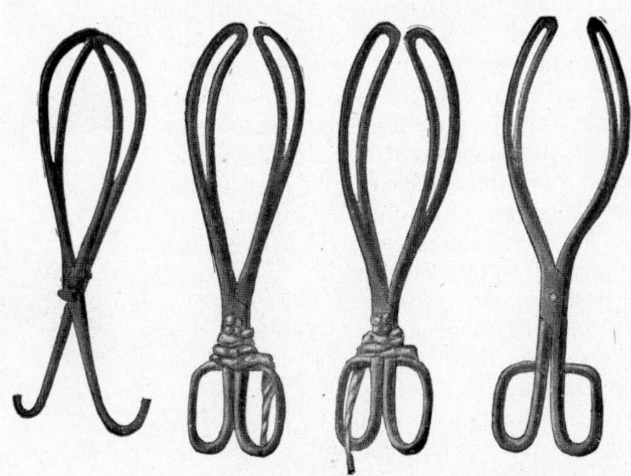

FIG. 546.—CHAMBERLEN'S FORCEPS.

Some years later he went to Holland and sold his secret to Roger Roonhuysen. Shortly afterward the Medico-Pharmaceutical College of Amsterdam was given the sole privilege of licensing physicians to practice in Holland, to each of whom, under the pledge of secrecy, was sold Chamberlen's invention for a large sum. This practice continued for a number of years, until Vischer and Van der Poll purchased and made public the secret, when it was found that the device consisted of one blade only of the forceps. Whether this was all that Chamberlen sold to Roonhuysen, or whether the Medico-Pharmaceutical College had swindled the purchasers, is not known.

Hugh Chamberlen left a considerable family, and one of his sons—Hugh (1664-1728)—practised medicine. He was a highly educated, respected, and philanthropic physician, and numbered among his clients members of the best families in England. He was an intimate friend of the Duke of Buckingham, and when he died the latter caused a statue to be erected in his honor in Westminster Abbey. During the later years of his life he allowed the family secret to leak out, and the instrument soon came into general use.

For more than one hundred years it was believed that the forceps was the invention of Dr. Peter Chamberlen, but in the year 1813 Mrs. Kemball, the mother of Mrs. Codd who was the occupant of Woodham Mortimer Hall at the time, found in the garret a trunk containing numerous letters and instruments, among the latter being four pairs of forceps, together with several levers and fillets. As is evident from the drawings, the forceps were in different stages of development, one pair being hardly applicable to the living woman, while the others were useful instruments. Aveling, who has carefully investigated the matter, believes that the three pairs of available forceps were used respectively by the three Peters, and that in all probability the first was devised by the elder Peter, son of the original William. Confirmation is lent to this view by the fact that Peter, on one occasion, at least, spoke of the invention of his uncle. Sänger and Budin, who have also investigated the subject, incline to the same belief.

The forceps came into general employment in England during the lifetime of Hugh

Chamberlen, the younger. The instrument was used by Drinkwater, who died in 1728, and was well known to Chapman and Giffard. The former, in "An Essay on the Improvement of Midwifery" published in London in 1733, says: "The secret mentioned by Dr. Chamberlen was the use of the forceps, now well-known by all the principal men of the profession, both in town and country."

In 1723, Palfyn, a physician of Ghent, exhibited before the Paris Academy of Medicine, a forceps which he designated as *mains de fer*. It was crude in shape and did not articulate. In the discussion following its presentation, De la Motte stated that it would be impossible to apply it to the living woman, and added that if by chance any one should happen to invent an instrument which could be so used, and kept it secret for his own

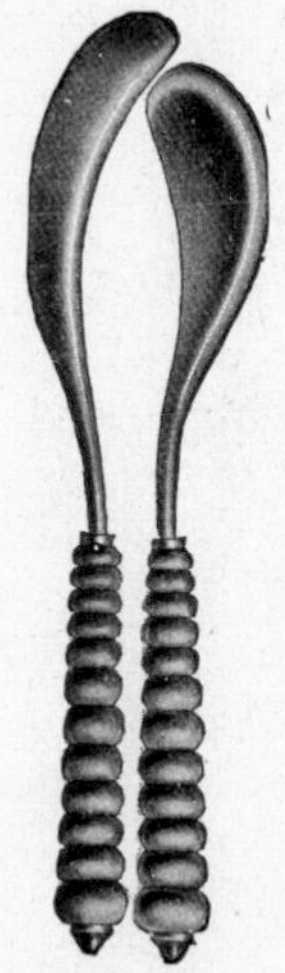

Fig. 547.—Palfyn's Forceps.

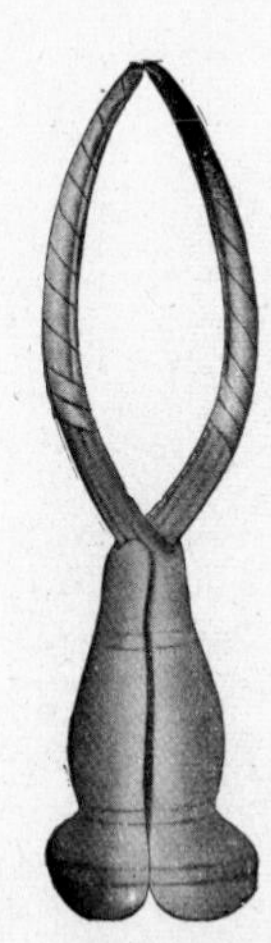

Fig. 548.—Smellie's Short Forceps.

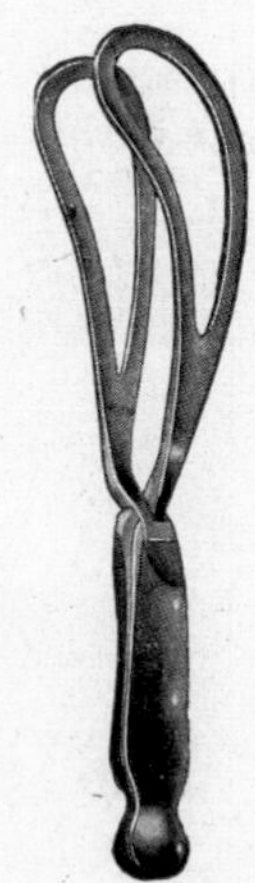

Fig. 549.—Short Forceps.

profit, he deserved to be exposed upon a barren rock and have his vitals plucked out by vultures, little knowing that at the time he spoke such an instrument had been in the possession of the Chamberlen family for nearly one hundred years.

The Chamberlen forceps was a short, straight instrument, which possessed only a cephalic curve, and is perpetuated in the short or low forceps of today. It was used, with but little modification, until the middle of the eighteenth century, when Levret, in 1747, and Smellie, in 1751, quite independently of one another, added the pelvic curve and increased the length of the instrument. Levret's forceps was longer and possessed a more decided pelvic curve than that of Smellie, and it is from these two instruments that the long forceps of the present day is descended—the long French forceps being the lineal descendant of the former, and that of Simpson of the latter.

As soon as the forceps became public property it was subjected to various modifications, so that Mulder, in an atlas published in 1798, was able to give illustrations of nearly 100 varieties. Some idea of the desire to modify and improve the instrument may be gained by glancing at Witkowski's Obstetrical Arsenal, in which are pictured several hundred forceps, which, after all, constitute only a small portion of those devised. The monographs of Poullet and Das contain excellent historical sketches of the development of the instrument. But, considering all the work done, it is surprising how little advance was made over the instruments of Levret and Smellie, until Tarnier, in 1877, clearly enunciated the principle of axis traction, which has since revolutionized our ideas upon the subject.

Definitions. Forceps operations are classified according to the level of the fetal head at the time the blades are applied, as follows:

Low forceps is the application of forceps when the head is visible, the skull is on the perineal floor and the sagittal suture is in the antero-posterior diameter of the pelvis.

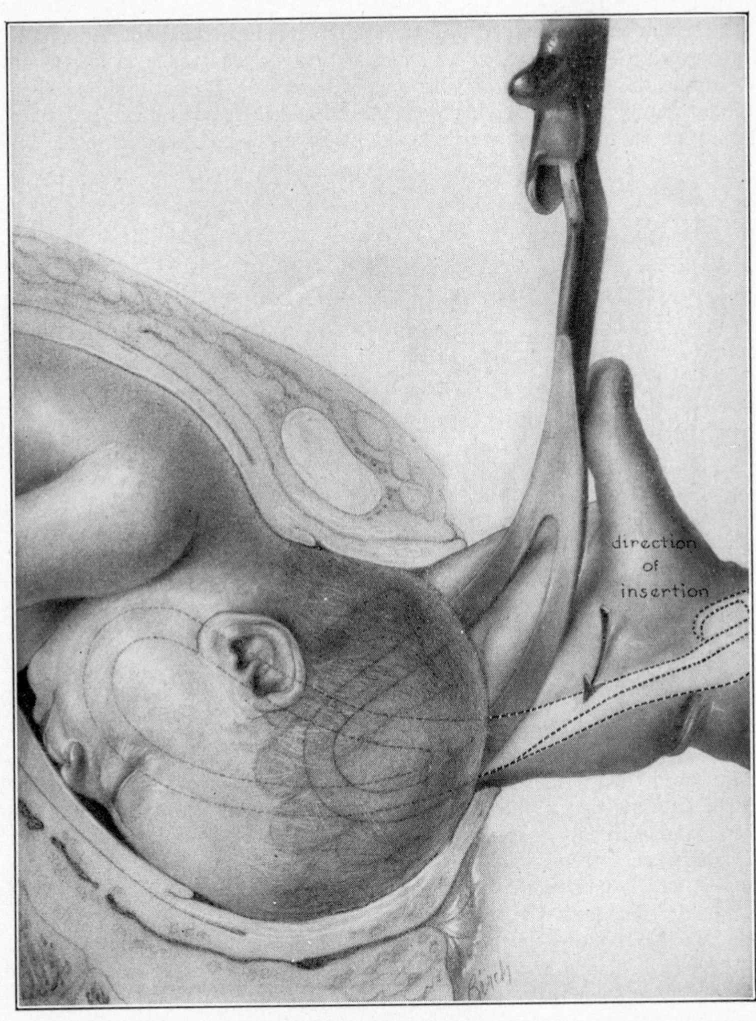

FIG. 550.—LOW FORCEPS.

The *left* blade is being introduced into the *left* side of the pelvis by the *left* hand of the operator. The fingers of the right hand are being used to protect the maternal soft parts, while the thumb helps guide the instrument into place.

Midforceps is the application of forceps before the criteria of low forceps have been met as stated above, but after engagement has taken place; that is, after the plane of the greatest cephalic diameter (biparietal) has passed the inlet. Clinical demonstration that engagement has occurred is afforded by the fact that the lowermost part of the skull is at or below the level of the ischial spines.

High forceps is the application of forceps before engagement has taken place. A subdivision of high forceps is "forceps on the floating head," that is, when the

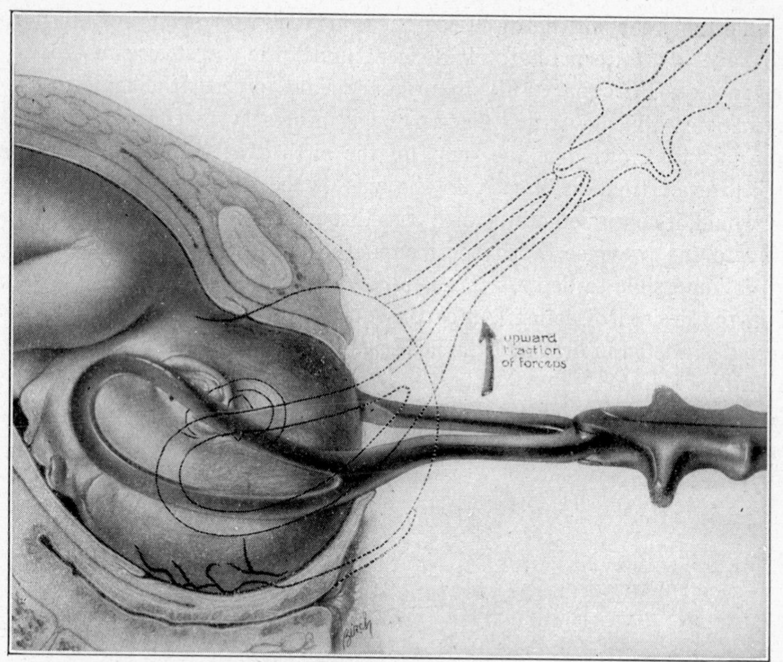

FIG. 551.—DIRECTION OF TRACTION IN LOW FORCEPS; NAMELY, OUTWARD AND UPWARD.
(SEE ALSO FIGS. 566 TO 568.)

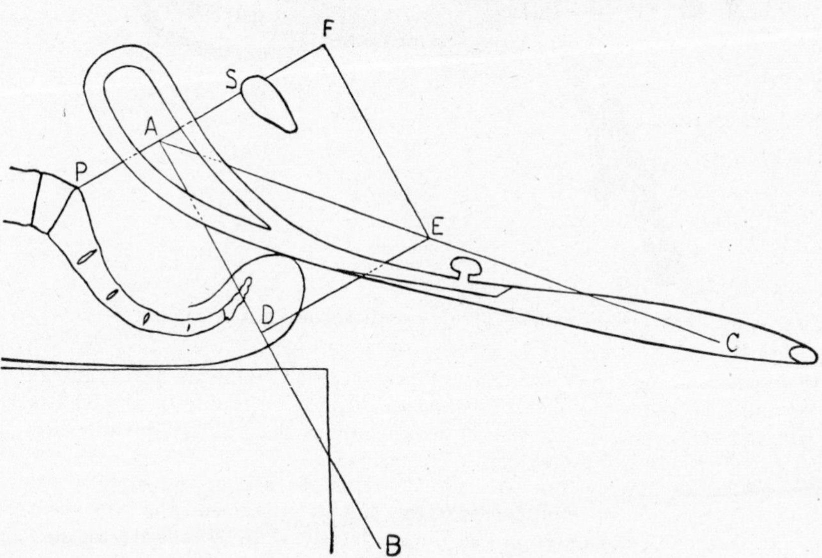

FIG. 552.—TARNIER'S DIAGRAM; SHOWING DEFECTS OF ORDINARY FORCEPS.

A E C, line of actual traction; *A D B,* line of desired traction; *A S F,* force wasted against symphysis pubis.

head is ballottable. As will be discussed subsequently, **no variety of high forceps has any place in modern obstetrics** except under the rarest circumstances.

Axis-traction Forceps. With an ordinary long forceps, the midforceps operation is sometimes difficult, strong traction being necessary to effect delivery. This is due to the fact that, owing to the shape of the birth canal and of the forceps, it is impossible to exert traction directly in the axis of the superior strait. The latter, as we know, would, if continued downward, pass through the lower portion of the sacrum; but, owing to the presence of the perineum, the extremity of the sacrum and the coccyx, it is impossible to depress the handles of the forceps sufficiently to permit of traction in the desired direction. As a consequence, a very considerable part of the force exerted is wasted in dragging the head against the symphysis, instead of bringing it downward.

Tarnier solved this problem by attaching a rod to each blade and connecting them with a traction bar. The forceps he eventually perfected is practically a long French forceps without a perineal curve, provided with short, detachable traction rods, one of which is

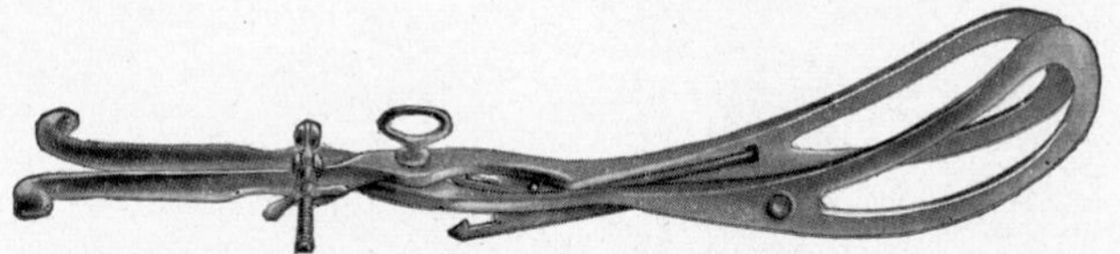

FIG. 553.—TARNIER'S FORCEPS; TRACTION RODS IN PLACE WITHOUT HANDLE BAR.

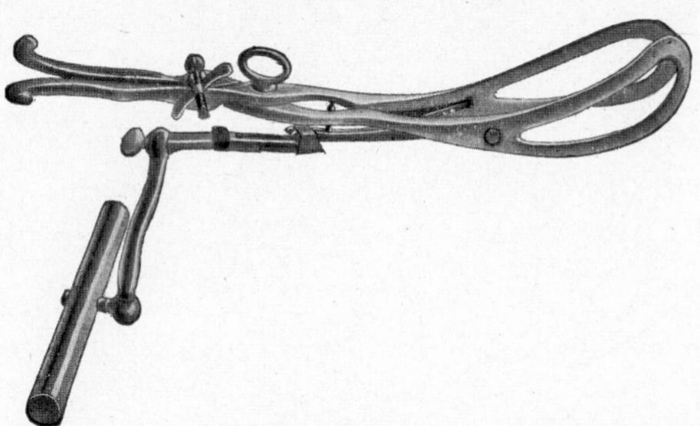

FIG. 554.—TARNIER'S FORCEPS WITH HANDLE BAR ATTACHED.

inserted just beyond the eye of each blade. When not in use, these are held in place by a pin upon the under surface of the shank, from which they can be readily freed, and attached by their free ends to a traction attachment which terminates in a handle bar which can be grasped by one or both hands (see Figs. 553 and 554).

With this device, traction can be made almost in the axis of the superior strait, and, owing to the presence of numerous joints in the traction attachment, the instrument can be used in any position. The handles of the forceps merely serve to indicate the direction in which traction should be made, the force being applied to the handle bar, which is held horizontally no matter what the position of the blades may be, the traction rods being kept about 1 cm. beneath the handles (Fig. 555).

Choice of Forceps. Any properly shaped instrument will give satisfactory results, provided it is used intelligently, but for general purposes the ordinary Simpson forceps is probably the best, though, if one expects to do much obstetrical work, a suitable axis-traction forceps becomes essential. In certain cases of *transverse arrest,* with the head well flexed, the Kielland forceps has definite advantages over most of the other types of forceps as discussed on page 1077.

Functions of the Forceps. The forceps may be used as a tractor, rotator, compressor, dilator, lever, or irritator.

Its most important function is *traction,* exercised for the purpose of drawing the head through the genital tract. In not a few cases, however, particularly in transverse and posterior occipital presentations, its employment as a rotator is attended by happy results.

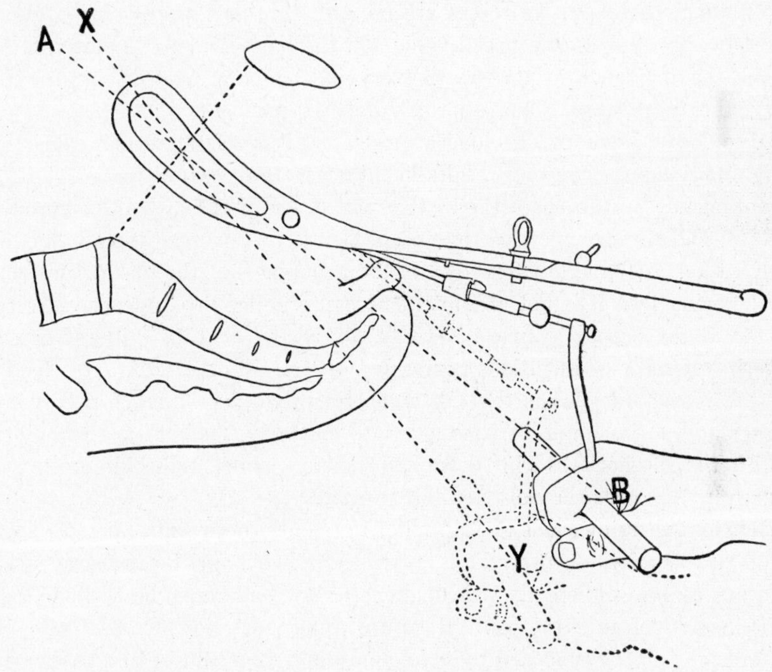

Fig. 555.—Diagram Showing Traction with Tarnier's Forceps.
A B in proper and *X Y* in improper manner (Ribemont-Dessaignes).

Indications for the Use of Forceps. Strictly speaking, the termination of labor by forceps, provided it can be accomplished without great danger, is indicated in any condition which threatens the life of the mother *or* child, and which offers a reasonable prospect of being relieved by delivery. On the part of the mother, such conditions are eclampsia, heart disease, acute edema of the lungs, hemorrhage from premature separation of the placenta, intrapartum infection, or exhaustion. Whenever there is question of interference for the last-named condition, definite objective symptoms should be present, the condition of the pulse being of especial importance. Likewise, it is generally advisable to relieve the strain upon a cicatrix resulting from a previous cesarean section.

As regards the child, the operation may be called for by prolapse of the umbilical cord, premature separation of the placenta, undue pressure exerted upon the head, and especially by changes in the rhythm of the heart beat and the escape of meconium in vertex presentations. A fetal pulse falling permanently below 100 indicates that the child is in danger and may perish if not promptly delivered. In vertex presentations the discharge of amniotic fluid tinged with meconium usually indicates interference with the placental circulation and imperfect oxygenation, manifesting itself by paralysis of the sphincter ani. In breech presentations, on the other hand, the escape of meconium is without significance, being due merely to pressure exerted upon the child's abdomen.

One of the most frequent indications is afforded by uterine inertia. Furthermore, in primiparae the amount of resistance offered by the perineum and the vaginal outlet may sometimes be so great as to oppose a serious obstacle to the passage of the child, even when the expulsive forces are normal. In this type of case a median or mediolateral episiotomy is of especial value. On the basis of definite maternal or fetal indications, the incidence of forceps delivery in the New York Lying-In Hospital service ("indicated forceps") was approximately 10 per cent.

Elective Low Forceps. Prolonged pressure of the fetal head against a more or less rigid perineum sometimes results in injury to the cerebral tissues. To forestall such a contingency and to spare the mother the strain of the last few minutes of the second stage, DeLee recommended the "prophylactic forceps operation." This is more commonly called "elective low forceps" on the grounds that the obstetrician elects to interfere knowing that it is not absolutely necessary since spontaneous delivery is to be expected in the natural course of events within the next 15 minutes or so. The vast majority of forceps operations performed in this country today are elective low forceps. One reason for this is that all analgesic programs, whether they consist of barbiturates and scopolamine or conduction technics, interfere to a greater or lesser degree with the mother's bearing-down efforts, and under these circumstances low forceps delivery becomes the most feasible procedure.

The fact that these methods of pain relief frequently necessitate forceps delivery is not an indictment of these procedures, provided the obstetrician adheres strictly to the definition of low forceps as stated above. The head must be visible, the skull on the perineal floor and the sagittal suture anteroposterior. Under these circumstances, forceps delivery preceded by episiotomy is a very simple and safe operation, gentle traction by the fingers and wrists being all that is necessary. By giving the patient ample time, these criteria for low forceps can usually be met despite the influence of analgesic medication. If, however, the head does not descend and rotate in keeping with these criteria, any forceps operation performed is not an elective low forceps but an indicated midforceps. It is true that in many instances the latter type of operation, especially in cases in which the rotation criterion is the only one not met, may also be easy in expert hands. Nevertheless, as a general rule an unrotated head is higher than one which is anteroposterior, and more traction is often required. Hence for optimal safety both for mother and infant, forceps should not be elected until conditions permit the performance of a low forceps operation as defined.

Prerequisites of Forceps Application. The following conditions must be present before the forceps can be applied with safety:

1. The head must be engaged, preferably deeply engaged. Application of the blades prior to engagement—that is, high forceps—is an extremely difficult operation, often entailing brutal trauma of the maternal tissues and killing a large proportion of the babies. Many years ago when cesarean section was also a highly dangerous operation, high forceps had a certain place in operative obstetrics, but it is rarely employed

today and it is mentioned here only to condemn it. Even after engagement occurs, the higher the station of the fetal head, the more difficult and traumatic forceps delivery becomes. Moreover, whenever the blades are applied before the head has reached the perineal floor, it is common experience to find the head decidedly higher than rectal or vaginal examination had indicated, extensive caput succedaneum formation having misled the examiner in regard to the actual level of the fetal skull.

These difficulties of midforceps operation when the head has not reached the perineal floor must be borne in mind even in cases in which there is a very valid

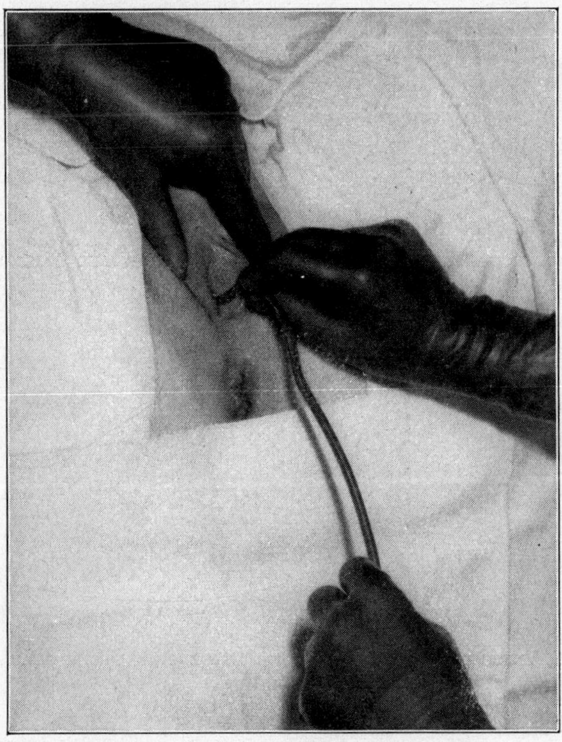

Fig. 556.—Catheterization of Bladder Prior to Application of Forceps.

maternal indication for forceps delivery. For instance, it is generally agreed that patients with rheumatic heart disease and preeclampsia should be spared the bearing-down efforts of the second stage if it is at all feasible to do so. However, such efforts may be much less harmful than a difficult midforceps, and in the presence of such an indication, forceps should not be used until the station of the head promises an easy operative procedure. The same generalization applies to forceps for fetal distress when the skull is not close to the perineal floor. Granted that the fetal heart rate in such a case may suggest that the infant is suffering from anoxia, it may still be judicious to allow more time for the head to descend rather than to superimpose the trauma of a difficult midforceps operation on an already distressed infant. Indeed, under the circumstances mentioned, more infants have been killed by operations to relieve fetal distress than have been saved. In sum, except for cases in which arrest of the fetal head has occurred in midpelvis because of maternal exhaustion or intractable inertia (and in which the obstetrician has little choice), it is best to defer the application of the blades until a low forceps operation is possible, even in the presence of maternal disease or fetal distress.

2. The child must present either by the vertex or by the face with the chin anterior. The forceps is not applicable, of course, to shoulder presentations, nor is it intended to be applied to the breech. Generally speaking, it should not be employed

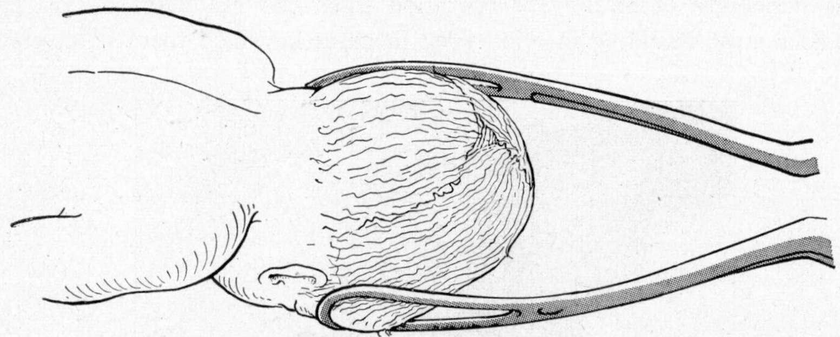

Fig. 557.—Incorrect Application of Forceps over Brow and Mastoid Region.

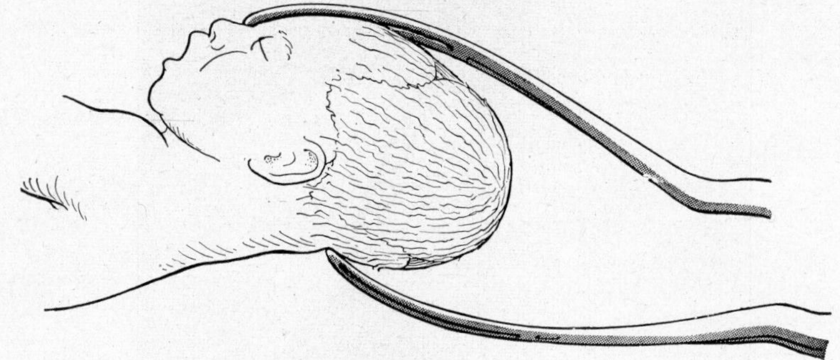

Fig. 558.—Incorrect Application of Forceps, One Blade over Occiput and Other over the Brow.

Note that the forceps cannot be locked.

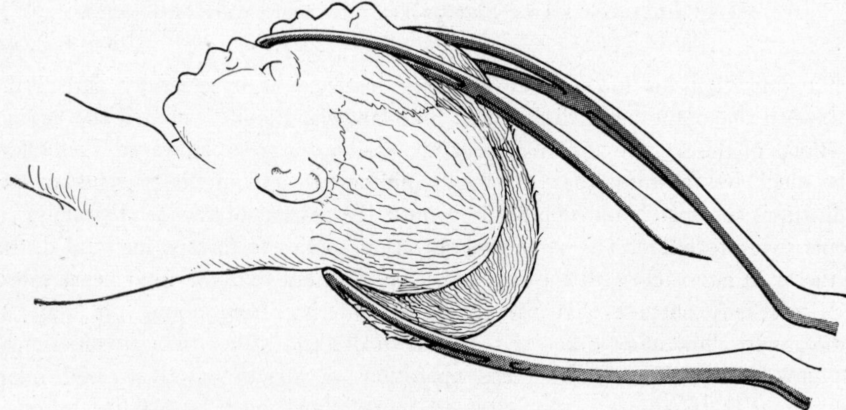

Fig. 559.—Forceps Applied Incorrectly as in Fig. 558.

Note extension of head and tendency of blades to slip off with traction.

in brow cases until after conversion into a vertex or face presentation has been brought about.

3. The cervix must be completely dilated before the application of forceps. Even the presence of a small rim of cervix offers surprising resistance to forceps traction and may result in extensive cervical lacerations which may also implicate the lower uterine segment. Accordingly, if prompt delivery becomes imperative before complete dilatation of the cervix, cesarean section or Dührssen's incisions are preferable, depending upon the circumstances of the case, as discussed on page 1080.

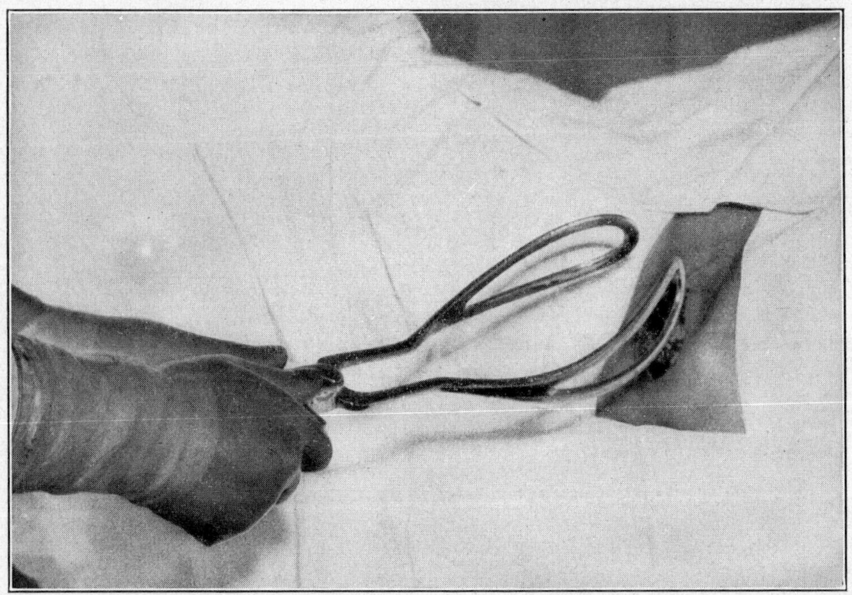

FIG. 560.—ORIENTATION FOR L.O.A. POSITION (Simpson Forceps).

4. The membranes must be ruptured. If the membranes intervene between the head and the forceps blades, the grasp is not so firm and there is a conceivable possibility that traction may bring about abruptio placentae.

5. There should be no advanced degree of disproportion between the size of the head and that of the midpelvis and/or outlet, as discussed on page 854. Since forceps should not be employed until after the head has passed through the inlet, the presence of inlet contraction as a contraindication to forceps is not pertinent to present-day practices.

Preparations for Operations. When anesthesia is complete, the patient's buttocks should be brought to the edge of the table, and her legs held in position by an appropriate leg holder, or by stirrups. The patient is then prepared for operation, as previously described. Catheterization is next done and is a most important preliminary procedure, since an empty bladder not only facilitates delivery but minimizes the danger of bladder injury.

Application of Forceps. The forceps is so constructed that its cephalic curve is best adapted to the sides of the child's head, the biparietal diameter corresponding to the line of greatest distance between the blades. Consequently, the head is grasped

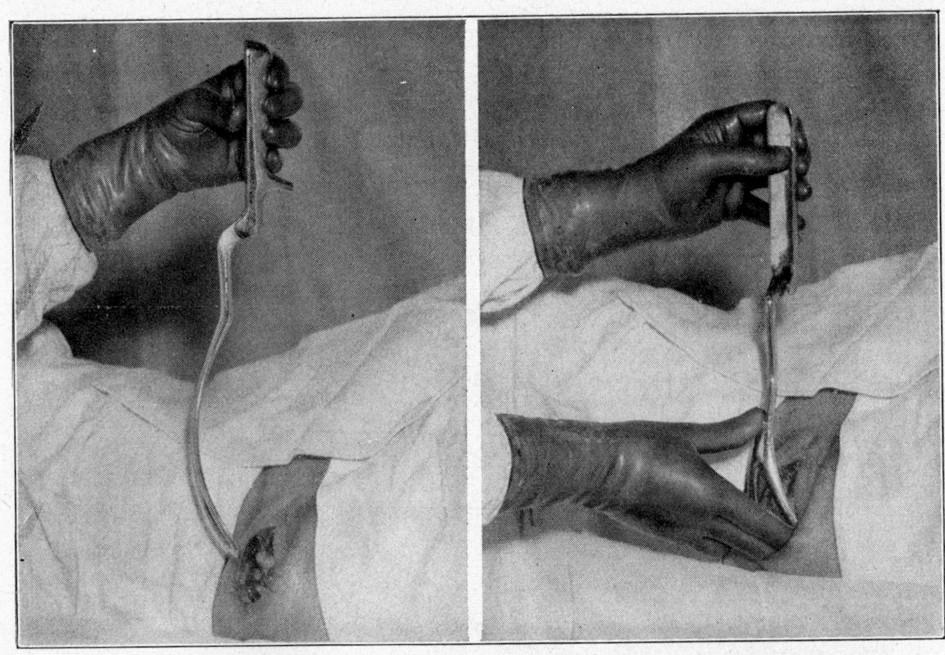

Fig. 561.—The Left Handle Held in the Left Hand. Simpson Forceps.

Fig. 562.—Introduction of Left Blade to Left Side of Pelvis.

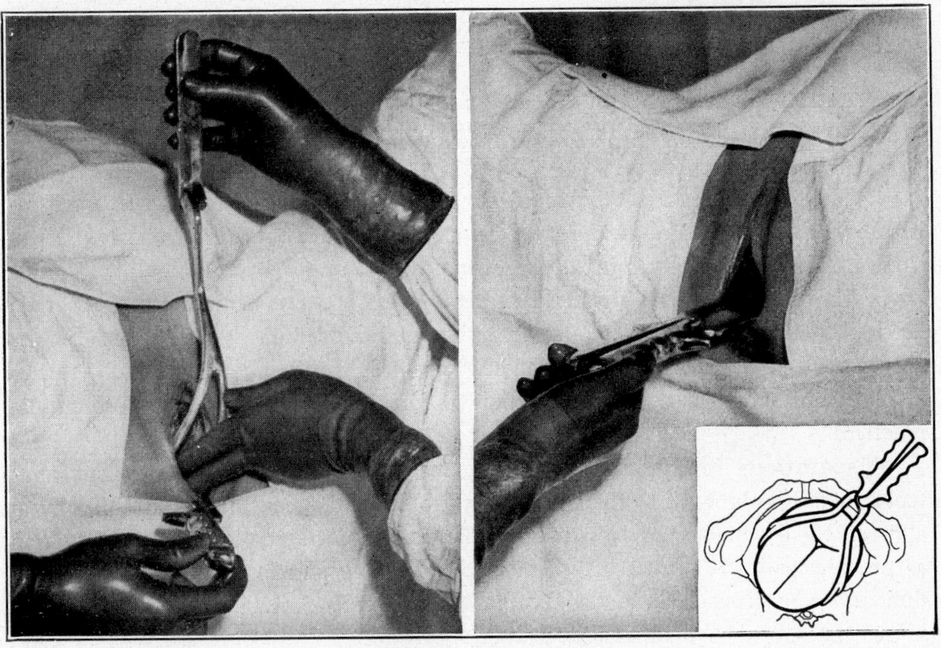

Fig. 563.—Left Blade in Place, Introduction of Right Blade by Right Hand.

Fig. 564.—Forceps Have Been Locked.

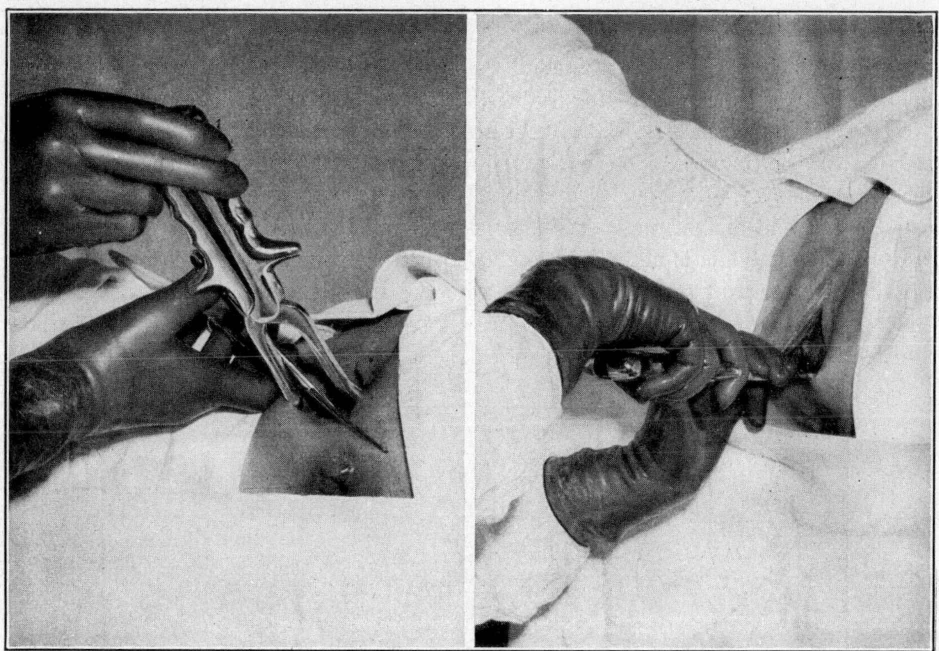

Fig. 565.—Left Mediolateral Episiotomy May Be Performed.

Fig. 566.—Horizontal Traction, Operator Seated.

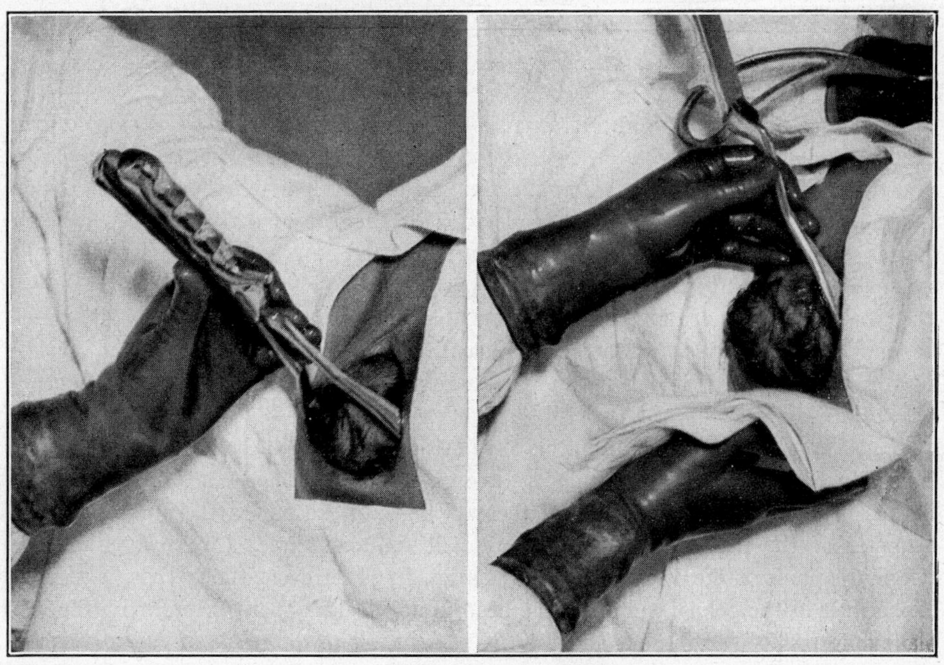

Fig. 567.—Upward Traction.

Fig. 568.—Disarticulation of Blades. Beginning Modified Ritgen Maneuver.

in an ideal manner only when the long axis of the blades corresponds to the occipitomental diameter, the fenestra including the parietal bosses and the tips lying over the cheeks, while the concave margins of the blades look toward either the occiput or the face. With such a grasp the forceps obtains a firm hold and cannot slip off, and traction can be made in the most advantageous manner. On the other hand, when the forceps is applied obliquely with one blade over the brow and the other over the opposite mastoid region, the grasp is less secure, and the head is exposed to injurious pressure. If one blade is accurately applied over the face and the other over the occiput, the instrument cannot be locked, while, if the blade over the face is slipped down so as to permit articulation, the grasp is very insecure and each traction tends to extend the head (Figs. 557 to 559).

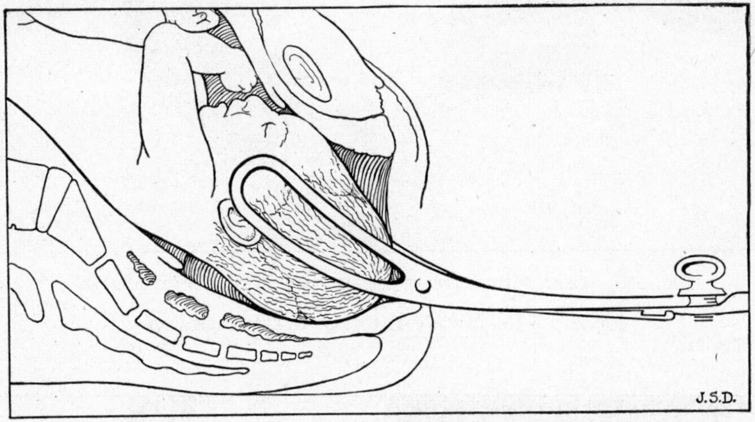

FIG. 569.—LOW FORCEPS. OCCIPUT DIRECTLY POSTERIOR; HORIZONTAL TRACTION.

For these reasons, then, the forceps should be applied directly to the sides of the head along its *occipitomental* or *jugoparietal diameter*. This is known as the *cephalic,* in contradistinction to the *pelvic application*. In the latter application, the left blade is applied to the left and the right blade to the right side of the mother's pelvis, no matter what the presentation, consequently the head is grasped satisfactorily only when the sagittal suture is directed anteroposteriorly.

An accurate idea of the exact position of the head is essential to the cephalic application. With the head low down, this can usually be obtained by examining the sagittal suture; but when it is higher up an absolute diagnosis can be made only by *locating the posterior ear.*

Low Forceps. With the head in this low position, as defined, the obstacle to delivery is usually due to insufficient expulsive force or to abnormal resistance on the part of the perineum. In such circumstances the sagittal suture occupies the anteroposterior diameter of the pelvic outlet, with the small fontanel directed toward either the symphysis pubis or the concavity of the sacrum. In either event the forceps, if applied to the sides of the pelvis, will grasp the head in an ideal manner. Accordingly, the left blade is introduced to the left and the right blade to the right side of the pelvis, the mode of procedure being somewhat as follows: Two fingers of the right hand are passed into the left and posterior portion of the vulva and carried up the vagina past the margins of the external os. The handle of the left branch is then seized between the thumb and two fingers of the left hand—just as in holding a pen—and the tip of the blade is gently passed into the vagina along the palmar surface of the fingers of the right hand which serve as a guide. As it is introduced, the handle is at first held almost vertically, but, as the blade adapts itself to the head, it is depressed, so that it eventually takes a horizontal position. The guiding fingers are then withdrawn, and the handle is left to itself or is held by an assistant. In the same manner, two fingers of the left hand are then introduced into the right and posterior portion of the birth canal to serve as a guide for the right blade, which is held in the right hand and introduced into the vagina. The guiding fingers are now removed and all that remains to be done is to articulate the branches. Usually they lie in such a manner that they can be locked without difficulty; but when this cannot be done, first one and then the other blade should be gently moved until the handles are brought into such a position as to be articulated with ease. As explained on page 410, episiotomy is performed routinely either just prior to the application of the blades or shortly afterward.

An examination is made to ascertain whether the blades have been correctly applied, or whether they inclose the lips of the cervix. In the latter case the forceps should be loosened and reapplied. When it is certain that the blades are satisfactorily placed, the handles are seized with one hand and gentle intermittent traction is made in a horizontal direction until the perineum begins to bulge. As soon as the vulva begins to be distended by the occiput, the handles are gradually elevated, and eventually point almost directly upward as the parietal bones emerge. During the latter maneuver, the four fingers should grasp the upper surface of the handles and shanks, while the thumb upon their lower surface exerts the necessary force, as shown in Figure 567.

In delivering the head, spontaneous delivery should be simulated as closely as possible, and the minimum amount of force employed. Accordingly, traction should be made intermittently, the head being allowed to recede in the intervals, as in spontaneous labor. Except when urgently indicated, it should be extracted so slowly as to give time for proper stretching and dilatation of the perineum, which in primiparous women cannot be satisfactorily accomplished in less than five minutes.

When the vulva is well distended by the head and the brow can be felt through the perineum, the mode of completing delivery varies. We often do so with the forceps in place, holding that in this way one has the greatest control over the advance of the head. On the other hand, the thickness of the blades may at times add to the distention of the vulva and thus increases its liability to laceration. In such cases, we remove the forceps and complete the delivery by Ritgen's maneuver—slowly expressing the head by making upward pressure upon the brow through the posterior portion of the perineum, the anal region being covered by a towel in order to prevent as far as possible any contamination from the bowel. Occasionally the forceps are removed too soon, and in this event Ritgen's maneuver proves a tedious and inelegant procedure.

When the occiput lies directly posteriorly, traction should be made in a horizontal direction until the forehead or root of the nose engages under the symphysis, after which the handles should be slowly elevated, until the occiput slowly emerges over the anterior margin of the perineum, and then, by imparting a downward motion to the instrument, the forehead, nose, and chin will successively emerge from the vulva.

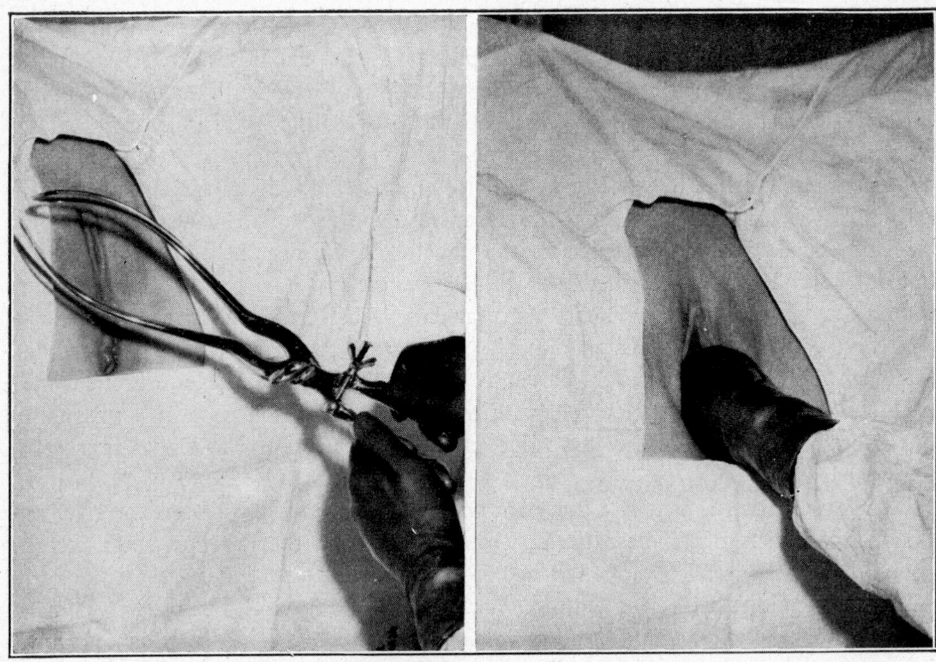

Fig. 570.—Orientation for Tranverse (R. O. T.) Position. Tarnier Forceps.

Fig. 571.—Hand in Vagina Seeking Posterior Ear.

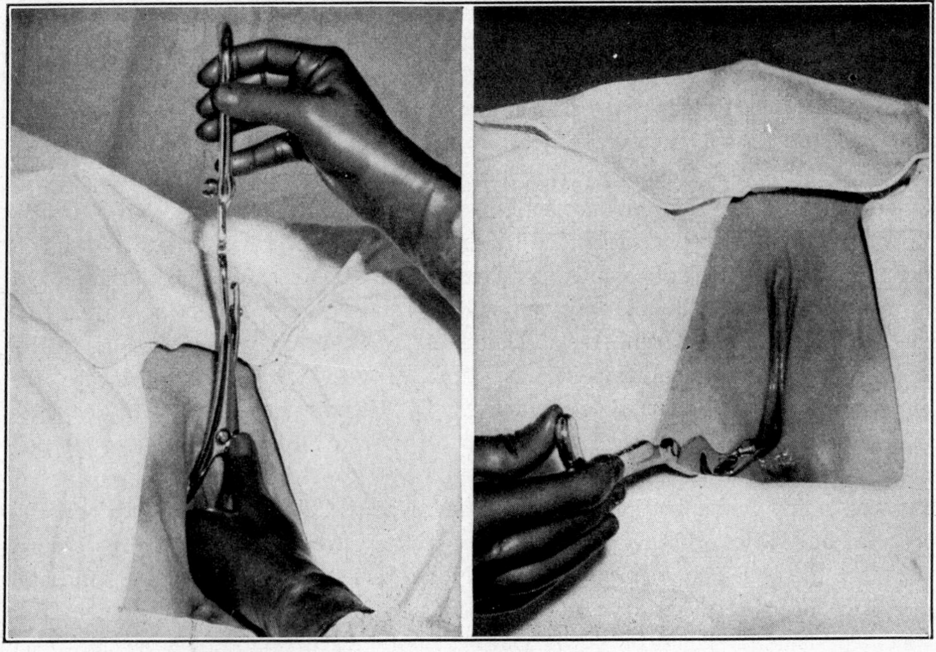

Fig. 572.—Introduction of Posterior Blade by Right Hand, Using Left Hand as a Guide.

Fig. 573.—Posterior Blade in Position.

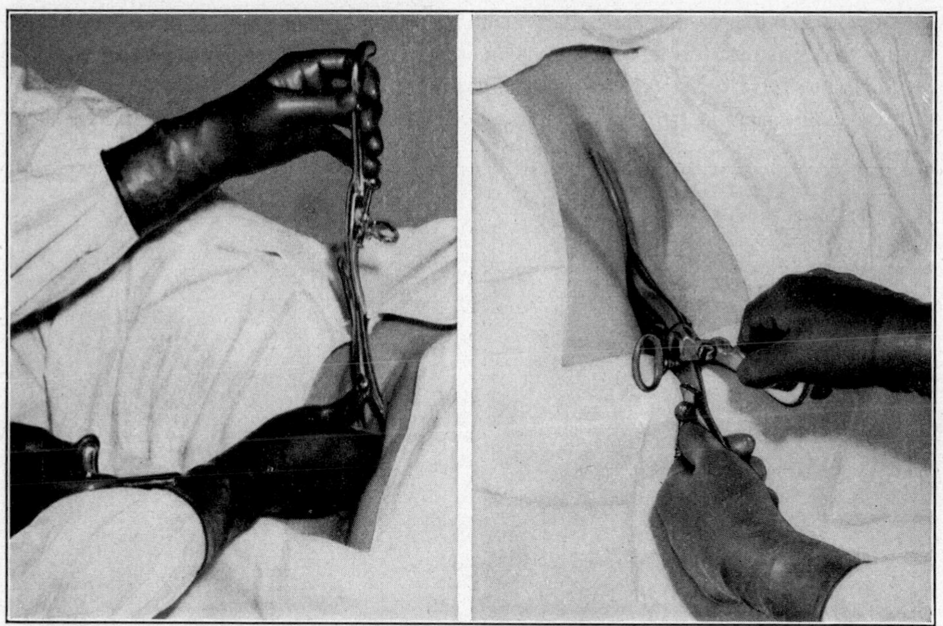

Fig. 574.—Introduction of Anterior Blade Which Is Wandered over Face.

Fig. 575.—Locking the Forceps.

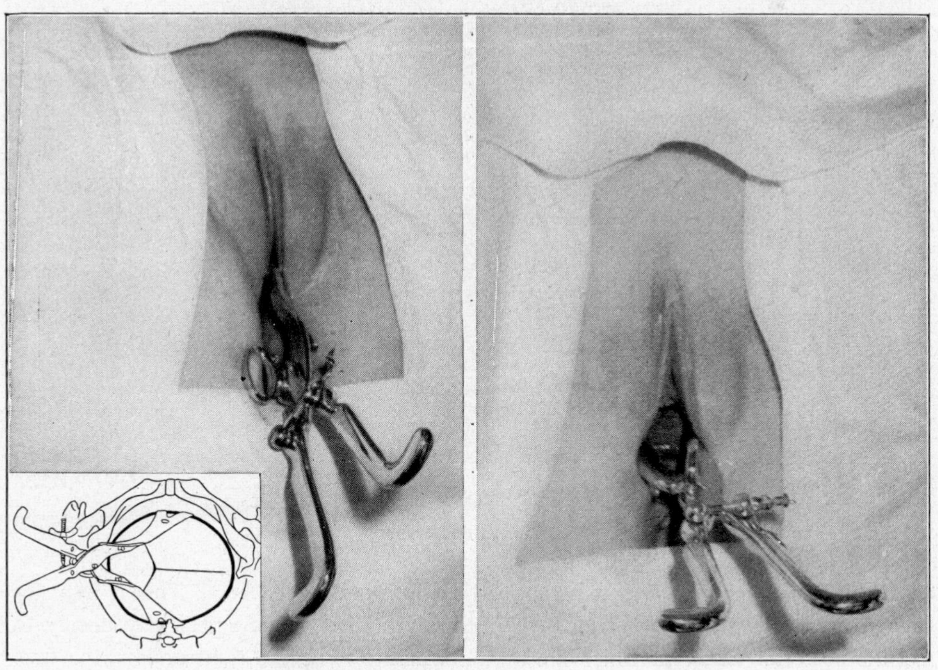

Fig. 576.—Application Now Complete for R. O. T. Position.

Fig. 577.—Rotation to Anterior Position.

This extraction is more difficult than when the occiput is anterior, and, owing to the greater distention of the vulva, perineal tears are more likely to occur (Fig. 569).

Mid Forceps Operations. When the head lies above the perineum, the sagittal suture usually occupies an oblique or transverse diameter of the birth canal. In such

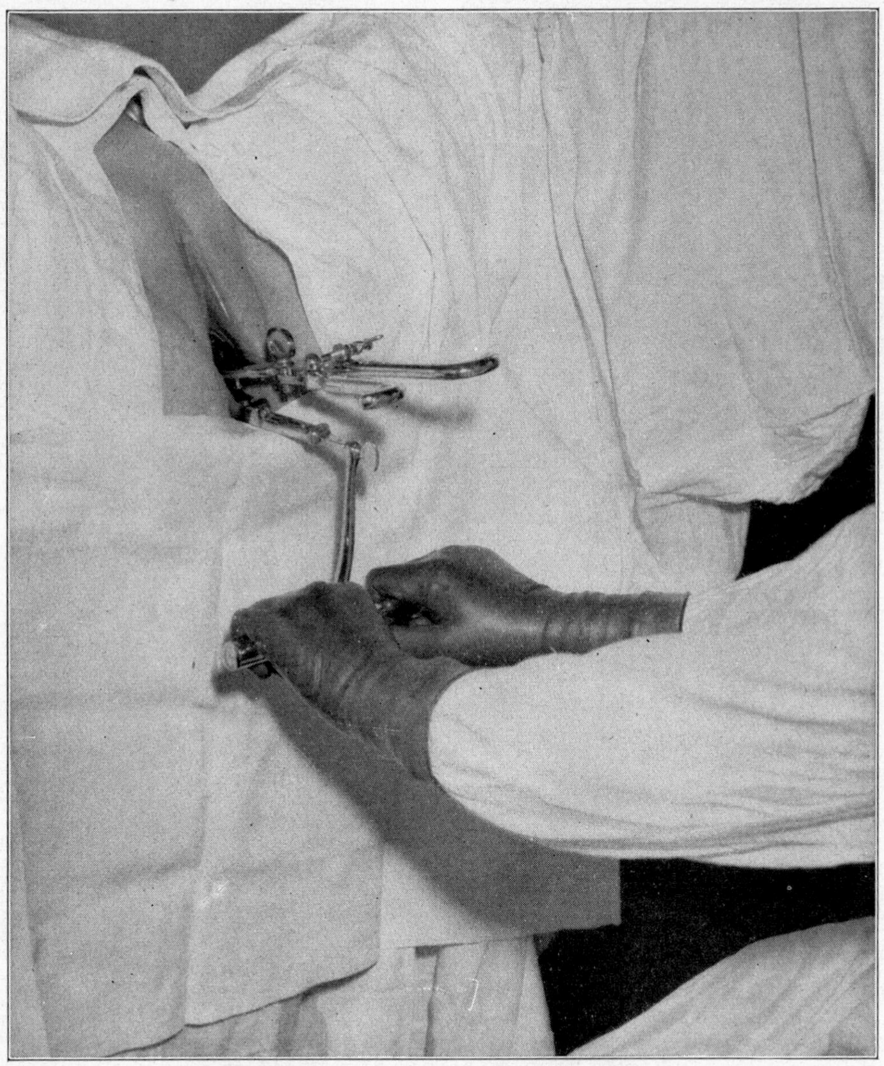

FIG. 578.—TRACTION ON HANDLE BAR. OPERATOR IS SEATED.

Note distance between forcep handles and traction rods.

cases the forceps should always be applied to the sides of the head. This is best accomplished by introducing two or more fingers into the vagina sufficiently deeply to feel the posterior ear, over which, no matter whether it be the right or left, the first blade should be applied (see Figs. 570 to 573).

In left occipito-anterior positions the entire right hand, introduced into the left posterior segment of the pelvis, should locate the posterior ear, and at the same time

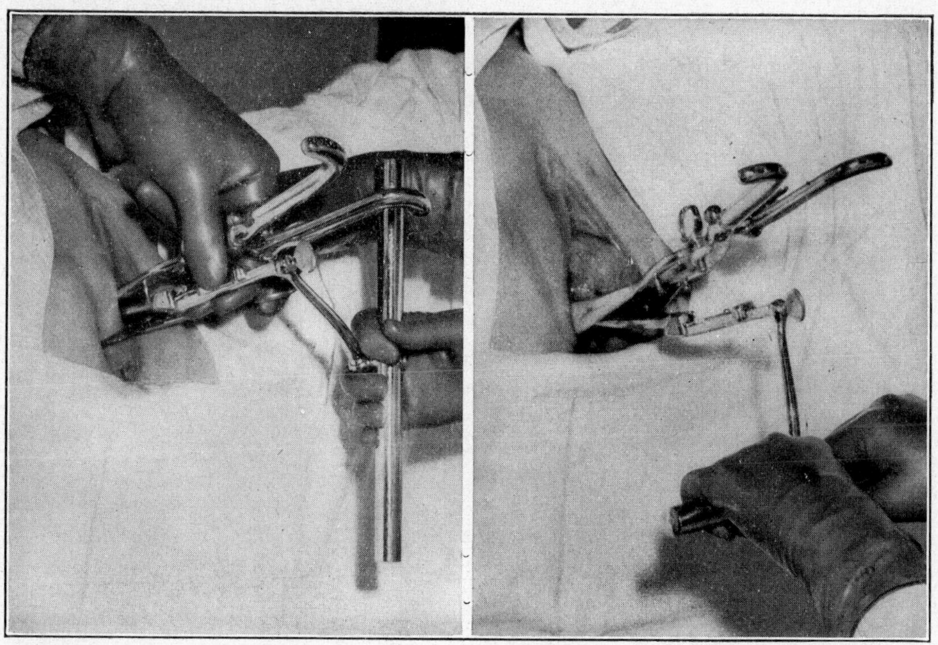

Fig. 579.—Right Mediolateral Episiotomy.

Fig. 580.—Further Traction, Head Is Emerging at the Vulva.

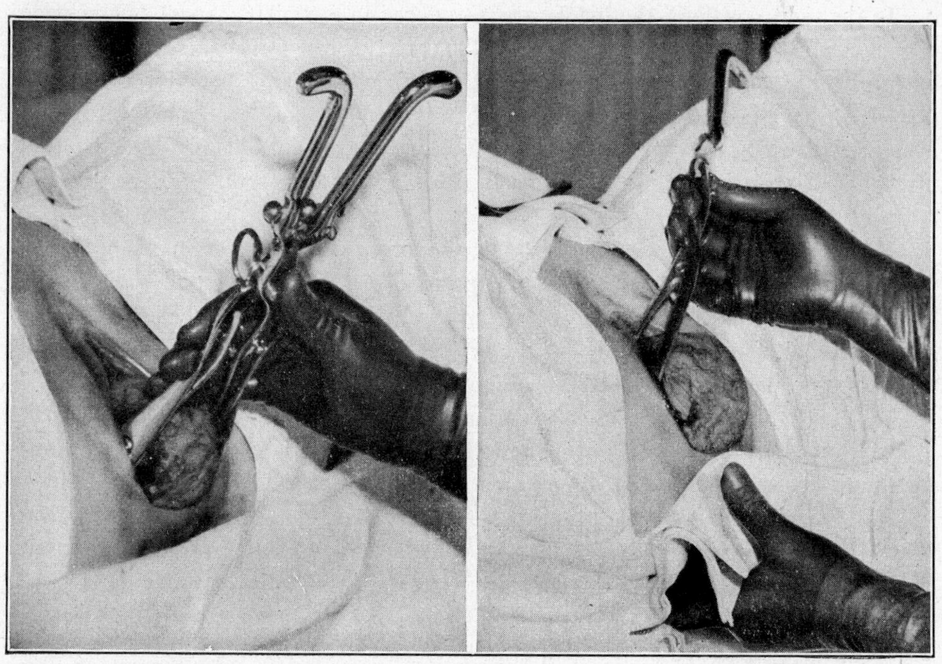

Fig. 581.—Upward Traction on Shank of Forceps, Bar Removed.

Fig. 582.—Removal of Forceps, Beginning Modified Ritgen Maneuver.

serve as a guide for the introduction of the left branch of the forceps, which is held in the left hand and applied over the posterior ear. The guide hand is then withdrawn, when the handle may be held by an assistant or left to itself, as the blade will usually retain its position without difficulty.

Two fingers of the left hand are then introduced into the right and posterior segment of the birth canal, no attempt being made to reach the anterior ear, which lies in the neighborhood of the right iliopectineal eminence. The right branch of the forceps, held in the right hand, is then introduced along the left hand as a guide. After its introduction it still remains to apply it over the anterior ear of the child. This is accomplished by gently sweeping it anteriorly until it comes to lie directly opposite the blade which was first introduced. The two branches being now articulated, one blade of the forceps occupies the posterior and the other the anterior extremity of the left oblique diameter.

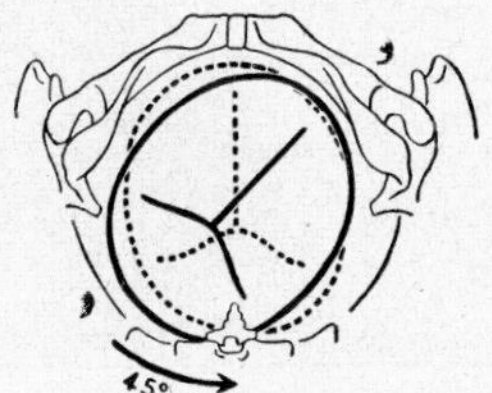

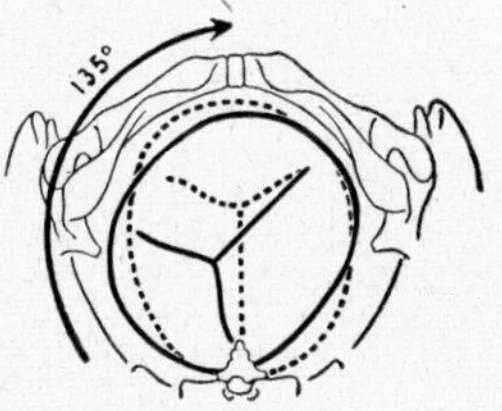

Fig. 583.—Diagrams Showing Rotation of Obliquely Posterior Occiput to Sacrum and Symphysis Pubis, Respectively.

In the right positions, the blades are introduced in a similar manner but in opposite directions, for in this case the right is the posterior ear, over which the first blade inserted must accordingly be placed. It should, however, be remembered that after the blades have been applied to the sides of the head the left handle and shank will lie above the right, and consequently the forceps will not immediately articulate, but this difficulty can be readily overcome by rotating the former around the latter so as to bring the lock into proper position.

If the occiput is in a *transverse position,* the forceps is introduced in a similar manner, the first blade being applied over the posterior ear, and the second being rotated anteriorly until it comes to lie opposite the first. In this case one blade lies in front of the sacrum and the other behind the symphysis. The Tarnier or Kielland forceps may be used as shown in Figs. 570 to 582 and Figs. 593 to 600.

Whatever the original position of the head may be, delivery is effected by making traction obliquely downward until the occiput appears at the vulva, the rest of the operation being completed in the manner already described. When the occiput is obliquely anterior, it gradually rotates spontaneously to the symphysis pubis as traction is made. But when it is directed transversely, in order to bring it to the front, it is sometimes necessary to impart a *rotary motion* to the forceps while making traction. The direction in which this rotary motion is to be imparted varies, of course, according to the position of the occiput, rotation from the left side toward the middle line being necessary when the occiput is directed toward the left, and in the reverse direction when it is directed toward the right side of the pelvis (see Figs. 575, 576, and 577).

In making traction, before the head appears at the vulva, *one or both hands* may be employed according to the amount of force required. When the Simpson forceps are used, one hand grasps the handles of the instrument, while the fingers of the other are hooked over the transverse projection at their upper ends. Care must be taken not to employ too much force. To avoid this error the operator should sit with his arms flexed and the elbows held closely against the thorax, as it is not permissible to make use of the body weight (see Fig. 578).

Application of Forceps in Obliquely Posterior Positions. Prompt delivery may become necessary if the small fontanel is directed toward one or the other sacro-iliac synchondrosis—namely, in R. O. P. and L. O. P. positions. When interference is required in either of these, the head is often imperfectly flexed. In many cases, when the hand is introduced to locate the posterior ear the occiput will rotate spontaneously to a transverse position, and delivery by forceps is then accomplished, as already described. If, however, rotation does not occur, the head should be seized, with four fingers over its posterior and the thumb over its anterior ear, and an attempt made to rotate the occiput to a transverse position. This can usually be accomplished with ease, and occasionally even rotation to an anterior position can be brought about. The forceps is then applied as described above. In other cases, after manual rotation has been effected, the head slips back into its original position before the forceps can be applied. Another method of internal manual rotation is that of Pomeroy or of Lackie, where the whole hand is introduced and passed beyond the head until the anterior shoulder is reached. Pressure on the shoulder with the head lying in the hollow of the hand usually brings about the desired rotation. We do not recommend this maneuver to the beginner or unskilled operator.

If manual rotation cannot be accomplished at once and easily, application of the blades to the head in posterior position and delivery as such is the next safest procedure in the hands of the average operator, as emphasized by Litzenberg, Louis H. Douglass and others. In many of these cases the cause of the persistent occiput posterior position and of the difficulty in accomplishing rotation is an anthropoid pelvis in which the pelvic architecture plainly predisposes to posterior delivery and opposes rotation. It is true that somewhat more traction is necessary with delivery of an occiput posterior head as such and that a liberal mediolateral episiotomy is advisable. But except in the hands of experts who have had extensive experience with manual rotation or the Scanzoni maneuver, it is conducive to less maternal and fetal injury than is a difficult rotation of the head.

Scanzoni Maneuver. Unfortunately, when it is desired to rotate the occiput forward by means of the forceps, an application to the sides of the head with the pelvic curvature directed upward results in the blades becoming inverted by the time rotation is completed, so that the pelvic curve then looks posteriorly, and an attempted delivery with the instrument in this position is likely to cause serious injury to the maternal soft parts. In order to avoid this, it is best to remove and reapply the instrument as described below.

The *double application of forceps,* which was first described by Smellie and rediscovered by Scanzoni nearly a century later, has given satisfactory results in some hands but it is rarely necessary, and is generally employed in only a small percentage of all obliquely posterior occipital positions. As the right posterior variety is much the more frequent, we shall describe the steps of the operation in some detail.

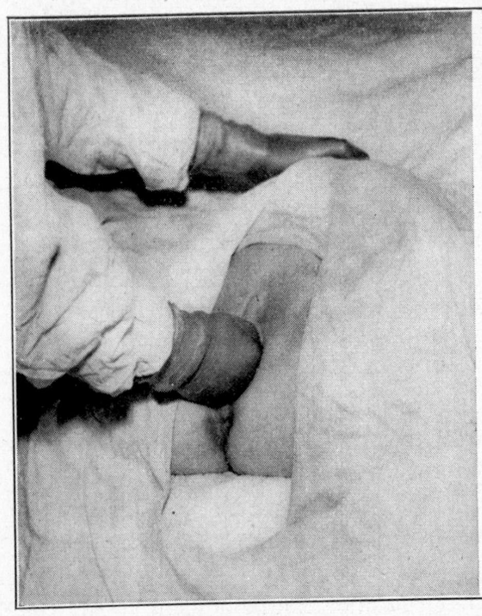

Fig. 584.—Vaginal Examination Seeking Posterior Ear.

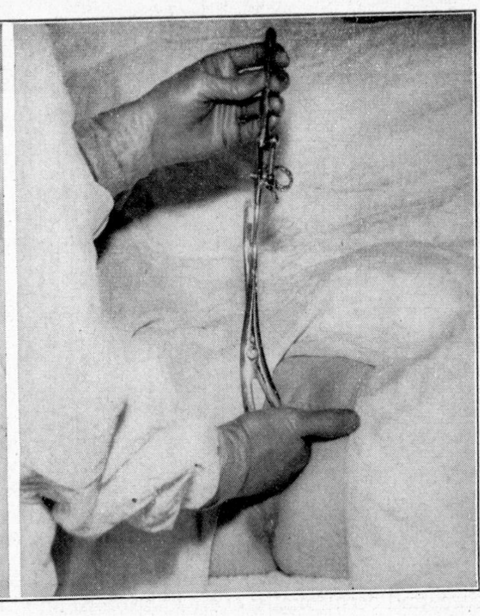

Fig. 585.—Introduction of Posterior Blade, Pelvic Application.

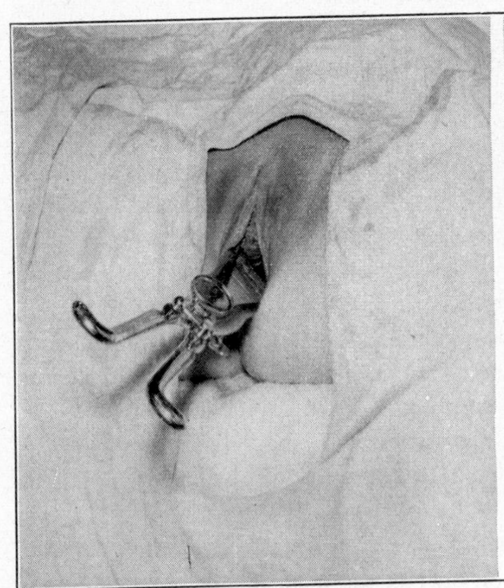

Fig. 586.—Forceps Locked in First Application, R.O.P.

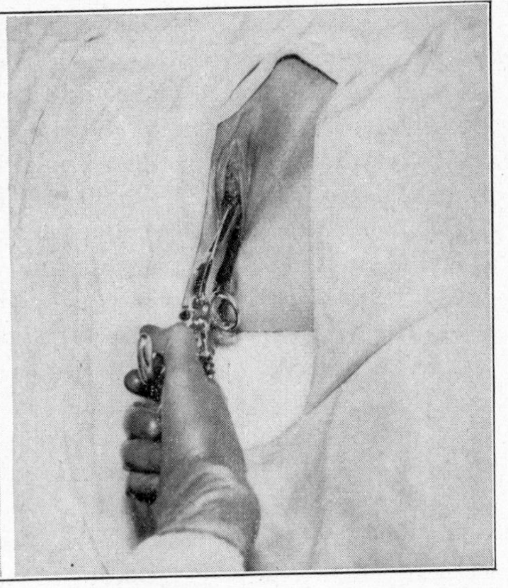

Fig. 587.—Rotation to R.O.T.

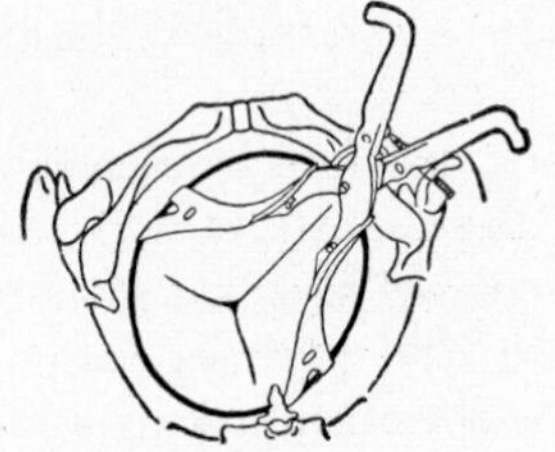

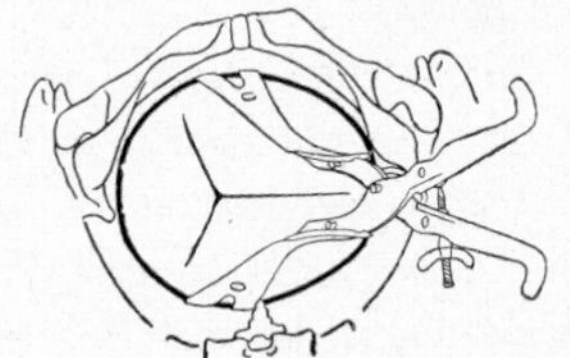

Fig. 588.—Rotation from R.O.P. to Transverse as Shown in Photographs, Figs. 586 and 587.

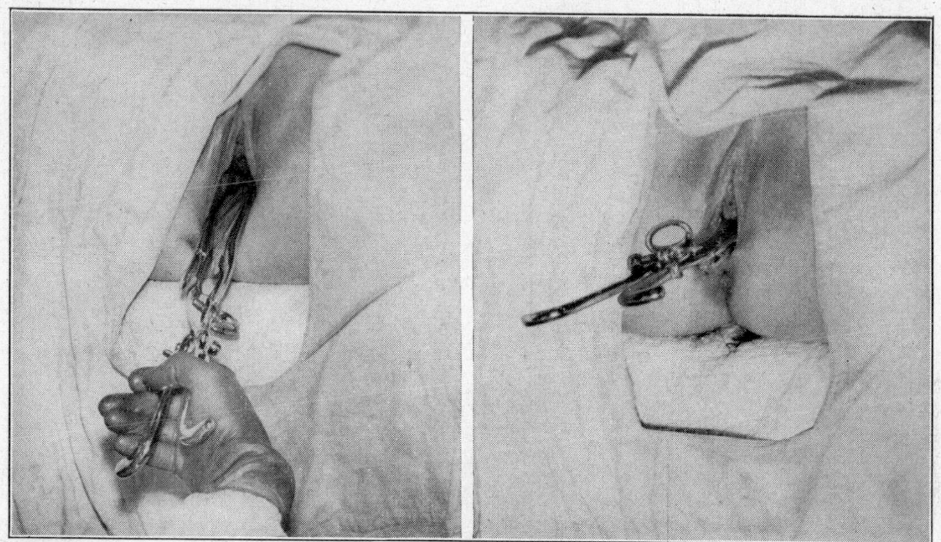

Fig. 589.—Rotation to R.O.A.

Fig. 590.—Forceps Reintroduced for R.O.A., Now a Cephalic and Pelvic Application.

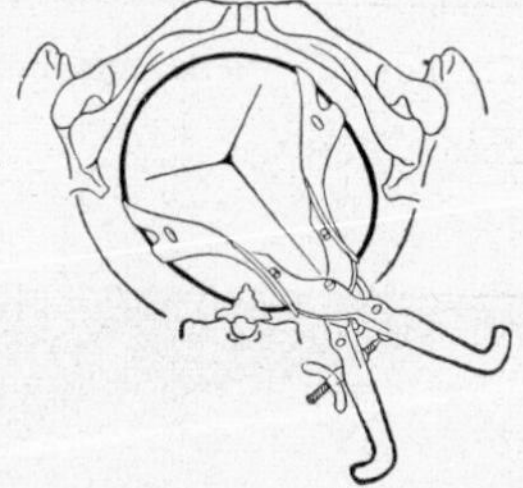

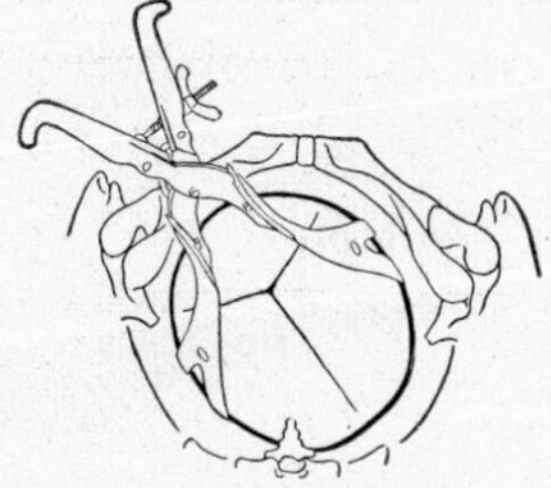

Fig. 591.—Forceps after Rotation to R.O.A. (Fig. 589) with Pelvic Curvature of Forceps Directed Downward; and the Reapplied Forceps for R.O.A. (Fig. 590) with Pelvic Curvature Upward and Properly Directed.

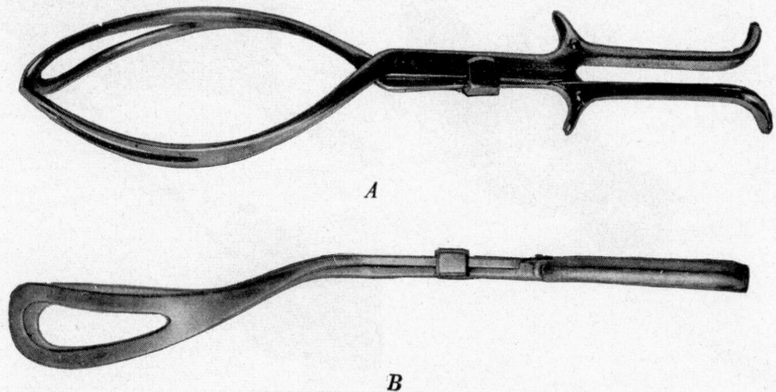

A

B

Fig. 592.—Kielland's Forceps.

A, front view; *B,* side view. × ¼.

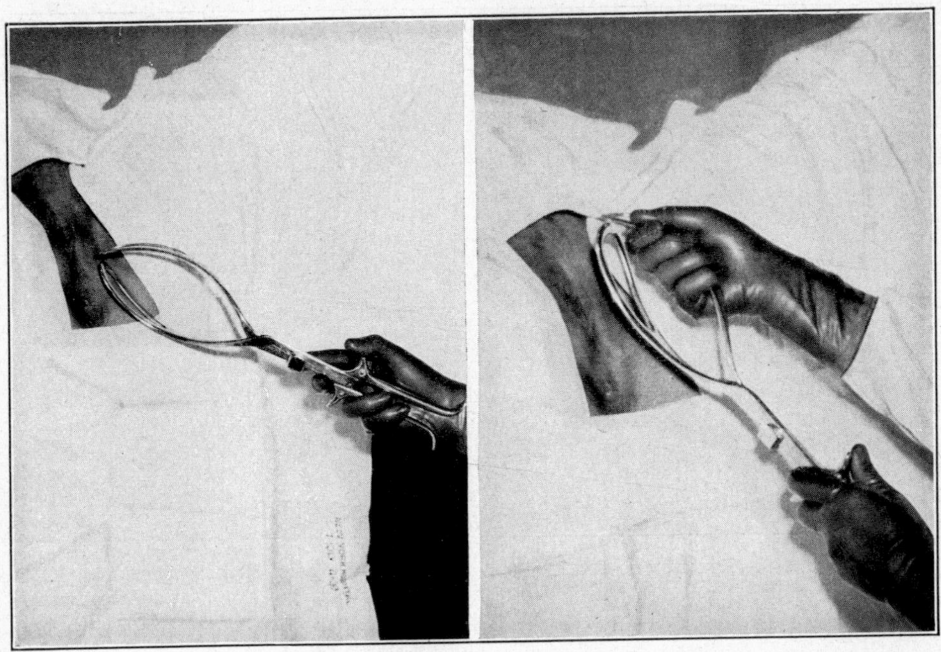

Fig. 593.—Orientation for Transverse (R. O. T.) Position. Kielland Forceps.

Fig. 594.—Grasping the Anterior Blade.

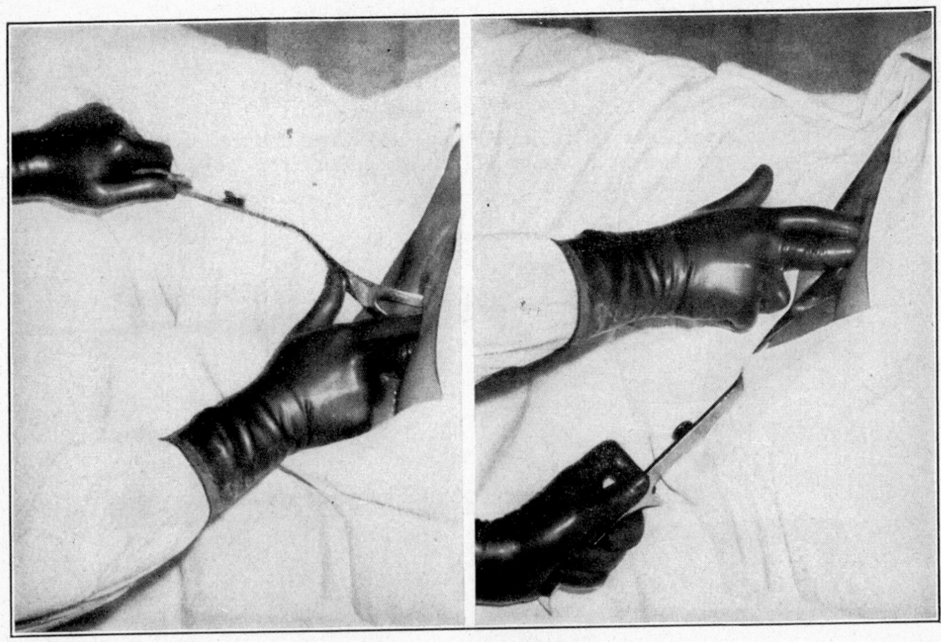

Fig. 595.—Introduction of Blade and Wandering It Anteriorly.

Fig. 596.—Further Wandering of Blade with Shank of Forceps against Buttock.

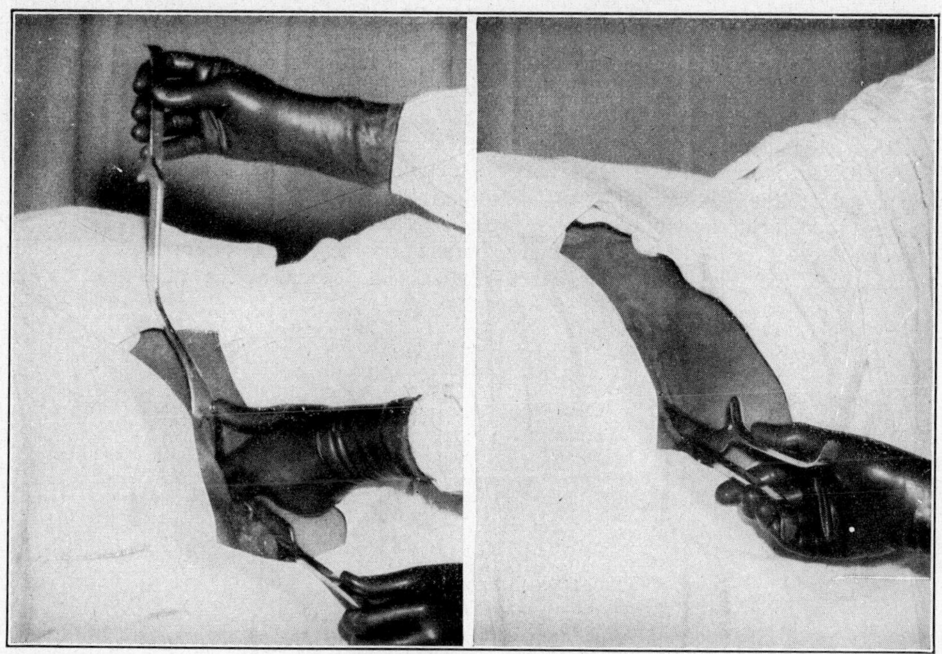

Fig. 597.—Introduction of Posterior Blade.

Fig. 598.—Forceps Are Locked.
Note overlapping of handles which sliding lock permits.

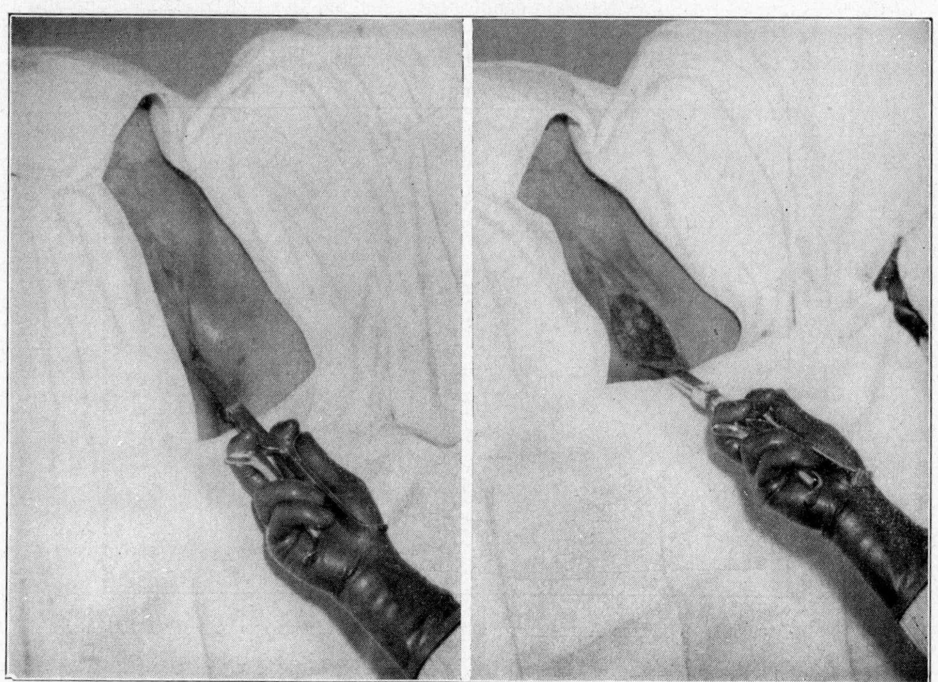

Fig. 599.—Rotation to Anterior Position Followed by Downward Traction.

Fig. 600.—Further Downward Traction. Occiput Emerging at Introitus.

In the first application the blades are applied to the sides of the head with the pelvic curve looking toward the face of the child, whereas in the second manipulation it looks toward the occiput. For the first application (Figs. 584 and 585) the right hand is passed into the left posterior segment of the genital tract, and the posterior (right) ear sought for. Over it the left blade is applied. This is held in position by an assistant, while the operator's left hand is passed into the right side of the vagina to control the introduction of the right blade, which is then rotated anteriorly until it comes to lie opposite the blade first introduced. The forceps is then locked, its blades now occupying the left and the sagittal suture the right oblique diameter of the pelvis. Downward traction is then made, and at the same time a rotary

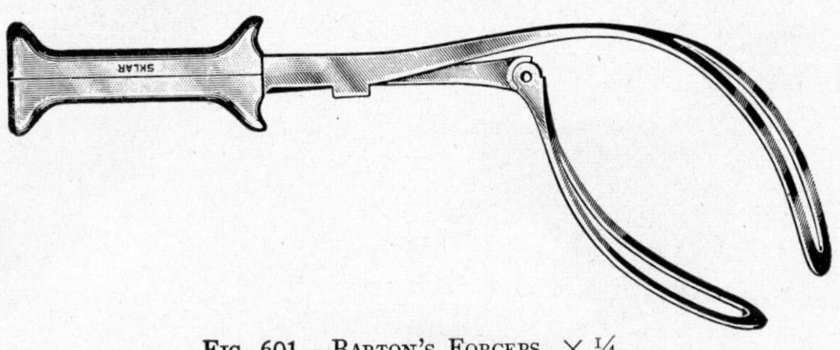

FIG. 601.—BARTON'S FORCEPS. × ¼.
(Courtesy of J. Sklar Mfg. Co.)

motion is imparted to the forceps when the head slowly descends and rotates to a right transverse, and later on when it impinges upon the pelvic floor further rotation occurs to an obliquely anterior position (see Figs. 587–589, 591).

The forceps having become inverted, must be taken off, and reapplied in the usual manner to the head, which now occupies a right anterior position, when delivery is readily accomplished. Some difficulty may arise in bringing about proper articulation, since the handle of the left branch lying above the right cannot be locked, but this can be readily overcome by rotating the former around the latter so as to bring the lock into proper position. In left positions the blades are applied in a similar manner, but in the reverse direction.

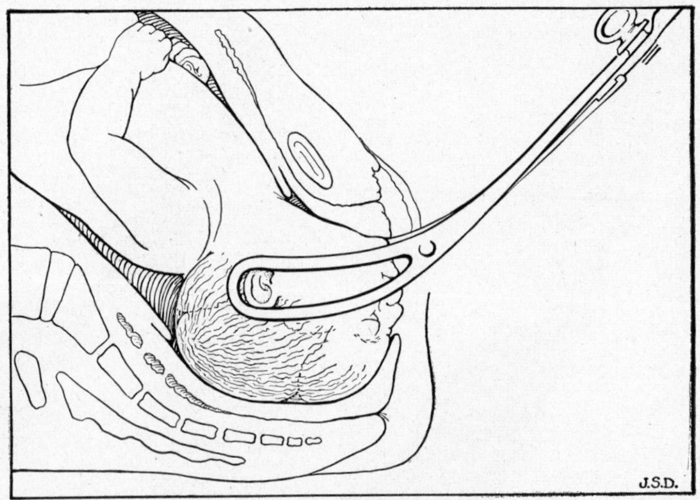

FIG. 602.—FORCEPS APPLIED TO FACE ALONG OCCIPITOMENTAL DIAMETER.

To avoid the necessity of constantly bearing in mind which is the left and which the right branch of the forceps, it is a good practical rule for a beginner, after having made an accurate diagnosis of the position of the head, to articulate the forceps and to hold them before the vulva of the patient. In this way he readily appreciates how they should be applied, and which blade is to go over the posterior ear (see Fig. 560). It is well to remember that the *left* blade of the forceps always goes to the *left* side of the mother and is introduced by the *left* hand of the operator.

Kielland of Christiania in 1916 described a forceps with narrow, somewhat bayonet-shaped blades, which he claimed could readily be applied to the sides of the head, and surpassed all other models as a *rotator*. He held that his forceps were particularly useful in high application and where the sagittal suture of the fetal head is directed transversely. These forceps have also been advocated as of particular value in the delivery of posterior positions. The Kielland forceps lack almost completely a pelvic curvature, have a sliding lock and are of very light construction. On each handle is a small knob which indicates the direction of rotation. In the application of these forceps the anterior blade is introduced first with its cephalic curvature directed forward, and, after it has entered sufficiently far into the uterine cavity, is turned through 180 degrees in order to adapt the cephalic curvature to the head. This rota-

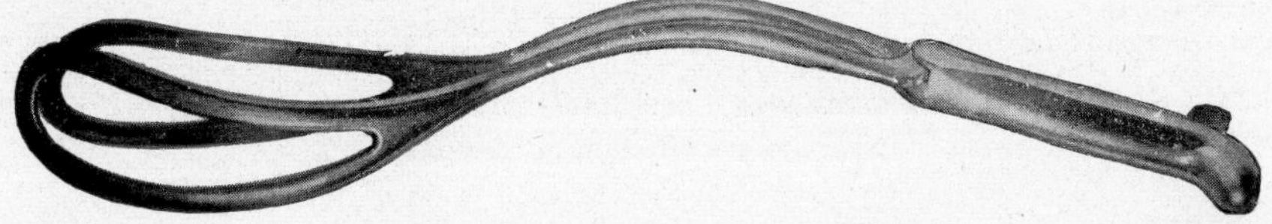

FIG. 603.—PIPER'S FORCEPS. × ¼.

tion of the anterior blade must take place in the direction of the side on which the concave margin of the blade points, as indicated by the small knob on the blade. The shank now rests on the perineum. The second blade is introduced posteriorly. When the blades are locked traction may be exerted downwards, in the direction in which the handles point. The head may be gently rotated to an anterior position. Rotation and traction are not performed at the same time.

Kielland advises a "gliding method" of application for the anterior blade where the uterus is tightly contracted about the head and the lower uterine segment stretched and thin. In such cases or where the pelvis is slightly contracted, it is dangerous to introduce the anterior blade with its cephalic curvature directed upwards to be followed by rotation of the blade. In the wandering or gliding method the anterior blade is introduced at the side of the pelvis over the brow or face of the child. It is made to glide over the child's face to an anterior position, the handle of the blade being held close to the opposite buttocks through this maneuver. The posterior blade is introduced in the manner already described.

In our experience the Kielland forceps are of particular value in transverse arrest of the head, as the anterior blade may be applied without undue difficulty. We prefer the gliding method of application to that in which the anterior blade is introduced with the cephalic curvature directed forward, as there is less risk of injury to the uterus or bladder associated with the former.

Figure 601 illustrates a type of forceps described by Barton and well spoken of by Caldwell, Studdiford, and Bachman. It differs from the usual types in that the anterior blade is hinged where it joins the shank. It appears to be particularly useful

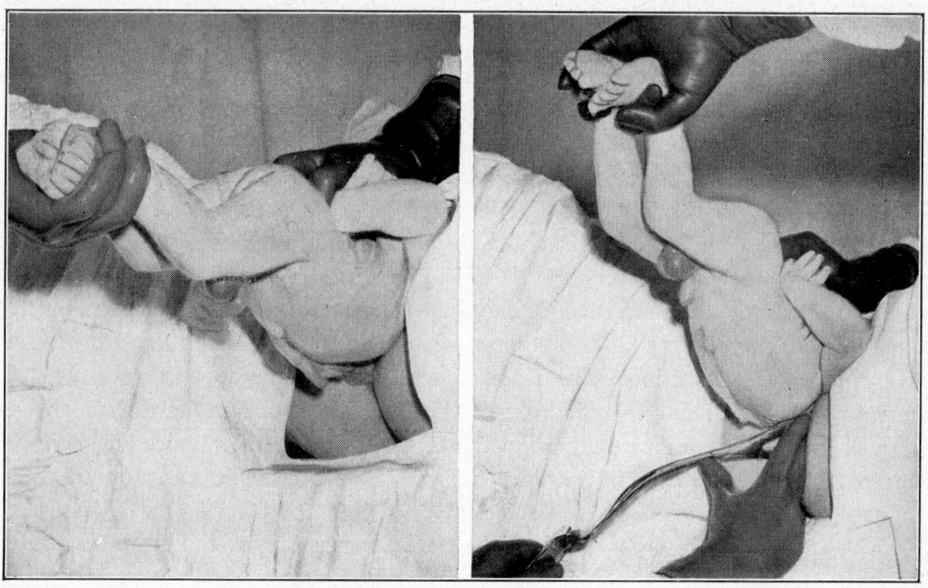

Fig. 604.—Position of Infant with Head in Pelvis Prior to Application of Piper's Forceps.

Fig. 605.—Introduction of Left Blade to Left Side of Pelvis.
Note upward direction of forceps.

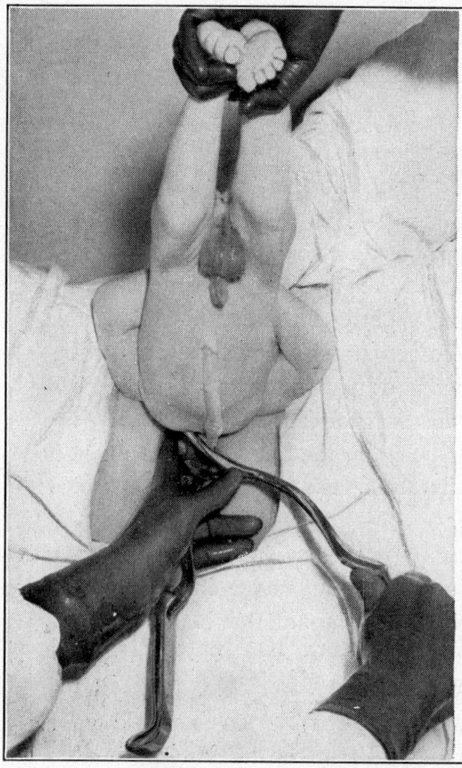

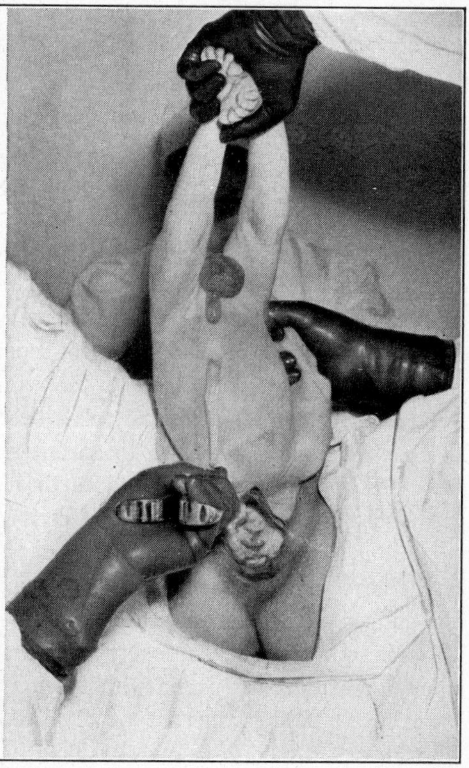

Fig. 606.—Introduction of Right Blade Completing Pelvic Application.

Fig. 607.—Forceps Locked and Traction Applied; Chin, Mouth, Nose Emerging over Perineum.

when the sagittal suture occupies the transverse diameter of the pelvic canal, and for such cases is used with satisfactory results in several clinics in this country.

Application of Forceps in Face Presentations. In face presentations the application of forceps occasionally becomes necessary, but is usually successful only in the transverse and anterior varieties, the blades being applied to the sides of the head along the mento-occipital diameter, with the pelvic curvature directed toward the neck. Traction is made in a downward direction until the chin appears under the symphysis; then by an upward movement the face is slowly extracted through the vulva, the nose, eyes, brow, and occiput appearing in succession over the anterior margin of the perineum (Fig. 602).

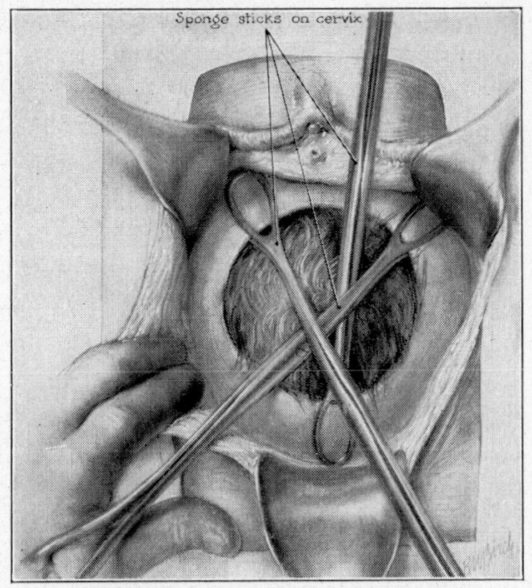

FIG. 608.—DÜHRSSEN'S INCISIONS.

Sponge forceps are applied to the cervix at 2, 6 and 10 o'clock; that is, at the sites where incisions are to be made. Once the first incision has been made, the remaining rim of cervix tends to retract and becomes more difficult to reach, unless it has been grasped previously and held by some such clamp as here shown. Although the two extra forceps are somewhat in the way when the first incision is made, experience shows that this practice is worth the trouble if the operation is to be a thorough one.

Forceps should not be applied when the chin is directed toward the hollow of the sacrum, as delivery cannot be effected in that position. In exceptional cases, if version is out of the question, and conversion into a vertex presentation cannot be effected, an expert operator may endeavor to rotate the chin to a transverse and later to an anterior position before resorting to pubiotomy or craniotomy, though such attempts are rarely successful.

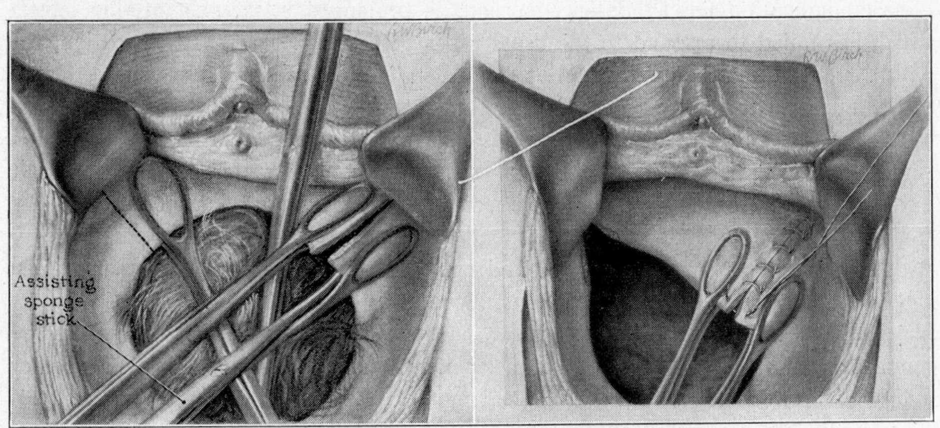

FIG. 609. FIG. 610.

FIG. 609.—DÜHRSSEN'S INCISIONS. THE FIRST INCISION HAS BEEN MADE.

FIG. 610.—DÜHRSSEN'S INCISIONS. REPAIR OF INCISION WITH INTERRUPTED SUTURES OF CHROMIC CATGUT.

Forceps to the Aftercoming Head. Forceps to the aftercoming head is a most valuable procedure in the management of breech presentations, as discussed on page 801. The infant is held up by an assistant as shown in Figs. 604 to 607, and the blades are introduced under it and to the sides of the head. Figure 603 illustrates a special type of forceps which Piper has devised for this purpose, and which is longer than the usual instrument and possesses a perineal curve. It is the instrument of choice for this operation.

Prognosis. The fetal mortality depends upon the condition of the child at the time the operation is undertaken, as well as upon the position of the head. It should be practically zero in low operations. On the other hand, the midforceps operation is attended by a fetal mortality which will be in direct proportion to the height of the skull above the perineal floor. In such cases the head may be subjected to injurious pressure, which may lead to intracranial hemorrhage and the subsequent death of the child.

OPERATIONS PREPARATORY TO FORCEPS

Dührssen's Incisions, or Hysterostomatomy. When immediate delivery appears desirable and the cervix is not yet fully dilated, multiple radial incisions may be made in the cervix and repaired by sutures after the completion of labor. They are usually called Dührssen's incisions, after the German obstetrician who first described them in 1890; the operation is sometimes referred to also as *hysterostomatomy.* The technic of the operation is comparatively simple, three incisions, roughly corresponding to the hours 2, 6, and 10 on the face of a clock, being made by scissors, as shown in Figs. 608 and 609. The incisions should extend to the junction of the cervix with the vaginal wall. Delivery is then effected by forceps or breech extraction, as the case may be.

The operation should never be done unless the cervix is fully effaced and more than 5 cm. dilated; if done before this time, profuse, even fatal, hemorrhage may result. The procedure is, of course, also contraindicated in placenta previa. The most common indication for Dührssen's incisions is prolonged intractable uterine inertia which has failed to respond to the usual types of therapy. Maternal exhaustion, the development of a pathologic retraction ring (Bandl's ring), fetal distress, and prolapse of the umbilical cord may also constitute occasional indications.

Although the making of the incisions is a relatively simple operation, the procedure carries with it major hazards and cesarean section is often preferable. For instance, in cases of uterine inertia in which the cervix is not yet fully dilated, the head is usually well above the pelvic floor and a difficult midforceps operation may be necessary with its attendant trauma to mother and child. Under such circumstances, maternal shock is common, even in cases in which blood loss is inconsequential. Moreover, the incisions heal satisfactorily in only about half the cases, so that the end results are often anatomically poor, the sites of the incisions being marked by deep crevices or adhesions between the cervix and vaginal mucosa. Despite these drawbacks, hysterostomatomy has an occasional place in operative obstetrics and, in any event, is much preferable to manual dilatation of the cervix.

Manual Dilatation of the Cervix. There is no such thing as "manual dilatation of the cervix." What actually happens, when this procedure is attempted, is manual laceration of the cervix. The operation has no place in modern obstetrics and has been superseded, when indicated, by Dührssen's incisions.

Vaginal Cesarean Section. Previous to and during the early years of this century, when abdominal cesarean section carried a very high maternal mortality, vaginal cesarean section was sometimes performed by separating the bladder from the anterior surface of the cervix and lower uterine segment and incising these structures lengthwise; delivery was then effected either by forceps or version and extraction, as seemed desirable. Vaginal cesarean section and manual dilatation of the cervix comprised the two main methods of accomplishing what used to be called *accouchement forcé,* that is, rapid vaginal delivery regardless of the status of the cervix. Accouchement forcé killed an untold number of women and, together with vaginal cesarean section, is today a matter of historical interest only.

Symphysiotomy and Pubiotomy. By *symphysiotomy* is meant the division of the pubic joint, by means of a wire saw, in order to bring about an increase in the capacity of a contracted pelvis sufficient to permit the passage of a living child. In the operation of *pubiotomy,* the pubic bone is severed a few centimeters lateral to the symphysis. Because of interference with subsequent locomotion, bladder injuries, and hemorrhage, and because of the greater safety of modern cesarean section, these two operations have long since been abandoned in the United States.

BIBLIOGRAPHY

Aveling, J. H. The Chamberlens and the Midwifery Forceps. London, 1882.

Bachman, C. The Barton Obstetrical Forceps. Surg., Gynec. & Obst., 1927, 45:805-812.

Barton, L. G., Caldwell, W. E., and Studdiford, W. E. A New Obstetrical Forceps. Am. J. Obst. & Gynec., 1928, 15:16-26.

Bill, A. H. Forceps Rotation of the Head in Persistent Occipito-posterior Positions. Am. J. Obst., 1918, 78:791.

Caldwell, W. E., Moloy, H. C., and Swenson, P. C. The Use of the Roentgen Ray in Obstetrics. Am. J. Roentgen., 1939, 41:305.

Das, K. The Obstetric Forceps, Its History and Evolution. Calcutta, 1929, p. 913.

DeLee, J. B. The Treatment of Obstinate Occipito-posterior Positions. J.A.M.A., 1920, 75:145-147.

——— The Prophylactic Forceps Operation. Am. J. Obst. & Gynec., 1920, 1:34-44.

Hunt, A. B., and McGee, W. B. Dührssen's Incisions. An Analysis of 592 Cases. Am. J. Obst. & Gynec., 1936, 31:598.

Kielland, C. Ueber die Anlegung der Zange am nicht rotierten Kopf mit Beschreibung eines neuen Zangenmodelles, etc. Monatschr. f. Geburtsh. u. Gynaek., 1916, 43:48.

Luikart, Ralph. A New Forceps Possessing a Sliding Lock, Modified Fenestra, with Improved Handle and Axis Traction Attachment. Am. J. Obst. & Gynec., 1940, 40:1058.

Piper, E. B., and Bachman, C. Prevention of Foetal Injuries in Breech Delivery. J.A.M.A., 1929, 92:217.

41

BREECH EXTRACTION AND VERSION

EXTRACTION IN BREECH PRESENTATIONS

Breech deliveries may be of three types:

A Spontaneous Breech Delivery is one in which the entire infant is expelled by natural forces without any traction being employed and without any manipulation other than support of the infant. This is uncommon.

A Partial Breech Extraction is one in which the infant is extruded as far as the umbilicus by natural forces, but the remainder of the body is extracted by the attendant.

A Total Breech Extraction is a breech delivery in which the entire body of the infant is extracted by the attendant.

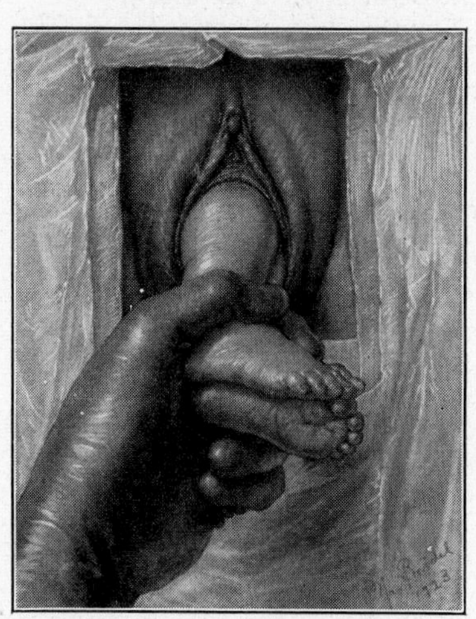

FIG. 611.—BREECH EXTRACTION; TRACTION UPON THE FEET.

Since the technic of breech extraction varies according to whether one has to deal with a complete or incomplete breech, or with a frank breech presentation, it will be necessary to consider the two conditions separately. In both the essential prerequisite for the successful performance of extraction lies in the complete dilatation of the cervix and the absence of any serious mechanical obstacle. It is true that extraction through an imperfectly dilated cervix is sometimes possible, but this is usually effected only at the cost of deep cervical tears with resulting hemorrhage. It should, furthermore, be realized that full dilatation of the cervix in relation to the presenting part in breech presentation does not necessarily imply that the cervix is sufficiently dilated to allow passage of the head without laceration of the cervix or further stretching. Moreover, the additional resistance offered to the passage of the head will generally lead to its extension, the arms at the same time becoming elevated over it, thereby so complicating and delaying delivery that the child is almost invariably lost.

Indications for Extraction. In all breech presentations, preparations should be made for extraction as soon as the feet or buttocks appear at the vulva, so that the operation can be promptly resorted to if, after the appearance of the umbilicus, the extrusion of the rest of the body does not promptly follow and the fetal circulation is interfered with as evidenced by the fetal heart rate. If the rate, as shown by the pulsations in the cord, falls below 100 per minute or reveals marked irregularity, extraction becomes necessary in the interests of the child. In a certain number of cases, no matter what the location of the breech, extraction may be called for by some condition which threatens the life of the mother or child, as in vertex presentations. It should, however, be realized that the passage of meconium is without significance, as it is

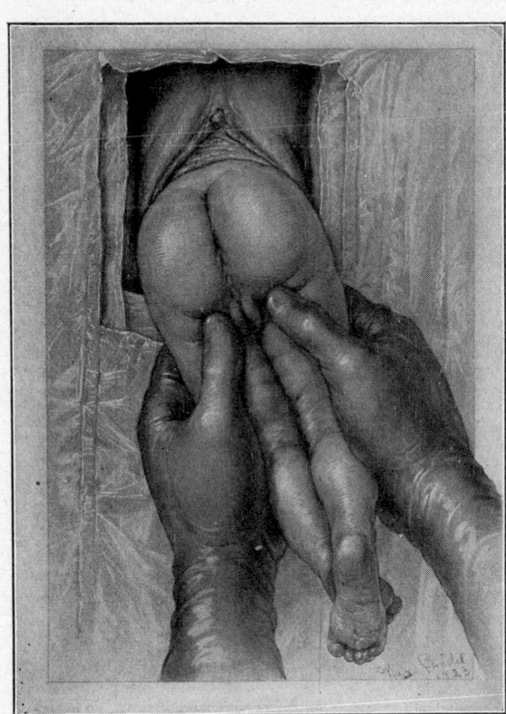

Fig. 612.—Breech Extraction; Traction upon the Thighs. Sterile Towel Not Illustrated.

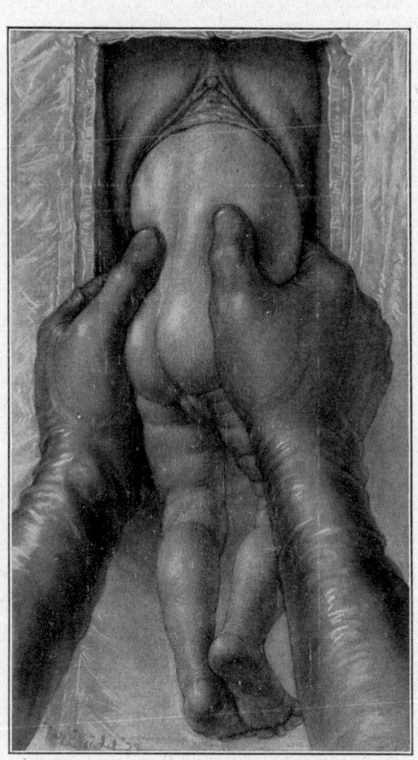

Fig. 613.—Breech Extraction; Extraction of Body, Thumbs over Sacrum.

simply the result of the compression to which the abdomen of the child is being subjected. Moreover, it should be remembered that extraction by the feet constitutes the usual method of completing delivery following internal podalic version, in which event the joint procedure is designated as version and extraction.

Extraction of Complete or Incomplete Breech. The patient should be placed upon a suitable operating table, but if one is not available she should be brought to the edge of the bed and subjected to the usual preliminary preparations. Complete anesthesia is desirable, even when the body of the child has already been born and only the head remains to be extracted.

As a rule, extraction is a simple operation when the breech has been born spontaneously (partial breech extraction); whereas it is less so when the feet are still within the uterus (total breech extraction). In the latter case, the entire hand should be introduced into the vagina and both feet seized, the ankles being grasped in such a manner that the second finger lies between them. The feet are then brought down into the vagina, and traction is made until they appear at the vulva. If, however, difficulty is experienced in seizing both feet, one should be brought down, and the hand immediately reintroduced in order to grasp and extract the other.

As soon as the feet have been drawn through the vulva, they should be wrapped in a sterile towel so that a firmer grasp may be obtained, since the vernix caseosa renders them so slippery that they are difficult to hold. Traction is then made in a downward direction (Fig. 611), and as the legs emerge they are grasped higher up, first by the calves and later by the thighs. When the breech appears at the vulva, traction is made in an upward direction until it is delivered. The thumbs are then applied over the sacrum and the fingers over the hips, and traction is continued in a downward manner until the costal margins, and later the scapulae, become visible

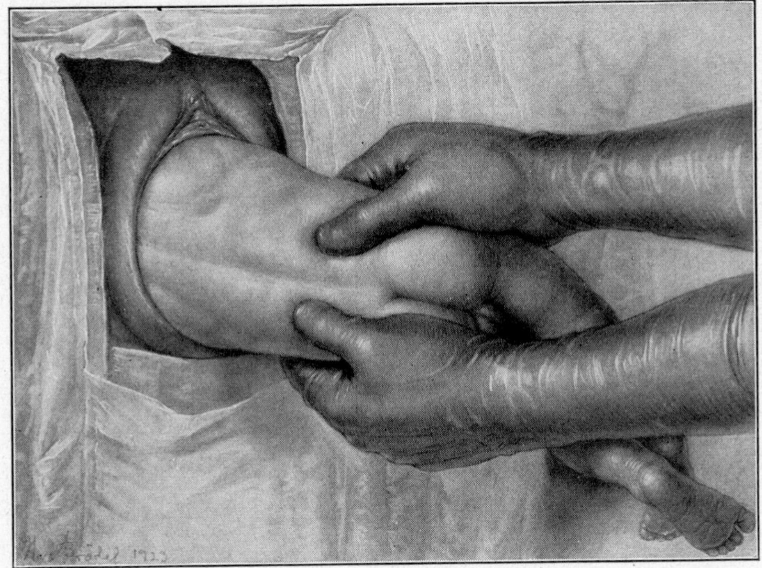

Fig. 614.—Breech Extraction; Scapulae Visible.

(Figs. 612 to 614). As the buttocks emerge the back of the child faces more or less upward, but as further traction is made it tends to turn spontaneously toward the side of the mother toward which it was originally directed. If, however, this does not occur, a slight rotary movement should be added to the traction with the object of bringing the bisacromial diameter of the child in approximation with the antero-posterior diameter of the outlet.

The cardinal point in successful extraction is to continue downward traction until at least the lower halves of the scapulae are outside of the vulva, and to give no thought to the birth of the shoulders and arms until one of the axillae becomes visible. Failure to observe this rule frequently renders difficult what would otherwise be a simple procedure. As soon as one axilla becomes visible, the time has arrived for the delivery of the shoulders, and so long as the arms maintain their normal flexed attitude, it makes little difference which shoulder is delivered first; for it sometimes happens, when it is planned to deliver one, the other is born spontaneously.

There are two methods by which the shoulders may be delivered. (1) With the scapulae visible, as shown in Fig. 614, the trunk is rotated in such a way that one shoulder and arm appear at the vulva and can easily be released, that is, the anterior shoulder is delivered first. Further reference to Fig. 614 will make this maneuver clear. Here the operator is rotating the trunk of the infant in a counter-clockwise direction in order to deliver the right shoulder and arm. With these delivered the body of the

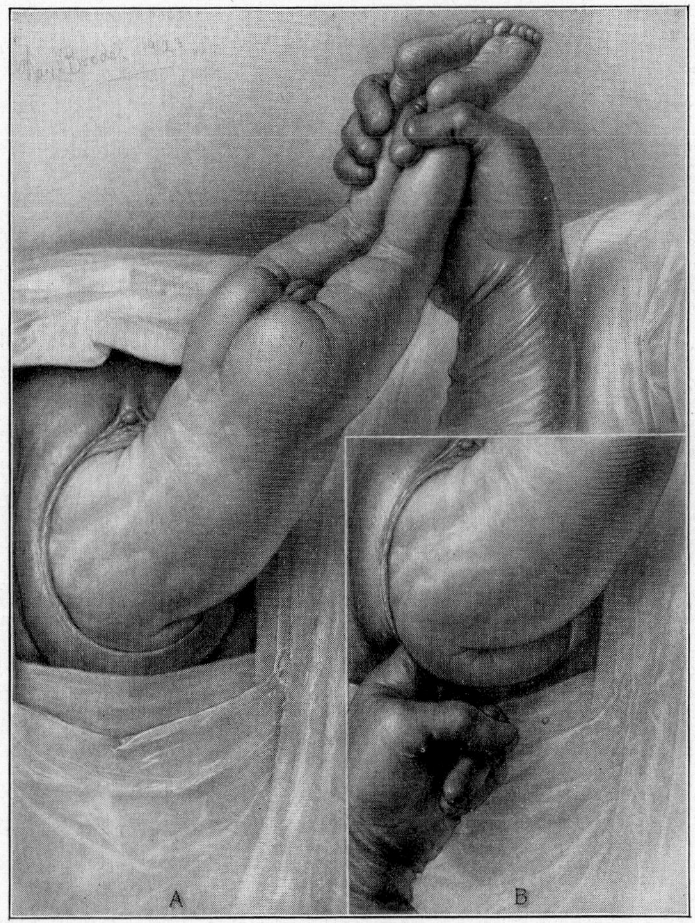

Fig. 615.—Breech Extraction; A, Upward Traction to Effect Delivery of Posterior Shoulder; B, Freeing Posterior Arm.

child is rotated in the reverse direction to deliver the other shoulder and arm. If this method is unsuccessful, the posterior shoulder must be delivered first. (2) To do this, the feet are grasped in one hand and drawn upward over the groin of the mother corresponding to the ventral surface of the child; in this way leverage is exerted upon the posterior shoulder which slips out over the perineal margin and is usually followed by the arm and hand (Fig. 615). Then by depressing the body of the child the anterior shoulder emerges beneath the pubic arch, the arm and hand usually following it spontaneously (Fig. 616). When this has occurred, the back tends to rotate spontaneously in such a way that it becomes directed more or less upward or, in case it fails to do so, it is brought about by rotating the body manually; then all is ready for the delivery of the head.

Unfortunately, however, the process is not always so simple and it sometimes becomes necessary to free and deliver the arms. This is much less frequently called for than in the past, and we attribute the change to following the admonition to continue traction without thought of the shoulders until an axilla becomes visible, instead of proceeding to free the arms shortly after the costal margins emerge, a procedure about which the beginner should be cautioned.

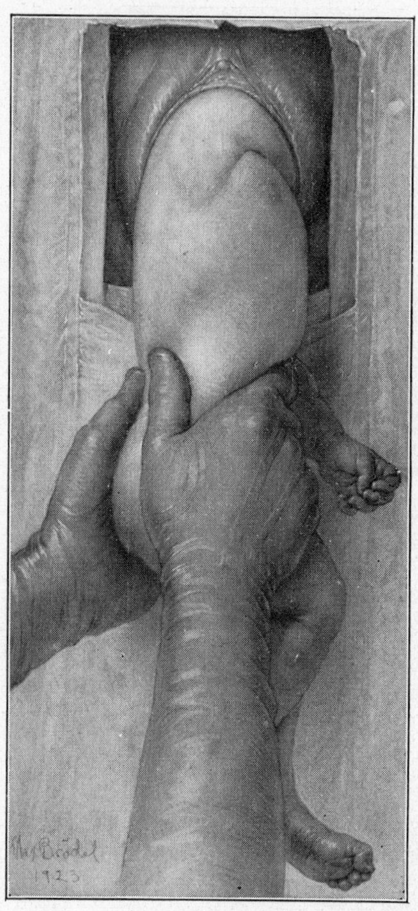

FIG. 616.—BREECH EXTRACTION; DELIVERY OF ANTERIOR SHOULDER BY DOWNWARD TRACTION.

Since there is more available space in the posterior and lateral segments of the pelvis than elsewhere, the posterior arm should be freed first. As the corresponding axilla is already visible, upward traction upon the feet is continued and two fingers of the other hand are passed along the humerus until the elbow is reached (Fig. 615). The fingers are now applied in such a way as to serve as a splint to the arm, which is swept downward and delivered from the vulva. To effect the delivery of the anterior arm, it is sometimes only necessary to depress the body of the child, when it slips out spontaneously; in other cases it can be wiped down over the thorax using two fingers as a splint, while occasionally the body must be seized with the thumbs over the scapulae and rotated so as to bring the undelivered shoulder into the neighborhood of the nearest sacrosciatic notch. The legs are then carried upward, so as to bring the ventral surface of the child to the opposite groin of the mother, after which the arm can be delivered as described above.

If the arms have become extended over the head, their delivery, although more difficult, can usually be accomplished by the maneuvers just described. In doing this, particular care must be taken to carry the fingers up to the elbow and to use them as a splint for, if they are merely hooked over the arm, the humerus or clavicle is exposed to great danger of fracture.

Very exceptionally the arm is found around the back of the neck (nuchal arm), when its delivery becomes still more difficult. If it cannot be freed in the manner just described, its extraction may be facilitated by rotating the child through half a circle in such a direction that the friction exerted by the birth canal will serve to draw the elbow toward the face. Should the arms be over the back of the neck and rotation of the child does not free them, it may be necessary to push the child upwards in the

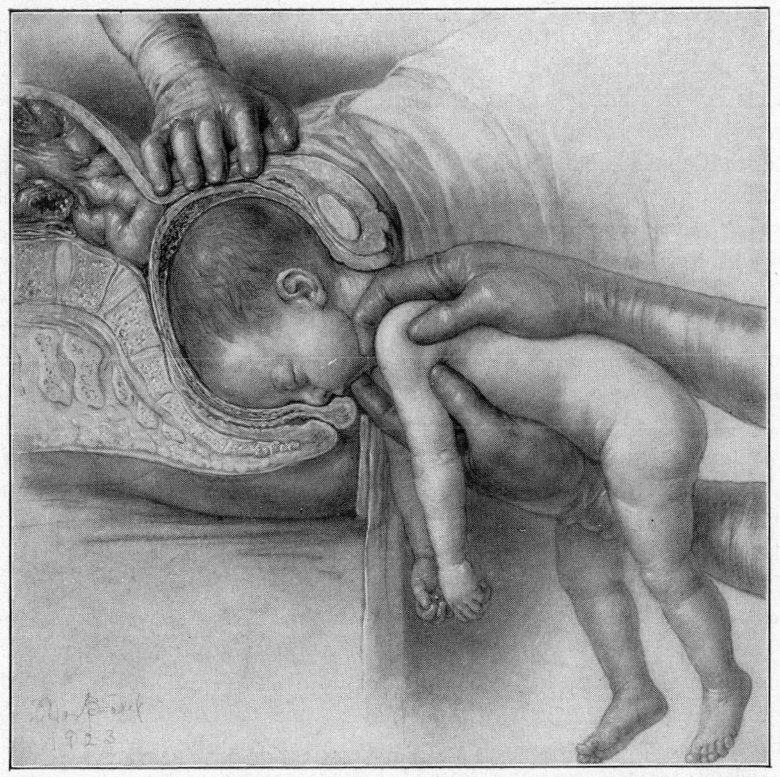

Fig. 617.—Breech Extraction; Suprapubic Pressure and Horizontal Traction Have Caused the Head to Enter the Pelvis. Mauriceau's Maneuver.

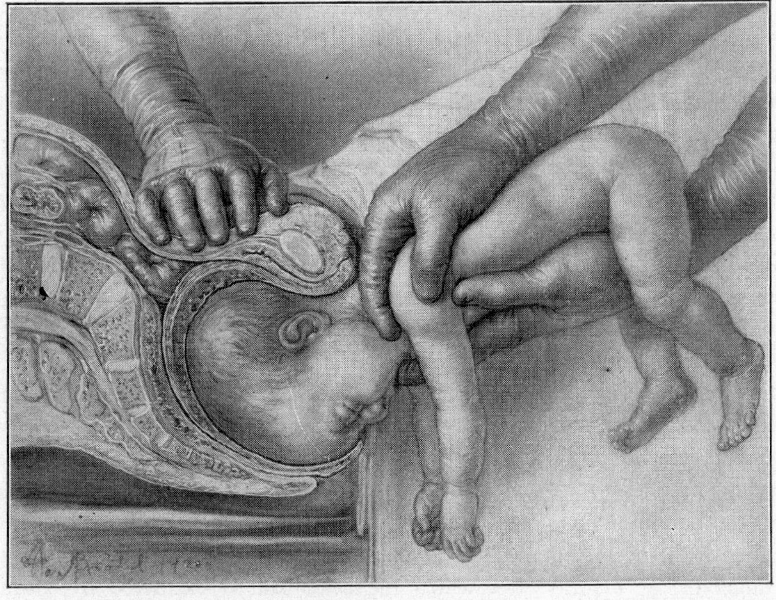

Fig. 618.—Breech Extraction; Mauriceau's Maneuver, Upward Traction.

attempt to release them. If the rotation maneuvers are unsuccessful, the arm must be forcibly extracted by hooking a finger over it. In this event, fracture of the humerus or clavicle is, unfortunately, very common. Such an accident, however, is not very serious, as good union can always be secured by appropriate treatment.

After the shoulders have been born, the head usually occupies an oblique diameter of the pelvis with the chin directed posteriorly, when its extraction may be effected by *Mauriceau's* maneuver (Fig. 618). For this purpose, the index finger of one hand is introduced into the mouth of the child and applied over the superior maxilla, while the body rests upon the palm of the hand and the forearm, with the legs straddling the latter. Two fingers of the other hand are then hooked over the neck, and, grasping the shoulders, make downward traction until the occiput appears under the symphysis. The body of the child is now raised up toward the mother's abdomen, and the mouth, nose, brow, and eventually the occiput successively emerge over the perineum. Traction should be exerted only by the fingers over the shoulders and not by the finger in the mouth, since the latter may slip from the superior maxilla and come to rest upon the inferior maxilla and base of the tongue, a consequence of which serious injury may be done to the child.

This maneuver was first practiced by Mauriceau in the seventeenth century, but for some reason fell into disfavor. Nearly a hundred years later Smellie described a similar procedure, but rarely made use of it, as he preferred the employment of forceps. In the meantime, other devices came into use until G. Veit in 1863 redirected attention to the inestimable advantages which Mauriceau's method of extraction possessed over all others. For this reason, in Germany the procedure is frequently called after Veit or, when greater accuracy is desired, it is designated as the Mauriceau-Smellie-Veit maneuver. Litzmann, however, correctly pointed out the impropriety of such a designation, and insisted that only the name of the original inventor—Mauriceau—should be used in describing it. A somewhat similar method is that of Wiegand, also known as the Wiegand-Martin maneuver, where pressure is applied above and over the symphysis by the operator's second hand, the first being under the child as in the original Mauriceau maneuver. Numerous other methods of extraction have been devised; Winckel in 1888 collected twenty-one different procedures from the literature, although none has proved as serviceable as that of Mauriceau. When the head does not deliver spontaneously a Mauriceau or a Wiegand-Martin maneuver usually suffices to deliver the aftercoming head. Should these simpler methods fail, the Piper forceps may be applied to the head or they may be used to advantage as an elective procedure instead of the Mauriceau procedure. Recent x-ray evidence indicates that when the pelvis is flat or platypelloid, it may be better to allow the aftercoming head to pass through the pelvis in a transverse position and then to rotate the occiput anteriorly on the perineum.

In the vast majority of cases the back of the child eventually rotates toward the front, no matter what its original position, but when it does not take place spontaneously, the movement may be inaugurated by making stronger traction upon the leg, which would naturally rotate anteriorly. If this does not bring about the desired result, and the back remains posterior after the birth of the shoulders, extraction must be begun with the occiput posterior. As a rule, rotation can still be effected by means of the finger in the mouth, after which the head can be extracted by Mauriceau's maneuver. When, however, this is not possible, delivery must be attempted, with the head in its abnormal position by the employment of a modified *Prague maneuver*, which is so-called for the reason that its advantages were strongly urged more particularly by Kiwisch of that city, although it had been described by Pugh a century earlier. The procedure is somewhat as follows: two fingers of one hand grasp the shoulders from below, while the other hand draws the feet up over the abdomen of the mother. As a result, the occiput is born first and the perineum is necessarily subjected to greater liability of rupture.

Extraction in Frank Breech Presentations. When indications for delivery in a frank breech arise, the extraction becomes somewhat more difficult. In such cases it is advisable to try to decompose the wedge and to bring down one or, better, both feet, which can be readily accomplished if the membranes have only recently ruptured, but becomes extremely difficult if a considerable time has elapsed after the escape of the liquor amnii, more particularly if the uterus has become tightly contracted over the child.

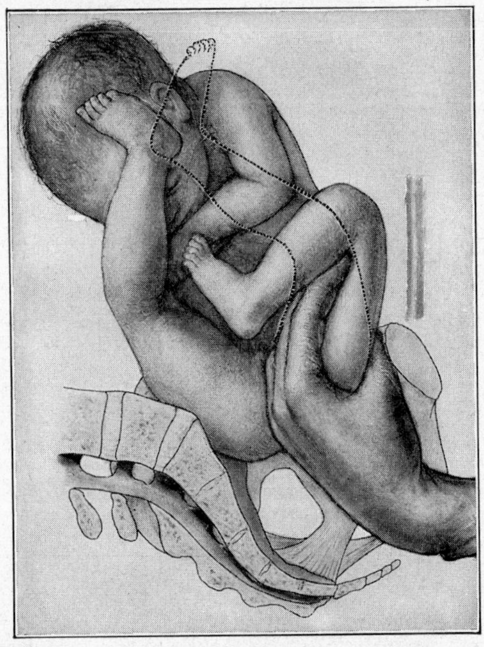

Fig. 619.—Pinard's Maneuver for Bringing Down a Foot in Frank Breech Presentation.

In many cases the employment of the following maneuver suggested by Pinard will aid materially in bringing down the foot: Two fingers are carried up along one leg to the knee and push it away from the middle line. This is usually followed by spontaneous flexion, and the foot of the child will be felt to impinge upon the back of the hand, when it can be readily seized and brought down (Fig. 619). As soon as the buttocks are born, first one leg and then the other is drawn out and extraction is accomplished as described above.

The Fillet. The older authors advocated making traction upon the groin by means of a fillet or metallic hook. These procedures should never be employed upon living children on account of their liability to cause fracture of the femur or injury to the soft parts. On the other hand, when the child is dead, and such an accident is a matter of indifference, the hook affords a convenient means of making traction.

Prognosis. In all forms of breech extraction the prognosis for the mother is good, although it is more serious in frank breech than in the other varieties. In the former the increased manipulation affords greater opportunity for infection, while the attempt to reach the posterior groin often gives rise to deep, and sometimes to complete, tears before the buttocks have reached the perineum. In extraction by the feet, on the other hand, the liability to perineal tears is no greater, than in head presentations. Moderate degrees of disproportion between the size of the head and the pelvis scarcely influence the maternal prognosis, since the pressure of the head upon the soft parts lasts but a few seconds, instead of being prolonged for hours as in head presentations.

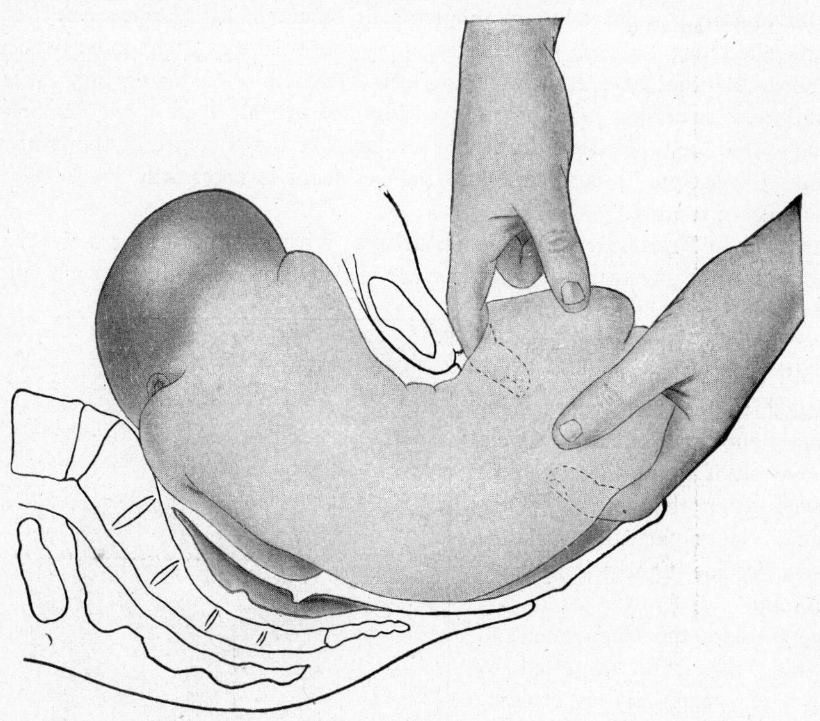

FIG. 620.—EXTRACTION OF FRANK BREECH; FINGERS IN GROINS.

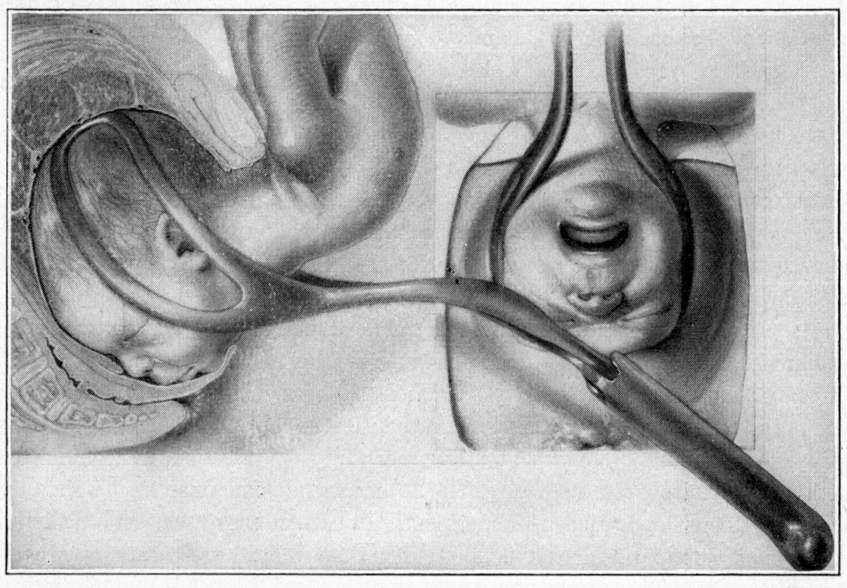

FIG. 621.—PIPER FORCEPS ON THE AFTERCOMING HEAD. (SEE ALSO FIGS. 603 TO 607.)

For the child, however, the outlook is not so favorable, and becomes more serious the higher the presenting part is situated at the beginning of the operation. In addition to the increased liability to tentorial tears and intracerebral hemorrhage, which Eardley Holland, Capon, and Crothers have shown are inherent to breech presentations, the fetal mortality is augmented by the greater probability of the occurrence of traumatism during extraction. In incomplete breech presentations, moreover, prolapse of the umbilical cord is much more common than in vertex presentations, and aggravates still more the prognosis for the infant.

As has already been said, fractures of the humerus and clavicle cannot always be avoided when freeing the arms, while fracture of the femur may occur in difficult frank breech extractions. Occasionally, hematomas of the sternocleidomastoid muscles develop after the operation, though they usually disappear spontaneously. More serious results, however, may follow separation of the epiphyses of the scapula, humerus or femur. Exceptionally, paralysis of the arm follows pressure upon the brachial plexus by the fingers in making traction, but more frequently it is due to overstretching the neck while freeing the arms. When the child is forcibly extracted through a contracted pelvis, spoon-shaped depressions or actual fractures of the skull may result, which generally prove fatal, while occasionally even the neck may be broken when great force is employed. In general, it may be said that in simple extractions the prognosis for the child is good, while in complicated ones it is dubious.

VERSION

Version, or turning, is an operation through which the presentation of the fetus is artificially altered, one pole being substituted for the other, or an oblique or transverse being converted into a longitudinal presentation.

According to whether the head or breech is made the presenting part, the operation is spoken of as cephalic or podalic version, respectively. It is also designated according to the method by which it is accomplished. Thus we speak of *external version* when the manipulations are made exclusively through the external abdominal wall; of *internal version* when the entire hand is introduced into the uterine cavity; and of *combined version* when one hand manipulates through the abdominal wall, while two or more fingers of the other are introduced through the cervix.

External Cephalic Version. The object of the operation is to substitute a vertex for a less favorable presentation.

Indications. If a breech or transverse presentation is diagnosed in the last weeks of pregnancy, its conversion into a vertex may be attempted by external maneuvers, provided there be no marked disproportion between the size of the child and the pelvis. Cephalic version is thought by many to be indicated by reason of the increased fetal mortality attending spontaneous delivery in breech presentation; while if the child lies transversely, a change of presentation is extremely desirable, inasmuch as a natural labor is out of the question, and if appropriate measures are not adopted, the lives of both mother and child may be lost.

External cephalic version can be accomplished only under the following conditions: (1) the presenting part must not be deeply engaged; (2) the abdominal wall must be sufficiently thin to admit of accurate palpation; (3) the abdominal and uterine walls must not be too irritable; (4) the uterus must contain a sufficient quantity of liquor amnii to permit the easy movement of the child. Given these essentials, it may be attempted.

In the early stages of labor, before the membranes have ruptured, the same indications hold good, and at this time may be extended to oblique presentations as well, though these usually right themselves spontaneously as labor progresses. On the other hand, external cephalic version can be effected but rarely after the cervix has become fully dilated and the membranes have ruptured.

Method. Cephalic version, in modern obstetrics, is performed solely by *external manipulations.* The technic is as follows: the patient's abdomen having been bared,

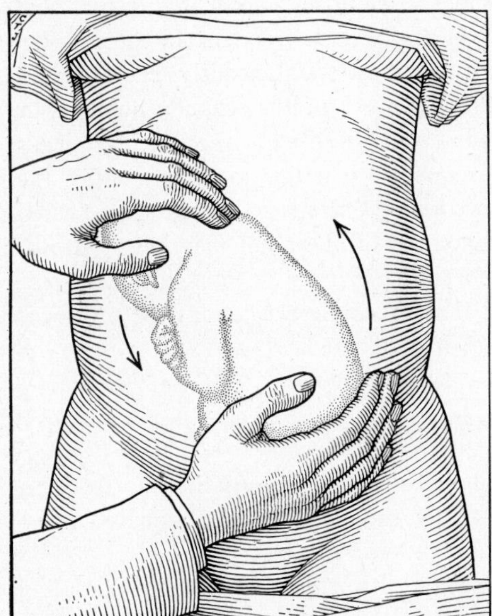

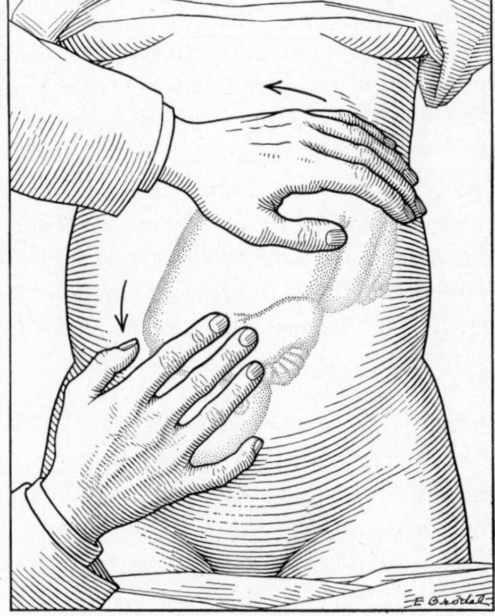

Fig. 622.—External Cephalic Version.

the presentation and position of the child are carefully mapped out. The fetal poles are then seized with either hand, and the one which we wish to present is gently stroked toward the pelvic inlet, while the other is moved in the opposite direction. After version has been completed, the child will tend to return to its original position unless engagement occurs; but at the time of labor the head may be pressed down into the superior strait and held firmly in position until it becomes fixed under the influence of the uterine contractions.

Podalic Version. By this is understood the turning of the child by seizing one or both feet and drawing them through the cervix, the operation being usually followed by extraction.

Indications. Podalic version is occasionally indicated in three types of cases, namely, in transverse or oblique presentations, in certain varieties of head presentations in which it is believed that delivery can be more safely and more rapidly accomplished after version, and in certain twin pregnancies for delivery of the second infant.

The most favorable time for performing podalic version is just after the cervix has become fully dilated but before the membranes have ruptured. In this event, the amniotic fluid will be still in utero and the child readily movable in any direction. It should never be attempted when the cervix is imperfectly dilated, except in certain cases of placenta previa, when the bipolar method of Braxton Hicks is employed. It sometimes happens that the patient is not seen until long after rupture of the membranes, and conditions may then be present which render the operation extremely difficult or even impossible. For example, the uterus may be tetanically contracted and so tightly applied to the body of the child as to render even the introduction of the hand extremely difficult. In other cases, the retraction ring may have risen to such an extent and the lower uterine segment be so stretched as to render the operation dangerous in the highest degree, as the attempt at version will probably lead to rupture of the uterus.

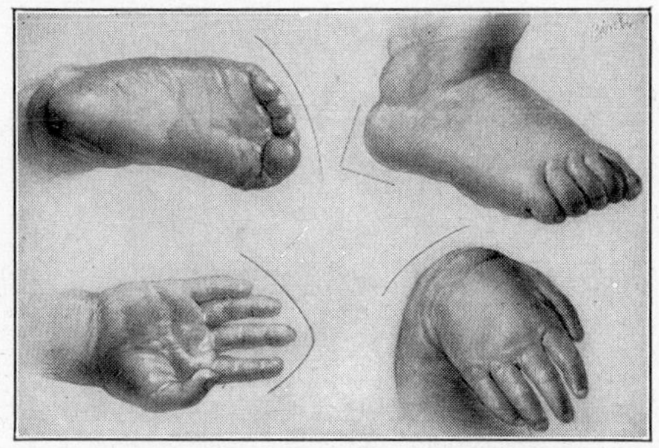

Fig. 623.—Internal Podalic Version.

Differentiation of a foot from a hand, parts that feel very much the same in the uterus unless one identifies the foot by its heel. A hand presents nothing which resembles a *heel,* and this fact will serve satisfactorily alone as a means of distinguishing between the two. To attempt to differentiate fingers from toes, as shown on the left, is less practical. At classical cesarean section, moreover, knowing to search for a heel will spare the inexperienced operator the embarrassment of pulling out many a hand.

Technic. For the performance of internal podalic version the patient should be placed in lithotomy position and the usual preoperative preparations carried out. Version should never be attempted without an accurate diagnosis as to the presentation and position of the child nor as to the existence of disproportion between its size and that of the pelvis. Its performance will be greatly facilitated by the use of long rubber gloves reaching to the elbow, as recommended by Potter, and by an extensive preliminary "ironing out" of the vaginal outlet and pelvic floor. Version is most easily effected while the membranes are intact, and becomes increasingly difficult with every half hour after their rupture. Uterine relaxation is of paramount importance for the satisfactory performance of version and hence the anesthetic of choice is ether, administered to the surgical level.

The operative technic varies somewhat, according to whether one has to do with a head or a transverse position. In the first instance the hand and arm must be introduced considerably farther into the birth canal than in the latter, which is facilitated by free lubrication of the operating hand and arm by albolene or green soap. It is usually taught that the choice of the hand to be employed depends upon the location of the small parts, and that if the back be directed to the left, the feet can be most conveniently seized with the left hand, and vice versa. Potter, however, has taught that the left hand can be used equally satisfactorily no matter what the position of the feet may be.

Accordingly, if the membranes are still intact, the left hand is passed through the cervix and carried up into the uterine cavity until it reaches the neighborhood of the feet. The membranes are then ruptured, and if possible both feet are seized and downward traction is made, as illustrated in Figs. 624 and 625. Ordinarily the child turns without difficulty, so that the feet are readily brought down into the vagina, and thence through the outlet. When the knees emerge, one knows that version has been effected, after which delivery is completed by extraction as already described.

If the membranes have already ruptured and the head is engaged, version is always more difficult. In this case, after pushing the head out of the pelvic brim, the hand should be introduced past it, when the feet are seized and brought down as before. Of course, if the amniotic fluid has long since drained off, and the uterus is tightly applied over the child, this may be difficult or impossible, and if persisted in after the lower uterine segment has become markedly stretched may result in rupture of the uterus.

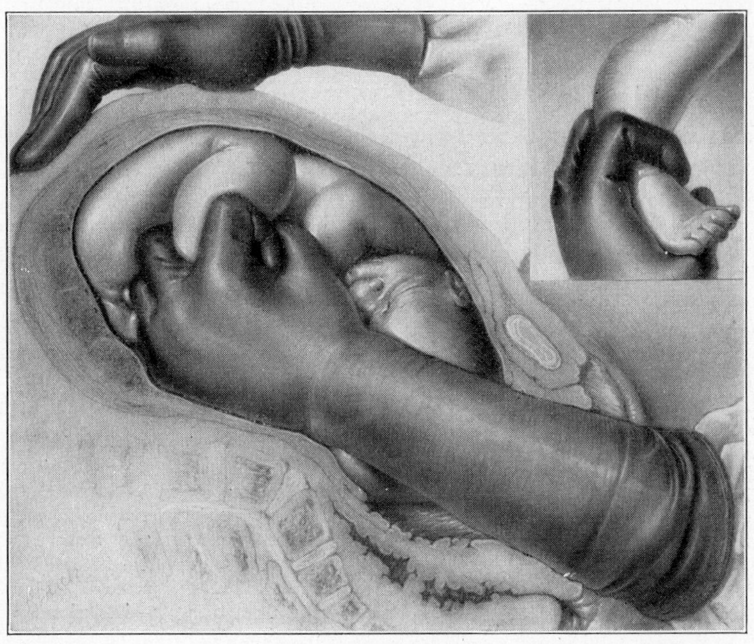

FIG. 624.—INTERNAL PODALIC VERSION.

Grasping feet, both if at all possible, since it makes the turning much easier. Note use of long version gloves.

In transverse presentation, it is desirable to bring down both feet, but in case this cannot readily be accomplished, one foot will suffice. In this event, however, the choice of the foot is a matter of very considerable importance. When the back is directed anteriorly, the lower one should be seized, for by so doing the back of the child is kept directed toward the symphysis, whereas, if the upper foot be seized, the back may turn in the opposite direction. On the other hand, when the back looks posteriorly, the upper is the foot of choice, since traction upon it will cause the back to rotate to the front, while if the lower foot be seized, although anterior rotation will usually occur, the upper buttock is liable to impinge upon the anterior portion of the pelvic brim, and great force may become necessary to effect its dislodgment. Version and extraction should always be followed by internal exploration of the uterus to make certain the common accident of rupture of the uterus has not been produced.

Prognosis. For the mother the prognosis following podalic version is good in properly selected cases, provided the patient is in good condition at the commencement of the operation. On the other hand, when attempted in the case of a tetanically contracted uterus, or when the lower uterine segment is overstretched, forcible attempts at version may lead to the rupture of the organ and death. In general, the most common cause of traumatic rupture of the uterus is version and extraction.

The prognosis for the child is uncertain, and depends upon the nature of the indication and the difficulty experienced in extraction. In the case of version and extraction used to deliver the second twin, the prognosis for the infant is excellent. On the other hand, in single pregnancies, if the operation is undertaken through an imperfectly dilated cervix, and the child's head is arrested by the external os, the time re-

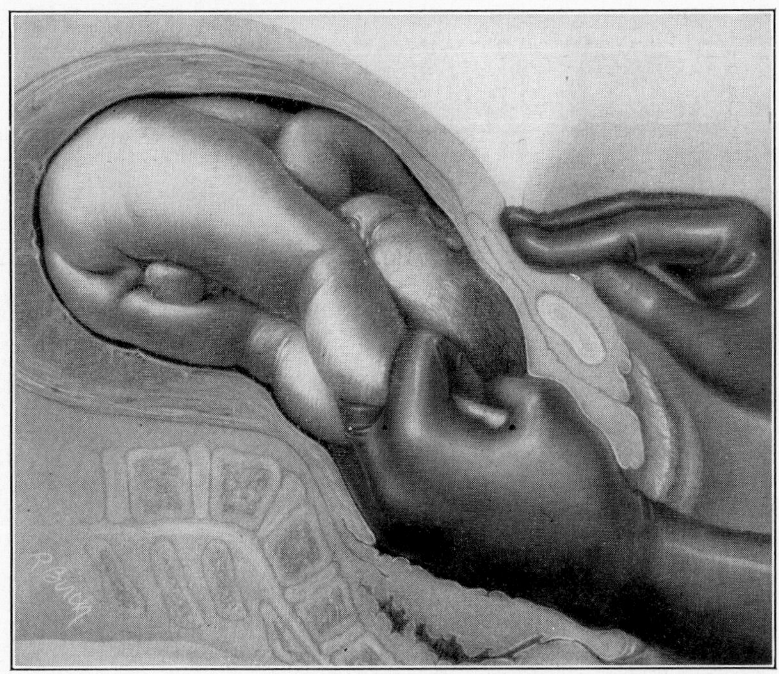

FIG. 625.—INTERNAL PODALIC VERSION.
Upward pressure on head is made as downward traction is exerted on feet.

quired for its extraction is usually so great that death from asphyxiation is inevitable. Moreover, in cases of marked pelvic contraction the fetal mortality is very high. In many such cases forcible traction may enable one to deliver the child but usually not until after the cord has been so long compressed as to have caused pronounced asphyxia and death, not to mention injuries to the head resulting from pressure and eventuating in death of the child either at the time of delivery or during the neonatal period.

BIBLIOGRAPHY

CAPON, N. B. Intracranial Traumata in the New-born. J. Obst. & Gynaec. Brit. Emp., 1922, 29:572-590.

CROTHERS, B. Injury to the Spinal Cord in Breech Extraction as an Important Cause of Foetal Deaths, etc. Am. J. M. Sc., 1923, 165:94.

FRAMM, W. Ueber die Anlegung der Kopfzange am Steiss, und eine neue Steisszange. Zentralbl. f. Gynäk., 1928, 52:609.

HICKS, J. B. On Combined External and Internal Version. London, 1864.

HOLLAND, E. Cranial Stress in the Foetus During Labor. J. Obst. & Gynaec. Brit. Emp., 1922, 29:549.

LITZMANN, C. C. Der Mauriceau-Levret'sche Handgriff. Arch. f. Gynaek., 1887, 31:102.

MAURICEAU. Le Moyen d'Accoucher la Femme, quand l'Enfant Présente Un ou Deux Pieds les Premiers. Traité des Maladies des Femmes Grosses, 6me éd., 1721, pp. 280-285.

MENGERT, W. F. The After-coming Head. J. Iowa M., 1938, 28:478.

MOORE, W. T., and STEPTOE, P. P. The Experience of the Johns Hopkins Hospital with Breech Presentation. South. M. J., 1943, 36:295.

POTTER, I. W. The Place of Version in Obstetrics. C. V. Mosby, St. Louis, 1922.

RYDER, G. H. Breech Presentations Treated by Cephalic Versions in the Consecutive Deliveries of 1,700 Women. Am. J. Obst. & Gynec., 1943, 45:1004.

42

CESAREAN SECTION

In this operation the child is removed from the uterus through an incision in the abdominal and uterine walls. The origin of the term has given rise to a great deal of discussion. It has been generally asserted that Julius Cæsar (100-44 B.C.) was brought into the world by this means and obtained his name from the manner in which he was delivered (*a caeso maturis utero*). This explanation, however, can hardly be correct as his mother, Julia, lived many years after her son's birth; and besides Julius was not the first of his name, since there is mention of a priest named Cæsar who lived several generations earlier. The following view, however, would appear to be more plausible. In the Roman law, as codified by Numa Pompilius (762-715 B.C.), it was ordered that the operation should be performed upon women dying in the last few weeks of pregnancy in the hope of saving the child. This *lex regia,* as it was called at first, under the emperors became the *lex cæsarea* and the procedure itself became known as the *cæsarean* operation.

History. The history of cesarean section may be said to extend over five periods; the first lasting from the earliest times to the beginning of the sixteenth century; the second extending from the year 1500 to 1876; the third beginning with the introduction by Porro of amputation of the body of the uterus; the fourth extending from 1882 to 1907, following the description by Sänger of an accurate technic for suturing the uterine incision; and the fifth beginning with 1907 when Frank devised the extraperitoneal technic. During the first period the operation was occasionally resorted to after the death of the mother in the hope of saving the child, but it is improbable that it was practiced upon the living woman although several authorities are inclined to believe that certain passages in the Talmud may be so interpreted. The fact that Felkin saw a cesarean section performed by the natives in Uganda renders it possible that it may have been employed upon the living woman at an early period by certain of the uncivilized races.

The second period begins with the year 1500, when, according to Casper Bauhin, Jacob Nufer, a castrator of pigs at Sigerhausen, Switzerland, operated successfully upon his own wife after she had been given up by the midwives and barbers in attendance. This operation is usually described as the first cesarean section to be performed upon a living woman, but in reality it probably consisted in the removal of an extra-uterine child from the abdominal cavity, as the fact that the woman had five spontaneous labors afterwards speaks strongly against the probability that the operation was necessitated by obstruction due to a contracted pelvis or to a tumor.

François Rousset, a contemporary of Paré, wrote a treatise in 1581, in which he gave the histories of a number of cesarean sections collected from various sources. Several of them were apocryphal while others, in all probability, were operations of advanced extra-uterine pregnancy. His article, however, had the merit of directing attention to the operation and to the possibility of performing it upon the living woman. The first authentic cesarean section was probably done in 1610 by Trautmann, of Wittenberg. Following this, it was occasionally performed until it became temporarily eclipsed by symphysiotomy, in 1777, to be taken up again after the latter operation had fallen into disrepute.

During this period, the uterus was simply incised and the child extracted. The uterine walls were not sutured, the contraction and retraction of the organ being relied upon to check hemorrhage. Most of the women perished from hemorrhage or infection. Sutures were first employed by Lebas (1769), but did not come into general use until after the appearance of Sänger's epoch-making article in 1882.

Before the work of Porro and Sänger, the mortality following the operation was appalling. Meyer (1867) collected 1,605 cases from the literature with a mortality of 54 per cent; while in 80 cases performed in the United States up to 1878, collected by Harris, 52.5 per cent of the women died. According to Budin, not a single successful cesarean section was performed in Paris between the years 1787 and 1876. Such poor results were obtained that Harris in 1887 pointed out that the operation was more successful when performed by the patient herself, or when the abdomen was ripped open by the horn of an infuriated bull. He collected nine such cases from the literature with five recoveries, and stated, that out of 11 cesarean sections performed in New York City during the same period, only one patient recovered.

The third period began with the year 1876, when Porro advised amputating the body of the uterus and stitching the cervical stump into the lower angle of the abdominal wound in order to lessen the danger from hemorrhage and infection. Certain writers claim that the credit for this intervention belongs to Storer of Boston, who, in 1861, amputated a myomatous pregnant uterus with fatal result. Inasmuch, however, as he did not appear to recognize the importance of the innovation, the credit for proposing it undoubtedly belongs to Porro. This procedure, being followed by satisfactory results, soon became quite popular so that in 1890 Harris was able to collect 264 operations from the literature. After the technic for supravaginal amputation of the myomatous uterus had become perfected, similar methods were applied to the Porro operation, the cervical stump being covered by a flap of peritoneum and dropped into the abdominal cavity; while in a small number of cases particularly when the cervix was carcinomatous, the entire organ was removed.

The fourth period began with Sänger, who, in 1882, revolutionized cesarean section by insisting upon the necessity for suturing the uterine incision and by describing an accurate technic for the purpose. As the uterus was not sacrificed in this operation, it was designated as the conservative, in contradistinction to the Porro, or radical, cesarean section. With increasing perfection of surgical technic, as well as with better knowledge of the indications for its performance, more and more satisfactory results have been obtained from it, while the radical operation has become less popular.

The fifth period began in 1907 when Frank, of Cologne, who had become dissatisfied with the results following the classical conservative section, particularly in women who had been exposed to the possibility of infection prior to the operation, described a new operative technic. In this procedure a transverse incision is made through the anterior abdominal wall several centimeters above the symphysis and the peritoneum separated from the posterior surface of the bladder and the anterior surface of the lower uterine segment. After proper exposure, the latter is then incised transversely, the child is extracted by forceps, the placenta removed manually, and the wound closed. By this method the entire operation is done extraperitoneally, and, according to its inventor, may be safely employed in such cases where conservative section would be contraindicated.

The extraperitoneal technic was enthusiastically taken up in Germany, and subjected to minor modifications by Latzko, Sellheim and others, while Döderlein resuscitated the operation of laparo-elytrotomy, which had been suggested by Philip Syng Physick and by Baudelocque in 1823, and rehabilitated by Gailard Thomas in 1871, to be afterward abandoned in favor of the classical cesarean section. After reporting 32 such operations, he in turn abandoned the procedure, as he found that the wound healing was complicated, that drainage was always required and that the operation was not available for use in infected patients. The historical aspects of the question were carefully considered by Küstner in his monograph which appeared in 1915. In general it may be said that, after a fair trial, the various methods of extraperitoneal section have somewhat fallen into disfavor, and have been replaced by the so-called low cervical operation. Recently, however, attention has again been directed to this operation, particularly because of the modifications introduced by Waters and by Ricci.

Krönig contended that the main advantage of the extraperitoneal technic consisted not so much in avoiding the peritoneal cavity, as in opening the uterus through its thin lower segment and then covering the incision by peritoneum. To accomplish this he cut through the vesical reflection of the peritoneum from one round ligament to the other, and separated it and the bladder from the lower uterine segment and cervix. The latter was then opened by a vertical median incision and the child extracted by forceps. The uterine incision was then closed and was buried under the vesical peritoneum. With minor modifications this low cervical technic has become popularized in this country by Beck, DeLee and others.

Gottschalk, in 1909, and Portes, in 1924, independently described a new type of cesarean section, which it is claimed is particularly adapted to infected cases in which it is important to preserve the uterus. In this procedure the unopened organ is delivered through the abdominal incision, but is not incised until after the peritoneum has been sutured about its cervical portion and the abdominal wound closed above it. After extracting the child, the uterine incision is sutured, and the exteriorized organ is covered with moist dressings. During convalescence the involution changes can be followed by the naked eye, and five or six weeks later when the uterus has returned to its usual size, the abdominal wound is reopened and the uterus restored to the pelvic cavity. This operation has been performed in a few isolated instances in this country. In 1927 Phaneuf reported two personal cases and stated that 16 such operations had been reported up to that time. He informs us that lately he has not had occasion to employ the Portes technic. In general it may be said that this operation has been discarded in favor of the extraperitoneal or low cervical operation for the infected as well as the potentially infected case.

Indications. The indications for cesarean section have been discussed in connection with the various conditions which sometimes call for the operation. A summary of the common indications for abdominal delivery in 1,000 cases in our clinic is shown in Table 30. Since this analysis is based on 1,000 cases, the absolute figure can be readily converted into percentages. The most common single indication was pelvic contraction, which was responsible for the operation in 27.3 per cent of the cases. This figure is weighted by the circumstance that almost one half of our clientele is made up of colored women in whom the high incidence of rachitic pelves is well known. As a consequence, in any representative cross section of the population, the relative frequency of pelvic contraction as an indication for cesarean section would doubtless be less than the one cited. The next most frequent indication for cesarean section was fear that a previous cesarean section scar might rupture, almost a quarter of the operations being done for this reason. In many clinics this is the most common indication for cesarean section.

It will be noted that the term "cephalo-pelvic disproportion" does not appear. It is true that in the cases of pelvic contraction, malpresentation, oversize baby and tumor blocking the birth canal, listed in the table, disproportion was thought to exist between the diameters of the infant which presented and the birth passage and that this was the actual reason for the operation. Nevertheless, clearer thinking about dystocia will result if the specific cause of the disproportion be stated. Actually, the term "cephalo-pelvic disproportion" is widely (but incorrectly) employed to designate almost any situation in which labor does not progress satisfactorily. A large proportion of such cases are the result of uterine inertia; and if so, we believe it preferable to say so rather than use the term "cephalo-pelvic disproportion" which obviously connotes inadequacy of space rather than inadequacy of the forces.

I. Pelvic contraction and mechanical dystocia		
Pelvic contraction		273
Uterine inertia		66
Malpresentations		44
Oversize baby		8
Tumor blocking birth canal		23
	Total	414
II. Previous cesarean section		240
III. Hemorrhagic complications		
Placenta previa		91
Abruptio placentae		49
	Total	140
IV. Toxemias		
Preeclampsia		70
Chronic hypertensive vascular disease		26
	Total	96
V. Intercurrent disease		
Diabetes mellitus		14
Other		12
	Total	26
VI. Miscellaneous		
Elderly primigravida		32
Other		52
	Total	84
	Grand total	1,000

TABLE 30. RELATIVE INCIDENCE OF COMMON INDICATIONS FOR CESAREAN SECTION.
(Based on 1,000 consecutive cases at Johns Hopkins Hospital, 1941-1949.)

Occasionally a cesarean section may be necessary because of several indications, no single one of which, in the degree present, would justify the operation. Thus, a preeclamptic patient with moderate pelvic contraction and an unengaged head, may have uterine inertia. It is our attitude, when several "partial indications" are present, that the hazards are additive and that when taken together, these "fractions" of an indication may sometimes make a whole; but this entails such nicety of judgment that any sweeping statements would be improper. In the preparation of Table 30, cases with multiple indications were carefully scrutinized and the main indication only used.

Another, and possibly more informative, way of analyzing cesarean section statistics is to establish in what proportion of cases of a given condition abdominal delivery was done. To this end, the cases in several groupings of Table 30 were correlated with the total number of cases of that particular complication which were managed in the clinic over the same period. In inlet contraction, cesarean section was performed in 9.3 per cent of the cases. (In midpelvic and outlet contraction, abdominal delivery is performed so rarely that a statistical statement about these groups would be meaningless.) In uterine inertia, as defined on page 782, the frequency of abdominal delivery was 8.6 per cent. In preeclampsia it was 4.7 per cent; in placenta previa, 43.3 per cent; in abruptio placentae, 37.9 per cent; in cases of previous cesarean section, 67.1 per cent; and in elderly primigravidae (over 35), 26.7 per cent.

The incidence of cesarean section in any given obstetrical clinic will depend in part on the extent to which applicants are screened in favor of those most needing specialists' care and to what extent the clinic is a referral center for complicated cases. The 1,000 cesarean sections discussed in the foregoing paragraphs were performed in the course of 21,739 deliveries, an incidence of 4.6 per cent. In most maternity hospitals this figure ranges between 2.0 and 6.0 per cent.

Statistics from various sources would seem to indicate that the incidence of cesarean section in the United States at large is about 2 per cent of all deliveries or slightly less. It is naturally higher in the metropolitan centers because many complicated cases from rural districts are sent there for management and because of other factors. Thus, a survey of cesarean section in Minneapolis for the year 1946 by Ehrenberg revealed an incidence of 2.6 per cent, while a five-year study of cesarean section in Ramsay County, Minnesota showed a frequency of 1.5 per cent. Through the courtesy of Dr. Buford Word of Birmingham, Alabama, and Mr. Ralph W. Roberts, State Registrar, Montgomery, Alabama, the following figures have been put at my disposal. In 242,438 total births which occurred in Alabama during the three-year period, 1945 to 1947, there were 3,205 cesarean sections, an incidence of 1.32 per cent. Of these total deliveries, slightly under one half took place in hospitals so that the incidence of abdominal deliveries in hospital obstetrics was 2.29 per cent.

Elderly Primigravidae. When a woman has her first pregnancy at the age of 35 or beyond, she is called an "elderly primigravida." The placing of such patients in a special category is justified on two scores. In the first place, certain complications inimical to successful childbearing are observed with greater frequency in this group of patients; notably, chronic hypertensive vascular disease, myomata, uterine inertia, and failure of the fetal head to engage at the onset of labor. As a consequence, the outlook for the baby is somewhat less favorable in elderly primigravidae. In the second place, since these women are in "the twilight of their reproductive period," as Davis and Seski phrase it, the number of future pregnancies which they can anticipate is often minimal; hence, a successful outcome for the present infant is of paramount importance. In other words, in these very cases in which a living child is most to be desired, the odds are a trifle against it because of the frequency of the several complications noted. Because of these circumstances, in elderly primigravidae, cesarean section is indicated more often than usual. It was performed in 26.7 per cent of such patients in the series shown in Table 30.

In 830 elderly primigravidae (35 years of age and over) delivered at the New York Hospital, Kuder and Johnson noted an increased incidence of toxemia, placenta previa, myomata uteri, occipitoposterior and arrested transverse positions, postpartum hemorrhage, operative delivery, and maternal and infantile mortality, as compared with the figures for the total clinic population. They noted, moreover, that the head of the child was unengaged at term in 53.5 per cent of the elderly primigravidae, in contrast to only 20.9 per cent in a control group of patients. Most studies of fetal loss in elderly primigravidae show rates three times the usual figure, or in the neighborhood of 12 per cent.

It must not be deduced, however, from what has been said that cesarean section is always indicated in elderly primigravidae or even in a majority of the cases. But when such a patient presents a substantial complication, cesarean section is indicated more often than is the case with younger women presenting the same complication.

Contraindications. Except in the presence of an absolute pelvic indication, abruptio placentae with the cervix closed, or in certain cases of placenta previa, cesarean section should never be performed when the child is dead or in serious danger. It is likewise contraindicated when the mother is in poor condition, or among surroundings which render an aseptic operation impossible. Again the classical operation is contraindicated when the patient is already infected, has been long in labor, or subjected to repeated vaginal examinations by those whose technic is questionable, even though no signs of infection are apparent at the time. If the patient is definitely infected, the body of the uterus should be amputated after delivery of the child or extraperitoneal cesarean section done depending on the parity of the patient and other factors.

Douglas has carried out bacteriologic studies at the New York Lying-In Hospital in over 500 patients at the time of cesarean section. He obtained cultures from the intra-ovular space after extraction of the child, as well as from the lower uterine segment after removal of the placenta. His bacteriologic findings, correlated with the clinical results, clearly show that a cesarean section performed prior to the onset of labor is relatively safe; that during the first eight hours of labor particularly with the membranes intact, the hazards are only slightly increased; but that after 12 hours of labor the risk from infection increases definitely and progressively with each hour of labor. The danger from infection thus increases not only with the period of ruptured membranes but also with the duration of labor. This danger, however, may be greatly reduced by the prophylactic administration of penicillin and one of the sulfonamides; but this protection should not be abused and, certainly, actual fever at the time of the operation is still a contraindication to any method of cesarean section other than extraperitoneal types and cesarean hysterectomy.

Operative Technic. *Classical Cesarean Section.* The operation will give almost ideal results if performed at an appointed time, a day or so prior to the end of pregnancy; whereas it preferably should not be performed after the onset of labor, as the prognosis becomes progressively worse with the duration of labor.

Our routine orders make it mandatory that blood be available from either the blood bank or a donor who is actually present prior to the commencement of the operation, in order that valuable time may not be lost when an indication for transfusion arises. For this same reason, the necessary grouping and matching of blood must be carried out before the operation is started.

When the operation can be performed at a fixed time, the patient should be prepared exactly as for an ordinary abdominal operation. The preoperative medication consists usually of 0.0004 gm. of atropine but no morphine. Special attention should be given to the type of anesthesia administered and the anesthetist should be specially versed in administering anesthesia for cesarean section. Just before the beginning of the operation, the bladder is catheterized and the abdomen disinfected by means of tincture of iodine and alcohol. A competent person should be charged with the reception and care of the child and receive careful instructions as to the best method of resuscitating it, if necessary.

An incision 12 to 15 cm. long should be made in the linea alba, extending from above the symphysis to just below the umbilicus. Care is, of course, exercised to check

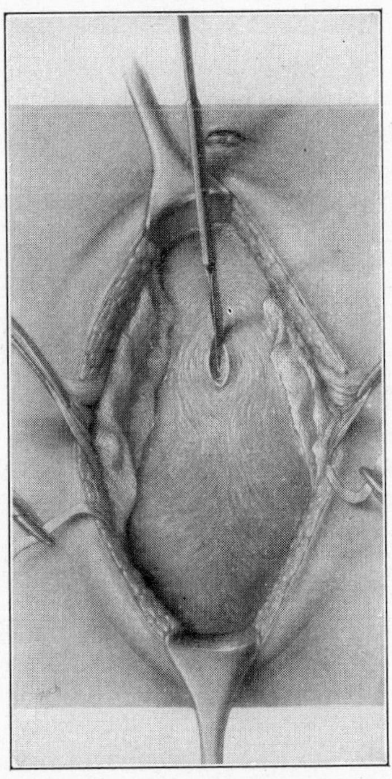

Fig. 626.

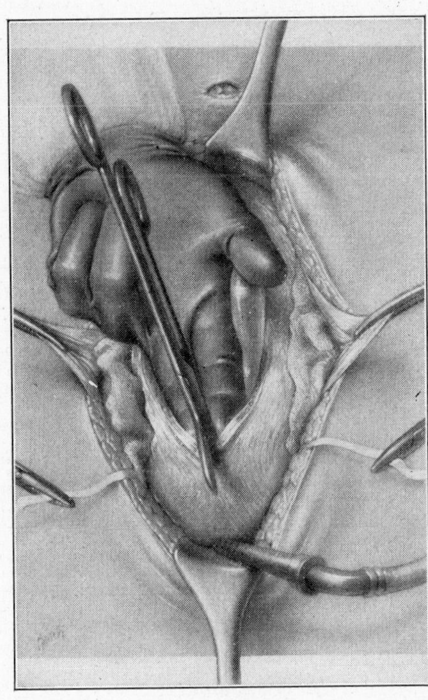

Fig. 627.

Fig. 626.—Classical Cesarean Section (the Umbilicus above, the Symphysis Pubis below). Beginning incision in uterus with scalpel.

Fig. 627.—Classical Cesarean Section.

Completing incision of uterus with bandage scissors. Note below, suction nozzle in place to remove blood and thus provide better exposure. The membranes are shown as still intact, but in an actual operation they are usually ruptured inadvertently before this juncture.

hemorrhage from the abdominal wound, as in any other laparotomy. The uterus is found directly beneath the incision, and with the index finger one can readily palpate one or both round ligaments. Where there is marked rotation of the uterus we prefer to retract that side of the abdominal wound to which such rotation has occurred, thus enabling the operator to incise the uterus approximately in the midline.

It is our practice to pack the abdominal cavity around the exposed part of the uterus, by starting at the lower angle of the abdominal incision and placing a moistened pack between the abdominal wall and the uterus. This prevents, to a large extent, any abdominal spill of amniotic fluid and blood and so ensures a smoother convalescence. The anterior surface of the uterus is now opened longitudinally along its midline with the lower end of the incision terminating just above the reflexion of the bladder peritoneum. This is best accomplished by making an incision a few centimeters long with a scalpel other than the one used for the abdominal incision and then rapidly enlarging it with the scissors to about 10 cm. The membranes are than ruptured and the whole hand of the operator inserted through the uterine incision in order to grasp one or both feet of the baby. In this manner the child can be readily extracted. Two clamps are applied to the cord, which is cut between them, and the child handed to an assistant. If the placenta lies under the incision, as it does in two cases out of five, it should be rapidly cut through or pushed to one side and the child extracted. This is accompanied by a slight increase of hemorrhage, but as the bleeding is only momentary, it is without significance. Shortly after the delivery of the child, the uterus usually contracts down and hemorrhage practically ceases. In order to insure satisfactory contraction of the uterus, and thus minimize the amount of bleeding, 0.2 mg. of ergonovine should be administered intramuscularly just as the child is being delivered.

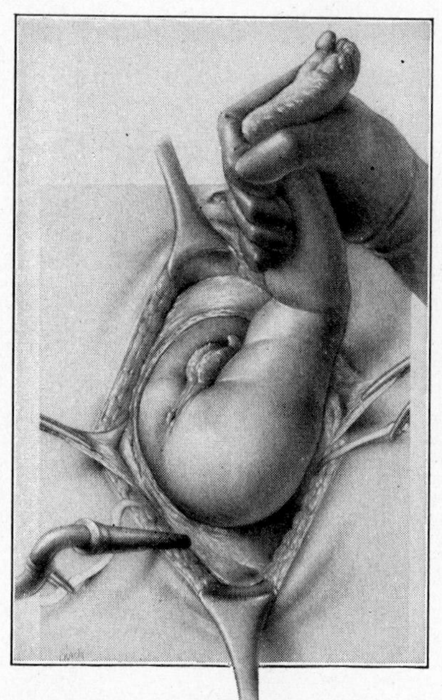

Fig. 628.—Classical Cesarean Section.

Delivery of the infant after version. The calf of the infant's leg should be grasped with a towel rather than with the bare gloved hand as shown, in order to secure better traction.

After extraction of the child, if excessive bleeding occurs or pelvic pathology is suspected, the uterus may be delivered through the abdominal incision, and the peritoneal cavity posterior to it protected by moist warm gauze packs. The exposed uterus should be covered with moist warm towels. If the placenta and membranes have not become separated spontaneously, they should be peeled off and removed with the hand, care being taken that no shreds of membranes are left behind. Disinfection of the uterine cavity is not necessary. Even when the operation is undertaken before the onset of labor, it is not necessary to dilate the cervix artificially as the canal is always sufficiently patulous to permit free drainage.

The uterine wound is now closed with a minimum of catgut material in such a manner that the cut edges are evenly and completely coapted and hemorrhage is adequately controlled. There are several ways of accomplishing these ends. Our practice is to employ one layer of interrupted chromic catgut to approximate the inner halves of the cut edges, followed by a continuous chromic catgut suture for the outer half and finally a continuous suture for the peritoneum and the muscle fibers immediately underlying it. The first deep layer of interrupted sutures should not penetrate the decidual lining of the cavity. Any blood which may have escaped into the pelvic cavity is then carefully sponged out, and the abdominal wound closed by suturing the peritoneum, fascia, and skin in separate layers. (See Figs. 626 to 630.)

Low Cervical Cesarean Section. This operation is also called laparotrachelotomy. While slightly more difficult than the classical operation, it is the procedure of choice in many cases and certainly whenever cesarean section is performed six or more hours after the onset of labor. If, however, the patient shows signs of actual infection, as indicated by elevation of temperature and rapid pulse, much better maternal results are obtained if the body of the uterus is amputated or by extraperitoneal cesarean section.

After emptying the bladder by catheter, the patient is placed in a moderate Trendelenburg posture, and the abdomen opened in the midline just as in the classical operation. The margins of the abdominal incision are then drawn apart by suitable

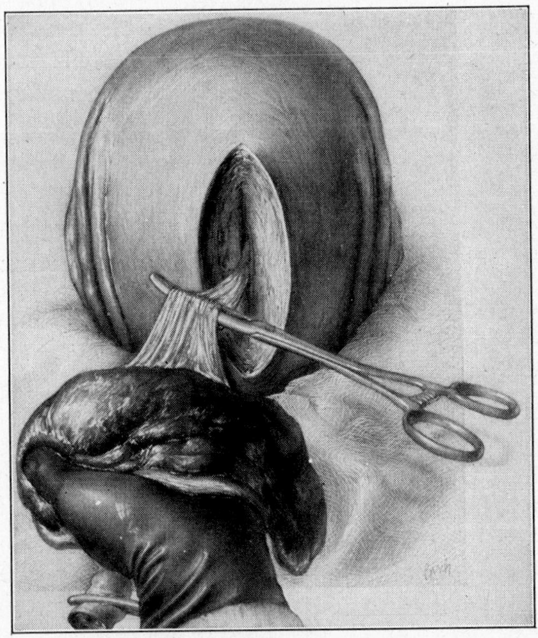

FIG. 629.—CLASSICAL CESAREAN SECTION.

Delivery of placenta and membranes. Care must be taken that *all* the membranes are removed.

retractors, and the lowermost portion of the uterus exposed. The loose peritoneum is seized by dissecting forceps just below its firm attachment to the anterior wall of the uterus and, together with the tissue just beneath, incised transversely by scissors for almost the entire distance between the round ligaments. Then, by means of a small sponge stick, or a finger covered with gauze, the peritoneum and posterior surface of the bladder are separated from the uterine wall. In this way two flaps are formed, a short upper one, which terminates where the peritoneum is firmly attached to the uterine body, and a longer lower one which consists of the vesical peritoneum and the posterior surface of the bladder. The midline of the lower flap is then caught with a suture or an Allis clamp and when the flap is drawn up against the symphysis by a suitable retractor, the entire lower uterine segment and upper part of the cervix become exposed. A small nick is then made in its midline with a scalpel and the incision is prolonged with scissors until sufficiently large to permit the passage of the child's head. By means of a finger in the mouth, the head of the child is rotated until the face comes to occupy the uterine incision, when delivery is effected by means of a short forceps, or by passing the hand under the occipital region, aided by pressure upon the fundus of the uterus.

As in classical section, ergonovine is administered intramuscularly just as the child is being delivered, and after its delivery the placenta is expressed or removed manually. An Allis clamp in the upper angle serves to make the incision taut, and its thin walls are brought together by a continuous catgut suture which it is well to reinforce by a second suture which does not penetrate the uterine wall. All clots are carefully removed by means of sponge sticks, the upper peritoneal flap is brought down and sometimes attached to the uterus by one or two interrupted sutures, after which the lower flap is brought into place and united to the upper by a continuous catgut suture, and the abdominal wall closed in layers without drainage.

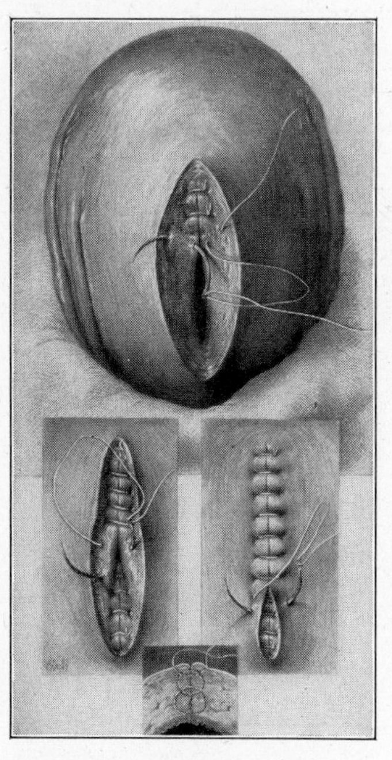

Fig. 630. — Classical Cesarean Section. Three-layer Closure.

Instead of incising the uterus vertically, Munro Kerr advocates making the incision transversely. We have tried both methods, and prefer the former incision. During the entire procedure the uterus remains in situ and, if the anesthetic is well given, the intestines and uterine-appendages at no time come into view. Ordinarily the hemorrhage is not excessive but occasionally, and particularly when the uterine incision diverges from the midline, it may prove troublesome. (See Figs. 631 to 638.)

Extraperitoneal Cesarean Section. The extraperitoneal operations most commonly used in this country today are those of Waters and Norton. The former is illustrated in Figs. 639 to 642 and the latter in Figs. 643 to 646. The main steps in both technics are described in the legends.

Cesarean Hysterectomy. After delivery of the child by classical or low cervical cesarean section, the same technic is employed as in an ordinary supravaginal hysterectomy with retention of the ovaries. After the uterus has been delivered from the abdominal cavity, the tubes, ovarian and round ligaments on either side are doubly clamped, severed and ligated. The broad ligament on either side is cut through down to its base. An elliptical incision is then made through the peritoneum on the anterior surface of the uterus, just above the bladder, and a peritoneal flap rapidly peeled off by means of a piece of gauze applied around the end of the finger or by the handle of a scalpel. The uteriné arteries are then isolated, ligated and severed, after which the body of the uterus is amputated. The cervical stump is brought together by the necessary number of catgut sutures, suspended by the round ligaments and covered by the peritoneal flap, with a continuous catgut suture which also closes the openings in the broad ligaments. The pelvic cavity is sponged out, and the abdominal wound closed. The operation is readily performed, and can be completed in as short a time as cesarean section. (See Figs. 647 and 648.)

Choice of Operation. When the operation is to be performed at an appointed time before labor upon patients who have not been exposed to the possibility of infection,

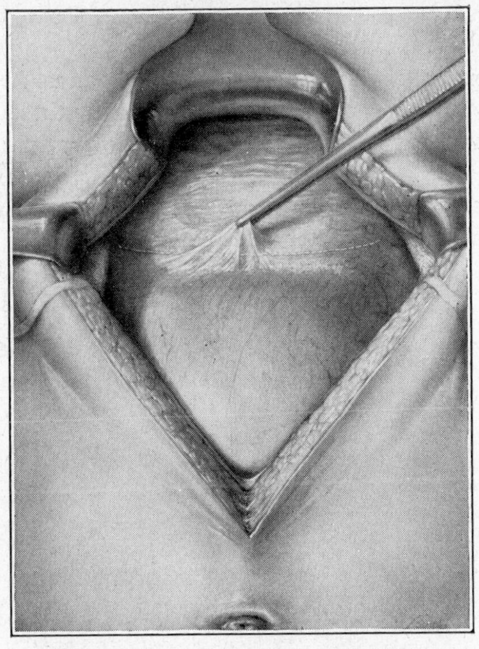

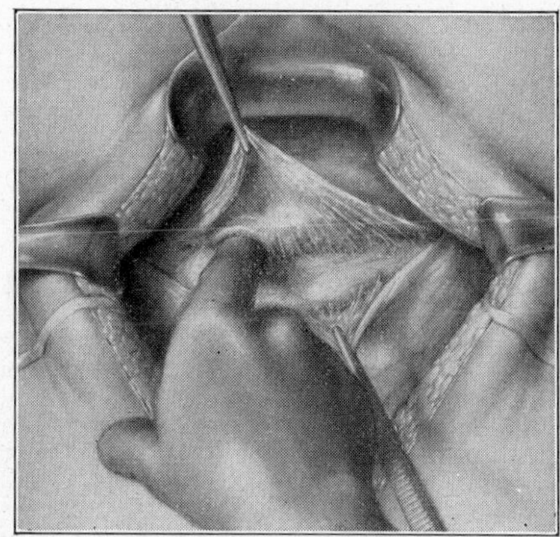

FIG. 631. FIG. 632.

FIG. 631.—LOW CERVICAL CESAREAN SECTION (THE UMBILICUS BELOW, THE SYMPHYSIS PUBIS ABOVE).

The transverse incision in the perineum is made about one inch below the point where the peritoneum is firmly attached to the uterus. Incision of the peritoneum as indicated by the dotted line, creates an upper and a lower flap of peritoneum.

FIG. 632.—LOW CERVICAL CESAREAN SECTION (LOOKING TOWARD SYMPHYSIS PUBIS).

Dissection of peritoneum and bladder off uterus to expose lower uterine segment.

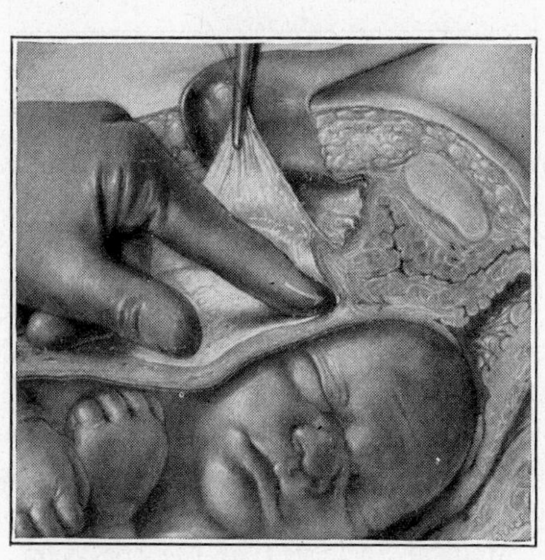

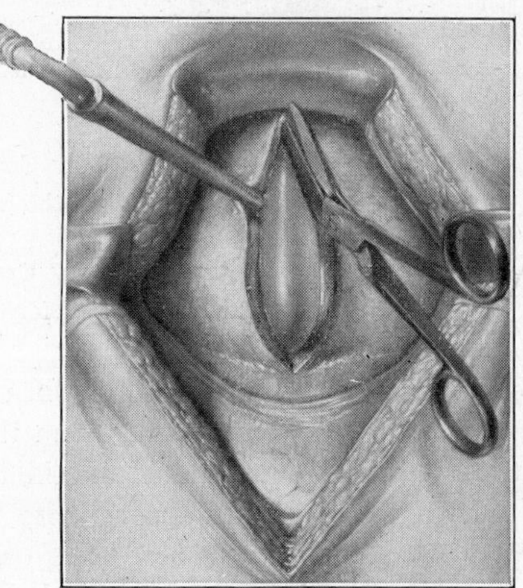

FIG. 633. FIG. 634.

FIG. 633.—LOW CERVICAL CESAREAN SECTION.

Cross section showing dissection of bladder off uterus to expose lower uterine segment.

FIG. 634.—LOW CERVICAL CESAREAN SECTION.

The bladder is protected by the retractor which at the same time helps expose the lower uterine segment while the incision is made.

the classical cesarean section is, in our opinion, the operation of choice; whereas, if the operation is undertaken later or upon women who have been examined by those whose technic is open to suspicion, better results will be obtained by the low cervical technic.

It should be pointed out that the low cervical operation is advocated by many to be the better procedure both for elective cases as well as for those patients already in

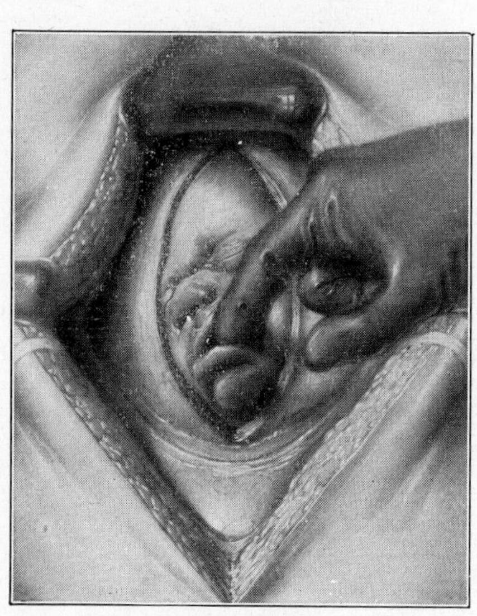

FIG. 635. 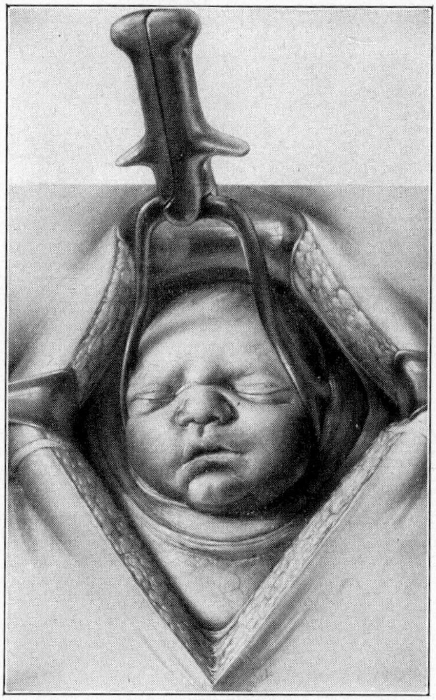 FIG. 636.

FIG. 635.—LOW CERVICAL CESAREAN SECTION.

A finger in the baby's mouth rotates the face anterior, and the chin is delivered over the upper edge of the wound.

FIG. 636.—LOW CERVICAL CESAREAN SECTION.

Delivery of infant's head *slowly* with forceps.

labor. This claim may be justified when the operation is performed in well-conducted hospitals and upon patients in whom the lower uterine segment is developed to the extent of allowing extraction of the child through it and not through the lower portion of the body of the uterus. Furthermore, we are convinced from investigations into the causes of maternal deaths now being conducted by such bodies as the Committee on Maternal Mortality of the New York County Medical Society, that the operation is not without danger, particularly from hemorrhage. In a critical study of the low cervical and classical operations, Falls comes to the conclusion that "the results obtained by the low cervical operation are hardly so superior to those following the classical operation as to justify the extravagant praise of some of its sponsors." On the basis of our own experience and results, as detailed below, we agree with him. It is our practice to perform the low cervical operation whenever the patient has had sufficient labor to develop a lower segment of the uterus permitting this technic. On the other hand, if the patient already presents signs of actual infection, as indicated by elevation of temperature, rapid pulse, and, possibly, a foul smelling vaginal discharge, many maternal lives will be saved by the extraperitoneal operation or by amputating the body of the uterus. Naturally, when the indication is afforded by myomata, cesarean hysterectomy may at times be indicated as well as in those cases in which uncontrollable hemorrhage resulting from uterine atony complicates the intended classical operation. We consider

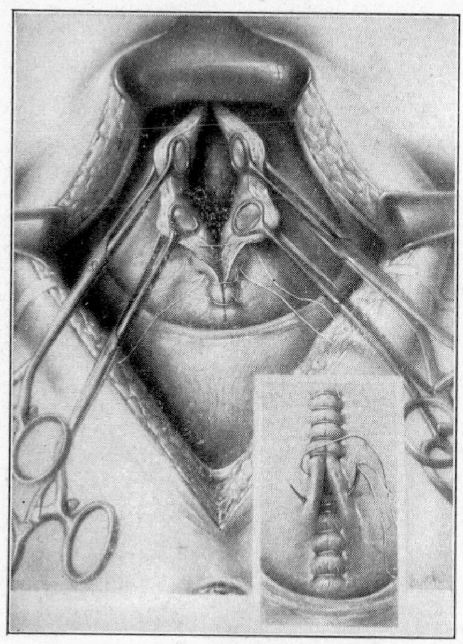

FIG. 637.

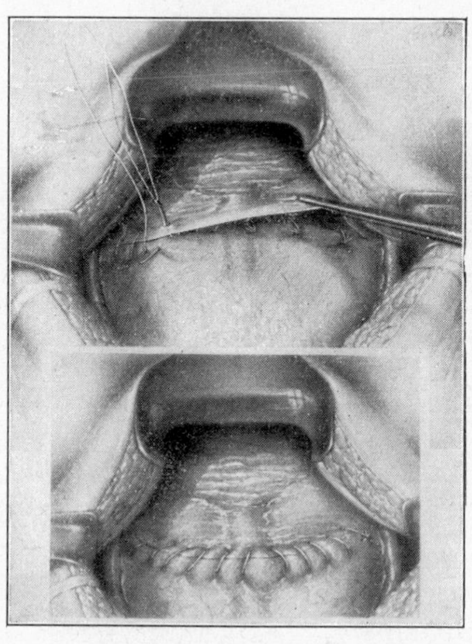

FIG. 638.

FIG. 637—LOW CERVICAL CESAREAN SECTION.
Closure of lower uterine segment in two layers.

FIG. 638.—LOW CERVICAL CESAREAN SECTION.
Overlapping of two flaps of peritoneum to seal off incision from peritoneal cavity.

myomectomy at the time of section contraindicated, unless the myoma be pedunculated or in the incision and thus easily removable.

Upon proper indications in frankly infected patients, the extraperitoneal cesarean operation is undoubtedly of great value especially when, due to the age or obstetrical history of the patient, sacrifice of the uterus is undesirable. This set of circumstances rarely occurs today, especially with the help of chemotherapy.

Prognosis. In 1937, Campbell reported 482 sections comprising 404 classical, 73 with hysterectomy, 4 vaginal and 1 low cervical, with a maternal mortality of 0.8 per cent. Daily, likewise, recorded a maternal mortality of 0.8 per cent in 1,000 sections. In the 1,000 consecutive cesarean sections in our clinic discussed above, there was one maternal death, due to extremely severe preeclampsia. Moreover, Lull has reported over 1,000 consecutive cesarean sections with one maternal death, due to leukemia. With the availability of a good blood bank, with chemotherapy and in competent, judicious hands, the maternal death rate from cesarean section should be under 1 per cent.

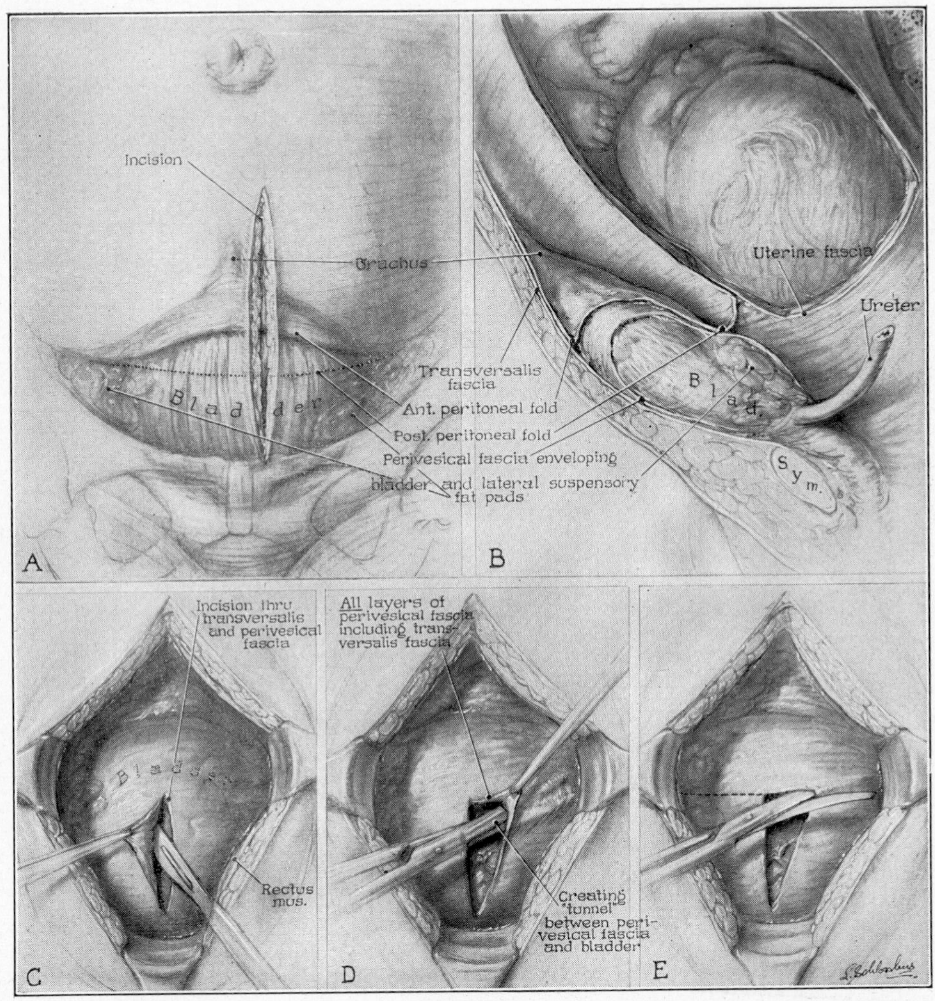

Fig. 639.—The Waters Extraperitoneal Cesarean Section.

A. Demonstration of the anatomy of the distended bladder, lateral suspensory fat pads, peritoneal folds and urachus at the time of operation.

B. Lateral view of the distended bladder, uterus, fascias and peritoneum.

C. The left rectus muscle has been freed from the underlying transversalis fascia and is retracted to the left. All fascial layers overlying the bladder are cut through. The appearance of the blood vessels and musculature of the bladder determines whether all fascial layers have been cut through.

D. The scissors are then placed between the fascial layers and the bladder, and by staying close to and pushing the bladder musculature downward and away from the fascia, a "tunnel" is created.

E. The fascia is then divided on the left. This "tunneling" is repeated on the right and the fascia is divided, as indicated by the dotted line. A T-shaped incision in the fascia has then been made.

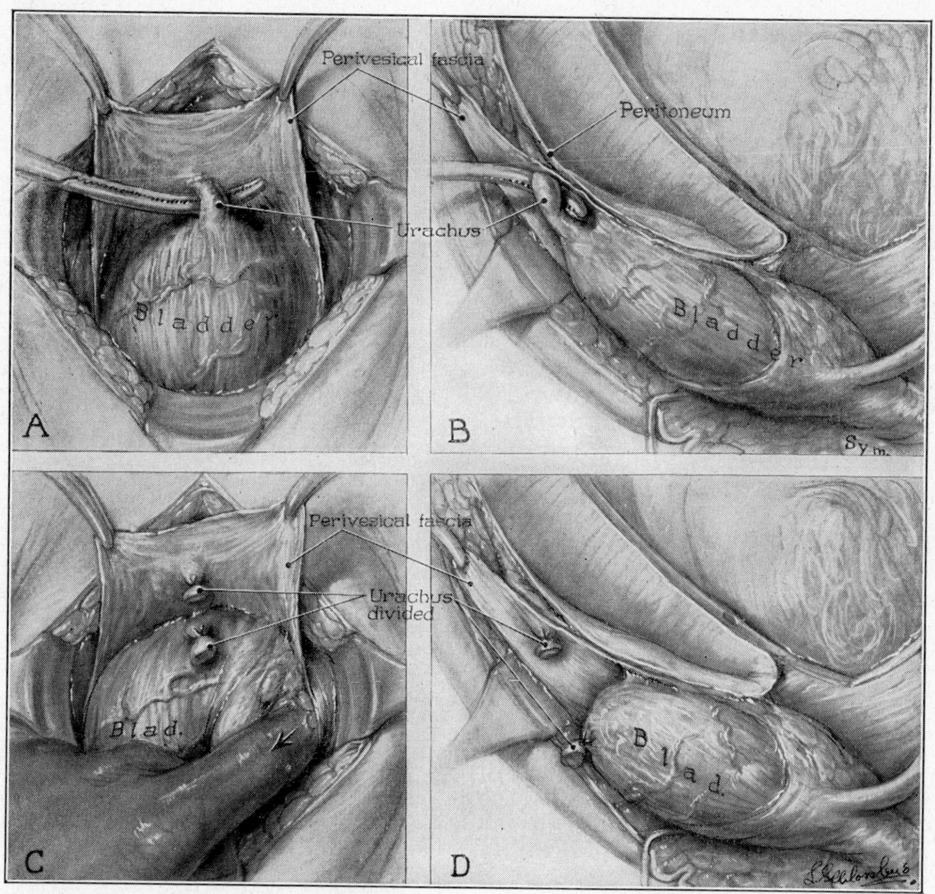

FIG. 640.—THE WATERS EXTRAPERITONEAL CESAREAN SECTION.

A,B. The perivesical fascia is dissected off the front and top of the bladder. The urachus and anterior peritoneum is in this region, and with gentle dissection the urachus is exposed and divided.

C. The left lateral fat is approached and the bladder is displaced medially and inferiorly.

D. Upper portion of the bladder is released and dropped downward following division of the urachus.

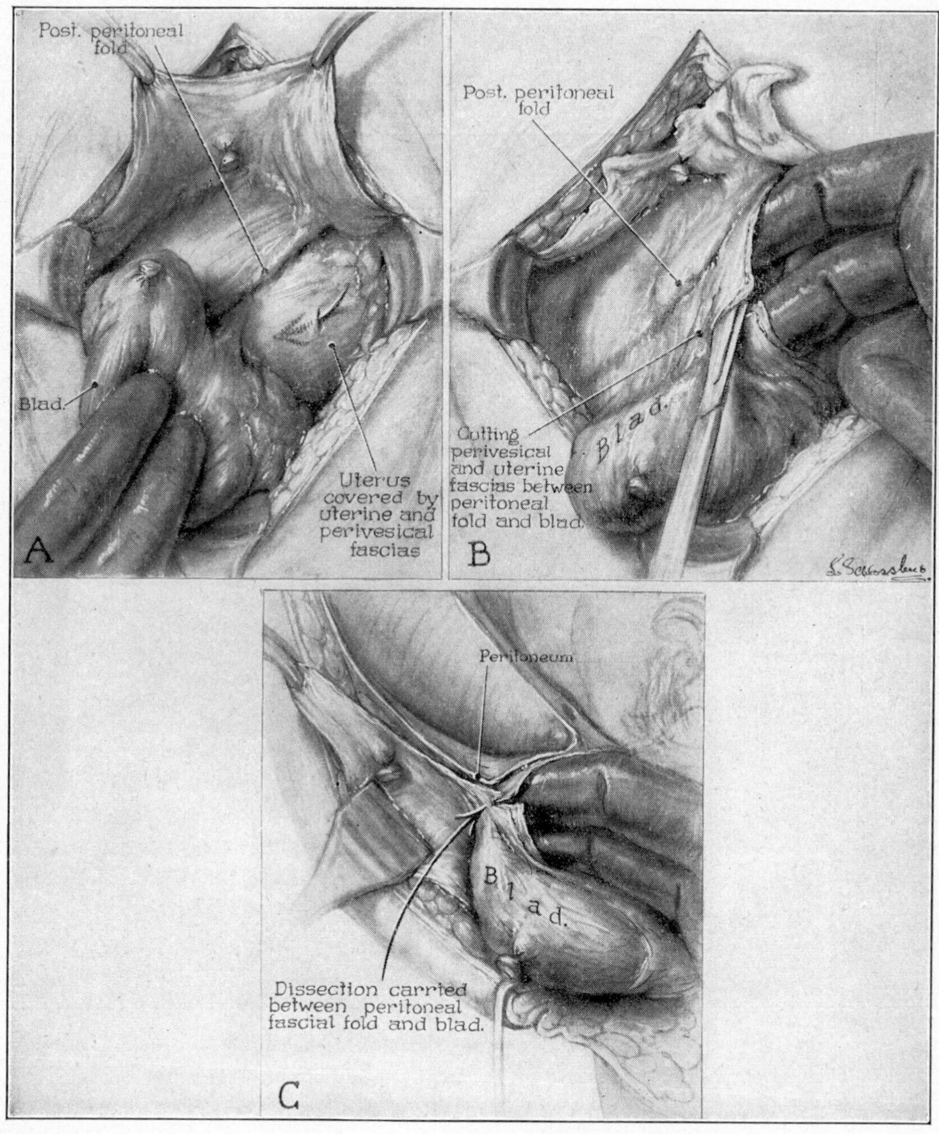

FIG. 641.—THE WATERS EXTRAPERITONEAL CESAREAN SECTION.

A. Bladder is emptied and drawn medially and inferiorly, exposing the uterus. This triangular uterine space is bordered above by the posterior peritoneal fold, medially and inferiorly by the bladder.

B. An incision is made in the perivesical and uterine fascias, and fingers are inserted elevating the fascias, peritoneal fold and bladder. The fascias are then divided. This dissection and division is carried close to the bladder.

C. Lateral view of elevation and division of fascias as shown in B.

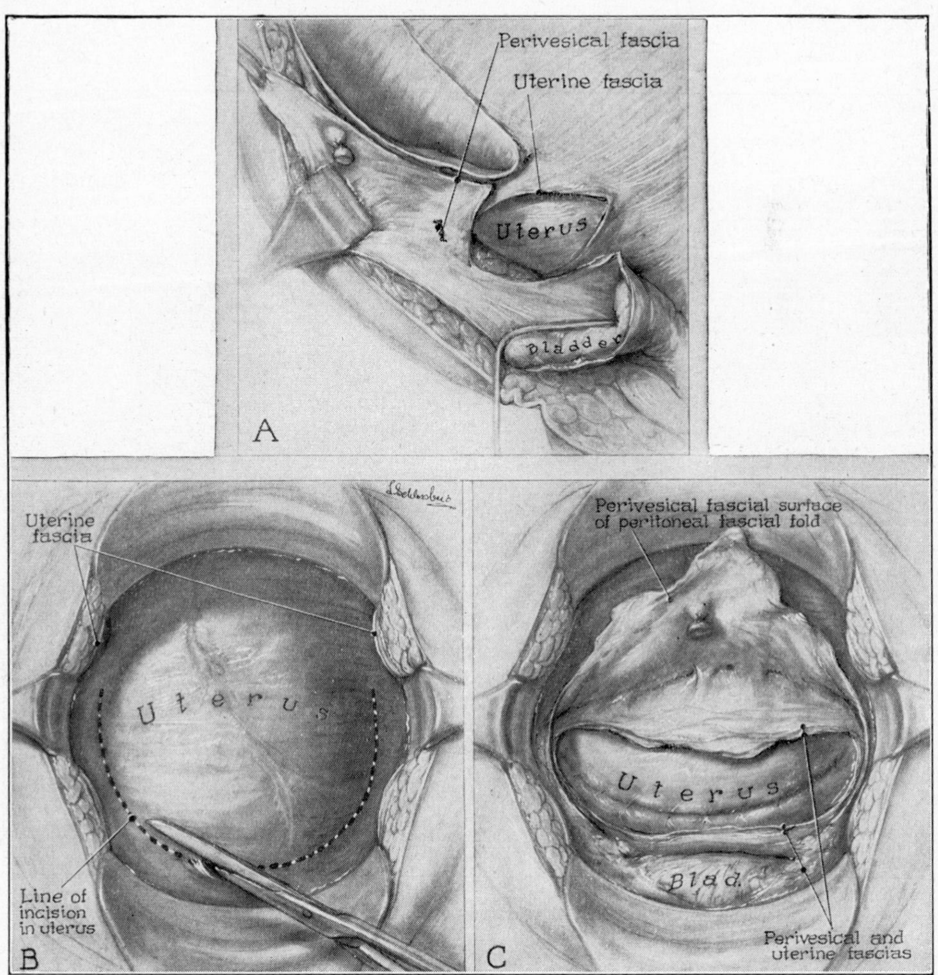

Fig. 642.—The Waters Extraperitoneal Cesarean Section.

A. Bladder is freed posteriorly and inferiorly.

B. Retractors are placed in the uterine fascial incision and with the lower uterine segment exposed, an incision is made in the uterus with bandage scissors.

C. Uterus is closed with two rows of sutures, using number 1 catgut. The first is a continuous suture and the second is a Cushing continuous stitch which completely buries the suture material.

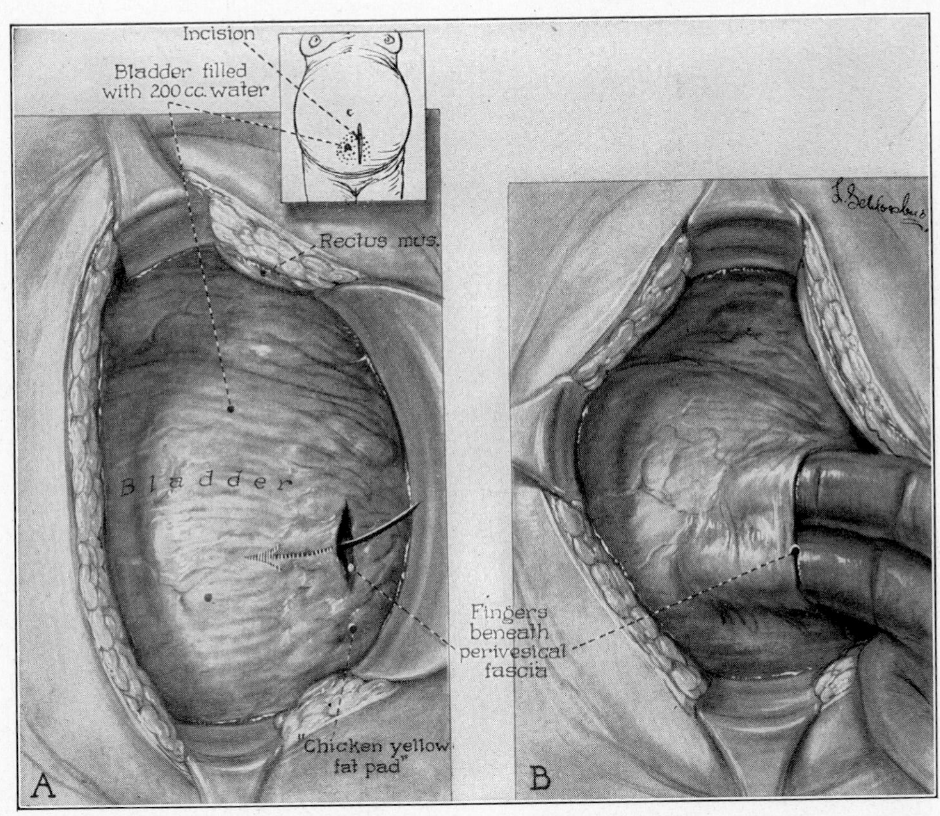

FIG. 643.—THE NORTON EXTRAPERITONEAL CESAREAN SECTION.

A. Bladder distended. Left rectus muscle has been freed from the underlying transversalis fascia and retracted to the left. Left lateral suspensory fat ("chicken") pad is exposed. Finger is "pushed" through the transversalis and perivesical fascias as indicated by the arrow. The entrance into the fascias should be over the lower region of the bladder in order to avoid injury to the anterior peritoneal fold.

B. Beginning separation of the fascias from the bladder.

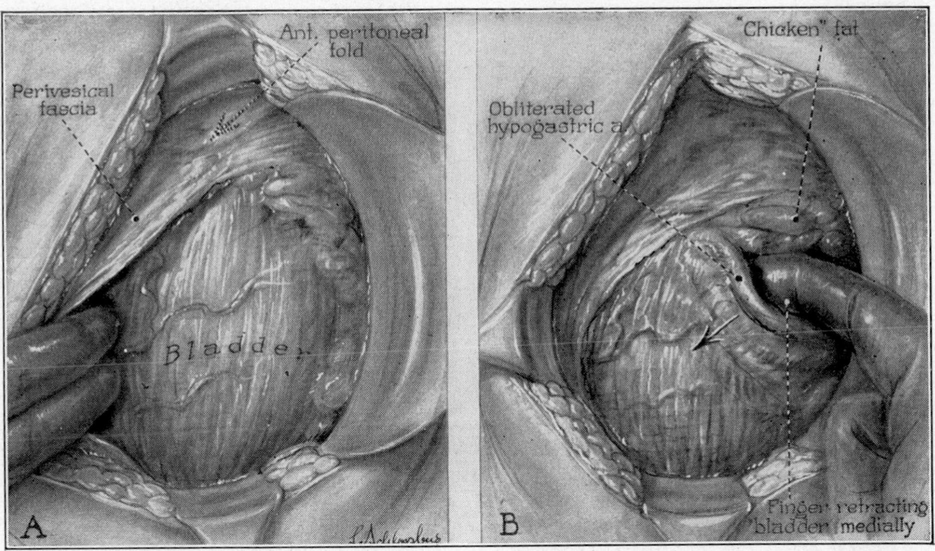

FIG. 644.—THE NORTON EXTRAPERITONEAL CESAREAN SECTION.

A. Perivesical fascia drawn medially, exposing the bladder. Anterior peritoneal fold in fatty mass above.

B. The obliterated hypogastric artery is located laterally in the "chicken" fat, and, with this as a landmark, the bladder is drawn medially.

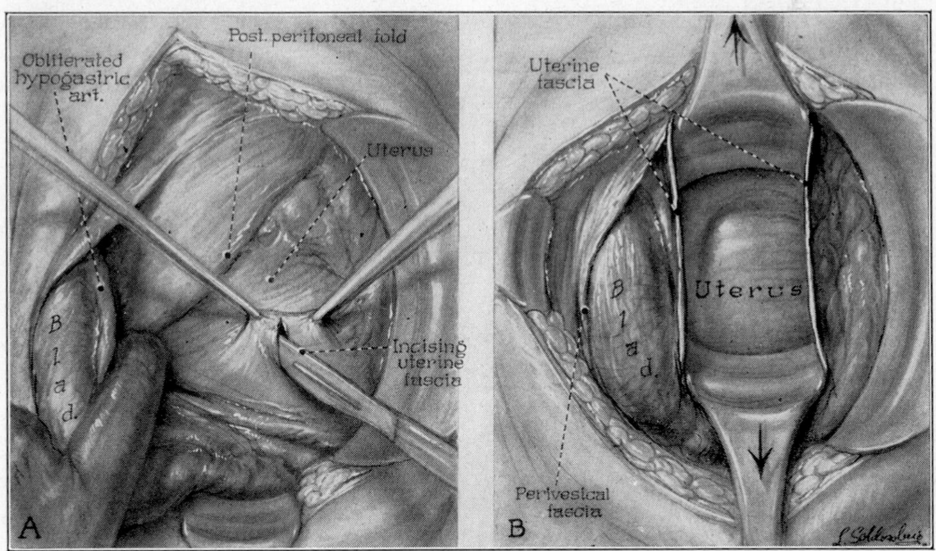

FIG. 645.—THE NORTON EXTRAPERITONEAL CESAREAN SECTION.

A. Bladder emptied and drawn medially. Triangle of exposed uterus is bordered above by the posterior peritoneal fold and medially and inferiorly by the bladder. An incision is made in the uterine fascia.

B. Retractors are placed in the uterine fascia incision, and traction is exerted. The uterine fascia acts as a buffer for the peritoneum during retraction.

Repeated Cesarean Section. The performance of conservative cesarean section does not interfere with future conception as is shown by the fact that even in preantiseptic times not a few instances were reported in which the same woman had repeatedly been subjected to the operation. Nor does it necessarily affect recovery at a subsequent operation. With the increased employment of the operation, repeated cesarean sections are frequently necessary. Koch reports an incidence of 21.8 per cent of repeated operations in a total of 289 sections. Contracted pelvis formed the indication for operation in 92 per cent of his 63 repeated sections. Among 944 sections per-

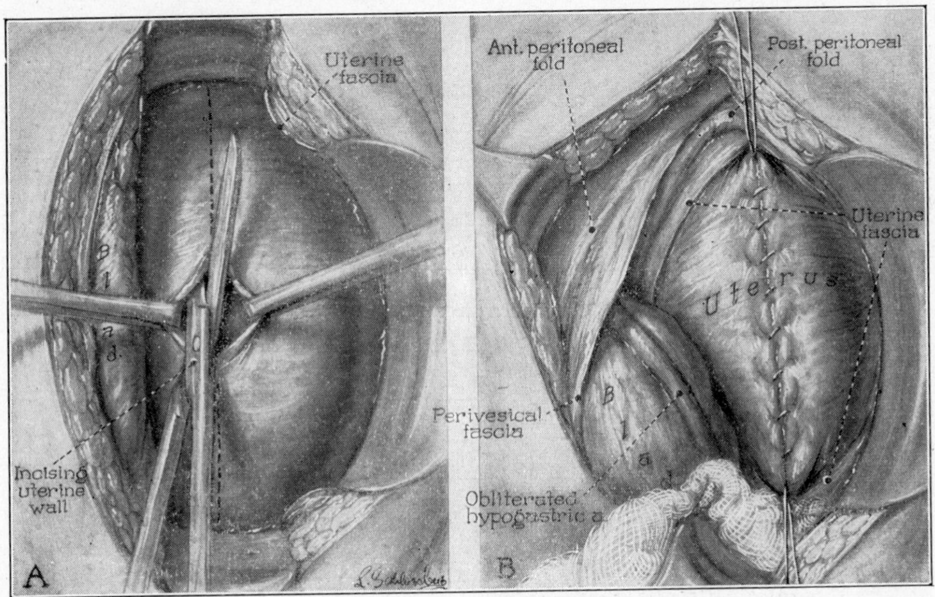

FIG. 646.—THE NORTON EXTRAPERITONEAL CESAREAN SECTION.

A. Uterus is incised with bandage scissors.

B. Closure of the uterus showing the intact posterior peritoneal fold well above the uterine incision. The anterior peritoneal fold is visible beneath the perivesical fascia.

formed in Stander's service from 1932 to 1943, 252 were repeat operations which were divided as follows: 186 second, 51 third, 10 fourth, 4 fifth and 1 sixth sections.

The occurrence of pregnancy after a cesarean section is not devoid of danger as the recent literature indicates that rupture occurs through the site of the previous incision in from 1 to 4 per cent of the subsequent gestations, and certain authors consider it so real a danger that they have laid down the dictum, "Once a cesarean, always a cesarean." This is an exaggeration and is in part based upon the belief that the uterine incision heals by the formation of scar tissue, whence the term cicatrix, and that the newly formed connective tissue stretches and sometimes yields when the uterus becomes distended. Williams was of the opinion that this belief is erroneous and that the uterus heals by regeneration of the muscle fibers and not by scar tissue. He based his conclusions on histologic examination of the site of the incision and on the following observations: First, inspection of the unopened uterus at the time of repeated sections usually shows no trace of the former incision, or, if present, it appears as an almost invisible linear scar. Second, when the body of the uterus has been amputated, no scar is visible after hardening, or at most a shallow vertical furrow is present upon the external and internal surfaces of the anterior uterine wall, while between them no trace of scar tissue is apparent. Schwarz and his associates, on the other hand, conclude that healing occurs mainly by the proliferation of fibroblasts. They studied the site of the incision in the human uterus, some days following cesarean section, as well as in the

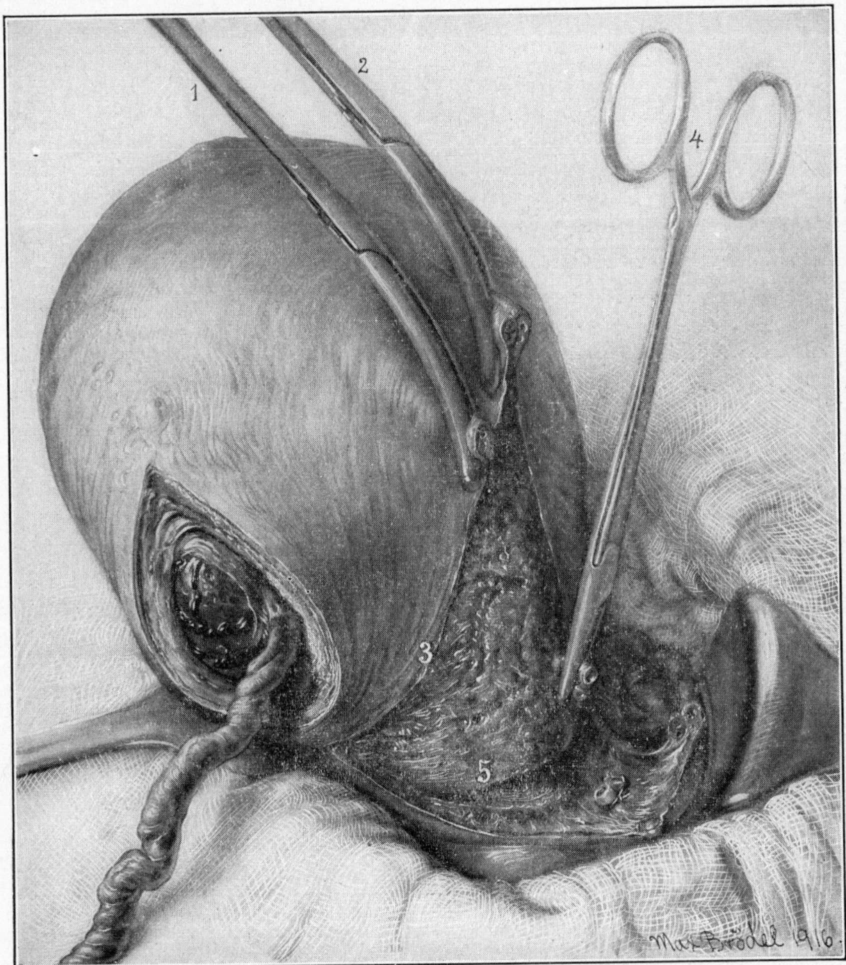

Fig. 647.—Supravaginal Hysterectomy Following Cesarean Section. Placenta in Utero.

1, Clamp applied to round ligament; 2, clamp applied to proximal end of tube and broad ligament; 3, anterior peritoneal flap; 4, clamp applied to proximal end of uterine artery; 5, transverse incision through cervix.

uteri of experimental animals, guinea pigs, rabbits and dogs. They observed that as the scar shrinks the proliferation of connective tissue becomes less perceptible, requiring special stains (van Gieson) for demonstration. It would appear that Schwarz's conclusions are justifiable on the basis of his histologic studies, particularly where there is inadequate approximation of the muscle edges of the uterine wound. Undoubtedly, if the cut surfaces are brought in close apposition, the amount of connective tissue proliferation must be minimal, and gradually the normal relationship of smooth muscle and connective tissue, as in the uninjured uterus, is re-established. This will account for the fact, mentioned above, that sometimes one finds no trace of a former incision, while at other times a definite scar is seen. It should be noted, however, that even when

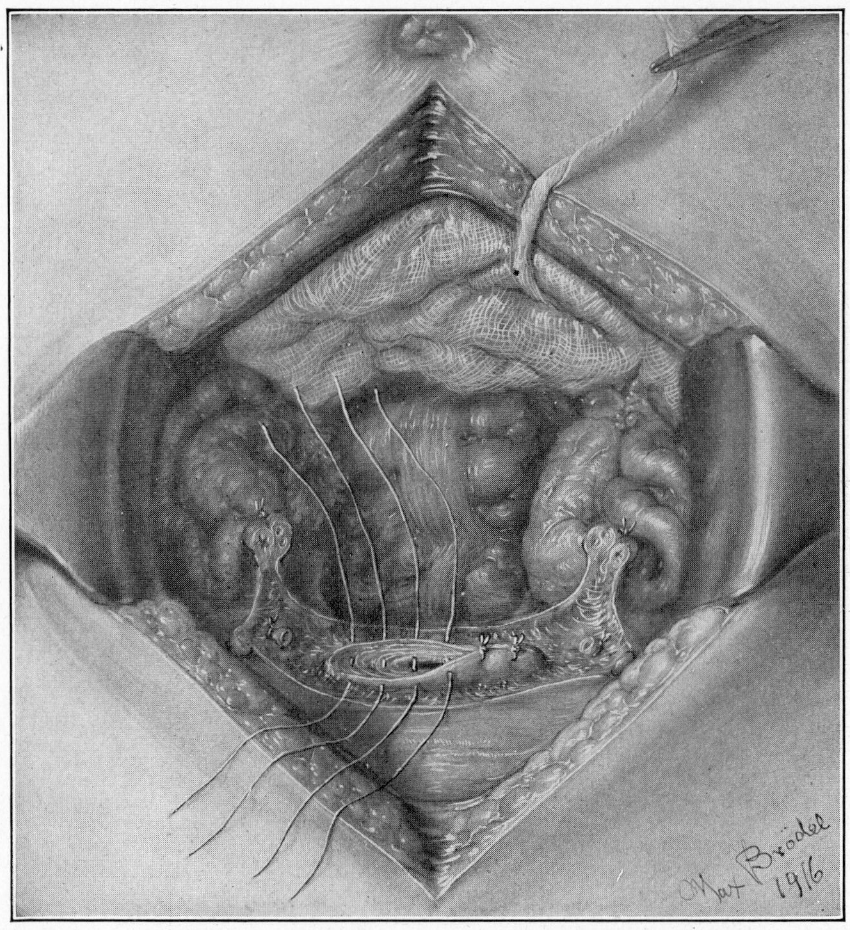

Fig. 648.—Cesarean Section Followed by Supravaginal Hysterectomy.

Note the tubes and ovaries in situ; the method of suturing the cervical stump, and the broad ligament wound which will later be closed by a continuous suture.

the healing has been so imperfect that marked thinning has resulted, the tissue which remains is often almost entirely muscular in character.

Rupture of the scar is probably less apt to follow low cervical section than to follow the classical operation. The possible occurrence of rupture should always be considered in connection with the employment of cesarean section for other than pelvic indications, as thereafter the uterus must be considered as a "locus minoris resistentiae." In such cases a normal spontaneous termination should be anticipated in subsequent labors, unless the puerperium had been febrile, but it is nevertheless advisable for the

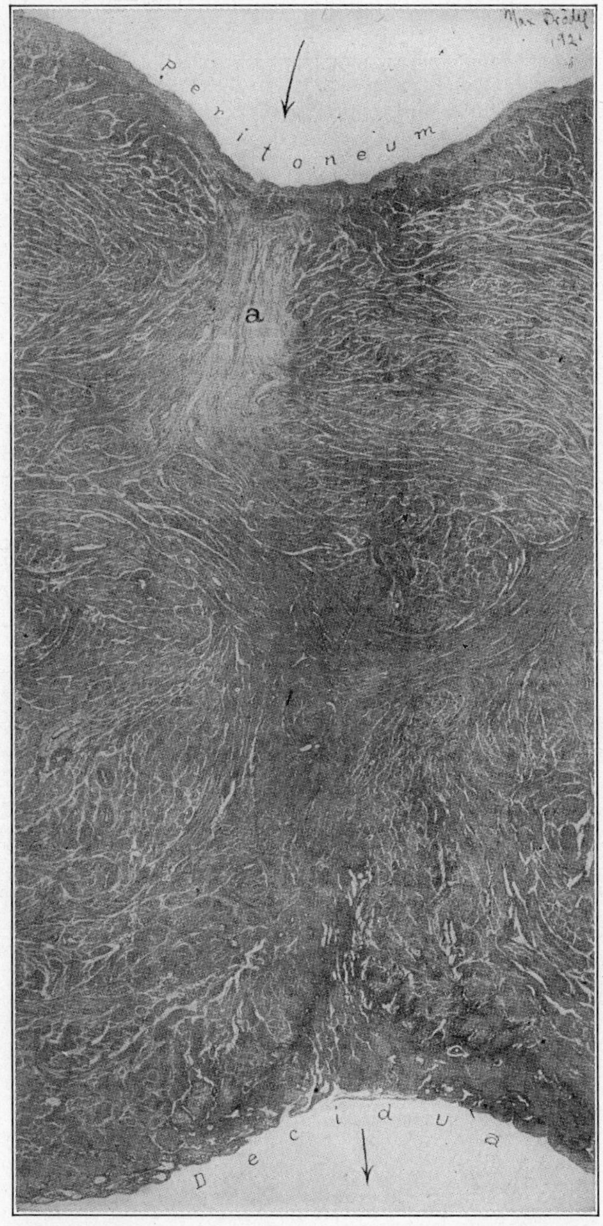

Fig. 649.—Ideal Healing of Cesarean Section Scar. Scar Tissue at *a*.

patient to be under observation in a hospital so that immediate laparotomy can be undertaken should rupture occur.

As shown in Table 31, in 624 deliveries on our service subsequent to a cesarean section and in whom the patients were under our care prior to any rupture, the incidence of rupture was 1.0 per cent in pregnancy and 1.1 per cent in labor, a total incidence of 2.1 per cent. This table also shows the percentage of patients who delivered vaginally.

	No.	%
Total deliveries	624	
Cesarean section because disproportion plus scar	316	50.7
Cesarean section—scar only indication	120	19.2
Delivered vaginally	188	30.1
Total pregnancies	624	
Ruptures in pregnancy	6	1.0
Total labors	188	
Ruptures in labor	2	1.1

TABLE 31. SHOWING INCIDENCE OF RUPTURE OF CESAREAN SECTION SCAR IN PATIENTS, UNDER OUR SURVEILLANCE, WHO HAD HAD ONE OR MORE ABDOMINAL DELIVERIES.

With increasing incidence of section, rupture of the scar has become the commonest cause of uterine rupture. A rational plan for the handling of patients with scarred uteri is, therefore, of importance. Obviously, when the indication for the first operation is still present or where there is the slightest possibility of mechanical dystocia, repeat section should be done. Unusual distention of the uterus as with hydramnios, multiple pregnancy, or excessive size of fetus should favor repeat section. In the remaining

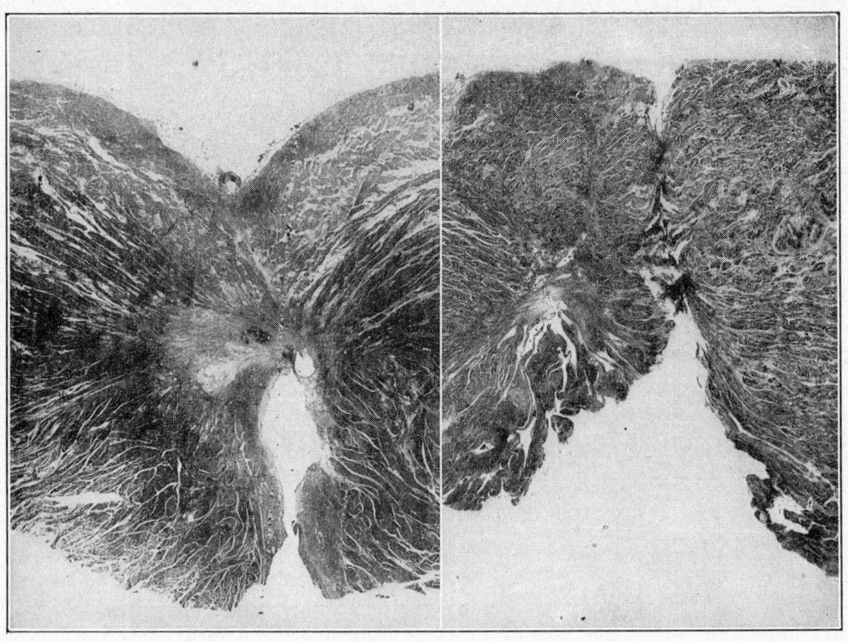

FIG. 650.—PHOTOMICROGRAPHS OF TWO POORLY HEALED CESAREAN SECTION SCARS.

cases in which there are no adverse factors present, we have found no reliable criteria for predicting which scars will rupture or when. For the mother vaginal delivery seems to offer safety almost equal to section. The incidence of rupture in pregnancy and labor being 2 per cent with 10 per cent mortality, the maternal risk is 0.2 per cent, as compared with an elective section mortality rate of 0.1 per cent in this clinic. However, the fetal loss is very high when rupture occurs and, in addition, hope of future

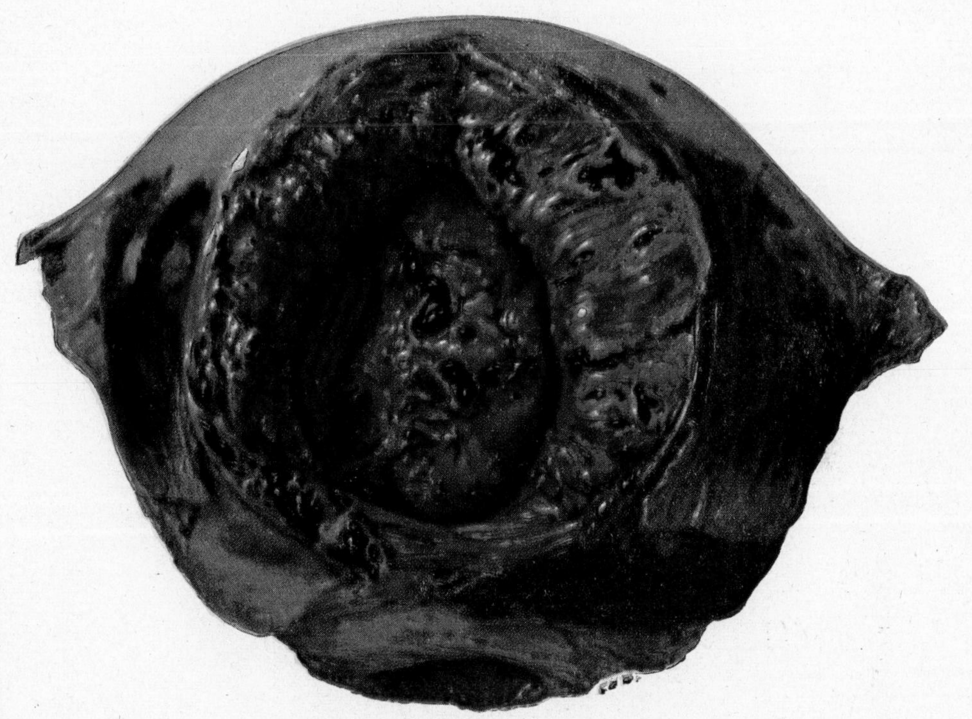

Fig. 651.—Rupture of Uterus through Scar of Previous Cesarean Section.

childbearing is usually sacrificed. Thus in patients who have no living children or where a future pregnancy may be strongly desired, section may be preferable. When repeat section is decided upon, it should be carried out two or three weeks before the expected date of confinement as many ruptures occur in the last weeks of gestation.

The occurrence of spontaneous rupture of the uterus may be reduced by recognition of the hazard of multiparity and by alertness for even minor degrees of disproportion in this vulnerable group. Traumatic rupture is decreasing in incidence with the decline in version and extraction and other traumatizing manipulations.

The excessive maternal mortality from rupture of the uterus in the past should be vastly improved with earlier diagnosis, support with blood transfusions and prompt operation.

Postmortem Cesarean Section. From the earliest times, when a patient died undelivered at nearly full term, cesarean section was sometimes performed immediately after the death in the hope of saving the life of the child. The number of children rescued by the procedure, however, has always been very small. Despite this fact, it is my opinion that it should be done provided the fetal heart is audible a few minutes before the mother's death and provided full written permission has been obtained from the patient's husband.

BIBLIOGRAPHY

Aldridge, A. H. Extraperitoneal (Latzko) Cesarean Section. With a Report of Cases and Suggested Modifications in Technic. Am. J. Obst. & Gynec., 1937, 33:788.

Barrett, R. L. A Fifteen-year Study of Cesarean Section in Women's Hospitals in the State of New York. Am. J. Obst. & Gynec., 1939, 37:434.

Beck, A. C. The Two-flap Low Incision Cesarean Section. Surg., Gynec. & Obst., Chicago, 1921, 33:290.

Brown, T. K. Bacteriology of the Uterus at Cesarean Section. Am. J. Obst. & Gynec., 1939, 38:969.

Butler, H. B. A Method of Performing Lower Segment Caesarean Section, with Special Reference to a New Compressor Instrument. J. Obst. & Gynaec. Brit. Emp., 1937, 44:1091.

Campbell, James V. An Analysis of 482 Cesarean Sections in Private Practice. Am. J. Obst. & Gynec., 1937, 33:451.

Cooke, W. R. Cesarean Section in Infected Cases. Am. J. Obst. & Gynec., 1938, 35:469.

Daichman, I., and Pomerance, W. A Review of Cesarean Sections. Am. J. Obst. & Gynec., 1939, 37:137.

——— Experience with the Supravesical Extraperitoneal Cesarean Section (Waters Operation). Am. J. Obst. & Gynec., 1944, 47:678.

Daily, Edwin F. Cesarean Section. An Analysis of 1,000 Consecutive Operations. Am. J. Obst. & Gynec., 1939, 37:348.

Davis, A. B. A Report of All Abdominal Cesarean Operations Performed in the Service of the Lying-In Hospital, Am. J. Obst., New York, 1915, 71:116.

Davis, M. E., and Seski, A. Childbearing in the Twilight of the Reproductive Period. Surg., Gynec. & Obst., 1948, 87:145.

DeLee, J. B. Low, or Cervical, Cesarean Section. J.A.M.A., Chicago, 1925, 84:741-798.

——— Nadelhoffer, L. E., and Greenhill, J. P. Repeated Laparo-trachelotomy. Am. J. Obst. & Gynec., St. Louis, 1928, 16:791.

DeMuth, O. An Improved Cesarean Section Technic. Am. J. Surg., 1939, 43:119.

DeNormandie, R. L. Cesarean Section in Massachusetts in 1937. New England J. Med., 1938, 219:871.

——— Five-Year Study of Cesarean Sections in Massachusetts. Int. Abst. Surg. (Surg., Gynec. & Obst.), 1943, 76:247.

Falls, Frederick. A Critical Study of the Low Cervical and Classical Cesarean Section Operations. Am. J. Obst. & Gynec., 1936, 32:989.

Fleischer, A. J., and Kushner, J. I. Experiences with the Latzko Cesarean Section. Surg., Gynec. & Obst., 1936, 62:238.

Gordon, C. A. A Survey of Cesarean Section in the Borough of Brooklyn. Am. J. Obst. & Gynec., 1928, 16:307-324.

Gordon, C. A., and Rosenthal, A. H. Cesarean Section. The Modern Operation. Am. J. Surg., 1941, 54:525.

Gustafson, G. W. An Evaluation of the Transverse Cervical Caesarean Section. A Report Based on a Study of 208 Cases. Am. J. Obst. & Gynec., 1943, 46:841.

Harris, J. W. A Study of the Results Obtained in 64 Cesarean Sections Terminated by Supravaginal Hysterectomy. Bull. Johns Hopkins Hosp., 1922, 33:318-321.

Harris, J. W., and Brown, J. H. The Bacterial Content of the Uterus at Cesarean Section. Am. J. Obst. & Gynec., 1927, 13:133-143.

Harris, R. P. Remarks on the Caesarean Operation. Am. J. Obst., 1878, 11:620.

——— Cattle-horn Lacerations of the Abdomen and Uterus in Pregnant Women. Am. J. Obst., 1887, 20:673-685, 1033.

——— Results of the Porro Caesarean Operation in All Countries. Brit. M. J., 1890, 1:68.

——— The Remarkable Results of Antiseptic Symphysiotomy. Tr. Am. Gynec. Soc., 1892, 17: 98-126.

——— The Porro Caesarean Section Tested by a Trial of Sixteen Years, etc. N. Y. J. Gynec. & Obst., 1893, 3:273-283.

Holland, E. The Results of a Collective Investigation into Caesarean Section Performed in Great Britain from the Years 1911 to 1920 Inclusive. J. Obst. & Gynec. Brit. Emp., 1921, 28:358-446.

——— Rupture of the Cesarean Scar in Subsequent Pregnancy and Labor. Proc. Roy. Soc. Med., 1920, 14 (Obst. & Gynaec. Sect.): 22-124.

Irwin, J. C. Extraperitoneal Cesarean Section. A Modification of the Latzko Technic with the Report of Thirty-Two Cases. West. J. Surg., 1941, 49:158.

Kerr, J. M. M. The Technic of Cesarean Section with Special Reference to the Lower Uterine Segment Incision. Am. J. Obst. & Gynec., 1926, 12:729.

Keyes, J. L., and Whitehouse, A. J. Portes Cesarean Section. Am. J. Obst. & Gynec., 1942, 44:705.

King, E. L. A Comparison of Two Cesarean Section Surveys Carried on in the City of New Orleans. Am. J. Obst. & Gynec., 1940, 40:860.

Koch, Roland. Der Wiederholte abdominale Kaiserschnitt. Indikation, Technik und Verlauf unter besonderer. Berucksichtigung der Indikation zur Sterilisierung bei wiederholtem Kaiserschnitt. Ztschr. f. Geburtsh. u. Gynak., 1939, 118:177.

Krönig. Transperitonealer, cervicaler Kaiserschnitt. Krönig-Döderlein, Operative Gynäkologie. III. Auf., 1912, ff. 879-886.

Kuder, K., and Johnson, D. G. The Elderly Primipara. Am. J. Obst. & Gynec., 1944, 47:794.

Latzko, W. Ueber den extra-peritonealen Kaiserschnitt. Zentralbl. f. Gynäk., 1909, 33:275.

La Vake, R. T. The Cesarean Problem. Minnesota Med., 1939, 22:437.

Lazard, E. M. An Analysis of 507 Consecutive Cases of Cesarean Section. Sixth Annual Meeting Pacific Coast Soc. of Obst. & Gynec., 1937, Nov. 4.

Lull, C. B. A Survey of Cesarean Sections in Philadelphia. Comparison between Years 1931 and 1941. Am. J. Obst. & Gynec., 1943, 46:314.

Manahan, C. P., Connally, H. F., Jr., and Eastman, N. J. The Experience of the Johns Hopkins Hospital with Cesarean Section. Am. J. Obst. & Gynec., 1942, 44:999.

Matthews, H. B., and Acken, H. S. A Critical Survey of 1066 Cesarean Sections. Am. J. Obst. & Gynec., 1939, 38:956.

Miller, J. R. Cesarean Sections at the Hartford Hospital, 1904-1927. New Eng. J. Med., 1928, 199: 651-656.

Montgomery, T. L. The Immediate and the Remote Effect of Abdominal Cesarean Section. Am. J. Obst. & Gynec., 1936, 31:968.

Phaneuf, Louis E. The Low or Cervical Cesarean Section. An Analysis of the End-results of an Additional 166 Operations. Am. J. Obst. & Gynec., 1936, 32:240.

——— Cesarean Section Followed by Temporary Exteriorization of the Uterus. Surg., Gynec. & Obst., 1927, 44:788-794.

Pickrell, K. L. An Inquiry into the History of Cesarean Section. Bull. Soc. Med. Hist., 1935, 4:414.

Quigley, J. K. Cesarean Section. A Ten Year Study Conducted in Rochester and Monroe County by the Committee on Maternal Welfare of the Medical Society of the County of Monroe. New York State J. Med., 1940, 40:699.

Report of Committee on Maternal and Infant Welfare of the Massachusetts Medical Society. Boston M. & S. J., 1923, 188:288-290.

Sänger, M. Der Kaiserschnitt bei Uterusmyomen, etc. Leipzig, 1882.

Schumann, Edward A. Cesarean Section. Evaluation of Types of Section and Their Indications. Am. J. Surg., 1943, 59:50.

Schwarz, Otto H., Paddock, Richard, and Bortnick, A. R. The Cesarean Scar. An Experimental Study. Am. J. Obst. & Gynec., 1938, 36:962.

SLEMONS, J. M. Hemorrhage Following Cesarean Section. Am. J. Obst. & Gynec., 1933, 26:656.

SMITH, David L. Mortality from Cesarean Section in Indianapolis and the Central States. J.A.M.A., 1937, 108:1334.

SOSA, A. I., y SANCHEZ, and NÖLTING, David E. Cesarean Section and Simultaneous Myomectomy. Am. J. Obst. & Gynec., 1944, 47:584.

SOULE, S. D. A Ten-year Study of Cesarean Section in the St. Louis Maternity Hospital. Am. J. Obst. & Gynec., 1938, 36:648.

TAMIS, A. B., and KLEIN, M. D. A Critical Analysis of Cesarean Section in a Large Municipal Hospital. Am. J. Obst. & Gynec., 1940, 40:250.

THOMAS, Rufus C. Cesarean Section under Spinal Analgesia. J. Obst. & Gynaec. Brit. Emp., 1942, 49:247.

VOGT, W. H., and VOGT, W. H., Jr. The Portes Cesarean Section with Report of a Case. Am. J. Obst. & Gynec., 1941, 42:499.

WATERS, Edward G. Supravesical Extraperitoneal Cesarean Section. Presentation of a New Technic. Am. J. Obst. & Gynec., 1940, 39:423.

WENTSLER, N. E., and STOUT, J. H. Cesarean Section at the University of Iowa. J. Iowa State Med. Soc., 1943, 33:166.

WILLIAMS, J. W. Pelvic Indications for the Performance of Caesarean Section. Tr. Am. Gynec. Soc., 1901, 26:260.

——— A Histological Study of 50 Uteri Removed at Cesarean Section. Bull. Johns Hopkins Hosp., 1917, 28:335.

——— A Critical Analysis of Twenty-one Years' Experience with Caesarean Section. Bull. Johns Hopkins Hosp., 1921, 32:173-184.

——— Cesarean Section at the Johns Hopkins Hospital. Northwest Med., Seattle, Oct., 1926.

WILLIAMSON, H. C., and GOLDBLATT, M. E. The "Latzko" Extraperitoneal Cesarean Section. A Report Based on a Study of Twenty-five Cases. Am. J. Obst. & Gynec., 1943, 45:103.

WILSON, K. M. A Clinical Study of 133 Pregnancies Following Cesarean Section. Am. J. Obst. & Gynec., 1916, 12:268.

43

DESTRUCTIVE OPERATIONS

CRANIOTOMY

The term *craniotomy,* as used in obstetrics, means any operation which brings about a decrease in the size of the fetal head for the purpose of rendering its delivery easier. It comprises puncture of the fetal skull and evacuation of the brain contents after which the skull collapses; this is followed by extraction of the infant by means of suitable tenaculum-like instruments applied to the collapsed cranial vault. Thanks to more widespread prenatal care, the more astute management of pelvic contraction, the availability of the sulfonamides and penicillin, and improvements in extraperitoneal cesarean section, craniotomy is the rarest of operations in modern obstetrics.

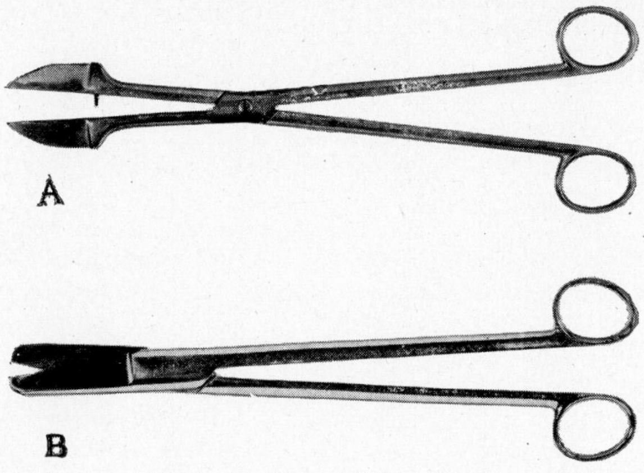

Fig. 652.—A, Smellie Scissors for Perforation of Skull; B, Dubois Scissors for Incision of Scalp.

In the presence of a dead child, craniotomy becomes indicated whenever delivery of the intact head by other means threatens to be difficult. It is never employed today on living infants except in cases of hydrocephalus. The operation is positively contraindicated in the extremely rare instances in which the obstetrical conjugate is less than 5.5 cm. because it is impossible to manipulate the instruments used in craniotomy through such a small aperture.

Hydrocephalus affords a positive indication for craniotomy, which is usually performed as soon as the cervix is completely dilated, but as stated on page 827, it may judiciously be performed slightly earlier if rupture of the distended lower segment seems imminent. In many instances extraction will not be necessary, as the mere evacuation of the fluid may be followed by the spontaneous extrusion of the child. In this condition a destructive operation is the more readily undertaken, as even a successful cesarean section will only give us a child that is doomed to die shortly or to remain an idiot. If, in a case of hydrocephalus, there are religious objections to the usual form of craniotomy, a spinal puncture needle may be inserted through the most accessible suture space and sufficient fluid withdrawn to allow descent of the head through the pelvis. In the few cases in which I have done this, delivery has been prompt and there have been no discernible effects of a harmful nature on the infant, but of course the hydrocephalic condition develops again subsequently.

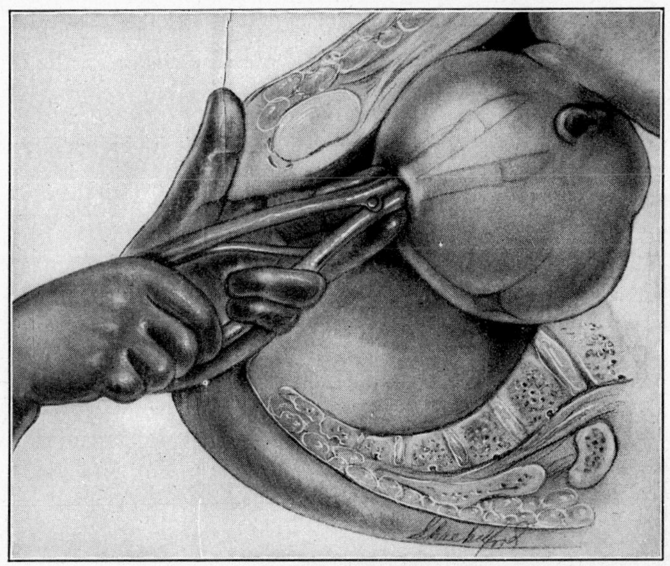

Fig. 653.—Craniotomy. Perforation of Head.

(From Titus, *Management of Obstetric Difficulties,* 2nd edition. Courtesy C. V. Mosby Company, St. Louis.)

With the exception noted above, craniotomy should not be performed upon the mature child until the external os has become completely dilated, as the imperfectly opened canal may offer a serious obstacle to its extraction. On the other hand, this caution does not apply when a dead child is immature, for in such conditions craniotomy affords a satisfactory means of delivery through a partially dilated cervix.

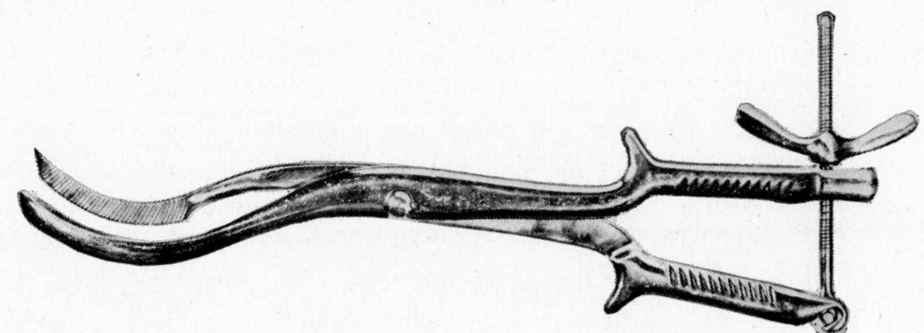

Fig. 654.—Braun's Cranioclast.

Operative Technic. The patient should be placed in the lithotomy position, and prepared as for other obstetrical operations. Craniotomy usually includes two steps: first, the perforation of the head and evacuation of its contents; and secondly, the extraction of the mutilated child.

Numerous instruments have been devised for perforating the head, the most suitable of which is *Smellie's scissors*. If the head is engaged and firmly fixed, perforation is accomplished with but little difficulty. With two fingers the large or small fontanel, whichever may be more convenient, is located, and the perforator plunged through it. The opening is then enlarged and the instrument briskly moved about within the skull so as to destroy the central ganglia, and to disintegrate the brain. As the result of the pressure to which the skull is subjected under these circumstances, the brain contents flow out spontaneously and there is no need to flush them out.

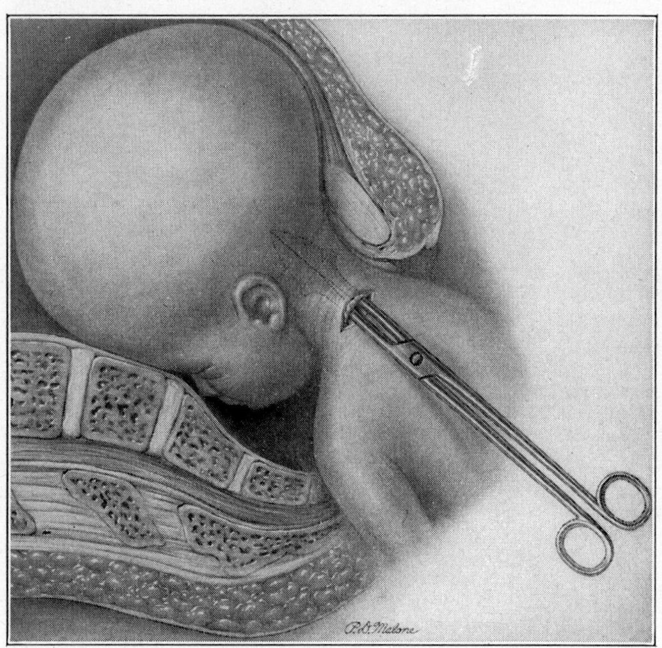

FIG. 655.—PERFORATION OF AFTERCOMING HEAD.

Note that the Smellie scissors are introduced under the skin of the infant's neck as a safeguard against injuring maternal soft parts, as recommended by Gustafson.

If the head is movable above the superior strait, it must be firmly fixed by means of pressure exerted by an assistant through the abdominal wall. Great care should be exercised to protect the maternal soft parts from injury by the sharp edges of the Smellie scissors. To this end, one hand should be introduced into the vagina and the fingers extended in such a way as to create an open pathway for the passage of the instrument to the skull. Moreover, this hand should remain in the same protecting position until all manipulations with the Smellie scissors have been completed and the instrument has been withdrawn from the vagina. In face presentations perforation should be effected through the frontal suture.

To pierce the aftercoming head, the body of the child should be depressed, and the instrument carried into the skull in the neighborhood of the occipital plate. This can be most safely performed as shown in Fig. 655. An incision in the skin of the neck is made and the Smellie scissors introduced under the skin to the region of the occipital plate. Here again, however, as an additional safeguard, the fingers of the operator should form a cone over the instrument to protect the maternal soft parts against any inadvertent slipping of the scissors. This injunction about protecting the maternal tissues applies to all destructive operations, especially to cleidotomy. If, as occasionally happens, this point cannot be reached, the body of the child should be carried up over the abdomen of the mother, and perforation effected through the mouth and base of the skull. When a hydrocephalic child presents by the breech, and the head is arrested at the pelvic brim, the fluid contents of the skull may be evacuated by cutting through the arch of one of the cervical vertebrae, after which a metallic catheter is passed through the opening and carried along the vertebral canal into the skull.

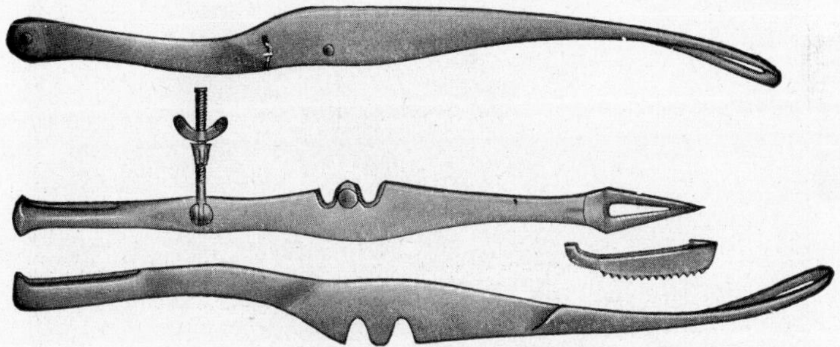

Fig. 656.—Tarnier's Basiotribe, Disarticulated.

After the brain has been evacuated, the collapsed head may be expelled by the uterine contractions alone, or may be extracted by means of heavy tenaculum forceps. It is usually advisable to make use of a special instrument for grasping and crushing the base of the skull. The *cranioclast,* invented by Simpson and modified by Carl Braun, serves the purpose most satisfactorily. Its solid blade is introduced through the perforation until its free end impinges upon the base of the skull, while the fenestrated

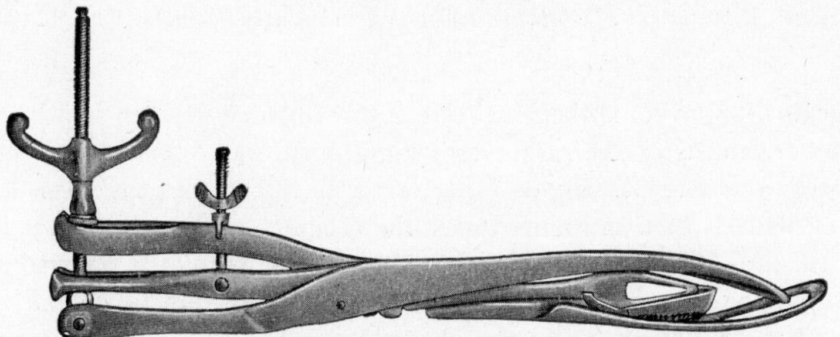

Fig. 657.—Tarnier's Basiotribe, Articulated.

blade is applied over the face or lower portion of the occiput. The vise at the end of the instrument is then tightened, and as a result not only is the base of the skull more or less compressed, but at the same time a firm hold is obtained for the extraction that is to follow.

Although the vault of the cranium collapses after craniotomy and the washing out of its contents, the base of the skull still remains unchanged and, as the bimastoid diameter measures between 7 and 7.5 cm., it is obvious that delivery cannot be effected through a pelvis presenting smaller measurements until the base of the skull has likewise been crushed. For this purpose many instruments have been devised, and formerly the cephalotribe, invented by Baudelocque the younger, was extensively employed. This is essentially a very heavy forceps, whose blades come closely together and forcibly compress the head, when the vise at the ends of the handles is tightened. At the same time, it labors under the disadvantage that it aims to accomplish two purposes, *i.e.*, crushing and extracting the head; and, unfortunately, whenever it is so constructed as to be an efficient crusher it is a poor tractor, and vice versa. For these reasons the cephalotribe, as such, is but little used.

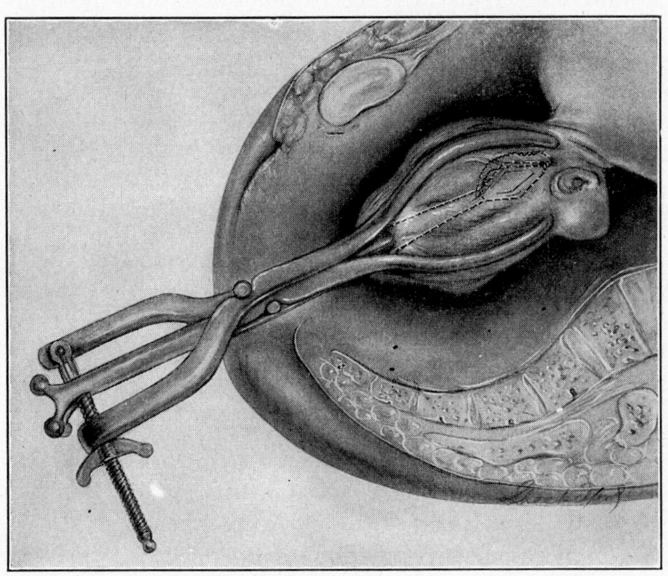

Fig. 658.—Craniotomy. Basiotribe Has Been Applied.

(From Titus, *Management of Obstetric Difficulties,* 2nd edition. Courtesy C. V. Mosby Company, St. Louis.)

Tarnier in 1883 invented the *basiotribe,* a three-bladed instrument which combines in one the advantages of the perforator, cranioclast, and cephalotribe. One blade is spear-pointed, and after serving as a perforator is forced into the base of the skull. The second blade is then introduced over the occiput and the third over the face of the child. All three are articulated, and the vise at the handles is screwed down, with the result that the base of the skull is fractured in many directions, and the head is compressed into an elongated and shapeless mass.

When perforating a hydrocephalic child, it is important to remember that the brain is spread out over the interior of the skull as a layer of tissue which may be only a few millimeters thick. When this is perforated, the fluid filling the dilated ventricles of the brain escapes and the skull collapses, after which delivery is readily effected. Unless especial precautions are taken, mere perforation occasionally does not result in the death of the child, which will cry after its birth. In order to guard against this distressing occurrence, the obstetrician should not be content with merely perforating the skull at one point, but should carry the instrument back to the base of the brain and stir it around so as to destroy effectually the upper portion of the medulla. Pernice reported the case of an infant who survived craniotomy and grew up an idiot.

In embryotomy the viscera are removed through an opening in the thorax or abdomen of the child, or the head is severed from the body. The former operation is known as evisceration, the latter as decapitation.

At present *evisceration* is rarely employed, though it occasionally becomes necessary in order to effect the delivery of certain monstrosities, or of children suffering from unusual enlargement of the thoracic or abdominal cavities resulting from tumor formation. It may likewise become necessary in rare cases of transverse presentation, when the thorax or abdomen of the child lies over the superior strait and the neck is not accessible. In such circumstances an opening is made by scissors through the thoracic or abdominal wall, as the case may be, sufficiently large to admit two fingers, with which the viscera are torn loose from their attachments and slowly extracted.

Decapitation is much more frequently employed, and is indicated more particularly in *neglected transverse presentations,* that is, when one shoulder has become firmly impacted in the pelvic canal and the lower uterine segment may have become so

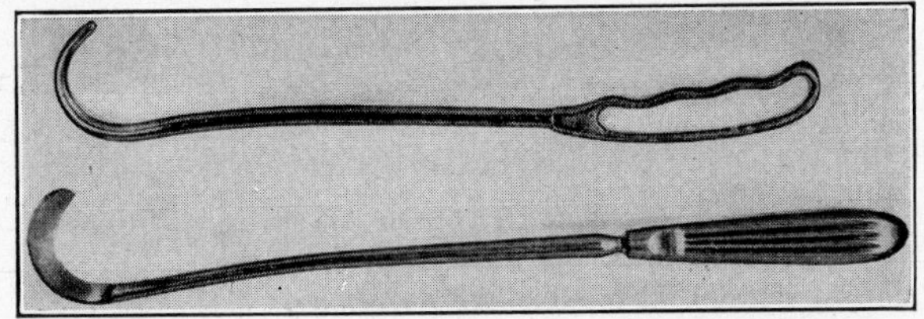

Fig. 659.—Blunt Hook, Above; Sickle Knife, Below.

stretched as to make an attempt at version practically synonymous with rupture of the uterus. Under such circumstances the child can be delivered only by decapitation or cesarean section. The former is the operation of choice in neglected cases, and should always be chosen if the child is dead. It can readily be accomplished by means of a sickle knife, which is illustrated in the lower half of Fig. 659.

Fortunately, in neglected shoulder presentations, decapitation is usually materially facilitated by the prolapse of one arm into the vagina. This having been seized and brought through the vulva, firm traction should be exerted upon it so as to put the neck on the stretch as much as possible. The index finger of one hand is then passed over the neck and used as a guide in applying the sickle knife as accurately as possible. When in position, the tip of the instrument is covered by the finger so as to avoid wounding the maternal soft parts. All being in readiness, strong traction is now made upon the handle of the instrument, which at the same time is rocked from side to side, by which motion the cervical vertebrae are disarticulated, and on continuation of the motion the neck is readily severed from the body. If any resistance is offered by the skin, it may be cut with scissors. After decapitation the body is extracted by traction upon the arm; or, if that be not available, by version. The head can frequently be expressed from the uterus by maneuvers similar to those employed for the delivery of the placenta, but if these prove unsuccessful a finger is inserted into the mouth of the child, after which, as a rule, extraction is readily effected by traction upon the lower jaw. If this is not effectual, delivery can be accomplished by means of a cephalotribe or after perforation.

Occasionally, in head presentations, the excessive size of the shoulders may prove a serious obstacle to labor. In such cases *cleidotomy* renders excellent service provided the child is dead. In this operation a pair of long curved scissors is introduced under the guidance of the hand and cuts through the clavicles on either side, after which the shoulder girdle collapses and delivery is more readily effected.

BIBLIOGRAPHY

Gustafson, G. W. Simple Technic for Craniotomy on the High Aftercoming Head. Am. J. Obst. & Gynec., 1939, 38:522.

Kerr, J. M. M., and Moir, J. C. Operative Obstetrics. Williams and Wilkins Co., Baltimore, 1950.

Marshall, C. McI. Neglected Shoulder Presentation: Decapitation by the Blond-Heidler Instrument. J. Obst. & Gynaec. Brit. Emp., 44:735.

INDEX

(Page numbers in italic type refer to illustrations, diagrams, or charts.)